Surgical Pathology of Non-neoplastic Gastrointestinal Diseases

Lizhi Zhang • Vishal S. Chandan • Tsung-Teh Wu
Editors

Surgical Pathology of Non-neoplastic Gastrointestinal Diseases

Springer

Editors
Lizhi Zhang
Mayo Clinic
Rochester, MN
USA

Vishal S. Chandan
University of California Irvine
Irvine, CA
USA

Tsung-Teh Wu
Mayo Clinic
Rochester, MN
USA

ISBN 978-3-030-15572-8 ISBN 978-3-030-15573-5 (eBook)
https://doi.org/10.1007/978-3-030-15573-5

This Springer imprint is published by the registered company Springer Nature Switzerland AG
The registered company address is: Gewerbestrasse 11, 6330 Cham, Switzerland

Preface

In the last few years, there have been significant additions and advances in both our knowledge and our concepts regarding many nonneoplastic gastrointestinal (GI) tract entities. The advances in endoscopic techniques have led to an increased number of GI tract biopsies being performed. New surgical techniques have also led to increased GI surgeries being performed with minimal morbidity. The pathology of these GI entities is intriguing, varied, and very important for most surgical pathologists. The proper diagnosis and classification of nonneoplastic GI pathology are vital for correct patient management decisions.

This book has been written for a broad target audience with the aim of it being of interest and benefit to pathologists who are already in practice to those who are just beginning their training in pathology. All of the authors are practicing GI/liver pathologists or gastroenterologists at the Mayo Clinic, where we are very fortunate to see an extensive number and a wide variety of cases in GI pathology. We are also grateful for the wealth of consult cases shared with us over the years by pathologists like you, and many of the rare cases illustrated in this book came from you! The chapters in this book reflect the current literature on the topics in the field of nonneoplastic GI pathology with important inputs from personal experiences of the authors.

This book includes chapters that provide an in-depth coverage of topics in GI pathology which we believe the readers will find useful. Each major/common entity within the chapters is described in detail with its definition, clinical features, pathological features (covering both the gross and microscopic details), differential diagnosis, and treatment/prognosis. All the chapters also highlight the use of special/immunohistochemical stains and other supporting studies as needed with a focus on providing a practical differential diagnosis rather than just a list of potential associations. This book has also been extensively illustrated with both gross and microscopic images to be an integral part of the information provided in the text.

We would also like to acknowledge the exceptional administrative support of Crystal Holtz, Amanda Rudat, Alison Smarzyk, Laurie Frazier, Monica Kendall, and Courtney Hyland for this book.

Finally, this book has been written for surgical pathologists by surgical pathologists who have a passion for GI pathology. We enjoy and love to read, talk, write, and sign out GI pathology cases. We hope that our zest for GI pathology comes through in this book and we would be able to contribute in some way to your understanding and enjoyment of GI pathology.

Rochester, MN, USA — Lizhi Zhang, MD
Irvine, CA, USA — Vishal S. Chandan, MD
Rochester, MN, USA — Tsung-Teh Wu, MD, PhD

Contents

Contributors

Editors

Lizhi Zhang, MD Department of Laboratory Medicine and Pathology, Mayo Clinic, Rochester, MN, USA

Vishal S. Chandan, MD Department of Pathology, University of California – Irvine, Irvine, CA, USA

Tsung-Teh Wu, MD, PhD Department of Laboratory Medicine and Pathology, Mayo Clinic, Rochester, MN, USA

Authors

Ferga C. Gleeson, MD Division of Gastroenterology and Hepatology, Mayo Clinic, Rochester, MN, USA

Murli Krishna, MD Department of Laboratory Medicine and Pathology, Mayo Clinic, Jacksonville, FL, USA

Jason T. Lewis, MD Department of Laboratory Medicine and Pathology, Mayo Clinic Florida, Jacksonville, FL, USA

Taofic Mounajjed, MD Department of Laboratory Medicine and Pathology, Mayo Clinic, Rochester, MN, USA

Bobbi S. Pritt, MD, MSc Department of Laboratory Medicine and Pathology, Mayo Clinic, Rochester, MN, USA

Samar Said, MD Department of Laboratory Medicine and Pathology, Mayo Clinic, Rochester, MN, USA

Audrey N. Schuetz, MD, MPH Department of Laboratory Medicine and Pathology, Mayo Clinic, Rochester, MN, USA

Sejal Subhash Shah, MD Department of Pathology, Kaiser Permanente Southern California, Irvine, CA, USA

Thomas C. Smyrk, MD Department of Laboratory Medicine and Pathology, Mayo Clinic, Rochester, MN, USA

Michael Torbenson, MD Department of Laboratory Medicine and Pathology, Mayo Clinic, Rochester, MN, USA

Saba Yasir, MBBS Department of Laboratory Medicine and Pathology, Mayo Clinic, Rochester, MN, USA

Part I

Introduction

Normal Histology of Gastrointestinal Tract

1

Vishal S. Chandan

Esophagus

Anatomy

The esophagus is a hollow muscular tube that connects the pharynx to the stomach. It begins in the neck region at the cricoid cartilage, traverses through the thorax in the posterior mediastinum, and extends past the diaphragm up to the stomach. In an adult, it measures approximately 25 cm in length. At endoscopy, usually the length of the esophagus is measured as the anatomic distance from the incisor teeth. This corresponds to the esophagus beginning at 15–18 cm from the incisor teeth and extending to the gastroesophageal junction (GEJ) which is located at approximately 40 cm. The adult human esophagus can be divided into cervical, thoracic, and abdominal parts. The upper esophageal sphincter is usually referred to as a 3 cm segment of the proximal esophagus at the level of the cricopharyngeus muscle. The lower esophageal sphincter is usually referred to as a 2–4 cm segment just proximal to the anatomic GEJ, at the level of the diaphragm. Of note, there are no well-established anatomic landmarks that outline these sphincters in relation to the esophageal musculature, though they may be recognized during endoscopy.

The normal esophagus has several points of constriction along its course. They are at the cricoid origin of the esophagus, at the aortic arch, at the crossing of the left main bronchus and left atrium, and at the passage through the diaphragm. These constrictions are clinically relevant as food or medication pills can become lodged at these sites of luminal narrowing resulting in contact mucosal injury to the esophagus [1, 2].

The GEJ is defined as the upper limit of the proximal gastric folds. The anatomic landmarks that can define the GEJ include the peritoneal reflection from the stomach onto the diaphragm or the incisura. Of note, the mucosal GEJ does not correspond to the muscular GEJ. The proximal margin of the gastric folds has been shown to closely correlate with the muscular GEJ and may provide a reasonable and reproducible anatomic landmark for the muscular GEJ [3]. The Z line represents the mucosal squamocolumnar junction seen at endoscopy or on gross examination.

Normal Histology

The esophageal wall consists of four layers: mucosa, submucosa, muscularis propria, and adventitia (Fig. 1.1). The esophagus does not have a distinct serosal lining. Hence, esophageal tumors tend to spread more easily and are difficult to treat surgically. The absence of a serosal layer also makes esophageal luminal disruptions more difficult to repair at surgery.

The mucosa consists of nonkeratinizing stratified squamous epithelium, lamina propria, and muscularis mucosae (Fig. 1.2). Almost the entire length of the esophagus is lined by squamous epithelium which can be divided into basal, prickle, and superficial layers (Fig. 1.3). The basal layer is usually 1 to 3 cells thick and occupies about 5–15% of the epithelial thickness. The prickle and superficial cell layers which lie above the basal layer are rich in glycogen and become flatter toward the surface. The most distal segment of the esophagus which is immediately below the squamous mucosa is normally lined by gastric cardiac-type mucosa and varies in length from a millimeter to about a centimeter. Rare endocrine cells and melanocytes may also exist within the squamous mucosa. Occasional intraepithelial lymphocytes can be seen as a normal finding and usually located in the suprabasal portion of the epithelium. Sometimes, the nuclei of the lymphocytes can become convoluted and may cause confusion with the nuclei of neutrophils (Fig. 1.4).

V. S. Chandan (✉)
Department of Pathology, University of California – Irvine, Irvine, CA, USA
e-mail: vchandan@uci.edu

L. Zhang et al. (eds.), *Surgical Pathology of Non-neoplastic Gastrointestinal Diseases*,
https://doi.org/10.1007/978-3-030-15573-5_1

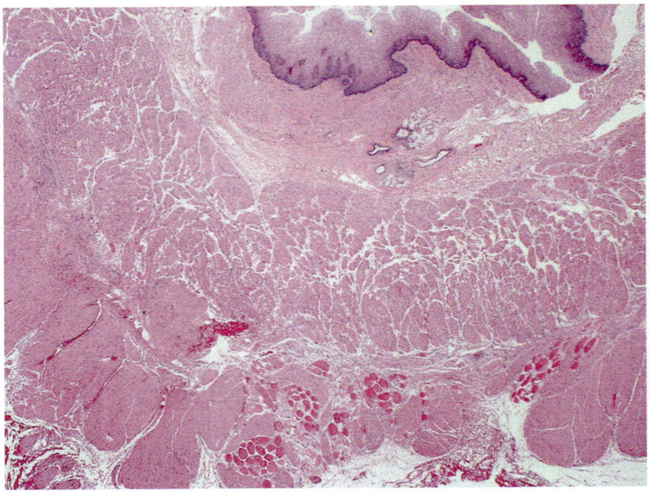

Fig. 1.1 Full-thickness section of esophagus showing four layers: mucosa, submucosa, muscularis propria, and adventitia

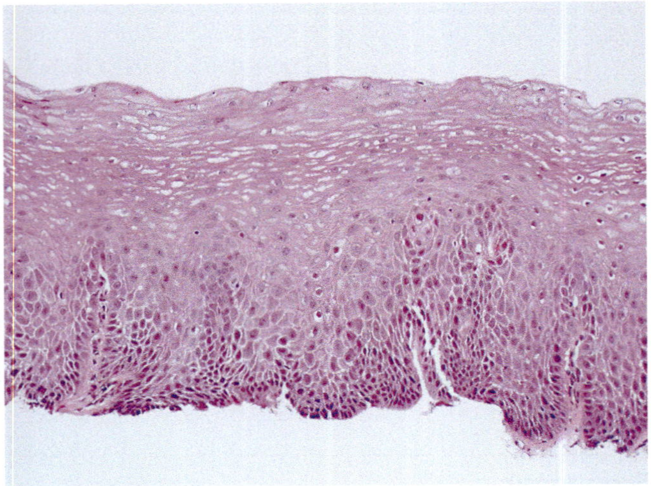

Fig. 1.3 Normal esophageal squamous epithelium, with basal, prickle, and superficial layers; and projections of the lamina propria extending into the overlying epithelium (< 2/3 of epithelial thickness) to form papillae

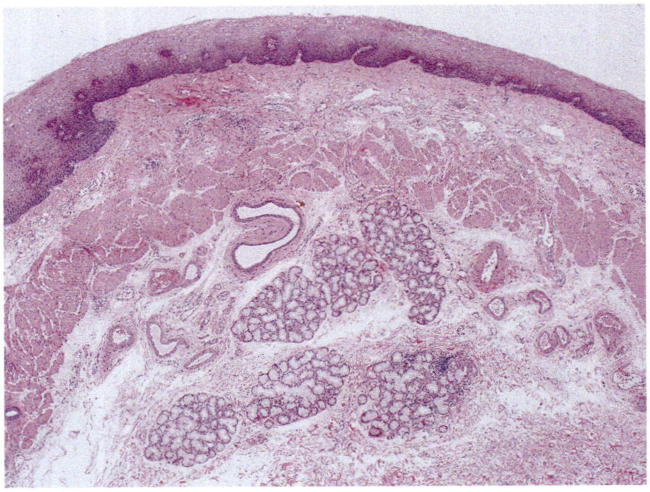

Fig. 1.2 Normal squamous mucosa, consisting of nonkeratinizing stratified squamous epithelium, lamina propria, and muscularis mucosae. The submucosa contains submucosal glands, ducts, and large caliber vessels, which are important anatomic land markers when evaluating submucosal invasion

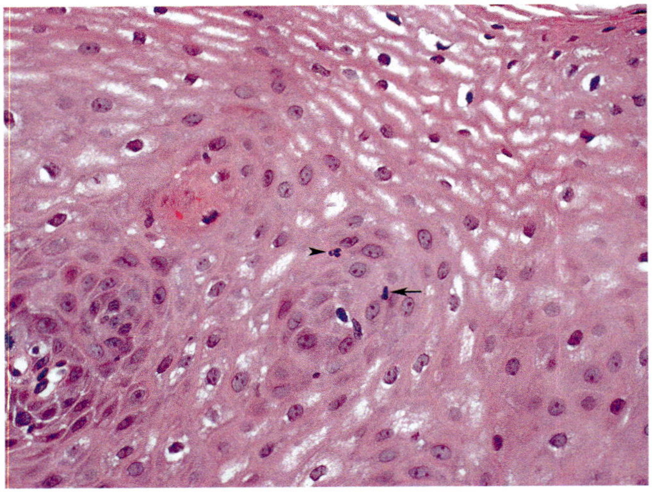

Fig. 1.4 Occasional intraepithelial lymphocytes (arrow) can be seen as a normal finding within the esophagus. Sometimes, the nuclei of the lymphocytes can become convoluted (arrowhead) and may cause confusion with the nuclei of neutrophil

The lamina propria lies beneath the epithelium and above the muscularis mucosae. It consists of connective tissue, vessels, scattered inflammatory cells such as lymphocytes as well as plasma cells, and mucous-secreting glands. Papillae are fingerlike projections of the lamina propria extending into the overlying epithelium, normally less than 2/3 of epithelial thickness (Fig. 1.3). The esophageal cardiac-type glands seen within the lamina propria are composed of cells secreting neutral mucins and resemble the gastric cardiac glands (Fig. 1.5). Their ducts are lined by simple mucus-producing cells. The muscularis mucosa is composed of longitudinally arranged smooth muscle fibers and may be traversed by the squamous epithelium-lined submucosal gland ducts. In cases of Barrett esophagus, the muscularis mucosae may become reduplicated (Fig. 1.6) [4].

The submucosa consists of loose connective tissue containing blood vessels, nerves, lymphatics and submucosal glands (Fig. 1.2). The submucosal glands consist of mucus cells and produce mucin which has a local protective effect (Fig. 1.7). The ducts lining these submucosal glands are proximally lined by a single layer of cuboidal epithelium which more distally becomes stratified squamous epithelium

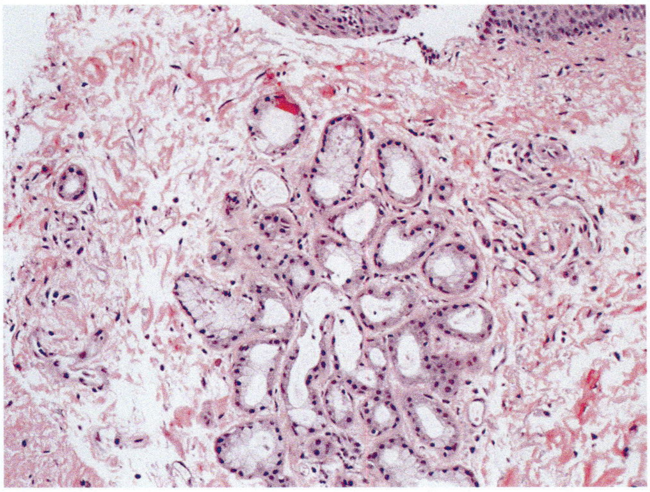

Fig. 1.5 Esophageal mucous-secreting glands in the lamina propria, similar to cardiac-type glands

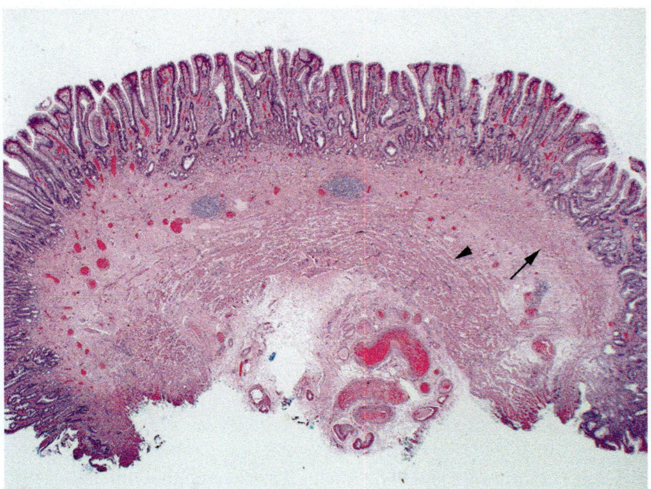

Fig. 1.6 Endoscopic mucosal resection showing duplication of the muscularis mucosae in a case of Barrett esophagus. The original muscularis mucosa is thicker and seen below (arrowhead). The duplicated, more delicate muscle layer is seen superficially (arrow). The fibroconnective tissue between these two layers should not be confused as submucosa

as it penetrates the muscularis mucosae and overlying epithelium to open into the esophageal lumen. Small periductal aggregates of lymphocytes and plasma cells can be seen adjacent to the ducts.

The muscularis propria of the esophagus has presence of both striated and smooth muscle. The Auerbach's plexus and its associated interstitial cells of Cajal are found between the two muscle layers. A short proximal segment of the muscularis propria (approximately 5%) is composed only of striated muscle [5]. Distal to the most proximal

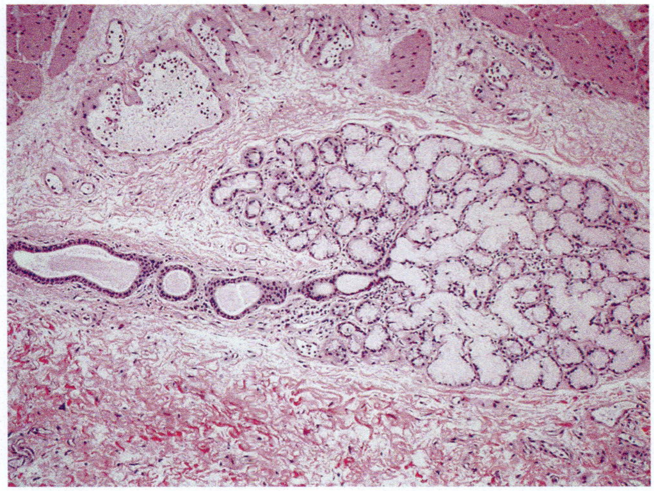

Fig. 1.7 Esophageal submucosal glands and ducts

segment, there is a mixture of smooth and striated muscle fibers. Greater than 50% of the distal muscularis propria is composed only of smooth muscles.

The majority of the esophagus is surrounded by fascia. The serosa lines only short segments of the thoracic and intra-abdominal esophagus derived from the pleura and peritoneum, respectively.

Lymphatic Drainage

The esophagus has a rich supply of lymphatic vessels which form anastomosing networks within the submucosa and connecting longitudinal channels in the muscularis propria. The cervical esophagus primarily drains into the internal jugular and paratracheal lymph nodes, while the thoracic esophagus drains into the mediastinal and bronchial lymph nodes and the abdominal esophagus into the subdiaphragmatic lymph nodes. Esophageal carcinomas can show wide nodal metastasis due to their rich lymphatic network. Unlike the colon, the esophageal mucosa contains lymphatics, accounting for the small but definite risk of lymph node metastasis for intramucosal esophageal carcinomas [6, 7].

Innervation

Both parasympathetic and sympathetic nerves supply afferent and efferent fibers to the esophagus. The vagus nerve supplies both parasympathetic and sympathetic fibers to the esophagus. Cervical and paravertebral sympathetic fibers also end at the esophagus. The esophagus also has its own intrinsic innervation system composed of Meissner's plexus (ganglion cells in the submucosa) and Auerbach's plexus (between the circular and longitudinal layers of the muscularis propria). The submucosal and muscle layers of the esophagus also contain widely distributed interstitial cells of Cajal.

Stomach

Anatomy

The stomach is an extremely distensible J-shaped organ located in the upper abdomen. At its upper end, it joins the esophagus, just left of the midline and below the diaphragm. Inferiorly, it connects to the duodenum, just right of the midline. Grossly, the stomach can be divided into four regions: cardia, fundus, body (corpus), and antrum [8]. The inferolateral margin of the stomach is known as the greater curvature, while the superomedial margin is known as the lesser curvature. The point where the tubular esophagus becomes the stomach is known as the GEJ. Generally, the GEJ is at the same level where the squamous esophageal mucosa transitions to the gastric mucosal folds. The gastric cardia is a small and ill-defined area found just distal to the lower end of the esophagus, extending approximately 1–3 cm from the GEJ. The gastric fundus is the portion of the stomach that lies above the GEJ, but just below the hemidiaphragm. The gastric antrum constitutes the distal 1/3 of the stomach, extending distal to the incisura and proximal from the pyloric sphincter. The remainder of the stomach is referred to as the gastric body (corpus). Of note, some do not distinguish between the corpus and the fundus and designate both parts of the stomach as fundus since they have the same type of mucosa. The term rugae applies to the thickened folds of the gastric mucosa. The incisura angularis is the angle along the lesser curvature which marks the approximate point at which the stomach narrows before joining the duodenum.

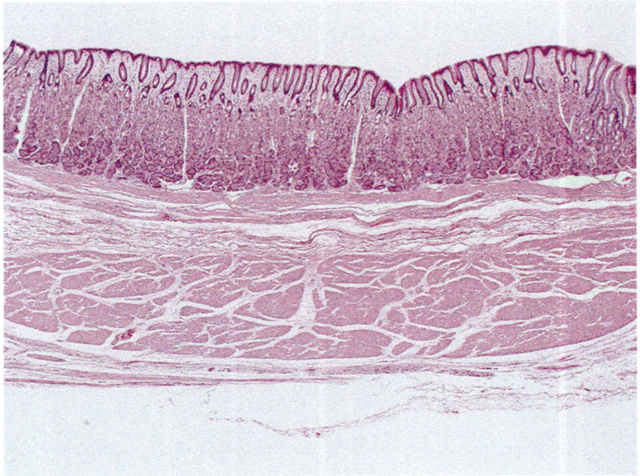

Fig. 1.8 Full-thickness section of stomach showing four layers: mucosa, submucosa, muscularis propria, and serosa

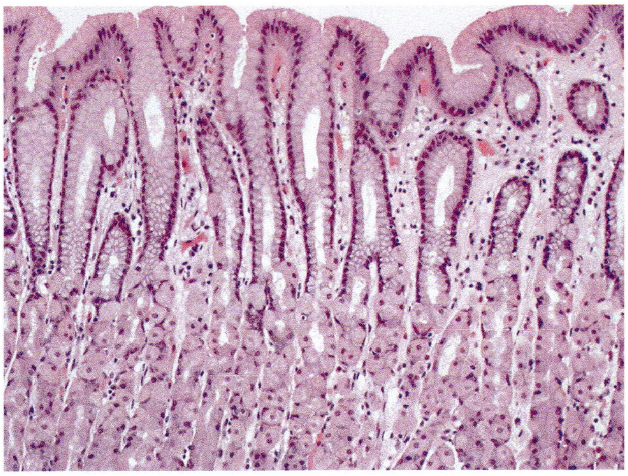

Fig. 1.9 Gastric foveolae. The mucosal surface epithelium and gastric pits are composed of tall, columnar, and mucous-secreting cells with basally situated nuclei and mucus-filled cytoplasm

Normal Histology

The gastric wall consists of four layers: mucosa, submucosa, muscularis propria, and serosa (Fig. 1.8). The gastric mucosa has two main epithelial components: the superficial foveolar component and the deeper glandular component (Figs. 1.9, 1.10, and 1.11). Throughout the entire stomach, the foveolar component is relatively uniform comprising tall, columnar, and mucous-secreting cells with basally situated nuclei and mucus-filled cytoplasm. These foveolar cells line the entire mucosal surface and gastric pits (foveolae) (Fig. 1.9). The deeper layer consists of coiled glands that empty into the base of these foveolae. However, the glandular layer of the stomach differs in structure and function depending on the individual gastric zone.

Within the gastric cardia, the foveolae occupy about half of the mucosal thickness (Fig. 1.10). It contains mucus-secreting

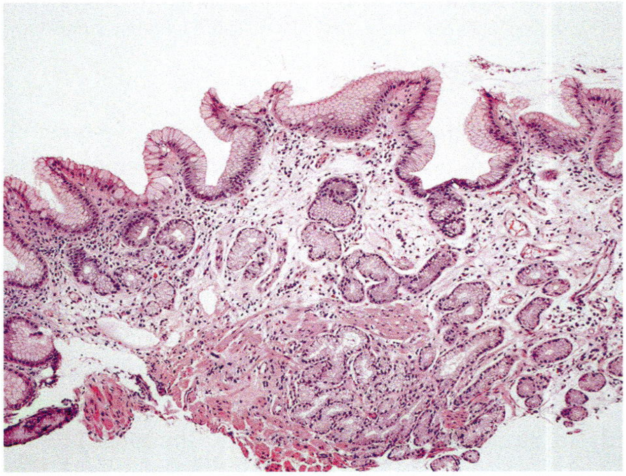

Fig. 1.10 Gastric cardiac mucosa. The foveolae are overlying mucus-secreting glands and occupying about half of the mucosal thickness. Inflammatory cells are typically present in the lamina propria

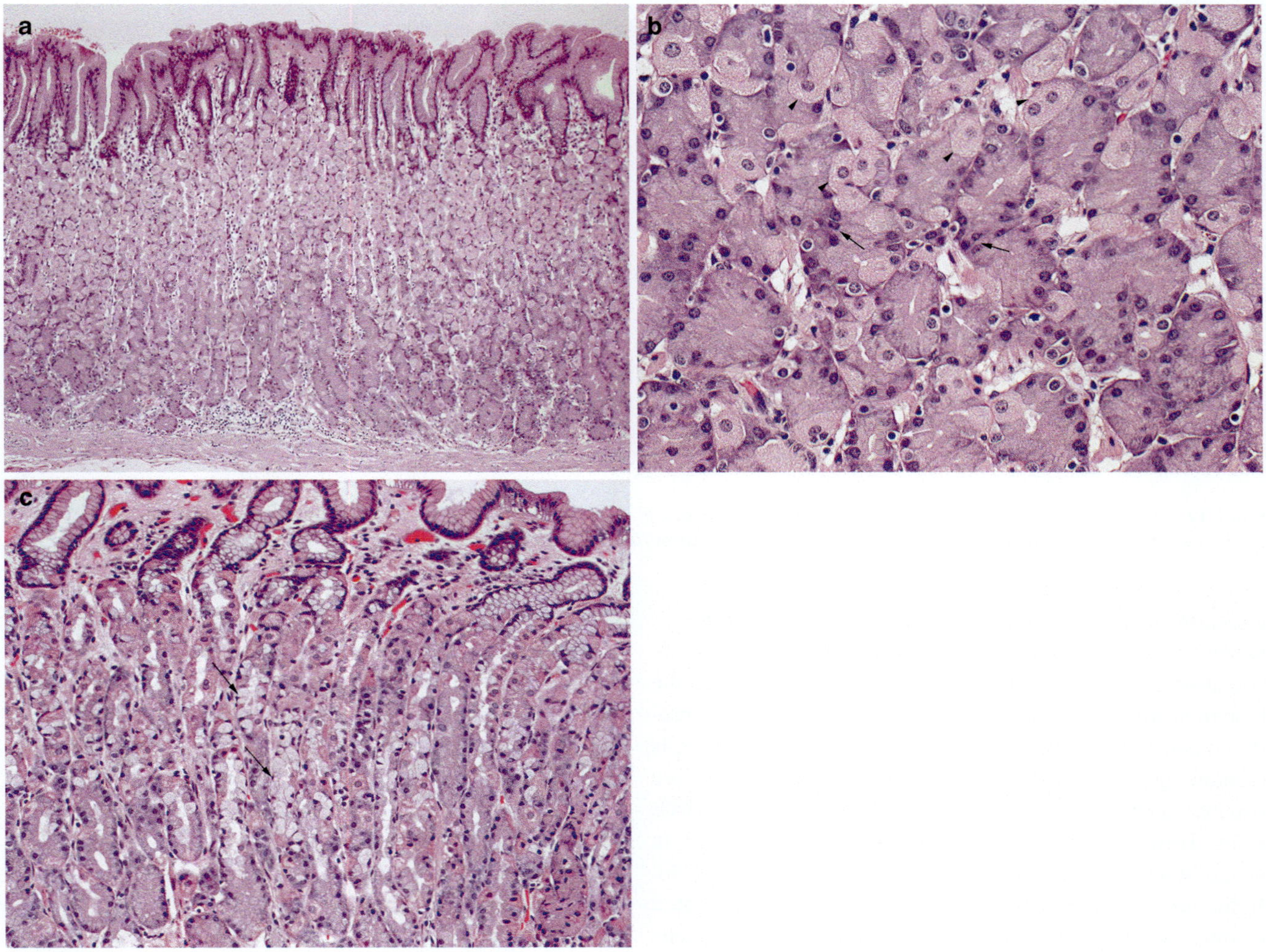

Fig. 1.11 Gastric fundic mucosa. (**a**) The oxyntic glands beneath the foveolae consist of tightly packed straight glands and are divided into three portions: base, neck, and isthmus. (**b**) Chief cells (black arrow) characterized by cuboidal shape with basophilic cytoplasm and basally situated nuclei; parietal cells (arrowhead) have a characteristic "fried-egg" appearance with acidophilic cytoplasm and centrally placed nuclei; endocrine cells (white arrow), sitting between the chief cells with a round shape, distinct cell border, and clear cytoplasm. (**c**) Mucous neck cells (arrows) intermixed with chief cells and parietal cells in the junctional region of the gastric pits and glands, characterized by clear or vacuolated cytoplasm with basal nuclei

glands that are loosely packed with abundant intervening lamina propria. The mucus cells have ill-defined borders and a bubbly cytoplasm. They secrete mucus and pepsinogen II. Single or small clusters of oxyntic cells may also be seen especially near the junctional zone with the fundus.

The fundic (oxyntic gland) mucosa found in the fundus and body shows tightly packed straight glands with little intervening lamina propria. They can be divided into three parts: base, neck, and isthmus (Fig. 1.11a). The chief/zymogenic cells (pepsinogen I and II secreting) are the major component of the basal portion. These cells are cuboidal with basophilic cytoplasm (due to the presence of a rough endoplasmic reticulum rich in ribosomal ribonucleic acid), basally situated nucleus with small nucleoli (Fig. 1.11b). The parietal cells (acid and intrinsic factor secreting) predominate in the isthmic portion of the glands [9]. These cells are triangular in shape with the base parallel to the basement membrane. They have a deep pink-colored (acidophilic) cytoplasm (due to abundant microcanaliculi composed of protein) with a centrally placed nucleus (Fig. 1.11b). They can be highlighted by the use of human milk fat globulin antibody [10]. The neck portion contains a mixture of zymogenic and parietal cells with admixed mucous neck cells. These mucous neck cells resemble the mucus cells in the pyloric region but can be difficult to appreciate on the H&E stain and can be highlighted on the PAS stain (Fig. 1.11c).

The antral and pyloric glands are identical with the foveolae occupying about half of the mucosal thickness (Fig. 1.12a). Both regions contain mucus-secreting glands that are loosely packed with abundant intervening lamina propria. Single or small clusters of oxyntic cells may also be seen especially near the junction with the gastric body (Fig. 1.12b).

The stomach also contains a variety of endocrine (hormone producing) cells. In the gastric antrum, the gastrin-producing G cells comprise approximately 50% of the entire

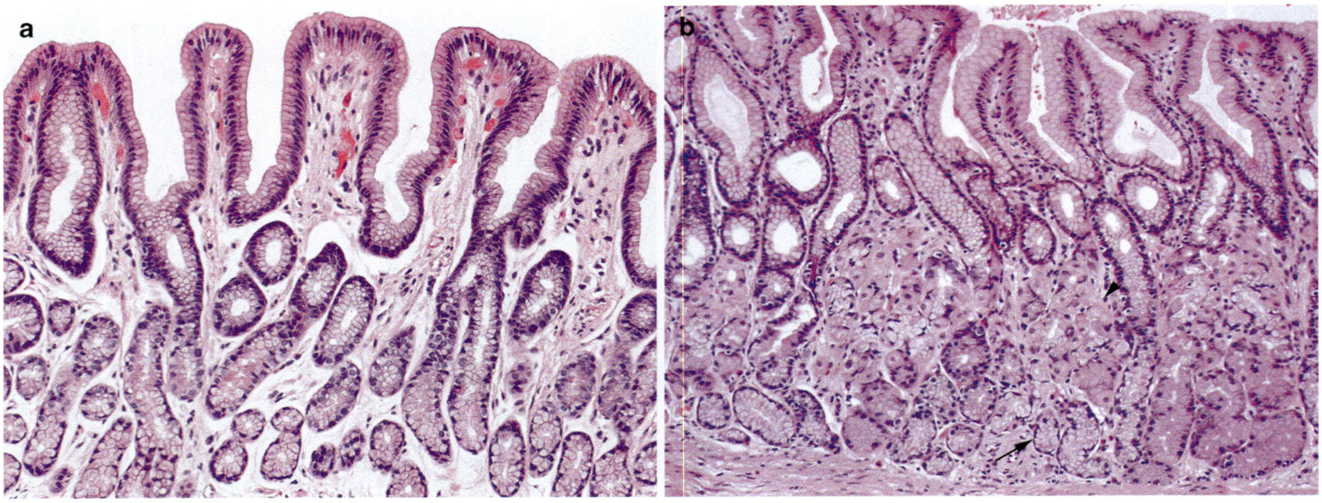

Fig. 1.12 (**a**) Gastric antral mucosa composed of foveolae and pyloric glands, with each occupying about half of the mucosal thickness. (**b**) Antral fundic transitional zone mucosa, containing both pyloric glands (arrow) and oxyntic glands (arrowhead)

endocrine cell population, approximately 30% are serotonin-producing enterochromaffin (EC) cells, and about 15% are somatostatin-producing D cells. In the fundic mucosa, the histamine-secreting enterochromaffin-like (ECL) cells predominate, with smaller numbers of EC cells and X cells (producing unknown secretion). These endocrine cells are usually inconspicuous and difficult to appreciate on H&E stain. However, on closer inspection, they are round in shape, with clear cytoplasm and small nuclei (Fig. 1.11b). In the fundic mucosa, the endocrine cells are mostly located toward the base of the glands and are range in 10–20 cells per crypt. However, in the antral mucosa, these endocrine cells are more numerous ranging between 20 and 50 cells per crypt, located in the neck region. Immunostains such as chromogranin and synaptophysin can be used to highlight these endocrine cells [11]. Individual hormones such as gastrin can also be demonstrated by specific antibodies.

The lamina propria consists of a fine meshwork of reticulin, collagen, and elastic fibers beneath the basement membrane, providing structural support to the overlying epithelium. A mixture of few lymphocytes, plasma cells, macrophages, and fibroblasts can be seen within the lamina propria. Occasional neutrophils and mast cells may also be present. The lamina propria also contains nerve fibers, capillaries, vessels, and lymphatics. Occasional small lymphoid aggregates composed of small lymphocytes (primary lymphoid follicles) can also be seen within the lamina propria in a normal stomach [12]. The muscularis mucosae consist of two layers: the inner circular and outer longitudinal.

The submucosa lies between the muscularis mucosae and muscularis propria. It is composed of loose connective tissues containing elastic fibers. A network of veins, arteries, and lymphatics as well as the Meissner's nerve plexus is found in the submucosa.

The muscularis propria is composed of three layers: outer longitudinal, inner circular, and the innermost oblique. The oblique layer is incomplete in nature and is present anterior to the circular layer and is most obvious in the cardiac region. At the pylorus, the inner circular layer forms the pyloric sphincter.

Lymphatic Drainage

The lymphatic drainage of the stomach has been identified into four main areas. The left gastric lymph nodes comprise the largest group, draining the lower end of the esophagus and most of the lesser curvature. The right gastric and hepatic nodes drain the pyloric region and the lesser curvature. The pancreaticosplenic nodes drain the proximal portion of the greater curvature, while the distal portion of the greater curvature drains into the right gastroepiploic and pyloric lymph nodes.

The gastric lamina propria immediately superficial to the muscularis mucosae has a network of lymphatics which penetrate the muscularis mucosae and communicate with the lymphatic channels present in the submucosa. Hence, intramucosal gastric adenocarcinomas that are even entirely superficial to the muscularis mucosae have a potential for lymph node metastasis.

Innervation

The celiac plexus supplies the sympathetic nerves to the stomach. The left and right phrenic nerves also innervate the stomach. The vagus nerve provides the parasympathetic supply to the stomach. Of note, either side of the subserosal layer of the stomach is devoid of true nerve plexus.

Small Bowel

Anatomy

The small bowel extends from the gastric pylorus to the cecum and measures approximately 6–7 m in adults [13]. It is divided into three parts: duodenum, jejunum, and ileum. The duodenum measures approximately 12 inches in length and is the most proximal portion of the small bowel, extending from the gastric pylorus into the duodeno-jejunal flexure. The duodenum itself is subdivided into four parts: The first portion known as the duodenal cap or bulb, the second or descending portion (into which the common bile duct and pancreatic ducts open), the third or horizontal portion; and the fourth or ascending portion which connects to the jejunum. The ligament of Treitz which consists of a strip of fibromuscular tissue marks the origin of the jejunum. Distal to the ligament of Treitz, the rest of the small bowel is subjectively subdivided into the jejunum (the proximal two-fifths) and the ileum (the distal three-fifths).

The duodenum is retroperitoneal, while the jejunum lies in the peritoneal cavity. The remainder of the small bowel is intraperitoneal until it ends at the ileocecal valve.

Normal Histology

The wall of the small bowel is divided into four basic layers: mucosa, submucosa, muscularis propria, and serosa (Fig. 1.13). The mucosal lining of the small bowel is designed to provide maximal surface area for the basic function of food absorption [14, 15]. The mucosa is composed of an epithelial layer, lamina propria, and muscularis mucosae. The entire luminal surface of the small bowel is composed of microscopic finger-like projections known as villi (Fig. 1.14). Each villous surface is lined by a single layer of epithelium composed of various cell types, beneath which lies the lamina propria containing a rich network of arteriovenous capillaries and lymphatic channels. The crypts of Lieberkuhn (pit-like crypts or depressions of the surface epithelium) lie beneath the villi in between the intervening regions. The normal villus-to-crypt ratio ranges between 3:1 and 5:1 [14].

Four main cell types are identified within the surface epithelium of the small bowel: absorptive cells, goblet cells, endocrine cells, and Paneth cells. The absorptive cells are the most common type seen within the surface epithelium. They are tall and columnar and have an eosinophilic cytoplasm and basally located round nucleus. A brush border composed of microvilli and glycocalyx is seen on their luminal surface. The microvilli are best seen on ultrastructural examination, and the brush border can also be highlighted on the PAS stain or CD10 immunostain (see Fig. 9.23). The goblet cells are scattered among the absorptive cells. They are characterized by presence of apical mucin droplet with an attenuated and basally situated nucleus. The numbers of goblet cells increase from the duodenum toward the ileum. Endocrine cells are more abundant within the crypts, but they can also be scattered within the villous epithelium. The cytoplasm of these endocrine cells contains abundant fine eosinophilic granules which contain secretory products. The main portion of the endocrine cell is located at the base of the epithelium. They have a small nucleus which is present on the luminal side of the cytoplasmic granules. The Paneth cells have bright coarse eosinophilic granules which are api-

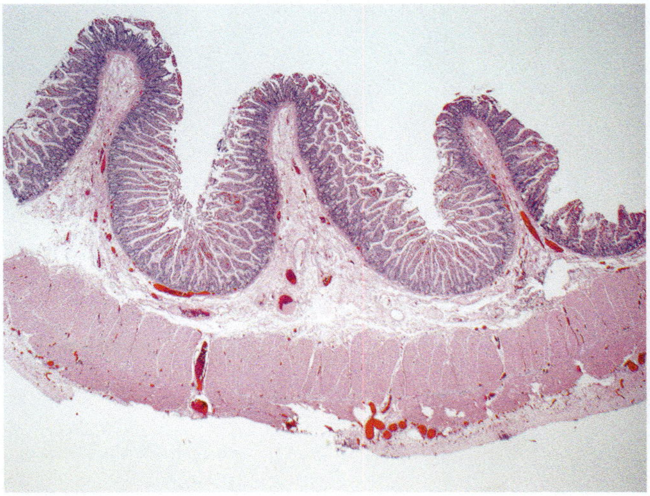

Fig. 1.13 Full-thickness section of small bowel showing four layers: mucosa, submucosa, muscularis propria, and serosa. Note the villi sitting on the mucosal circular folds (plicae circulares)

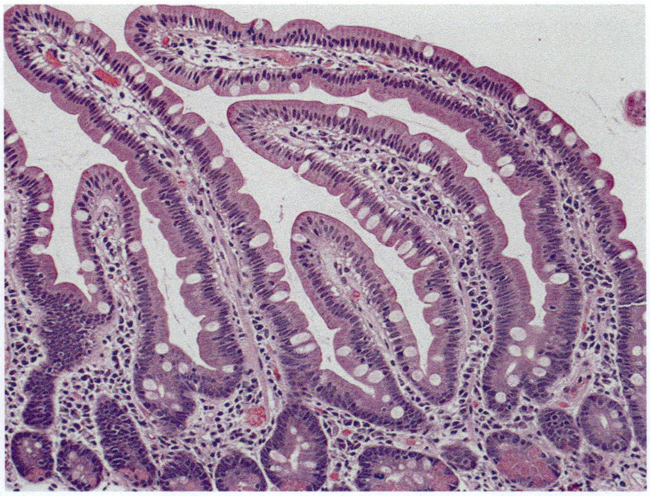

Fig. 1.14 Normal small bowel villi. Finger-like projections lined by a single layer of absorptive epithelium interspersed with goblet cells lying on lamina propria containing some inflammatory cells, a rich network of arteriovenous capillaries and lymphatics. Note the Paneth cells at the base of the crypts

cally oriented. The Paneth cells secrete growth factors and antimicrobial proteins which play a role in immunity against bacterial infections. The size as well as color of the eosinophilic cytoplasmic granules and the position of the nucleus help in the histologic distinction between endocrine cells and Paneth cells. The Paneth cell granules are larger, coarser, brightly eosinophilic, and apical relative to the basally located cell nucleus. In contrast, the endocrine cell granules are smaller, finer, deeply eosinophilic, and basally oriented relative to the apically displaced nucleus. Of note, it may be difficult to appreciate the Paneth cells on H&E-stained sections if the tissue is fixed in fixatives containing picric acid (like Hollande's or Bouin's) as they mask the eosinophilic staining of the granules [16].

There are two specific structures in the second portion of the duodenum: major and minor duodenal papilla. The major duodenal papilla is the landmark separating foregut and midgut, where common bile duct and pancreatic duct open into the duodenum, and the minor duodenal papilla is the opening of the accessory pancreatic duct which is typically located 2 cm proximal to the major papilla. The histology of the major papilla is different from the adjacent duodenal mucosa. It is surrounded by thin smooth muscle bundles, the sphincter of Oddi, and contains ampulla of Vater where the pancreatic duct and the distal common bile duct unite (Fig. 1.15). The epithelium at the major papilla tends to be flat and often has focal gastric mucinous metaplasia. There is no muscularis mucosae and submucosal tissue in the papilla. The ampulla of Vater is lined by cuboidal to low columnar pancreaticobiliary-type epithelium with occasional goblet cells, but no absorptive-type cells. The epithelium may form papillary structures. There are peribiliary glands and pancreatic acini in the vicinity. Understanding the local anatomy and normal histology is important when evaluating carcinoma arising around the papilla, ampulla, distal common bile duct, or pancreatic head.

Small nodules of lymphoid tissue can be seen within the mucosa of the small bowel. Few scattered intraepithelial lymphocytes (one lymphocyte for every four to five epithelial cells) can also be seen within the normal small bowel [17–19]. These intraepithelial lymphocytes are CD3 positive, and majority of them also express CD8 [20, 21]. The intraepithelial lymphocytes usually decrease in number from the base toward the tip within the normal small bowel (Fig. 1.16; also see Fig. 9.2).

The framework of the lamina propria is composed of interweaving collagen bundles and other connective tissue fibers. A network of blood capillaries, lymphatics, and nerve fibers courses through the lamina propria. The lamina propria of the small bowel also contains numerous lymphocytes, plasma cells, and eosinophils. A few histiocytes, dendritic cells, and mast cells may also be present. The lamina propria rests upon a thin fibromuscular layer known as the muscularis mucosae, which separates the mucosa from the underlying submucosa.

The submucosa which lies between the muscularis mucosae and muscularis propria is composed of a mixture of collagenous and elastic fibers with fibroblasts. Few scattered inflammatory cells such as histiocytes, lymphocytes, and plasma cells can be seen within the submucosa along with adipose tissue. The submucosa also contains a rich network of large arterials, venules, and lymphatics. Neural structures are also present in the submucosa, including the Meissner's plexus.

The submucosa of the duodenum contains the Brunner's glands. They are most concentrated in the gastroduodenal

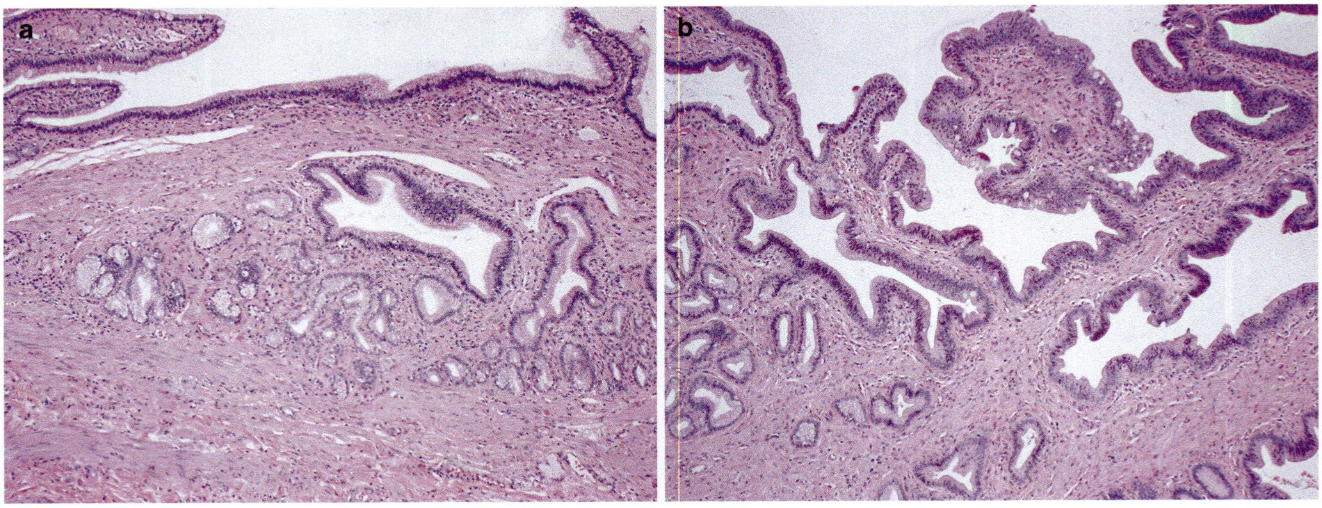

Fig. 1.15 Major papilla and ampulla of Vater. (**a**) The major papilla is lined by flat epithelium showing gastric mucinous metaplasia and surrounded by thin smooth muscle bundles of sphincter of Oddi. (**b**) The ampulla of Vater is lined by cuboidal to low columnar pancreaticobiliary-type epithelium with occasional goblet cells, with a papillary appearance and scattered peribiliary glands

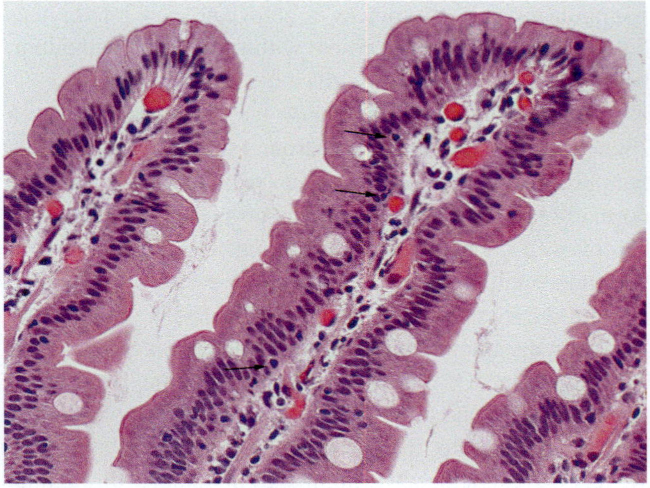

Fig. 1.16 Scattered intraepithelial lymphocytes (arrows) within the normal small bowel mucosa (one lymphocyte for every four to five epithelial cells)

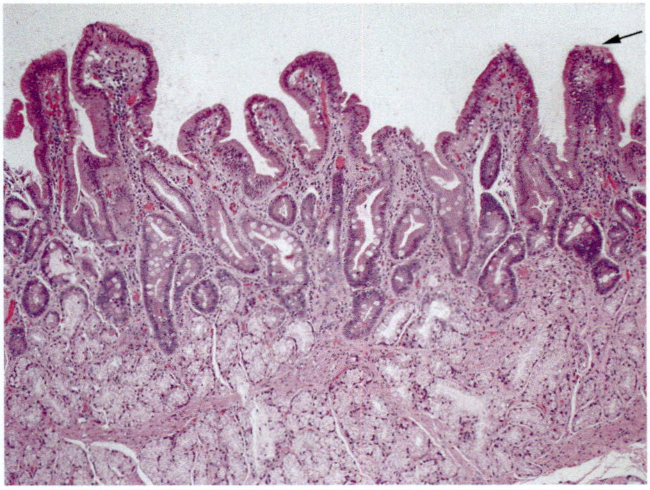

Fig. 1.17 Duodenal bulb mucosa containing abundant Brunner's glands. Note the focal gastric foveolar metaplasia (arrow)

junction and gradually decrease in quantity along the length of duodenum. They serve as microscopic landmark for duodenum. Brunner's glands are lobular collections of glands lined by cuboidal to columnar cells with uniform pale appearing cytoplasm with an oval basally located nucleus (Fig. 1.17). They contain neutral mucin which is PAS positive and diastase resistant. Their ducts are lined by similar epithelium.

The ileum shows prominent well-defined lymphoid tissue including Peyer's patches and isolated lymphoid follicles (Fig. 1.18). Peyer's patches can be seen within the submucosa and also within the mucosa. The follicles within Peyer's patches are composed predominantly of B lymphocytes with admixed follicular dendritic cells and macrophages. Most follicles also contain a germinal center

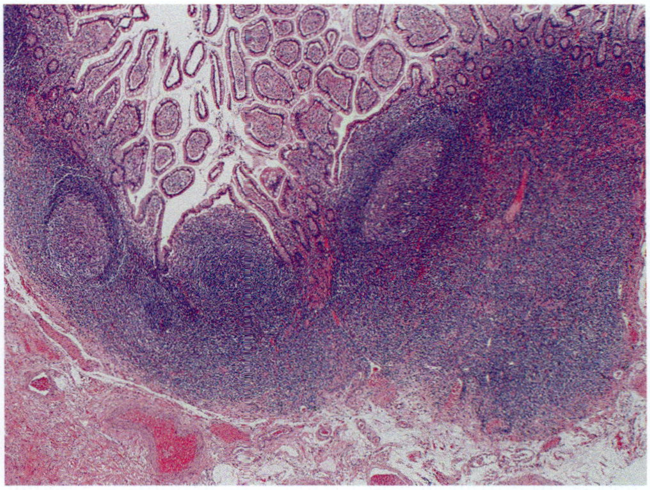

Fig. 1.18 Peyer's patches in terminal ileum containing prominent reactive lymphoid aggregates/follicles in mucosa and submucosa

composed of CD10-positive and bcl-2-negative B cells. The germinal center is surrounded by a mantle zone of small IgD-positive and IgM-positive B cells.

The muscularis propria is the outer smooth muscle layer surrounding the submucosa. It consists of an outer longitudinal layer and inner circular area. Blood vessels, lymphatics, and nodes traverse through the muscularis propria. The myenteric plexus of Auerbach lies between the outer longitudinal and inner circular muscle layers. Interstitial cells of Cajal form a network around the Auerbach's plexus and within the circular muscle layer.

The serosa envelopes the outermost surface of the small bowel. It consists of a single layer of cuboidal mesothelial cells, beneath which lies a thin layer of loose connective tissue.

Lymphatic Drainage

The lymphatic drainage of the duodenum occurs to the peripancreaticoduodenual lymph nodes consisting of the retropancreatic, hepatic artery, inferior pancreaticoduodenal, and superior mesenteric lymph nodes. The rest of the small bowel drains along the mesentery to the cecal, ileocolic, superior mesenteric, and mesenteric lymph nodes.

Innervation

The celiac and superior mesenteric plexuses provide the sympathetic nerves to the small bowel. The parasympathetic nerve supply to the small bowel is provided by the vagus nerve.

Appendix

Anatomy

Appendix is a slender tubular structure that protrudes from the posteriomedial aspect of the cecum, originating within about 2 cm below the insertion of the ileum into the cecum. The length of the appendix is quite variable, but on average measures 7–10 cm [22]. It measures approximately 0.3–0.5 cm in diameter. The appendix is covered by the peritoneum along almost its entire external surface.

The exact role of the appendix in the human body is uncertain. Some believe it to be a functionless vestigial structure. However, others have suggested that the lymphocytes derived from the appendix migrate to other sites within the GI tract and help in immunity [23].

Normal Histology

Histologically the appendix is similar to the colon, consisting of four layers, namely, mucosa, submucosa, muscularis propria, and serosa. However, the most prominent feature is the abundance of organized lymphoid tissue which is circumferentially arranged within both the lamina propria and submucosa (Fig. 1.19).

The surface epithelium of the appendix consists of absorptive cells which are tall and columnar with eosinophilic cytoplasm and round basally situated nucleus. These absorptive cells are admixed with goblet cells, neuroendocrine cells, and scattered Paneth cells. The crypts of the appendix are more irregular in shape, length, and distribution when compared to the colon. The crypts may even be absent in areas where the lymphoid tissue is prominent or abundant. Few intraepithelial lymphocytes may be present within the crypt epithelium, but neutrophils and plasma cells are normally absent.

The lamina propria surrounds the crypts and forms a connective tissue framework around them. Plasma cells, lymphocytes, macrophages, eosinophils, and mast cells are normally present within the lamina propria. A varying number of well-defined lymphoid aggregates may be present within the lamina propria, and they may even extend beneath the muscularis mucosae into the underlying submucosa. However, the amount of lymphoid tissue within the appendix varies with age. Of note, in newborns, there may be scant or no lymphoid tissue present. The amount of lymphoid tissue within the appendix increases with age, peaking at around 10 years. Then, it steadily diminishes in quantity throughout the rest of the life. The lamina propria also contains a rich network of blood capillaries, lymphatics, and nerve fibers.

The muscularis mucosae lie beneath the lamina propria, and in the appendix, it may be attenuated, poorly developed, or even focally absent in the areas of prominent lymphoid aggregates.

The submucosa lies between the mucosa and muscularis propria. It consists of a meshwork of elastic and collagenous fibers with admixed fibroblasts. A few lymphocytes, plasma cells, macrophages, and mast cells may be present within the submucosa. Prominent vessels including arterioles, venules, and lymphatics along with the Meissner's plexus are also present within the submucosa.

The muscularis propria of the appendix consists of an inner circular layer and an outer longitudinal layer. The Auerbach's (myenteric) plexus lies between these two muscle layers. The subserosa lies external to the outer longitudinal layer of the muscularis propria. It consists of loose

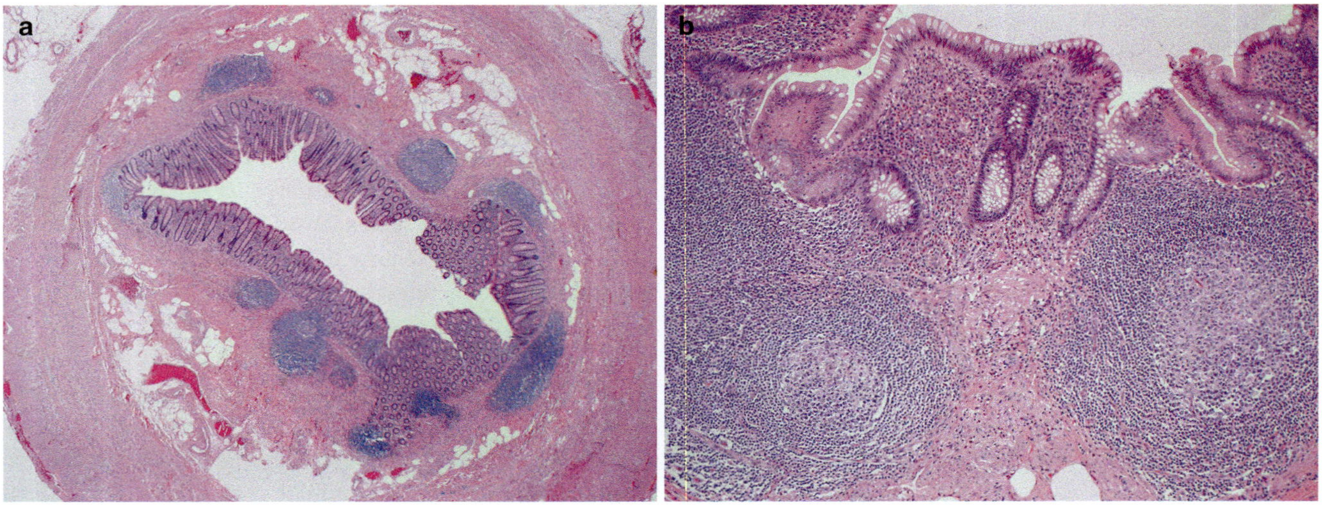

Fig. 1.19 Normal appendix. (**a**) Four layers of appendix: mucosa, submucosa, muscularis propria, and serosa. Scattered lymphoid aggregates circumferentially arranged within both the lamina propria and submucosa. (**b**) Appendiceal mucosa, similar to colonic mucosa, but with irregular crypts and prominent lymphoid aggregates and follicles

connective tissue with intermixed blood vessels, lymphatics, and nerve fibers. The serosa is the outermost layer composed of cuboidal mesothelial cells. Of note, the attachment of the fibrofatty mesoappendix lacks the serosa.

Lymphatic Drainage

The appendix drains into the ileocolic chain of lymph nodes.

Innervation

The parasympathetic nerves to the appendix are derived from the vagus nerve, while the sympathetic nerves come from the superior mesenteric plexus.

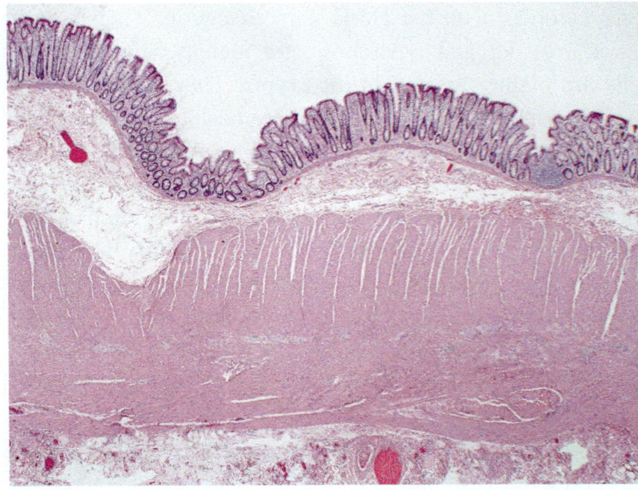

Fig. 1.20 Full-thickness section of colon showing four layers: mucosa, submucosa, muscularis propria, and serosa

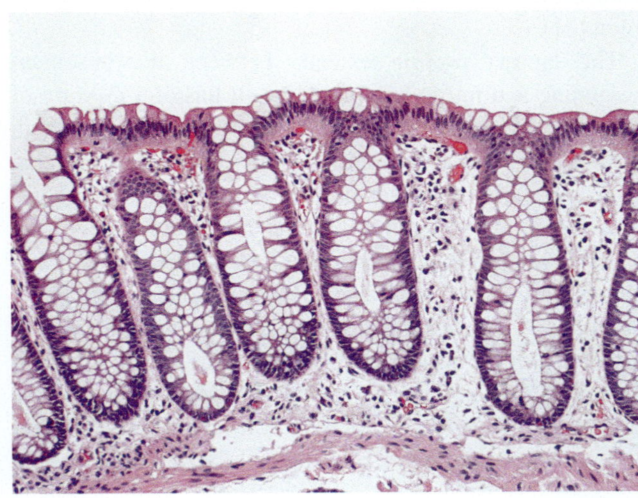

Fig. 1.21 Normal colonic mucosa. Regularly and parallelly arranged crypts perpendicular to the muscularis mucosae consisting of absorptive cells, goblet cells, and endocrine cells. Paneth cells are normally present in proximal colon. The lamina propria contains a variable number of inflammatory cells and a rich network of capillaries, venules, and lymphatics

Colon

Anatomy

The colon connects the terminal ileum to the anal canal and measures about 1.0–1.5 m in an adult [24, 25]. The major regions of the colon consist of cecum, ascending colon, hepatic flexure, transverse colon, splenic flexure, descending colon, sigmoid colon, and rectum. The cecum is bulbous and along with the ascending colon constitutes the colon on the right side of the abdomen. The ventral surfaces of the cecum and ascending colon are covered by the peritoneum, while their dorsal aspect lies directly on the posterior abdominal wall. The transverse colon extends between the hepatic flexure and splenic flexure and is suspended by the lesser omentum. The descending colon is attached to the left posterior abdominal wall. The sigmoid colon starts around the pelvic rim and is suspended entirely by the mesentery, leading to its increased susceptibility for volvulus. The sigmoid colon connects to the rectum which passes between the peroneal muscles to exit the abdominal cavity.

Normal Histology

Histologically, the colon consists of four distinct compartments: mucosa, submucosa, muscularis propria, and serosa (Fig. 1.20).

The mucosa consists of columnar epithelium lining the colonic crypts that extend deep into the lamina propria up to the muscularis mucosae (Fig. 1.21). These crypts are arranged perpendicular to the muscularis mucosae running parallel to each other and imparting a "rack of test tubes" appearance. The epithelial cells identified within the mucosa consist of absorptive cells, goblet cells, endocrine cells, and Paneth cells. The basement membrane provides support to the overlying epithelial cells. Normally, it is 3–5 μm in thickness with a regular outline. Basement membrane irregularity, with entrapment of the capillaries within the superficial lamina propria and thickness greater than 10 μm, is considered pathological [26, 27].

The absorptive cells compose majority of the surface epithelium. They are columnar in shape with lightly eosinophilic cytoplasm and basally placed oval nucleus. The luminal surface shows tightly packed apical microvilli. The goblet cells can be seen both within the surface epithelium and crypts. They are oval to round in shape with relatively clear cytoplasm on the H&E-stained section. They have a dense, irregular, and hyperchromatic nucleus. The endocrine cells are mainly located in the crypts. They contain small, deeply eosinophilic granules that are basally oriented [28]. They have a small nucleus that is pushed toward the lumen. The Paneth cells are pyramidal in shape with apical densely eosinophilic granules and basally located oval nucleus and can be present in proximal colon but normally absent in distal colon and rectum [29]. They are usually seen at the base of the crypts (Fig. 1.22). Of note, the Paneth cell granules are autofluorescent on H&E-stained sections [30].

Few intraepithelial lymphocytes can be seen within normal colon and range from one to five lymphocytes per 100 epithelial cells. However, 20 or more lymphocytes per 100 epithelial cells are considered pathological. Increased intraepithelial lymphocytes can be seen within the epithelium overlying lymphoid aggregates, and this should not be misinterpreted as pathological in nature. Rare intraepithelial eosinophils may also be occasionally seen within the normal colon [31].

The lamina propria extends between the basement membrane and muscularis mucosae. It has of a mixture of inflammatory and mesenchymal cells organized within an extracellular matrix. The entire length of the colonic lamina propria contains thousands of well-defined lymphoid aggregates, especially prominent within the cecum. In addition to these lymphoid aggregates, the lamina propria also contains a mixture of lymphocytes, plasma cells, eosinophils, mast cells, and macrophages. The density of the inflammatory cells within the lamina propria varies within different segments of the colon. The cecum and right colon are more cellular than the other segments of the colon. There is usually a progressive decrease in the cellularity of the lamina propria from the right to the left colon. Muciphages are macrophages with ingested mucin. They are normal constituents of the lamina propria and commonly seen within the left colon and rectum (Fig. 1.23). The lamina propria also contains a rich network of capillaries, venules, and lymphatics. The muscularis mucosae is formed by a thin layer of smooth muscle, forming the deep boundary of the lamina propria. It also contains vascular channels and nerve twiglets.

The submucosa consists of loosely arranged smooth muscle and fibroadipose tissue with a rich network of angiolymphatic and neural tissue. Scattered inflammatory cells and few lymphoid aggregates may also be seen within the submucosa. The amount of adipose tissue within the submucosa varies significantly among individuals and also between the right and left colon. The ileocecal valve and cecal regions show abundance of mature adipose tissue within the submucosa, often times even resembling a lipoma. The submucosa contains two neural plexuses, namely, the plexus of Meissner which is located immediately beneath the muscularis mucosae and the deeper Henle's plexus. These neural plexuses consist of neurons, glial cells, ganglion cells, and stromal components (Fig. 1.24). The interstitial cells of Cajal are also present within the submucosa and play an important role in the gut motor activity [32–34].

The muscularis propria of the colon consists of an inner circular layer and outer longitudinal layer. Blood vessels and lymphatics are seen within the muscularis propria. The interstitial cells of Cajal are also present between the muscle layers and around the nerve plexuses. The subserosal fibroadipose tissue lies beyond the muscularis propria, which is limited by the serosa consisting of a mesothelial lining and adjacent fibroelastic tissue.

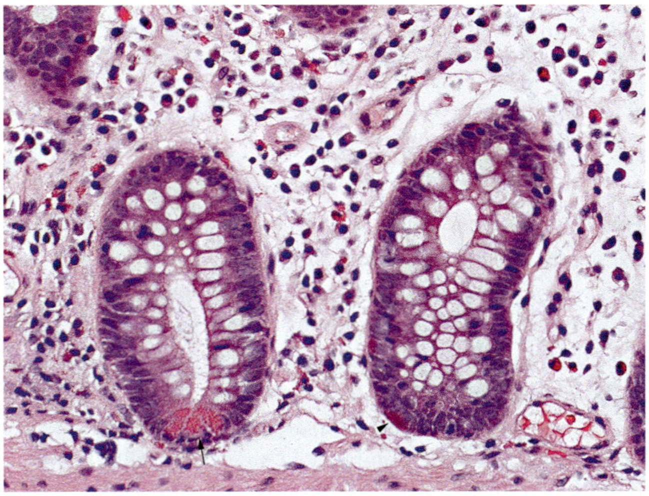

Fig. 1.22 Paneth cells (arrow) versus endocrine cells (arrowhead) in colonic mucosa

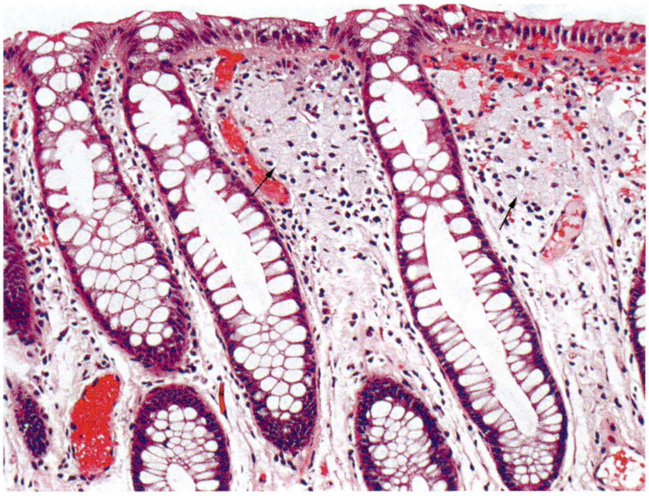

Fig. 1.23 Muciphages (arrows) in lamina propria are a common finding within the left colon and rectum

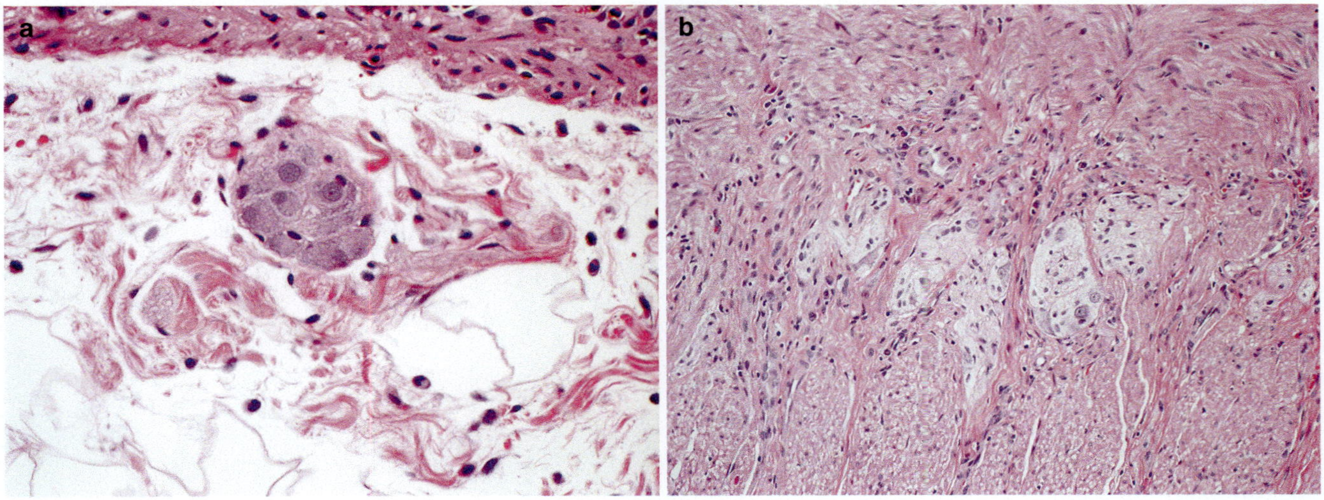

Fig. 1.24 Colonic neural plexuses. (**a**) The submucosal plexus of Meissner, consisting of neurons, glial cells, ganglion cells, and stromal components. (**b**) The myenteric plexus (or Auerbach's plexus) located between the longitudinal and circular layers of muscularis propria

Lymphatic Drainage

The cecum, ascending colon, and hepatic flexure drain into the pericolic, ileocolic, and right colic lymph nodes. The transverse colon and splenic flexure drain into the pericolic, middle colic, and left colic lymph nodes. The descending and sigmoid colon drain into the pericolic, left colic, sigmoid, and inferior mesenteric lymph nodes.

Innervation

The ascending colon and proximal two-thirds of the transverse colon receive their sympathetic, parasympathetic, and sensory supply via nerves from the superior mesenteric plexus. The distal one-third of the transverse colon, descending colon, and sigmoid colon receive their sympathetic, parasympathetic, and sensory supply via nerves from the inferior mesenteric plexus, composed of parasympathetic innervation via the pelvic splanchnic nerves and sympathetic innervation via the lumbar splanchnic nerves.

Anal Canal

Anatomy

The anal canal is the most terminal part of the large intestine connecting the rectum to the anus. It extends from the level of the pelvic floor (anorectal ring) to the anal opening (anus). In an adult, the anal canal measures around 3–4 cm in length [35, 36]. The sequence of epithelial zones from the rectum to the perianal skin is divided into four different areas: (1) zone covered by colorectal type of mucosa; (2) anal transitional zone; (3) zone covered by squamous epithelium; and (4) perianal skin lined by keratinized squamous epithelium, skin appendages, and hair follicles. The muscles of the anal canal (from inside out) consist of musculus submucosae ani, internal anal sphincter, anal longitudinal muscle, and external anal sphincter.

Normal Histology

The colorectal zone of the anal canal is a continuation of the rectal mucosa [37]. The anal transitional zone is lined by small basal cells whose nuclei are arranged perpendicular to the basement membrane (Fig. 1.25). The superficial cells can be flattened to columnar in shape. The anal transitional zone may also show small areas of mature squamous epithelium and simple columnar epithelium. The squamous epithelium just distal to the anal transitional zone is nonkeratinized. Toward the distal end of the anal canal, keratinization becomes apparent as it blends with the perianal skin containing hair and skin appendages.

The anal glands open into the anal transitional zone. They are present within the submucosa and extend into the internal sphincter with some even penetrating the external sphincter [38]. The lining epithelium of these anal glands is similar to the epithelium lining the anal transitional zone (Fig. 1.26a, b). Intraepithelial microcysts and goblet cells may also be seen within the anal glands. The anal glands are surrounded by myoepithelial cells and may also show few lymphocytes around them. Within the perianal skin, an additional type of glands known as the anogential mammary-like glands is also seen. They are lined by a simple columnar

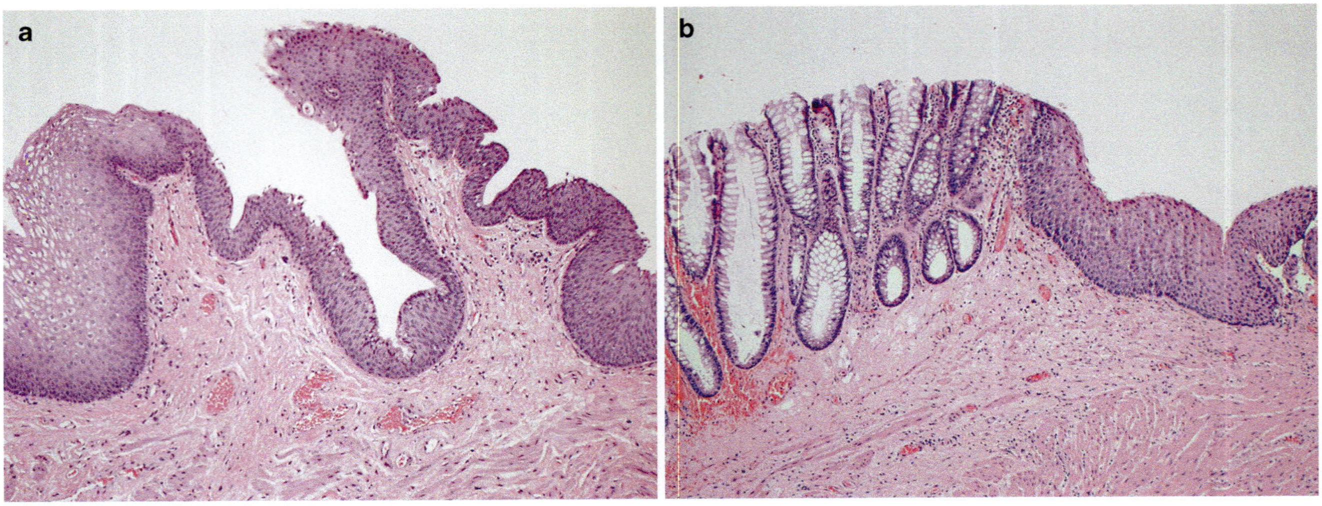

Fig. 1.25 (a) The anal transitional zone mucosa (right), lined by multilayered small basal cells, in comparison to the anal squamous epithelium (left). (b) Transition from the columnar colonic epithelium to anal transitional zone mucosa

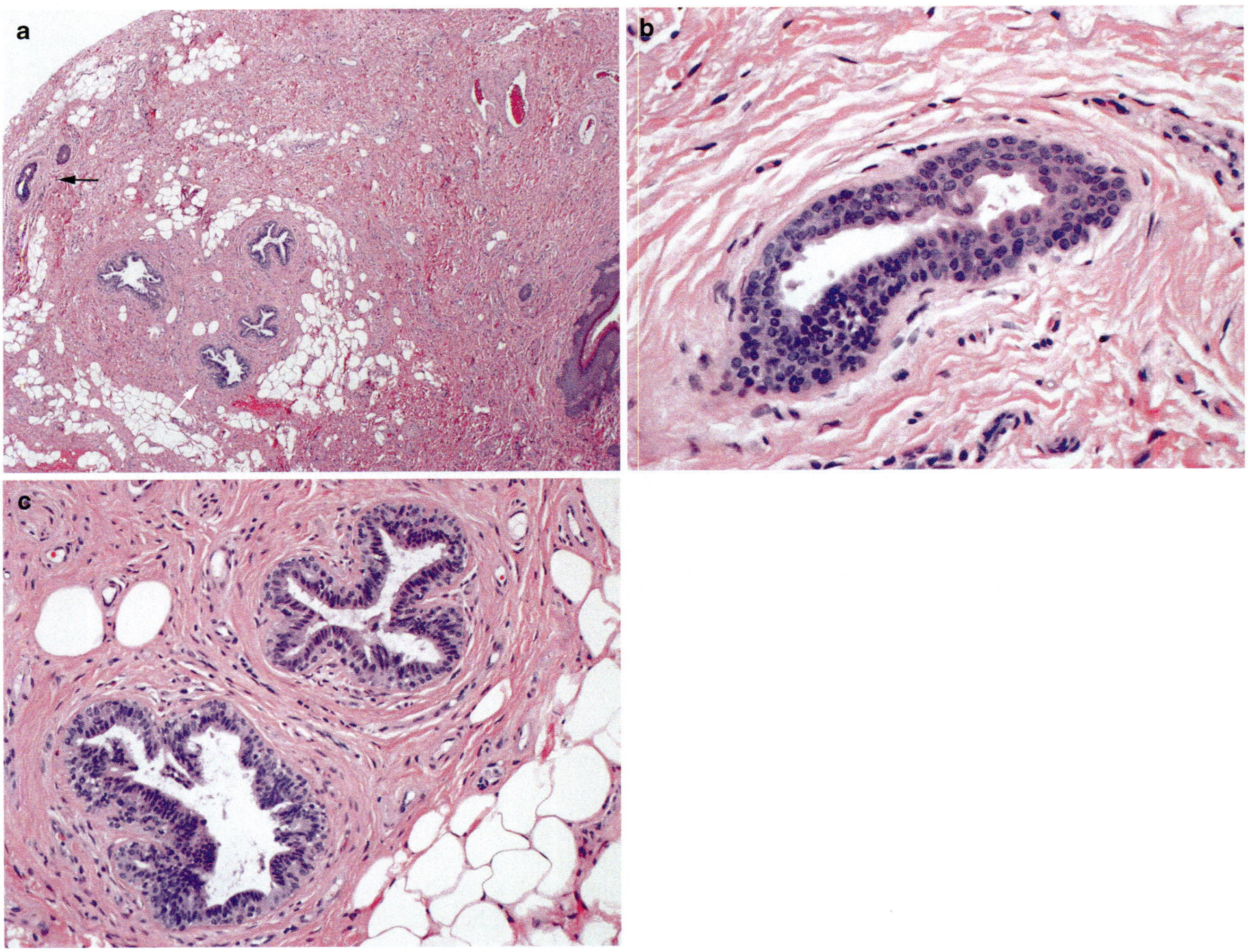

Fig. 1.26 Anal glands and anogenital mammary-like glands. (a) Two distinct structures in this section: anal gland ducts (black arrow) and anogenital mammary-like glands (white arrow). (b) An anal gland duct lined by transitional zone epithelium. (c) Transverse section of anogenital mammary-like glands lined by one layer of low columnar epithelial cells surrounded by myoepithelial cells and loose connective tissue, with small acini formation (arrow)

epithelium with cytoplasmic projections protruding into the glandular lumen and surrounded by an outer myoepithelial layer (Fig. 1.26a, c).

The lamina propria consists of loose connective tissue containing a variable number of mast cells and lymphocytes. The muscularis mucosae of the rectum continue into the proximal anal canal and can also be found in the proximal anal transitional zone. Few interstitial cells of Cajal may be seen in the internal anal sphincter but not in the external sphincter [39].

Lymphatic Drainage

The upper part of the anal canal drains to the hypogastric, obturator, and internal iliac lymph nodes. The lower part of the anal canal and perianal skin drain into the superficial inguinal nodes.

Innervation

Sympathetic fibers from the superior rectal and hypogastric plexuses innervate the internal anal sphincter. The pudendal and fourth sacral nerves provide the innervation to the external anal sphincter.

References

1. Abid S, Mumtaz K, Jafri W, Hamid S, Abbas Z, Shah HA, et al. Pill-induced esophageal injury: endoscopic features and clinical outcomes. Endoscopy. 2005;37(8):740–4. https://doi.org/10.1055/s-2005-870129.
2. McCullough RW, Afzal ZA, Saifuddin TN, Alba LM, Khan AH. Pill-induced esophagitis complicated by multiple esophageal septa. Gastrointest Endosc. 2004;59(1):150–2.
3. McClave SA, Boyce HW Jr, Gottfried MR. Early diagnosis of columnar-lined esophagus: a new endoscopic diagnostic criterion. Gastrointest Endosc. 1987;33(6):413–6.
4. Abraham SC, Krasinskas AM, Correa AM, Hofstetter WL, Ajani JA, Swisher SG, et al. Duplication of the muscularis mucosae in Barrett esophagus: an underrecognized feature and its implication for staging of adenocarcinoma. Am J Surg Pathol. 2007;31(11):1719–25. https://doi.org/10.1097/PAS.0b013e318093e3bf.
5. Meyer GW, Austin RM, Brady CE 3rd, Castell DO. Muscle anatomy of the human esophagus. J Clin Gastroenterol. 1986;8(2):131–4.
6. Shimada H, Nabeya Y, Matsubara H, Okazumi S, Shiratori T, Shimizu T, et al. Prediction of lymph node status in patients with superficial esophageal carcinoma: analysis of 160 surgically resected cancers. Am J Surg. 2006;191(2):250–4. https://doi.org/10.1016/j.amjsurg.2005.07.035.
7. Eguchi T, Nakanishi Y, Shimoda T, Iwasaki M, Igaki H, Tachimori Y, et al. Histopathological criteria for additional treatment after endoscopic mucosal resection for esophageal cancer: analysis of 464 surgically resected cases. Mod Pathol. 2006;19(3):475–80. https://doi.org/10.1038/modpathol.3800557.
8. Lewin KJ, Riddell RH, Weinstein WM. Normal structure of the stomach. In: Lewin KJ, Riddell RH, Weinstein WM, editors. Gastrointestinal pathology and its clinical implications. New York: Igaku-Shoin; 1992. p. 496–505.
9. Rubin W, Ross LL, Sleisenger MH, Jefries GH. The normal human gastric epithelia. A fine structural study. Lab Invest. 1968;19(6):598–626.
10. Walker MM, Smolka A, Waller JM, Evans DJ. Identification of parietal cells in gastric body mucosa with HMFG-2 monoclonal antibody. J Clin Pathol. 1995;48(9):832–4.
11. Rindi G, Buffa R, Sessa F, Tortora O, Solcia E. Chromogranin A, B and C immunoreactivities of mammalian endocrine cells. Distribution, distinction from costored hormones/prohormones and relationship with the argyrophil component of secretory granules. Histochemistry. 1986;85(1):19–28.
12. Genta RM, Hamner HW, Graham DY. Gastric lymphoid follicles in Helicobacter pylori infection: frequency, distribution, and response to triple therapy. Hum Pathol. 1993;24(6):577–83.
13. Ahrens EH Jr, Blankenhorn DH, Hirsch J. Measurement of the human intestinal length in vivo and some causes of variation. Gastroenterology. 1956;31(3):274–84.
14. Rubin W. The epithelial "membrane" of the small intestine. Am J Clin Nutr. 1971;24(1):45–64. https://doi.org/10.1093/ajcn/24.1.45.
15. Holmes R, Hourihane DO, Booth CC. The mucosa of the small intestine. Postgrad Med J. 1961;37:717–24.
16. Goldman H, Antonioli DA. Mucosal biopsy of the esophagus, stomach, and proximal duodenum. Hum Pathol. 1982;13(5):423–48.
17. Dobbins WO 3rd. Human intestinal intraepithelial lymphocytes. Gut. 1986;27(8):972–85.
18. Ferguson A, Murray D. Quantitation of intraepithelial lymphocytes in human jejunum. Gut. 1971;12(12):988–94.
19. Hayat M, Cairns A, Dixon MF, O'Mahony S. Quantitation of intraepithelial lymphocytes in human duodenum: what is normal? J Clin Pathol. 2002;55(5):393–4.
20. Selby WS, Janossy G, Bofill M, Jewell DP. Lymphocyte subpopulations in the human small intestine. The findings in normal mucosa and in the mucosa of patients with adult coeliac disease. Clin Exp Immunol. 1983;52(1):219–28.
21. Cerf-Bensussan N, Schneeberger EE, Bhan AK. Immunohistologic and immunoelectron microscopic characterization of the mucosal lymphocytes of human small intestine by the use of monoclonal antibodies. J Immunol. 1983;130(6):2615–22.
22. Buschard K, Kjaeldgaard A. Investigation and analysis of the position, fixation, length and embryology of the vermiform appendix. Acta Chir Scand. 1973;139(3):293–8.
23. Bjerke K, Brandtzaeg P, Rognum TO. Distribution of immunoglobulin producing cells is different in normal human appendix and colon mucosa. Gut. 1986;27(6):667–74.
24. Smith ME, Morton D. The colon. In: Smith ME, Morton D, editors. The digestive system. Edinburgh: Churchill Livingstone; 2001. p. 175–86.
25. Guyton A. The digestive and metabolic systems. In: Guyton A, editor. Anatomy and physiology. Philadelphia: WB Saunders; 1984. p. 643–700.
26. Gledhill A, Cole FM. Significance of basement membrane thickening in the human colon. Gut. 1984;25(10):1085–8.
27. Anagnostopoulos I, Schuppan D, Riecken EO, Gross UM, Stein H. Tenascin labelling in colorectal biopsies: a useful marker in the diagnosis of collagenous colitis. Histopathology. 1999;34(5):425–31.
28. Schonhoff SE, Giel-Moloney M, Leiter AB. Minireview: development and differentiation of gut endocrine cells. Endocrinology. 2004;145(6):2639–44. https://doi.org/10.1210/en.2004-0051.
29. Porter EM, Bevins CL, Ghosh D, Ganz T. The multifaceted Paneth cell. Cell Mol Life Sci. 2002;59(1):156–70.
30. Rubio CA, Nesi G. A simple method to demonstrate normal and metaplastic Paneth cells in tissue sections. In Vivo. 2003;17(1):67–71.

31. Rothenberg ME, Mishra A, Brandt EB, Hogan SP. Gastrointestinal eosinophils. Immunol Rev. 2001;179:139–55.
32. Rumessen JJ, Peters S, Thuneberg L. Light- and electron microscopical studies of interstitial cells of Cajal and muscle cells at the submucosal border of human colon. Lab Invest. 1993;68(4):481–95.
33. Ward SM, Sanders KM. Interstitial cells of Cajal: primary targets of enteric motor innervation. Anat Rec. 2001;262(1):125–35.
34. Takayama I, Horiguchi K, Daigo Y, Mine T, Fujino MA, Ohno S. The interstitial cells of Cajal and a gastroenteric pacemaker system. Arch Histol Cytol. 2002;65(1):1–26.
35. Fenger C. The anal transitional zone. Location and extent. Acta Pathol Microbiol Scand A. 1979;87A(5):379–86.
36. Nivatvongs S, Stern HS, Fryd DS. The length of the anal canal. Dis Colon Rectum. 1981;24(8):600–1.
37. Wendell-Smith CP. Anorectal nomenclature: fundamental terminology. Dis Colon Rectum. 2000;43(10):1349–58.
38. Seow-Choen F, Ho JM. Histoanatomy of anal glands. Dis Colon Rectum. 1994;37(12):1215–8.
39. Hagger R, Gharaie S, Finlayson C, Kumar D. Distribution of the interstitial cells of Cajal in the human anorectum. J Auton Nerv Syst. 1998;73(2–3):75–9.

2 Endoscopy, Tissue Processing, Stains, and Special Tests

Ferga C. Gleeson and Lizhi Zhang

Endoscopy

Introduction of Endoscopy

Flexible endoscopes to visualize the upper gastrointestinal tract were pioneered in 1957 by Hirschowitz and colleagues [1]. There have been numerous innovations in endoscopic technology since that time, to improve upon mucosal visualization. Improved lesion detection has allowed the endoscopist to provide a real-time optical diagnosis. Such advances in image acquisition technologies including magnification endoscopy; autofluorescence imaging; electronic chromoendoscopy techniques such as narrow-band imaging, i-scan, or flexible spectral imaging color enhancement; and confocal laser micro endoscopy have all enabled visualization of the mucosa and subsurface structures such as the vasculature in greater detail (Figs. 2.1a, b and 2.2a, b). With the evolution and the variations of this optimized visualization technology, the emphasis has been placed upon characterizing subtle flat and depressed lesions harboring precancerous changes or early cancer.

Colonoscopy Bowel Preparation and Historical Impact on Colonic Epithelium

Colonoscopy can evaluate mucosal changes and prevent colorectal cancer by the detection and removal of premalignant lesions. The combination of dietary restriction and cathartics has proven to be safe and effective for colonic cleansing in preparation for colonoscopy. However, up to 25% of all such procedures are reported to have an inadequate bowel cleansing preparation [2, 3]. The ideal preparation should reliably empty the colon of all fecal matter with no gross or histological alteration of the colonic mucosa. In the 1970s, the effect of laxatives and enemas on normal human rectal mucosa was reported by Meisel and colleagues, noting sloughing of the surface epithelium leading to a possible misdiagnosis from rectosigmoid biopsy specimens [4]. Then, in the 1980s, the effects of lavage and laxative preparations on colonic mucosal histology in a prospective, randomized study noted that a standard preparation (48-hour clear liquid diet, 240 ml of magnesium citrate and a senna derivative) flattened the surface epithelial cells, depleted goblet cells, and increased edema of the lamina propria in contrast to a 3–4 l of colonic lavage with Golytely, a polyethylene glycol–electrolyte lavage solution [5]. Regimens for FDA-approved colonic cleansing preparations now include polyethylene glycol–electrolyte lavage solution (PEG-ELS)-based cleansing agents and sodium phosphate solutions. The routine use of adjunctive agents for bowel cleansing before colonoscopy is not recommended. The use of sodium phosphate-containing preparations can be associated with the development of superficial mucosal abnormalities that may resemble features of early inflammatory bowel disease. In a prospective study of patients without known inflammatory bowel disease, mucosal lesions secondary to the effect of sodium phosphate were reported in 3.3% [6]. Another prospective, randomized, single-blinded trial in 634 patients reported that colonoscopy preparation-induced mucosal inflammation was ten times greater with sodium phosphate when compared to PEG solutions [7]. In another trial of 97 patients, aphthoid-like mucosal lesions were reported in 2.3% of patients receiving PEG compared with 24.5% of patients who received sodium phosphate solution [8]. Although these mucosal changes may mimic the changes of Crohn's disease, the histologic appearance is distinctive and thought to permit differentiation from inflammatory bowel disease.

F. C. Gleeson
Division of Gastroenterology and Hepatology, Mayo Clinic, Rochester, MN, USA

L. Zhang (✉)
Department of Laboratory Medicine and Pathology, Mayo Clinic, Rochester, MN, USA
e-mail: Zhang.Lizhi@mayo.edu

L. Zhang et al. (eds.), *Surgical Pathology of Non-neoplastic Gastrointestinal Diseases*,
https://doi.org/10.1007/978-3-030-15573-5_2

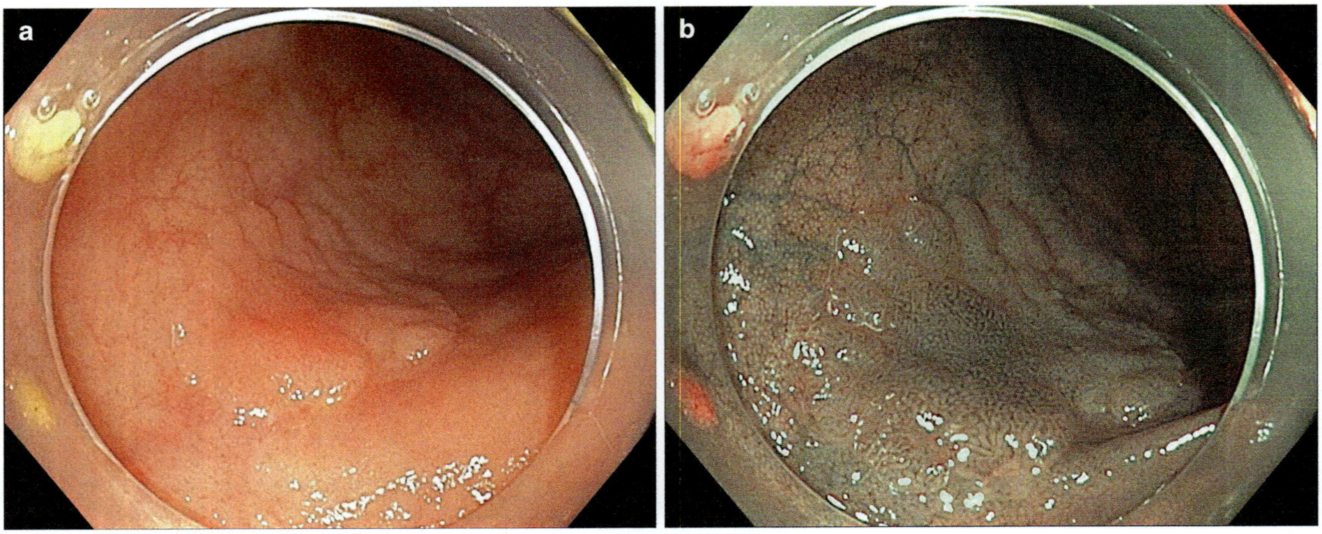

Fig. 2.1 A 40 mm sessile polyp at the hepatic flexure viewed by white light (**a**) and narrow band imaging (**b**) revealing a central depression. On subsequent EMR, the flat polyp was histologically established to be a tubulovillous adenoma with focal high-grade dysplasia

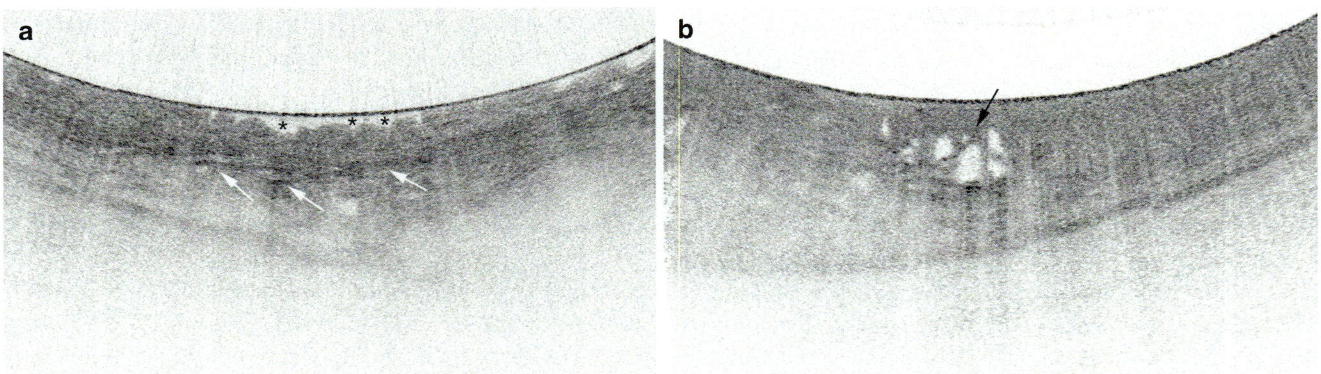

Fig. 2.2 Volumetric laser endomicroscopy image of (**a**) nondysplastic Barrett's esophagus showing a partially effaced layered architecture (white arrows) and villiform epithelium (asterisks) and (**b**) Barrett's esophagus with high-grade dysplasia showing lack of a layered architecture with a cluster of atypical glands (black arrow) characterized by their cribriform appearance and presence of intraluminal debris

Mechanisms of Acquiring Cellular and Histological Material

Cytosponge Cytosponge is a nonendoscopic cell collection device composed of a polyurethane sponge within a gelatin capsule attached to a string. The capsule is swallowed and dissolves in the proximal stomach and retrieved 5 minutes later. The subsequent sample has the potential to retrieve more than 500,000 cells from the esophageal lining. The immunohistochemical biomarker, trefoil factor 3 (TFF3) has been shown to distinguish Barrett's esophagus cells from normal squamous epithelium and gastric cardia with a sensitivity and specificity of 80% and 92%, respectively [9]. A methylation marker panel may also have promise as a diagnostic biomarker for Barrett's esophagus [10]. Cytosponge may also provide an accurate method to assess eosinophilic esophagitis histologic activity (Fig. 2.3) [11].

Endoscopic Biopsy and Polypectomy Polypectomy is the basis for cancer prevention during colonoscopy. Cold snaring is now the primary technique for the resection of polyps up to 10 mm in size [12]. Hot forceps is no longer used or recommended. Although large-capacity cold forceps can be used to remove tiny polyps (1–2 mm) in a single piece, cold snaring is thought to be more effective and efficient than cold forceps resection for diminutive lesions (<5 mm). The technique of cold snaring is fundamentally different from hot snare resection [13]. Hot snare polypectomy may be used following submucosal injection for sessile polyps sized 10–19 mm. For scenarios to include 10–19 mm polyps in the cecum or ascending colon, or patients with increased risk of post-polypectomy bleeding, a piecemeal cold snare polypectomy, with or without prior submucosal injection, may be performed.

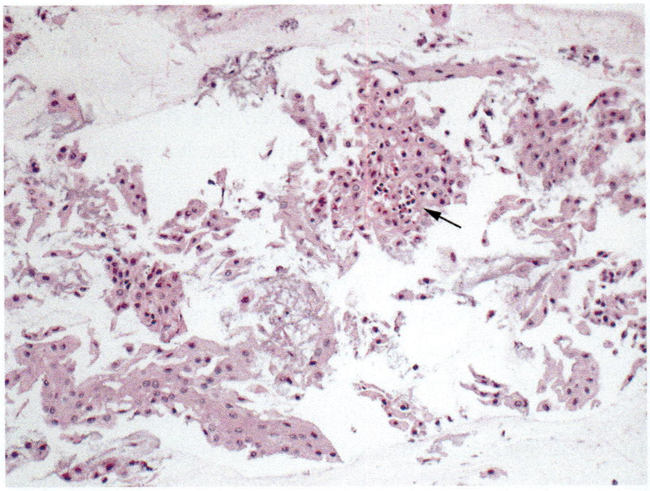

Fig. 2.3 Detection of intraepithelial eosinophils (arrow) in the superficial layer of esophageal squamous epithelium obtained using cytosponge in eosinophilic esophagitis

Endoscopic Mucosal Resection Endoscopic mucosal resection (EMR) was developed for minimally invasive, organ-sparing endoscopic removal of benign and early malignant lesions confined to the mucosa and submucosa in the GI tract. It is commonly used for Barrett's esophagus-associated neoplasia. It has also been reported to be effective in resecting type 1 gastric carcinoids <10 mm and is widely used for the resection of large or flat colonic lesions. EMR is a single section of tissue excision limited to a maximum of 20–25 mm. The commonly used techniques can be categorized as injection-, cap-, and ligation-assisted or under-water EMR. The injection-assisted EMR is also often called saline solution lift-assisted polypectomy developed in the 1950s. A solution is placed into the submucosal space under the lesion to create a safety cushion, thereby lifting the lesion, facilitating capture using a snare. The cap method uses a dedicated mucosectomy device using a clear plastic cap affixed to the endoscope that comes prepared with an electrocautery snare that must be opened and positioned on an internal ridge at the tip of the cap (Fig. 2.4). The endoscope is positioned over the target lesion, and suction is applied to retract the mucosa into the cap, after which the snare is closed to capture the lesion. In ligation-assisted EMR, a band ligation device is attached to the endoscope, and the banding cap is positioned over the target lesion with or without previous submucosal injection. As per the cap-assisted EMR technique, suction is applied to retract the lesion into the banding cap, and a band is deployed to capture the lesion, thereby creating a pseudo polyp. An electrocautery snare is then used to resect the pseudo polyp either above or below the band.

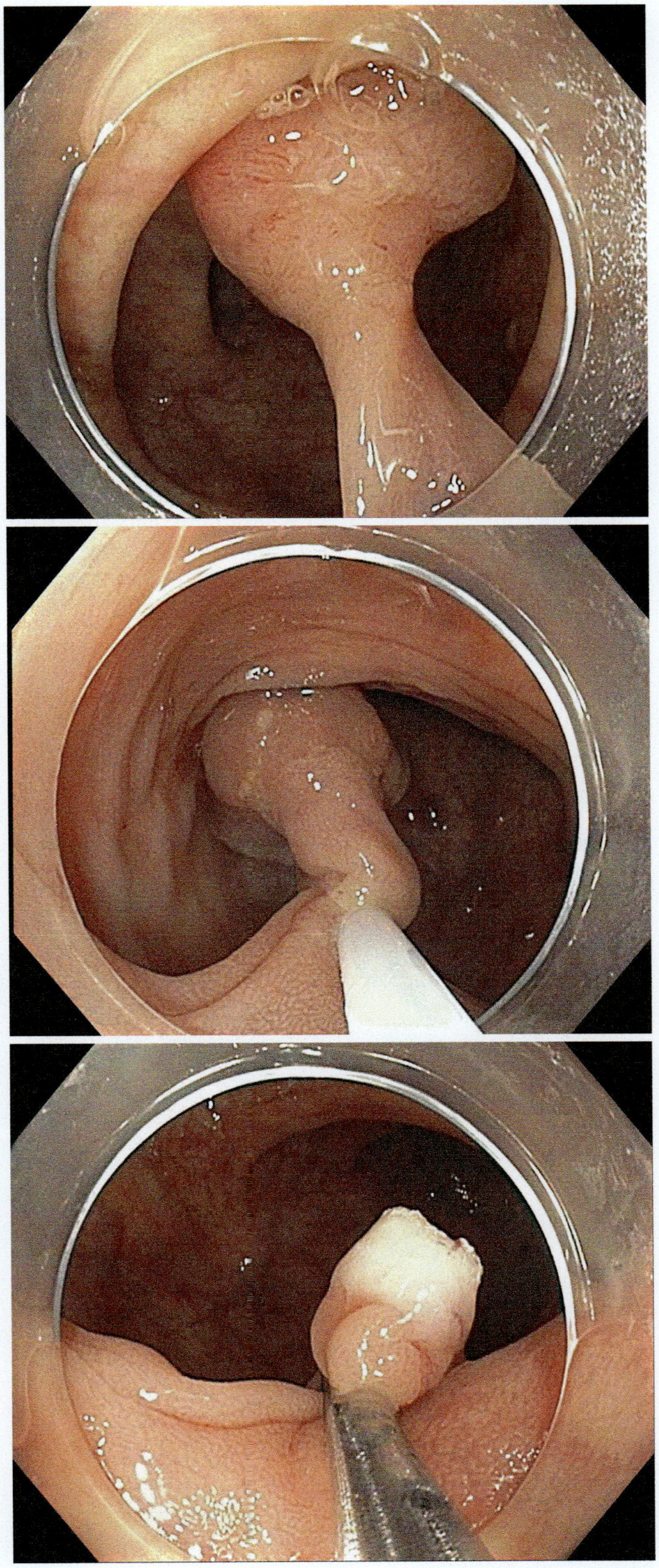

Fig. 2.4 Snare resection of a pedunculated polyp (upper), with a snare (middle) and post polypectomy (low)

Endoscopic Submucosal Dissection In contrast to EMR, with endoscopic submucosal dissection (ESD), the submucosa is dissected under the lesion with a specialized knife which in turn enables removal of larger and potentially deeper lesions with a curative intent. For larger sized lesions, an "en bloc" resection technique is necessary based on the oncologic principle that an "en bloc" excision of the neoplasm with free macroscopic and microscopic margins should be achieved. It was pioneered in Japan as a treatment for "en-bloc" excision of early gastric cancer. It also has an emerging role in Barrett's neoplasia, particularly in bulky disease and lesions predicted to have low-risk submucosal invasive cancers.

ESD is accomplished in a stepwise manner with a variety of devices (Fig. 2.5). Typically, the ESD steps include that the perimeter of the target lesion is demarcated with electrocautery, followed by a lifting agent into the submucosa around the perimeter of the target. The mucosa is then incised and cut circumferentially around the target using a specialized knife. The submucosa deep to the target is injected and then dissected in a free-hand manner using a knife until the specimen has been completely resected [14].

Full-Thickness Resection Conventional endoscopic resection techniques such as EMR or ESD are powerful endoscopic techniques for lesions restricted to the superficial layers of the GI tract. Endoscopic full-thickness resection (EFTR) is an evolving technique. It naturally results in a GI wall defect that will require secure defect closure. In the upper GI tract, subepithelial lesions arising from (or infiltrating) the muscularis propria are the most frequent indication for EFTR. In the lower GI tract, the technique may be used for recurrent adenomas with negative lifting sign,

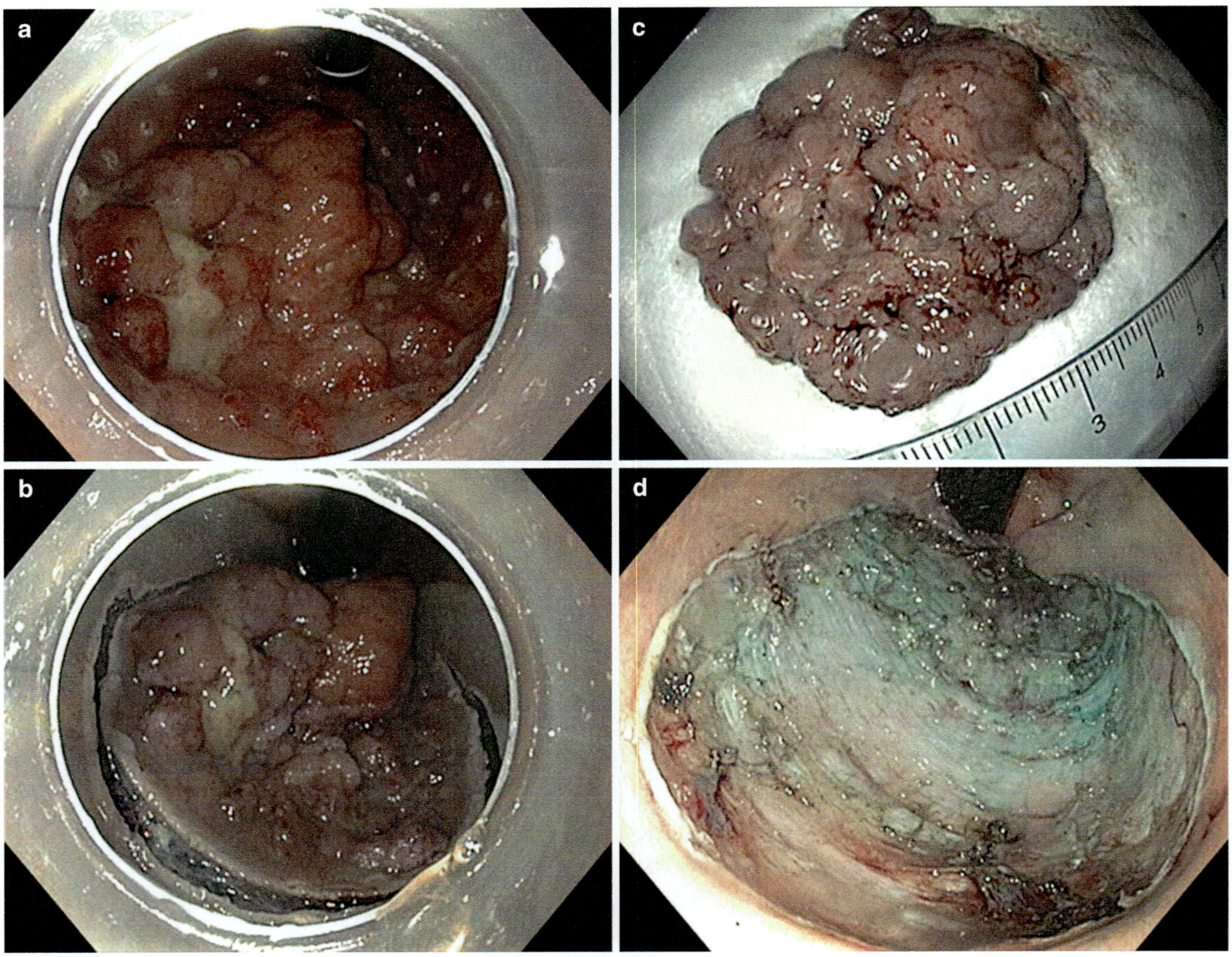

Fig. 2.5 A large laterally spreading 5 cm distal rectal polyp revealing a tubulovillous adenoma with focal high-grade dysplasia following ESD: (**a**) cautery demarcation marks around the perimeter of the lesion; (**b**) post electrocautery knife; (**c**) en bloc resection specimen; (**d**) post ESD mucosal defect

incompletely resected nonlifting adenomas, treatment-naïve nonlifting adenomas, re-resection of T1 carcinomas, adenomas in challenging anatomic locations not suitable for standard endoscopic resection, and subepithelial lesions and, although unusual, maybe to obtain a diagnostic yield in patients with suspected motility disorders such as Hirschsprung's disease.

EUS-Guided Biopsy Endoscopic ultrasound tissue acquisition via fine-needle aspiration (FNA) cytology or fine-needle biopsy (FNB) using specialized core needles designed to obtain histological specimens has become a central technique in the assessment of GI and non-GI malignancies. The use of FNB may provide tissue architecture and facilitate immunohistochemical staining necessary for various diagnosis to include lymphoma, GI stromal tumors, and metastasis. Diagnostic yields for EUS-FNA in assessing GI subepithelial lesions have ranged from 46% to 93% but are improved with the use of FNB. This is an area where EUS will have a role in personalized medicine as the acquired material may be used for therapeutic purposes, for example, scoring PD-L1 expression in pancreatic carcinoma on EUS-FNB specimens staining (Fig. 2.6) [15, 16].

Endoscopy- and Bowel Preparation-Related Histological Changes

The procedures of endoscopy, biopsy, and bowel preparation may create some artifacts and tissue damages. Knowing these changes can help pathologists to better interpret the biopsy and to avoid an incorrect diagnosis. Some of them are introduced in this section and also summarized in Table 2.1.

Endoscopy-Induced Injury

Scope Trauma This is referred to the mechanical mucosal injury secondary to the direct contact of the endoscope with the mucosa during the procedure, especially when the biopsies are taken at the last after visual inspection of the gut. Microscopically, the mucosa can present with congestion, edema, and hemorrhage in lamina propria (Fig. 2.7). Surface flattening, epithelial sloughing, or pneumatosis intestinalis can occur in more severe cases.

Pneumatosis Intestinalis Gas or air can be iatrogenically introduced into the wall of the intestine secondary to air insufflation and increased intraluminal pressure during endoscopy but rarely can it cause any signs or symptoms [17]. Biopsy tissue may occasionally show changes of pneumatosis intestinalis characterized by empty spaces in lamina propria or submucosa, which resemble fat cells (Fig. 2.8). Therefore, it is also known as pseudolipomatosis. However, the absence of nuclear structures at the peripheral of the open spaces should distinguish them from fat cells. In addition, adipose tissue should not normally present in lamina propria. For chronic cases, it may be associated with eosinophils, histiocytes, or multinucleated giant cells. Pneumatosis intestinalis may also mimic intestinal lymphangiectasia which is characterized by diffuse or patchy dilated lymphatics involving mucosa and submucosa. But the dilated lymphatics are usually much larger than the air spaces, and they often contain light eosinophilic lymphatic protein in the lumens.

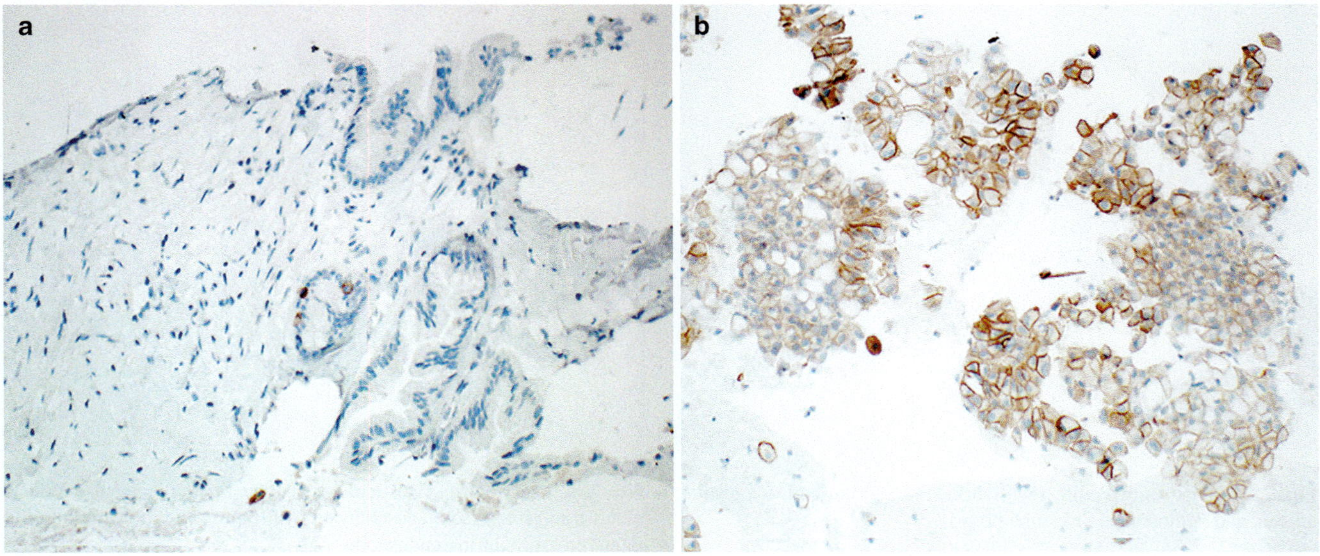

Fig. 2.6 Scoring PD-L1 expression on EUS-FNB specimens. Tumor proportion score of (**a**) 1% and (**b**) 80% in treatment-naïve pancreas ductal adenocarcinoma

Table 2.1 Common histological changes and artifacts related to endoscopy and tissue processing

Cause	Histological changes	Comment
Scope trauma	Mucosal congestion, edema, and hemorrhage	Epithelial sloughing in severe injury
Pneumatosis intestinalis	Open spaces in mucosa and submucosa	Mimicking fat cells or dilated lymphatics
Postbiopsy site changes	Hemorrhage and inflammation, re-epithelialization with underlying granulation tissue reaction and scar formation, proliferative crypts, and minimal crypt architectural changes	Complete mucosal healing typically in 1–2 weeks Larger biopsy needs more healing time and shows significant glandular architectural distortion with fibrosis, mimicking chronic colitis
Bowel perforation	Bowel wall defect with associated inflammation	Clinicians should be alerted of the risk of perforation if muscularis propria is identified on biopsy
Bowel preparation artifacts	Mild changes: surface flattening, goblet cell and mucin depletion, edema, extravasated red blood cells and neutrophils in lamina propria, apoptosis; Severe changes: epithelial sloughing, hemorrhage, aphthous lesions, cryptitis, and acute colitis	Oral sodium phosphate causes more severe tissue injury than PEG solutions and has been withdrawn Preparation-related aphthous lesions do not show chronicity
Crush artifact	Mucosal hemorrhage, tissue distortion, rearrangement of tissue morphology, and loss of cytological details	Inflammatory and tumor cells are most susceptible Pseudoinvasion by misplacing epithelium in submucosa
Cautery artifact	Nuclei spindling and palisading; opaque and amorphous appearance of fibrous connective tissue, fat, and muscle	Inadequate specimen for evaluating dysplasia Help identifying stalk margin
Freezing artifact	Interstitial and intracytoplasmic vacuoles	Rarely used for biopsy
Air-drying artifact	Eosinophilic staining and tissue shrinkage	Immerse tissue in fixative as quickly as possible Do not deliver tissue on tissue paper or saline-soaked gauze
Inadequate fixation	Tissue autolysis; altered staining quality of cells; cell shrunken	Immerse tissue in fixative as quickly as possible Tissue/formalin ratio of at least 1:10 Other fixatives such as alcohol are not recommended
Floaters	A tissue fragment with different histology from that of other pieces or a type that would not be expected	Small biopsy tissue fragments are more susceptible for tissue contamination
Improper tissue orientation	Artificial structural and architectural changes	Although orientation is not required, embedding in edge to ensure vertical cut is necessary, especially for polypoid tissue to include the margins
Improper H&E staining	Lack of contrast or overstaining	Difficult to differentiate from dysplasia
Foreign materials and pigments	Stain deposits, formalin pigment, etc.	May mimic microorganisms

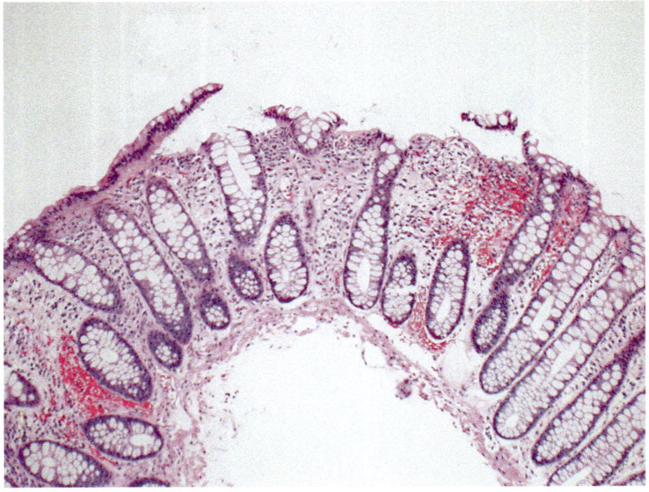

Fig. 2.7 Scope injury, with focal surface sloughing and congestion, edema, and hemorrhage in lamina propria

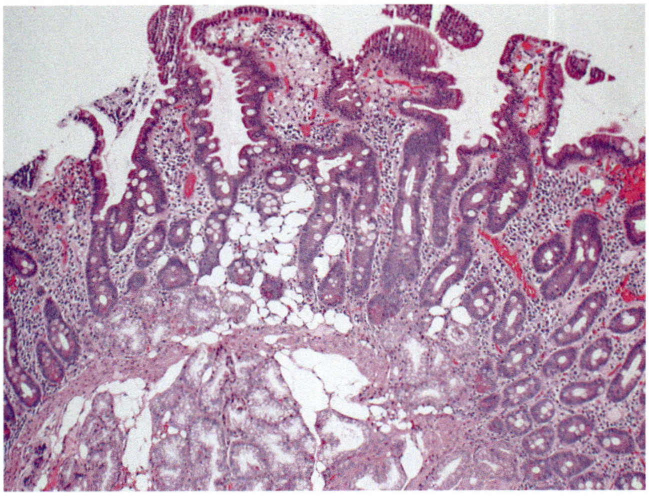

Fig. 2.8 Pneumatosis intestinalis. Irregular open spaces in duodenal mucosa and submucosa caused by air insufflation and increased intraluminal pressure during endoscopy

Perforation Gastrointestinal perforation after diagnostic or therapeutic endoscopic procedures is a rare but potentially life-threatening complication. The incidence of iatrogenic perforation is increasing worldwide because of the more frequent use of endoscopy for screening and more widespread use of endoscopic therapy [18, 19]. Pathologists should recognize the presence of muscularis propria in the biopsy tissue and alert clinicians of the potential risk of perforation.

Endoscopic Biopsy Artifact

Crush Artifact This can occur when pressing the biopsy forceps, removing tissue with forceps, or cutting tissue especially when using a blunt blade. Crushing can squeeze the chromatin out of nuclei resulting in loss of cytological details. Inflammatory and tumor cells are most susceptible. The force also produces mucosal hemorrhage, tissue distortion, and rearrangement of tissue morphology. For example, the surface epithelium may be forced through the connective tissue and misplaced in submucosa resembling invasion; crushed Brunner's glands in duodenal biopsy may mimic a neural or myxoid/mucinous neoplasm (Fig. 2.9).

Cautery Artifact This is produced as a result of electrocautery. It is commonly seen in the polypoid tissue undergoing endoscopic electrosurgical cutting such as hot snare polypectomy. The mucosal biopsy for non-neoplastic diseases is usually obtained using cold biopsy with no such artifact. The heat generated damages the tissue and alters the morphology of both epithelium and connective tissue. The epithelium is detached from basement membrane. The epithelial cells have an "explosion" appearance. The nuclei are spindling and palisading with hyperchromasia, which makes it impossible to differentiate from dysplasia (Fig. 2.10). The fibrous connective tissue, fat, and muscle have an opaque and amorphous appearance. In fact, these changes may be helpful for determining stalk margins when examining endoscopic resection specimens.

Postbiopsy Site Changes The routine endoscopic biopsy typically causes minor mucosal damage that can heal quickly after procedures. The earliest changes at the biopsy site are coagulation and acute inflammatory reaction. Re-epithelialization starts from the adjacent epithelium with underneath granulation tissue reaction and early scar formation within 1–2 days after biopsy. Complete mucosal healing typically needs 1–2 weeks, but deeper biopsy or mucosal resection takes longer time to heal. The healed biopsy sites may display minimal abnormal morphology such as increased inflammatory cells in lamina propria, crypts with proliferative changes such as increased proliferative zone and budding, and minimal crypt architectural change. Larger biopsy or mucosal biopsy sites may demonstrate significant glandular architectural distortion with fibrosis and disrupted muscularis mucosae, which may mimic chronic mucosal injury secondary to ischemia or chronic colitis (Fig. 2.11).

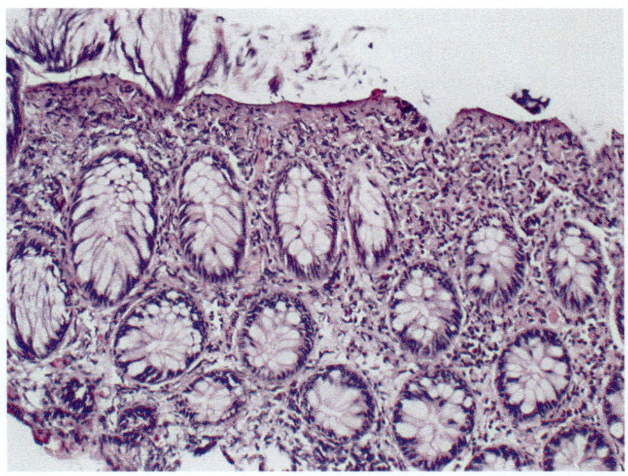

Fig. 2.10 Cautery artifact. Note dysplasia-like nuclear changes

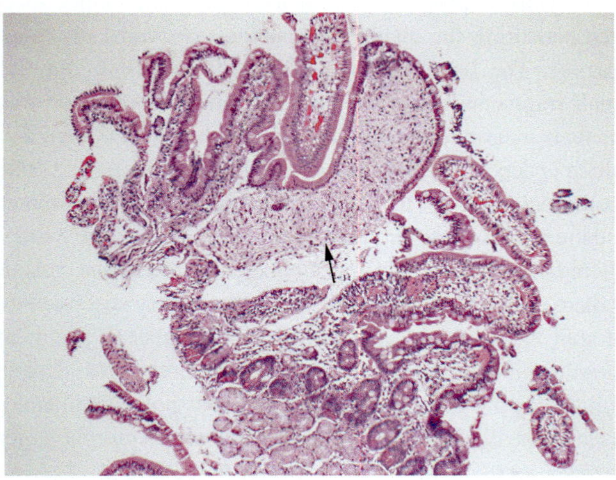

Fig. 2.9 Crushed Brunner's glands (arrow) showing a neural or myxoid/mucinous appearance

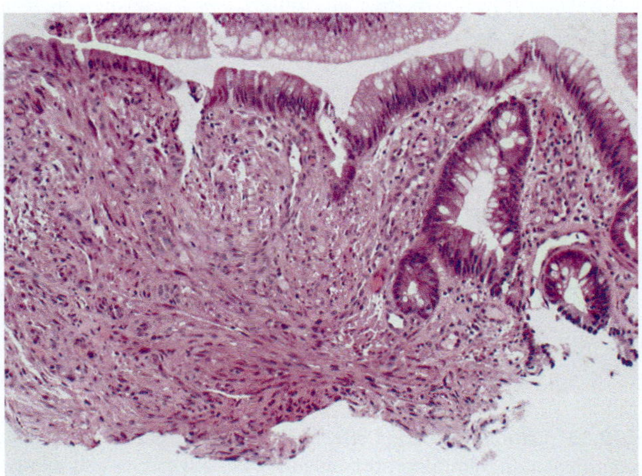

Fig. 2.11 Postbiopsy site change. The glandular architectural distortion with fibrosis resembling chronic mucosal injury

Bowel Preparation Effect

Bowel preparation-related changes are mainly seen in colonic biopsy since the preparation of upper gastrointestinal endoscopy only needs no drinking and eating 4–8 hours before the procedure without using any laxative. Nowadays, PEG-based solutions are the main agents used for preparation [3]. Although a variety of mucosal changes have been described, including surface epithelial damage (flattening, goblet cell and mucin depletion, cytoplasmic vacuolization, and sloughing), lamina propria edema and congestion, extravasated red blood cells, presence of neutrophil cells in lamina propria or even cryptitis, and increased crypt proliferation (Fig. 2.12), studies have found that PEG agents only occasionally cause those damages which are typically minimal and insignificant [8, 20–22]. Preparation-related aphthous lesions may be found endoscopically which mimic those in Crohn's disease, but these lesions are not friable and not associated with other mucosal changes in chronic colitis. More importantly, the mucosa does not show chronic changes microscopically. Once pathologists are familiar with these physiological artifacts, they can neglect these changes and do not need to report them which may cause unnecessary confusion and concerns for clinicians or patients who may consider these features being pathologic.

Sodium phosphate could cause more severe tissue injury than PEG solutions such as epithelial sloughing, increased crypt apoptosis, hemorrhage, or even colitis mimicking pseudomembranous colitis or inflammatory bowel disease [8, 23, 24]. It should not be used for patients in evaluation of graft-versus-host disease since the increased apoptosis caused by the preparation can mimic mild graft-versus-host disease (Fig. 2.13). Oral sodium can also induce serious adverse events such as renal injury and electrolyte abnormalities, and it has been withdrawn from the market since 2008. Other hyperosmotic agents such as oral sodium sulfate are also occasionally used, with no significant side effects [25].

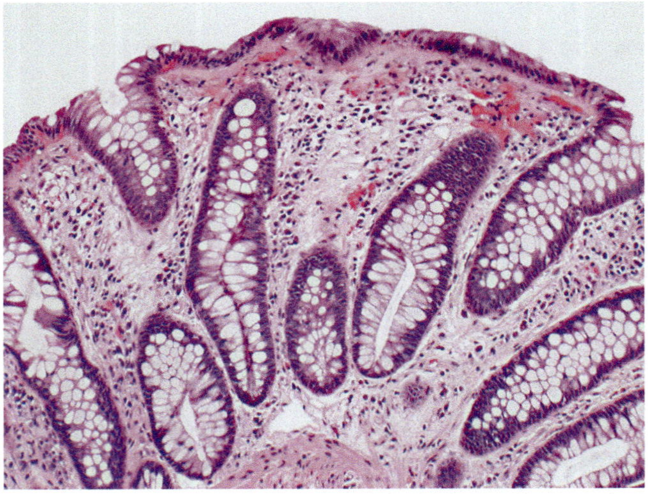

Fig. 2.12 Bowel preparation effect, with surface epithelial flattening, mucin depletion, lamina propria edema and congestion, and extravasated red blood cells

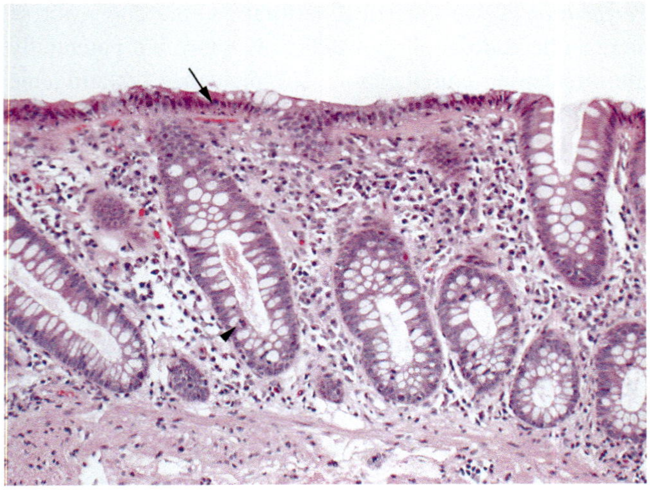

Fig. 2.13 Bowel preparation induced apoptosis, predominantly in surface epithelium (arrow) and rarely in crypts (arrowhead)

Tissue Processing, Stains, and Special Tests

Proper tissue processing and staining are essential for the subsequent morphology assessment. The commonly encountered pitfalls and artifacts created during these processes are summarized in Table 2.1. It is important for pathologists to recognize and avoid these pitfalls during diagnosis.

Gross Evaluation and Tissue Processing

Biopsy Specimens

A majority of histopathological evaluations for non-neoplastic gastrointestinal disorders is based on endoscopic biopsy specimens. Thus, to properly process the endoscopic biopsy specimens, assuring the quality of histology is critical in clinical practice. The biopsy specimens usually consist of multiple small fragments with variable sizes. The size of tissue fragments is measured as a range (typically less than 0.3 cm each which is dependent upon the size of biopsy forceps and endoscopic techniques). The number of tissue fragments is counted. If there are less than ten fragments in each biopsy, the tissue is filtered into a biopsy bag and submitted en toto in one cassette. If there are more than ten fragments, the biopsy specimen can be split into multiple cassettes, and the number of fragments submitted in each cassette is also recorded in the gross description. Inking the tissue fragments is generally not recommended, because the thick ink may obscure some subtle morphological changes, especially for smaller biopsy tissue (Fig. 2.14).

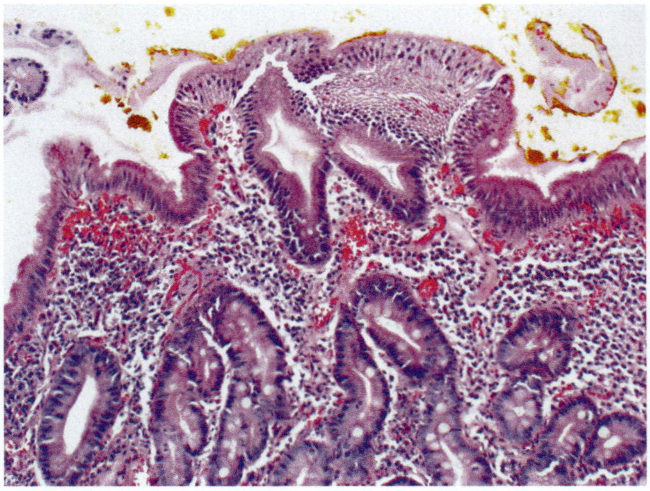

Fig. 2.14 The yellow ink on the surface may obscure the gastric foveolar metaplasia in this duodenal biopsy sample

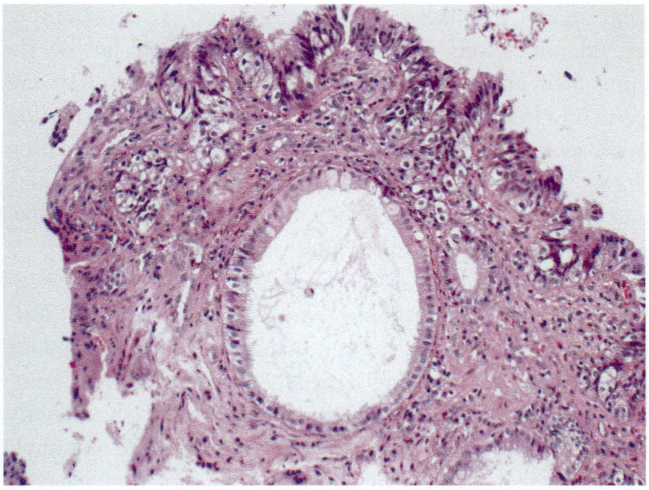

Fig. 2.15 Bouin's fixation revealing striking nuclear details mimicking epithelial dysplasia in the Barrett's mucosa

Fixation using 10% neutral buffered formalin is standard in histology labs. Sections cut from well-fixed gastrointestinal mucosal biopsy tissue can be used for routine hematoxylin and eosin (H&E) stain, immunohistochemistry, most histochemical stains, and RNA or DNA tests. The tissue should be immersed in a large volume of formalin fixative as rapidly as possible. The ratio of fixative to tissue should be at least 10:1 [26]. Do not put the tissue on tissue paper or saline-soaked gauze to delivery to histology labs because marked dry artifact can be created, and this jeopardizes the morphological examination. Fixation time is critical for obtaining appropriate morphology. Under-fixed tissue can produce artifacts from dehydrating alcohols used in subsequent tissue processing. Formalin penetrates the tissue at a rate of approximately 1.0 mm per hour at room temperature. Therefore, at least 1 hour is needed for a tissue fragment with a size of 1.0 mm. Increased temperatures using microwave can accelerate fixation, but this may influence the quality of histological and molecular studies [27, 28]. Nowadays, most labs use automated tissue processors which only need 10-minute fixation in 10% neutral-buffered formalin at 50 °C and can produce adequate tissue specimens, and the turnaround time of the whole tissue processing for biopsy specimens, including fixation, dehydration, clearing, and tissue infiltration, is usually less than 2 hours. Frozen sections are rarely required for evaluation of non-neoplastic gastrointestinal diseases except for few specific conditions such as identifying ganglion cells in rectal biopsy in Hirschsprung's disease.

Other fixatives such as Bouin's solution and B5 have been used in some labs. These fixatives can produce excellent nuclear morphology compared to formalin-fixed tissue, but they are usually only recommended for fixation of hematopoietic and lymphoid tissue. Gastrointestinal biopsy tissue fixed in Bouin's or B5 solution may reveal striking nuclear details mimicking nuclear atypia seen in epithelial dysplasia (Fig. 2.15). They can also highlight lymphoid cells that could be overestimated when evaluating inflammatory disorders (Fig. 2.16). Furthermore, these fixatives contain heavy metal that can interfere with nucleic acid extraction and create biohazard disposal problems.

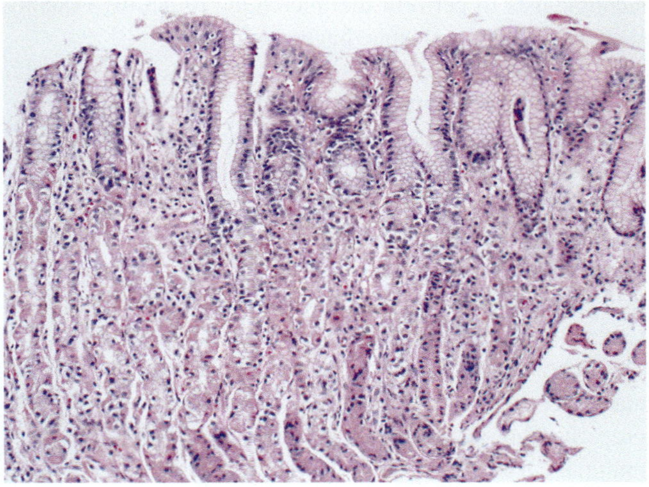

Fig. 2.16 B5 fixation making lymphocytes so prominent that it seems intraepithelial lymphocytosis mimicking lymphocytic gastritis

Paraffin embedding is the standard method used in histology labs to produce blocks of tissue for cutting. Although tissue orientation is not required, properly oriented tissue is important in evaluating mucosal biopsy, especially for structural and architectural assessment such as villous atrophy in celiac disease or submucosal invasion in an adenoma. Improperly orientated tissue may increase the difficulties for pathologists to interpret the biopsy and sometimes may lead to misdiagnoses. Therefore, the histology technologists who embed the tissue should understand tissue sampling and identification. The tissue fragments should be orderly embedded on edge to ensure that the mucosa will be cut vertically to show the full thickness of mucosa. A dissecting microscope is rarely used to determine the tissue orientation during embedding nowadays because multiple fragments and sections of small biopsy material can generally allow proper tissue orientation for microscopic examination.

The embedded biopsy tissue is cut in a ribbon of consecutive sections in a microtome. Two sections for routine H&E stain are generated per cassette, and each section contains multiple levels which are dependent on the size and number of the tissue fragments. Deeper sections are occasionally required when the initial sections are not adequate or pathologists suspect more informative morphological changes in deeper levels. The sections are typically cut at 3–5 μm thickness for routine stains including immunohistochemistry, but some special stains may need thicker cut such as Congo red stain at 10 μm. It is critical to have well-trained histology technologists to perform the microtome to get high-quality sections and save valuable diagnostic tissue.

Polypoid Specimens

Polypoid specimens are usually obtained during endoscopic treatment for neoplastic lesions such as large polyps or early cancer, which include EMR and ESD. They are larger in size than biopsy tissue. After measuring the three dimensions, identifying the base or stalk and inking its margin are necessary. The polypoid tissue should be bisected (if >0.3 cm), trisected (if <1.0 cm), or serially sectioned (if >1.0 cm). The cuts should be made vertically along the long axis of the stalks to make sure that the surgical margins are included and sectioned properly. The specimens can be submitted entirely in one or multiple cassettes. For piecemeal polypectomy, tissue orientation to identify the margins is not practical, and the tissue fragments can be counted or measured in aggregate and then submitted en toto. Longer fixation time is required for polypoid specimens which may need overnight in formalin. The tissue sections are embedded on edge to include the margins.

Resection Specimens

Surgical resections are occasionally performed for non-neoplastic gastrointestinal disorders. Appendectomy and bowel resections for inflammatory bowel disease are probably the two most commonly seen specimens in surgical pathology. Gross examination and tissue processing are introduced in the corresponding chapters in this book.

Stains

Hematoxylin and Eosin Stain

H&E stain is the standard for morphological examination and is routinely performed on all tissues submitted for histopathological evaluation. The principle and importance of H&E stains are needless to be introduced here. Most labs use automated slide stainers that can provide a standardized process that ensures reproducible and consistent staining. However, we have noticed significant variation of the quality of H&E stains among different labs in our daily consultation practice. We have to request additional H&E sections performed in our lab for a significant number of send-in cases. The most common problems are lack of contrast and overstaining. The staining may be too "blue" to examine the detailed histocytological features. For example, the overstained sections can create artificial nuclear hyperchromasia which makes it difficult when evaluating dysplasia (Fig. 2.17). Undissolved stain particles can sometimes incorporate into the tissue

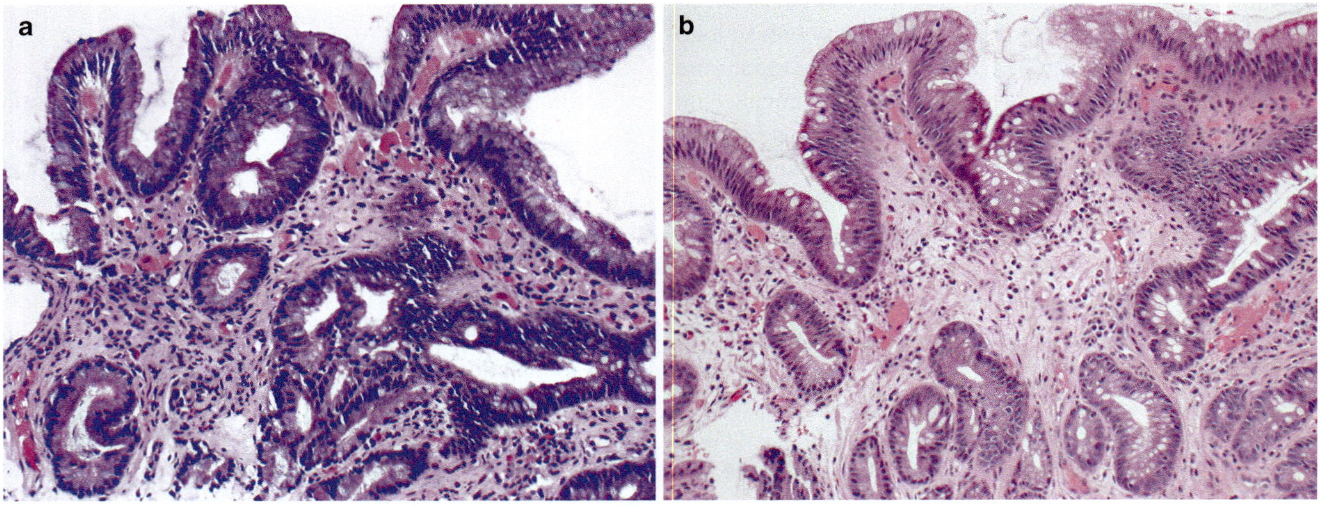

Fig. 2.17 Inappropriate H&E staining. (**a**) Overstained Barrett's mucosa with nuclear atypia and hyperchromasia raising concern for dysplasia; (**b**) A repeated H&E staining with proper contrast ruling out this possibility

leading to precipitation which can mimic microorganisms. Therefore, maintenance and quality control are critical for the labs to produce reliable stains that can satisfy microscopic examination.

Histochemical Stains

Besides routine H&E stains, special histochemical stains are also often used in daily practice. Most of these stains are used to demonstrate microorganism. Understanding the principle and usage of these stains are important for pathologists, and to properly choose the stains can provide diagnostic value in some cases. The commonly used special histochemical stains are listed below:

Warthin–Starry Stain It is a silver stain that is commonly used to identify *Helicobacter pylori* and spirochetes. The bacteria stain black. However, the background is usually dirty, which makes it hard to read. Hence, immunohistochemical stains for *Helicobacter pylori* and *T. pallidum* are preferred. This stain is particularly helpful in confirming intestinal spirochetosis which shows densely packed filamentous spirochetes on the epithelial surface (Fig. 2.18).

Periodic Acid–Schiff (PAS) Stain PAS stain with or without diastase (PAS-D) is used to detect polysaccharides and mucosubstances such as mucins in tissue. It stains neutral mucin in normal esophageal glands, stomach, and anal glands. It can also highlight fungal organisms. However, PAS stain is most commonly used to detect *Tropheryma whipplei* in Whipple's disease in duodenal biopsy. The foamy histiocytes in the lamina propria are filled with PAS-D positive intracytoplasmic microorganisms (Fig. 2.19).

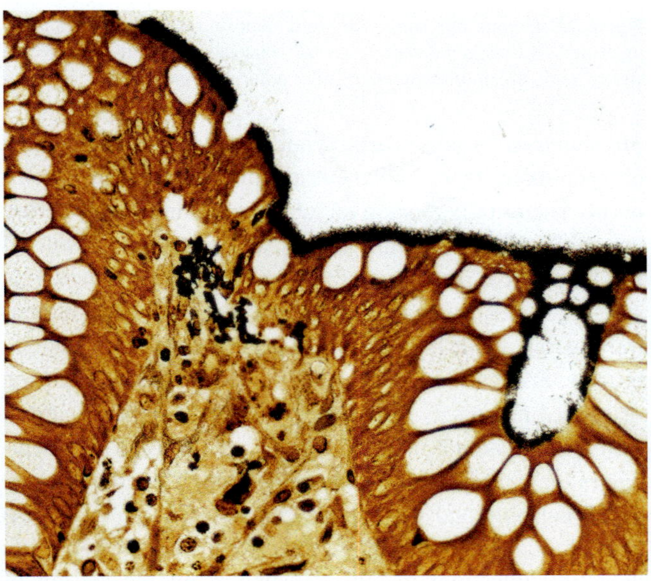

Fig. 2.18 Warthin–Starry stain, showing filamentous spirochetes on colonic epithelial surface

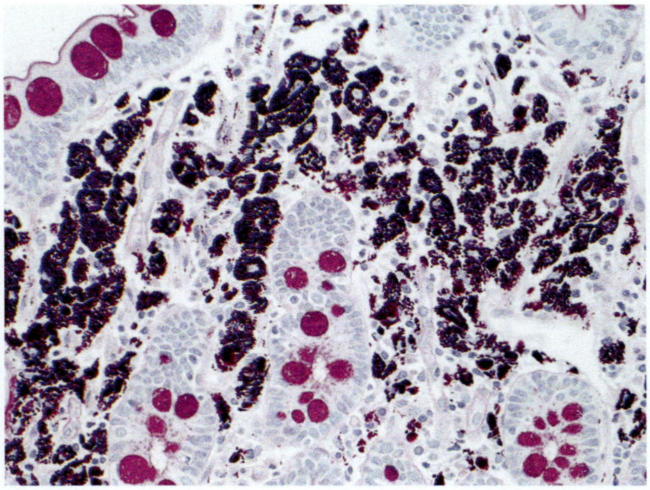

Fig. 2.19 Periodic acid–Schiff (PAS) stain. PAS stain with diastase (PAS-D) highlights mucin in goblet cells and PAS-D positive intracytoplasmic microorganisms in histiocytes in duodenal mucosa, consistent with *Tropheryma whipplei*

Grocott's Methenamine Silver (GMS) Stain This silver stain is the most commonly used stain for identifying fungal organisms in gastrointestinal biopsies. The organisms are outlined by black-stained cell walls which allow further classification of the species in most cases (Fig. 2.20a, b).

Gram Stain It is occasionally used to identify bacterial infection. Gram stain on paraffin-embedded tissue typically has dirty background and nonspecific staining that limits its usage. Of note, normal luminal flora is also often stained.

Ziehl–Neelsen (AFB) Stain It is commonly used for detecting acid-fast bacteria in tissue when granulomas present, especially if they are caseating. The AFB stain should be examined carefully because the bacteria are typically sparse (Fig. 2.21). If there is strong clinical suspicion, examining under 60×, or oil objective, and a repeat stain can be helpful if the first set of stain is negative. Even though PCR test for mycobacteria using paraffin-embedded tissue is available, the AFB stain should still be performed because of the low sensitivity of the PCR.

Congo Red Stain Apple green birefringence under polarization following Congo red staining is considered the most specific technique for the demonstration of amyloid (Fig. 2.22). However, false-positive staining can occasionally occur. The amyloid stains deep pink to red under light microscopy, while the elastic and fibrotic tissue stains pale pink. Furthermore, the elastic and fibrotic tissues show bright sliver birefringence under polarization rather than apple green.

Iron (Gomori's Prussian Blue) Stain It is used to demonstrate iron deposition in gastrointestinal mucosa. For example, it can confirm iron pill-induced mucosal injury

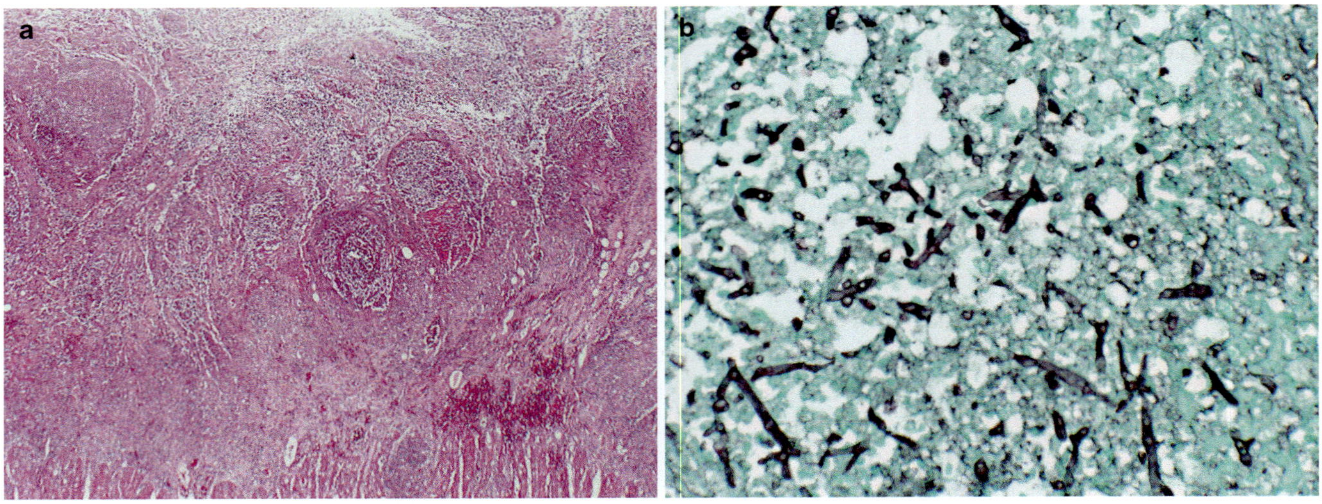

Fig. 2.20 Grocott's Methenamine Silver (GMS) stain. Necrotizing enteritis (**a**) caused by mucormycosis shown on a GMS stain (**b**)

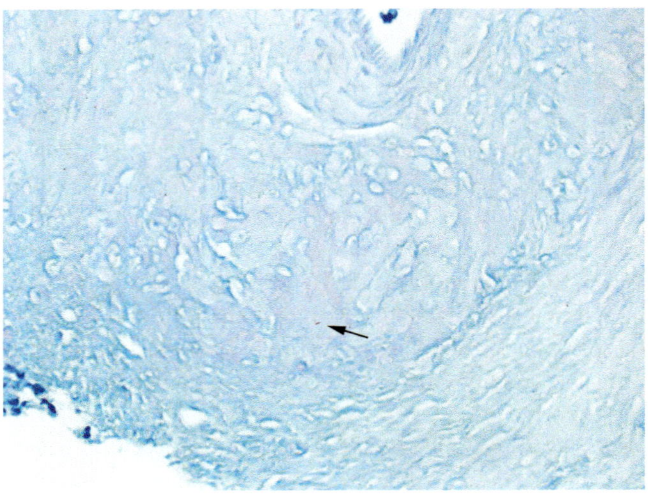

Fig. 2.21 Ziehl–Neelsen (AFB) stain. A single acid-fast bacterium detected in the tissue

(Fig. 2.23a, b) or hemosiderin-laden macrophages in melanosis duodeni.

Von Kossa and Alizarin Red S Stains They are used to detect abnormal deposits of calcium in tissue such as mucosal calcinosis. Alizarin red S stain works best to identify small amounts of calcium such as Michaelis–Gutmann bodies in malakoplakia.

Verhoeff's Elastic Van Gieson (V-VG) Stain It is used to demonstrate elastic fibers (black) in tissue and highlight vessel walls. The collagen stains pink–red, while other tissues stain yellow. It is most used when evaluating vascular disorders such as vasculitis.

Mucin Stains There are several methods to demonstrate different types of mucins in gastrointestinal epithelial cells.

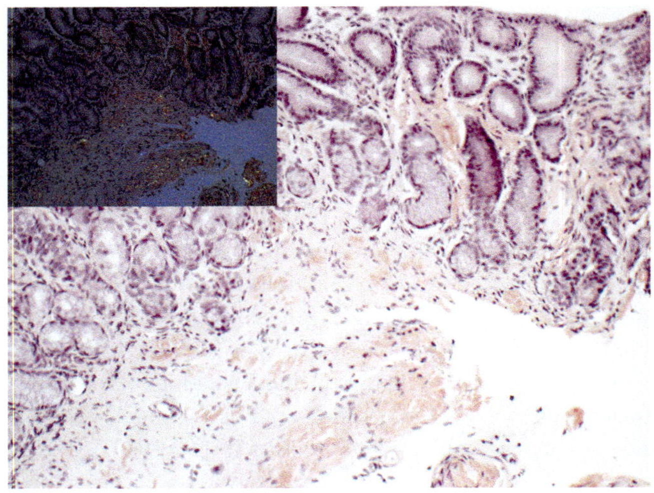

Fig. 2.22 Congo red stain. Amyloid deposit (red–orange staining) identified on Congo red stain in gastric mucosa and submucosa, which shows apple green birefringence under polarization (inset)

Mucicarmine stains carboxylated and sulfated mucins (deep pink–red), but not neutral mucins. It is more commonly used in diagnosing an adenocarcinoma by detecting mucin production by tumor cells. It also stains capsule of the fungus *Cryptococcus neoformans*. *Alcian blue* stains acid mucosubstances and acetic mucins (blue) and not neutral mucins, while Alcian blue at pH 2.5 only detects acidic mucins. *PAS stain* is particularly sensitive for the detection of neutral mucins as well as acid mucins (bright magenta). Cells that contain both neutral and acidic mucins may demonstrate a dark blue or purple coloration. The combination of Alcian blue and PAS stains can be used to distinguish neutral mucins from acid mucins; and this can be helpful in detecting intestinal metaplasia such as in the setting of Barret's esophagus (Fig. 2.24a, b). In intestinal metaplasia, acid mucins replace the original gastric neutral mucins and

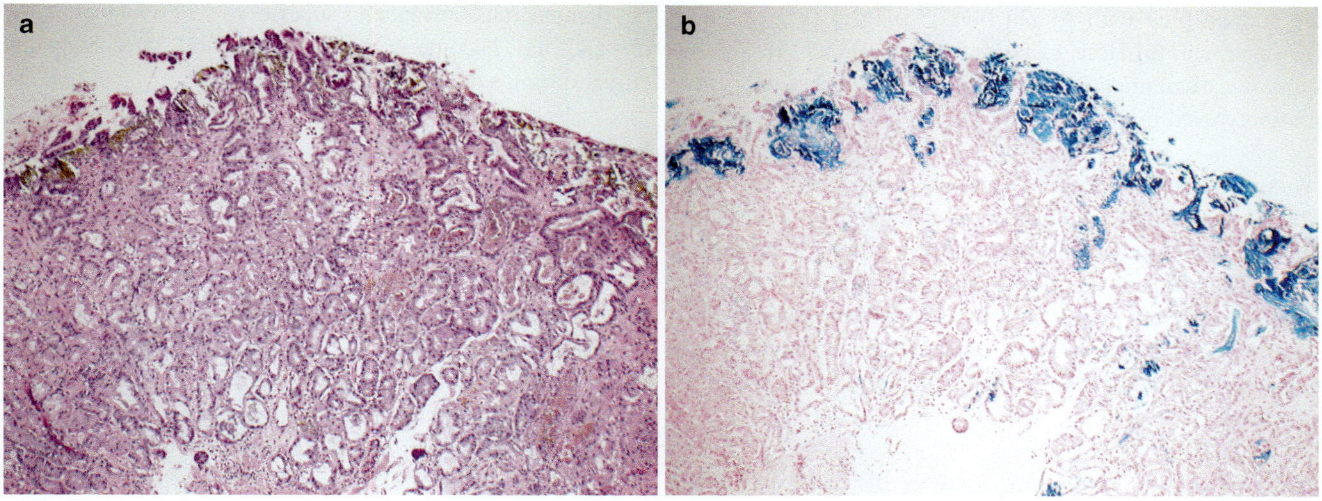

Fig. 2.23 Iron stain (Gomori's Prussian Blue). Iron pill-induced erosive gastropathy (**a**) with a large amount of iron deposition (**b**)

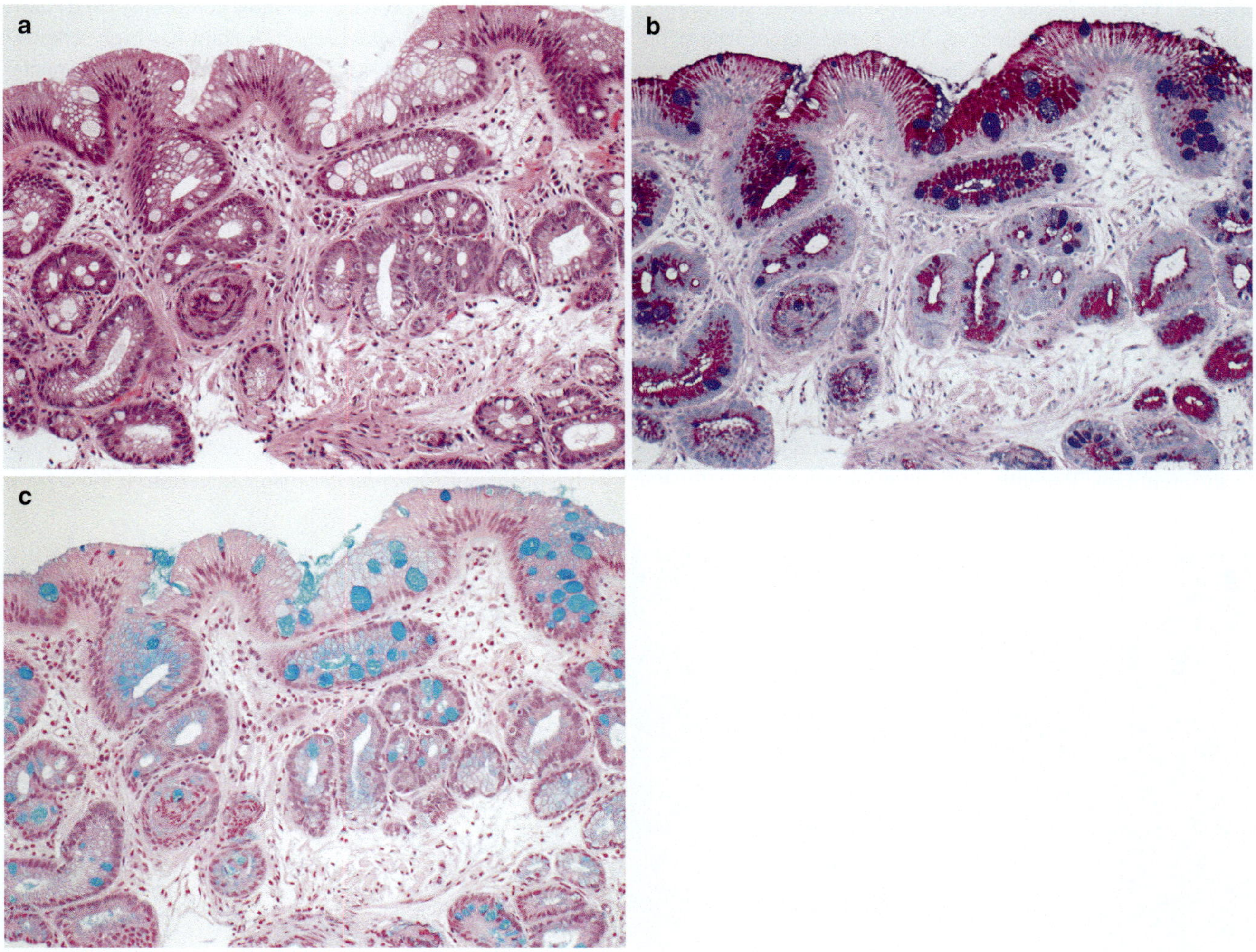

Fig. 2.24 Mucin stains. Goblet cell metaplasia in Barrett's esophagus (**a**) is highlighted by an Alcian blue/PAS stain (**b**, goblet cell-containing acid mucin stained blue by Alcian blue and gastric foveolar cells with neutral mucin stained magenta by PAS) and Alcian blue stain at pH 2.5 (**c**)

are stained blue with Alcian blue at pH 2.5 (Fig. 2.24c). However, careful H&E examination is sufficient in identifying intestinal metaplasia, and hence, this technique is not routinely used in most labs.

Masson's Trichrome Stain This stain is used for evaluating fibrosis such as collagenous colitis, but it is only ordered for questionable cases and not as a routine method for determining the thickness of subepithelial collagen bands. Trichrome stain also plays an important role for evaluating motility disorder which can demonstrate fibrosis in submucosa and muscular layers. It is also useful in identifying parasitic structures.

Reticulin Stain It is rarely used in the gastrointestinal biopsy. The reticular fibers and basement membrane material are stained black to outline the gland architecture. One potential usage of this stain is to distinguish benign signet ring cell change (pseudo-signet ring cell) from signet ring cell carcinoma in the mucosa. The pseudosignet ring cells are still confined by the basement membrane with an intact glandular contour (Fig. 2.25a, b), while the signet ring carcinoma cells show infiltrate growth [29].

Acetylcholinesterase (AChE) Histochemistry In Hirschsprung's disease, the cholinergic nerve fibers of the aganglionic segment are prominent and contain an increased amount of AChE, which can be revealed with AChE histochemistry. Although the sensitivity and specificity of this method in the diagnosis of Hirschsprung's disease were over 90% [30], there are some limitations for AChE histochemistry such as requiring immediately frozen sections, experience in reading the staining patterns, and limited availability in different labs. Recently, calretinin immunohistochemistry has demonstrated advantages superior to AChE histochemistry and has become a preferred method in diagnosing Hirschsprung's disease [31].

Immunohistochemistry

Although the usage of immunohistochemistry in evaluating non-neoplastic disorders is not as wide as it is in tumor evaluation in surgical pathology, some stains are essential to confirm the diagnoses, especially for infectious diseases. The commonly used immunohistochemistry in different conditions are listed in Table 2.2 for quick reference. New immunohistochemical stains emerge every day, such as immunohistochemistry for mycobacterial infection [32], but validation by multiple studies is necessary before they can become truly useful clinical tests.

It is important for pathologists to be aware of some pitfalls or unusual staining patterns when reading immunostains to avoid wrong diagnoses. Immunostains for *Helicobacter pylori* and CMV are probably the most commonly used stains on a daily base. *Helicobacter pylori* stain has high sensitivity and specificity, and it is easier to read than other special stains such as Warthin–Starry or Giemsa stains because of clean background. Of note, *Helicobacter heilmannii* is also positive on *Helicobacter pylori* immunostain, and this can be readily distinguished on H&E sections based on their long tight spiral appearance. *Helicobacter pylori* may not always have a curved bacillary morphology, and they can transform to a coccoid form under certain circumstances such as treatment effect [33]. Immunohistochemistry is very helpful in this setting, but pathologists have to know this phenomenon in order to recognize the positive staining (Fig. 2.26a, b). Some plasma cells and macrophages in lamina propria can show dotted cytoplasmic staining, especially for patients with a history of *Helicobacter pylori* infection. If these posi-

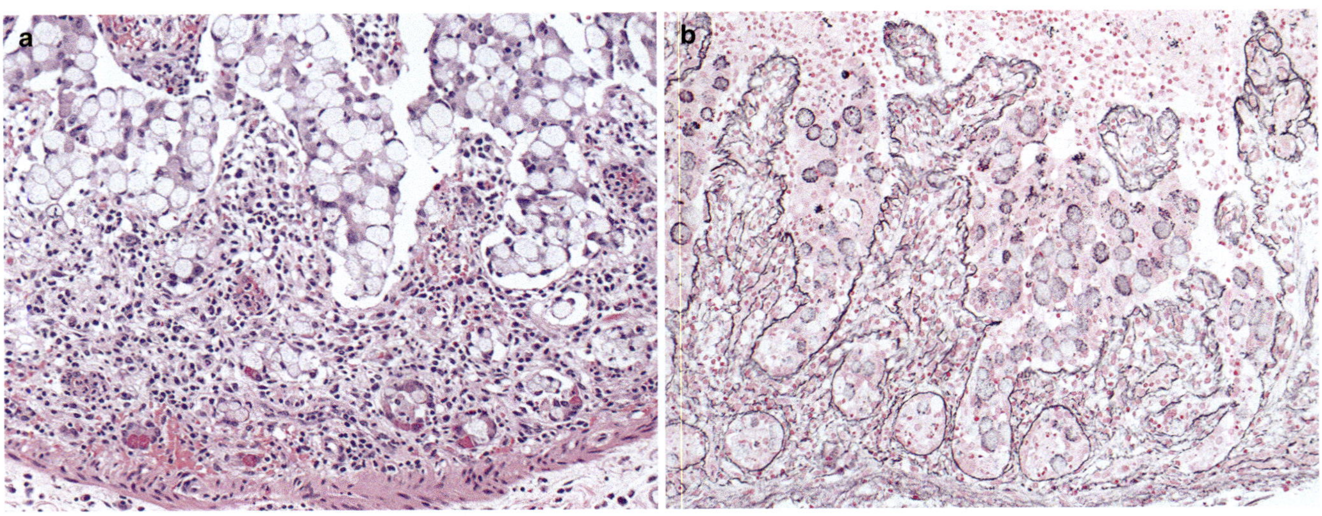

Fig. 2.25 Reticulin stain. Pseudosignet ring cell changes in ischemic enteritis mimicking signet ring cell carcinoma (**a**), but the cells are still confined within the basement membrane shown on reticulin stain (**b**)

Table 2.2 Commonly used immunohistochemistry in evaluating non-neoplastic gastrointestinal disorders

Disorders	Immunohistochemistry (IHC)	Comment
Infections Bacteria Virus Parasites	*Helicobacter pylori*; *Treponema pallidum* (syphilis); *Tropheryma whipplei* (Whipple's disease); *Mycobacterium tuberculosis* complex CMV; adenovirus; herpes simplex virus Varicella zoster virus Toxoplasma; KIT (for giardia)	*Helicobacter pylori* IHC can also stain *Helicobacter heilmannii* *Treponema pallidum* IHC has cross reaction with spirochete and other bacteria CMV IHC may have high background staining leading to false positivity Nonspecific staining of giardia on KIT IHC
Atrophic gastritis	Gastrin (G-cells) and chromogranin (endocrine cell hyperplasia)	Gastrin IHC highlights G-cells to distinguish antrum from body/fundus mucosa G-cells present in the intestinal metaplastic area in body/fundus mucosa
Motility disorder Colonic dismobility/chronic constipation Hirschsprung disease	KIT; smooth muscle actin; CD3 (ganglionitis) Calretinin; NSE	KIT recognizes interstitial cells of Cajal but no standard for quantification Calretinin IHC is a preferred method
Mast cell disorder	Tryptase; KIT; CD25	Tryptase is more specific than KIT and is preferred. CD25 distinguishes neoplastic from reactive mast cells
Refractory sprue	CD3;CD8;TCR beta; TCR delta	Often in combination with T-cell receptor gene rearrangement test to identify a monoclonal T-cell population
Miscellaneous Intraepithelial lymphocytosis Gastric antral vascular ectasia Microvillus inclusion disease Dysplasia CVID Schwann cell hyperplasia Langerhans cell histiocytosis Xanthomatous inflammation	CD3 CD61 (fibrin thrombi) CD10 (brush border) p53 IgG, IgM, IgA s100; Glut1; Claudin-1; EMA CD1a, Langerin, s100 CD68	The number of intraepithelial lymphocytes often overestimated on CD3 stain Brush border may have losses in CD10 staining in active enteritis p53 is not routinely used in evaluating high-grade dysplasia and be aware of p53 null mutation with completely negative staining s100/Glut1/Claudin-1/EMA used to differentiate perineurioma and neurofibroma

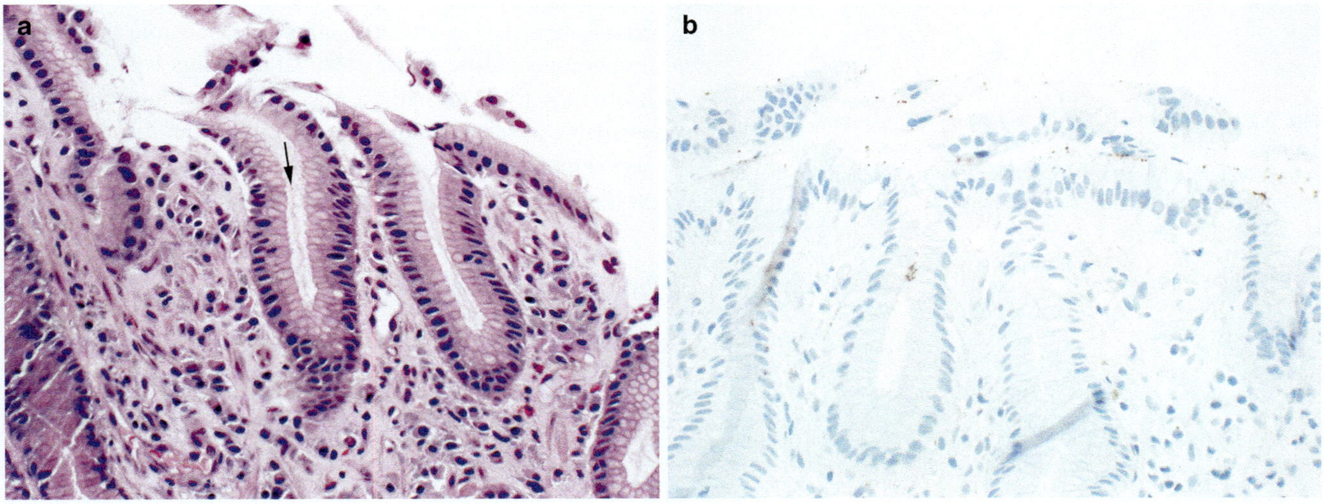

Fig. 2.26 *Helicobacter pylori* immunostain. A coccoid form of *Helicobacter pylori* (arrow) which is difficult to be recognized on the H&E staining (**a**) but confirmed by an immunostain (**b**)

tively stained cells are too close to the pits, it may be misinterpreted as positive (Fig. 2.27).

The CMV immunostain also has similar issue of nonspecific staining in plasma cells and macrophages (Fig. 2.28a, b). Only the cells with distinct dark nuclear staining should be considered positive. Correlation with H&E sections to find the CMV-infected cells is necessary to confirm the diagnosis sometimes. This rule is also applied for other viral immunohistochemistry such as adenovirus and herpes simplex virus. Another important issue of CMV immunostain is the density of CMV infection because the viral load is related to the severity of colitis in inflammatory bowel disease and steroid resistance [34–36]. There is no standardized quantitative or semi-quantitative method to report the severity of CMV infection identified on the biopsy. Kuwabara et al. [34] proposed > 10 inclusions per histological section as dense CMV disease. Nguyen et al. [35] defined "high-grade CMV infection" if the viral inclusions could be identified on both H&E and immunohistochemical stains while the "low-grade infection" as the absence of viral inclusions on H&E stains but the presence of positive CMV immunostains. A recent study from our group defined high-grade CMV density by the presence of five or more inclusions in a single tissue fragment and those patients benefitted from antiviral treatment [36]. Regardless of which criteria is used for defining high-grade CMV infection, recent evidence suggests reporting the number of inclusions per biopsy specimen for patients with inflammatory bowel disease. More accurate quantitative methods to determine the CMV load in biopsy tissue such as real-time PCR tests have been developed, but they have not been widely used yet [37, 38].

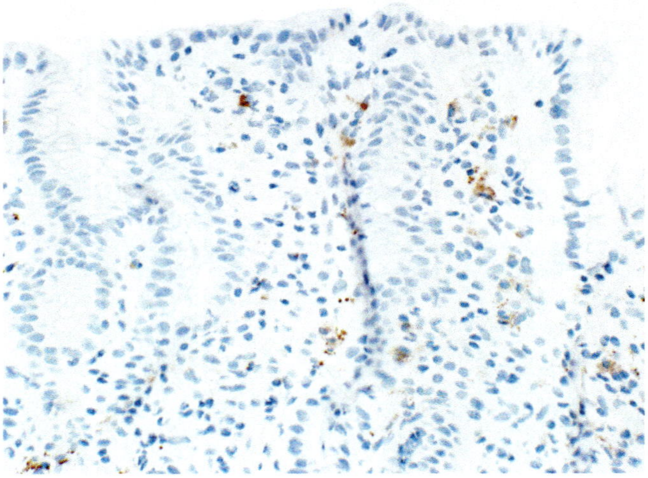

Fig. 2.27 Artifact in *Helicobacter pylori* immunostain. False-positive staining in plasma cells and macrophages mimicking *Helicobacter pylori*. Note the false-positive staining within the tissue rather than on the epithelium surface as shown in Fig. 2.26

Besides identifying infectious pathogens, immunohistochemistry is also occasionally used in evaluating other non-neoplastic disorders such as motility disorder, refractory sprue, autoimmune gastritis, microscopic colitis, etc. They will be discussed in the corresponding sections in this book.

In Situ Hybridization

This method has limited value in non-neoplastic gastrointestinal diseases. The most commonly used in situ hybridization test is for Epstein–Barr virus when evaluating a lymphoproliferative disorder. CMV in situ hybridization is essentially replaced by immunohistochemistry. In situ hybridization may be potentially useful to distinguish different species of fungal organisms in tissue sections such as *Aspergillus*, *Fusarium*, and *Pseudallescheria*, but the tests were developed mainly for research purposes [39].

Special Tests

Molecular Tests

Although molecular and genetic tests have become more and more important in modern pathology, their role in evaluating non-neoplastic gastrointestinal disorders is still limited. Currently, there are only a few PCR-based molecular tests available which are mainly used for infectious disorders such as Whipple's disease and mycobacterial infection. They generally face similar issues of low sensitivity and specificity.

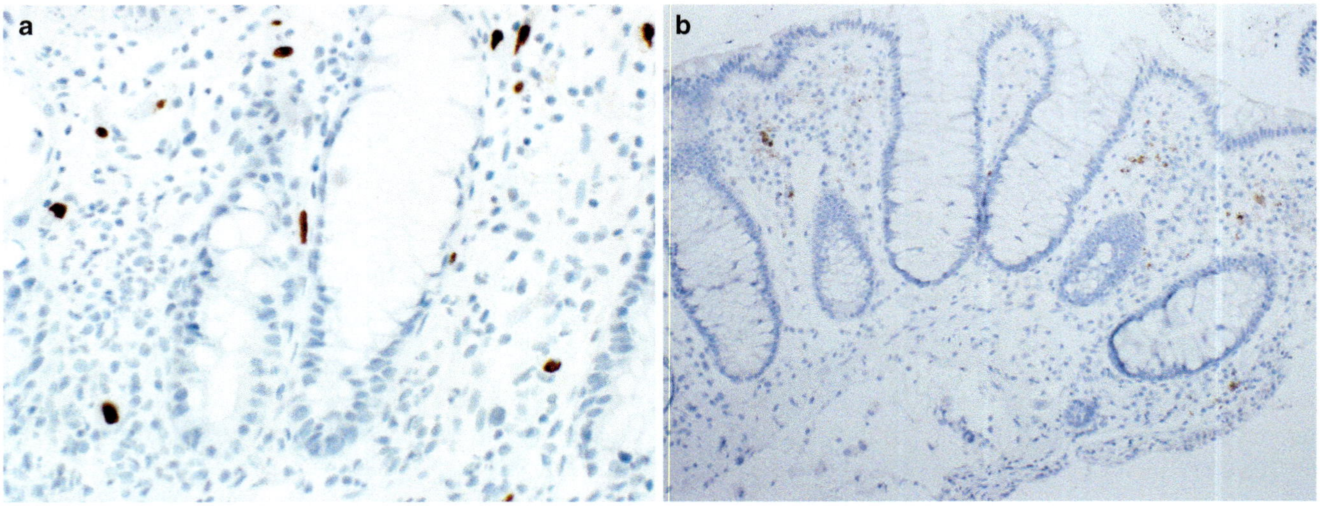

Fig. 2.28 CMV immunostain. The CMV-positive cells show discrete strong nuclear staining (**a**), in contrast to the false-positive, granular cytoplasmic staining in plasma cells and macrophages (**b**)

Therefore, these tests must be used in combination with histology and clinical information. The pros and cons of these tests will be discussed in the corresponding chapter.

Electron Microscopy

The usage of electron microscopy for non-neoplastic gastrointestinal disorders is limited, especially with the rise of immunohistochemistry, molecular, and serological tests. However, ultrastructural analysis is still the key for certain congenital disorders such as microvillus inclusion disease (Fig. 2.29) or tufting enteropathy. If the clinician or pathologist has deemed that a small bowel biopsy may require ultrastructural evaluation, adequate tissue submission and processing is essential at the time of the biopsy. A small specimen (no larger than 1 mm^3 for optimal fixative penetration) should be submitted separately for electron microscopy. The biopsy tissue should be immediately immersed in 1.5–2.5% buffered glutaraldehyde fixative for at least 1–2 hours at room temperature. The fixed tissue is then cut into small pieces no larger than 1 mm in the greatest dimension each. Toluidine blue-stained thick sections are commonly used for determining the quality of the tissue and choosing the most representative tissue for further detailed study by transmission electron microscopy.

Formalin fixation can not only result in poor tissue preservation but also alter some ultrastructure which is generally not recommended for electron microscopy. However, some reports have shown well-preserved fine structures, viruses, and other microorganisms identified by transmission electron microscopy in formalin-fixed paraffin-embedded tissue [40–42]. In our practice, formalin-fixed paraffin-embedded tissue is occasionally used for transmission electron microscopy if separately submitted tissue in glutaraldehyde is not available, but detailed examination of the delicate structure of organelles is difficult.

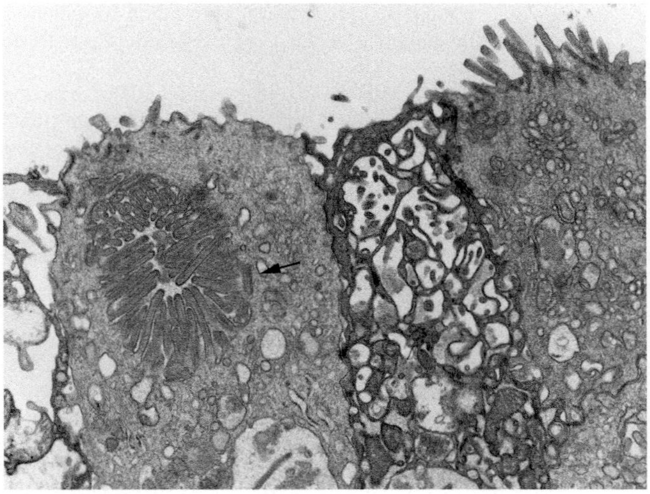

Fig. 2.29 Electron microscopy. Abnormal microvillus structures at luminal border and apical intracytoplasmic microvillus inclusion (arrow) identified in microvillus inclusion disease

Tissue Culture

Tissue culture to identify a certain infectious disorder on gastrointestinal biopsy is less frequently used because of the availability of non-invasive methods, technical difficulties, and time-consumption. But, it is still an important axillary test, and sometimes can be confirmative, if clinician or pathologist has suspicion for a specific infection such as tuberculosis. Tissue culture can also provide information on the antibiotic susceptibility profile when managing refractive infectious patients such as antibiotic-resistant *Helicobacter pylori* gastritis [43]. In addition, jejunal fluid aspirate or unwashed endoscopic jejunal mucosal biopsy culture is considered as the standard for establishing the diagnosis of small intestinal bacterial overgrowth [44, 45]. The biopsy tissue for culture is usually obtained at first during the endoscopy and should be sent to the microbiology labs within 30 minutes. Specimens can be placed in sterile physiological solutions such as 0.9% NaCl or on sterile saline-soaked gauze in the container. For anaerobic bacteria, tissue is placed in anaerobic ("vacuum-containing CO_2") sterile tubes immediately.

Spectrometry-Based Amyloid Typing

Amyloid deposition is commonly seen in gastrointestinal biopsies, which can represent either a secondary change to known amyloidosis or a new diagnosis. Laser microdissection with mass spectrometry is the preferred method for amyloid subtyping with a 100% specificity and a sensitivity of 98% [46]. This method is particularly useful because it can be performed with a very small amount of tissue and uses formalin-fixed paraffin-embedded tissue instead of fresh tissue, frozen tissue, or other specially stored tissue samples. Mass spectrometry also can be helpful in histologically difficult cases, such as those with equivocal Congo red staining or less common forms of amyloid [47].

Enzyme Tests

Disaccharidases enzyme test on small bowel biopsy is the gold standard in establishing the diagnosis of disaccharidase deficiency [48]. This test using spectrophotometry measures the activities of four types of disaccharidases: lactase, maltase, palatinase, and sucrase. A tissue sample (5 mg required) is obtained from the distal duodenum or proximal jejunum at the time of endoscopy, and the tissue should be frozen within 2 hours of collection at −20 °C and delivered to the lab on dry ice. An additional small bowel biopsy is also taken at the same time to evaluate structural abnormalities.

Quantitative assessment of acetylcholinesterase activity in rectal mucosal biopsies was used as a complementary test in diagnosing Hirschsprung's disease [49]. With the availability of other more convenient and reliable methods, this assay has no value in clinical practice nowadays.

Acknowledgments We thank Dr. Cadman Leggett and Dr. Louis Michel Wong Kee Song for providing endoscopic images of their respective cases, Mayo Clinic, Rochester, MN.

References

1. Hirschowitz BI, Peters CW, Curtiss LE. Preliminary report on a long fiberscope for examination of stomach and duodenum. Med Bull (Ann Arbor). 1957;23(5):178–80.
2. Johnson DA, Barkun AN, Cohen LB, Dominitz JA, Kaltenbach T, Martel M, et al. Optimizing adequacy of bowel cleansing for colonoscopy: recommendations from the U.S. multi-society task force on colorectal cancer. Gastrointest Endosc. 2014;80(4):543–62. https://doi.org/10.1016/j.gie.2014.08.002.
3. Committee ASoP, Saltzman JR, Cash BD, Pasha SF, Early DS, Muthusamy VR, et al. Bowel preparation before colonoscopy. Gastrointest Endosc. 2015;81(4):781–94. https://doi.org/10.1016/j.gie.2014.09.048.
4. Meisel JL, Bergman D, Graney D, Saunders DR, Rubin CE. Human rectal mucosa: proctoscopic and morphological changes caused by laxatives. Gastroenterology. 1977;72(6):1274–9.
5. Pockros PJ, Foroozan P. Golytely lavage versus a standard colonoscopy preparation. Effect on normal colonic mucosal histology. Gastroenterology. 1985;88(2):545–8.
6. Rejchrt S, Bures J, Siroky M, Kopacova M, Slezak L, Langr F. A prospective, observational study of colonic mucosal abnormalities associated with orally administered sodium phosphate for colon cleansing before colonoscopy. Gastrointest Endosc. 2004;59(6):651–4.
7. Lawrance IC, Willert RP, Murray K. Bowel cleansing for colonoscopy: prospective randomized assessment of efficacy and of induced mucosal abnormality with three preparation agents. Endoscopy. 2011;43(5):412–8. https://doi.org/10.1055/s-0030-1256193.
8. Zwas FR, Cirillo NW, el-Serag HB, Eisen RN. Colonic mucosal abnormalities associated with oral sodium phosphate solution. Gastrointest Endosc. 1996;43(5):463–6.
9. Ross-Innes CS, Debiram-Beecham I, O'Donovan M, Walker E, Varghese S, Lao-Sirieix P, et al. Evaluation of a minimally invasive cell sampling device coupled with assessment of trefoil factor 3 expression for diagnosing Barrett's esophagus: a multi-center case-control study. PLoS Med. 2015;12(1):e1001780. https://doi.org/10.1371/journal.pmed.1001780.
10. Chettouh H, Mowforth O, Galeano-Dalmau N, Bezawada N, Ross-Innes C, MacRae S, et al. Methylation panel is a diagnostic biomarker for Barrett's oesophagus in endoscopic biopsies and non-endoscopic cytology specimens. Gut. 2017; https://doi.org/10.1136/gutjnl-2017-314026.
11. Katzka DA, Smyrk TC, Alexander JA, Geno DM, Beitia RA, Chang AO, et al. Accuracy and safety of the cytosponge for assessing histologic activity in eosinophilic esophagitis: a two-center study. Am J Gastroenterol. 2017;112(10):1538–44. https://doi.org/10.1038/ajg.2017.244.
12. Kawamura T, Takeuchi Y, Asai S, Yokota I, Akamine E, Kato M, et al. A comparison of the resection rate for cold and hot snare polypectomy for 4–9 mm colorectal polyps: a multicentre randomised controlled trial (CRESCENT study). Gut. 2017; https://doi.org/10.1136/gutjnl-2017-314215.
13. Moss A, Nalankilli K. Standardisation of polypectomy technique. Best Pract Res Clin Gastroenterol. 2017;31(4):447–53. https://doi.org/10.1016/j.bpg.2017.05.007.
14. Committee AT, Maple JT, Abu Dayyeh BK, Chauhan SS, Hwang JH, Komanduri S, et al. Endoscopic submucosal dissection. Gastrointest Endosc. 2015;81(6):1311–25. https://doi.org/10.1016/j.gie.2014.12.010.
15. Wani S, Muthusamy VR, McGrath CM, Sepulveda AR, Das A, Messersmith W, et al. AGA white paper: optimizing endoscopic ultrasound-guided tissue acquisition and future directions. Clin Gastroenterol Hepatol. 2018;16(3):318–27. https://doi.org/10.1016/j.cgh.2017.10.020.
16. Gleeson FC, Zhang L, Roden AC, Levy MJ. Endoscopic ultrasound-guided fine-needle biopsies from pancreatic ductal adenocarcinomas can be used to quantify PD-L1. Clin Gastroenterol Hepatol. 2018;16:1535–6. https://doi.org/10.1016/j.cgh.2018.01.001.
17. Heng Y, Schuffler MD, Haggitt RC, Rohrmann CA. Pneumatosis intestinalis: a review. Am J Gastroenterol. 1995;90(10):1747–58.
18. Bielawska B, Day AG, Lieberman DA, Hookey LC. Risk factors for early colonoscopic perforation include non-gastroenterologist endoscopists: a multivariable analysis. Clin Gastroenterol Hepatol. 2014;12(1):85–92. https://doi.org/10.1016/j.cgh.2013.06.030.
19. Burgess NG, Bassan MS, McLeod D, Williams SJ, Byth K, Bourke MJ. Deep mural injury and perforation after colonic endoscopic mucosal resection: a new classification and analysis of risk factors. Gut. 2017;66(10):1779–89. https://doi.org/10.1136/gutjnl-2015-309848.
20. Fa-Si-Oen PR, Penninckx F. The effect of mechanical bowel preparation on human colonic tissue in elective open colon surgery. Dis Colon Rectum. 2004;47(6):948–9. https://doi.org/10.1007/s10350-004-0515-1.
21. Bingol-Kologlu M, Senocak ME, Talim B, Kale G, Ocal T, Buyukpamukcu N. A comparative histopathologic evaluation of the effects of three different solutions used for whole bowel irrigation: an experimental study. J Pediatr Surg. 2000;35(4):564–8. https://doi.org/10.1053/jpsu.2000.0350564.
22. Parente F, Marino B, Crosta C. Bowel preparation before colonoscopy in the era of mass screening for colo-rectal cancer: a practical approach. Dig Liver Dis. 2009;41(2):87–95. https://doi.org/10.1016/j.dld.2008.06.005.
23. Driman DK, Preiksaitis HG. Colorectal inflammation and increased cell proliferation associated with oral sodium phosphate bowel preparation solution. Hum Pathol. 1998;29(9):972–8.
24. Chlumska A, Benes Z, Mukensnabl P, Zamecnik M. Histologic findings after sodium phosphate bowel preparation for colonoscopy. Diagnostic pitfalls of colonoscopic biopsies. Cesk Patol. 2010;46(2):37–41.
25. Rex DK, DiPalma JA, McGowan J, Cleveland M. A comparison of oral sulfate solution with sodium picosulfate: magnesium citrate in split doses as bowel preparation for colonoscopy. Gastrointest Endosc. 2014;80(6):1113–23. https://doi.org/10.1016/j.gie.2014.05.329.
26. Thavarajah R, Mudimbaimannar VK, Elizabeth J, Rao UK, Ranganathan K. Chemical and physical basics of routine formaldehyde fixation. J Oral Maxillofac Pathol. 2012;16(3):400–5. https://doi.org/10.4103/0973-029X.102496.
27. Durgun-Yucel B, Dere F, Yucel AH, Oguz O. Rapid fixation of whole organ specimens and attendant problems. Acta Med Okayama. 1992;46(2):75–81. https://doi.org/10.18926/AMO/32649.
28. Looi LM, Loh KC. Microwave-stimulated formaldehyde fixation of experimental renal biopsy tissues: computerised morphometric analysis of distortion artefacts. Malays J Pathol. 2005;27(1):23–7.
29. Boncher J, Bronner M, Goldblum JR, Liu X. Reticulin staining clarifies florid benign signet ring cell change with mitotic activity in a penetrating gastric ulcer. Am J Surg Pathol. 2011;35(5):762–6. https://doi.org/10.1097/PAS.0b013e318213f833.

30. Agrawal RK, Kakkar N, Vasishta RK, Kumari V, Samujh R, Rao KL. Acetylcholinesterase histochemistry (AChE)—a helpful technique in the diagnosis and in aiding the operative procedures of Hirschsprung disease. Diagn Pathol. 2015;10:208. https://doi.org/10.1186/s13000-015-0443-5.
31. Guinard-Samuel V, Bonnard A, De Lagausie P, Philippe-Chomette P, Alberti C, El Ghoneimi A, et al. Calretinin immunohistochemistry: a simple and efficient tool to diagnose Hirschsprung disease. Mod Pathol. 2009;22(10):1379–84. https://doi.org/10.1038/modpathol.2009.110.
32. Solomon IH, Johncilla ME, Hornick JL, Milner DA Jr. The utility of immunohistochemistry in mycobacterial infection: a proposal for multimodality testing. Am J Surg Pathol. 2017;41(10):1364–70. https://doi.org/10.1097/PAS.0000000000000925.
33. Azevedo NF, Almeida C, Cerqueira L, Dias S, Keevil CW, Vieira MJ. Coccoid form of Helicobacter pylori as a morphological manifestation of cell adaptation to the environment. Appl Environ Microbiol. 2007;73(10):3423–7. https://doi.org/10.1128/AEM.00047-07.
34. Kuwabara A, Okamoto H, Suda T, Ajioka Y, Hatakeyama K. Clinicopathologic characteristics of clinically relevant cytomegalovirus infection in inflammatory bowel disease. J Gastroenterol. 2007;42(10):823–9. https://doi.org/10.1007/s00535-007-2103-3.
35. Nguyen M, Bradford K, Zhang X, Shih DQ. Cytomegalovirus reactivation in ulcerative colitis patients. Ulcers. 2011;2011:282507. https://doi.org/10.1155/2011/282507.
36. Jones A, McCurdy JD, Loftus EV Jr, Bruining DH, Enders FT, Killian JM, et al. Effects of antiviral therapy for patients with inflammatory bowel disease and a positive intestinal biopsy for cytomegalovirus. Clin Gastroenterol Hepatol. 2015;13(5):949–55. https://doi.org/10.1016/j.cgh.2014.09.042.
37. Roblin X, Pillet S, Oussalah A, Berthelot P, Del Tedesco E, Phelip JM, et al. Cytomegalovirus load in inflamed intestinal tissue is predictive of resistance to immunosuppressive therapy in ulcerative colitis. Am J Gastroenterol. 2011;106(11):2001–8. https://doi.org/10.1038/ajg.2011.202.
38. Mills AM, Guo FP, Copland AP, Pai RK, Pinsky BA. A comparison of CMV detection in gastrointestinal mucosal biopsies using immunohistochemistry and PCR performed on formalin-fixed, paraffin-embedded tissue. Am J Surg Pathol. 2013;37(7):995–1000. https://doi.org/10.1097/PAS.0b013e31827fcc33.
39. Hayden RT, Isotalo PA, Parrett T, Wolk DM, Qian X, Roberts GD, et al. In situ hybridization for the differentiation of Aspergillus, Fusarium, and Pseudallescheria species in tissue section. Diagn Mol Pathol. 2003;12(1):21–6.
40. Wang NS, Minassian H. The formaldehyde-fixed and paraffin-embedded tissues for diagnostic transmission electron microscopy: a retrospective and prospective study. Hum Pathol. 1987;18(7):715–27.
41. Johannessen JV. Use of paraffin material for electron microscopy. Pathol Annu. 1977;12(Pt 2):189–224.
42. Rossi GL, Luginbuhl H, Probst D. A method for ultrastructural study of lesions found in conventional histological sections. Virchows Arch A Pathol Pathol Anat. 1970;350(3):216–24.
43. De Francesco V, Giorgio F, Hassan C, Manes G, Vannella L, Panella C, et al. Worldwide H pylori antibiotic resistance: a systematic review. J Gastrointestin Liver Dis. 2010;19(4):409–14.
44. Chandra S, Dutta U, Noor MT, Taneja N, Kochhar R, Sharma M, et al. Endoscopic jejunal biopsy culture: a simple and effective method to study jejunal microflora. Indian J Gastroenterol. 2010;29(6):226–30. https://doi.org/10.1007/s12664-010-0072-6.
45. Rubio-Tapia A, Barton SH, Rosenblatt JE, Murray JA. Prevalence of small intestine bacterial overgrowth diagnosed by quantitative culture of intestinal aspirate in celiac disease. J Clin Gastroenterol. 2009;43(2):157–61. https://doi.org/10.1097/MCG.0b013e3181557e67.
46. Vrana JA, Gamez JD, Madden BJ, Theis JD, Bergen HR 3rd, Dogan A. Classification of amyloidosis by laser microdissection and mass spectrometry-based proteomic analysis in clinical biopsy specimens. Blood. 2009;114(24):4957–9. https://doi.org/10.1182/blood-2009-07-230722.
47. Sethi S, Vrana JA, Theis JD, Leung N, Sethi A, Nasr SH, et al. Laser microdissection and mass spectrometry-based proteomics aids the diagnosis and typing of renal amyloidosis. Kidney Int. 2012;82(2):226–34. https://doi.org/10.1038/ki.2012.108.
48. Dahlqvist A, Auricchio S, Semenza G, Prader A. Human intestinal disaccharidases and hereditary disaccharide intolerance. The hydrolysis of sucrose, isomaltose, palatinose (isomaltulose), and a 1,6-alpha-oligosaccharide (isomalto-oligosaccharide) preparation. J Clin Invest. 1963;42:556–62. https://doi.org/10.1172/JCI104744.
49. Patrick WJ, Besley GT, Smith II. Histochemical diagnosis of Hirschsprung's disease and a comparison of the histochemical and biochemical activity of acetylcholinesterase in rectal mucosal biopsies. J Clin Pathol. 1980;33(4):336–43.

Part II

Non-neoplastic Diseases of the Esophagus

Reflux Esophagitis and Barrett Esophagus

3

Jason T. Lewis

Reflux Esophagitis

Definition

Reflux esophagitis is a term which comprises a constellation of histologic changes in the esophagus representing a reaction to injury caused by gastroesophageal reflux.

Introduction

There is a complex mechanism in place which keeps harmful gastric contents safely confined to the stomach. The lower esophageal sphincter (LES), in conjunction with the crural folds of the diaphragm and gastric sling muscles, works in unison to form a mechanical barrier to the retrograde reflux of gastric contents [1]. Transient relaxation of the LES allows swallowed air to vent from the stomach into the esophagus, and a mild degree of "physiologic" reflux is to be expected, especially within the most distal 1–2 cm of the esophagus [1].

The symptoms of heartburn and acid regurgitation are common, affecting every human at some point. It is no surprise that a strict definition of gastroesophageal reflux disease (GERD) remained elusive until 2006, when the Montreal consensus defined it as a syndrome which produces "troublesome symptoms and/or complications" [2]. GERD can therefore be considered a derangement of a normal process.

It has become clear that GERD is not a single diagnostic entity but instead represents several different diseases which present with the symptoms of heartburn/acid regurgitation. GERD may produce endoscopically visible changes—termed erosive reflux disease (ERD) or appear endoscopically normal—termed nonerosive reflux disease (NERD) [3]. The pathologist's role lies in the identification of objective features which support the diagnosis of ERD/NERD or their sequelae, specifically esophagitis or specialized Barrett mucosa.

Clinical Features

The most frequent gastrointestinal diagnosis rendered in the outpatient setting is GERD [4]. Studies demonstrate prevalence rates as low as 3.5% to nearly 30% depending upon the geographic population and definition of GERD [3, 5–7]. Certain trends are apparent, with GERD more common in the West than in East Asia [8]. Studies in North America demonstrate ranges between 18.1% and 27.8% [8]. These numbers are consistent with those obtained in the Mayo Clinic's Olmsted County population-based study, which revealed a prevalence of 19.8% in adults aged 25–74 years of age for weekly symptoms of GERD [7].

The prevalence of GERD is increasing [9]. While the cause is likely multifactorial, possible drivers for this include an aging population and rising levels of obesity. There is an age-related increase in acid exposure to the distal esophagus, a sequela of shorter LES length and decreased esophageal peristalsis which occurs with the aging process [10]. Becher and Dent performed a review of population-based studies looking at the association between age and GERD-related symptoms and complications and determined that "aging is associated with more severe patterns of acid reflux and reflux esophagitis, but that there is probably a paradoxical reduction in the severity of heartburn and regurgitation with age" [11]. A meta-analysis of nine studies demonstrated that obesity is associated with increased GERD symptoms, erosive esophagitis, and risk of esophageal adenocarcinoma [12]. Using a cohort of 10,545 female registered nurses, Jacobson et al. further characterized the association between BMI and GERD [13]. Their analysis showed that GERD symp-

J. T. Lewis (✉)
Department of Laboratory Medicine and Pathology, Mayo Clinic Florida, Jacksonville, FL, USA
e-mail: lewis.jason@mayo.edu

L. Zhang et al. (eds.), *Surgical Pathology of Non-neoplastic Gastrointestinal Diseases*,
https://doi.org/10.1007/978-3-030-15573-5_3

toms increased with rising BMI, and this was true in both normal-weight and overweight individuals. In other words, the risk of reflux symptoms increases in a given person with an elevation in BMI.

While black and white populations in the United States have similar prevalence rates with respect to GERD symptoms, in patients with weekly heartburn or acid regurgitation, white individuals are more likely to develop erosive esophagitis than black individuals (50% vs. 24%, respectively) [14]. In addition, erosive esophagitis is more likely to occur in male than in female patients [15].

There is an inverse relationship between inflammation in the stomach and reflux esophagitis. Specifically, patients with gastric ulcers, duodenal ulcers, or gastritis appear to have lower risk of developing reflux esophagitis [15, 16]. Chronic gastritis involving the body of the stomach is postulated to damage the acid-producing parietal cells, which results in less acidic gastric fluid. In spite of the apparent protective role of gastric inflammation, the relationship between *Helicobacter pylori* infection and reflux esophagitis is less clear. It appears that the region of the stomach involved by inflammation (i.e., the body) is more of a factor than the presence or absence of *H. pylori* [16]. The fact that *H. pylori* eradication does not result in increased relapse rates for GERD symptoms is supportive of this hypothesis [17]. Hiatus hernia has also been shown to be a risk factor for the development of reflux esophagitis [15, 18].

Heart burn and acid regurgitation are the most common symptoms of GERD. Other esophageal symptoms include dysphagia and chest pain [19, 20]. In the study of 11,945 patients with erosive esophagitis, dysphagia was identified in 37% of subjects. However, many times, patients are asymptomatic or present with extraesophageal complaints [19, 21]. If the refluxate reaches the level of the larynx, patients may experience chronic cough, hoarseness, throat clearing, and dysphonia [19, 21, 22].

Pathological Features

Gross Findings

GERD may or may not cause grossly visible changes to the mucosa which are detectable at the time of upper endoscopy. In 1999, the Los Angeles system was officially adopted by gastrointestinal societies as a formal set of criteria for the endoscopic grading of esophagitis. The goal was to create a "clinically relevant stratification of the severity of esophagitis" [23]. In the Los Angeles classification, erosions or ulcerations are defined as endoscopic mucosal breaks, and the length and circumferential involvement of these breaks are quantified in a four-tier system [23]. While some of the features evaluated are subjective, this remains the most widely used and reproducible schema for scoring erosive esophagitis. Grades A and B, in which breaks do not extend between the tops of two mucosal folds, are considered low-grade disease. Once the breaks begin to bridge between mucosal folds (grades C and D), the findings are considered high grade (Fig. 3.1).

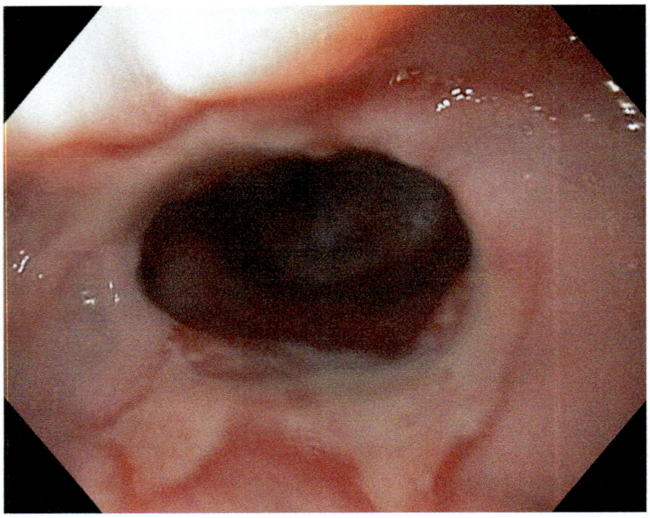

Fig. 3.1 Los Angeles grade D esophagitis, characterized by continuous mucosal breaks involving greater than 75% of the esophageal circumference. Image courtesy of Dr. Michael Wallace

Interestingly, approximately 70% of patients with reflux symptoms do not have grossly visible lesions at the time of endoscopy [24–26]. In other words, the majority of patients with GERD symptoms do not have erosive esophagitis. These patients are classified as having NERD [27]. In spite of the negative endoscopic findings, patients with NERD have an abnormal acid exposure time (AET) on pH testing which helps distinguish them from functional disorders [28].

Microscopic Findings

Whether from direct toxicity to the surface epithelial cells or a cytokine-mediated process secondary to recruitment of inflammatory cells in the lamina propria, GERD induces an injury response in the squamous epithelium. Studies have shown that histology suffers from lower sensitivity and specificity than clinical and endoscopic findings [29]. In individuals with ERD, a biopsy is not essential since these patients have endoscopically visible lesions. However, tissue sampling may provide support for the diagnosis of NERD as well as identify features of esophageal inflammation in the setting of extraesophageal disease [30, 31]. Biopsy is also performed to exclude other etiologies (e.g., infectious and eosinophilic esophagitis) and to screen for complications, such as Barrett esophagus.

The features detailed below are not specific for reflux esophagitis and may be seen in several disorders (see section "Differential Diagnosis"). Reflux esophagitis is characterized by (1) dilated intercellular spaces, (2) basal cell hyperplasia, (3) papillary elongation, (4) increased epithelial thickness, (5) inflammation, and (6) erosions. Pathologists demonstrate the greatest agreement when assessing papillary elongation, intraepithelial eosinophils, increased epithelial thickness, and erosions [32–34]. Formal measurements of these features are not typically taken, and the overall appearance of the biopsy is assessed at both low- and high-power magnifications to arrive at a diagnosis. Basal cell hyperplasia, papillary length, and dilated intercellular spaces demonstrate sensitivities and specificities of 70–89% for GERD [30, 35]. Dilated intercellular spaces and total epithelial thickness are thought to be the most sensitive indicators of NERD [30, 36]. The six features are defined below:

Dilated Intercellular Spaces The cells of normal squamous mucosa are tightly approximated to one another. Intercellular edema, alternatively known as spongiosis, is characterized by gaps between adjacent squamous epithelial cells, typically measuring greater than 2.5 μm [37]. These may be diffusely present within the tissue or in the form of irregular, round spaces between adjacent cells (Fig. 3.2a) [33, 36, 38]. In clinical practice, determining the presence or absence of spongiosis is typically a subjective evaluation.

Basal Cell Hyperplasia The basal, proliferative cell layer of normal squamous mucosa typically involves only the first one to four cell layers [33, 34]. Injury results in an increased turnover and proliferative activity within the basal zone. Basal cells have high nuclear/cytoplasmic ratios, which are seen as a dark blue band on scanning magnification. Because of this, the nuclei of basal cells are typically separated from one another by a distance less than the diameter of basal cell nucleus [34, 39]. The upper limit of the basal cell layer has been defined as the point when either (1) nuclei are separated by a distance greater than nuclear diameter or (2) 50% of cells are separated by a distance less than one nucleus [30, 34, 39]. Practically speaking, one usually performs a subjective assessment of basal layer thickness, measuring up from the basement membrane in well-oriented sections. Hyperplasia occurs when the basal cell layer involves >15% of the squamous epithelial thickness (Fig. 3.2b) [35, 39]. It is straightforward to orient sections from surgical or autopsy resections such that the squamous epithelium is perpendicular to the epithelial basement membrane, allowing the pathologists to obtain an accurate measurement of basal cell thickness. However, biopsy fragments are often tangentially embedded, which hinders the ability to accurately measure basal cell thickness in many cases (Fig. 3.2c) [40].

Papillary Elongation Papillary elongation is defined as an extension of the lamina propria vessels beyond 50% the thickness of the squamous epithelium, measured from the base of the papilla to the upper limit of the vessel wall in well-oriented sections (Fig. 3.2b) [30, 33, 35, 39]. As with basal cell hyperplasia, it is often difficult to obtain an accurate measurement of papillary elongation due to tangential embedding (Fig. 3.2c) [35, 40].

Epithelial Thickness Total epithelial thickness, measured at 0.5 and 2.0 cm proximal to the Z line, has been shown to be an excellent marker for reflux esophagitis. Using a cutoff of 430 μm, the sensitivity and specificity for GERD have been shown to be 76% and 48%, respectively [2, 31, 32].

Inflammation Inflammatory cells including lymphocytes, neutrophils, and eosinophils may be seen in reflux esophagitis (Fig. 3.2d). Cases of reflux esophagitis may show an increase in lymphocytes within the lamina propria and surface epithelium, often in a diffuse distribution [41]. Neutrophils may be seen, especially in the setting of erosion. However, neutrophilic inflammation is not specific and may be seen in other conditions, such as infection and pill esophagitis [35]. The eosinophil is the inflammatory cell most often associated with reflux esophagitis (Fig. 3.2e) [40, 42]. Typical cases contain a scattering of eosinophils within the squamous epithelium. Unlike papillary elongation and basal layer thickness, identification of eosinophils does not require a well-oriented section. It should be noted that some patients with GERD do not demonstrate eosinophils and some asymptomatic patients may contain eosinophils in their mucosa [34, 43]. There are two caveats with respect to identification and counting of eosinophils: (1) eosinophils within the lamina propria of rete pegs should be ignored, and (2) degranulated cells lacking a nucleus should not be counted.

Erosions If the reflux damage is significant enough, the surface epithelial component may undergo necrosis with formation of erosion.

Differential Diagnosis

Conditions that enter the differential diagnosis of reflux esophagitis are outlined in Table 3.1 and detailed below. As mentioned above, no feature is pathognomonic for reflux esophagitis. Instead, it is necessary to evaluate a constellation of histologic findings to arrive at the diagnosis.

Eosinophilic Esophagitis

Eosinophils play an integral role in the diagnosis of both eosinophilic esophagitis (EoE) (see also Chap. 4) and reflux esophagitis. Both reflux esophagitis and EoE may show basal hyperplasia, dilated intercellular spaces, and elongated papillae. However, the basal cell hyperplasia in EoE is typically greater than in reflux esophagitis, and on low power, the biopsy fragments often appear very dark [44]. One diag-

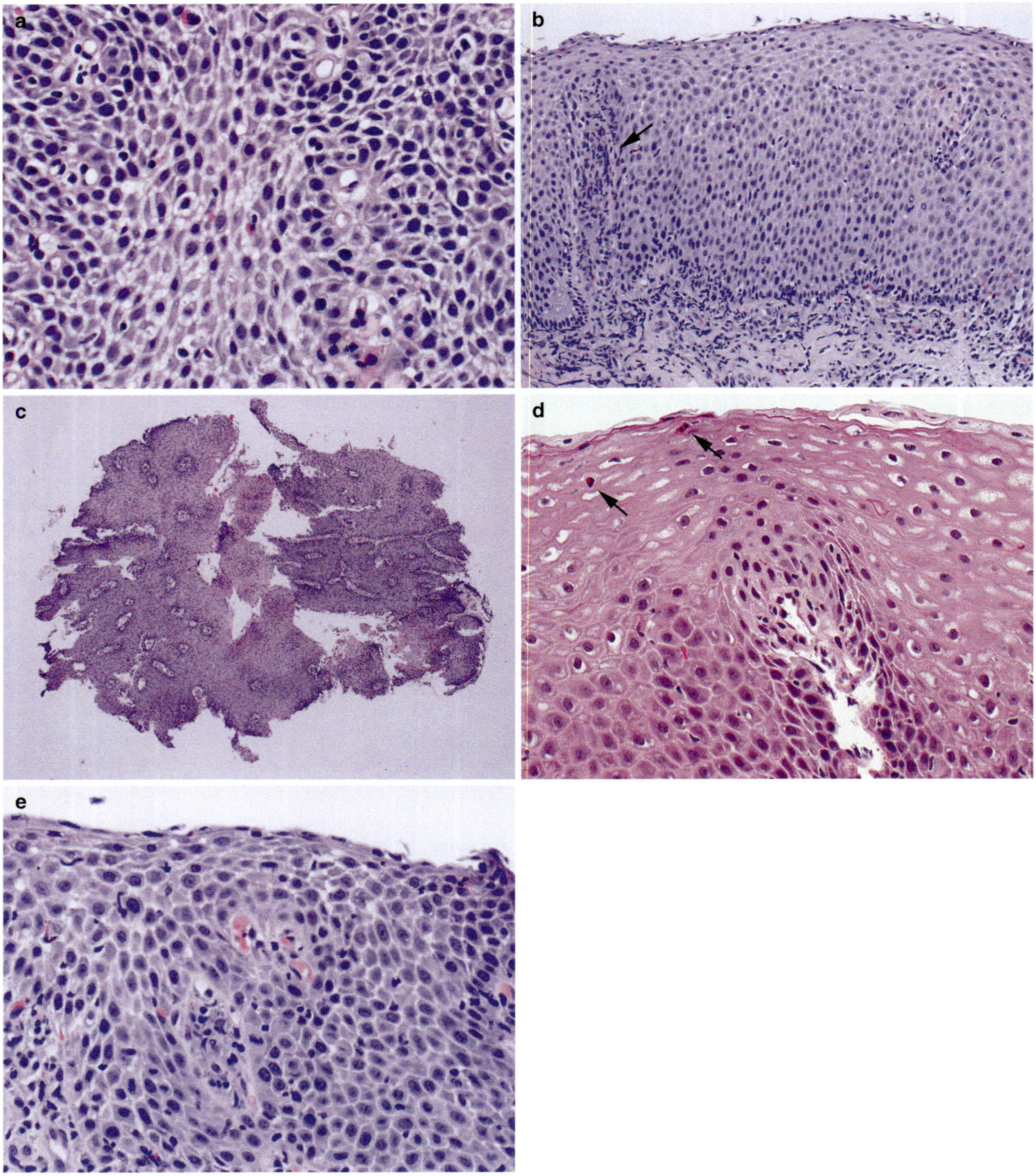

Fig. 3.2 Histological features of reflux esophagitis. (**a**) Dilated intercellular spaces (spongiosis) characterized by optically clear gaps between squamous epithelial cells. Intercellular bridges can often be seen spanning these spaces. The edema may diffusely involve the epithelium (as in this example) or take the form of irregular, spherical structures. Notice the eosinophils in the center of the image. (**b**) Papillary elongation (arrow) and basal cell hyperplasia are present in this example of severe reflux esophagitis. The rete peg in the left of the field extends almost to the surface of the epithelium, and the basal zone involves over half the thickness of the surface epithelium. Spongiosis is present as scattered, round spheres between epithelial cells. (**c**) Tangentially embedded mucosal biopsy imparting a dark appearance to the entire fragment. It would be impossible to assess papillary elongation or basal cell hyperplasia in such a fragment. (**d**) Typical finding in a case of mild reflux esophagitis. Mild edema and occasional eosinophils (arrows) are present. (**e**) Severe reflux esophagitis. Lymphocytes are scattered about in the form of "squiggle" cells intercalating between epithelial cells. Eosinophils, basal cell hyperplasia, and dilated intercellular spaces are present

nostic criterion for EoE is the presence of ≥15 intraepithelial eosinophils in a single high-power field (hpf) (Fig. 3.3a) [45]. This is not specific, however, as cases of severe reflux esophagitis may show eosinophil counts >15/hpf. Eosinophilic microabscesses are more typical of EoE (Fig. 3.3b).

EoE is a clinicopathologic diagnosis, requiring symptoms of esophageal dysfunction and esophageal eosinophilia on biopsy. While initially it was thought that EoE was restricted to the proximal or mid esophagus, it is now apparent that it may involve the distal esophagus as well. As such, the American College of Gastroenterology (ACG) recommends sampling of both the proximal and distal esophagus [45]. Endoscopically, EoE characteristically demonstrates rings, furrows, and strictures [46]. There is a subset of patients who meet the clinical and pathologic criteria for EoE but respond to proton-pump inhibitor (PPI) therapy. This condition is referred to as PPI-responsive esophageal eosinophilia. At present, this is considered neither a subgroup of EoE nor a type of reflux esophagitis [45].

Table 3.1 Differential diagnoses of reflux esophagitis

Diagnosis	Histology
Reflux esophagitis	Eosinophils typical (usually <15 eosinophils/hpf) Basal cell hyperplasia and papillary elongation (less than that in eosinophilic esophagitis) Neutrophils present in areas of erosion
Pill esophagitis	Neutrophil-predominant inflammation May have crystalline pill fragments along the surface No viral inclusions
Eosinophilic esophagitis	Eosinophils present (>15 eosinophils/hpf) Eosinophilic abscesses Marked basal cell hyperplasia and papillary elongation
Candida esophagitis	Neutrophil-predominant inflammation (surface band of neutrophils) Detached necrotic squamous cells *Candida* yeast and pseudohyphal forms visible (special stains)
Viral esophagitis	Neutrophil-predominant inflammation Viral inclusions present Ulcers present Immunostains confirmatory

Infectious Esophagitis

Candida Esophagitis Reflux esophagitis and Candida esophagitis (see also Chap. 5, section "Fungal (Candida) Esophagitis") share some histologic features, including basal cell hyperplasia and elongation of stromal rete pegs. The majority of Candida esophagitis cases reveal some degree of an inflammatory response within the squamous epithelium, with only 11% demonstrating no inflammatory infiltrates in a recent study [41]. In addition, *Candida* organisms are often visible on routine H&E slides (Fig. 3.4a). Many cases contain aggregates of necrotic squamous epithelial cells, either along the surface of the mucosa or detached and separated from the main tissue fragments (Fig. 3.4b). *Candida* pseudohyphae and yeast forms are often identified in these clusters of necrotic cells (Fig. 3.4c). When they are not detected at first review, there are some histologic clues which should trigger the pathologists to perform a more diligent search for organisms, as well as histochemical stains (periodic acid-Schiff [PAS] or GMS) to aid in identification. Martin et al. demonstrated that the concurrent presence of neutrophils and lymphocytes was more common in Candida (61%) than reflux (2%) esophagitis [41]. In particular, the presence of a superficial band of neutrophils was very suggestive of *Candida* infection, present in 75% of Candida esophagitis cases and only 14% of reflux esophagitis cases [41]. Even though the squamous epithelium in both Candida and reflux esophagitis may contain intraepithelial lymphocytes, their distribution seems to vary by etiology. Lymphocytes are

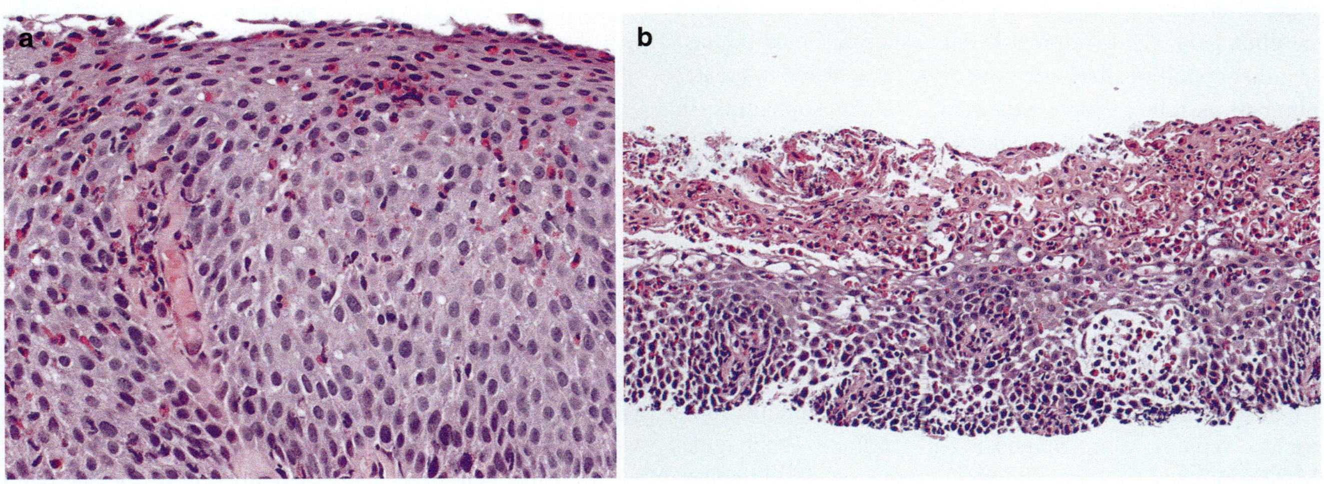

Fig. 3.3 Eosinophilic esophagitis. (**a**) Marked intraepithelial eosinophilia in excess of 15 eosinophils/hpf. (**b**) Eosinophilic microabscesses, typical of eosinophilic esophagitis

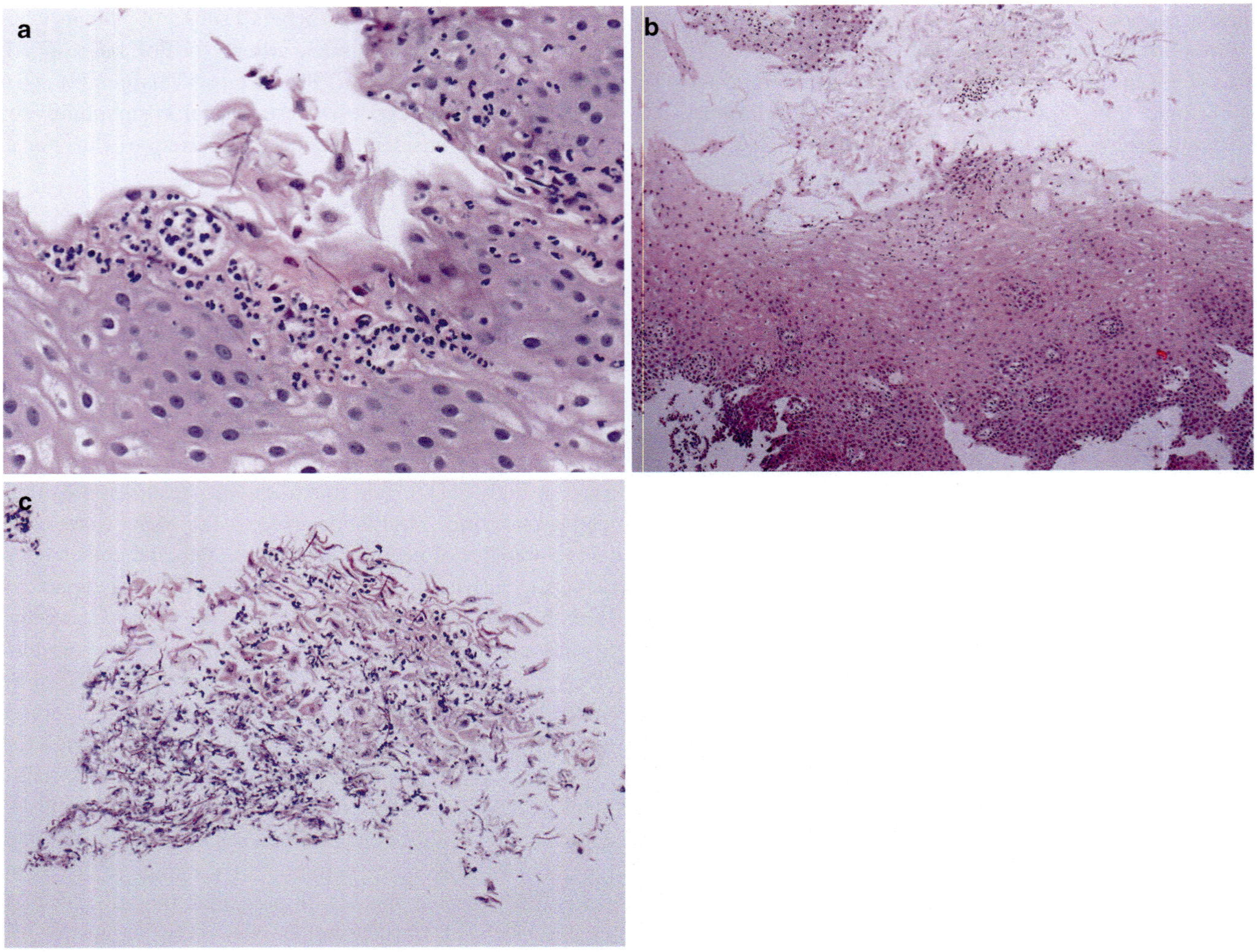

Fig. 3.4 Candida esophagitis. (**a**) *Candida* pseudohyphae are easily appreciated on routine H&E within the surface epithelial cells. Note the band-like accumulation of neutrophils underlying the fungal structures. Active esophagitis, characterized by neutrophilic infiltrates, is typical of *Candida*. (**b**) *Candida* is often associated with detached aggregates of necrotic epithelial cells (upper center of image) which have become separated from the mucosal biopsy fragment. Neutrophils are present in this necrotic cluster and within the underlying mucosa. (**c**) Detached, necrotic squamous epithelium containing *Candida* organisms and acute inflammation

more often peripapillary in Candida and diffusely distributed in reflux [41]. While intraepithelial eosinophils may be seen in either condition, they are more often present and in greater numbers in reflux esophagitis than Candida esophagitis. In the study by Martin et al., eosinophils were identified in 75% of reflux cases, while they were found in only 34% of the Candida cases [41].

Viral Esophagitis Both herpes simplex virus (HSV) and cytomegalovirus (CMV) may induce inflammation and ulceration within the esophagus. It is only cases of severe reflux esophagitis with ulceration that are likely to be confused with these two infectious processes. Eosinophilic infiltrates support the diagnosis of reflux esophagitis. Identification of characteristic inclusions is required to diagnose CMV or HSV esophagitis. Immunostains for CMV and HSV can be also be used to confirm these organisms as the etiology of esophageal ulcerations.

CMV preferentially infects stromal and endothelial cells, sparing the squamous epithelium (see also Chap. 5, section "Cytomegalovirus Esophagitis"). As such, inclusions are typically found within granulation tissue of the ulcer bed. There may be nuclear and/or cytoplasmic inclusions. Cowdry type A inclusions are characteristic, with an enlarged, amphophilic nuclear inclusion surrounded by a clear halo, resulting in the classic owl's eye morphology. Cytoplasmic inclusions are typically granular and eosinophilic.

HSV has a predilection for epithelial cells and is often identified in the squamous epithelium adjacent to the ulcer edge (see also Chap. 5, section "Herpes Esophagitis"). The cytologic nuclear changes can be remembered by the 3 Ms: (1) multinucleation, (2) margination, and (3) molding. Infected cells are characteristically multinucleated, with smudgy, basophilic inclusions that compress the chromatin against the nuclear membrane (margination), with nuclei closely approximated against one another (molding).

Pill Esophagitis Numerous medications may injure the esophageal mucosa, with nonsteroidal anti-inflammatory drugs (NSAIDs), antibiotics, iron, and bisphosphonates as the most common causal agents [47, 48]. While some affect the lower esophageal sphincter causing secondary acid exposure, others appear to exert a direct effect on the mucosa. Typically, pill esophagitis is characterized by a nonspecific pattern of inflammation consisting predominantly of neutrophils with or without ulceration and occasionally superficial epithelial necrosis (esophagitis dissecans superficialis). The crystals of certain drugs, such as sodium polystyrene sulfate, may be identifiable in the exudate which aids in diagnosis (see also Chap. 5, section "Miscellaneous Drugs").

Reflux esophagitis may also result in erosions/ulcers and have a neutrophilic inflammatory component. While eosinophils are not present in all cases of reflux, their identification is suggestive of reflux and argues against pill esophagitis.

Treatment

Therapy for reflux esophagitis may be either medical or surgical, and outcome studies have demonstrated conflicting results. It appears that laparoscopic reflux surgery (LARS) is more effective at lowering acid exposure of the distal esophagus [49, 50]. However, a subset of patients who undergo surgical intervention will need continued medical therapy [51, 52]. It should be noted that some patients who continue with antisecretory medication after LARS do not have pH monitoring performed to document continued acid exposure within the esophagus [53]. The LOTUS randomized clinical trial in Europe demonstrated remission rates of 92% and 86% at 5 years for esomeprazole (a PPI) and LARS, respectively [54]. They concluded that both forms of treatment were "effective in achieving and maintaining a reduction in distal esophageal acid exposure to a normal level" [54].

Due to the side effects associated with surgery, medical therapy and lifestyle changes are typically the first line of treatment for reflux esophagitis. Symptomatic improvement with PPIs in patients with heart burn or acid regurgitation empirically supports the diagnosis of GERD. Given the strong association between BMI and reflux, weight loss is also recommended for patients who have had weight gain or in those with an elevated BMI [55]. In those with nocturnal reflux, other lifestyle changes include elevating the head of bed and avoidance of evening meals within 2–3 hours of reclining. The ACG does not recommend "global elimination of food that can trigger reflux," but does recommend selective elimination if there is a documented correlation with symptoms [55]. There are no randomized or case-controlled trials to support this however.

Nissen fundoplication, in which a portion of the stomach is wrapped around the LES, has historically been the laparoscopic surgical intervention for refractory GERD. As mentioned above, it provides excellent control of reflux-related symptoms in the majority of patients, with satisfaction rates >85% [56]. However, it is associated with side effects such as the gas bloat syndrome, characterized by dysphagia, flatulence, and bloating secondary to the inability to belch or vomit [57]. Consequently, several endoscopic procedures have been developed recently, which include transoral incisionless fundoplication (using the EsophyX device), endoscopic stapling of the stomach to the esophagus (the Medigus SRS Endoscopic Stapling System), and the administration of radiofrequency (RF) energy to the LES (the Stretta procedure), as well as augmentation of the LES with a magnetic implant (magnetic sphincter augmentation device) or pacing using an implanted pacemaker (EndoStim) [57].

Prognosis

Esophageal complications of reflux include erosions, stricture formation, and Barrett esophagus [4]. If the refluxate is significant enough, injury and inflammation may develop within the larynx and/or trachea. Symptoms of laryngopharyngeal reflux include chronic cough, hoarseness, and dysphonia [19, 21, 22].

The majority of patients with esophagitis experience a resolution of erosions upon treatment with acid suppression [4]. A meta-analysis of 134 trials by Khan et al. demonstrated healing rates for PPI therapy and H2 blockers of 83% and 52%, respectively [4, 58]. Interestingly, the subjective symptoms of chronic reflux are more resistant to therapy than are objective findings at endoscopy. Resolution of the symptom of heartburn is seen in only 40% of patients on PPI therapy [4].

The most significant complication of chronic reflux esophagitis is the development of Barrett esophagus with its attendant risk of developing into esophageal adenocarcinoma. However, the majority of patients with GERD do not develop Barrett esophagus. Current estimates place the risk at 10–15% in patients with GERD [59]. As stated above, patients do not always have symptoms of heartburn/acid regurgitation, and esophageal adenocarcinoma can develop in patients without a history of GERD.

Barrett Esophagus

Definition

Barrett esophagus is defined as the presence of metaplastic columnar mucosa containing goblet cells (intestinal metaplasia) within the tubular esophagus.

Introduction

The normal lining of the esophagus is stratified squamous epithelium, while the stomach is lined by columnar foveolar cells overlying mucous or oxyntic glands. The gastroesophageal junction (GEJ) is the anatomic location at which the distal end of the esophagus meets the most proximal extent of the gastric folds [60]. The GEJ is a dynamic region and its precise location in situ varies with gastric distension, insufflation, motility, and respiration [60].

The squamocolumnar junction (SCJ; Z line) is a mucosal junction which forms a grossly visible line where the squamous mucosa and columnar mucosa meet. These mucosal types appear grossly distinct: squamous mucosa is pink-colored, while columnar mucosa is salmon-colored. When the SCJ does not coincide with the GEJ, there is by definition a segment of metaplastic columnar mucosa within the tubular esophagus. Endoscopically, this appears as an abrupt transition of pink, squamous-lined mucosa with salmon-colored columnar mucosa, located proximal to the anatomic GEJ.

Intestinal metaplasia (defined as the presence of goblet cells) has historically been requisite for the diagnosis of Barrett esophagus because it was considered the best "surrogate marker" for neoplastic transformation and malignancy [61]. Several studies published within the past decade have demonstrated the development of esophageal adenocarcinoma in the setting of columnar metaplasia without intestinal metaplasia [62–64].

However, other studies appear to confirm the role of intestinal metaplasia in the development of esophageal adenocarcinoma [65, 66]. Their conclusions suggested that the absence of intestinal metaplasia in relation to neoplasia (dysplasia or esophageal adenocarcinoma) within the esophagus is merely a reflection of sampling. For example, Smith et al. were unable to identify intestinal metaplasia in 37% of 27 endoscopic mucosal resection (EMR) specimens for esophageal adenocarcinoma [66]. However, a more detailed analysis of the ten cases without intestinal metaplasia in the index EMRs demonstrated intestinal metaplasia in either a concurrent, second EMR (three cases), prior biopsy (four cases), or follow-up esophagectomy (two cases). The single patient without intestinal metaplasia had been undergoing Barrett's surveillance for >20 years.

Allanson et al. were able to identify intestinal metaplasia in 79% of EMRs from 139 patients with esophageal neoplasia (91 EMRs contained intramucosal adenocarcinoma or esophageal adenocarcinoma; 19 contained dysplasia only) [65]. However, intestinal metaplasia was identified in prior samples of seven patients and in follow-up specimens of three patients. Ultimately, intestinal metaplasia was detected in 86% of patients at some point in surveillance or treatment. All 42 cases in which neoplasia were limited to either dysplasia or intramucosal adenocarcinoma with lamina propria invasion (considered early disease) were associated with intestinal metaplasia. The cases without intestinal metaplasia contained more aggressive lesions, with invasion at least into the inner layer of duplicated muscularis mucosae, suggesting that the intestinal metaplasia had been overrun by carcinoma [65].

Clinical Features

Chronic GERD results in damage to the squamous lining of the esophagus, with subsequent columnar metaplasia. This metaplastic change is thought to be a protective mechanism. One estimate puts the prevalence of Barrett esophagus at 5.6% of the adult population in the United States [59]. Barrett esophagus is diagnosed in 10%–15% of patients with symptoms of GERD who undergo endoscopy [67]. Studies have shown that there is an association between the length of Barrett esophagus and the severity of GERD [68]. While there is a strong association between GERD and Barrett esophagus, up to half of patients with Barrett esophagus report no symptoms of GERD [55].

Barrett esophagus is more common in men than in women, with a 2–3:1 male-to-female ratio [55, 59, 60]. It preferentially occurs in Caucasians over 50 years of age [59, 60]. Other risk factors include central adiposity, tobacco usage, hiatal hernia, and history of erosive esophagitis [59, 60]. Interestingly, the presence of *H. pylori* infection appears to be protective [60]. This is hypothesized to be related to the decreased acid content which results from gastritis within the stomachs of patients with *H. pylori* infection. There is no association between EtOH consumption and Barrett esophagus, and wine may be protective [59, 60].

The incidences of Barrett esophagus and EAC have both increased over the past few decades, though esophageal adenocarcinoma has shown a much steeper rise in frequency [59, 69]. The cause of this disparate increase is unclear.

Pathological Features

Gross Findings

The normal, stratified squamous lining of the esophagus is pink-colored. Endoscopically, Barrett esophagus appears as salmon-colored mucosa which extends proximally from the GEJ to involve the tubular esophagus. Barrett esophagus is divided into long-segment Barrett esophagus (LSBE) and short-segment Barrett esophagus (SSBE) based upon the length of involvement. LSBE is defined as Barrett esophagus which extends >3 cm from the GEJ, while SSBE is defined as Barrett esophagus which extends <3 cm from the GEJ (Fig. 3.5a, b) [60]. According to the ACG guidelines, this salmon-colored extension of columnar mucosa must extend

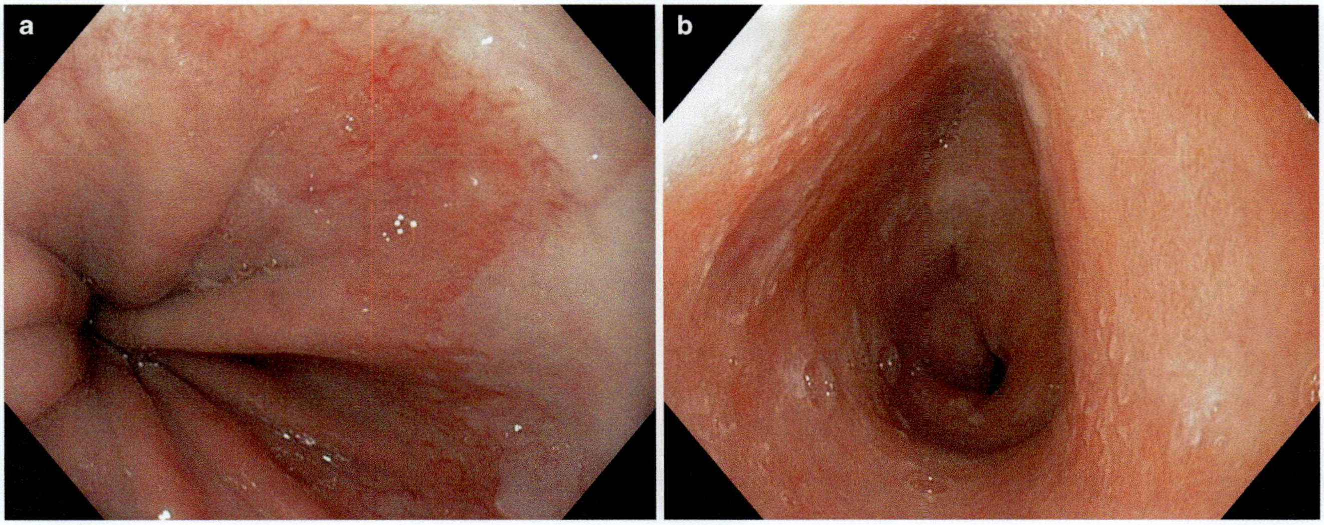

Fig. 3.5 Endoscopic appearance of Barrett esophagus. (**a**) Short-segment Barrett esophagus. The pink-colored mucosa of the esophagus (at right) interfaces with the salmon-colored columnar mucosa of columnar metaplasia within 3 cm of the anatomic GE junction. Rugal folds of the stomach are present at the left. (**b**) Long-segment Barrett esophagus. Salmon-colored columnar mucosa is present in the tubular esophagus. No gastric folds are visible. Images courtesy of Dr. Michael Wallace

at least 1 cm into the esophagus [60]. An irregular Z line describes the situation in which there are very short tongues (<1 cm) of columnar mucosa which extend into the esophagus (i.e., the distance between the GEJ and SCJ is <1 cm) [60]. Approximately 5–20% of patients undergoing endoscopy will have an irregular Z line [70].

Microscopic Findings

It remains unclear what should be considered "normal" GEJ mucosa. Historically, cardiac-type gastric mucosa was thought to line the most proximal stomach for several centimeters [71]. However, studies over the past two decades have challenged this dogma. At present, most, if not all, cardiac mucosa is considered to be a metaplastic lining which develops secondary to chronic reflux (Fig. 3.6) [61, 72–74]. The presence of cardiac mucosa in the distal esophagus thus represents a nonintestinal columnar metaplasia, which may represent a precursor to Barrett esophagus.

Barrett esophagus is a form of metaplasia in which the stratified squamous lining of the esophagus is replaced by a mosaic of many cell types, including goblet cells, pseudoabsorptive intestinal cells, gastric foveolar cells, glands (cardiac and oxyntic), and Paneth cells (Fig. 3.7a, b). The histologic changes one can see in BE are outlined in Table 3.2. Goblet cells are a requirement for the diagnosis and are the defining element of "intestinal metaplasia." Without the goblet cells, any metaplastic change would constitute columnar metaplasia, which appears identical endoscopically to intestinal metaplasia. In routine H&E-stained slides, the apical aspect of the goblet cell is markedly expanded by mucin-filled secretory granules which distend the upper portion of the cell. The nucleus is displaced into the narrow base of the cell, along with the remaining organelles. Unlike the neutral mucin in the foveolar cells, the mucus of true goblet cells is acidic and stains gray-blue on H&E. This form of metaplasia, consisting of secretory cells with acidic mucin and absorptive cells lacking a brush border, was historically known as incomplete intestinal metaplasia or specialized columnar epithelium (specialized Barrett mucosa) [75, 76].

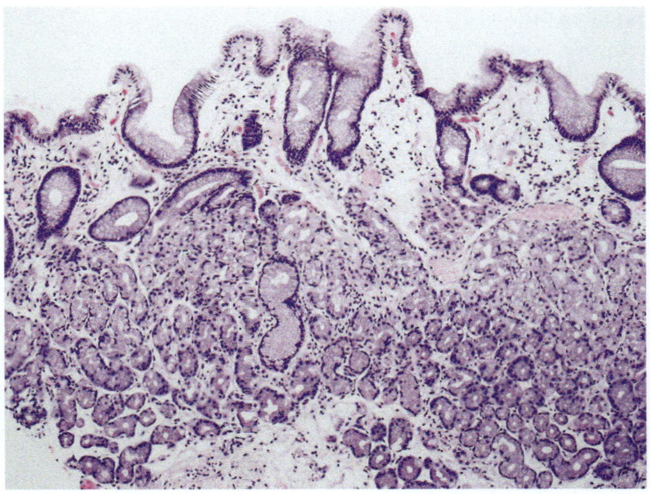

Fig. 3.6 Cardio-oxyntic mucosa, representing a form of columnar metaplasia, within the esophagus. The surface foveolar compartment rests upon a glandular compartment which consists of a mixture of mucous and oxyntic glands. No goblet cells are present, so this would not be classified as Barrett esophagus

Barrett esophagus also contains a zone of surface columnar cells which differentiate toward either gastric foveolar-type cells or intestinal-type cells. This surface columnar zone overlies a deeper, glandular compartment which is

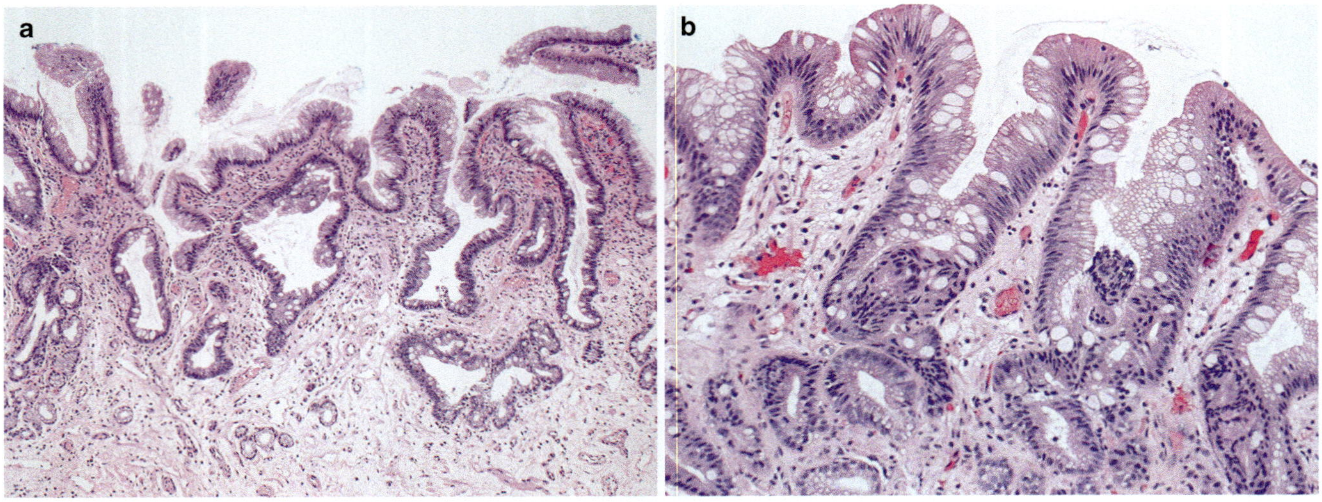

Fig. 3.7 Histological appearance of Barrett esophagus. (**a**) Columnar cells are intermixed with randomly distributed goblet cells (clear to light-blue staining). The mucus droplets fill the cytoplasm, compressing the nuclei to the base of the cells, imparting the appearance of a goblet. The lamina propria has a loose appearance, with variable inflammation. Note the mucous glands at the base of the image, some of which merge with the intestinal metaplasia. (**b**) A high-power view of Barrett mucosa with goblet cells

Table 3.2 Histologic components which may be seen in Barrett esophagus

Histologic components of Barrett esophagus
Goblet cells[a]
Intestinal pseudo-absorptive cells
Foveolar mucinous cells
Mucinous or oxynto-mucinous glands
Multilayered epithelium
Duplication of muscularis mucosae
Musculofibrous anomaly

[a]Required for the diagnosis

composed of mucous glands, oxyntic glands, or a mixture of the two [61].

Barrett esophagus is associated with a unique microanatomy, including multilayered epithelium, duplication of the muscularis mucosae, and the fibromuscular anomaly. Multilayered epithelium is a special type of epithelium consisting of columnar epithelial cells (Fig. 3.8a, b) that contain an acidic mucin (Fig. 3.8c) which rest upon a foundational layer of squamous cells [77]. Multilayered epithelium is often identified in the region of the SCJ in patients with Barrett esophagus or GERD and is thought to possibly represent a precursor or intermediate step in the development of Barrett esophagus [78].

A duplicated layer of muscularis mucosae can be identified beneath Barrett esophagus in just over 90% of esophagectomy specimens and roughly 2/3 of EMRs [79, 80]. When one has the entire field of Barrett esophagus to evaluate from esophagectomy, it becomes apparent that this muscularis mucosae duplication can be patchy in its distribution, involving anywhere from 5% to 90% of the Barrett esophagus segment [80]. The outer layer of duplicated muscularis mucosae is in continuity with the single layer of muscularis mucosae which underlies the squamous mucosa, indicating that it is the inner layer which is the "neo"-muscle (Fig. 3.9a) [80]. There is a network of lymphatics in the loose connective tissue between the duplicated layers of muscle, affording a risk of metastatic disease if the tumor reaches this layer (Fig. 3.9b). Evaluating 30 esophagectomy cases with adenocarcinoma that involved the duplicated muscularis mucosae, Abraham et al. identified lymphovascular invasion in 17% of cases and lymph node metastases in 10% [80].

The musculofibrous anomaly describes the prolapse-type changes associated with Barrett esophagus, in which there is an overgrowth and replacement of the loose, lamina propria connective tissue by smooth muscle fibers and collagen [81]. The former arises from the muscularis mucosae and extends as tendrils and arms of smooth muscle into the lamina propria [81]. The muscle and collagen can entrap and distort glands which, if dysplastic, can be mistaken for invasive adenocarcinoma. This can be especially problematic in biopsy specimens. As detailed below, histologic features present in the submucosa include fat, large muscular arteries, and submucosal glands [82].

Dysplasia in Barret Esophagus

From a histologic perspective, dysplasia represents the phenotypic expression of various clonal mutations within the metaplastic epithelial cells. While subjective, the presence and grade of dysplasia remain the best markers of progression risk in Barrett esophagus [61, 83]. Dysplasia may arise within the intestinal-type cells, gastric foveolar-type cells, or a mixture of these two, and it may begin in the crypt bases (crypt dysplasia) and migrate upward to eventually involve the surface [84]. Three primary subtypes of dysplasia have been described in Barrett esophagus: (1) intestinal-type, (2) foveolar-type, and (3) serrated-type [61, 85–87]. Criteria

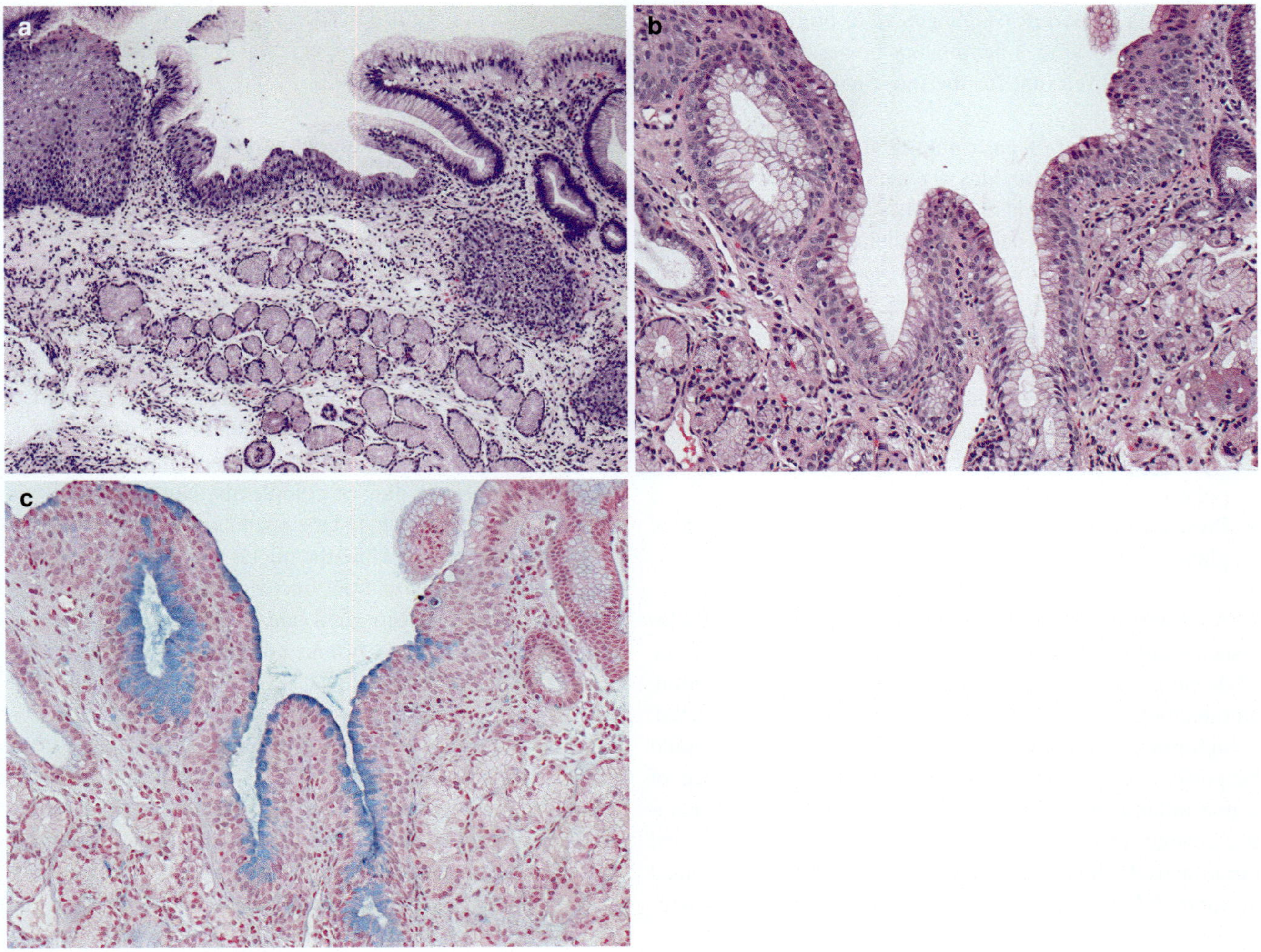

Fig. 3.8 Multilayered epithelium. (**a**) The multilayered epithelium occupies the center of the field, connecting squamous epithelium (at the left) and columnar epithelium (at the right). A variable layer of columnar cells overlies a couple of layers of squamous epithelial cells. Mucous glands involve the lower half of the field. No goblet cells are seen, which precludes a diagnosis of Barrett esophagus. (**b**) A high-power view of multilayered epithelium. (**c**) The columnar cells within the multilayered epithelium contain acidic mucin and are positive on Alcian blue stain

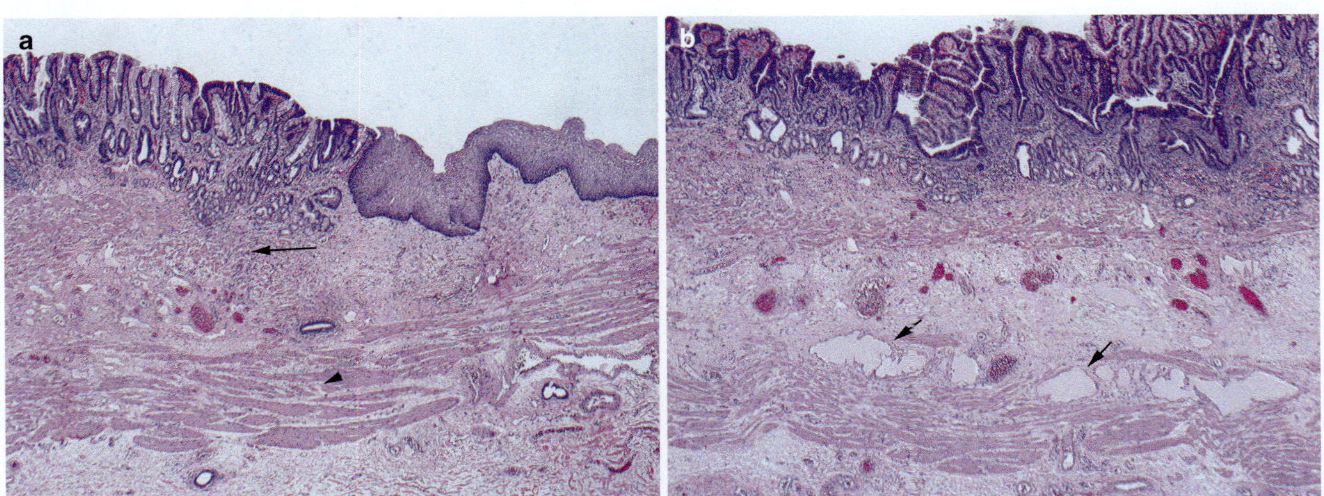

Fig. 3.9 Duplicated layer of muscularis mucosae in Barrett esophagus. (**a**) Duplicated inner layer of muscularis mucosae (arrow) is present in Barrett mucosa. The outer layer of duplicated muscularis mucosae (arrowhead) is in continuity with the single layer of muscularis mucosae underlying the squamous mucosa. (**b**) The loose connective tissue with a network of lymphatics (arrows) between the duplicated layers of muscle

for dysplasia in Barrett esophagus were originally adopted from those utilized in inflammatory bowel disease, making them implicitly relevant for the intestinal type of dysplasia [85, 88].

In 2001, a panel of gastrointestinal pathologists created an algorithm which provides a practical framework to use when assessing dysplasia in Barrett esophagus [86]. The four features assessed in this algorithm include:

1. Surface maturation—comparison of the tinctorial staining of the deeper glands with the surface epithelium in well-oriented tissue sections
2. Gland architecture—number, density, and shape of glands in relation to the lamina propria
3. Cytology of the cells—nuclear size, shape, staining, and polarity
4. Presence of inflammation—ulceration or infiltration of glands by neutrophils.

As noted in the study by Montgomery et al., pathologists should begin with a low-power, scanning surveillance of the slide looking for abnormalities in surface maturation, architecture, or ulceration [86]. If any areas are detected, a high-power evaluation of the cytologic features should be performed, paying careful attention to the presence of active inflammation which could lead to reactive/regenerative changes [86]. There are four categories of dysplasia and intramucosal adenocarcinoma, detailed below and outlined in Table 3.3. The following descriptions represent a distillation of commonly used criteria obtained from consensus papers and the practices of experts in the field of Barrett esophagus [61, 85, 86, 89–93].

Table 3.3 Differentiating features of intestinal-type dysplasia in Barrett esophagus

Histologic feature	Negative for dysplasia	Indefinite for dysplasia	Low-grade dysplasia	High-grade dysplasia
Surface maturation[a]	+	+/−	−	−
Architectural complexity	−	−	+/−	+
Inflammation[b]	+/−	+	−	−
Nuclear pleomorphism	−	−	+	+
Loss of nuclear polarity	−	−	−	+
Surface mitoses	−	+/−	+/−	+
Nuclear stratification	−	+/−	+	+
Nucleoli	−	−	+/−	+

+, present; −, absent; +/−, feature may or may not be present

[a]Tangential sectioning may make it impossible to evaluate for surface maturation. Indefinite for dysplasia may be the most prudent categorization of such cases

[b]Low- and high-grade dysplasia may be diagnosed in the setting of inflammation if the changes are unequivocal. Otherwise, Barrett esophagus associated with significant inflammation is better categorized as indefinite for dysplasia

Negative for Dysplasia Since Barrett esophagus is a metaplastic process, a mild degree of cytologic atypia is normally present and most pronounced in the basal layer of proliferating cells. At low-power scanning magnification, this proliferative zone appears as a dark band along the base of the glands. There is a gradual transition to lighter staining as nuclear/cytoplasmic ratios diminish, with relatively more cytoplasm per cell as they approach the surface, referred to as surface maturation (Fig. 3.10). Nuclei are typically darker in the deeper portions of the glands and may contain occasional mitoses, restricted to the basal zone. Glands are evenly spaced without crowding or complexity. Nuclear polarity is normal, with the long axis of the nucleus perpendicular to the basement membrane, while the nuclei maintain an even distribution in the cells without nuclear stratification. There is minimal pleomorphism, and any nucleoli are small. If inflammation is present, it does not significantly impact the above features.

Indefinite for Dysplasia This category is reserved for cases in which there is atypia, but it is impossible to determine if the changes are reactive or truly neoplastic. In some situations, there is a degree of atypia within the deep crypts that does not reach the threshold for low-grade dysplasia in either quantity or quality (Fig. 3.11a). At other times, the pathologist may be concerned about low-grade dysplasia but is unable to assess for surface maturation due to tangential sectioning, surface sloughing, or overlying by squamous

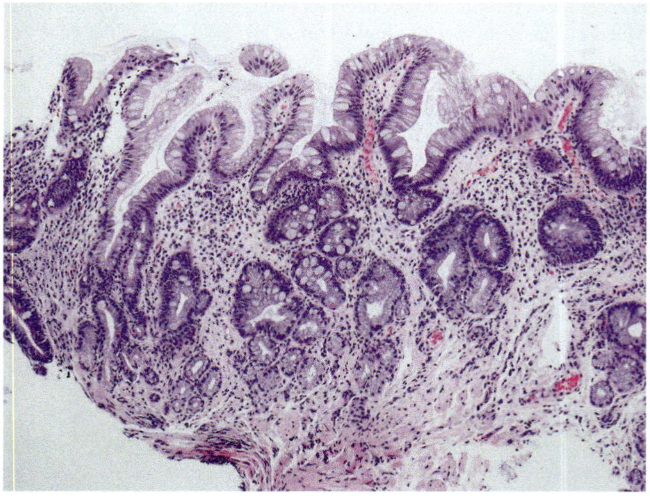

Fig. 3.10 Barrett mucosa, negative for dysplasia. A typical low-power appearance of non-dysplastic Barrett mucosa with nuclear hyperchromasia being restricted to the basal aspect of the glands, with maturation toward the surface. Architecture is preserved, with minimal distortion or crowding. The lamina propria is mildly inflamed

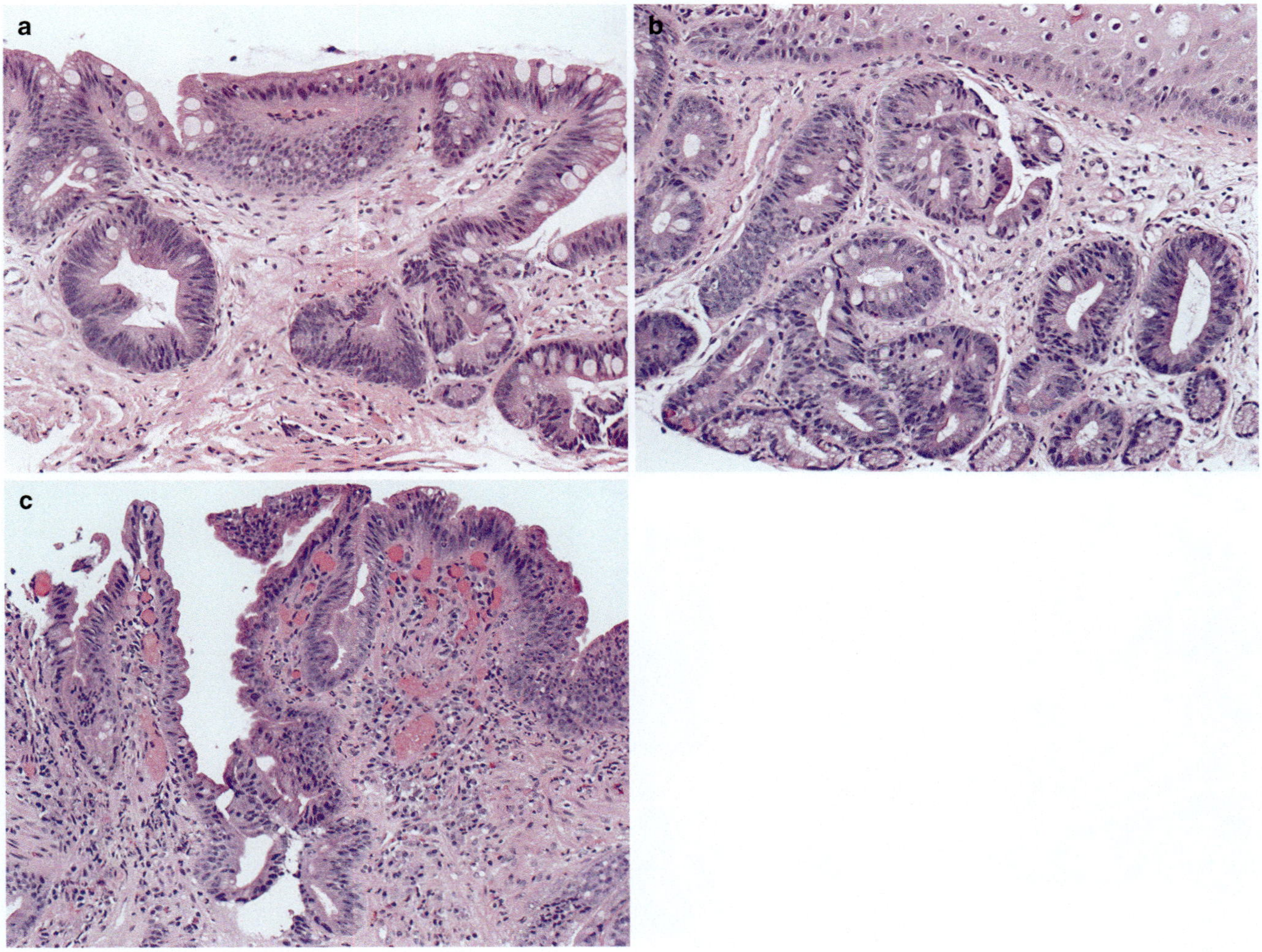

Fig. 3.11 Barrett mucosa, indefinite for dysplasia. (**a**) There is a hyperchromatic gland underlying the surface epithelium. While atypical, there are quantitatively insufficient glands involved to designate this as dysplastic. In addition, no significant surface atypia is appreciated. (**b**) The glands in the lower aspect of the field are atypical but are present beneath the squamous epithelium, making it impossible to assess for surface maturation. Indefinite for dysplasia is the best classification in this setting. (**c**) Epithelial atypia is present in the background of active inflammation. In the absence of incontrovertible features of dysplasia, indefinite for dysplasia is the most prudent categorization

epithelium (so-called "buried Barrett esophagus") (Fig. 3.11b). While it is possible to diagnose dysplasia restricted to the basal crypts (see "Low-Grade Dysplasia" section below), the inability to evaluate the surface may make the pathologist uncomfortable diagnosing dysplasia unless all of the features of dysplasia are present in the deeper crypts. Lastly, active inflammation or ulceration can induce architectural changes or significant cytologic atypia (Fig. 3.11c). In this setting, it may be impossible to determine if the changes are regenerative in nature or representative of true dysplasia. Designating these cases as indefinite for dysplasia provides adequate follow-up without labeling the patient as having progressed to true dysplasia.

Low-Grade Dysplasia Low-grade dysplasia typically shows abnormalities in surface maturation and nuclear cytology with minimal to mild changes in architecture. Low-grade dysplasia is reminiscent of a colonic tubular adenoma with low-grade dysplasia. Surface maturation is usually absent, and the deep glands and surface have a similar tinctorial appearance on scanning magnification (Fig. 3.12a). In general, gland architecture is preserved with only mild crowding or distortion. On high-power evaluation, the nuclei demonstrate mild hyperchromasia, increased nuclear/cytoplasmic ratios with nuclear stratification confined to the lower half of the cell cytoplasm (Fig. 3.12b). Mucin depletion and mitotic figures outside the basal proliferative zone are present. Nuclear polarity with respect to the basement membrane is maintained. These changes typically involve the surface (conventional low-grade dysplasia), though if the findings are significant enough, one may render a diagnosis of low-grade dysplasia in the deep crypts alone (crypt dysplasia) (Fig. 3.12c) [84]. The latter is based upon nuclear and cytologic changes which have a clonal appearance distinctive

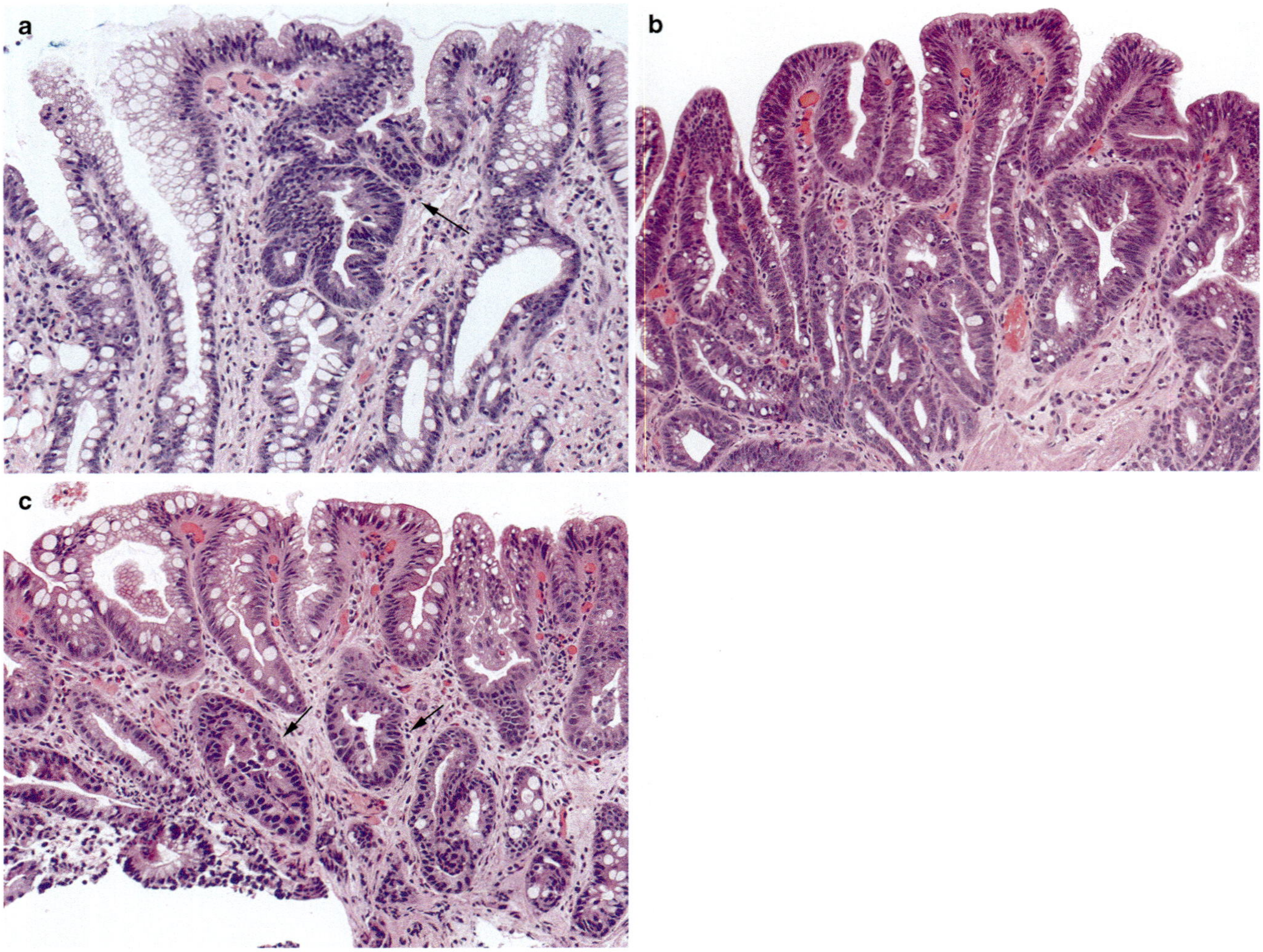

Fig. 3.12 Barrett mucosa, low-grade dysplasia. (**a**) At low-power scanning magnification, low-grade dysplasia (arrow) typically appears darker than the adjacent, non-dysplastic mucosa. This imparts a "clonal" appearance to the dysplastic glands. Hyperchromasia and atypia involve the surface (lack of maturation). (**b**) Intestinal-type low-grade dysplasia, characterized by hyperchromatic nuclei with pseudostratification typically restricted to the lower half of the cell. The nuclei are oval-shaped and maintain a perpendicular orientation with respect to the basement membrane (referred to as normal polarity). There is mild crowding, but no marked architectural distortion. (**c**) Barrett esophagus with crypt dysplasia (arrows). Even though the changes do not involve the surface, the atypical appearance is distinct from the adjacent glands. There is nuclear hyperchromasia and pseudostratification

from the adjacent, non-dysplastic crypts and in excess of those seen in proliferative atypia. However, the concept of crypt dysplasia is not universally accepted by gastrointestinal pathologists, and instead indefinite for dysplasia may be used in this setting. Cytologic changes suggestive of low-grade dysplasia in the setting of marked inflammation, whether it involves only the crypts or both the crypts and surface, may be better categorized as indefinite for dysplasia.

High-Grade Dysplasia High-grade dysplasia may demonstrate a combination of architectural and cytologic abnormalities or be diagnosed purely on cytologic features. A single focus with features of high-grade dysplasia warrants the designation, without a minimal number of glands required for the diagnosis [61]. As with low-grade dysplasia, there is usually no surface maturation at scanning magnification. Glandular architecture is typically more distorted than in low-grade dysplasia, with marked crowding and distorted arrangement of glands (Fig. 3.13a). Some intervening lamina propria should be present. Nuclear/cytoplasmic ratios are increased with nuclear enlargement, hyperchromasia, clumped nuclear chromatin, and irregularity. Stratification involves the full thickness of the cell. Loss of nuclear polarity with respect to the basement membrane is a defining feature of high-grade dysplasia, characterized by an irregular and uneven distribution of nuclei within the gland, imparting a jumbled appearance (Fig. 3.13b). Mitoses are frequent and may be present in the surface epithelium. The presence of cribriform architecture or dilated glands containing intralu-

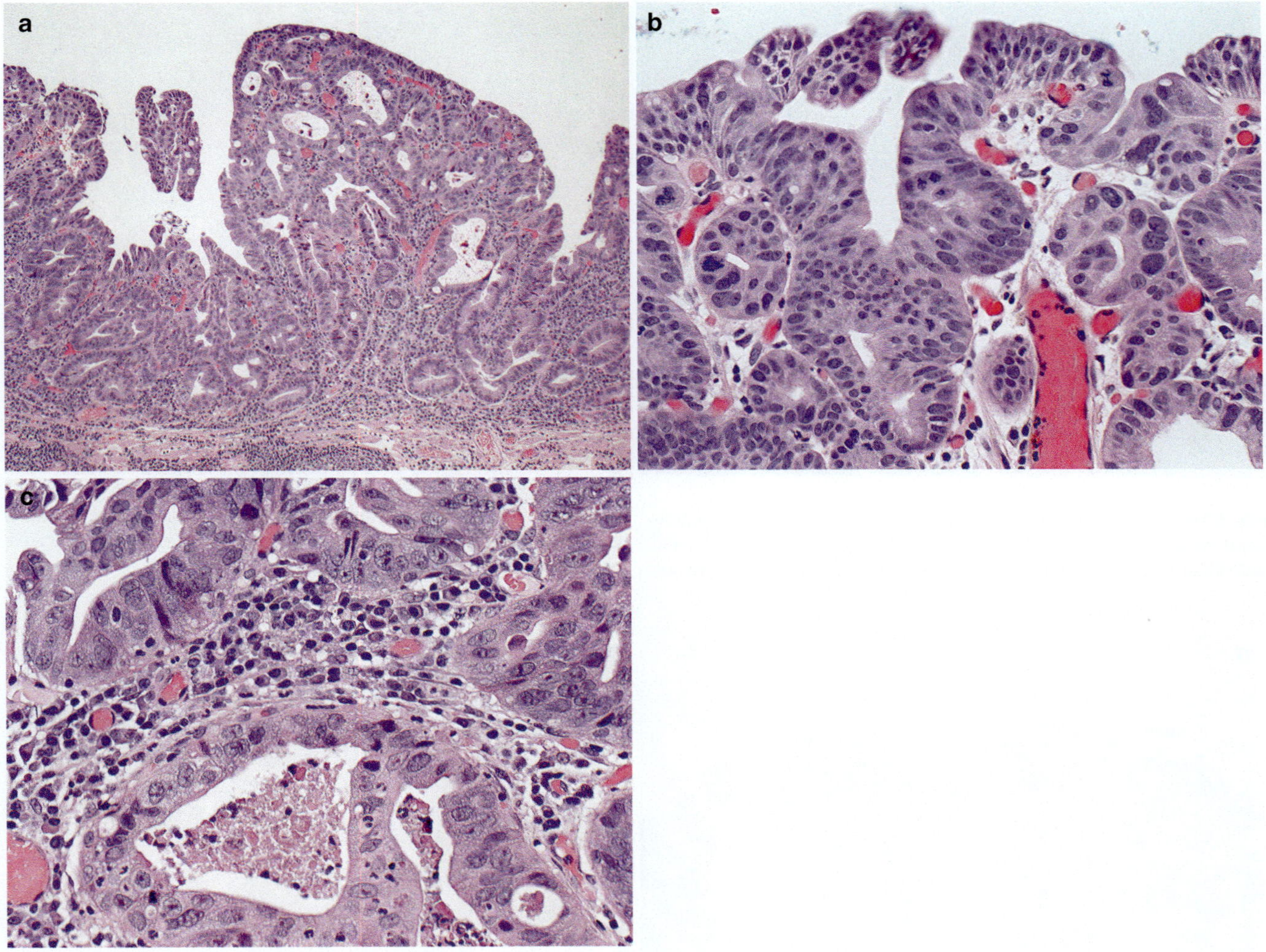

Fig. 3.13 Barrett mucosa, high-grade dysplasia. (**a**) A low-power view of high-grade dysplasia with marked gland crowding is present. Nuclear abnormalities are more pronounced than in low-grade dysplasia. (**b**) High-power view shows jumbled, disorganized appearance of nuclei (loss of polarity), prominent nucleoli, high nuclear/cytoplasmic ratios, and irregular nuclear contour features typically seen in high-grade dysplasia. (**c**) High-grade dysplasia with foci of intraluminal necrosis

minal necrotic debris imparts an increased risk of carcinoma in resection specimens (Fig. 3.13c) [94].

Intramucosal Adenocarcinoma Intramucosal adenocarcinoma is defined by penetration of neoplastic cells through the basement membrane into the lamina propria. Distinguishing high-grade dysplasia from intramucosal adenocarcinoma may at times be highly subjective, as marked architectural changes are part of the diagnostic criteria for high-grade dysplasia [93]. Lack of a desmoplastic reaction in intramucosal adenocarcinoma further compounds the problem. Nevertheless, the following four features have been used as criteria for intramucosal adenocarcinoma: (1) individual cells present within the lamina propria in more than one focus; (2) sheets of cells which obliterate the intervening lamina propria; (3) small angulated, abortive glands; or (4) a "never-ending/anastomosing" pattern of glands (Fig. 3.14a, b) [93]. In some situations, it may not be possible to be definitive. Stating that there is "high-grade dysplasia with foci suspicious for intramucosal adenocarcinoma" is adequate as high-grade dysplasia and intramucosal adenocarcinoma are managed similarly (section "Treatment").

Foveolar Dysplasia Foveolar dysplasia represents a non-adenomatous type of dysplasia of the gastric foveolar component of Barrett esophagus [87, 91, 95, 96]. In biopsy material, foveolar dysplasia constitutes 6–8% of dysplastic Barrett esophagus cases [61]. Foveolar dysplasia is morphologically distinct from intestinal-type dysplasia. Both low- and high-grade foveolar dysplasia are characterized by round-oval, basally located, non-stratified nuclei with open chromatin; nuclear stratification is not a feature of foveolar-type dysplasia (Fig. 3.15a, b) [61, 96]. While goblet cells may be inconspicuous, they

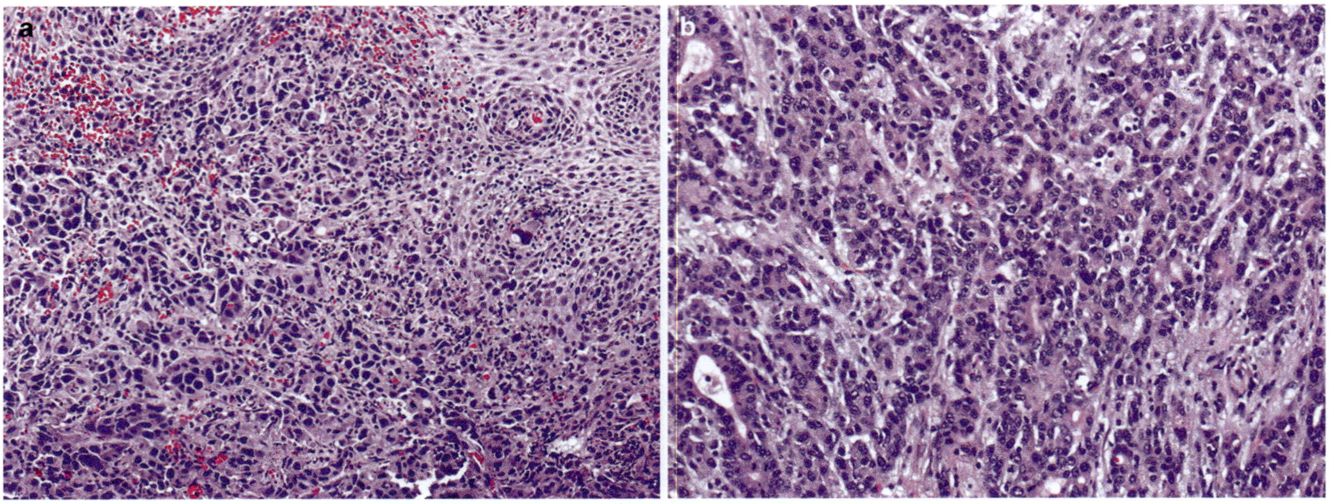

Fig. 3.14 Intramucosal adenocarcinoma. (**a**) Intramucosal adenocarcinoma undermining squamous epithelium. There are cords of cells and individual cell infiltration into the lamina propria, indicating invasion through the basement membrane. (**b**) Intramucosal adenocarcinoma characterized by an anastomosing pattern of malignant cells indicative of invasion through the basement membrane

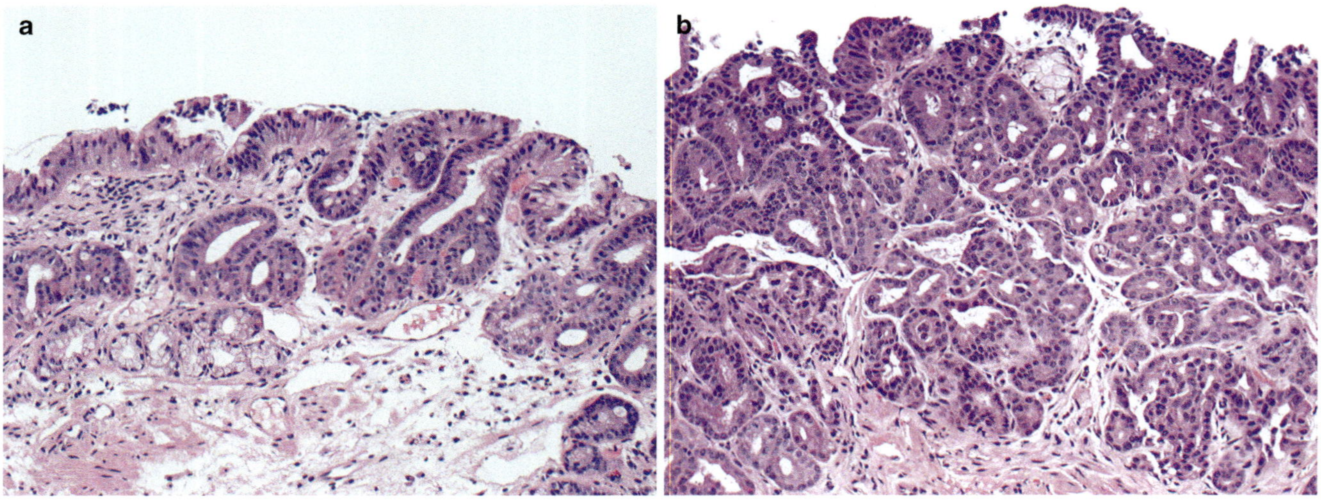

Fig. 3.15 Barrett mucosa, foveolar-type dysplasia. (**a**) Low-grade foveolar dysplasia is characterized by atypical, basally localized nuclei within mucinous, foveolar cells. Goblet cells are often inconspicuous. Note the back-to-back arrangement of the glands. (**b**) High-grade foveolar dysplasia demonstrating surface involvement and back-to-back glands. Marked mucin depletion and nuclear enlargement are readily appreciated

are usually present indicating the setting of Barrett esophagus [96]. Foveolar dysplasia invariably involves the surface epithelium. Nuclear size, presence of nucleoli, and gland architecture help differentiate low-grade from high-grade foveolar dysplasia. The gland architecture of low-grade dysplasia is overall preserved, with minimal crowding and no villiform architecture (Fig. 3.15a) [61, 96]. In contrast, high-grade foveolar dysplasia is defined as the presence of back-to-back glands with extensive branching, complexity, and occasional villiform growth (Fig. 3.15b) [96]. The nuclei of low-grade dysplasia are two to three times the size of a mature lymphocyte without prominent nucleoli, while the nuclei of high-grade dysplasia measure three to four times the size of a mature lymphocyte and typically contain prominent nucleoli [96]. Architectural crowding and complexity, high nuclear/cytoplasmic ratios, and mucin depletion are helpful in distinguishing high-grade from low-grade foveolar dysplasia [61, 96]. The natural history of foveolar-type dysplasia is as yet poorly defined. However, several studies have demonstrated that it likely behaves more aggressively than intestinal-type dysplasia [61].

Serrated Dysplasia Serrated changes may be observed in some cases of Barrett esophagus without dysplasia [90]. There are examples in the literature of dysplasia having a serrated appearance, akin to a serrated adenoma of the colon (Fig. 3.16a, b). Criteria for dysplasia are less well-defined

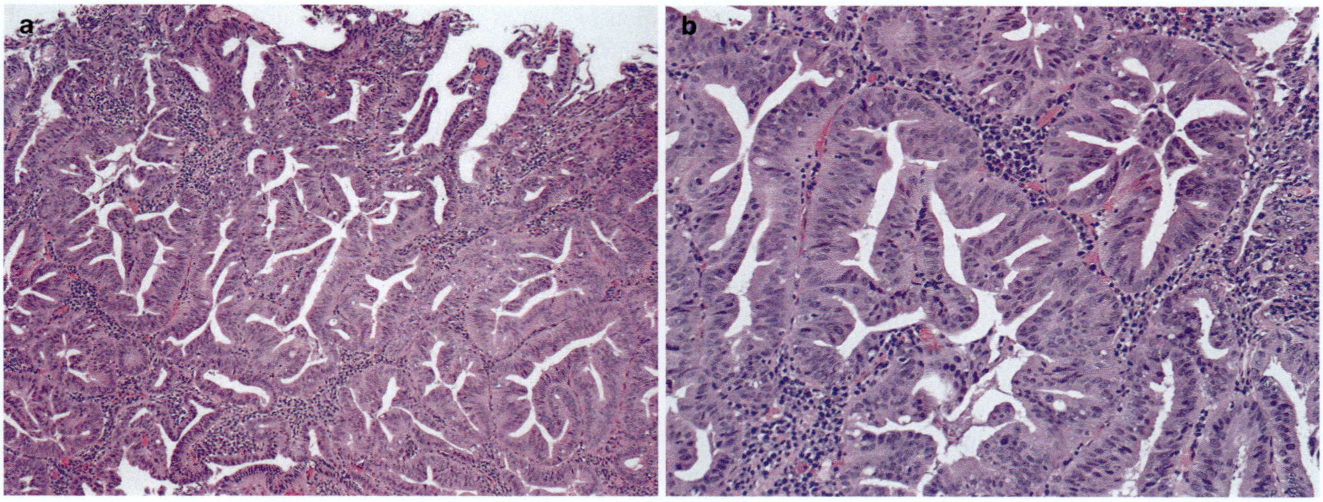

Fig. 3.16 Barrett mucosa, serrated dysplasia. (**a**) Serrated dysplasia is characterized by a sawtooth architecture and eosinophilic cytoplasm similar to serrated adenoma in the colon. Rare goblet cells are seen. (**b**) High-power view of serrated dysplasia

than the intestinal type of dysplasia [61, 90]. As with foveolar dysplasia, some suggest that serrated dysplasia confers elevated risk of progression [61, 90].

Histochemical and Immunohistochemical Findings

Numerous studies have been performed analyzing histochemical and immunohistochemical stains which may aid in the identification of Barrett esophagus, grading of dysplasia, or predicting risk of progression to a higher grade of dysplasia or esophageal adenocarcinoma. The presence and grade of dysplasia remain the best biomarkers for the progression of disease and serve as the only criterion for surveillance and treatment guidelines [60, 61]. A panel of experts from the Rodger C. Haggitt Gastrointestinal Pathology Society recently released a set of recommendations concerning the role of histochemical and immunohistochemical stains in Barrett esophagus [83].

Goblet Cell Identification

Histochemical Stains Alcian blue (at pH 2.5) will stain the acidic mucin of goblet cells blue-purple. It can be combined with the PAS stain which marks the neutral mucin of foveolar cells with a magenta color (Fig. 3.17). The Alcian blue/PAS cocktail can be used to highlight goblet cells and distinguish them from pseudogoblet cells (see "Differential Diagnosis" section below). Unfortunately, Alcian blue lacks specificity as columnar cells containing variable amounts of acidic mucin (columnar blue cells) will also stain blue-purple [83]. This may lead to false positives if the diagnosis is based solely upon histochemical staining alone.

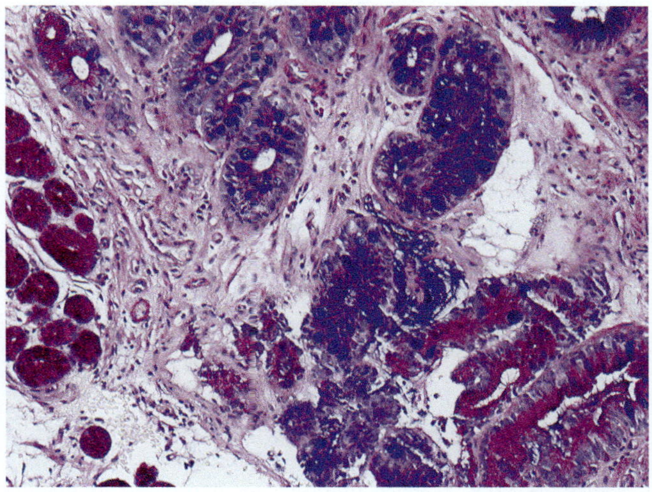

Fig. 3.17 Alcian blue-PAS stain in which the acidic mucin of goblet cells is stained blue, while the neutral mucin of foveolar cells appears magenta in color

At one point, it was hypothesized that columnar blue cells might represent an important histologic finding, possibly a precursor or early form of Barrett esophagus [76, 83, 97, 98]. However, subsequent studies have shown that columnar blue cells are not specific for Barrett esophagus and may be seen in a variety of situations, including submucosal ducts and cardiac-type mucosa unaffiliated with Barrett esophagus [83, 99]. Given the lack of specificity of Alcian blue/PAS, the routine use of this stain for diagnosing Barrett esophagus is not recommended, though judicious use in select cases may prove helpful if the diagnosis is in question [83].

Immunohistochemical Stains Immunostains targeting mucin glycoprotein subtypes (MUCs) or markers of intestinal differentiation have been extensively studied. Of the former, MUC2 is the best marker of intestinal phenotype and is consistently expressed in goblet cells [100–102]. MUC5AC on the other hand is expressed in metaplastic gastric foveolar cells [100, 102]. MUC2 can also be detected in the columnar cells of patients with intestinal metaplasia. McIntire et al. demonstrated MUC2 expression in non-goblet columnar cells of 78% of patients with intestinal metaplasia elsewhere, while it was only detected in columnar cells of 4% of those without intestinal metaplasia [101]. Given that MUC2-positive columnar cells were more often present close to goblet cells, they hypothesized that goblet cells may develop from MUC2-positive columnar cells [101]. However, MUC2 lacks the sensitivity and specificity needed to be used in the clinical setting for predicting the development of Barrett esophagus. Zhang et al. identified MUC2 expression in only 40% of non-goblet columnar mucosa cases which were found to have Barrett esophagus on subsequent biopsy [103]. It was also expressed in 9% of non-goblet columnar mucosa cases which remained negative for goblet cells on subsequent biopsy [103]. As noted in the recommendation paper by Srivastava et al., at present the use of MUC stains to confirm, diagnose, or predict development of Barrett esophagus is not indicated in the literature [83].

Evidence of intestinal differentiation can be provided by antibodies to nuclear transcription factors involved in intestinal columnar differentiation or to markers expressed by intestinal columnar cells [83, 103, 104]. Caudal-type homeobox 2 (CDX2) and SRY (sex-determining region) box 9 (SOX9) are the best-studied examples of the former, while Das-1, villin, and Hep Par 1 represent the latter [83, 103, 105]. CK7/CK20 profile expression has also been studied, especially in the context of distinguishing Barrett esophagus from intestinal metaplasia of the gastric cardia [106–108].

As with MUC2, these markers are expressed in intestinal metaplasia and are often identified in non-goblet columnar mucosa in the setting of Barrett esophagus, providing evidence that goblet cells may arise from a subset of non-goblet columnar epithelium [83]. Expression of the hedgehog ligand occurs in response to acid or bile and has been documented in Barrett esophagus [109]. This results in the induction of Hedgehog signaling pathway and activation of the Hedgehog stromal target gene bone morphogenetic protein 4 (BMP4), which subsequently induces expression of SOX9 [109]. SOX9, a nuclear transcription factor present in the intestinal crypt cells, is consistently expressed in Barrett epithelium [109].

SOX9, along with other cell signaling molecules, has been shown to result in the differentiation of squamous epithelium to columnar epithelium, suggesting that it plays a critical role in Barrett esophagus formation [104, 110]. Zhang et al. determined that the expression of either SOX9 or CDX2 in non-goblet columnar metaplasia could predict the identification of Barrett esophagus in a subsequent biopsy material with a sensitivity and specificity of 85% (positive predictive value, 73%) [103]. However, they noted that the study suffered from small sample size, with 13 cases that developed Barrett esophagus (test group) and 26 cases that did not develop Barrett esophagus on subsequent biopsy (control group) [103]. More studies are necessary to determine the role of SOX9 in the diagnosis (prevalent or incident) of Barrett esophagus.

Markers of Dysplasia and/or Risk Progression

Identifying Barrett esophagus is relatively straightforward in the majority of cases. However, determining whether or not there is dysplasia and grading it accurately are subjective and fraught with extensive interobserver variability. In addition to search for biomarkers of dysplasia, much work has been done in an attempt to identify markers that predict risk of progression among subsets of patients with and without dysplasia. p53 immunohistochemistry is the most extensively studied.

Srivastava et al. have compiled a comprehensive summary of p53 studies and its use in grading dysplasia and predicting disease progression [83]. Wild-type expression appears as "faint scattered p53 positivity within nuclei" [83]. Mutations which result in aberrant expression may take the form of upregulation and overexpression (diffuse positivity) (Fig. 3.18a, b) or truncating mutations which result in complete negativity (null pattern) [83]. Like grading dysplasia, distinguishing normal expression (scattered positivity) from overexpression of p53 is a subjective endeavor. The prevalence of abnormal p53 expression increases across the spectrum of dysplasia. Non-dysplastic Barrett esophagus patients show aberrant expression in 0–10% of cases [83]. Kastelein et al. identified abnormal expression in 38% of low-grade dysplasia cases, 83% of high-grade dysplasia cases, and 100% of esophageal adenocarcinoma cases [111]. Kaye et al. demonstrated higher interobserver agreement for p53 evaluation than grading of dysplasia when the latter was divided into negative for dysplasia, indefinite for dysplasia, low-grade dysplasia, and high-grade dysplasia [112]. However, kappa values were similar when dysplasia was also placed into a two-tier system of present or absent [112]. Studies also indicated that aberrant p53 expression was a risk factor for progression to high-grade dysplasia/esophageal adenocarcinoma. For example, the study by Kastelein et al. demonstrated aberrant p53 expression in 49% of cases that progressed to high-grade dysplasia/esophageal adenocarcinoma and 14% of controls which did not progress [83, 111].

While the British Society of Gastroenterology recommends the use of p53 in some cases, no gastrointestinal societies in the USA recommend the use of p53 in clinical practice. Similarly, the consensus panel of the Gastrointestinal Pathology Society does not presently endorse the use of p53 for evaluating dys-

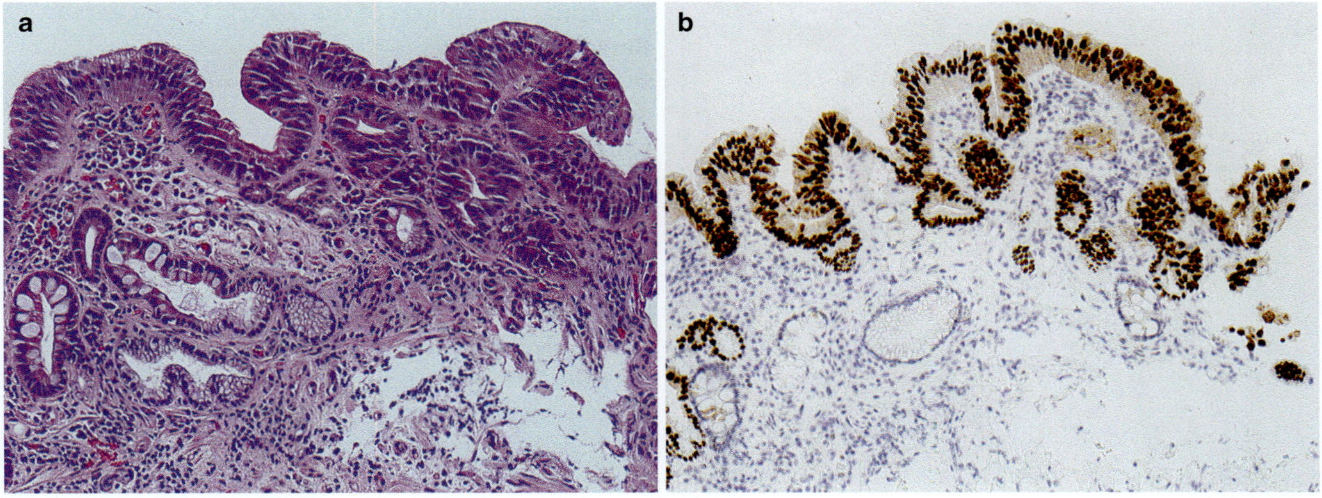

Fig. 3.18 Aberrant p53 expression in dysplastic Barrett mucosa. (**a**) Barrett mucosa shows low-grade dysplasia with surface involvement. (**b**) Aberrant p53 expression characterized by strong and diffuse positivity in dysplastic nuclei. Note the absence of staining in the non-dysplastic glands at the bottom left and bottom right

plasia in Barrett esophagus until studies develop more precise criteria for assessment and grading of the stain, including more precise definitions of minimal staining and how many biopsies to stain [83]. Surveillance guidelines are currently based upon the grade of dysplasia, and no recommendations exist on how to combine histologic grade with p53 expression profile or how that should affect surveillance intervals.

CyclinD1, AMACR, IMP3, and SOX2 have also been studied, albeit less extensively than p53 [83]. While the first three show trends of increased expression across the dysplasia spectrum, and SOX2 loss is more common in dysplasia, none are sufficiently sensitive or specific enough to be utilized as an adjunct for grading dysplasia or predicting risk of progression [83]. Dysplasia remains a morphologic diagnosis [83]. While p53 appears to show greater aberrant expression in patients at risk of progression, there is at present not enough data to recommend its routine use as a prognostic marker [83].

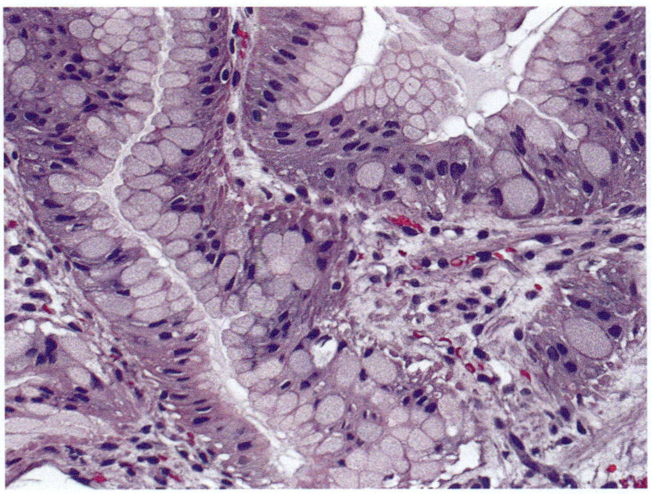

Fig. 3.19 Pseudogoblet cells have the morphology of true goblet cells. However, they contain neutral mucin which stains pink on H&E, and they are not randomly distributed like goblet cells. Instead, they are usually arranged in a continuous, linear manner

Differential Diagnosis

Pseudogoblet Cells Versus Goblet Cells

Pseudogoblet cells are foveolar cells which contain a voluminous amount of mucin, imparting a barrel-shaped appearance reminiscent of a goblet cell (Fig. 3.19). However, the mucus is neutral, and thus the cells maintain a lightly eosinophilic staining quality on H&E [113]. In addition, pseudogoblet cells are typically arranged in a continuous and linear fashion, while goblet cells are scattered irregularly among foveolar cells [83]. When an isolated finding and not associated with intestinal metaplasia, pseudogoblet cells confer no increased risk of dysplasia or malignancy [113].

Foveolar Blue Cells Versus Goblet Cells

Some foveolar cells contain enough acid mucin to have a bluish cytoplasmic tinge on H&E. However, these cells do not have a barrel-shaped morphology but instead maintain their normal, columnar shape (Fig. 3.20). Like pseudogoblet cells, foveolar blue cells have a continuous, linear arrangement which is distinct from the irregular distribution of goblet cells. As above, these cells are not associated with an increased risk of dysplasia or malignancy [113]. Their significance relates solely to being misinterpreted as intestinal metaplasia.

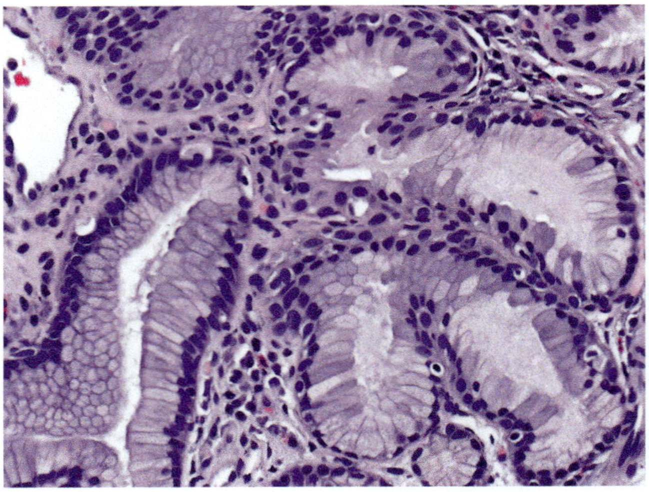

Fig. 3.20 Foveolar blue cells contain acidic mucin and are thus light blue on H&E. However, they do not have the barrel shape of goblet cells but rather maintain a columnar configuration with nondistended apical mucin, typical of foveolar cells

Table 3.4 Reactive gastric cardia versus foveolar-type dysplasia

Histologic feature	Gastric cardiac mucosa	Foveolar dysplasia
Architectural crowding	Absent to minimal	Present with back-to-back glands (high grade)
Full-thickness atypia	Absent	Present
Villiform architecture	Usually present	Usually absent (may be present in high-grade dysplasia)
Nuclear arrangement	Some degree of stratification	Basally located

Gastric Cardiac Mucosa Versus Foveolar Dysplasia

Gastric cardiac mucosa may be difficult to distinguish from Barrett esophagus with foveolar dysplasia, especially if the former is inflamed by GERD and the latter is low grade. The study by Patil et al. identified several features which aid in the distinction between these two types of mucosa [114]. Table 3.4 contains an outline of the most pertinent features. Foveolar dysplasia demonstrates architectural crowding with back-to-back glands, full-thickness atypia (surface and crypts), and non-villiform architecture, especially in the low-grade form [114]. In contrast, the glands of gastric cardiac mucosa are not abnormally crowded, and the surface foveolar compartment often shows hyperplastic, villoglandular proliferation [114]. Lastly, the nuclei of foveolar dysplasia are basally located, while the reactive surface cells of gastric cardia mucosa typically demonstrate some degree of nuclear stratification [114].

Intestinal Metaplasia of the Gastric Cardia Versus Barrett Esophagus

Intestinal metaplasia of the gastric cardia behaves less aggressively than Barrett esophagus, with a lower risk of progression to dysplasia and adenocarcinoma [83, 115]. It is therefore important to distinguish between these two whenever possible. Challenges with the gross anatomy at endoscopy (accurate identification of the GEJ), in conjunction with other structural issues such as hiatus hernia, may make it difficult for the endoscopists to identify important landmarks, leading to sampling of one region when another was intended. The pathologists must look for other clues which indicate sampling from the tubular esophagus. Srivastava et al. identified a set of histologic findings which suggest Barrett esophagus: (1) the presence of squamous epithelium overlying crypts with intestinal metaplasia; (2) crypt atrophy or disarray; (3) incomplete intestinal metaplasia; (4) diffuse intestinal metaplasia; (5) hybrid glands, with intestinal metaplasia restricted to the superficial aspect of the mucous glands; (6) multilayered epithelium; and (7) esophageal ducts [77]. As noted above, immunostains for CK7 and CK20 are not specific enough to be utilized on an individual case to distinguish these two lesions [83].

Treatment

The goal of treatment is the prevention of disease progression. Surveillance strategies attempt to maximize detection of intestinal metaplasia and dysplasia. There are several issues which mitigate the screening of the general population. To begin, up to half of patients with GERD are asymptomatic, and roughly 40% of patients with esophageal adenocarcinoma provide no antecedent history of GERD [59]. The low prevalence of Barrett esophagus, in conjunction with the cost and risks associated with endoscopy, precludes widespread screening. However, patients with chronic GERD and other risk factors (e.g., male, age >50 years, Caucasian race, central obesity, etc.) may undergo screening for Barrett esophagus [60]. Of note, the ACG recommends that patients who are negative for Barrett esophagus on screening examination do not undergo follow-up endoscopy to search for Barrett esophagus [60]. One look is enough.

If Barrett esophagus is detected, surveillance guidelines recommend four-quadrant biopsies every 1 cm in patients with a history of dysplasia and every 2 cm in patients without dysplasia [60]. Esophagitis is often a confounding factor, and these areas should not be biopsied. After an initial diagnosis of Barrett esophagus, if there is no dysplasia, patients do not need repeat endoscopy for 3–5 years [60]. It is recommended that those with histology that is indefinite for dysplasia undergo follow-up in 3–6 months after maximization of PPI therapy [60].

Once dysplasia of any grade is identified, the ACG recommends treatment by endoscopic therapy, though regular surveillance with a 12-month interval may be utilized in patients with low-grade dysplasia [60]. Endoscopic therapies include resection and ablation. EMR is recommended as the diagnostic and therapeutic modality of choice for patients who have a grossly visible area of nodularity. If the EMR contains dysplasia or esophageal adenocarcinoma confined to the mucosa, then the remaining Barrett esophagus should be ablated [60]. If no grossly visible lesion is present, then the patient should undergo ablation [60].

EMR is a technique which samples the mucosa and superficial submucosa, providing a much larger piece of tissue than routine biopsy. Endoscopic submucosal dissection (ESD) allows en bloc resection of even larger neoplastic lesions to achieve higher R0 resection rates. Both EMR and ESD are highly effective, but ESD is more time-consuming and may cause severe adverse events. EMRs may be injection, ligation, or CAP-assisted. Regardless of the exact technique, they all aim to separate the mucosa from the muscularis propria in the plane of the submucosa. The larger specimens obtained with EMR allow the procedure to serve both diagnostic and therapeutic roles (Fig. 3.21a). Studies have shown that the majority of EMRs (88–89%) include a sampling of submucosa, and they have been shown to increase diagnostic

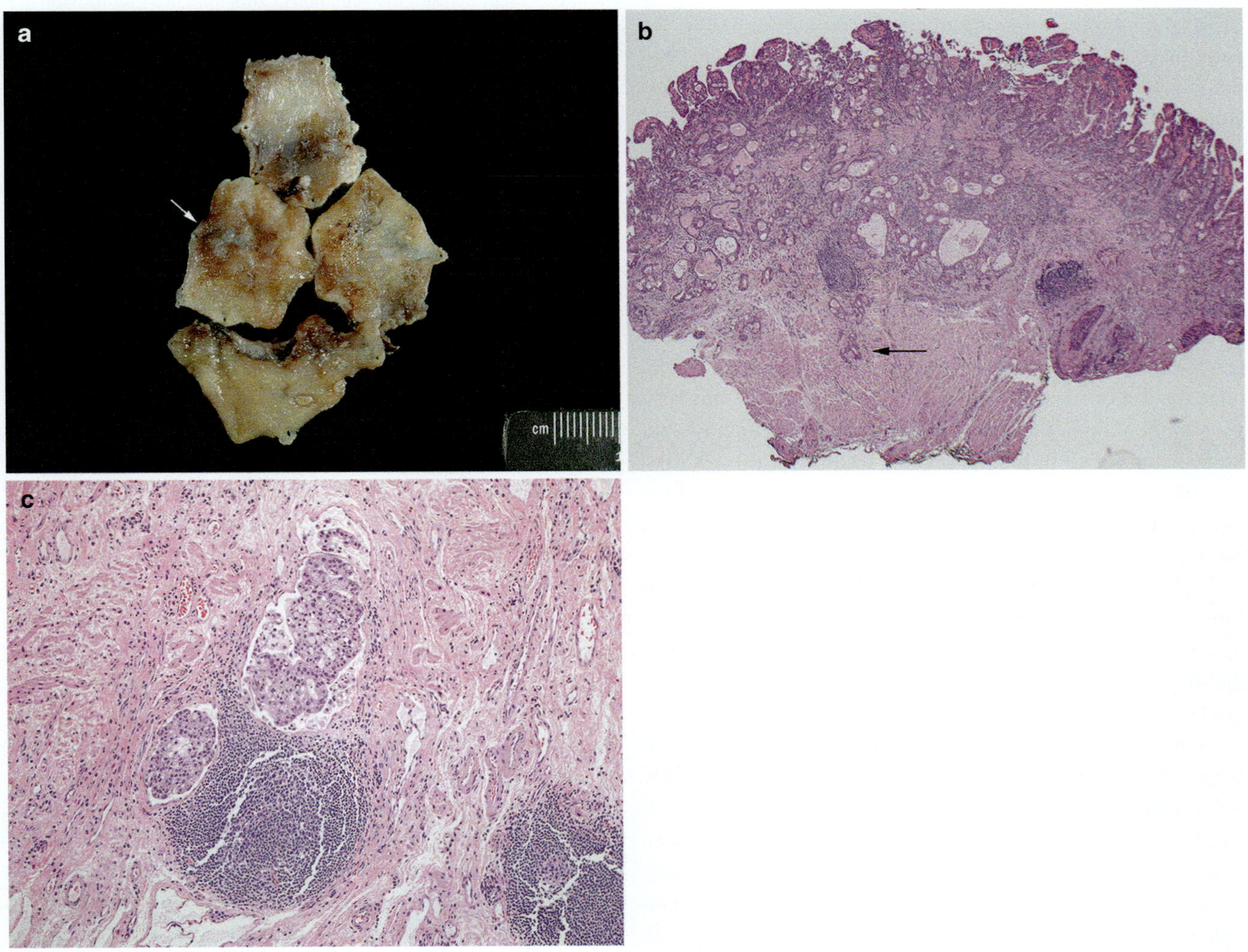

Fig. 3.21 Intramucosal adenocarcinoma on endoscopic mucosal resection (EMR). (**a**) EMR specimens of Barrett esophagus with nodular lesion of intramucosal adenocarcinoma (arrow). In this case, four EMRs have been performed. (**b**) Intramucosal adenocarcinoma with invasion into the outer layer of duplicated muscularis mucosae (arrow). (**c**) High-power view highlights a focus of lymphovascular invasion which is present within the space between duplicated layers of muscularis mucosae in a case of intramucosal adenocarcinoma

accuracy and interobserver agreement in grading of dysplasia [79, 116]. The depth of tissue obtained by EMR is especially helpful in the setting of adenocarcinoma, allowing the pathologists to clarify if the tumor is confined to the mucosa (i.e., intramucosal) (Fig. 3.21b) or demonstrates submucosal invasion. Unequivocal evidence of the latter includes tumor adjacent to fat, submucosal glands, or thick-walled muscular arteries, all of which are structures present in the true submucosa [82]. Gland entrapment within changes of the musculofibrous anomaly has been identified in 56% of EMR specimens [79]. Fortunately, the tissue landmarks present in the larger samples of EMR allow ready distinction between the musculofibrous anomaly and submucosal invasion [82]. As described above, glands associated with fat, thick-walled muscular arteries, or submucosal glands represent invasive adenocarcinoma as these three structures are confined to the submucosa.

In the setting of intramucosal adenocarcinoma, the pathologist should clarify whenever possible what level of the mucosa is involved by tumor. If duplication of the muscularis mucosae is present, the levels can be subdivided as follows: (1) lamina propria invasion, (2) invasion into the inner layer of muscularis mucosae, (3) invasion into space between duplicated layers of muscularis mucosae, or (4) invasion into the outer layer of muscularis mucosae. These distinctions are important as there is a network of lymphatics within the loose connective tissue between duplicated layers of muscularis mucosae. Lymphovascular invasion (Fig. 3.21c) may be seen in approximately 10% of EMRs once the tumor reaches this space [79]. Because of this risk, we comment upon the presence or absence of lymphovascular invasion for all intramucosal adenocarcinomas on EMRs. The pathologist should also comment upon the status of the lateral and deep margins whenever there is dysplasia and/or esophageal adenocarcinoma.

Radiofrequency ablation (RFA) involves the application of a high-frequency alternating current to the mucosa using an electrode or balloon, depending upon the size of the Barrett esophagus. After one to four treatments, low-grade dysplasia is completely eradicated in approximately 90% of patients, while eradication of high-grade dysplasia is achieved in approximately 80% of patients [117]. Roughly 3/4 of patients demonstrate complete eradication of intramucosal adenocarcinoma as well [117]. In the study by Shaheen et al., 25.2% of patients had subsquamous intramucosal adenocarcinoma before RFA, and this had decreased substantially to only 5.1% of participants (Fig. 3.22) at 12-month follow-up [117].

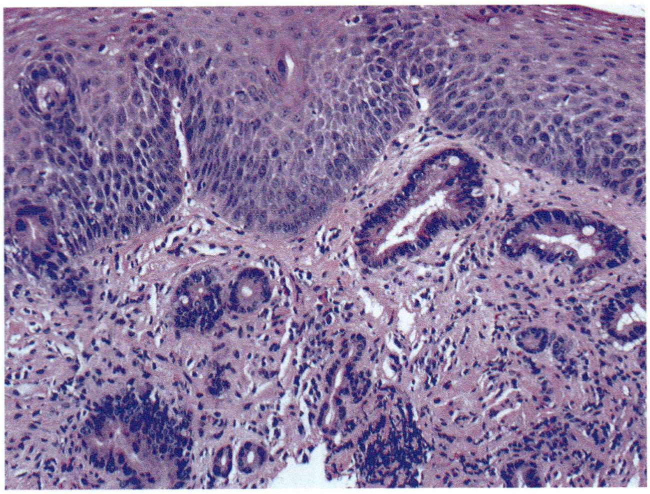

Fig. 3.22 Barrett mucosa after radiofrequency ablation. Barrett epithelium is present beneath the squamous epithelium after radiofrequency ablation

Prognosis

The retrospective nature of most studies, with the attendant variability in biopsy protocol, definition of Barrett esophagus, and subjectivity of grading dysplasia, makes it difficult to define the natural history of Barrett esophagus. Most patients with Barrett esophagus do not die from the disease or its complications [118].

Irregular Z Line (Intestinal Metaplasia <1 cm in Length)

Thota et al. compared 167 patients with an irregular Z line in 1624 patients with Barrett esophagus >1 cm and demonstrated that none of the patients with an irregular Z line developed high-grade dysplasia or adenocarcinoma over a median follow-up of 4.8 years [70]. These results are similar to those of Jung et al., who identified no increased risk of dysplasia or adenocarcinoma in patients with intestinal metaplasia of the GEJ, as opposed to those with Barrett esophagus >1 cm [119]. Given the similar outcomes for these two groups (i.e., patients with intestinal metaplasia of the GEJ and those with an irregular Z line), the ACG recommends including cases of intestinal metaplasia within an irregular Z line into the category of intestinal metaplasia of the GEJ [60]. They recommend not routinely sampling a normal appearing GEJ or an irregular Z line (columnar metaplasia of <1 cm) so that patients are not incorrectly assigned the diagnosis of Barrett esophagus [60].

Barrett Esophagus Negative for Dysplasia

The consensus is that non-dysplastic Barrett esophagus confers a risk of 0.1–0.5% per year of developing adenocarcinoma [59, 120]. A meta-analysis of 57 studies (11,434 patients) restricted to patients with Barrett esophagus (intestinal metaplasia) and no dysplasia demonstrated a pooled incidence of esophageal adenocarcinoma of 1 per 300 patients (0.33%) per year [121]. When restricted to patients with short-segment Barrett esophagus, the risk of esophageal adenocarcinoma decreased to 0.2% per year [121].

Barrett Esophagus Indefinite for Dysplasia

The risk of progression from indefinite dysplasia to high-grade dysplasia/esophageal adenocarcinoma ranges from 0.86–1.4% per year [83]. Several studies have demonstrated this rate, once prevalent disease was excluded. For example, in the study by Ma et al., 8% of patients diagnosed as indefinite for dysplasia were found to have dysplasia or esophageal adenocarcinoma within 1 year (designated prevalent disease) [122]. However, the incident rate of progression developing >1 year after initial diagnosis of indefinite for dysplasia was 1.4/100 person-years and for high-grade dysplasia/esophageal adenocarcinoma was 0.9/100 person-years [122]. These results are similar to those by Kestens et al., who identified an incidence rate for high-grade dysplasia/esophageal adenocarcinoma of 1.4 cases/100 person-years in 842 patients diagnosed as indefinite for dysplasia [123].

Barrett Esophagus with Low-Grade Dysplasia

The exact risk of progression of low-grade dysplasia to high-grade dysplasia/esophageal adenocarcinoma remains a subject of controversy. It can be very difficult to reliably diagnose low-grade dysplasia, with only fair agreement ($K = 0.32$) among expert gastrointestinal pathologists [86]. Variability in the reported natural history of low-grade dysplasia likely reflects this difficulty, with many studies having populations of patients which are artificially diluted with patients actually negative for dysplasia/indefinite for dysplasia.

A meta-analysis of 24 studies found a pooled incidence rate of esophageal adenocarcinoma development of 0.5% in patients with low-grade dysplasia [124]. The rate of developing high-grade dysplasia and/or esophageal adenocarcinoma was 1.7% per year [124]. However, when using a low-grade dysplasia/Barrett esophagus ratio as a surrogate marker for pathology quality, the individual studies showed significant heterogeneity. Wani et al. demonstrated similar findings, with a risk of 1.8% per year for developing high-grade dysplasia/esophageal adenocarcinoma in 210 patients with low-grade dysplasia [125]. They found no risk factors, such as duration or extent of low-grade dysplasia, which would predict a greater risk of progression in some patients [125]. However, other studies suggest that persistence of low-grade dysplasia and confirmation of the diagnosis by expert review do increase the risk of progression [126–128]. In a study of 255 patients with low-grade dysplasia, Duits et al. showed that the risk of progression to high-grade dysplasia/esophageal adenocarcinoma increased when the diagnosis was confirmed by a gastrointestinal pathologist, and the risk increased with the number of pathologists who confirmed the diagnosis of low-grade dysplasia (one pathologist confirmation, 10-fold; two pathologist confirmations, 27-fold; three pathologist confirmations, 47-fold) [128]. They also demonstrated that the persistence of low-grade dysplasia in follow-up biopsy yielded a ninefold risk of progression to high-grade dysplasia/esophageal adenocarcinoma [128]. It seems logical that these two factors (persistence of low-grade dysplasia and pathologist agreement) would minimize the chances of overcalling a sample as low-grade dysplasia, which is a common occurrence. In a separate study, Duits et al. showed that only 27% of 293 cases signed out as low-grade dysplasia in community practice were confirmed as low-grade dysplasia by expert consensus review [127]. This subgroup of confirmed low-grade dysplasia demonstrated a progression rate to high-grade dysplasia/esophageal adenocarcinoma of 9.1% per patient-year. Krishnamoorthi et al. also demonstrated that low-grade dysplasia may be overdiagnosed in a substantial subset of patients [129]. In their study of 203 patients diagnosed with low-grade dysplasia, 29% were downgraded to negative for dysplasia based upon consensus expert review [129].

Barrett Esophagus with High-Grade Dysplasia

It is difficult to distinguish prevalent vs. incident disease in patients with high-grade dysplasia, making outcome studies problematic [83]. As with low-grade dysplasia, risk of developing esophageal adenocarcinoma in patients with high-grade dysplasia varies by study, the annual rates range from 7–19% [60, 130]. Investigators have shown that the risk of progression also varies with the extent, or amount, of dysplasia [131].

References

1. Kahrilas PJ. Anatomy and physiology of the gastroesophageal junction. Gastroenterol Clin N Am. 1997;26(3):467–86.
2. Vakil N, van Zanten SV, Kahrilas P, Dent J, Jones R. The Montreal definition and classification of gastroesophageal reflux disease: a global evidence-based consensus. Am

J Gastroenterol. 2006;101(8):1900–20; quiz 43. https://doi.org/10.1111/j.1572-0241.2006.00630.x.
3. Gyawali CP, Kahrilas PJ, Savarino E, Zerbib F, Mion F, Smout A, et al. Modern diagnosis of GERD: the Lyon consensus. Gut. 2018;67(7):1351–62. https://doi.org/10.1136/gutjnl-2017-314722.
4. Kahrilas PJ. Clinical practice. Gastroesophageal reflux disease. N Engl J Med. 2008;359(16):1700–7. https://doi.org/10.1056/NEJMcp0804684.
5. Cho YS, Choi MG, Jeong JJ, Chung WC, Lee IS, Kim SW, et al. Prevalence and clinical spectrum of gastroesophageal reflux: a population-based study in Asan-si, Korea. Am J Gastroenterol. 2005;100(4):747–53. https://doi.org/10.1111/j.1572-0241.2005.41245.x.
6. Kennedy T, Jones R. The prevalence of gastro-oesophageal reflux symptoms in a UK population and the consultation behaviour of patients with these symptoms. Aliment Pharmacol Ther. 2000;14(12):1589–94.
7. Locke GR 3rd, Talley NJ, Fett SL, Zinsmeister AR, Melton LJ 3rd. Prevalence and clinical spectrum of gastroesophageal reflux: a population-based study in Olmsted County, Minnesota. Gastroenterology. 1997;112(5):1448–56.
8. El-Serag HB, Sweet S, Winchester CC, Dent J. Update on the epidemiology of gastro-oesophageal reflux disease: a systematic review. Gut. 2014;63(6):871–80. https://doi.org/10.1136/gutjnl-2012-304269.
9. El-Serag HB. Time trends of gastroesophageal reflux disease: a systematic review. Clin Gastroenterol Hepatol. 2007;5(1):17–26. https://doi.org/10.1016/j.cgh.2006.09.016.
10. Lee J, Anggiansah A, Anggiansah R, Young A, Wong T, Fox M. Effects of age on the gastroesophageal junction, esophageal motility, and reflux disease. Clin Gastroenterol Hepatol. 2007;5(12):1392–8. https://doi.org/10.1016/j.cgh.2007.08.011.
11. Becher A, Dent J. Systematic review: ageing and gastro-oesophageal reflux disease symptoms, oesophageal function and reflux oesophagitis. Aliment Pharmacol Ther. 2011;33(4):442–54. https://doi.org/10.1111/j.1365-2036.2010.04542.x.
12. Hampel H, Abraham NS, El-Serag HB. Meta-analysis: obesity and the risk for gastroesophageal reflux disease and its complications. Ann Intern Med. 2005;143(3):199–211.
13. Jacobson BC, Somers SC, Fuchs CS, Kelly CP, Camargo CA Jr. Body-mass index and symptoms of gastroesophageal reflux in women. N Engl J Med. 2006;354(22):2340–8. https://doi.org/10.1056/NEJMoa054391.
14. El-Serag HB, Petersen NJ, Carter J, Graham DY, Richardson P, Genta RM, et al. Gastroesophageal reflux among different racial groups in the United States. Gastroenterology. 2004;126(7):1692–9.
15. Avidan B, Sonnenberg A, Schnell TG, Sontag SJ. Risk factors for erosive reflux esophagitis: a case-control study. Am J Gastroenterol. 2001;96(1):41–6. https://doi.org/10.1111/j.1572-0241.2001.03449.x.
16. El-Serag HB, Sonnenberg A, Jamal MM, Inadomi JM, Crooks LA, Feddersen RM. Corpus gastritis is protective against reflux oesophagitis. Gut. 1999;45(2):181–5.
17. Moayyedi P, Bardhan C, Young L, Dixon MF, Brown L, Axon AT. Helicobacter pylori eradication does not exacerbate reflux symptoms in gastroesophageal reflux disease. Gastroenterology. 2001;121(5):1120–6.
18. Mittal RK, Balaban DH. The esophagogastric junction. N Engl J Med. 1997;336(13):924–32. https://doi.org/10.1056/nejm199703273361306.
19. Richter JE. Typical and atypical presentations of gastroesophageal reflux disease. The role of esophageal testing in diagnosis and management. Gastroenterol Clin N Am. 1996;25(1):75–102.
20. Vakil NB, Traxler B, Levine D. Dysphagia in patients with erosive esophagitis: prevalence, severity, and response to proton pump inhibitor treatment. Clin Gastroenterol Hepatol. 2004;2(8):665–8.
21. Koufman JA. The otolaryngologic manifestations of gastroesophageal reflux disease (GERD): a clinical investigation of 225 patients using ambulatory 24-hour pH monitoring and an experimental investigation of the role of acid and pepsin in the development of laryngeal injury. Laryngoscope. 1991;101(4 Pt 2 Suppl 53):1–78.
22. Kahrilas PJ, Altman KW, Chang AB, Field SK, Harding SM, Lane AP, et al. Chronic cough due to gastroesophageal reflux in adults: CHEST guideline and expert panel report. Chest. 2016;150(6):1341–60. https://doi.org/10.1016/j.chest.2016.08.1458.
23. Lundell LR, Dent J, Bennett JR, Blum AL, Armstrong D, Galmiche JP, et al. Endoscopic assessment of oesophagitis: clinical and functional correlates and further validation of the Los Angeles classification. Gut. 1999;45(2):172–80.
24. van Malenstein H, Farre R, Sifrim D. Esophageal dilated intercellular spaces (DIS) and nonerosive reflux disease. Am J Gastroenterol. 2008;103(4):1021–8. https://doi.org/10.1111/j.1572-0241.2007.01688.x.
25. Spechler SJ. Epidemiology and natural history of gastro-oesophageal reflux disease. Digestion. 1992;51(Suppl 1):24–9. https://doi.org/10.1159/000200911.
26. Gyawali CP, Azagury DE, Chan WW, Chandramohan SM, Clarke JO, de Bortoli N, et al. Nonerosive reflux disease: clinical concepts. Ann N Y Acad Sci. 2018;1434:290. https://doi.org/10.1111/nyas.13845.
27. Modlin IM, Hunt RH, Malfertheiner P, Moayyedi P, Quigley EM, Tytgat GN, et al. Diagnosis and management of non-erosive reflux disease—the Vevey NERD Consensus Group. Digestion. 2009;80(2):74–88. https://doi.org/10.1159/000219365.
28. Aziz Q, Fass R, Gyawali CP, Miwa H, Pandolfino JE, Zerbib F. Functional esophageal disorders. Gastroenterology. 2016;150:1368. https://doi.org/10.1053/j.gastro.2016.02.012.
29. Dent J, Brun J, Fendrick A, Fennerty M, Janssens J, Kahrilas P, et al. An evidence-based appraisal of reflux disease management—the Genval Workshop Report. Gut. 1999;44(Suppl 2):S1–16.
30. Krugmann J, Neumann H, Vieth M, Armstrong D. What is the role of endoscopy and oesophageal biopsies in the management of GERD? Best Pract Res Clin Gastroenterol. 2013;27(3):373–85. https://doi.org/10.1016/j.bpg.2013.06.010.
31. Tripathi M, Streutker CJ, Marginean EC. Relevance of histology in the diagnosis of reflux esophagitis. Ann N Y Acad Sci. 2018;1434:94. https://doi.org/10.1111/nyas.13742.
32. Vieth M, Mastracci L, Vakil N, Dent J, Wernersson B, Baldycheva I, et al. Epithelial thickness is a marker of gastroesophageal reflux disease. Clin Gastroenterol Hepatol. 2016;14(11):1544–51.e1. https://doi.org/10.1016/j.cgh.2016.06.018.
33. Yerian L, Fiocca R, Mastracci L, Riddell R, Vieth M, Sharma P, et al. Refinement and reproducibility of histologic criteria for the assessment of microscopic lesions in patients with gastroesophageal reflux disease: the Esohisto project. Dig Dis Sci. 2011;56(9):2656–65. https://doi.org/10.1007/s10620-011-1624-z.
34. Grin A, Streutker CJ. Esophagitis: old histologic concepts and new thoughts. Arch Pathol Lab Med. 2015;139(6):723–9. https://doi.org/10.5858/arpa.2014-0132-RA.
35. Ismail-Beigi F, Horton PF, Pope CE 2nd. Histological consequences of gastroesophageal reflux in man. Gastroenterology. 1970;58(2):163–74.
36. Caviglia R, Ribolsi M, Maggiano N, Gabbrielli AM, Emerenziani S, Guarino MP, et al. Dilated intercellular spaces of esophageal epithelium in nonerosive reflux disease patients with physiological esophageal acid exposure. Am J Gastroenterol. 2005;100(3):543–8. https://doi.org/10.1111/j.1572-0241.2005.40978.x.
37. Tobey NA, Carson JL, Alkiek RA, Orlando RC. Dilated intercellular spaces: a morphological feature of acid reflux—damaged human esophageal epithelium. Gastroenterology. 1996;111(5):1200–5.

38. Schneider NI, Plieschnegger W, Geppert M, Wigginghaus B, Hoess GM, Eherer A, et al. Validation study of the Esohisto consensus guidelines for the recognition of microscopic esophagitis (histoGERD trial). Hum Pathol. 2014;45(5):994–1002. https://doi.org/10.1016/j.humpath.2013.12.013.
39. Fiocca R, Mastracci L, Riddell R, Takubo K, Vieth M, Yerian L, et al. Development of consensus guidelines for the histologic recognition of microscopic esophagitis in patients with gastroesophageal reflux disease: the Esohisto project. Hum Pathol. 2010;41(2):223–31. https://doi.org/10.1016/j.humpath.2009.07.016.
40. Brown LF, Goldman H, Antonioli DA. Intraepithelial eosinophils in endoscopic biopsies of adults with reflux esophagitis. Am J Surg Pathol. 1984;8(12):899–905.
41. Martin IW, Atkinson AE, Liu X, Suriawinata AA, Lefferts JA, Lisovsky M. Mucosal inflammation in Candida esophagitis has distinctive features that may be helpful diagnostically. Mod Pathol. 2018;31(11):1653–60. https://doi.org/10.1038/s41379-018-0060-4.
42. Winter HS, Madara JL, Stafford RJ, Grand RJ, Quinlan JE, Goldman H. Intraepithelial eosinophils: a new diagnostic criterion for reflux esophagitis. Gastroenterology. 1982;83(4):818–23.
43. Tummala V, Barwick KW, Sontag SJ, Vlahcevic RZ, McCallum RW. The significance of intraepithelial eosinophils in the histologic diagnosis of gastroesophageal reflux. Am J Clin Pathol. 1987;87(1):43–8.
44. Steiner SJ, Kernek KM, Fitzgerald JF. Severity of basal cell hyperplasia differs in reflux versus eosinophilic esophagitis. J Pediatr Gastroenterol Nutr. 2006;42(5):506–9. https://doi.org/10.1097/01.mpg.0000221906.06899.1b.
45. Dellon ES, Gonsalves N, Hirano I, Furuta GT, Liacouras CA, Katzka DA. ACG clinical guideline: evidenced based approach to the diagnosis and management of esophageal eosinophilia and eosinophilic esophagitis (EoE). Am J Gastroenterol. 2013;108(5):679–92; quiz 93. https://doi.org/10.1038/ajg.2013.71.
46. Croese J, Fairley SK, Masson JW, Chong AK, Whitaker DA, Kanowski PA, et al. Clinical and endoscopic features of eosinophilic esophagitis in adults. Gastrointest Endosc. 2003;58(4):516–22.
47. Tutuian R. Adverse effects of drugs on the esophagus. Best Pract Res Clin Gastroenterol. 2010;24(2):91–7. https://doi.org/10.1016/j.bpg.2010.02.005.
48. De Petris G, Gatius Caldero S, Chen L, Xiao SY, Dhungel BM, Wendel Spizcka AJ, et al. Histopathological changes in the gastrointestinal tract due to drugs: an update for the surgical pathologist (part I of II). Int J Surg Pathol. 2014;22(2):120–8. https://doi.org/10.1177/1066896913502229.
49. Hatlebakk JG, Zerbib F, des Varannes SB, Attwood SE, Ell C, Fiocca R, et al. Gastroesophageal acid reflux control 5 years after antireflux surgery, compared with long-term esomeprazole therapy. Clin Gastroenterol Hepatol. 2016;14(5):678–85.e3. https://doi.org/10.1016/j.cgh.2015.07.025.
50. Mahon D, Rhodes M, Decadt B, Hindmarsh A, Lowndes R, Beckingham I, et al. Randomized clinical trial of laparoscopic Nissen fundoplication compared with proton-pump inhibitors for treatment of chronic gastro-oesophageal reflux. Br J Surg. 2005;92(6):695–9. https://doi.org/10.1002/bjs.4934.
51. Spechler SJ, Lee E, Ahnen D, Goyal RK, Hirano I, Ramirez F, et al. Long-term outcome of medical and surgical therapies for gastroesophageal reflux disease: follow-up of a randomized controlled trial. JAMA. 2001;285(18):2331–8.
52. Grant AM, Cotton SC, Boachie C, Ramsay CR, Krukowski ZH, Heading RC, et al. Minimal access surgery compared with medical management for gastro-oesophageal reflux disease: five year follow-up of a randomised controlled trial (REFLUX). BMJ. 2013;346:f1908. https://doi.org/10.1136/bmj.f1908.
53. Dassinger MS, Torquati A, Houston HL, Holzman MD, Sharp KW, Richards WO. Laparoscopic fundoplication: 5-year follow-up. Am Surg. 2004;70(8):691–4; discussion 4–5
54. Galmiche JP, Hatlebakk J, Attwood S, Ell C, Fiocca R, Eklund S, et al. Laparoscopic antireflux surgery vs esomeprazole treatment for chronic GERD: the LOTUS randomized clinical trial. JAMA. 2011;305(19):1969–77. https://doi.org/10.1001/jama.2011.626.
55. Katz PO, Gerson LB, Vela MF. Guidelines for the diagnosis and management of gastroesophageal reflux disease. Am J Gastroenterol. 2013;108(3):308–28; quiz 29. https://doi.org/10.1038/ajg.2012.444.
56. Cowgill SM, Arnaoutakis D, Villadolid D, Al-Saadi S, Arnaoutakis D, Molloy DL, et al. Results after laparoscopic fundoplication: does age matter? Am Surg. 2006;72(9):778–83; discussion 83–4
57. Ganz RA. A review of new surgical and endoscopic therapies for gastroesophageal reflux disease. Gastroenterol Hepatol. 2016;12(7):424–31.
58. Khan M, Santana J, Donnellan C, Preston C, Moayyedi P. Medical treatments in the short term management of reflux oesophagitis. Cochrane Database Syst Rev. 2007;(2):CD003244. https://doi.org/10.1002/14651858.CD003244.pub2.
59. Spechler SJ, Souza RF. Barrett's esophagus. N Engl J Med. 2014;371(9):836–45. https://doi.org/10.1056/NEJMra1314704.
60. Shaheen NJ, Falk GW, Iyer PG, Gerson LB. ACG clinical guideline: diagnosis and management of Barrett's esophagus. Am J Gastroenterol. 2016;111(1):30–50; quiz 1. https://doi.org/10.1038/ajg.2015.322.
61. Naini BV, Souza RF, Odze RD. Barrett's esophagus: a comprehensive and contemporary review for pathologists. Am J Surg Pathol. 2016;40(5):e45–66. https://doi.org/10.1097/pas.0000000000000598.
62. Takubo K, Aida J, Naomoto Y, Sawabe M, Arai T, Shiraishi H, et al. Cardiac rather than intestinal-type background in endoscopic resection specimens of minute Barrett adenocarcinoma. Hum Pathol. 2009;40(1):65–74. https://doi.org/10.1016/j.humpath.2008.06.008.
63. Lavery DL, Martinez P, Gay LJ, Cereser B, Novelli MR, Rodriguez-Justo M, et al. Evolution of oesophageal adenocarcinoma from metaplastic columnar epithelium without goblet cells in Barrett's oesophagus. Gut. 2016;65(6):907–13. https://doi.org/10.1136/gutjnl-2015-310748.
64. Riddell RH, Odze RD. Definition of Barrett's esophagus: time for a rethink—is intestinal metaplasia dead? Am J Gastroenterol. 2009;104(10):2588–94. https://doi.org/10.1038/ajg.2009.390.
65. Allanson BM, Bonavita J, Mirzai B, Khor TS, Raftopoulos SC, de Boer WB, et al. Early Barrett esophagus-related neoplasia in segments 1 cm or longer is always associated with intestinal metaplasia. Mod Pathol. 2017;30(8):1170–6. https://doi.org/10.1038/modpathol.2017.36.
66. Smith J, Garcia A, Zhang R, DeMeester S, Vallone J, Chandrasoma P. Intestinal metaplasia is present in most if not all patients who have undergone endoscopic mucosal resection for esophageal adenocarcinoma. Am J Surg Pathol. 2016;40(4):537–43. https://doi.org/10.1097/pas.0000000000000601.
67. Sharma P. Clinical practice. Barrett's esophagus. N Engl J Med. 2009;361(26):2548–56. https://doi.org/10.1056/NEJMcp0902173.
68. Fass R, Hell RW, Garewal HS, Martinez P, Pulliam G, Wendel C, et al. Correlation of oesophageal acid exposure with Barrett's oesophagus length. Gut. 2001;48(3):310–3.
69. Coleman HG, Bhat SK, Murray LJ, McManus DT, O'Neill OM, Gavin AT, et al. Symptoms and endoscopic features at Barrett's esophagus diagnosis: implications for neoplastic progression risk. Am J Gastroenterol. 2014;109(4):527–34. https://doi.org/10.1038/ajg.2014.10.
70. Thota PN, Vennalaganti P, Vennelaganti S, Young P, Gaddam S, Gupta N, et al. Low risk of high-grade dysplasia or esophageal

adenocarcinoma among patients with Barrett's esophagus less than 1 cm (irregular Z line) within 5 years of index endoscopy. Gastroenterology. 2017;152(5):987–92. https://doi.org/10.1053/j.gastro.2016.12.005.
71. Spechler SJ. Cardiac metaplasia: follow, treat, or ignore? Dig Dis Sci. 2018;63(8):2052–8. https://doi.org/10.1007/s10620-018-5063-y.
72. Chandrasoma PT, Der R, Ma Y, Peters J, Demeester T. Histologic classification of patients based on mapping biopsies of the gastroesophageal junction. Am J Surg Pathol. 2003;27(7):929–36.
73. Chandrasoma PT, Der R, Ma Y, Dalton P, Taira M. Histology of the gastroesophageal junction: an autopsy study. Am J Surg Pathol. 2000;24(3):402–9.
74. Chandrasoma P. Controversies of the cardiac mucosa and Barrett's oesophagus. Histopathology. 2005;46(4):361–73. https://doi.org/10.1111/j.1365-2559.2005.02088.x.
75. Jauregui HO, Davessar K, Hale JH, Kessimian N, Cenoz C. Mucin histochemistry of intestinal metaplasia in Barrett's esophagus. Mod Pathol. 1988;1(3):188–92.
76. Gottfried MR, McClave SA, Boyce HW. Incomplete intestinal metaplasia in the diagnosis of columnar lined esophagus (Barrett's esophagus). Am J Clin Pathol. 1989;92(6):741–6.
77. Srivastava A, Odze RD, Lauwers GY, Redston M, Antonioli DA, Glickman JN. Morphologic features are useful in distinguishing Barrett esophagus from carditis with intestinal metaplasia. Am J Surg Pathol. 2007;31(11):1733–41. https://doi.org/10.1097/PAS.0b013e318078ce91.
78. Glickman JN, Chen YY, Wang HH, Antonioli DA, Odze RD. Phenotypic characteristics of a distinctive multilayered epithelium suggests that it is a precursor in the development of Barrett's esophagus. Am J Surg Pathol. 2001;25(5):569–78.
79. Lewis JT, Wang KK, Abraham SC. Muscularis mucosae duplication and the musculo-fibrous anomaly in endoscopic mucosal resections for Barrett esophagus: implications for staging of adenocarcinoma. Am J Surg Pathol. 2008;32(4):566–71. https://doi.org/10.1097/PAS.0b013e31815bf8c7.
80. Abraham SC, Krasinskas AM, Correa AM, Hofstetter WL, Ajani JA, Swisher SG, et al. Duplication of the muscularis mucosae in Barrett esophagus: an underrecognized feature and its implication for staging of adenocarcinoma. Am J Surg Pathol. 2007;31(11):1719–25. https://doi.org/10.1097/PAS.0b013e318093e3bf.
81. Rubio CA, Riddell R. Musculo-fibrous anomaly in Barrett's mucosa with dysplasia. Am J Surg Pathol. 1988;12(11):885–9.
82. Kaye PV, O'Donovan M, Mapstone N, Disep B, Novelli M, Ragunath K. Pathologists are able to differentiate reliably the lamina propria associated with Barrett's musculofibrous anomaly from submucosa in oesophageal endoscopic resections. Histopathology. 2015;67(6):914–7. https://doi.org/10.1111/his.12736.
83. Srivastava A, Appelman H, Goldsmith JD, Davison JM, Hart J, Krasinskas AM. The use of ancillary stains in the diagnosis of Barrett esophagus and Barrett esophagus-associated dysplasia: recommendations from the Rodger C. Haggitt gastrointestinal pathology society. Am J Surg Pathol. 2017;41(5):e8–e21. https://doi.org/10.1097/pas.0000000000000819.
84. Lomo LC, Blount PL, Sanchez CA, Li X, Galipeau PC, Cowan DS, et al. Crypt dysplasia with surface maturation: a clinical, pathologic, and molecular study of a Barrett's esophagus cohort. Am J Surg Pathol. 2006;30(4):423–35.
85. Reid BJ, Haggitt RC, Rubin CE, Roth G, Surawicz CM, Van Belle G, et al. Observer variation in the diagnosis of dysplasia in Barrett's esophagus. Hum Pathol. 1988;19(2):166–78.
86. Montgomery E, Bronner MP, Goldblum JR, Greenson JK, Haber MM, Hart J, et al. Reproducibility of the diagnosis of dysplasia in Barrett esophagus: a reaffirmation. Hum Pathol. 2001;32(4):368–78. https://doi.org/10.1053/hupa.2001.23510.
87. Rucker-Schmidt RL, Sanchez CA, Blount PL, Ayub K, Li X, Rabinovitch PS, et al. Nonadenomatous dysplasia in Barrett esophagus: a clinical, pathologic, and DNA content flow cytometric study. Am J Surg Pathol. 2009;33(6):886–93. https://doi.org/10.1097/PAS.0b013e318198a1d4.
88. Riddell RH, Goldman H, Ransohoff DF, Appelman HD, Fenoglio CM, Haggitt RC, et al. Dysplasia in inflammatory bowel disease: standardized classification with provisional clinical applications. Hum Pathol. 1983;14(11):931–68.
89. Goldblum JR. Controversies in the diagnosis of Barrett esophagus and Barrett-related dysplasia: one pathologist's perspective. Arch Pathol Lab Med. 2010;134(10):1479–84. https://doi.org/10.1043/2010-0249-ra.1.
90. Vieth M, Montgomery EA, Riddell RH. Observations of different patterns of dysplasia in Barrett's esophagus—a first step to harmonize grading. Cesk Patol. 2016;52(3):154–63.
91. Odze RD. Diagnosis and grading of dysplasia in Barrett's oesophagus. J Clin Pathol. 2006;59(10):1029–38. https://doi.org/10.1136/jcp.2005.035337.
92. Sangle NA, Taylor SL, Emond MJ, Depot M, Overholt BF, Bronner MP. Overdiagnosis of high-grade dysplasia in Barrett's esophagus: a multicenter, international study. Mod Pathol. 2015;28(6):758–65. https://doi.org/10.1038/modpathol.2015.2.
93. Downs-Kelly E, Mendelin JE, Bennett AE, Castilla E, Henricks WH, Schoenfield L, et al. Poor interobserver agreement in the distinction of high-grade dysplasia and adenocarcinoma in pretreatment Barrett's esophagus biopsies. Am J Gastroenterol. 2008;103(9):2333–40; quiz 41. https://doi.org/10.1111/j.1572-0241.2008.02020.x.
94. Zhu W, Appelman HD, Greenson JK, Ramsburgh SR, Orringer MB, Chang AC, et al. A histologically defined subset of high-grade dysplasia in Barrett mucosa is predictive of associated carcinoma. Am J Clin Pathol. 2009;132(1):94–100. https://doi.org/10.1309/ajcp78ckiojwovfn.
95. Brown IS, Whiteman DC, Lauwers GY. Foveolar type dysplasia in Barrett esophagus. Mod Pathol. 2010;23(6):834–43. https://doi.org/10.1038/modpathol.2010.59.
96. Mahajan D, Bennett AE, Liu X, Bena J, Bronner MP. Grading of gastric foveolar-type dysplasia in Barrett's esophagus. Mod Pathol. 2010;23(1):1–11. https://doi.org/10.1038/modpathol.2009.147.
97. Chen YY, Wang HH, Antonioli DA, Spechler SJ, Zeroogian JM, Goyal R, et al. Significance of acid-mucin-positive nongoblet columnar cells in the distal esophagus and gastroesophageal junction. Hum Pathol. 1999;30(12):1488–95.
98. Offner FA, Lewin KJ, Weinstein WM. Metaplastic columnar cells in Barrett's esophagus: a common and neglected cell type. Hum Pathol. 1996;27(9):885–9.
99. Genta RM, Huberman RM, Graham DY. The gastric cardia in Helicobacter pylori infection. Hum Pathol. 1994;25(9):915–9.
100. Guillem P, Billeret V, Buisine MP, Flejou JF, Lecomte-Houcke M, Degand P, et al. Mucin gene expression and cell differentiation in human normal, premalignant and malignant esophagus. Int J Cancer. 2000;88(6):856–61.
101. McIntire MG, Soucy G, Vaughan TL, Shahsafaei A, Odze RD. MUC2 is a highly specific marker of goblet cell metaplasia in the distal esophagus and gastroesophageal junction. Am J Surg Pathol. 2011;35(7):1007–13. https://doi.org/10.1097/PAS.0b013e318218940d.
102. Hahn HP, Blount PL, Ayub K, Das KM, Souza R, Spechler S, et al. Intestinal differentiation in metaplastic, nongoblet columnar epithelium in the esophagus. Am J Surg Pathol. 2009;33(7):1006–15. https://doi.org/10.1097/PAS.0b013e31819f57e9.
103. Zhang X, Westerhoff M, Hart J. Expression of SOX9 and CDX2 in nongoblet columnar-lined esophagus predicts the

detection of Barrett's esophagus during follow-up. Mod Pathol. 2015;28(5):654–61. https://doi.org/10.1038/modpathol.2014.157.

104. Minacapelli CD, Bajpai M, Geng X, Cheng CL, Chouthai AA, Souza R, et al. Barrett's metaplasia develops from cellular reprograming of esophageal squamous epithelium due to gastroesophageal reflux. Am J Physiol Gastrointest Liver Physiol. 2017;312(6):G615–g22. https://doi.org/10.1152/ajpgi.00268.2016.
105. Moskaluk CA, Zhang H, Powell SM, Cerilli LA, Hampton GM, Frierson HF Jr. Cdx2 protein expression in normal and malignant human tissues: an immunohistochemical survey using tissue microarrays. Mod Pathol. 2003;16(9):913–9. https://doi.org/10.1097/01.mp.0000086073.92773.55.
106. Ormsby AH, Goldblum JR, Rice TW, Richter JE, Falk GW, Vaezi MF, et al. Cytokeratin subsets can reliably distinguish Barrett's esophagus from intestinal metaplasia of the stomach. Hum Pathol. 1999;30(3):288–94.
107. Younes M. What is the role of cytokeratins in Barrett/cardia differentiation? Arch Pathol Lab Med. 2005;129(2):181–2. https://doi.org/10.1043/1543-2165(2005)129<181:witroc>2.0.co;2.
108. Coban S, Ormeci N, Savas B, Ekiz F, Ensari A, Kuzu I, et al. Evaluation of Barrett's esophagus with CK7, CK20, p53, Ki67, and COX2 expressions using chromoendoscopical examination. Dis Esophagus. 2013;26(2):189–96. https://doi.org/10.1111/j.1442–2050.2012.01352.x.
109. Wang DH, Clemons NJ, Miyashita T, Dupuy AJ, Zhang W, Szczepny A, et al. Aberrant epithelial-mesenchymal Hedgehog signaling characterizes Barrett's metaplasia. Gastroenterology. 2010;138(5):1810–22. https://doi.org/10.1053/j.gastro.2010.01.048.
110. Clemons NJ, Wang DH, Croagh D, Tikoo A, Fennell CM, Murone C, et al. Sox9 drives columnar differentiation of esophageal squamous epithelium: a possible role in the pathogenesis of Barrett's esophagus. Am J Physiol Gastrointest Liver Physiol. 2012;303(12):G1335–46. https://doi.org/10.1152/ajpgi.00291.2012.
111. Kastelein F, Biermann K, Steyerberg EW, Verheij J, Kalisvaart M, Looijenga LH, et al. Aberrant p53 protein expression is associated with an increased risk of neoplastic progression in patients with Barrett's oesophagus. Gut. 2013;62(12):1676–83. https://doi.org/10.1136/gutjnl-2012–303594.
112. Kaye PV, Haider SA, Ilyas M, James PD, Soomro I, Faisal W, et al. Barrett's dysplasia and the Vienna classification: reproducibility, prediction of progression and impact of consensus reporting and p53 immunohistochemistry. Histopathology. 2009;54(6):699–712. https://doi.org/10.1111/j.1365–2559.2009.03288.x.
113. Younes M, Ertan A, Ergun G, Verm R, Bridges M, Woods K, et al. Goblet cell mimickers in esophageal biopsies are not associated with an increased risk for dysplasia. Arch Pathol Lab Med. 2007;131(4):571–5. https://doi.org/10.1043/1543-2165(2007)131[571:gcmieb]2.0.co;2.
114. Patil DT, Bennett AE, Mahajan D, Bronner MP. Distinguishing Barrett gastric foveolar dysplasia from reactive cardiac mucosa in gastroesophageal reflux disease. Hum Pathol. 2013;44(6):1146–53. https://doi.org/10.1016/j.humpath.2012.10.004.
115. Sharma P, Weston AP, Morales T, Topalovski M, Mayo MS, Sampliner RE. Relative risk of dysplasia for patients with intestinal metaplasia in the distal oesophagus and in the gastric cardia. Gut. 2000;46(1):9–13.
116. Wani S, Mathur SC, Curvers WL, Singh V, Alvarez Herrero L, Hall SB, et al. Greater interobserver agreement by endoscopic mucosal resection than biopsy samples in Barrett's dysplasia. Clin Gastroenterol Hepatol. 2010;8(9):783–8. https://doi.org/10.1016/j.cgh.2010.04.028.
117. Shaheen NJ, Sharma P, Overholt BF, Wolfsen HC, Sampliner RE, Wang KK, et al. Radiofrequency ablation in Barrett's esophagus with dysplasia. N Engl J Med. 2009;360(22):2277–88. https://doi.org/10.1056/NEJMoa0808145.
118. Milind R, Attwood SE. Natural history of Barrett's esophagus. World J Gastroenterol. 2012;18(27):3483–91. https://doi.org/10.3748/wjg.v18.i27.3483.
119. Jung KW, Talley NJ, Romero Y, Katzka DA, Schleck CD, Zinsmeister AR, et al. Epidemiology and natural history of intestinal metaplasia of the gastroesophageal junction and Barrett's esophagus: a population-based study. Am J Gastroenterol. 2011;106(8):1447–55; quiz 56. https://doi.org/10.1038/ajg.2011.130.
120. Hvid-Jensen F, Pedersen L, Drewes AM, Sorensen HT, Funch-Jensen P. Incidence of adenocarcinoma among patients with Barrett's esophagus. N Engl J Med. 2011;365(15):1375–83. https://doi.org/10.1056/NEJMoa1103042.
121. Desai TK, Krishnan K, Samala N, Singh J, Cluley J, Perla S, et al. The incidence of oesophageal adenocarcinoma in non-dysplastic Barrett's oesophagus: a meta-analysis. Gut. 2012;61(7):970–6. https://doi.org/10.1136/gutjnl-2011–300730.
122. Ma M, Shroff S, Feldman M, DeMarshall M, Price C, Tierney A, et al. Risk of malignant progression in Barrett's esophagus indefinite for dysplasia. Dis Esophagus. 2017;30(3):1–5. https://doi.org/10.1093/dote/dow025.
123. Kestens C, Leenders M, Offerhaus GJ, van Baal JW, Siersema PD. Risk of neoplastic progression in Barrett's esophagus diagnosed as indefinite for dysplasia: a nationwide cohort study. Endoscopy. 2015;47(5):409–14. https://doi.org/10.1055/s-0034–1391091.
124. Singh S, Manickam P, Amin AV, Samala N, Schouten LJ, Iyer PG, et al. Incidence of esophageal adenocarcinoma in Barrett's esophagus with low-grade dysplasia: a systematic review and meta-analysis. Gastrointest Endosc. 2014;79(6):897–909.e4; quiz 83.e1, 83.e3. https://doi.org/10.1016/j.gie.2014.01.009.
125. Wani S, Falk GW, Post J, Yerian L, Hall M, Wang A, et al. Risk factors for progression of low-grade dysplasia in patients with Barrett's esophagus. Gastroenterology. 2011;141(4):1179–86, 86.e1. https://doi.org/10.1053/j.gastro.2011.06.055.
126. Curvers WL, ten Kate FJ, Krishnadath KK, Visser M, Elzer B, Baak LC, et al. Low-grade dysplasia in Barrett's esophagus: overdiagnosed and underestimated. Am J Gastroenterol. 2010;105(7):1523–30. https://doi.org/10.1038/ajg.2010.171.
127. Duits LC, Phoa KN, Curvers WL, Ten Kate FJ, Meijer GA, Seldenrijk CA, et al. Barrett's oesophagus patients with low-grade dysplasia can be accurately risk-stratified after histological review by an expert pathology panel. Gut. 2015;64(5):700–6. https://doi.org/10.1136/gutjnl-2014–307278.
128. Duits LC, van der Wel MJ, Cotton CC, Phoa KN, Ten Kate FJW, Seldenrijk CA, et al. Patients with Barrett's esophagus and confirmed persistent low-grade dysplasia are at increased risk for progression to neoplasia. Gastroenterology. 2017;152(5):993–1001.e1. https://doi.org/10.1053/j.gastro.2016.12.008.
129. Krishnamoorthi R, Lewis JT, Krishna M, Crews NJ, Johnson ML, Dierkhising RA, et al. Predictors of progression in Barrett's esophagus with low-grade dysplasia: results from a multicenter prospective BE registry. Am J Gastroenterol. 2017;112(6):867–73. https://doi.org/10.1038/ajg.2017.84.
130. Rastogi A, Puli S, El-Serag HB, Bansal A, Wani S, Sharma P. Incidence of esophageal adenocarcinoma in patients with Barrett's esophagus and high-grade dysplasia: a meta-analysis. Gastrointest Endosc. 2008;67(3):394–8. https://doi.org/10.1016/j.gie.2007.07.019.
131. Buttar NS, Wang KK, Sebo TJ, Riehle DM, Krishnadath KK, Lutzke LS, et al. Extent of high-grade dysplasia in Barrett's esophagus correlates with risk of adenocarcinoma. Gastroenterology. 2001;120(7):1630–9.

Eosinophilic Esophagitis

4

Thomas C. Smyrk

Introduction

The primary allergy-related eosinophilic conditions affecting the gut are grouped under the rubric "eosinophilic gastrointestinal disease" (EGID). All of the EGIDs depend on three elements for diagnosis: appropriate clinical symptoms, documentation of increased tissue eosinophils, and exclusion of other causes for tissue eosinophils. It should be noted here that because some EGIDs involve only layers of the intestinal wall deep into the mucosa, a negative biopsy in the setting of suspected EGID does not necessarily rule out the diagnosis. Eosinophilic esophagitis (EoE) is about as prevalent as inflammatory bowel disease, at least in the United States, Europe, and Australia, and both its incidence and prevalence are increasing. Histologic criteria for EoE are established and validated. Eosinophilic gastritis, eosinophilic gastroenteritis, and eosinophilic colitis are all rare; histologic criteria have been proposed based on findings derived from case series, but there are no validated criteria.

Eosinophils populate the tubular gut in numbers varying by site. They are rare to absent in the esophagus, sparse in the stomach, and more numerous in the small bowel and colon. Such generalities do not help much when it comes to deciding how many eosinophils are too many. Paying attention to eosinophil distribution can provide useful clues: eosinophils that infiltrate the epithelium or clump together to form mucosal aggregates are abnormal. Eosinophils in the muscularis mucosa or the submucosa are also abnormal.

Biopsies from patients with eosinophilic gastritis, enteritis, or colitis will often be impressively and obviously abnormal, with eosinophils filling the lamina propria in sheets and extending into submucosa. There may be extensive infiltration of gland/crypt epithelium and even gland/crypt abscesses. At some point though, the sense of what is normal or abnormal will depend on the density of the eosinophil infiltrate, usually expressed as eosinophils per high-power field (hpf), and diagnostic criteria will include a numerical cut point. Expert consensus has settled on 15 or more eosinophils/hpf as providing histologic support for EoE, and that cut point has been validated [1]. In the stomach, eosinophil counts of more than 30 in at least five high-power fields or more than 70 in at least three high-power fields have been proposed [2, 3]. In the small bowel, Collins suggests that numbers in excess of twice normal are sufficient to suggest a diagnosis of eosinophilic gastroenteritis; she gives a range of 50–60 eosinophils/hpf as an estimate of twice normal [4]. As eosinophil density in the colon varies by site (decreasing from right to left), proposed diagnostic cut points also vary: 50/hpf in the right colon, 35/hpf in the transverse colon, and 25/hpf in the left colon [5].

Pathologists may be reluctant to mention eosinophils when they seem numerically abnormal but do not form sheets, infiltrate crypts, etc., and there is not an obvious cause for the increase. Turner et al. argue that pathologists should report such increases [5]. This author agrees that a diagnosis of "increased eosinophils in otherwise normal colonic mucosa," for example, may be a helpful clue for the clinicians.

This chapter describes EoE in detail. The other EGIDs are covered in other chapters: sections "Eosinophilic Gastritis" in Chap. 7; "Eosinophilic Duodenitis/Enteritis" in Chap. 10; and "Eosinophilic Colitis" in Chap. 16.

Eosinophilic Esophagitis

Definition

EoE is a chronic inflammatory disease characterized by increased tissue eosinophils and a T-helper type 2 immune response. While eosinophils are necessary for the diagnosis, they are not sufficient; clinicopathologic correlation is

T. C. Smyrk (✉)
Department of Laboratory Medicine and Pathology, Mayo Clinic, Rochester, MN, USA
e-mail: Smyrk.Thomas@mayo.edu

L. Zhang et al. (eds.), *Surgical Pathology of Non-neoplastic Gastrointestinal Diseases*,
https://doi.org/10.1007/978-3-030-15573-5_4

required. The diagnostic criteria are symptoms of esophageal dysfunction, increased tissue eosinophils (at least 15 in at least one hpf), and exclusion of alternative explanations for the eosinophil infiltrate [6].

The first clinical guidelines for EoE included a fourth diagnostic criterion: failure to respond to proton pump inhibitors (PPI) [7]. Over the ensuing decade, it became apparent that some patients with otherwise typical EoE do respond to PPIs [8]. A diagnostic category called PPI-responsive eosinophilic esophagitis was created [9], but patients with PPI-responsive EoE proved to be identical to those with EoE in every way except the PPI response [10]. "Failure to respond to PPIs" has been dropped as a criterion for EoE, and all patients who meet the three existing criteria are considered to be EoE regardless of their clinical response to PPIs [11].

Clinical Features

Epidemiology

EoE has been reported in nearly every part of the world, with sub-Saharan Africa and India being the only exceptions thus far [12]. It affects infants, children, and adults. Adults with EoE are most likely to be diagnosed between the ages of 20 and 50, but the range is very broad [6]. Male patients outnumber females by a ratio of 3:1. Caucasians predominate in the large series reported thus far [13]. A population-based study using medical records of 30,301,440 US patients found that 89.3% of EoE patients were Caucasian, 6.1% African-American, and 5.6% Asian [14]. Small studies from centers with diverse patient populations have challenged the idea that Caucasians predominate. A retrospective chart review of 50 consecutive pediatric patients diagnosed with EoE at the Children's National Medical Center Allergy Clinic in Washington, DC, found that most were nonwhite (42% white, 42% African American, 4% Asian, and 12% others) [15]. It is probably best at this point to say that EoE can affect patients of either sex and any race and that the epidemiologic profile is still evolving.

A 2016 meta-analysis based on 13 pooled studies from Europe, the USA, and Australia calculated an incidence of 3.7/100,000, with incidence rates in individual studies ranging from 0.28 to 19.6/100,000 [16]. The same paper found an overall prevalence of 22.7/100,000, range 2.30–56.30. Not included in the meta-analysis was the US population-based study referenced above, which found a prevalence of 25.9/100,000 [14].

The incidence and prevalence are both increasing, and the increase is independent of confounders such as increased awareness and increased use of endoscopy [17, 18]. The 2016 meta-analysis found an incidence of 7.2/100,000 in studies conducted after 2008, compared to 3.7 for all studies combined [16].

Pathogenesis

EoE is a chronic atopic disease; that is, an allergic condition with a genetic component. Compared to the general population, EoE patients have much higher rates of other atopic diseases, including allergic rhinitis, atopic dermatitis, and asthma. EoE is driven by exposure to food antigens, with milk, egg, wheat, and soy being the most commonly implicated food groups [19]. Aeroallergens (inhaled, then swallowed) probably contribute as well; this may account for the observed seasonal variability in EoE diagnoses [20].

The interaction of allergens with esophageal epithelium in predisposed individuals activates production of cytokines IL-33 and thymic stromal lymphopoietin (TSLP), inducing a cascade of T-helper type 2 inflammation. The resulting increase in cytokines such as IL-4, IL-13, IL-5, and TGF-beta contributes to eosinophil infiltration and damage to the epithelial barrier [21]. The same cytokine stew has been implicated in esophageal fibrosis and altered muscle motility [22].

Predisposing factors may be genetic or epigenetic. Genome-wide association studies have identified several genetic risk loci, one of which is TSLP, encoded in the region of 5q22 [23]. The receptor for TSLP has also been found to have a coding variant, which is associated with EoE risk in men only [23]. There is strong association with risk at 2p23, which encodes a protease called CAPN14 [24]. Variants in this protein, which is produced only in the esophagus, may impair barrier function. Upregulation of CCL26 in EoE, which encodes for the eosinophil attractant eotaxin-3, is under epigenetic control [25].

All of the genes mentioned above belong to a portion of the human genome termed the EoE transcriptome, which is consistently dysregulated in EoE but not in reflux esophagitis [26]. Gene expression profiling focused on this region led to the development of an esophageal diagnostic panel, which utilizes a set of 96 genes expressed in the esophagus to show a characteristic pattern of dysregulation in EoE [27]. The authors reported that the diagnostic panel applied to esophageal biopsies from EoE patients and controls identified EoE patients with 96% sensitivity and 98% specificity.

While EoE clearly has a genetic component, environmental factors seem to play a significant role in disease risk. In a study of twins with EoE, Alexander et al. found 58% concordance in monozygotic twins versus 36% in dizygotic twins and calculated that genetics can explain only 14.5% of increased familial risk [28]. The rapidly increasing incidence and the fact that disease prevalence declines after age 45 or so have suggested to some that an environmental change starting 40–50 years ago contributes to disease development [29, 30]. One idea is that there is a loss of immune tolerance among individuals raised in clean environments; this concept could also explain the higher disease prevalence in developed countries [31]. One component of a "clean" environment is fewer *Helicobacter pylori* infections, and in fact, there does seem to be an inverse association between that infection and EoE [32]. Some early-life events have also been implicated in risk for EoE, including antibiotic use during the first year of life and Cesarean delivery [33, 34]. Risk for EoE is also higher for individuals living in rural rather than urban areas and cold or arid climates as opposed to temperate or tropical zones [35, 36].

EoE is an allergic condition characterized by increased tissue eosinophils, but it seems not to be mediated by IgE [37]. IgE depletion with omalizumab does not alter symptoms or esophageal histology [37, 38]. IgE-specific skin testing has some success in identifying trigger foods in children but is less successful in adults [39, 40]. IgG subclasses, IgA, and IgM are all increased in esophageal tissue of EoE patients, but not IgE [41].

Clayton et al. documented increased tissue IgG4 in EoE patients [37]. Serum IgG4 was approximately twice normal in these patients, but serum IgG4 antibodies reactive to the common trigger foods (wheat, milk, egg, and nuts) were markedly elevated. Others have also documented food-specific IgG4 in EoE [42]. Rosenberg et al. used esophageal tissue from pediatric EoE patients to demonstrate that IgG4 is increased and that the increase correlates with eosinophil numbers [41]. That study also demonstrated that increased tissue IgG4 also correlated with dysregulation of genes in the EoE transcriptome, including those involved in cell adhesion, epithelial barrier, and cytokines [41]. The significance of tissue IgG4 with regard to diagnosis, treatment, and assessment of treatment response has not been elucidated.

Clinical Presentation

The symptoms of EoE vary with the age of the patient. Infants present with failure to thrive, nausea, vomiting, poor feeding, and abdominal pain. Older children are often slow eaters complaining of chest pain or heartburn, while adult symptomatology is dominated by solid food dysphagia, food impaction, and non-swallowing-associated chest pain [6]. These generalizations make the diagnosis sound simple, but it is not; many patients report a long interval between symptom onset and diagnosis, and that delay does not seem to be decreasing despite increased awareness of the condition [43]. Delay in diagnosis increases the likelihood of stricture formation [44].

While 60–100% of adolescents and adults with EoE experience dysphagia, it may be intermittent and of varying intensity. Gradually acquired compensatory behaviors can mean that the patient will note only a history of eating slowly, chewing excessively, using liquids to lubricate each bite, or the necessity for repeated swallows. Dysphagia is an important symptom to elicit because approximately 20% of patients undergoing endoscopy for dysphagia will have EoE [12].

Food bolus impaction means either food sticking for an extended period of time before passing or sticking and requiring endoscopic removal. More than one quarter of adults with EoE have a history of food bolus impaction [45, 46]. Approximately half of all patients undergoing endoscopy for this indication will have EoE [12].

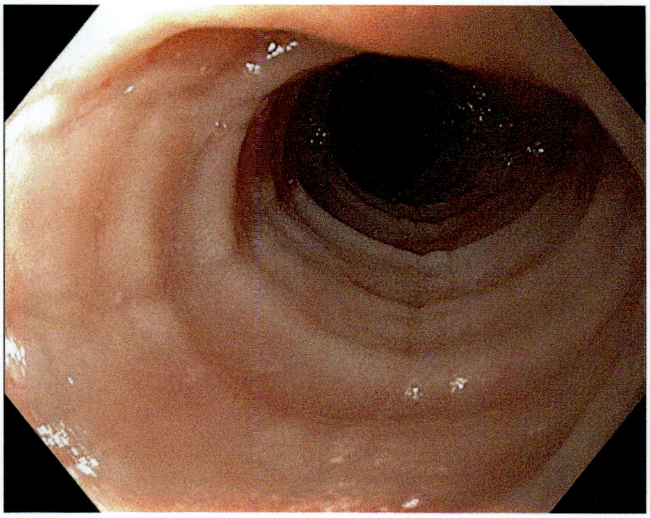

Fig. 4.1 Endoscopic view of the esophagus in eosinophilic esophagitis

Endoscopic Findings

Endoscopy is normal in less than 5% of EoE patients [47]. Edema, linear furrows, and exudates (generally visualized as white specks) are considered to be characteristic inflammatory changes in these patients, while rings and strictures are taken as evidence of fibrosis (Fig. 4.1). A standard scoring system for assessing edema, rings, exudates, furrows, and stricture (EREFS) has been proposed and appears to discriminate between patients with and without EoE [47]. Still, endoscopic findings alone do not establish a diagnosis of EoE [6].

Radiological Findings

The strictures of EoE may be lengthy and tapered. Barium swallow is a useful study in adolescents and adults, as it is much better than endoscopy at detecting these subtle narrowings [48].

Pathological Features

Esophageal biopsies typically have a striking increase in intraepithelial eosinophils (Fig. 4.2). Eosinophils can be found throughout the length of the esophagus, although the distribution is sometimes patchy, particularly after treatment, meaning that diagnostic yield is increased by sampling multiple areas. Updated guidelines advise at least six biopsies, taken from different locations, focusing on areas with endoscopic mucosal abnormalities [6].

How many eosinophils must there be to support a diagnosis of EoE? The first published report of the clinicopathologic disease now known as EoE had 12 patients with a mean of 56 eosinophils/hpf, range 21–110 [49]. Among 90 control patients with a positive 24-hour pH study, 47 had no eosinophils in

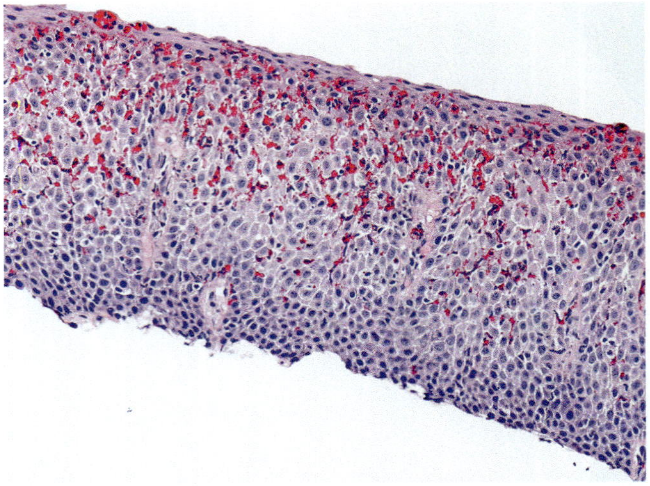

Fig. 4.2 Eosinophilic esophagitis. One does not need to spend too much time counting eosinophils here; they are markedly increased, as is almost always the case in untreated EoE

biopsy tissue and the remaining 43 had few (mean 3.3, range 1–19). While these data suggested 20 eosinophils/hpf as a cut point for separating reflux esophagitis from EoE, the paper did not claim that the two clinical populations could never have overlapping eosinophil counts or that there is a magic number of eosinophils entirely specific for EoE. Subsequent larger studies proposed slightly different cut points as having the best combination of sensitivity and specificity, with suggestions ranging from 10 to 30/hpf. Finally, an expert consensus conference settled on 15 eosinophils/hpf as the histologic criterion which would best support a diagnosis of EoE if other criteria were met [7]. Dellon et al. later found that this cut point gave a sensitivity of 100% and a specificity of 96% for establishing the diagnosis of EoE [1].

As has been noted by many, the area of a hpf varies according to the field number on the microscope eyepieces. If the field number is 20, for example, the area of a hpf (40× objective lens) is 0.196 mm^2. Eyepieces with a field number of 22 have an hpf area of 0.237 mm^2. Ideally, all published studies on EoE histology should either give a field area or report eosinophil counts in a standard unit, such as 1 mm^2. For the practicing surgical pathologist, reporting eosinophils/hpf is acceptable. There are several justifications for this admittedly unscientific opinion: First, the initial consensus recommendations did not specify a field size [7]. Even the most recent guidelines are no more stringent than "15 eosinophils/hpf or approximately 60/mm^2" [50]. Second, eosinophil counts do not correlate with severity of symptoms, nor do they help direct treatment options or predict response to treatment. There is little point in spending time assessing whether a given biopsy has a maximum density of 86 or 93 eosinophils and then spending additional time converting the count to a standard unit. Given current guidelines, it would not be wrong to simply report, as some pathologists do, "greater than 15" in all cases with increased eosinophils; a better option is to provide some sense of maximum density by doing a quick estimation of the maximum density. If the density looks to be near 15/hpf, some careful searching and counting will be necessary, but it should be noted that the 15/hpf threshold is a guideline only—if clinical features strongly suggest EoE and the pathologist reports 12 eosinophils/hpf, EoE will not be eliminated from consideration. As the updated European guidelines note, the 15 eosinophils/hpf threshold is "somewhat arbitrary and clinical judgment is required to interpret the significance of borderline counts" [6]. In support of that statement, there are reports of EoE patients with lower eosinophil density [51] or even no eosinophils at all [52]. Finally, there is a lot more to the histology of EoE than a peak eosinophil count; one should not let an emphasis on a precise eosinophil count detract from a more global assessment of the histology.

In addition to having increased EoE, eosinophils are abnormally distributed. They tend to be situated in the upper half of the epithelium, where they may cluster to form microabscesses (collections of eosinophils that disrupt the normal architecture) (Fig. 4.3). At times, the superficial distribution takes the form of surface layering (a line of eosinophils on the epithelial surface); pronounced layering produces a surface crust (Fig. 4.4). The intraepithelial eosinophils are often

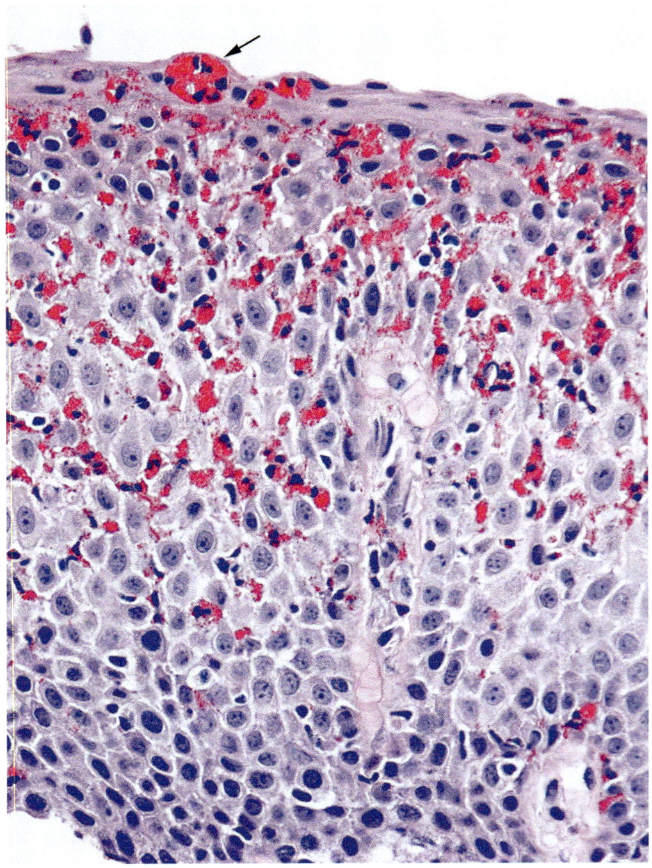

Fig. 4.3 Eosinophilic esophagitis. There is a microabscess (arrow) near the epithelial surface

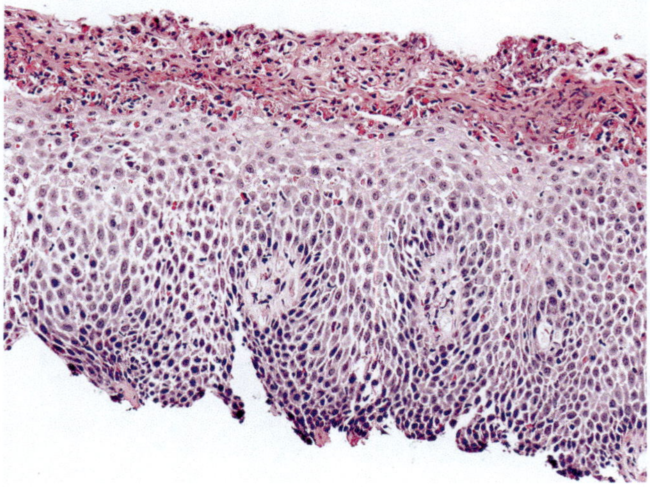

Fig. 4.4 Eosinophilic esophagitis with a surface crust of eosinophils and keratinous debris. This crust is visible endoscopically as a green-white membrane

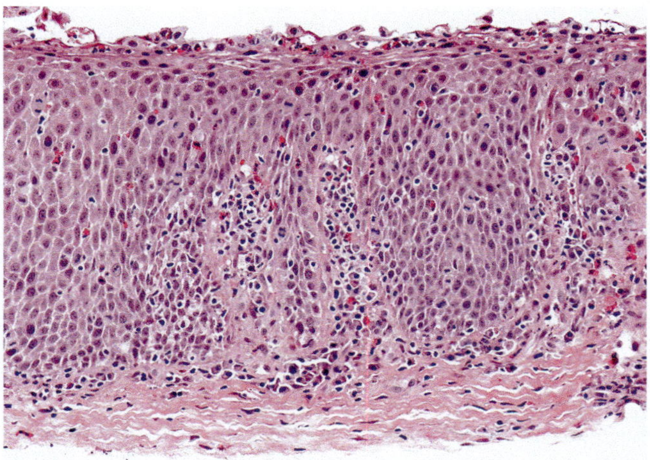

Fig. 4.5 Basal zone hyperplasia, with basal zone occupying 80% of the epithelial thickness. Note occasional eosinophils in the subepithelial papillae and many plasma cells in the lamina propria

degranulated, although it is not clear whether this is a pathologic feature or an artifact of biopsy/processing.

EoE shows signs of epithelial damage in the form of basal zone hyperplasia and dilated intercellular spaces. In the normal esophagus, the basal zone (roughly defined as the region in which epithelial nuclei are closer together than one nuclear diameter) occupies no more than 15% of the epithelial thickness. In EoE, the basal zone expands to fill the majority of the epithelium (Fig. 4.5). Intercellular spaces, not visible in normal esophagus, become dilated, a change also known as spongiosis (Fig. 4.6a). Intercellular bridges are often visible spanning the dilated spaces; at times, the bridges are disrupted and small vacuoles form in the epithelium (Fig. 4.6b, c). These histologic changes correlate with the impaired barrier function that characterizes the pathophysiology of EoE.

When lamina propria is present, it is often fibrotic. It may seem unreasonable to assess fibrosis in this setting, but even with scanty tissue, one can learn to see the difference between the slender, loosely arranged collagen fibers of normal lamina propria and the thick, tightly paced fibers one typically sees in EoE (Fig. 4.7a, b). It should be noted here that eosinophils (and other inflammatory cells) are often present in the lamina propria, but the limited sampling typical of most esophageal biopsies makes that difficult to quantify [53].

Collins et al. have combined all of these features (eosinophil count, eosinophil abscess, surface layering, dilated intercellular spaces, and lamina propria fibrosis) and two others (surface epithelial alteration and dyskeratotic epithelial cells) in an EoE scoring system that aims to provide an objective assessment of EoE histology [54]. All criteria are scored for severity and extent. The authors indicate that the system is easily learned and is reproducible.

While eosinophils are the defining cell in EoE, other cells are involved in the process. As noted above, IgG4 is associated with EoE, and tissue IgG4-positive plasma cells can be identified in most EoE biopsies. IgG4-positive plasma cells congregate in the lamina propria, and there is often granular IgG4 deposited in the dilated spaces of the epithelium (Fig. 4.8). This is a marker of Th2 response and is not specific for EoE; IgG4 has also been documented, for example, in esophageal lichen planus [55]. T-lymphocytes are also increased; they are distributed diffusely, not in a lichenoid pattern (Fig. 4.9a, b). Mast cells are increased as well. Interestingly, they seem to be limited to the epithelium and may persist after treatment reduces the number of epithelial eosinophils (Fig. 4.10) [56, 57]. Basophils, which share a common progenitor with eosinophils, have also been implicated in EoE pathogenesis [58]. Neutrophils are not a feature of uncomplicated EoE; unless there is a superimposed candidiasis, the presence of more than rare neutrophils should prompt a search for a different diagnosis.

Patients undergoing treatment for EoE may be re-biopsied, either because of persistent symptoms or to assess mucosal healing. Here, the pathologist is asked to do a little more than report only whether eosinophils are present or absent. If an infiltrate is present, it is reasonable to describe whether it is diffuse or patchy, perhaps even enumerating the eosinophil density in each tissue fragment. It is also reasonable to report the presence or absence of squamous hyperplasia and dilated intercellular spaces.

Follow-up sampling is often done on a protocol basis in patients undergoing dietary elimination therapy. There is interest in minimally invasive ways of sampling esophageal mucosa in these patients. The cytosponge is a swallowed gelatin capsule attached to a string, which dissolves in the

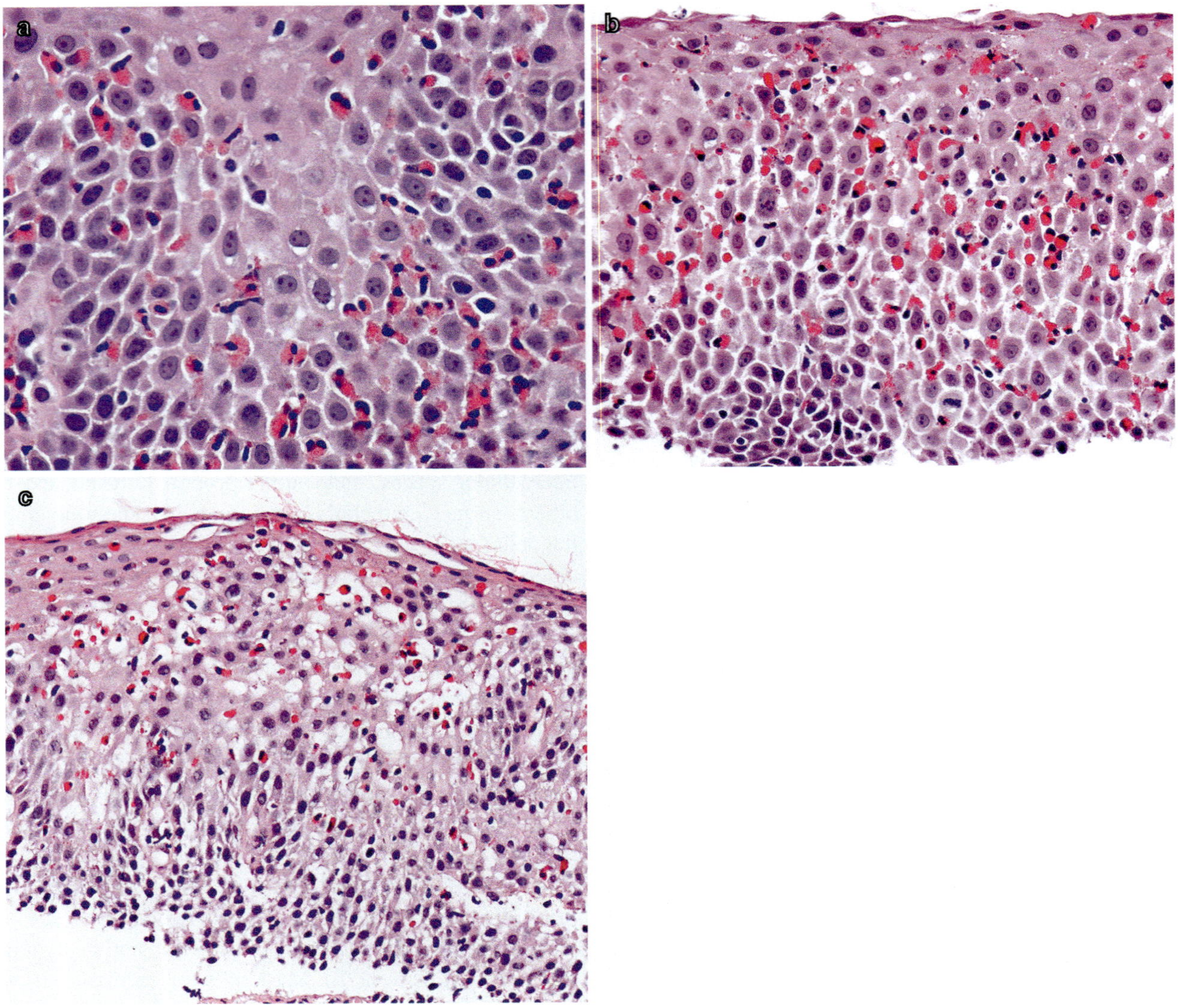

Fig. 4.6 Dilated intercellular spaces of varying severity. (**a**) Intercellular bridges are just visible in dilated intercellular spaces. (**b**) More extensive dilation gives a loose, disorganized look to the epithelium. (**c**) Some intercellular spaces have coalesced, forming vacuoles

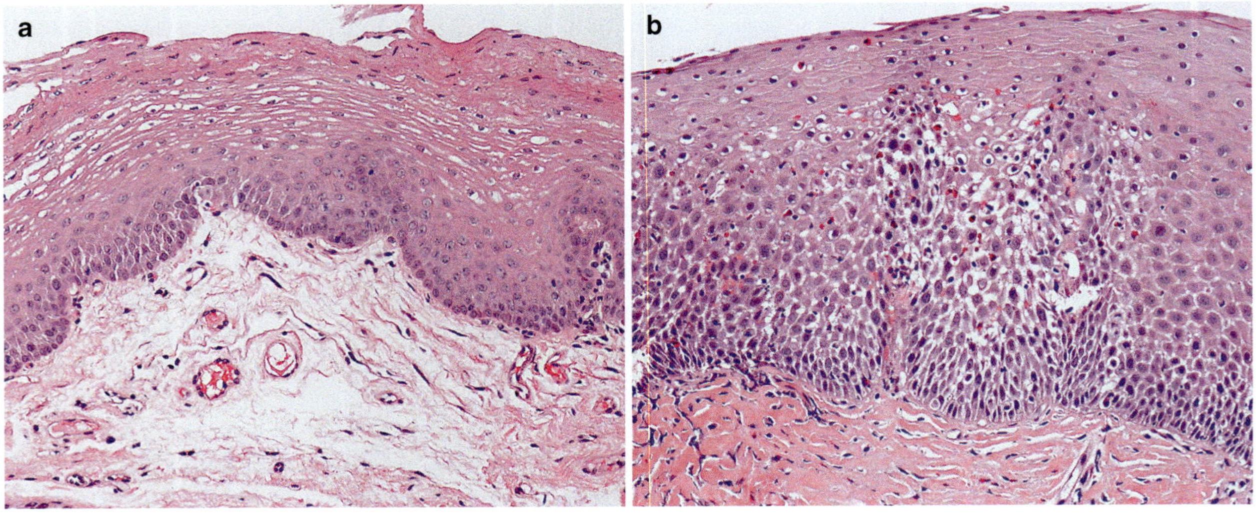

Fig. 4.7 Subepithelial fibrosis. (**a**) The lamina propria of the normal esophagus has a loose collection of slender collagen fibers. (**b**) In EoE, the lamina propria is often more dense, with thick fibers

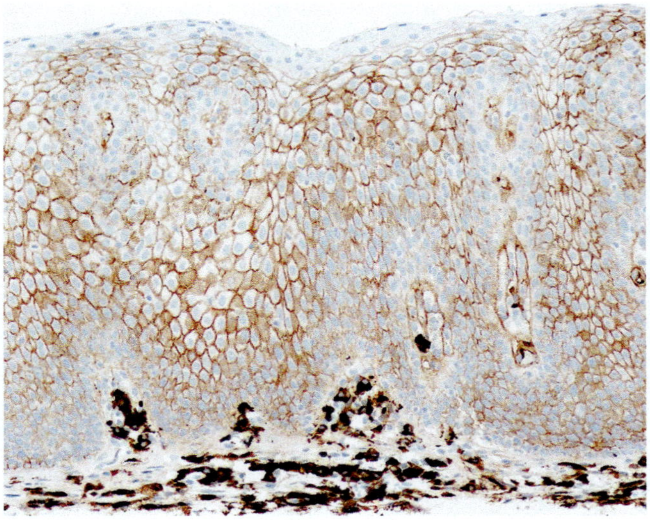

Fig. 4.8 IgG4 in eosinophilic esophagitis (IgG4 immunostain). Subepithelial plasma cells are positive. There is granular IgG4 in the intercellular spaces of the epithelium

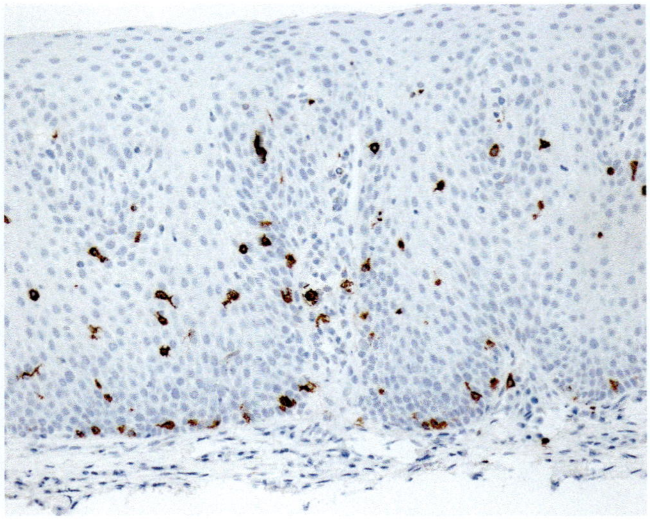

Fig. 4.10 Mast cells in eosinophilic esophagitis (CD117 immunostain). Note that they are confined to the epithelium

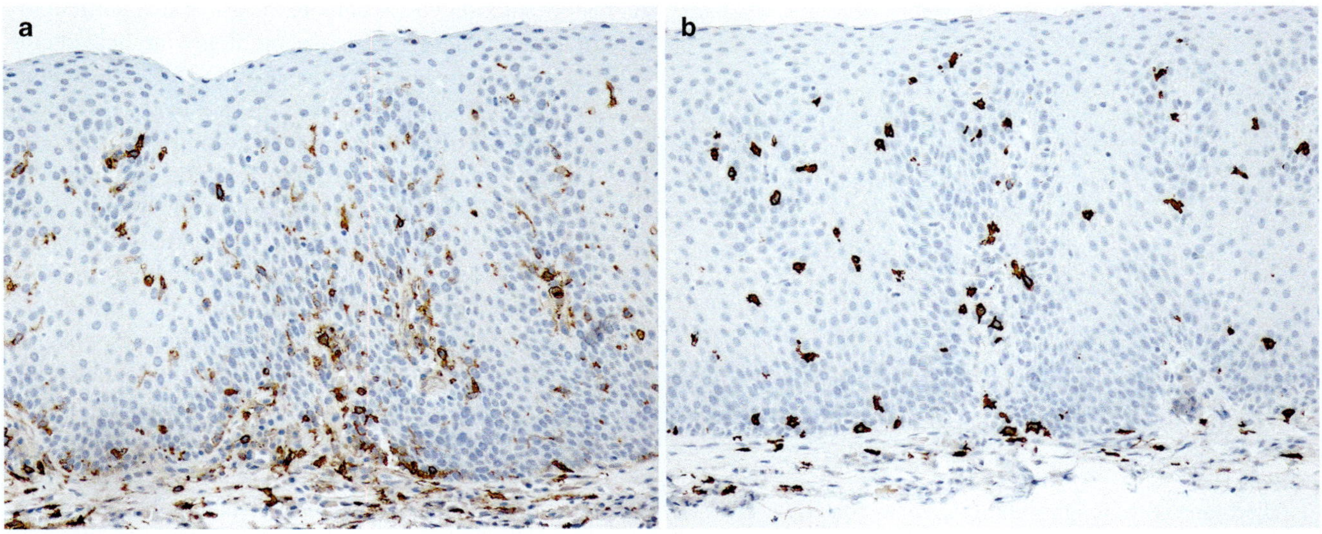

Fig. 4.9 Intraepithelial T cells in eosinophilic esophagitis. (**a**) CD4 immunostain highlights T helper cells. (**b**) CD8 immunostain highlights T suppressor cells

stomach and opens to release a 3 cm diameter mesh sponge. The mesh is withdrawn and submitted for cytology processing [59]. The cell block from retrieved material generally holds 50 or so small tissue fragments comprising superficial esophageal epithelium (Fig. 4.11a). Eosinophils, eosinophil abscesses, surface layering, squamous hyperplasia, and dilated intercellular spaces can all be detected (Fig. 4.11b).

Differential Diagnosis

Table 4.1 lists conditions that can involve the esophagus and can sometimes feature eosinophils. Most of them are unlikely to be confused with EoE. Gastroesophageal reflux disease (GERD) is the primary consideration in the differential diagnosis. The entity formerly known as PPI-responsive EoE deserves special comment here. When it became apparent that PPIs induced resolution in some patients with symptoms and histology typical of EoE, a period of diagnostic nihilism ensued. The consensus was that histology could not differentiate between EoE and GERD and that the only role for the pathologist was to provide a peak eosinophil count. Now that PPI-responsive EoE is no longer viewed as a separate entity, there is a revived role for pathology input into this sometimes difficult differential.

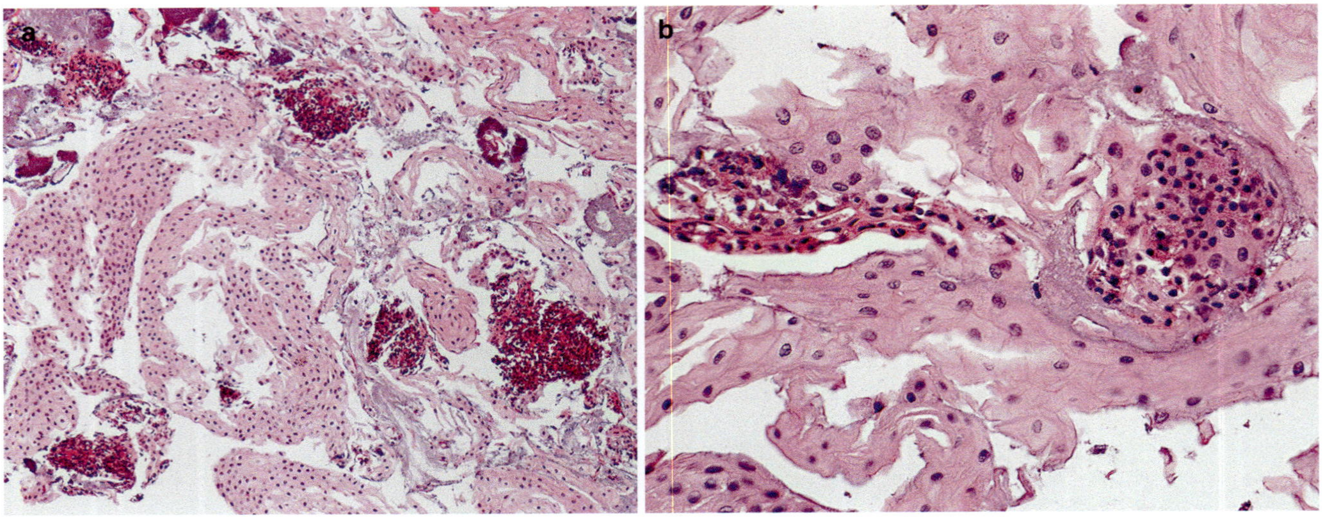

Fig. 4.11 Esophageal sampling via cytosponge. In this example, most of the eosinophils were present as surface crust. (**a**) Multiple collections of eosinophils in a background of normal esophageal epithelium. (**b**) High-power view shows two groups of eosinophils surrounded by the surface esophageal epithelium

Table 4.1 Conditions sometimes affecting the esophagus, which can elicit an eosinophilic response

Gastroesophageal reflux disease
Infection
Connective tissue disease
Crohn's disease
Achalasia
Pill esophagitis
Drug hypersensitivity
Neoplasm, e.g., granular cell tumor
Vasculitis
HIV-related esophageal ulcers
Esophageal involvement by eosinophilic gastroenteritis
Hypereosinophilic syndrome

There are no pathognomonic features for either EoE or GERD, but EoE generally has more eosinophils, more basal hyperplasia, more dilated intercellular spaces, and more subepithelial fibrosis. Because GERD changes tend to be more pronounced in the distal esophagus, biopsies from the mid esophagus reduce the chance of histologic overlap between the two conditions. Neutrophils are often present in reflux esophagitis and should be absent in EoE. IgG4 may prove to be a help in the differential as well, since IgG4 seems not to be present in reflux esophagitis [60, 61]. Adding to the difficulty of the differential diagnosis, some patients have both allergic EoE and acid reflux, with the latter possibly contributing to barrier dysfunction.

The commonly encountered fungal and viral infections of the esophagus usually have no or few eosinophils. Helminthic infections, well known to produce eosinophil infiltrations in the stomach, small bowel, and colon, rarely involve the esophagus, schistosomiasis being one possible exception. Connective tissue disease is a rare cause of increased mucosal eosinophils in the gut and is particularly rare in the esophagus. The most commonly implicated conditions are systemic lupus erythematosus (35%) and rheumatoid arthritis (20%) [62]. Crohn's disease of the esophagus is also a relatively rare diagnosis; neutrophils, lymphocytes, and granulomas usually predominate. The epithelium in achalasia is thickened, but the basal zone is not thickened as dramatically as in EoE, and the mixed inflammation that one can see in achalasia is dominated by lymphocytes and neutrophils. Pill injury may produce erosions or ulcers with a few eosinophils in the ulcer base. Sloughing esophagitis, another common pattern of drug injury, does not feature eosinophils. Drug hypersensitivity, in contrast, can involve any part of the gut; clinical history will be required to support this diagnosis. Granular cell tumor is notorious for inducing pseudoepitheliomatous squamous hyperplasia, but eosinophils can sometimes be part of the reactive process as well. The eosinophilic vasculitis of Churg-Strauss syndrome is reported to involve the gut in 30% of affected patients [63]. The idiopathic esophageal ulcers that can affect patients with HIV often have a significant eosinophil component. Approximately 20% of patients with eosinophilic gastroenteritis will have more than 15 eosinophils/hpf in the esophagus [64]. Hypereosinophilic syndrome is a systemic illness (defined as peripheral eosinophil counts of greater than 1500/μl for greater than 1 month, without other identifiable cause) which could be confused with EoE in an esophageal biopsy.

Treatment and Prognosis

EoE is a chronic disease. If untreated, symptoms and inflammation will likely persist, leading to stricture formation [65].

The goals of treatment are to control esophageal eosinophilia, control symptoms, and prevent or reverse esophageal fibrosis. Treatment options include PPIs, topical corticosteroids, and dietary modification. Dilation can be used to improve dysphagia in adults with esophageal stricture or narrowing [66].

PPIs, topical steroids, and elimination diet can all be offered as first-line therapy; the choice should be individualized for each patient. Each therapy can be used interchangeably over time. A typical treatment protocol might start with PPIs, using twice the standard dose for reflux.

Approximately 50% of EoE patients will have improvements in symptoms and inflammation on PPIs [8]. The reasons for this are not entirely clear; it may be that control of gastric acid helps protect barrier function. PPIs also block STAT6 activation and IL-13 activation and may have an antieosinophilic effect [67, 68]. In PPI responders, long-term therapy may maintain remission, although the recent European consensus guidelines for EoE characterized the evidence for this as "low" [6]. For those not responding to PPIs, either topical steroids or elimination diet would be a reasonable option. There is strong evidence that topical steroids induce histologic remission and that long-term therapy can maintain therapy in a subset of patients. Approximately 10% of those treated with topical steroids develop esophageal candidiasis.

Various dietary elimination protocols have been applied to patients with EoE. Spergel et al. analyzed 11 studies (some children and some adults; 702 patients in total) and listed the food groups most often implicated in EoE as: milk (66%), egg (24%), wheat (27%), peanuts/tree nuts (4%), soy/legumes (12%), and fish/shellfish (2%) [19]. Some patients react to more than one food group, and that sensitivity may have a genotype correlation; Fahey et al. found that individuals carrying the risk allele for TSLP variants were more likely to have three or more EoE food triggers [69]. The six-food elimination diet begins with eliminating all of these food groups and, assuming symptoms improve, reinstating the groups one-by-one over a multiweek period. A 2014 meta-analysis of seven studies evaluating this approach found 72.1% efficiency in producing histologic remission [70]. Four-group and two-group plans have also been assessed and found to be helpful in some patients. An elemental diet should only be considered after other treatment options have failed [6].

With insights into the pathophysiology of EoE, molecular therapies may become useful. Anti-IgE therapy (omalizumab) has not proved useful in EoE. Therapies directed against IL-5 (mepolizumab, reslizumab) have been equivocal [71, 72]. Biological therapies targeting IL-13, CRTH2, TSLP, eotaxin, and TGF-beta1 are also being trialed. See Weschler et al. for a 2018 update of this rapidly evolving field [73].

References

1. Dellon ES, Speck O, Woodward K, Covey S, Rusin S, Shaheen NJ, et al. Distribution and variability of esophageal eosinophilia in patients undergoing upper endoscopy. Mod Pathol. 2015;28(3):383–90. https://doi.org/10.1038/modpathol.2014.110.
2. Lwin T, Melton SD, Genta RM. Eosinophilic gastritis: histopathological characterization and quantification of the normal gastric eosinophil content. Mod Pathol. 2011;24(4):556–63. https://doi.org/10.1038/modpathol.2010.221.
3. Ko HM, Morotti RA, Yershov O, Chehade M. Eosinophilic gastritis in children: clinicopathological correlation, disease course, and response to therapy. Am J Gastroenterol. 2014;109(8):1277–85. https://doi.org/10.1038/ajg.2014.166.
4. Collins MH. Histopathologic features of eosinophilic esophagitis and eosinophilic gastrointestinal diseases. Gastroenterol Clin N Am. 2014;43(2):257–68. https://doi.org/10.1016/j.gtc.2014.02.007.
5. Turner KO, Sinkre RA, Neumann WL, Genta RM. Primary colonic eosinophilia and eosinophilic colitis in adults. Am J Surg Pathol. 2017;41(2):225–33. https://doi.org/10.1097/PAS.0000000000000760.
6. Lucendo AJ, Molina-Infante J, Arias A, von Arnim U, Bredenoord AJ, Bussmann C, et al. Guidelines on eosinophilic esophagitis: evidence-based statements and recommendations for diagnosis and management in children and adults. United European Gastroenterol J. 2017;5(3):335–58. https://doi.org/10.1177/2050640616689525.
7. Furuta GT, Liacouras CA, Collins MH, Gupta SK, Justinich C, Putnam PE, et al. Eosinophilic esophagitis in children and adults: a systematic review and consensus recommendations for diagnosis and treatment. Gastroenterology. 2007;133(4):1342–63. https://doi.org/10.1053/j.gastro.2007.08.017.
8. Lucendo AJ, Arias A, Molina-Infante J. Efficacy of proton pump inhibitor drugs for inducing clinical and histologic remission in patients with symptomatic esophageal eosinophilia: a systematic review and meta-analysis. Clin Gastroenterol Hepatol. 2016;14(1):13–22.e1. https://doi.org/10.1016/j.cgh.2015.07.041.
9. Liacouras CA, Furuta GT, Hirano I, Atkins D, Attwood SE, Bonis PA, et al. Eosinophilic esophagitis: updated consensus recommendations for children and adults. J Allergy Clin Immunol. 2011;128(1):3–20.e6; quiz 1–2. https://doi.org/10.1016/j.jaci.2011.02.040.
10. Molina-Infante J, Bredenoord AJ, Cheng E, Dellon ES, Furuta GT, Gupta SK, et al. Proton pump inhibitor-responsive oesophageal eosinophilia: an entity challenging current diagnostic criteria for eosinophilic oesophagitis. Gut. 2016;65(3):524–31. https://doi.org/10.1136/gutjnl-2015-310991.
11. Dellon ES, Liacouras CA, Molina-Infante J, Furuta GT, Spergel JM, Zevit N, et al. Updated international consensus diagnostic criteria for eosinophilic esophagitis: proceedings of the AGREE conference. Gastroenterology. 2018;155(4):1022–33.e10. https://doi.org/10.1053/j.gastro.2018.07.009.
12. Dellon ES, Hirano I. Epidemiology and natural history of eosinophilic esophagitis. Gastroenterology. 2018;154(2):319–32.e3. https://doi.org/10.1053/j.gastro.2017.06.067.
13. Dellon ES. Epidemiology of eosinophilic esophagitis. Gastroenterol Clin N Am. 2014;43(2):201–18. https://doi.org/10.1016/j.gtc.2014.02.002.
14. Mansoor E, Cooper GS. The 2010–2015 prevalence of eosinophilic esophagitis in the USA: a population-based study. Dig Dis Sci. 2016;61(10):2928–34. https://doi.org/10.1007/s10620-016-4204-4.
15. Weiler T, Mikhail I, Singal A, Sharma H. Racial differences in the clinical presentation of pediatric eosinophilic esophagitis. J Allergy Clin Immunol Pract. 2014;2(3):320–5. https://doi.org/10.1016/j.jaip.2014.01.011.

16. Arias A, Perez-Martinez I, Tenias JM, Lucendo AJ. Systematic review with meta-analysis: the incidence and prevalence of eosinophilic oesophagitis in children and adults in population-based studies. Aliment Pharmacol Ther. 2016;43(1):3–15. https://doi.org/10.1111/apt.13441.
17. Prasad GA, Alexander JA, Schleck CD, Zinsmeister AR, Smyrk TC, Elias RM, et al. Epidemiology of eosinophilic esophagitis over three decades in Olmsted County, Minnesota. Clin Gastroenterol Hepatol. 2009;7(10):1055–61. https://doi.org/10.1016/j.cgh.2009.06.023.
18. Hruz P, Straumann A, Bussmann C, Heer P, Simon HU, Zwahlen M, et al. Escalating incidence of eosinophilic esophagitis: a 20-year prospective, population-based study in Olten County, Switzerland. J Allergy Clin Immunol. 2011;128(6):1349–50.e5. https://doi.org/10.1016/j.jaci.2011.09.013.
19. Spergel J, Aceves SS. Allergic components of eosinophilic esophagitis. J Allergy Clin Immunol. 2018;142(1):1–8. https://doi.org/10.1016/j.jaci.2018.05.001.
20. Reed CC, Iglesia EGA, Commins SP, Dellon ES. Seasonal exacerbation of eosinophilic esophagitis histologic activity in adults and children implicates role of aeroallergens. Ann Allergy Asthma Immunol. 2019;122:296–301. https://doi.org/10.1016/j.anai.2018.12.013.
21. O'Shea KM, Aceves SS, Dellon ES, Gupta SK, Spergel JM, Furuta GT, et al. Pathophysiology of eosinophilic esophagitis. Gastroenterology. 2018;154(2):333–45. https://doi.org/10.1053/j.gastro.2017.06.065.
22. Rieder F, Nonevski I, Ma J, Ouyang Z, West G, Protheroe C, et al. T-helper 2 cytokines, transforming growth factor beta1, and eosinophil products induce fibrogenesis and alter muscle motility in patients with eosinophilic esophagitis. Gastroenterology. 2014;146(5):1266–77.e1–9. https://doi.org/10.1053/j.gastro.2014.01.051.
23. Sherrill JD, Gao PS, Stucke EM, Blanchard C, Collins MH, Putnam PE, et al. Variants of thymic stromal lymphopoietin and its receptor associate with eosinophilic esophagitis. J Allergy Clin Immunol. 2010;126(1):160–5.e3. https://doi.org/10.1016/j.jaci.2010.04.037.
24. Kottyan LC, Davis BP, Sherrill JD, Liu K, Rochman M, Kaufman K, et al. Genome-wide association analysis of eosinophilic esophagitis provides insight into the tissue specificity of this allergic disease. Nat Genet. 2014;46(8):895–900. https://doi.org/10.1038/ng.3033.
25. Lim EJ, Lu TX, Blanchard C, Rothenberg ME. Epigenetic regulation of the IL-13-induced human eotaxin-3 gene by CREB-binding protein-mediated histone 3 acetylation. J Biol Chem. 2011;286(15):13193–204. https://doi.org/10.1074/jbc.M110.210724.
26. Blanchard C, Wang N, Stringer KF, Mishra A, Fulkerson PC, Abonia JP, et al. Eotaxin-3 and a uniquely conserved gene-expression profile in eosinophilic esophagitis. J Clin Invest. 2006;116(2):536–47. https://doi.org/10.1172/JCI26679.
27. Wen T, Stucke EM, Grotjan TM, Kemme KA, Abonia JP, Putnam PE, et al. Molecular diagnosis of eosinophilic esophagitis by gene expression profiling. Gastroenterology. 2013;145(6):1289–99. https://doi.org/10.1053/j.gastro.2013.08.046.
28. Alexander ES, Martin LJ, Collins MH, Kottyan LC, Sucharew H, He H, et al. Twin and family studies reveal strong environmental and weaker genetic cues explaining heritability of eosinophilic esophagitis. J Allergy Clin Immunol. 2014;134(5):1084–92 e1. https://doi.org/10.1016/j.jaci.2014.07.021.
29. van Rhijn BD, Verheij J, Smout AJ, Bredenoord AJ. Rapidly increasing incidence of eosinophilic esophagitis in a large cohort. Neurogastroenterol Motil. 2013;25(1):47–52 e5. https://doi.org/10.1111/nmo.12009.
30. Dellon ES, Jensen ET, Martin CF, Shaheen NJ, Kappelman MD. Prevalence of eosinophilic esophagitis in the United States. Clin Gastroenterol Hepatol. 2014;12(4):589–96.e1. https://doi.org/10.1016/j.cgh.2013.09.008.
31. Garcia-Compean D, Gonzalez-Gonzalez JA, Gonzalez-Moreno EI, Maldonado-Garza HJ. Eosinophilic esophagitis. The north against the south? A bio-economic-social mechanistic approach and clinical implications. Rev Gastroenterol Mex. 2017;82(4):328–36. https://doi.org/10.1016/j.rgmx.2017.02.007.
32. Dellon ES, Peery AF, Shaheen NJ, Morgan DR, Hurrell JM, Lash RH, et al. Inverse association of esophageal eosinophilia with Helicobacter pylori based on analysis of a US pathology database. Gastroenterology. 2011;141(5):1586–92. https://doi.org/10.1053/j.gastro.2011.06.081.
33. Jensen ET, Kappelman MD, Kim HP, Ringel-Kulka T, Dellon ES. Early life exposures as risk factors for pediatric eosinophilic esophagitis. J Pediatr Gastroenterol Nutr. 2013;57(1):67–71. https://doi.org/10.1097/MPG.0b013e318290d15a.
34. Jensen ET, Bertelsen RJ. Assessing early life factors for eosinophilic esophagitis: lessons from other allergic diseases. Curr Treat Options Gastroenterol. 2016;14(1):39–50. https://doi.org/10.1007/s11938-016-0083-1.
35. Hurrell JM, Genta RM, Dellon ES. Prevalence of esophageal eosinophilia varies by climate zone in the United States. Am J Gastroenterol. 2012;107(5):698–706. https://doi.org/10.1038/ajg.2012.6.
36. Jensen ET, Hoffman K, Shaheen NJ, Genta RM, Dellon ES. Esophageal eosinophilia is increased in rural areas with low population density: results from a national pathology database. Am J Gastroenterol. 2014;109(5):668–75. https://doi.org/10.1038/ajg.2014.47.
37. Clayton F, Fang JC, Gleich GJ, Lucendo AJ, Olalla JM, Vinson LA, et al. Eosinophilic esophagitis in adults is associated with IgG4 and not mediated by IgE. Gastroenterology. 2014;147(3):602–9. https://doi.org/10.1053/j.gastro.2014.05.036.
38. Rocha R, Vitor AB, Trindade E, Lima R, Tavares M, Lopes J, et al. Omalizumab in the treatment of eosinophilic esophagitis and food allergy. Eur J Pediatr. 2011;170(11):1471–4. https://doi.org/10.1007/s00431-011-1540-4.
39. Lucendo AJ, Arias A, Gonzalez-Cervera J, Yague-Compadre JL, Guagnozzi D, Angueira T, et al. Empiric 6-food elimination diet induced and maintained prolonged remission in patients with adult eosinophilic esophagitis: a prospective study on the food cause of the disease. J Allergy Clin Immunol. 2013;131(3):797–804. https://doi.org/10.1016/j.jaci.2012.12.664.
40. Philpott H, Nandurkar S, Royce SG, Thien F, Gibson PR. Allergy tests do not predict food triggers in adult patients with eosinophilic oesophagitis. A comprehensive prospective study using five modalities. Aliment Pharmacol Ther. 2016;44(3):223–33. https://doi.org/10.1111/apt.13676.
41. Rosenberg CE, Mingler MK, Caldwell JM, Collins MH, Fulkerson PC, Morris DW, et al. Esophageal IgG4 levels correlate with histopathologic and transcriptomic features in eosinophilic esophagitis. Allergy. 2018;73(9):1892–901. https://doi.org/10.1111/all.13486.
42. Wright BL, Kulis M, Guo R, Orgel KA, Wolf WA, Burks AW, et al. Food-specific IgG4 is associated with eosinophilic esophagitis. J Allergy Clin Immunol. 2016;138(4):1190–2 e3. https://doi.org/10.1016/j.jaci.2016.02.024.
43. Reed CC, Koutlas NT, Robey BS, Hansen J, Dellon ES. Prolonged time to diagnosis of eosinophilic esophagitis despite increasing knowledge of the disease. Clin Gastroenterol Hepatol. 2018;16(10):1667–9. https://doi.org/10.1016/j.cgh.2018.01.028.
44. Schoepfer AM, Safroneeva E, Bussmann C, Kuchen T, Portmann S, Simon HU, et al. Delay in diagnosis of eosinophilic esophagitis increases risk for stricture formation in a time-dependent manner. Gastroenterology. 2013;145(6):1230–6 e1–2. https://doi.org/10.1053/j.gastro.2013.08.015.

45. Sperry SL, Crockett SD, Miller CB, Shaheen NJ, Dellon ES. Esophageal foreign-body impactions: epidemiology, time trends, and the impact of the increasing prevalence of eosinophilic esophagitis. Gastrointest Endosc. 2011;74(5):985–91. https://doi.org/10.1016/j.gie.2011.06.029.
46. Hiremath GS, Hameed F, Pacheco A, Olive A, Davis CM, Shulman RJ. Esophageal food impaction and eosinophilic esophagitis: a retrospective study, systematic review, and meta-analysis. Dig Dis Sci. 2015;60(11):3181–93. https://doi.org/10.1007/s10620-015-3723-8.
47. Hirano I, Moy N, Heckman MG, Thomas CS, Gonsalves N, Achem SR. Endoscopic assessment of the oesophageal features of eosinophilic oesophagitis: validation of a novel classification and grading system. Gut. 2013;62(4):489–95. https://doi.org/10.1136/gutjnl-2011-301817.
48. Podboy A, Katzka DA, Enders F, Larson JJ, Geno D, Kryzer L, et al. Oesophageal narrowing on barium oesophagram is more common in adult patients with eosinophilic oesophagitis than PPI-responsive oesophageal eosinophilia. Aliment Pharmacol Ther. 2016;43(11):1168–77. https://doi.org/10.1111/apt.13601.
49. Attwood SE, Smyrk TC, Demeester TR, Jones JB. Esophageal eosinophilia with dysphagia. A distinct clinicopathologic syndrome. Dig Dis Sci. 1993;38(1):109–16.
50. Spergel JM, Dellon ES, Liacouras CA, Hirano I, Molina-Infante J, Bredenoord AJ, et al. Summary of the updated international consensus diagnostic criteria for eosinophilic esophagitis: AGREE conference. Ann Allergy Asthma Immunol. 2018;121(3):281–4. https://doi.org/10.1016/j.anai.2018.05.035.
51. Ravi K, Talley NJ, Smyrk TC, Katzka DA, Kryzer L, Romero Y, et al. Low grade esophageal eosinophilia in adults: an unrecognized part of the spectrum of eosinophilic esophagitis? Dig Dis Sci. 2011;56(7):1981–6. https://doi.org/10.1007/s10620-011-1594-1.
52. Straumann A, Blanchard C, Radonjic-Hoesli S, Bussmann C, Hruz P, Safroneeva E, et al. A new eosinophilic esophagitis (EoE)-like disease without tissue eosinophilia found in EoE families. Allergy. 2016;71(6):889–900. https://doi.org/10.1111/all.12879.
53. Schoepfer AM, Simko A, Bussmann C, Safroneeva E, Zwahlen M, Greuter T, et al. Eosinophilic esophagitis: relationship of subepithelial eosinophilic inflammation with epithelial histology, endoscopy, blood eosinophils, and symptoms. Am J Gastroenterol. 2018;113(3):348–57. https://doi.org/10.1038/ajg.2017.493.
54. Collins MH, Martin LJ, Alexander ES, Boyd JT, Sheridan R, He H, et al. Newly developed and validated eosinophilic esophagitis histology scoring system and evidence that it outperforms peak eosinophil count for disease diagnosis and monitoring. Dis Esophagus. 2017;30(3):1–8. https://doi.org/10.1111/dote.12470.
55. Podboy AJ, Alexander JA, Smyrk TC, Halland M, Ravi K, Geno DM, et al. Occurrence of IgG4 in esophageal lichen planus. Clin Gastroenterol Hepatol. 2017;15(12):1975–7. https://doi.org/10.1016/j.cgh.2017.06.008.
56. Tappata M, Eluri S, Perjar I, Hollyfield J, Betancourt R, Randall C, et al. Association of mast cells with clinical, endoscopic, and histologic findings in adults with eosinophilic esophagitis. Allergy. 2018;73(10):2088–92. https://doi.org/10.1111/all.13530.
57. Strasser DS, Seger S, Bussmann C, Pierlot GM, Groenen PMA, Stalder AK, et al. Eosinophilic oesophagitis: relevance of mast cell infiltration. Histopathology. 2018;73(3):454–63. https://doi.org/10.1111/his.13653.
58. Noti M, Wojno ED, Kim BS, Siracusa MC, Giacomin PR, Nair MG, et al. Thymic stromal lymphopoietin-elicited basophil responses promote eosinophilic esophagitis. Nat Med. 2013;19(8):1005–13. https://doi.org/10.1038/nm.3281.
59. Katzka DA, Smyrk TC, Alexander JA, Geno DM, Beitia RA, Chang AO, et al. Accuracy and safety of the cytosponge for assessing histologic activity in eosinophilic esophagitis: a two-center study. Am J Gastroenterol. 2017;112(10):1538–44. https://doi.org/10.1038/ajg.2017.244.
60. Zukerberg L, Mahadevan K, Selig M, Deshpande V. Oesophageal intrasquamous IgG4 deposits: an adjunctive marker to distinguish eosinophilic oesophagitis from reflux oesophagitis. Histopathology. 2016;68(7):968–76. https://doi.org/10.1111/his.12892.
61. Pope AE, Stanzione N, Naini BV, Garcia-Lloret M, Ghassemi KA, Marcus EA, et al. Esophageal IgG4: clinical, endoscopic, and histologic correlations in eosinophilic esophagitis. J Pediatr Gastroenterol Nutr. 2018:1. https://doi.org/10.1097/MPG.0000000000002227.
62. Lecouffe-Desprets M, Groh M, Bour B, Le Jeunne C, Puechal X. Eosinophilic gastrointestinal disorders associated with autoimmune connective tissue disease. Joint Bone Spine. 2016;83(5):479–84. https://doi.org/10.1016/j.jbspin.2015.11.006.
63. Baldini C, Talarico R, Della Rossa A, Bombardieri S. Clinical manifestations and treatment of Churg-Strauss syndrome. Rheum Dis Clin N Am. 2010;36(3):527–43. https://doi.org/10.1016/j.rdc.2010.05.003.
64. Prussin C. Eosinophilic gastroenteritis and related eosinophilic disorders. Gastroenterol Clin N Am. 2014;43(2):317–27. https://doi.org/10.1016/j.gtc.2014.02.013.
65. Dellon ES, Kim HP, Sperry SL, Rybnicek DA, Woosley JT, Shaheen NJ. A phenotypic analysis shows that eosinophilic esophagitis is a progressive fibrostenotic disease. Gastrointest Endosc. 2014;79(4):577–85.e4. https://doi.org/10.1016/j.gie.2013.10.027.
66. Schoepfer AM, Gonsalves N, Bussmann C, Conus S, Simon HU, Straumann A, et al. Esophageal dilation in eosinophilic esophagitis: effectiveness, safety, and impact on the underlying inflammation. Am J Gastroenterol. 2010;105(5):1062–70. https://doi.org/10.1038/ajg.2009.657.
67. Rothenberg ME. Molecular, genetic, and cellular bases for treating eosinophilic esophagitis. Gastroenterology. 2015;148(6):1143–57. https://doi.org/10.1053/j.gastro.2015.02.002.
68. Zhang X, Cheng E, Huo X, Yu C, Zhang Q, Pham TH, et al. Omeprazole blocks STAT6 binding to the eotaxin-3 promoter in eosinophilic esophagitis cells. PLoS One. 2012;7(11):e50037. https://doi.org/10.1371/journal.pone.0050037.
69. Fahey LM, Chandramouleeswaran PM, Guan S, Benitez AJ, Furuta GT, Aceves SS, et al. Food allergen triggers are increased in children with the TSLP risk allele and eosinophilic esophagitis. Clin Transl Gastroenterol. 2018;9(3):139. https://doi.org/10.1038/s41424-018-0003-x.
70. Arias A, Gonzalez-Cervera J, Tenias JM, Lucendo AJ. Efficacy of dietary interventions for inducing histologic remission in patients with eosinophilic esophagitis: a systematic review and meta-analysis. Gastroenterology. 2014;146(7):1639–48. https://doi.org/10.1053/j.gastro.2014.02.006.
71. Stein ML, Collins MH, Villanueva JM, Kushner JP, Putnam PE, Buckmeier BK, et al. Anti-IL-5 (mepolizumab) therapy for eosinophilic esophagitis. J Allergy Clin Immunol. 2006;118(6):1312–9. https://doi.org/10.1016/j.jaci.2006.09.007.
72. Spergel JM, Rothenberg ME, Collins MH, Furuta GT, Markowitz JE, Fuchs G 3rd, et al. Reslizumab in children and adolescents with eosinophilic esophagitis: results of a double-blind, randomized, placebo-controlled trial. J Allergy Clin Immunol. 2012;129(2):456–63, 63.e1–3. https://doi.org/10.1016/j.jaci.2011.11.044.
73. Wechsler JB, Hirano I. Biological therapies for eosinophilic gastrointestinal diseases. J Allergy Clin Immunol. 2018;142(1):24–31.e2. https://doi.org/10.1016/j.jaci.2018.05.018.

Drug-induced Injury, Infections, and Congenital and Miscellaneous Disorders

5

Taofic Mounajjed

Drug-Induced Injury

Pill-induced Esophagitis

Definition

Pill-induced esophagitis is a type of esophageal mucosal damage caused by the direct injurious effect of certain medications on the mucosal lining.

Clinical Features

Pills, including capsules and tablets, can cause esophageal injury by direct contact with the mucosa. Most pills causing injury are large in size [1–7], and women and the elderly are most commonly affected [8, 9]. Iron deposition in the upper gastrointestinal tract is common in patients taking iron tablets and is frequently associated with mucosal disruption in the esophagus, manifesting as erosions [10]. Patients most often present with retrosternal pain, dysphagia, and odynophagia. In most cases, the pill intake occurs before sleep and is accompanied by minimal or no fluid intake. Medications that most frequently cause injury include antibiotics (most commonly tetracycline and clindamycin), iron supplements (see below), nonsteroidal anti-inflammatory drugs (NSAIDs), bisphosphonates, potassium chloride, quinidine, and ascorbic acid [1, 2, 8]. Although esophageal motility is most often normal, some patients have had history of external esophageal compression (such as due to cardiac enlargement), or esophageal entrapment by fixed mediastinal structures and adhesions after thoracic surgery [4].

Gross Findings

Grossly, pill-induced esophagitis manifests in mucosal ulcerations surrounded by normal or near-normal esophageal mucosa. The ulcers are most frequently found in the proximal esophagus, at the junction of the middle and proximal tthirds of the esophagus; this part of the esophagus is externally compressed by the aortic arch. The ulcers vary in depth but often extend deep into the esophageal muscularis mucosae. Occasionally, severe cases can cause very deep ulcerations, resulting in esophageal perforation.

Microscopic Findings

Histologically, the findings are nonspecific; they include esophageal epithelial hyperplasia, spongiosis, and infiltration of the epithelium by inflammatory cells, with a prominent eosinophilic component, epithelial necrosis, and ulceration (Fig. 5.1). In the case of alendronate-induced injury, a polarizable crystalline material may be seen [1]. In iron pill-induced esophagitis, a brown granular material (Fig. 5.2a) can sometimes be identified overlying the eroded epithelium, in ulcer/erosion beds, in the superficial layers of the squamous epithelium, and sometimes in the lamina propria [11]. Perls' iron staining (Fig. 5.2b) confirms that this material represents iron.

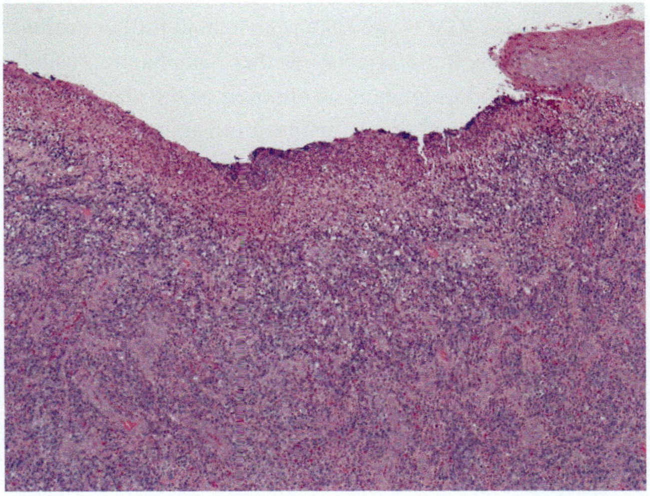

Fig. 5.1 Ulcerative pill-induced esophagitis. The histologic findings of pill-induced esophagitis are nonspecific; they often include mucosal ulceration featuring epithelial necrosis and granulation tissue

T. Mounajjed (✉)
Department of Laboratory Medicine and Pathology, Mayo Clinic, Rochester, MN, USA
e-mail: Mounajjed.taofic@mayo.edu

L. Zhang et al. (eds.), *Surgical Pathology of Non-neoplastic Gastrointestinal Diseases*,
https://doi.org/10.1007/978-3-030-15573-5_5

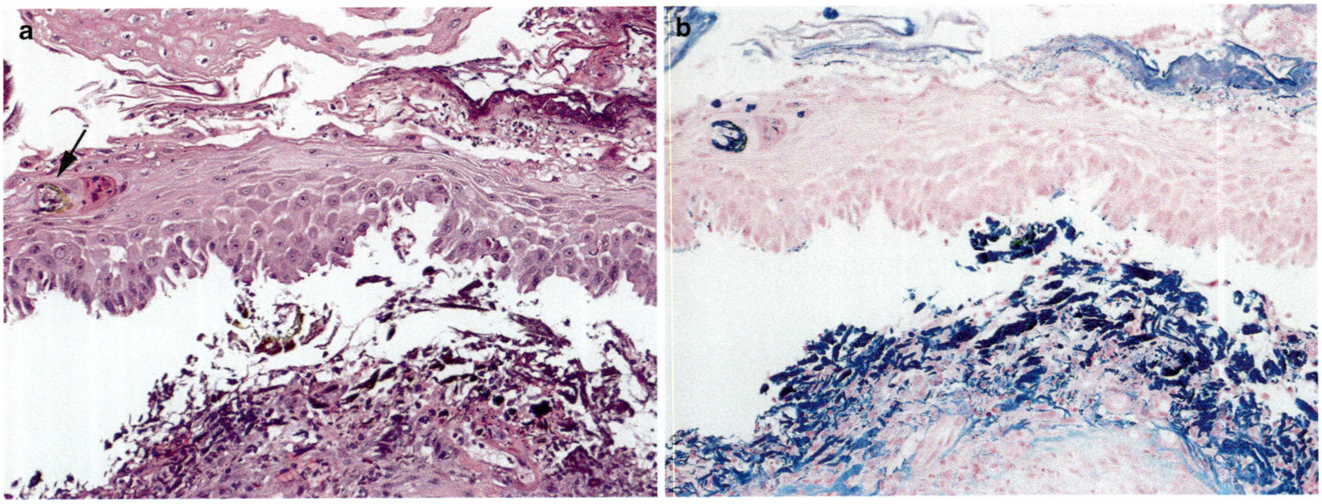

Fig. 5.2 Iron pill-induced esophagitis. By H&E staining, this acute erosive esophagitis shows refractile brown granular material in the squamous epithelium (arrow) and granulation tissue (**a**). Perls' iron staining confirms that the brown material represents iron (**b**)

Differential Diagnosis

Histologically, the main differential diagnoses include infectious esophagitis and reflux esophagitis. Infection can mimic pill-induced esophagitis clinically and pathologically. Identification of viral cytopathic inclusions (such as herpes or CMV inclusions) or other causative organisms (such as *Candida*) can help distinguish infection from pill-induced esophagitis. The clinical history, including history of intake of commonly implicated pills (which favors pill-induced esophagitis) or immune suppression (which raises consideration for infection), can also be helpful. The presence of a polarizable crystalline material, as can be seen in alendronate-induced injury, favors pill-induced esophagitis. In the absence of obvious H&E clues to the etiology, special stains for fungal organisms and immunohistochemical stains for viral organisms (CMV and HSV) can help to further evaluate for occult infectious agents. Reflux esophagitis usually affects the distal esophagus as opposed to the characteristic proximal esophageal involvement in pill-induced esophagitis; however, the histologic features of these two entities are significantly overlapping, and distinction between them is often not possible on histologic grounds alone; clinical distinction, on the other hand, is often possible.

Of note, though rare in the esophagus, mucosal iron deposition can be associated with iron overload disorders. In these patients, the iron deposits are confined to the lamina propria and submucosal glandular epithelium rather than the luminal epithelial surface and lack epithelial erosion, which is almost always present in iron pill-induced esophagitis. Furthermore, patients with erosive iron pill-induced injury are significantly older than those with mucosal iron deposits due to iron overload [11].

Miscellaneous Drugs

Medication resins can be encountered in the tissue samples of patients taking certain drugs such as Kayexalate, Welchol, and Renvela. Kayexalate is usually associated with mucosal injury, has a "fish-scale" appearance (Fig. 5.3a, b) and a purple color, and stains black with AFB. The crystals are most frequently adherent to ulcerated mucosa or admix with inflammatory exudates. Upper gastrointestinal tract injury due to Kayexalate is infrequent; gastrointestinal bleeding is the most common indication for a biopsy [12]. Welchol, which creates bright orange crystals, is unusually associated with mucosal injury (Fig. 5.4a, b) [13] and usually lacks fish-scale appearance; AFB stain renders the crystals dull yellow. Finally, Renvela can be associated with mucosal injury [14] and can appear as fish scales, but it has a two-toned pink/yellow color (Fig. 5.5), which turns magenta with AFB stain.

Colchicine, an alkaloid often used in gout treatment, causes toxicity due to its interference of tubulin polymerization into microtubules, thereby affecting cell mitosis and neutrophil degranulation and chemotaxis. Colchicine toxicity can cause esophageal mucosal injury. The main histologic feature is the presence of numerous metaphase mitoses including "ring-like" mitoses [15, 16]. Other histologic features encountered in the esophagus are apoptosis, nuclear swelling, dyskeratotic keratinocytes, nuclear pseudostratification, and some reduction in the squamous epithelial cell layers [15]. The latter changes, along with the increased mitotic activity, can be mistaken for dysplasia or Paget's disease. The clinical history, in conjunction with preserved surface epithelial maturation, should provide hints to the etiology of the mucosal changes. Taxol effects/toxicity

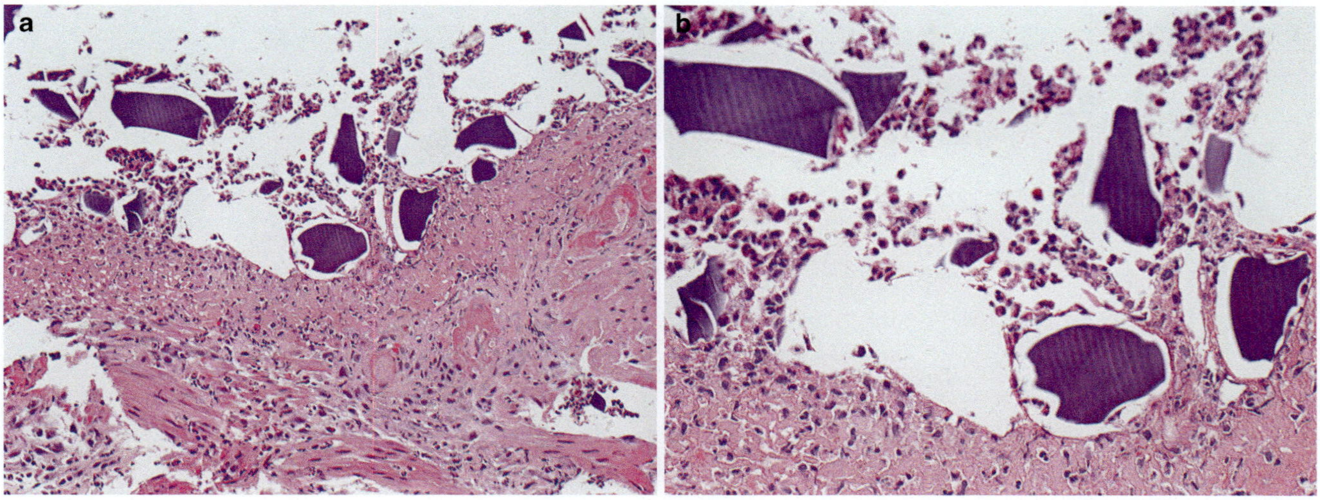

Fig. 5.3 Kayexalate. Kayexalate crystals can be associated with mucosal ulceration (**a**) and have a "fish-scale" appearance and a purple color (**b**)

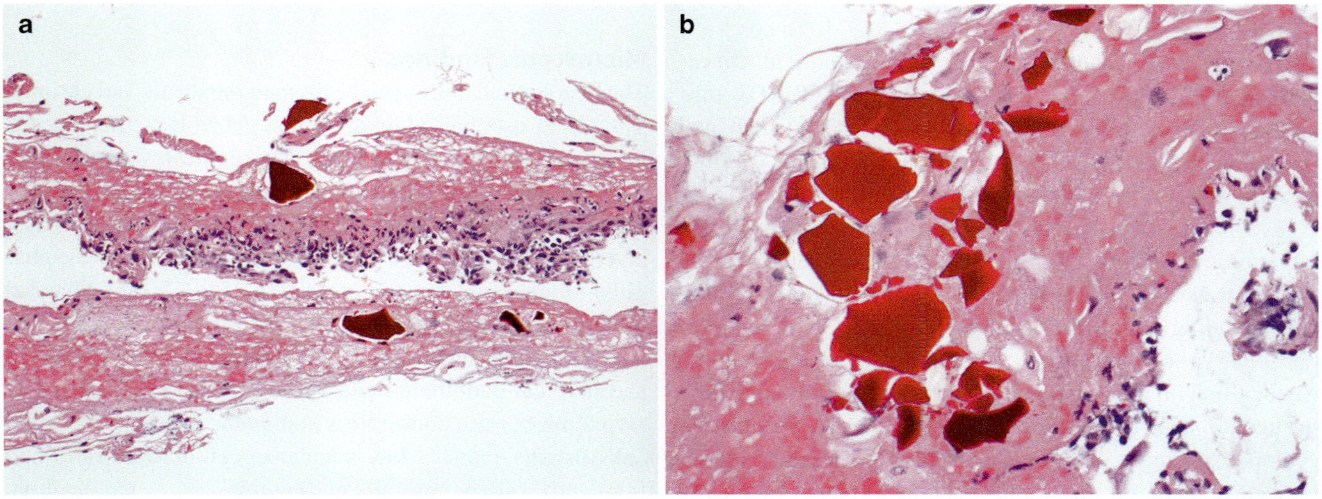

Fig. 5.4 Welchol. (**a**) Welchol crystals can be associated with mucosal damage (ulceration). (**b**) They lack "fish-scale" appearance and have a bright reddish orange color

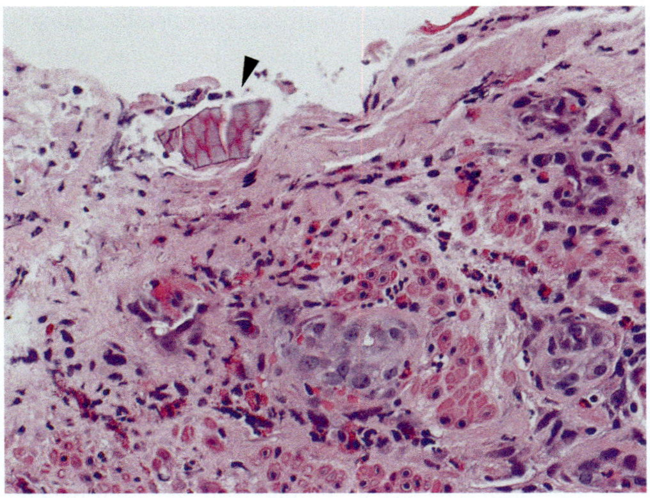

Fig. 5.5 Renvela. Renvela crystals, like Kayexalate crystals, have a "fish-scale" appearance, but they differ in their color; they have a two-toned pale pink/yellow color (arrowhead)

(Fig. 5.6a, b), which frequently affects the esophagus [17, 18], also causes mitotic arrest and produces histologic features similar to those seen in colchicine, including the presence of "ring-like" mitoses.

Chemotherapy- and Radiation-Induced Esophageal Injury

Definition

Chemotherapy- and radiation-induced esophageal injury is an esophageal damage as a result of the cytotoxic effects of chemotherapy and radiation therapy utilized for cancer treatment.

Clinical Features

Esophagitis in patients with cancer can be caused by the cytotoxic effects of chemotherapy and radiation or by opportunistic infections with viral, fungal, or bacterial organisms.

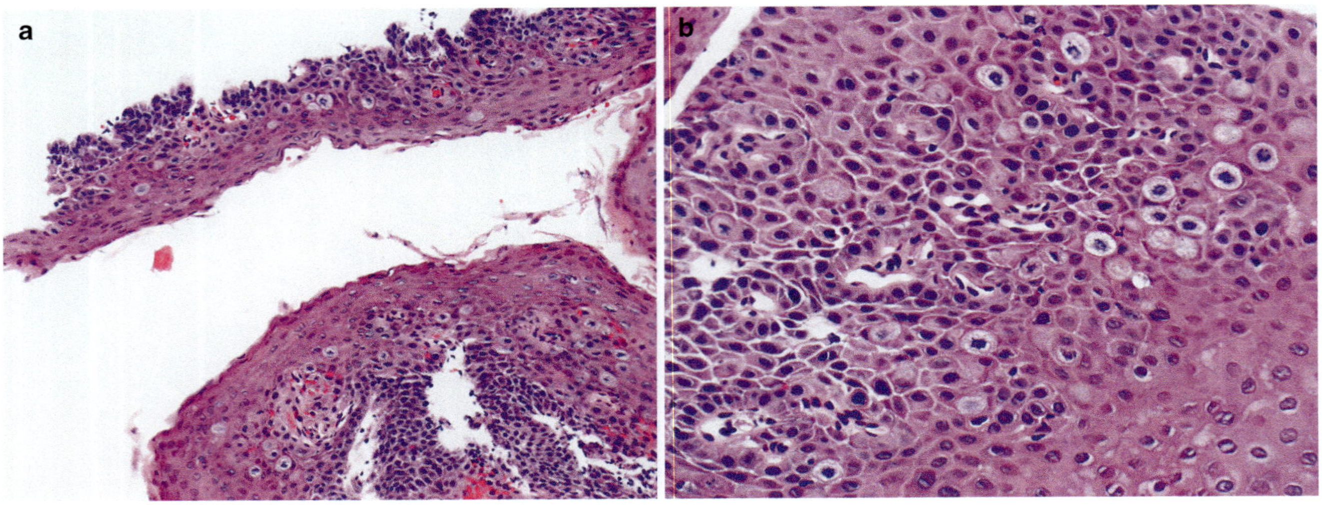

Fig. 5.6 Taxol effects/toxicity. The squamous esophageal epithelium contains numerous metaphase mitoses, including "ring-like" mitoses (**a**). A higher-power view of numerous "ring-like" mitoses (**b**)

Other causes of esophagitis that are common in cancer patients are gastroesophageal reflux disease (GERD), pill-induced injury, and graft-versus-host-disease in stem cell transplant recipients. We hereby discuss esophageal injury directly related to chemotherapy and/or radiation.

Esophagitis is a common side effect of chemotherapy and radiation therapy [19, 20]; it occurs most frequently during treatment of lung, esophageal, and other thoracic malignancies including lymphomas. The esophagitis is generally proportional in severity to the radiation dose and occurs more frequently with the combined use of certain chemotherapeutic agents such as doxorubicin hydrochloride, bleomycin, cyclophosphamide, and cisplatin [21–23]. In patients with lung cancer, significant esophageal injury is most frequently associated with concurrent chemotherapy and a maximal esophageal point dose ≥60 Gy [24].

Although acute injury, largely limited to the mucosa, can develop within the first 2 weeks of therapy, most changes occur later than 3 months following initiation of treatment and result in nerve and muscle damage, which can lead to stricture formation [25, 26]. Symptoms include burning sensation, dysphagia, and odynophagia. Frequent long-term complications include stricture and/or fistula formation.

Radiation-induced esophagitis is treated by viscous lidocaine hydrochloride and proton pump inhibitors to prevent further acid-related injury. Strictures are managed by endoscopic dilation and, if refractory, by the placement of self-expanding plastic stents (SEPS).

Gross Findings

The endoscopic features are variable and include erythema, edema, and friability of the mucosa. Ulceration and stricture formation can also be observed.

Microscopic Findings

The histologic features can be divided into acute and chronic. The acute esophageal injury mostly involves the mucosa with some submucosal edema. The earliest sign of acute mucosal injury is the occurrence of many apoptotic/dyskeratotic keratinocytes, which are most frequent in the basal layer. This is followed by the development of acute esophagitis, often with erosion/ulceration (Fig. 5.7a). Mucosal inflammation and erosion can be seen in chronic injury but also frequently found in the chronic phase as enlarged bizarre and atypical endothelial and stromal cells (Fig. 5.7b). The atypia might raise concern for malignancy, but the abnormal cells usually retain a low nuclear-to-cytoplasmic ratio and frequently show prominent cytoplasmic vacuolization. Furthermore, the atypical nuclei frequently have a smudged appearance and do not usually show mitotic activity. Chronic phase changes also include telangiectasia (Fig. 5.7c), atrophy of the submucosal glands, thick-walled submucosal arteries (Fig. 5.7d), intimal foam cell arteriopathy, and submucosal fibrosis. All these changes can persist indefinitely.

Differential Diagnosis

Because patients undergoing chemotherapy and radiation are immunocompromised, infectious esophagitis should be excluded. Viral esophagitis should be excluded by searching for viral cytopathic changes and inclusions and by the use of immunohistochemistry. Likewise, if no fungal elements are identified by H&E, fungal stains should be used to exclude fungal esophagitis. It is important to recognize that infectious and chemoradiation-induced esophagitis can coexist and that more than one infection can develop in these immunosuppressed patients.

The atypical cells seen in chronic chemoradiation-induced esophagitis can mimic malignant cells. However, the bizarre

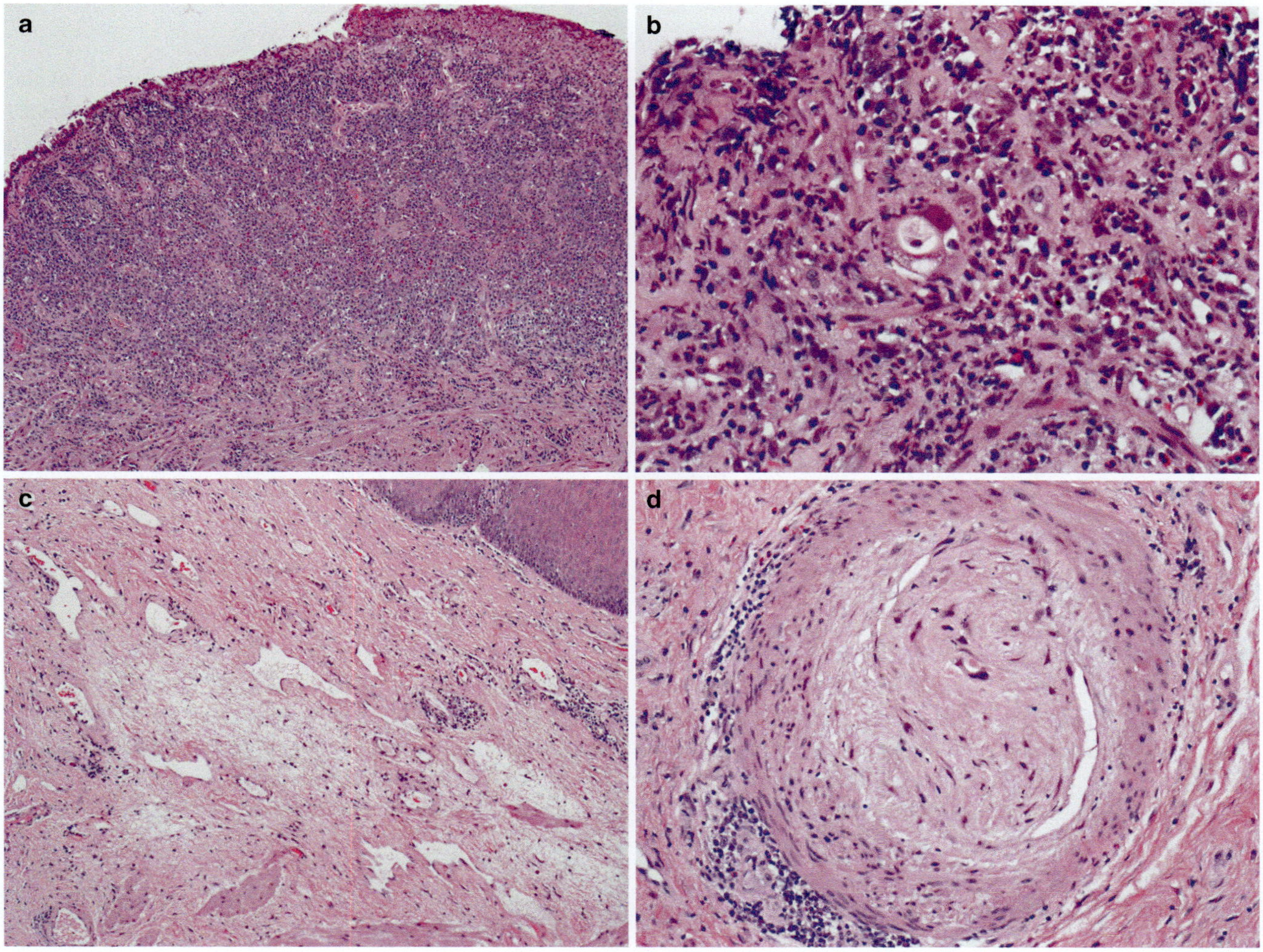

Fig. 5.7 Chemoradiation-induced esophageal injury. Acute esophagitis with ulceration is a common finding in chemoradiation-induced esophageal injury (**a**). Atypical stromal cells are frequently encountered in chemoradiation-induced esophageal injury. The atypical cell has a "smudged" nucleus, low nucleus-to-cytoplasmic ratio, and cytoplasmic vacuolization (**b**). In the chronic phase of chemoradiation-induced esophageal injury, capillary telangiectasia can develop (**c**), and abnormal thick-walled submucosal arteries are frequently encountered (**d**)

cells seen in chemoradiation-induced esophagitis, in contrast to malignant cells, have a low nuclear-to-cytoplasmic ratio and frequently show prominent cytoplasmic vacuolization and multinucleation. Furthermore, the atypical nuclei frequently have a smudged appearance and do not usually show mitotic activity.

Lymphocytic Esophagitis

Definition

Lymphocytic esophagitis is defined histologically by squamous epithelial spongiosis and infiltration of the peripapillary esophageal squamous epithelium by small T lymphocytes in the absence of a significant infiltration by other inflammatory cells (neutrophils or eosinophils) [27–29].

Clinical Features

If one adheres to the abovementioned strict histologic definition, the condition is rare (estimated to affect 1 in 1000 individuals) [29]. Most patients are symptomatic, most often complaining of dysphagia or odynophagia [29]. The clinical significance of this histologic pattern is still unclear, and several studies have shown conflicting results; associations with a variety of clinical conditions including Crohn's disease, celiac disease, *H. pylori* gastritis, and duodenal lymphocytosis have been postulated [27, 28, 30, 31]. Although the clinical significance remains to be fully understood, the few studies investigating this entity suggest that "lymphocytic esophagitis" is a histologic pattern that can arise in a response to a variety of esophageal insults, and some have suggested an autoimmune process as a possible etiology.

Gross Findings

The endoscopic findings associated with this histologic pattern are variable and include strictures (found in two-thirds of patients), rings and furrows reminiscent to eosinophilic esophagitis, and white mucosal plaques [29].

Microscopic Findings

The peripapillary esophageal squamous epithelium is infiltrated by small lymphocytes and shows spongiosis. Aside from lymphocytes, the inflammatory infiltrate lacks a significant component of other inflammatory cells (neutrophils or eosinophils) (Fig. 5.8). The intraepithelial small T lymphocytes express CD3 and CD4 or CD8.

Differential Diagnosis

Increased intraepithelial lymphocytes can be seen in a variety of esophageal mucosal injuries including GERD, but the inflammatory infiltrate in these other conditions also contains other inflammatory cells (neutrophils and/or eosinophils); in contrast, the inflammatory infiltrate in lymphocytic esophagitis is purely or almost purely lymphocytic.

Corrosive Esophagitis

Definition

Corrosive esophagitis is a form of esophageal injury caused by ingestion of caustic substances, which cause direct tissue damage.

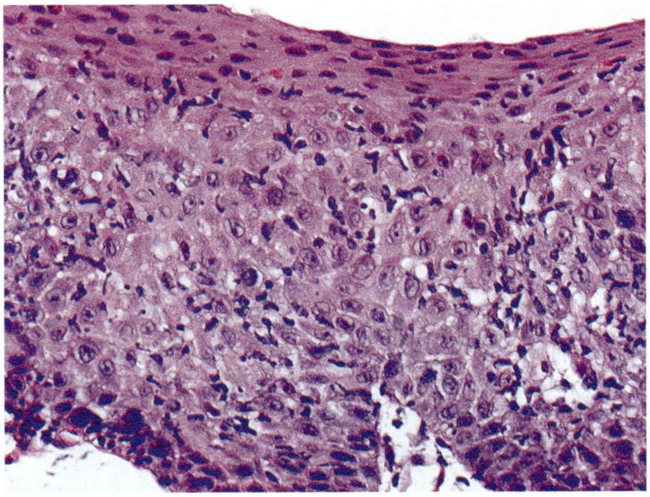

Fig. 5.8 Lymphocytic esophagitis. The esophageal squamous epithelium is infiltrated by an inflammatory infiltrate consisting purely of small lymphocytes; there is absence of infiltration by other inflammatory cells

Clinical Features

Corrosive or caustic esophagitis occurs as a result of the ingestion (accidental or suicidal) of corrosive substances (household cleaners, lye, washing soda, bleaches) which can be alkaline (lye) or acid (nitric) [32–34]. This esophageal injury can occur in children or adults and is often accompanied by injury to the stomach and duodenum. Patients present with a variety of symptoms, including dysphagia, vomiting, cough, drooling, and pain (in mouth and/or chest) following the ingestion of the corrosive agent. Patients often refuse to ingest food or fluids following the injury. Potential complications include glottic edema and airway obstruction, which can result in respiratory distress and stridor [35, 36]. Other long-term complications include stricture formation and, rarely, squamous cell carcinoma [37].

Gross Findings

The endoscopic findings are typically those of mucosal erythema, edema, hemorrhage, and necrosis. The mucosa is often sloughing, with frequent formation of circumferential ulcers. The severity of the endoscopic findings depends on the type, concentration, and amount of the ingested corrosive substance.

Microscopic Findings

Diagnostic tissue is not frequently obtained, as the diagnosis is usually evident based on the clinical history and endoscopic picture. The histologic findings are not entirely specific, mostly featuring tissue necrosis and ensuing inflammation. Initially, the inflammation is mainly neutrophilic. Vascular thrombosis and abundant granulation tissue formation usually follow. Some cases also show bacterial invasion into necrotic tissue. The histologic picture is somewhat dependent on the causative agent. For instance, alkaline substances cause liquefactive necrosis with associated fat and protein digestion. On the other hand, acid substances cause coagulative necrosis, with associated eschar formation, somewhat containing the depth of injury. Because an eschar is usually lacking in alkaline injury, alkaline substances usually cause deeper tissue necrosis than acid substances and are more frequently associated with esophageal perforation [33].

Differential Diagnosis

The histologic picture in corrosive esophagitis, especially in mild forms, is not entirely specific; there is histologic overlap with other forms of esophagitis, including reflux and infectious esophagitis. The distinction relies mainly on clinical and endoscopic grounds; a history of caustic agent ingestion is typical.

Esophagitis Dissecans Superficialis

Definition

Esophagitis dissecans superficialis is a rare condition characterized by sloughing of large portions of the esophageal epithelium, sometimes followed by expulsion of the sloughed tissue (by vomiting or regurgitation), often in the form of a tubular cast [38].

Clinical Features

Esophagitis dissecans superficialis has been associated with the intake of various substances including hot beverages, chemical irritants, and medications (NSAIDs [39], bisphosphonates [40], and potassium chloride). Other reported clinical associations include traumatic injury, heavy cigarette smoking, and autoimmune disorders including celiac disease [41] and autoimmune bullous dermatoses (pemphigus and pemphigoid) [40, 42]. Affected patients tend to be older adults with chronic debilitating conditions who take multiple medications [43]. Patients typically present with dysphagia, upper gastrointestinal bleeding, heartburn, and odynophagia [39]. Vomiting or coughing of esophageal epithelial casts can also occur [44]. The outcome is typically excellent despite the alarming clinical presentation. Patients are treated by discontinuing any suspected causative ingested substance alongside with acid suppression.

Gross Findings

Grossly, esophagitis dissecans superficialis usually features sloughing of large portions of squamous esophageal epithelium in the form of pseudomembranes or casts [45]. The lesions are usually identified in the middle and distal thirds of the esophagus, but diffuse involvement of the entire esophageal mucosa can occur in severe cases [39]. This endoscopic picture is dominated by the presence of white patches of sloughed mucosa (Fig. 5.9), which can be accompanied by mucosal cracks, fissures, and linear breaks. Bleeding can be either present or absent.

Microscopic Findings

Esophageal biopsies show detached superficial fragments of squamous epithelium (separated from the underlying basement membranes) with intraepithelial cracks of various sizes (Fig. 5.10a–c). The intraepithelial splitting can occur at different depths within the epithelium and can result in bullae formation [39]. Inflammation is not usually prominent, but occasional lymphocytes, neutrophils, and eosinophils can be seen. Some of the squamous epithelial fragments are completely necrotic; these can be colonized by bacterial and/or fungal elements. The viable detached squamous epithelial fragments usually show marked parakeratosis and/or orthokeratosis.

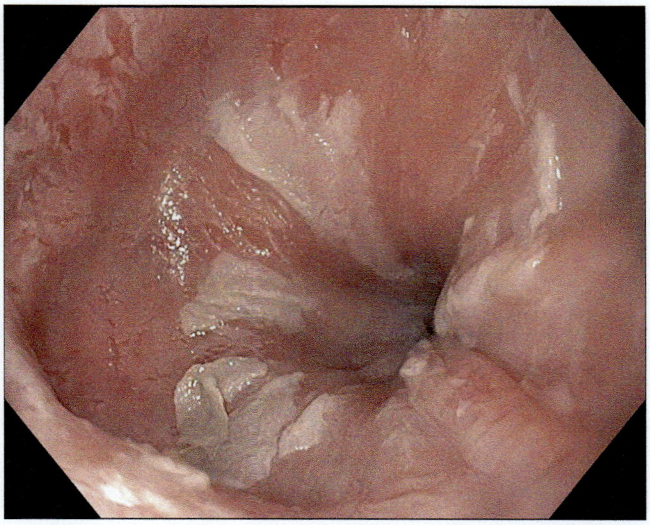

Fig. 5.9 Esophagitis dissecans superficialis. Endoscopic picture shows presence of white patches of sloughed mucosa

Differential Diagnosis

The main histologic differential diagnosis to consider is esophageal involvement by dermatologic bullous diseases such as pemphigus, bullous pemphigoid, or Stevens-Johnson syndrome. Clinical distinction, however, is usually clear; cutaneous and other mucosal lesions are absent in esophagitis dissecans superficialis and present in dermatologic bullous diseases. Furthermore, dermatologic bullous diseases show complement and immunoglobulin deposits by direct immunofluorescence and anti-desmoglein antibodies by enzyme-linked immunosorbent assay [46]; these findings are absent in esophagitis dissecans superficialis.

Another possibility to consider in the differential diagnosis is infectious esophagitis. A prominent inflammatory infiltrate is typical in infectious (viral or fungal) esophagitis; in contrast, inflammation is usually minimal in esophagitis dissecans superficialis. Furthermore, mucosal splitting and prominent parakeratosis/orthokeratosis are not features of infectious esophagitis. In difficult cases, special stains (immunohistochemistry for viral infection and GMS/PAS for fungal infection) can be helpful, but it is important to recognize that

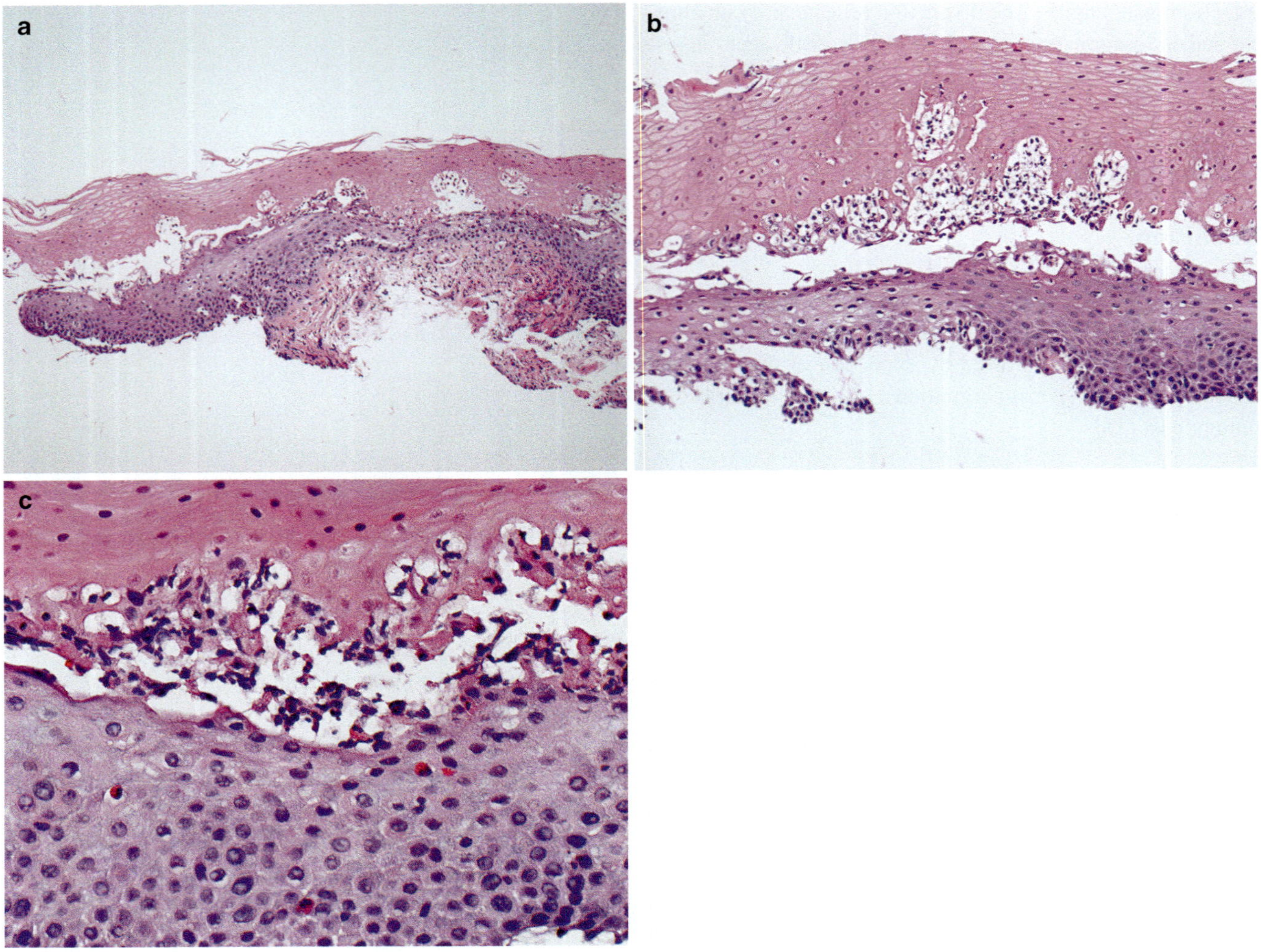

Fig. 5.10 Esophagitis dissecans superficialis. This biopsy shows detached squamous epithelium with some separation from the underlying basement membranes. The squamous epithelium shows discontinuous splitting with bullae formation (**a**), and higher-power view of bullae formation (**b**). The intraepithelial cracks can be associated with inflammatory cells including neutrophils and eosinophils (**c**)

bacterial and fungal colonization can involve some squamous epithelial fragments that are completely necrotic in esophagitis dissecans superficialis. Finally, mucosal mechanical trauma related to endoscopy can mimic esophagitis dissecans superficialis histologically. Mechanical injury has been reported to result from scope trauma associated with repeated attempts to obtain mucosal biopsies, which can cause detachment of squamous epithelial layers from the underlying mucosa, mimicking bullae [47, 48]. Correlation with a history of mechanical endoscopic trauma can help in the differential diagnosis. Furthermore, unlike esophagitis dissecans superficialis, the epithelial fragments seen in cases of mechanical trauma lack necrosis, parakeratosis/orthokeratosis, and inflammation.

Infectious Esophagitis

Viruses and fungi cause most forms of acute infectious esophagitis. Bacterial esophagitis occurs in some patients with systemic or upper respiratory infection, but this condition is rarely sampled histologically.

Herpes Esophagitis

Definition

Herpes esophagitis is an esophageal viral infection caused by herpes simplex viruses (HSV).

Clinical Features

Type 1 and type 2 HSV can both cause herpes esophagitis, but esophagitis due to HSV type 1 is far more common. In approximately 25% of patients, oral/oropharyngeal infection accompanies esophageal involvement [49, 50]. Although immunocompetent individuals can be affected, this infection primarily affects immunocompromised patients. Common causes of immunosuppression include bone marrow and solid organ transplantation, cancer (e.g., leukemia), chemotherapy, autoimmune diseases (such as lupus), and acquired immunodeficiency syndrome due to human immunodeficiency virus [51]. The disease can be severe in immunocompromised patients but is usually self-limited in immunocompetent individuals, usually resolving spontaneously within 14 days [50, 52, 53]. Although the infection can occasionally be asymptomatic, patients most commonly present with dysphagia, odynophagia, and fever [51]. Upper gastrointestinal bleeding sometimes occurs. The diagnosis of herpes esophagitis is usually based on endoscopic findings, which can be confirmed by pathologic examination of esophageal biopsies. Antiviral treatment (such as acyclovir) is indicated in all immunosuppressed patients and can be commenced based on clinical/endoscopic suspicion only. Antiviral treatment helps healing of active disease, but does not prevent future recurrences.

Gross Findings

Endoscopically, herpetic lesions usually affect the distal esophagus. The typical lesions are small (less than 2 cm), shallow, well-circumscribed, punched-out (volcano-like) ulcers, usually separated by normal-appearing mucosa [51]. Sometimes, the typical lesions can be accompanied by exudates and/or plaques. A diffuse form of erosive esophagitis is rare.

Microscopic Findings

Herpes ulcers contain necrotic debris and acute inflammatory exudate. It was suggested that a prominence of mononuclear cells with aggregates of macrophages with convoluted nuclei adjacent to inflamed epithelium is a characteristic finding of herpes esophagitis [54], However, similar cells can be found in other types of esophageal ulcers and are therefore nonspecific.

The histologic hallmark of herpes esophagitis is the presence of viral cytopathic changes (Fig. 5.11a, b) which are typically found in squamous epithelial cells at the lateral margins of the ulcers. For this reason, the most diagnostic biopsies are those that sample the immediate ulcer edge, which is the richest area in viral changes; some endoscopic biopsies may not contain viral changes. The characteristic viral cytopathic changes include:

- Cowdry type A inclusions: dense eosinophilic to amphophilic intranuclear inclusions that are surrounded by a clear halo, separating them from the nuclear membrane.
- Characteristic "ground-glass" appearance of affected nuclei; ground-glass nuclei have a smudged, homogeneous, and smooth chromatin pattern.
- Multinucleation of the affected epithelial cells.
- Nuclear molding and margination.
- Ballooning degeneration of affected epithelial cells.

Immunohistochemical stains (Fig. 5.11c) and in situ hybridization are available for HSV types 1 and 2 and can be very helpful in the detection of the infection, specifically in cases that do not contain conspicuous viral cytopathic changes. These stains are most useful in cases that are clinically suspected to represent herpes esophagitis, but the H&E examination reveals no obvious viral cytopathic changes.

Differential Diagnosis

As mentioned above, HSV type I is by far the most common cause of herpes esophagitis, but HSV type 1 cannot be distinguished morphologically from HSV type 2 or Varicella-Zoster virus (Fig. 5.12a, b); such distinction requires clinical correlation. The differential diagnosis for herpes esophagitis includes other types of infectious esophagitis (most specifically CMV esophagitis). Endoscopically, the punched-out (volcano-like) ulcers of herpes esophagitis differ from CMV esophageal ulcers, which tend to be linear or longitudinal and deeper. Furthermore, in contrast to herpetic inclusions, CMV inclusions primarily affect endothelial and stromal cells rather than epithelial cells and are not associated with multinucleation, ground-glass appearance, and nuclear molding and margination. Nevertheless, concurrent infection with CMV and herpes may occur, and one should evaluate for different inclusion types in the same sample.

Other conditions can mimic viral cytopathic changes of herpes esophagitis. For instance, squamous epithelial cells can show multinucleated giant cell transformation in reflux esophagitis or other types of reparative epithelial processes (Fig. 5.13a, b); this, however, is not associated with Cowdry A inclusions, ground-glass appearance, and nuclear molding and margination. Radiation-induced esophagitis can also cause marked enlargement of squamous epithelial cells with multinucleation and nucleolar prominence, which can occasionally mimic herpes esophagitis. Likewise, however,

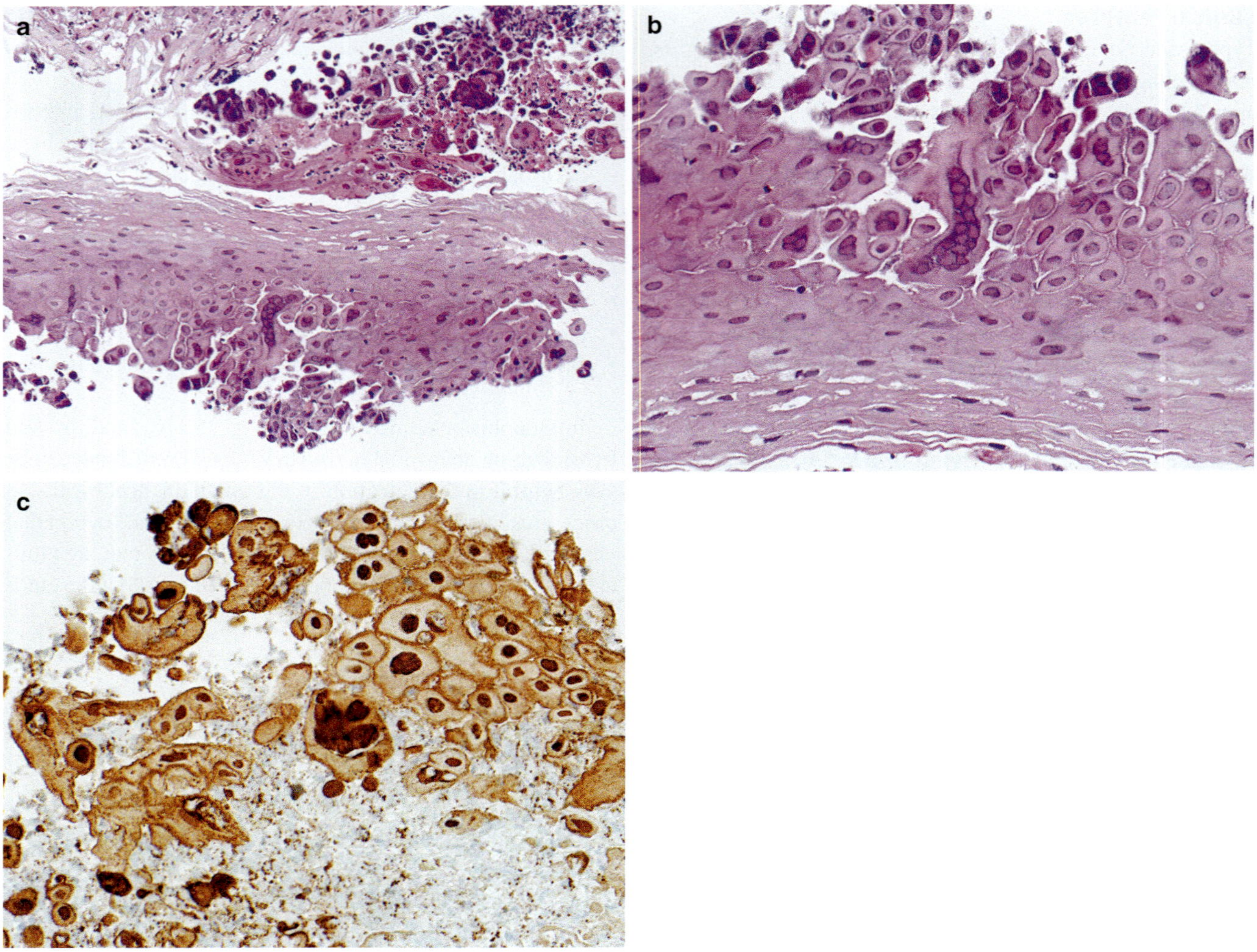

Fig. 5.11 Herpes simplex virus esophagitis. Viral cytopathic changes are typically found in squamous epithelial cells at the lateral margins of the ulcers (**a**). Characteristic viral cytopathic changes include multinucleation, "ground-glass" appearance of affected nuclei, nuclear molding, and margination (**b**). Immunohistochemical staining for herpes highlights infected epithelial cells (**c**)

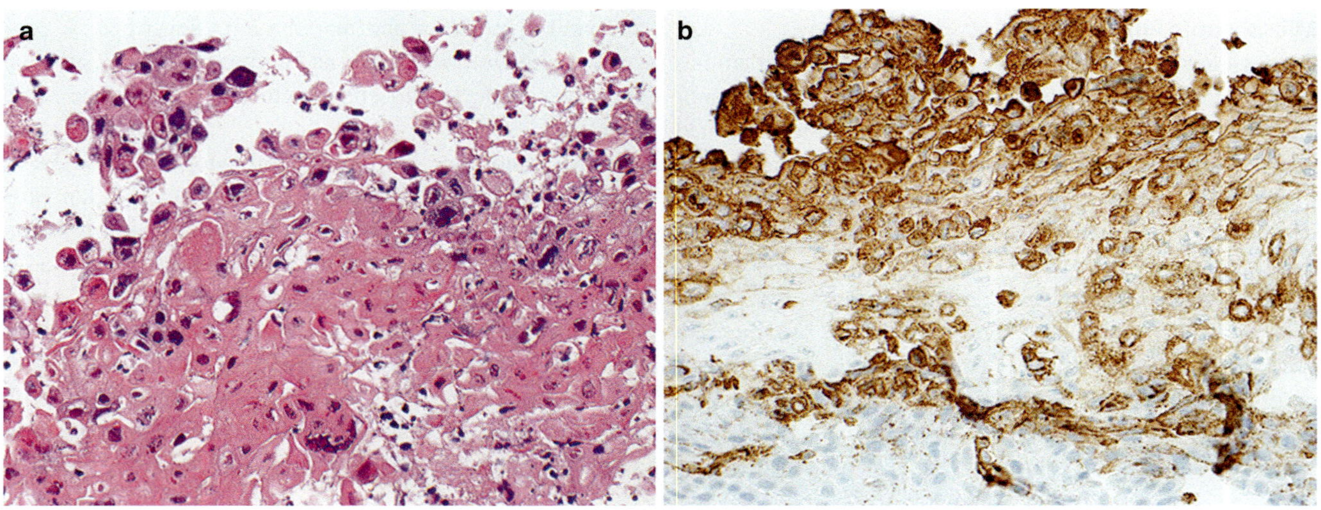

Fig. 5.12 Varicella-Zoster virus esophagitis. Viral cytopathic changes including multinucleation, "ground-glass" appearance of affected nuclei, and nuclear molding similar to herpes simplex virus are identified (**a**). Immunohistochemical staining for Varicella-Zoster virus highlights infected epithelial cells (**b**)

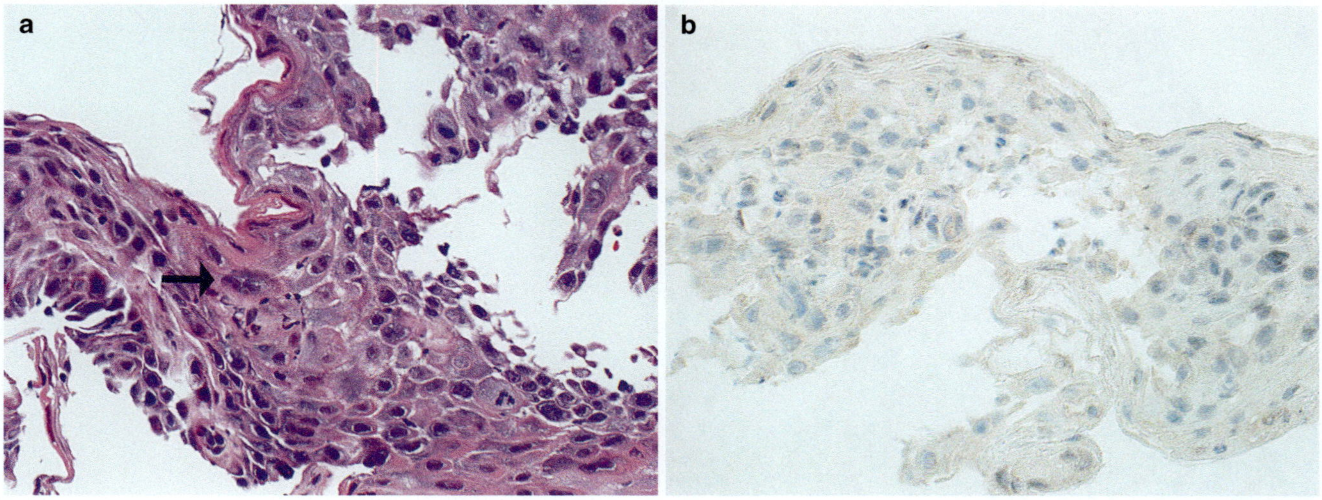

Fig. 5.13 Squamous epithelial multinucleated giant cell change. Reactive squamous epithelial cells can show multinucleated giant cell transformation (arrow) in reflux esophagitis or other types of reparative epithelial processes, mimicking herpes esophagitis. Notice the absence of ground-glass appearance, nuclear molding, and margination (**a**). Immunohistochemical staining for herpes is negative, ruling out herpes esophagitis (**b**)

Cowdry A inclusions, ground-glass change, and nuclear molding and margination are absent.

Viral cytopathic changes, specifically Cowdry A inclusions, can be mistaken for "macronucleoli," misleading the pathologist to suspect a malignant or dysplastic process. Neoplastic "macronucleoli," however, lack the clear halo typical of Cowdry A inclusions. Furthermore, although malignant processes can also have multinucleated cells, they lack ground-glass change and nuclear molding and margination.

Cytomegalovirus Esophagitis

Definition

Cytomegalovirus (CMV) esophagitis is an esophageal viral infection caused by CMV, a member of the human herpes virus family.

Clinical Features

CMV esophagitis is less common than herpes esophagitis but still represents the second most common gastrointestinal site of CMV infection after the colon. CMV esophagitis only rarely affects immunocompetent individuals [55]; most patients are immunocompromised due to bone marrow or solid organ transplantation, long-term renal dialysis, malignant neoplasia (most affected cancer patients undergoing chemoradiotherapy), or acquired immunodeficiency syndrome due to human immunodeficiency virus (especially with CD4 counts below 50 cells/μl) [56, 57]. CMV infection in such patients represents a major cause of morbidity and mortality. CMV infection can often co-exist with other forms of infectious esophagitis (herpes and *Candida*) [58]. Males are more frequently affected than females. Patients usually present with odynophagia, epigastric pain, and fever [59]. Confirmation of active infection often requires tissue biopsy evaluation because detection of the virus by other methods (viral culture) does not necessarily indicate an active infection. Antiviral treatment (e.g., ganciclovir) is indicated for treatment of CMV esophagitis, most critically in immunosuppressed patients [60].

Gross Findings

CMV most frequently causes multiple ulcers in the lower esophagus, but diffuse esophagitis has also been described [59, 61]. CMV esophageal ulcers are multiple, well-circumscribed, and tend to be deep, linear, or longitudinal [59]. Less frequently, the diffuse form of CMV esophagitis can cause erythema and diffuse erosions [62].

Microscopic Findings

The histologic hallmark of CMV esophagitis is the viral inclusions, which typically involve the endothelial and stromal cells, characteristically found at the ulcer base. Columnar epithelial cells are rarely infected, but squamous epithelium is not. For this reason, the biopsies with the largest diagnostic yield are those that sample the esophageal ulcers [63]. The infected cells (Fig. 5.14a) show marked cytomegaly and nucleomegaly and basophilic cytoplasm and often have coarse intracytoplasmic granular inclusions (eosinophilic to basophilic). Their nuclei also have prominent intranuclear basophilic inclusions that are separated from the nuclear membrane by a clear halo. Similar to herpes esophagitis, some have reported that perivascular aggregates of macrophages are suggestive of CMV or herpes esophagitis [62],

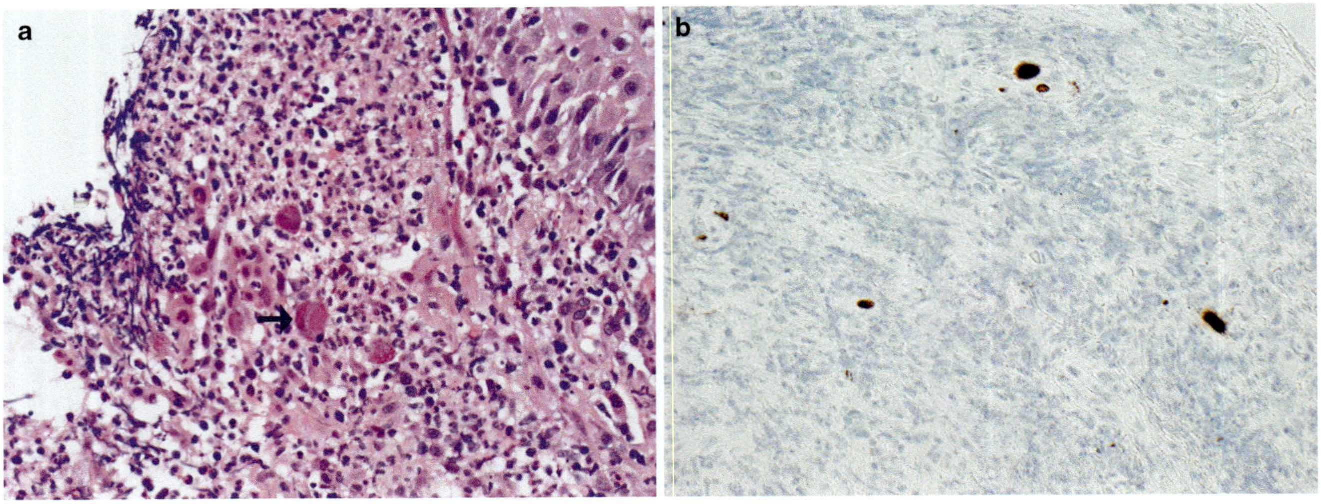

Fig. 5.14 Cytomegalovirus esophagitis. Viral inclusions typically involve endothelial and stromal cells. The infected cells (arrow) show marked cytomegaly and nucleomegaly, basophilic cytoplasm with coarse intracytoplasmic granular inclusions (**a**). Immunohistochemical staining for cytomegalovirus highlights infected epithelial cells (**b**)

but this feature seems nonspecific and is less prominent in patients who have received antiviral therapy.

Immunohistochemical stains (Fig. 5.14b) and in situ hybridization for CMV are available and very helpful in highlighting cells infected by CMV. These stains are more sensitive than routine H&E stains for viral detection and are most useful in cases that are clinically suspected to represent CMV esophagitis, but careful examination of H&E sections fails to reveal obvious cytomegalovirus inclusions.

Differential Diagnosis

The main differential diagnosis for CMV esophagitis includes other types of infectious esophagitis (most specifically herpes esophagitis). Endoscopically, the linear/longitudinal and deep ulcers of CMV esophagitis differ from the punched-out (volcano-like) ulcers of herpes esophagitis. Herpes affects squamous epithelial cells; in contrast, CMV affects endothelial and stromal cells. Although Cowdry type A inclusions in herpes esophagitis can mimic nuclear CMV inclusions, cells infected in herpes esophagitis also typically feature a characteristic "ground-glass" appearance, multinucleation, and nuclear molding and margination. That being said, concurrent infection with CMV and herpes may occur (most commonly in transplant and acquired immunodeficiency syndrome) [53], and one should evaluate for different inclusion types in the same sample.

Fungal (*Candida*) Esophagitis

Definition

Candida esophagitis is an esophageal fungal infection caused by *Candida*, most commonly *Candida albicans* or *Candida tropicalis* [58, 64].

Clinical Features

Although it occasionally affects otherwise healthy individuals [65], esophageal candidiasis is most common in immunosuppressed individuals, such as HIV-infected patients, in whom it is an AIDS-defining infection typically occurring at CD4 cell counts below 200 cells/μl, in patients with hematologic malignancies, and in patients taking corticosteroids [66], in diabetes, and in patients taking certain medications including broad-spectrum antibiotics and acid-suppressive therapy [67]. Clinically, the hallmark of *Candida* esophagitis is odynophagia or retrosternal/epigastric pain on swallowing. Some patients (especially the elderly) are asymptomatic, with the infection discovered incidentally upon upper endoscopy. The diagnosis of *Candida* esophagitis is usually suspected clinically and then further supported when white mucosal plaque-like lesions are noted on endoscopy. Confirmation of diagnosis requires tissue identification of organisms by histologic examination of tissue biopsy or by culture identification of *Candida* if a culture is performed. *Candida* esophagitis is usually successfully treated with antifungal agents (most frequently fluconazole), which are generally safe and well tolerated [68, 69], but if azole compounds fail, treatments with amphotericin B and echinocandins (used in randomized trials) can be used [70, 71].

Gross Findings

The endoscopic appearance of *Candida* esophagitis is very characteristic, featuring white plaques overlying erythematous esophageal mucosa; the underlying mucosa appears ulcerated if the plaques are removed. The plaques can be localized or confluent and are often covered by fibrinous/purulent exudate.

Microscopic Findings

The diagnosis of *Candida* esophagitis is achieved histologically by identification of *Candida* organisms, which grow in pseudohyphae and budding yeast forms and are most frequently found in squamous debris (Fig. 5.15a), fibrinopurulent exudate, or necrotic debris. The squamous esophageal mucosa itself typically shows acute esophagitis, with various amounts of intraepithelial neutrophils; the inflammation may be inconspicuous in immunocompromised patients. The squamous epithelium may become hyperplastic with parakeratosis. Indeed, the mere identification of fungal elements in an esophageal biopsy is insufficient to render a diagnosis of *Candida* esophagitis; *Candida* organisms are normal constituents of the gastrointestinal tract flora. Therefore, the diagnosis of *Candida* esophagitis can only be made when organisms (particularly pseudohyphae) are identified within esophageal tissue [72]. In fact, tissue invasion can be quiet deep into the esophageal wall (as deep as muscularis propria) in untreated *Candida* esophagitis affecting HIV patients [73]. The fungal organisms are often easily visible by H&E alone. However, silver stain (such as GMS stain) (Fig. 5.15b) or PAS stain should be used to identify the organisms in biopsies containing only rare fungal elements. In fact, many pathologists routinely order fungal stains on biopsies showing acute esophagitis in order to detect such rare fungal elements. Special stains allow morphologic evaluation and identification of the genus *Candida* based on the fungal morphology, but further identification of the species (*Candida albicans* vs. *Candida tropicalis* vs. other *Candida* spp.) cannot be accomplished by histology and can be achieved only by culture.

Differential Diagnosis

Glycogenic acanthosis or ectopic sebaceous glands, which are also characterized by the presence of multiple white mucosal plaques or elevations [74, 75], can occasionally be endoscopically mistaken for esophageal candidiasis. These entities, however, are easily distinguished from *Candida* esophagitis histologically. Glycogenic acanthosis is characterized by thickened squamous epithelium containing large squamous cells packed with glycogen and lacking significant inflammation. The glycogenic content is PAS positive, diastase sensitive [76]. Ectopic sebaceous glands, as their name indicates, consist of sebaceous glands morphologically identical to dermal sebaceous glands, aberrantly located in the esophageal mucosa. Special stains are negative for fungal organisms in both conditions.

As mentioned above, *Candida* organisms are normal constituents of the gastrointestinal tract flora; therefore, simple identification of *Candida* yeast forms may not represent true *Candida* esophagitis. Confirmation of a diagnosis of *Candida* esophagitis requires identification of fungal organisms (particularly pseudohyphae) within esophageal tissue.

Finally, *Candida* esophagitis should be distinguished from viral esophagitis. Both show acute inflammation involving the squamous esophageal mucosa, erosion, and/or ulceration. *Candida* esophagitis lacks viral inclusions and viral esophagitis lacks fungal organisms. Nevertheless, esophageal mucosal ulcers and/or erosions caused by other injurious (including infectious) agents can be colonized by *Candida* organisms [77]. Therefore, co-infection with *Candida* and another agent (herpes or CMV) should always be considered; biopsies affected by *Candida* esophagitis should be evaluated for viral inclusions.

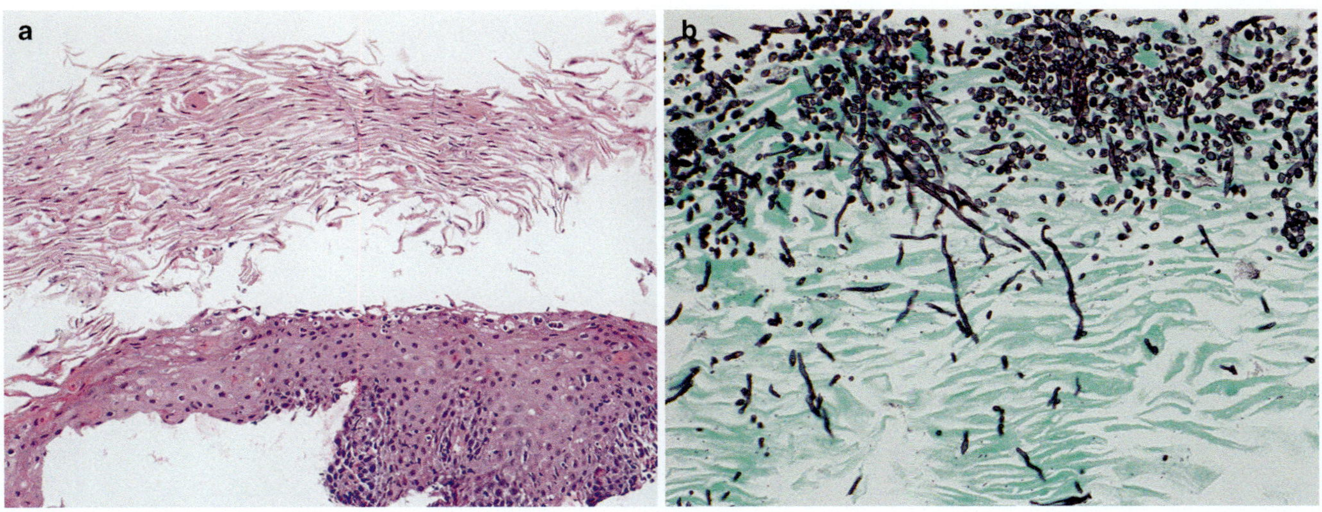

Fig. 5.15 *Candida* esophagitis. The fungal organisms are most frequently encountered in squamous debris (**a**). Grocott's methenamine staining shows numerous fungal yeast forms and pseudohyphae, morphologically consistent with *Candida* species (**b**)

Bacterial Esophagitis

Definition

Bacterial esophagitis is an esophageal bacterial infection evidenced by histopathologically demonstrable bacterial invasion into the esophageal mucosa and/or deeper layers of esophageal wall.

Clinical Features

Primary bacterial esophagitis in the absence of a concomitant viral or fungal infection, involvement by malignancy, or involvement of a site of prior esophageal surgery, is rare. Primary bacterial esophagitis most commonly affects immunosuppressed individuals [78], often suffering from hematologic malignancies or aplastic anemia, and many are profoundly neutropenic [79]. Most cases of bacterial esophagitis are secondary, involving areas of prior ulceration. Patients usually present with odynophagia [78]. The most common causative bacteria are normal constituents of oral or respiratory tract flora (*Staphylococcus aureus*, *Staphylococcus epidermidis*, and *Bacillus* species). Other bacteria have also been reported to cause esophagitis; for instance, *Actinomyces* can infect areas of prior tissue injury; *Actinomyces* colonies (sulfur granules) are seen at the center of an inflammatory response, composed of basophilic radiating filaments. Finally, rare cases of esophagitis caused by *Mycobacterium*, *Histoplasma*, and *Toxoplasma* species have been reported [80, 81]. In immunosuppressed patients, bacterial esophagitis can be complicated by bacteremia and sepsis.

Microscopic Findings

Bacterial esophagitis is histologically characterized by the presence of numerous bacterial elements (Fig. 5.16a, b), invading into the esophageal mucosa and/or deeper layers of esophageal wall. This is associated with ulceration and inflammatory tissue response. A diagnosis of bacterial esophagitis can be established when sheets of confluent bacteria invade the subepithelial tissue [49]. The number of bacteria appears to be inversely related to the intensity of the inflammatory reaction [79]. Because most cases of bacterial esophagitis are secondary, it is important to seek other infectious organisms (fungal or viral) in biopsies showing features of bacterial esophagitis.

Differential Diagnosis

Oral contaminants containing bacterial flora are sometimes encountered in esophageal biopsies. The bacteria, however, do not invade the esophageal wall and are not associated with an inflammatory response.

Parasitic Esophagitis: Chagas Disease

Definition

Chagas disease, also known as American trypanosomiasis, is a tropical parasitic disease caused by *Trypanosoma cruzi*.

Clinical Features

As of 2015, Chagas disease is estimated to affect approximately 6.6 million people, mostly in Central and South America, causing approximately 8000 annual deaths [82]. Humans are accidental hosts, and the disease is also known to affect more than 150 other animals [83]. Although predominantly a disease of Central and South America, population movements have resulted in more widespread disease, with cases now being reported in Europe and the United States. The infection most frequently spreads via contact with Triatominae insects but can

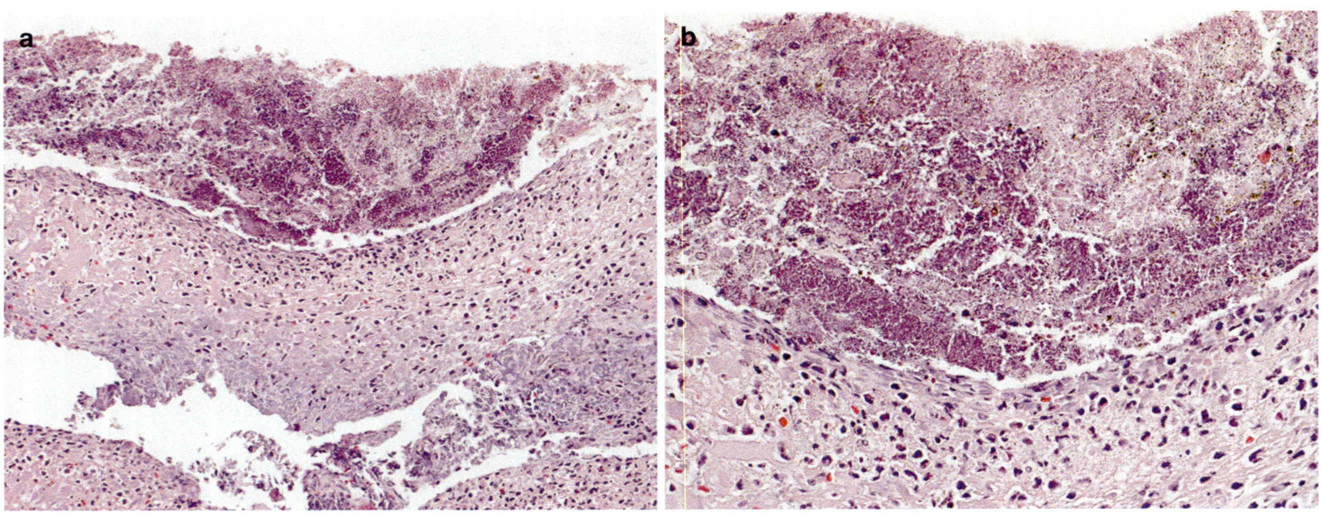

Fig. 5.16 Bacterial esophagitis. Bacterial elements are identified in the esophageal wall, with associated ulceration and inflammatory tissue response (**a**). A higher-power view shows the presence of numerous bacterial elements (**b**)

also spread congenitally or via blood transfusions [84, 85]. The infection has an early stage, which is either asymptomatic or presents with fever, conjunctivitis, lymphadenopathy, and headache. After a period of clinical latency, 30%–40% of patients develop a chronic infection, with symptoms developing up to 30 years after the initial infection; the most frequently affected organs are the heart (20%–30% of patients, leading to heart failure) and gastrointestinal tract (the esophagus and colon are affected in 10% of patients) [86]. Megaesophagus develops in approximately 3% of patients [84, 87–89]. Esophageal injury results from destruction of neuron plexuses in the esophagus by the inflammatory reaction induced by *Trypanosoma cruzi*. Patients with esophageal involvement typically develop dysphagia and odynophagia [84], which results in severe weight loss and malnutrition [90–92]. Other symptoms include cough, hiccups, and food/drink regurgitation. The infection can be treated effectively with nifurtimox and benznidazole [93–95] if initiated before long-term complications have developed. Patients with megaesophagus can benefit from endoscopic dilatation techniques of the gastroesophageal junction. Surgery (cardiotomy) is indicated in some patients.

Gross Findings

Esophageal injury in Chagas disease manifests in gradual narrowing of the distal esophagus, accompanied by proximal dilatation; severe cases of the latter are also known as "Chagasic megaesophagus."

Microscopic Findings

The main histologic findings of Chagas disease are dense mononuclear inflammatory infiltrates targeting the submucosal and myenteric plexuses of the esophagus, associated with morphologic features of neuronal injury [96, 97]. Other findings include muscular hypertrophy of the distal esophagus, associated with a mononuclear inflammatory infiltrate affecting the muscularis propria. Patients with Chagasic megaesophagus are reported to have a significant decrease in S100 and glial fibrillary acidic protein-positive enteroglial cells [88].

Esophagus Involved in Systemic Disease

Crohn's Disease

Clinical Features

The esophagus is rarely involved by Crohn's disease (<1%–11% of patients have esophageal involvement) [98, 99]. Most patients (88%) with esophageal involvement by Crohn's disease have extraesophageal disease, and about one third have oral ulcers at the time of esophageal symptom onset [98, 100]. Isolated esophageal Crohn's disease is extremely rare, and extraesophageal involvement usually follows. The majority of patients have esophageal specific symptoms (dysphagia and odynophagia) [100]. Inflammatory esophageal Crohn's disease shows good response to prednisone, topical budesonide, and biologics, whereas stricturing esophageal Crohn's disease requires a combination of biologic therapy, immunomodulators, and serial dilations with/without steroid injections [100].

Gross Findings

The endoscopic appearance of esophageal Crohn's disease is highly variable and may not correlate well with the clinical presentation [101]. The mid or distal esophagus is the most common site of esophageal involvement. The endoscopy shows superficial ulcerations (58% of patients), erythema and/or erosion (50% of patients), strictures (17% of patients), deep ulcerations (13% of patients), and fistulas (4% of patients) [100].

Microscopic Findings

Histologically, nonspecific chronic inflammation is seen in most (83%) cases, and approximately 7%–21% of patients have associated granulomas on biopsy (Fig. 5.17) [100, 102]. A "lymphocytic esophagitis" pattern can be seen (see section "Lymphocytic Esophagitis" above), and eosinophils can be particularly prominent. Acute inflammation is often present, particularly in cases with ulceration. In resection specimens, transmural inflammation is usually seen. Due to the superficial nature of mucosal biopsy specimens, Crohn's disease of the esophagus cannot be definitely diagnosed histologically in many cases. Nevertheless, when characteristic histologic features are present (transmural inflammation, granulomas, mural fibrosis, strictures, and deep ulcerations), especially in the presence of known extraesophageal Crohn's disease, a definitive diagnosis can be rendered.

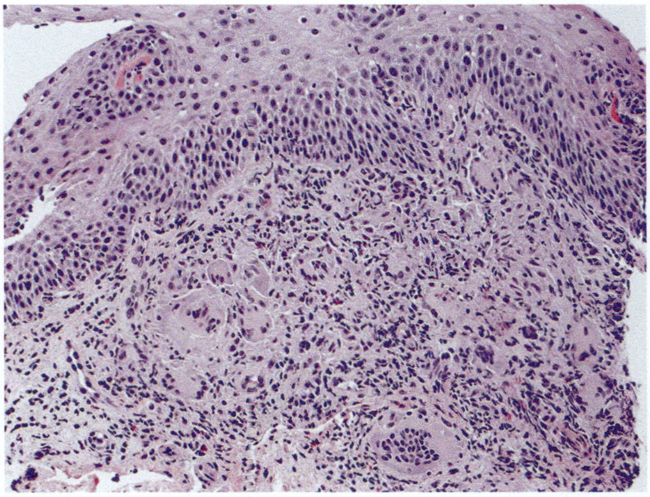

Fig. 5.17 Crohn's disease involving the esophagus. The lamina propria shows non-necrotizing granulomatous inflammation with multinucleated giant cells. The overlying squamous epithelium shows occasional intraepithelial lymphocytes

Differential Diagnosis

As mentioned above, due to the superficial nature of mucosal biopsies, the histologic features are often nonspecific and can mimic reflux esophagitis, infectious esophagitis, and even eosinophilic esophagitis (if eosinophils are particularly prominent). Distinguishing esophageal Crohn's disease from these other entities usually requires correlation with the endoscopic and clinical findings; the presence of extraesophageal Crohn's disease in most cases provides a clue to the correct diagnosis. Performing special (fungal, mycobacterial, and viral) stains in cases with acute inflammation, granulomas, and/or ulceration can also be helpful in the differential diagnosis and to exclude a superimposed infection. Finally, although "lymphocytic esophagitis" pattern can be seen in esophageal Crohn's disease [27], it is not specific for it and can be seen in a variety of other conditions (see section "Lymphocytic Esophagitis" above).

Esophageal Amyloidosis

Clinical Features

Esophageal involvement is present in approximately 72% of patients with gastrointestinal amyloidosis. On the other hand, isolated esophageal amyloidosis is very rare in the absence of systemic disease. In such cases, amyloid can be mass forming (amyloid tumor, aka amyloidoma) [103]. Most patients have AL-type amyloid deposition [103]. Rarely, esophageal amyloidosis can be complicated by perforation or hematemesis.

Microscopic Findings

Histologically, amyloid deposition in the esophagus is similar to amyloid seen elsewhere (Fig. 5.18), featuring extracellular deposition of amorphous eosinophilic material that is congophilic with Congo red stain and shows green birefringence under polarized light after Congo red staining. Because amyloid is usually seen in the deeper layers of the esophageal wall, biopsy specimens often fail to detect it.

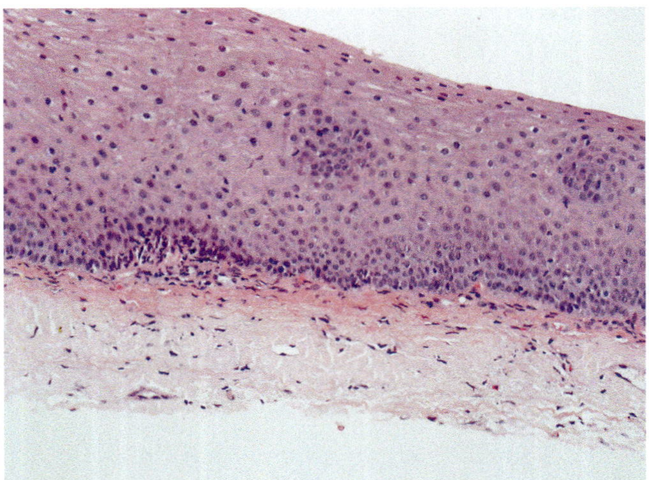

Fig. 5.18 Esophageal amyloidosis. This biopsy shows extracellular deposition of amorphous eosinophilic material underneath the esophageal squamous epithelium. This material showed green birefringence under polarized light after Congo red staining (not shown)

Differential Diagnosis

From a clinical standpoint, significant esophageal amyloid deposits can cause motor disorders of the esophagus, mimicking achalasia (clinically and radiologically) [103]. Histologic distinction between amyloidosis and achalasia, however, is easy; amyloidosis shows extracellular amorphous eosinophilic Congo red-positive deposits, whereas achalasia does not show extracellular deposits and instead shows marked reduction or complete absence of myenteric ganglion cells with associated nerve inflammation and reactive mucosal changes.

Esophageal Involvement in Autoimmune and Collagen Vascular Disorders

The esophagus can show involvement by various collagen vascular disorders including scleroderma [104], rheumatoid arthritis [105], systemic lupus erythematosus [106], mixed connective tissue disorders, polymyositis, dermatomyositis [107], and Sjögren syndrome, [108, 109]. Esophageal involvement in these conditions can be a direct result of the collagen vascular disease, manifesting as dysmotility and/or GERD, or an indirect result such as drug-induced injury from immunosuppressive therapy or infectious complication of the patients' immunocompromised status.

Scleroderma deserves some focus as it commonly involves esophagus. Esophageal damage results from fibrosis and atrophy of the muscularis propria and particularly affects the inner circular layer. This causes hypomotility, aperistalsis, and failure of the lower esophageal sphincter [110]. As a result, scleroderma is commonly associated with GERD; histologic evidence of reflux esophagitis can be seen in more than half of the patients [111]. Consequently, Barrett esophagus develops in up to 37% of scleroderma patients, and its neoplastic complications including adenocarcinoma have been documented [112, 113].

Cystic Fibrosis

Cystic fibrosis is known to affect the gastrointestinal tract, pancreas, and hepatobiliary tree [114]. Among the upper gastrointestinal tract manifestations, a common manifestation results from gastroesophageal reflux. Children with cystic fibrosis have an increased incidence of GERD, affecting up to 80% of cystic fibrosis patients [115, 116]; the disease is symptomatic in over 25% of patients younger than 5 years [117]. Gastroesophageal reflux can be a significant cause of morbidity in cystic fibrosis patients [118], and some adolescents have been reported to develop Barrett esophagus [119]. Possible contributing factors to the increased gastroesophageal reflux in cystic fibrosis include diaphragm depression due to pulmonary hyperinflation, increased abdominal pressure associated with cough, increased volume of swallowed secretions, and medications [115, 118]. In children with cystic fibrosis, reflux episodes are predominantly acidic [116, 120], and reflux reaching the proximal esophagus is common, generating a risk for aspiration [116]. The pathologic features of reflux esophagitis in cystic fibrosis are similar to those seen in patients without cystic fibrosis.

Graft-Versus-Host Disease Involving the Esophagus

Definition

Graft-versus-host disease is an alloiummune disorder that occurs after organ transplantation as a result of donor immune cells from the graft recognizing and attacking recipient tissue.

Clinical Features

Graft-versus-host disease is a common complication of organ transplantation (most commonly after bone marrow transplantation). Esophageal involvement occurs in less than 15% of bone marrow transplantation patients [121]. Patients usually have other gastrointestinal and/or cutaneous signs and symptoms related to graft-versus-host disease, but esophageal manifestation presents with dysphagia and odynophagia [122].

Gross Findings

Esophageal involvement by graft-versus-host disease most commonly manifests as a vesiculobullous, ulcerative, or desquamative process, rarely producing mucosal casts reminiscent to esophagitis dissecans superficialis [123–126]. A stricturing process, also associated with mucosal sloughing, has also been described [122].

Microscopic Findings

The histologic picture in graft-versus-host disease does not always correlate well in its severity with the clinical picture, and in some cases, the biopsy can appear almost normal, likely due to sampling error (very focal lesions). Therefore, evaluating multiple levels of esophageal biopsies in cases suspected for graft-versus-host disease is recommended if the initial levels appear normal [127]. The microscopic findings of esophageal involvement by graft-versus-host disease are similar to those seen elsewhere in the gastrointestinal tract. Apoptosis in the squamous esophageal epithelium manifests as dyskeratotic keratinocytes (Fig. 5.19a, b). A lichenoid inflammatory infiltrate is often present. In more severe and advanced histologic presentations, mucosal ulceration (Fig. 5.19c) and submucosal fibrosis occur.

Differential Diagnosis

The presence of a lichenoid inflammatory infiltrate and dyskeratotic keratinocytes can histologically mimic esophageal involvement by lichen planus. The clinical history of transplantation and absence of known dermatologic lichen planus should direct the pathologist to the correct diagnosis.

Esophageal Involvement in Dermatological Disease

Definition

This section describes esophageal involvement by primary dermatologic conditions including lichen planus, bullous diseases (including pemphigus vulgaris, as bullous pemphigoid, benign mucous membrane pemphigoid, and epidermolysis bullosa acquisita), erythema multiforme, and Stevens-Johnson syndrome [128–131]. Other rare skin disorders can also affect the esophagus but are beyond the scope of this chapter.

Clinical Features

Although most of these disorders occur in conjunction with a skin disorder, it is important to note that esophageal disease can sometimes occur in the absence of skin lesions (e.g., lichen planus). One common feature of these disorders is a predilection to involve the proximal esophagus.

Lichen planus most commonly affects middle-aged adults. Clinically, it is characterized by eruptions of violaceous, scaling pruritis, and skin plaques. In contrast to cutaneous lichen planus, which has an equal gender distribution, esophageal lichen planus almost exclusively affects middle-aged and older females. Esophageal lichen planus is more strongly associated with oral lichen planus (affecting 1% up to 26% of patients) than it is with cutaneous lichen planus; almost all patients with esophageal lichen planus had oral disease (prior, concurrent, or subsequent) [132–137]. Although patients with esophageal lichen planus can be asymptomatic, they typically present with dysphagia and odynophagia.

Pemphigus vulgaris, as its name implies, is the most prevalent form of pemphigus. It is an autoimmune mucocutaneous disease characterized by the formation of superficial flaccid bulla of various sizes. The bulla results from antibod-

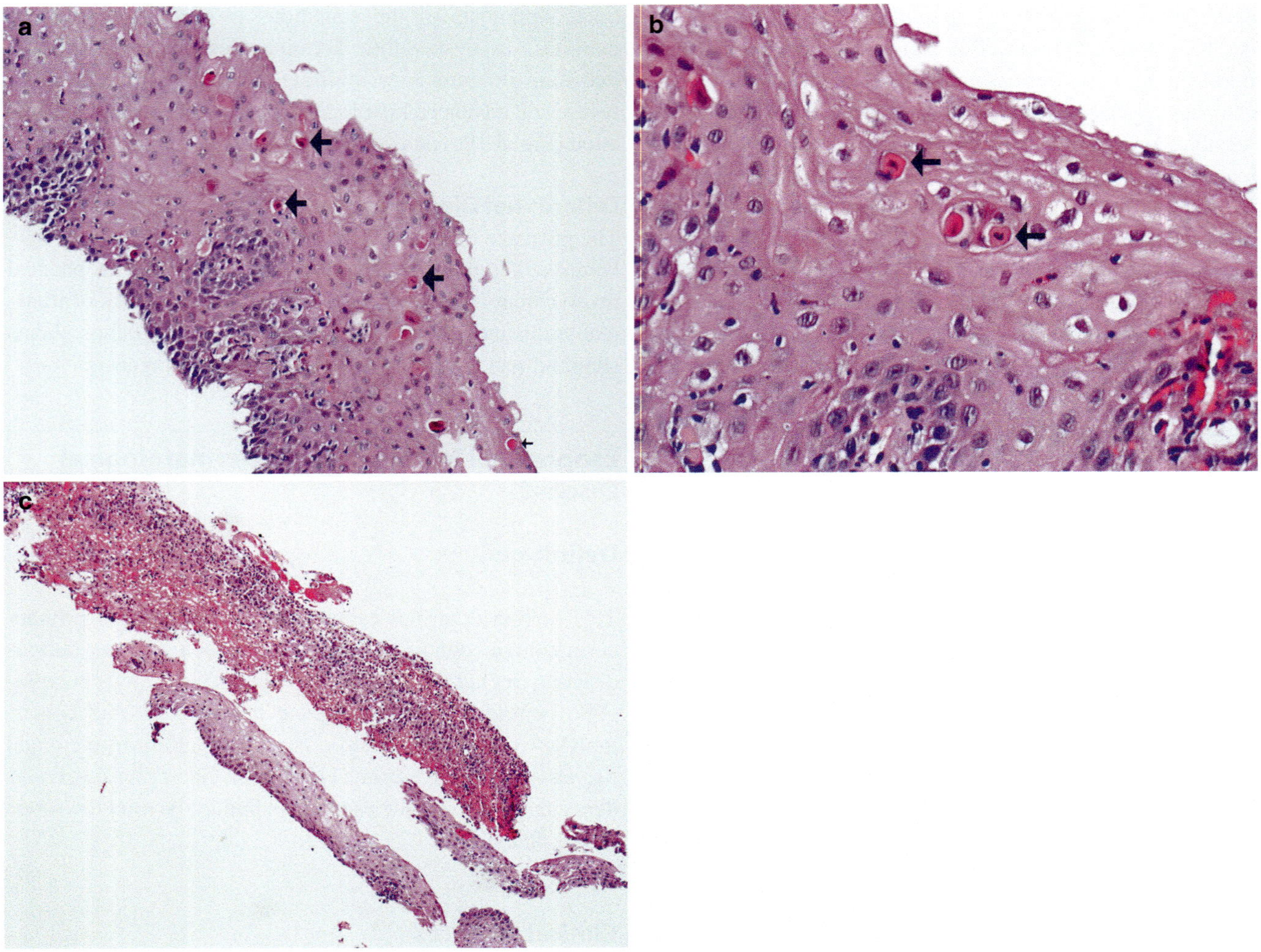

Fig. 5.19 Graft-versus-host disease involving the esophagus. Apoptosis in the squamous esophageal epithelium manifests as dyskeratotic keratinocytes (arrows), low-power view (**a**) and high-power view (**b**). In severe cases, mucosal ulceration can occur (**c**)

ies directed to desmoglein 3, which cause disruption of intercellular attachments between squamous epithelial cells [137, 138]. Most patients are middle-aged and older adults, and the disease has a predilection to affect individuals of Jewish [139] or Mediterranean descent. Studies indicate that most patients (up to 80%) with pemphigus vulgaris have endoscopic evidence of esophageal involvement [140, 141].

Bullous pemphigoid is an autoimmune subepidermal bullous disease characterized by the development of large tense blisters affecting the skin and less commonly the mucous membranes [139, 142]. Up to 4% of patients develop esophageal involvement [139]. The bullae develop as a result of IgG autoantibodies directed to the basement membrane, causing complement activation. Benign mucous membrane pemphigoid (cicatrical pemphigoid) is another autoimmune bullous disease related to bullous pemphigoid, which also affects the esophagus in approximately 4% of patients [143]. The circulating autoantibodies in this disease are directed to bullous pemphigoid antigen 2 (BPAC2) [143].

Epidermolysis bullosa represents a group of inherited disorders characterized by the formation of blisters, vesicles, and bullae on all surfaces lined by squamous epithelium [144] following pressure or minor trauma [145]. The disease is caused by mutations affecting genes that encode structural proteins located at the dermal-epidermal junction. Epidermolysis bullosa is classified into different subtypes (dystrophic, simplex, and junctional) based on the inheritance pattern, the immunohistochemical features, and the specific epidermal or dermal-epidermal level of disruption. Esophageal involvement most frequently develops in the dystrophic form of this disease [146]; it is caused by trauma resulting from boluses of food, which can be traumatic to the mucosa. Esophageal bullae can lead to ulceration and subsequent scarring, stricture, and web formation [147]. Epidermolysis bullosa aquisita is a rare acquired disorder with clinical characteristics that are similar to those of epidermolysis bullosa; in contrast to epidermolysis bullosa, however, epidermolysis bullosa aquisita lacks a family history, affects adults, and causes milder skin disease. A subset of patients with epidermolysis bullosa aquisita has circulating IgG autoantibodies that recognize collagen IV.

Erythema multiforme is an immune-mediated reaction that usually develops following infection (such as *Mycoplasma*) or drug exposure, characterized by the development of erythematous mucocutaneous lesions. The mucosal lesions usually involve the lip and oral cavity, with only rare cases of esophageal involvement [148]. The lesions are caused by the deposition of immune complexes in the superficial microvasculature of the skin and mucous membranes. The lesions typically regress. Stevens-Johnson syndrome (macular trunk lesions with mucosal involvement) is a severe form of erythema multiforme [149], characterized by acute eruption of bullous skin lesions, fever, and mucosal involvement.

Gross Findings

The endoscopic findings of lichen planus include elevated lacy white papules, esophageal webs, pseudomembranes, desquamation, and superficial pin-point erosions with and without stenosis, usually involving the proximal esophagus. Strictures of the cervical esophagus develop in up to two-thirds of patients [150].

Endoscopy of patients with esophageal involvement by pemphigus vulgaris reveals blisters, erosions, scattered red spots, white spots, and longitudinal erythematous streaks. A cast resembling those seen in esophagitis *dissecans superficialis* can occasionally develop [129].

In rare cases of bullous pemphigoid with esophageal involvement, endoscopy shows bullae, mucosal friability, and small erosions surrounded by erythema. Benign mucous membrane pemphigoid has similar endoscopic features, but because bullae develop as a result of endoscopy in this disease, it should be performed with caution.

In esophageal involvement by epidermolysis bullosa, endoscopy shows bullae, strictures, and web formations. Endoscopic interventions should also be done with caution as such techniques can cause bullae with further scarring.

In erythema multiforme, the esophagus endoscopically shows small white patches similar to those caused by *Candida* esophagitis. In Stevens-Johnson syndrome, the endoscopic appearance varies from scattered erosions to large areas of reddened, denuded mucosa with overlying white plaques.

Microscopic Findings

Biopsies of esophageal bullae can be challenging to interpret because the bullae often rupture before or during sampling. Histologically, the esophageal lesions are similar to those in the skin. In bullous diseases, clinical information and the skin findings (including skin biopsy findings) are critical for diagnosis. For bullous diseases, the most important histologic characteristics are the level of intraepithelial or epithelial/subepithelial separation, the presence or absence of acantholysis, and the nature of the inflammatory infiltrate [129, 137].

The histologic features of esophageal lichen planus differ from those in the skin and more closely resemble those of oral lesions. The skin lesions are characterized by hyperkeratosis, hypergranulosis, acanthosis, and "saw-tooth" elongation of the rete pegs. In contrast, as the normal esophageal mucosa lacks a granular layer, esophageal lesions usually lack hypergranulosis and show parakeratosis rather than orthohyperkeratosis. Furthermore, the esophageal epithelium tends to be atrophic rather than acanthotic or it can show alternating atrophy and acanthosis. The histologic hallmark of esophageal lichen planus is a band-like or "lichenoid" lymphocytic infiltrate consisting predominantly of mature T cells and associated with basal keratinocyte degeneration (Fig. 5.20a). Anucleated apoptotic keratinocytes (known as civatte bodies) are also a characteristic feature (Fig. 5.20b, c).

Endoscopic biopsies in pemphigus vulgaris are often superficial and therefore nondiagnostic [151]. The histology of pemphigus vulgaris is characterized by the presence of acantholysis (loss of intercellular cohesion) causing suprabasal separations and bullae formation. Acantholytic keratinocytes are dishesive and more rounded in contour. The basal layer of the squamous epithelium can remain attached to the underlying basement membrane, producing a "tombstone-like" appearance [152]. Mixed inflammation is usually present and eosinophils can be particularly prominent, particularly around bullae.

Esophageal histology is not well characterized in bullous pemphigoid, but skin lesions are characterized by subepidermal bullae and marked eosinophilic inflammatory infiltrate. The esophageal inflammatory infiltrate is also characteristically rich in eosinophils. In epidermolysis bullosa, esophageal lesions are characterized by the presence of subepithelial bullae separating the basal layer of the squamous epithelium from the underlying lamina propria, with little or no inflammatory infiltrate.

The esophageal lesions of erythema multiforme are characterized by mucosal erosions and superficial ulcerations and frequent dyskeratotic keratinocytes, most commonly found in the basal cell layer but sometimes involving the entire epithelial thickness. Inflammation is present and often characterized by increased intraepithelial lymphocytes. Stevens-Johnson syndrome features more extensive epithelial necrosis.

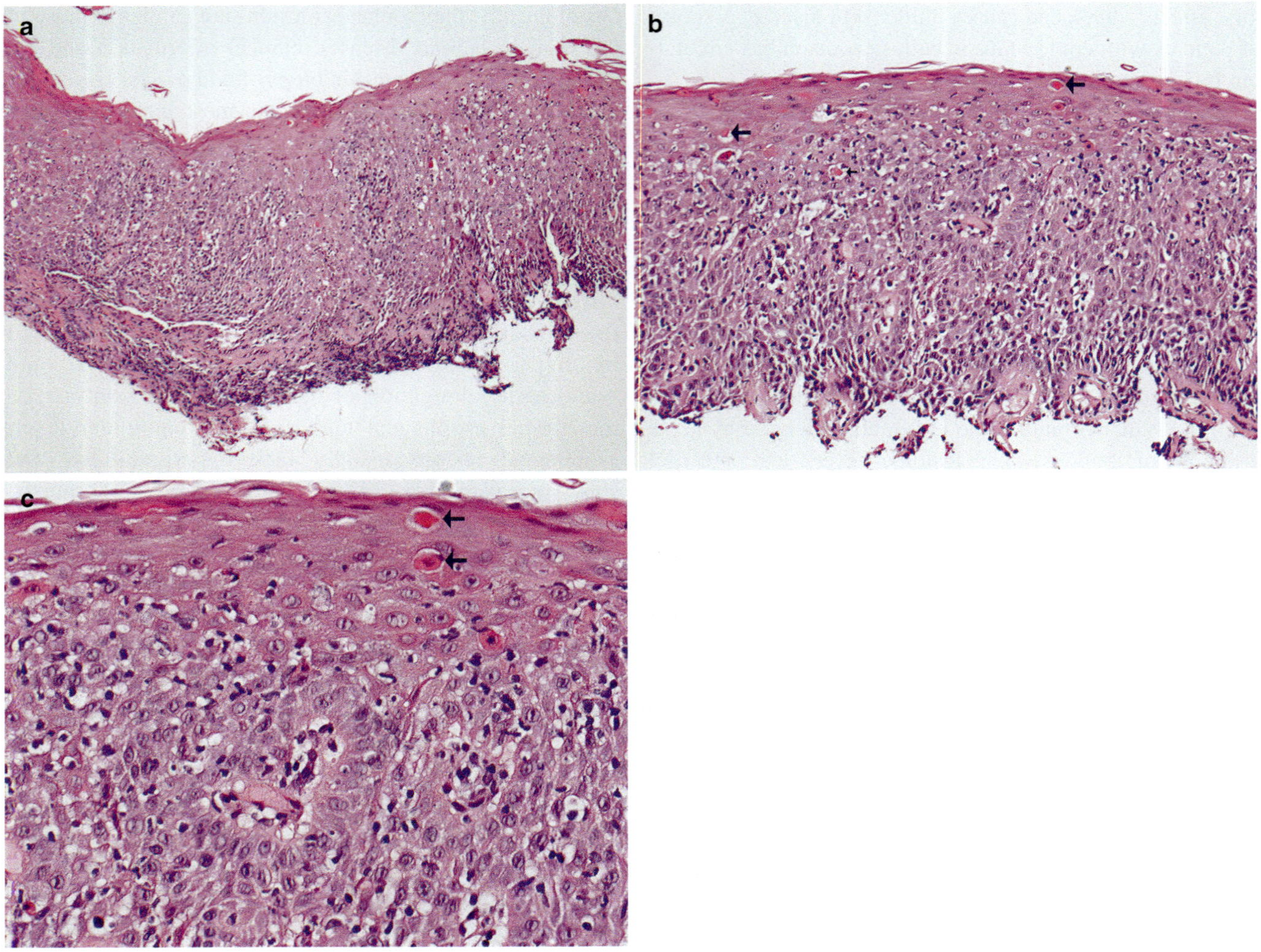

Fig. 5.20 Lichen planus. The squamous esophageal mucosa shows a lichenoid lymphocytic inflammatory infiltrate and parakeratosis (**a**), and numerous civatte bodies (arrows) (**b**) are the characteristic features of esophageal involvement by lichen planus. A high-power view of anucleated apoptotic keratinocytes (civatte bodies, arrows) (**c**)

Immunofluorescence Features

Immunofluorescence is critical for confirming the diagnosis and classification of bullous diseases, but a detailed description of immunofluorescence is beyond the scope of this chapter; such studies are typically done on skin biopsies and are therefore better characterized in dermatopathology textbooks. In brief, dermal lesions of pemphigus vulgaris are positive by direct immunofluorescence for deposits of IgG and complement component C3, localizing in the epidermal intercellular spaces [153]. Esophageal lesions show similar immunofluorescence findings [138]. In bullous pemphigoid, direct immunofluorescence shows linear IgG and C3 deposits at the level of the esophageal basement membrane [139]. Similar deposits are observed in benign mucous membrane pemphigoid (cicatrical pemphigoid). Epidermolysis bullosa acquisita also shows linear deposits of IgG and complement in the basement membrane of the esophagus, similar to those found in the skin [142].

Differential Diagnosis

Several patterns of esophageal mucosal injury can appear "lichenoid." Medications such as gold, thiazides, and antimalarial agents can produce lichen planus-like lesions; such medications need to be excluded clinically when considering lichen planus. The esophageal mucosa adjacent to ulcer sites of various etiologies (e.g., infectious, pill-induced esophagitis, or caustic injury) often shows nonspecific lymphocytic infiltrates that can mimic lichen planus. Viral inclusions and fungal elements, however, are absent in lichen planus. Furthermore, pill-induced esophagitis and caustic injury are excluded by correlation with the clinical and endoscopic findings. Likewise, reflux esophagitis can focally show prominent lymphocytic infiltrates, raising consideration for lichen planus. However, the other histologic criteria for reflux esophagitis, including intraepithelial eosinophils, are usually absent in esophageal lichen planus. In addition, lichen planus typically involves the proximal esophagus, in contrast to distal esophageal involvement in reflux esophagitis. Finally, patients with esophageal lichen planus do not respond to medications for reflux esophagitis. Graft versus host disease can show a lichenoid inflammatory infiltrate and dyskeratotic keratinocytes also mimicking esophageal involvement by lichen planus. The clinical history of transplantation and absence of known dermatologic or oral lichen planus should direct the pathologist to the correct diagnosis.

The main histologic differential diagnosis for esophageal involvement by dermatologic bullous diseases is esophagitis dissecans superficialis. Clinical distinction, however, is usually clear; cutaneous and other mucosal lesions are absent in esophagitis dissecans superficialis and present in dermatologic bullous diseases. Furthermore, dermatologic bullous diseases show complement and immunoglobulin deposits by direct immunofluorescence and anti-desmoglein antibodies by enzyme-linked immunosorbent assay [46]; these findings are absent in esophagitis dissecans superficialis. The presence of a prominent mucosal eosinophilic infiltrate is frequent in bullous diseases (e.g., pemphigus vulgaris and bullous pemphigoid) and can raise consideration for reflux esophagitis and eosinophilic esophagitis; the bullae and presence of dermatologic disease should help in this distinction.

Achalasia

Definition

Esophageal achalasia is an esophageal motility disorder characterized by incomplete lower esophageal sphincter relaxation, which results in increased lower esophageal sphincter tone and lack of peristalsis of the esophagus [154–156]. Achalasia results from destruction of ganglion cells in the esophageal wall, affecting the lower esophageal sphincter, which impairs lower esophageal sphincter relaxation. The exact mechanism of ganglion cell destruction in achalasia is unknown, but autoimmune, viral, and degenerative etiologies have been proposed [157].

Clinical Features

Most cases of achalasia are primary, but a small proportion of cases is secondary to a number of conditions including an obstructing esophageal malignancy, Chagas disease, amyloidosis, functional obstruction due to fundoplication or by gastric banding procedures, or Triple-A syndrome [158]. The annual incidence of achalasia is approximately 100,000 cases per year [158, 159]. Patients present with progressively worsening dysphagia, chest pain, odynophagia, food/drink regurgitation, and weight loss [160, 161]. Dysphagia first appears with solid foods but typically progresses to arise from liquids as well. Retained esophageal contents can be aspirated into the lungs. Esophagography with barium swallow typically shows tapering of the distal esophagus and the so-called "bird's beak" sign at the level of the esophageal hiatus (Fig. 5.21a); this study is sensitive and specific for the diagnosis of achalasia [162]. Achalasia can be managed medically, with injections of botulinum toxin into the lower esophageal sphincter, with endoscopic dilatation techniques, or with Heller's myotomy [163–166].

Gross Findings

The diagnosis of achalasia is typically obtained via esophagographic and manometric techniques; endoscopy is usually only performed to rule out other potential causes for obstruction of the lower esophageal sphincter (biopsies often obtained for this purpose). Grossly, the esophagus is typically dilated with narrowing of the lower esophageal sphincter (Fig. 5.21b).

Microscopic Findings

In the early stages of the disease, an inflammatory infiltrate, consisting predominantly of CD3-positive T lymphocytes [167–169], accompanied by some eosinophils, involves the esophageal myenteric plexus. The lymphocytic infiltrate can form follicles with germinal centers. The esophageal submucosal glands often show a lymphocytic infiltrate with variable degrees of glandular atrophy. With disease progression, ganglion cells in the myenteric plexus begin to disappear (Fig. 5.21c, d); this is the histologic hallmark of achalasia [168, 170]; as myenteric ganglion cells are destroyed, they become replaced by fibrosis. Hypertrophy of muscularis propria (Fig. 5.21e) also occurs at this point. The overlying squamous esophageal mucosa becomes hyperplastic, with associated papillomatosis and basal cell hyperplasia, resembling reflux esophagitis [171]. In some cases, the mucosal changes can closely resemble lymphocytic esophagitis.

Differential Diagnosis

The mucosal histologic features seen in achalasia are nonspecific; endoscopic mucosal biopsies in achalasia often resemble reflux esophagitis, infection, and sometimes lymphocytic esophagitis [172, 173]. It is important to recognize that such endoscopic biopsies are not usually obtained to arrive at a diagnosis of achalasia but are rather performed to rule out other potential causes of the lower esophageal

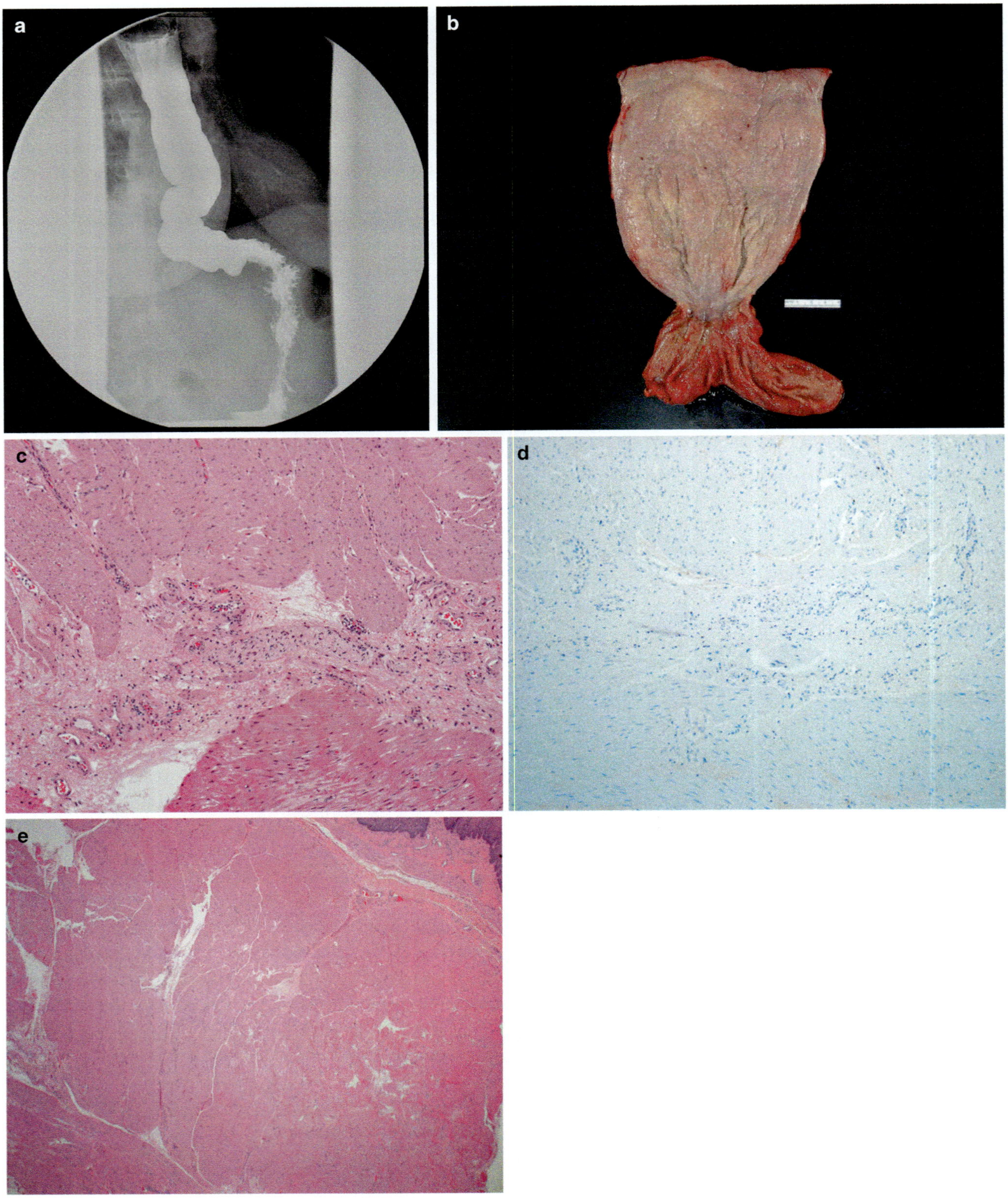

Fig. 5.21 Achalasia. Esophagography with barium swallow shows pneumatic dilatation of the esophagus with narrowing of the distal esophagus, producing the so-called "bird's beak" sign (**a**). Grossly, the esophagus is typically dilated with narrowing of the lower esophageal sphincter (**b**). The histologic hallmark of achalasia is the absence of ganglion cells in the myenteric plexus (**c**). Immunostaining for calretinin confirms the absence of ganglion cells in the myenteric plexus (**d**). Hypertrophy of muscularis propria is often seen in esophageal involvement by achalasia (**e**)

sphincter obstruction; the actual diagnosis of achalasia relies more heavily on esophagographic and manometric findings than on endoscopic and histologic features. Therefore, correlation with the findings of barium swallow and manometric studies can help pathologists better understand the purpose of the endoscopic biopsy and avoid misinterpretation of the etiology of mucosal changes.

Mallory-Weiss Syndrome and Boerhaave's Syndrome

Definition

Mallory-Weiss syndrome or tear is laceration of the mucosa near the gastroesophageal junction, which usually leads to bleeding/hematemesis. This is usually caused by severe violent vomiting and retching.

Boerhaave's syndrome represents a full-thickness tear in the esophageal wall due to a sudden increase in intraesophageal pressure combined with relatively negative intrathoracic pressure.

Clinical Features

Most patients affected by Mallory-Weiss syndrome are men (average age above 60 years). Hiatal hernia is present in many patients and is considered a risk factor for Mallory-Weiss syndrome [174, 175]. Triggers of the mucosal tear include violent vomiting/retching in individuals with heavy alcohol use or eating disorders (bulimia) or in any condition that can cause severe vomiting/retching such as food poisoning [176–178]. Other precipitating factors include violent coughing, blunt abdominal trauma, and violent cardiopulmonary resuscitation [179]. Hyperemesis gravidarum (severe morning sickness associated with vomiting and retching in pregnant women), is another known cause of Mallory-Weiss syndrome [180].

Patients present with hematemesis or less commonly melena. Presentation is most frequently associated with violent retching or vomiting, but the latter is not present in all cases. Definitive diagnosis is reached by endoscopy. The prognosis is good, and bleeding stops spontaneously in most cases within 48–72 hours. In a minority of severe cases, which can rarely be fatal, endoscopic and/or surgical treatments are indicated.

The term "Boerhaave's syndrome" is reserved to cases of full-thickness esophageal tear related to retching/vomiting (approximately 10% of all esophageal perforations); most esophageal perforations are nowadays caused by esophageal instrumentation (such as endoscopy or thoracic surgery) [181, 182]. Esophageal perforation in Boerhaave's syndrome results from sudden increase in intraesophageal pressure combined with relatively negative intrathoracic pressure caused by straining or retching/vomiting.

The classic clinical presentation of Boerhaave's syndrome is that of severe retching/vomiting followed by acute onset of excruciating retrosternal thoracic and upper abdominal pain. This can be followed by fever, tachypnea, dyspnea, cyanosis, and shock. The chest pain can sometimes radiate to the left shoulder, mimicking myocardial infarction. Mackler's triad (chest pain, vomiting, and subcutaneous emphysema) is relatively specific for Boerhaave's syndrome but is only detected in a minority of patients [183]. Typically, acute upper gastrointestinal bleeding is not seen in this condition, which helps distinguish it from the more common Mallory-Weiss syndrome.

The diagnosis of Boerhaave's syndrome is suggested by thoracic and cervical plain radiography and can be confirmed by chest computed tomography (CT) scan or contrast esophagography [184, 185]. Esophagoscopy has no role in the diagnosis of Boerhaave's syndrome; the endoscope and insufflation of air can extend the perforation and introduce air into the mediastinum [186].

Boerhaave's syndrome is associated with high morbidity and mortality and is fatal without treatment. The vast majority of patients will require some type of surgical intervention, which is usually dictated by the location and extent of esophageal injury.

Gross Findings

Mallory-Weiss tears involve the mucosa and submucosa and are located in the distal esophagus, gastroesophageal junction, and/or proximal stomach. The muscularis propria is intact in Mallory-Weiss syndrome. In contrast, the tear involves the full thickness of the esophageal wall in Boerhaave's syndrome. Boerhaave's perforations are most often located in the left posterolateral aspect of the distal esophagus (2–3 cm proximal to the gastroesophageal junction) and can extend up to several centimeters in length [187, 188].

Microscopic Findings

Specimens are not usually obtained for surgical pathology evaluation in patients with Mallory-Weiss and Boerhaave's syndromes; the diagnosis is typically made clinically and by endoscopic and imaging techniques. Histologic examination in both conditions reveals longitudinal tears, associated with inflammation, hemorrhage, and organizing fibrin; the tears are limited to the mucosa and submucosa in Mallory-Weiss syndrome, and involve the full thickness of the esophageal wall in Boerhaave's syndrome.

Differential Diagnosis

Clinically, the symptoms can be misleading, and both conditions can be misdiagnosed; for instance, Boerhaave's syndrome can be mistaken for myocardial infarction, pancreatitis, pericarditis, or spontaneous pneumothorax. The pathology, on the other hand, is relatively specific in the clinical context of both conditions.

Congenital Disorders

Esophageal Webs and Rings

Definition

An esophageal web is a thin (<2 mm) eccentric membrane of tissue in the esophagus. An esophageal ring is a concentric thin (2–5 mm) diaphragm of tissue growing into the esophageal lumen.

Clinical Features

Esophageal webs are most common in the anterior proximal esophagus. Most patients are asymptomatic; therefore, the exact prevalence of esophageal webs is not known but is found in 5%–15% of patients with dysphagia [189]. When patients are symptomatic, they present with dysphagia. If esophageal webs are associated with iron-deficiency anemia, glossitis, and koilonychia, the terms Plummer-Vinson or Paterson-Kelly syndrome can be used [190]. Webs seen in this setting respond to treatment of the underlying iron-deficiency state [189, 190]. Esophageal webs are also associated with other conditions, including thyroid disease, Zenker's diverticula, esophageal duplication cysts, blistering skin diseases, Stevens-Johnson syndrome, psoriasis, and idiopathic eosinophilic gastroenteritis [189]. The etiology of esophageal webs is unknown, but they likely represent remnants of incomplete vacuolation of the esophageal columnar epithelium during the early embryonic stage.

Esophageal rings (Fig. 5.22) most commonly involve the distal esophagus. "A" rings (also known as lower esophageal muscular rings) are located 1.5 cm proximal to the squamocolumnar junction. "B" rings (also known as a Schatzki's ring) involve the squamocolumnar junction at the proximal border of a hiatal hernia. Like esophageal webs, most esophageal rings are asymptomatic, and the true prevalence is therefore unknown, but esophageal rings are found in 6%–14% of routine barium radiographs [189]. Multiple esophageal rings (ringed esophagus) are rare and have been

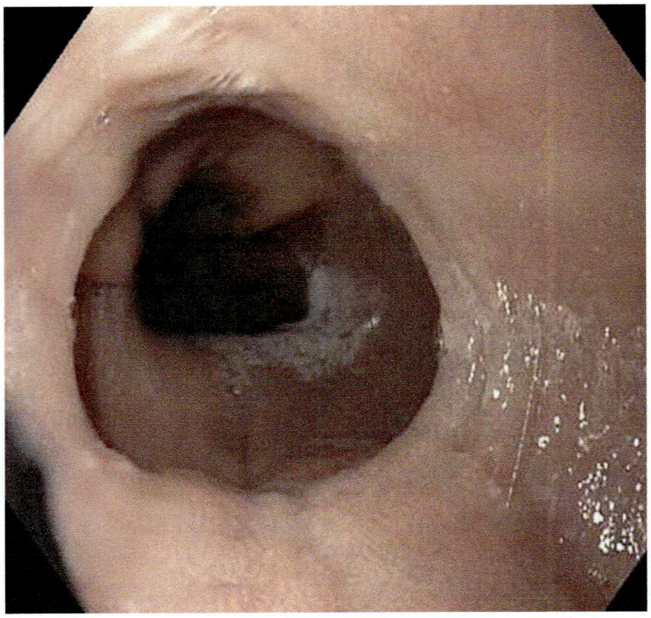

Fig. 5.22 Esophageal ring. This endoscopic image shows a concentric thin diaphragm of tissue growing into the esophageal lumen consistent with an esophageal ring

found in association with gastroesophageal reflux and asthma in the small number of reported cases. Although many patients are asymptomatic, when symptoms occur, they include dysphagia, regurgitation, and aspiration. The etiology of esophageal rings is unknown; they are thought to be congenital, but pill-induced esophageal inflammation may also play a role in the development and/or progression of esophageal rings [189].

Microscopic Findings

Microscopically, esophageal webs are composed of mucosa and submucosa with chronic inflammation, covering fibroconnective tissue. Esophageal rings likewise consist of mucosa and submucosa. The squamous mucosa in esophageal rings shows basal cell hyperplasia, hyperkeratosis, chronic inflammation, and increased intraepithelial eosinophils, which can be very prominent, representing a subtype of eosinophilic esophagitis. Mucosal chronic inflammatory changes can extend to short distances above and below the rings.

Differential Diagnosis

From a clinical standpoint, the differential diagnosis of an esophageal web includes inflammatory stenosis, postcricoid carcinoma, and postcricoid impression due to ventral venous plexus [189].The diagnosis of esophageal webs and rings is made on clinical, radiologic, and endoscopic grounds; endoscopic biopsies are not of diagnostic utility, and their histology is not specific. In esophageal rings, there is histologic overlap with reflux and eosinophilic esophagitis; review of the radiologic and endoscopic findings should direct the pathologist to the correct diagnosis.

Esophageal Diverticula

Definition

Esophageal diverticula represent full-thickness outpouchings of the esophagus encompassing all layers of the esophageal wall.

Clinical Features

Esophageal diverticula are uncommon and occur most commonly in elderly men. There are three types of esophageal diverticula. First, cervical diverticula (Zenker's diverticula), the most common type of esophageal diverticula, occur in the area of the cricopharyngeous muscle [191]; their prevalence in the general population is between 0.01% and 0.11% and 1.8%–2.3% in patients with dysphagia. Second, midesophageal diverticula (epiphrenic diverticula) arise in the middle third of the esophagus, most often at the level of the bifurcation of the trachea. Most midesophageal diverticula are thought to occur because of esophageal dysmotility, wherein high luminal pressure produces an outpouching in weak areas of the esophageal wall [192]. Third, epiphrenic diverticula arise from the distal esophagus proximal to the lower esophageal sphincter; they also likely represent pulsion diverticula and can also be associated with manometric abnormalities, including "nutcracker" esophagus, diffuse esophageal spasm, achalasia, hypertensive lower esophageal sphincter, and other esophageal motility disorders [189].

Microscopic Findings

Pathologically, esophageal diverticula are outpouchings of the esophagus that contain all the layers of the esophageal wall. In Zenker's diverticulum, cricopharyngeous muscle fibers can show degenerative changes and replacement by fibroadipose tissue [189].

Esophageal Pseudodiverticulosis

Definition

Esophageal pseudodiverticula are intramural outpouchings that consist of dilated and inflamed submucosal gland ducts. Because they do not consist of true outpouchings of all esophageal wall layers, they do not represent true diverticula.

Clinical Features

Esophageal pseudodiverticulosis is uncommon and typically develops in the elderly. It is almost always associated with an esophageal stricture involving the upper or middle esophagus. About one third of patients have associated *Candida* esophagitis; another association is esophageal dysmotility disorders, including achalasia [189]. Patients present with dysphagia, usually secondary to the underlying esophageal stricture. The diagnosis can be made by barium radiography (the most sensitive diagnostic method), which shows numerous small, flask-shaped outpouchings in the esophageal wall. Patients might have an increased risk of esophageal carcinoma, but this still needs to be confirmed by further studies [189]. Treatment of esophageal pseudodiverticulosis aims at the underlying obstruction and associated inflammation; symptoms usually respond to dilation of the underlying stricture. Patients with evidence of *Candida* esophagitis should be treated medically. The condition appears to remain stable over long periods of time [193, 194]. The underlying pathogenesis of esophageal pseudodiverticulosis is unclear, but the condition does not appear to be pulsion related. Possible etiologies include primary glandular secretory dysfunction, abnormal esophageal motility, or chronic recurrent inflammatory conditions [189, 193].

Gross Findings

Although the small outpouchings can occasionally be seen during upper endoscopy, this method is not usually helpful for diagnosis because the orifices are difficult to recognize and are usually concealed by nonspecific mucosal inflammatory changes.

Microscopic Findings

Histologic examination of resected specimens with esophageal pseudodiverticulosis reveals cystically dilated submucosal glands and gland ducts, lined by cuboidal or squamous epithelium, with a prominent surrounding inflammatory infiltrate consisting of lymphocytes, plasma cells, and eosinophils (Fig. 5.23a, b). Ruptured pseudodiverticula can also have an associated foreign body giant cell reaction. Sometimes, the squamous epithelium lining the pseudodiverticula can be quite abundant, entirely replacing the entire submucosal glands and gland ducts. The overall well-rounded glandular contour, however, is preserved. These histologic features are best appreciated in resection specimens; on the other hand, endoscopic mucosal biopsies are usually not helpful because they do not provide good representation of the pseudodiverticula that area seated deep in the submucosal [195].

Differential Diagnosis

The squamous epithelium lining the pseudodiverticula can become proliferative, entirely replacing the entire submucosal glands and gland ducts and raising consideration for invasive squamous cell carcinoma. In esophageal pseudodiverticulosis, however, the overall well-rounded glandular contour is preserved, and there is no infiltrative growth pattern. This, along with the lack of overlying squamous dyspla-

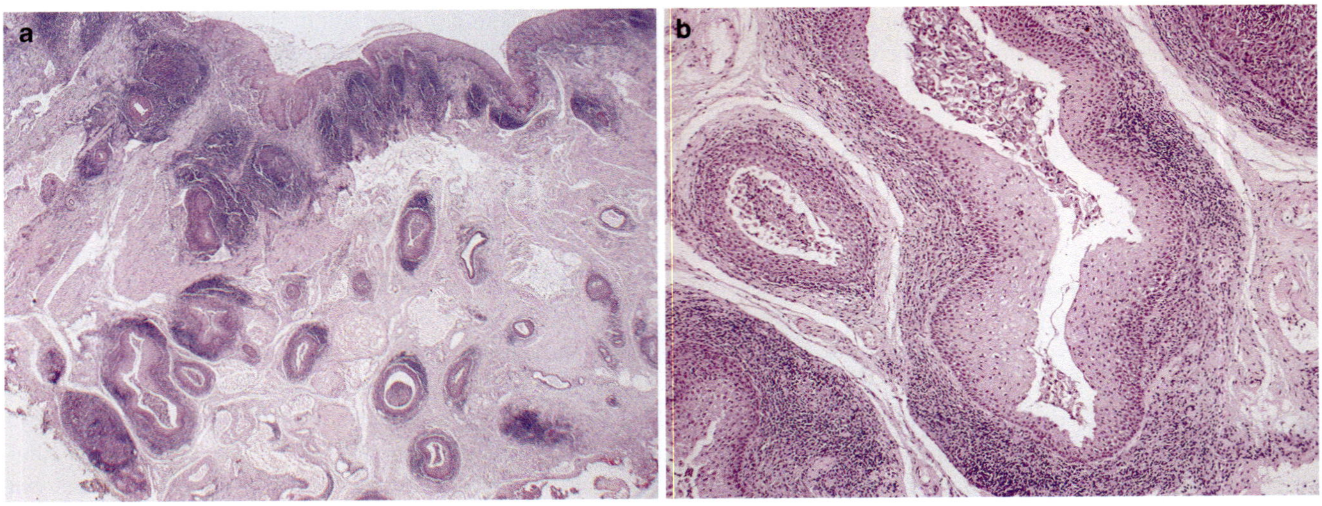

Fig. 5.23 Esophageal pseudodiverticulosis. The esophagus shows cystically dilated submucosal glands and gland ducts, lined by squamous epithelium (**a**), with a prominent surrounding inflammatory infiltrate consisting of lymphocytes, plasma cells, and eosinophils (**b**)

sia, should help distinguish pseudodiverticula from invasive squamous cell carcinoma.

Heterotopic and Ectopic Tissue

Definition

Inlet patches (gastric heterotopia) are islands of heterotopic gastric mucosa present in the esophagus, completely separated from the gastric mucosa by normal squamous esophageal mucosa. Ectopic sebaceous glands consist of sebaceous glands, morphologically identical to dermal sebaceous glands, aberrantly located in the squamous esophageal mucosa.

Clinical Features

Gastric heterotopia ("inlet patch") is the most common type of heterotopia found in the esophagus; they are present in 2%–11% of the general population [196–198]. They can be identified in individuals of all ages but are most frequently detected in individuals in the mid-50s [199]. Based on autopsy studies, ectopic sebaceous glands are identified in approximately 2% of individuals. Gastric heterotopia, which are believed to be congenital [200], are most often found in the upper third of the esophagus, usually in the proximal 3 cm, just distal to the upper esophageal sphincter [201–203]. Most patients are asymptomatic. When symptoms occur, they result from acidic secretions of the heterotopic mucosa and/or associated inflammation/erosion, which can cause heartburn and dysphagia. Potential complications include bleeding, perforation, and stricture formation [204, 205]. In addition, adenocarcinomas may rarely arise from inlet patches [206, 207]. Interestingly, if the stomach is infected by *Helicobacter pylori* gastritis, the heterotopic mucosa shows concurrent colonization by the organisms in 19%–73% of patients [208–210]. The diagnosis is usually made endoscopically, based on visual inspection alone. If there is doubt, however, biopsies can be obtained. Inlet patches are only treated if complications develop.

Gross Findings

In gastric heterotopia, the lesions are red, velvety patches in the esophageal mucosa that are usually flat but can occasionally be polypoid [211]. They range in greatest dimension from 2 to 5 mm and can be solitary or multiple [209, 212]. Ectopic sebaceous tissue endoscopically appears as yellow bumps.

Microscopic Findings

Histologically, inlet patches feature gastric-type mucosa, most commonly of fundic type (Fig. 5.24a), but antral phenotype can also occur (Fig. 5.24b). Although most cases contain both gastric glands and foveolar epithelium, superficial biopsies can only contain foveolar epithelium. Most inlet patches have associated inflammation. Pancreatic acinar tissue can be seen occasionally in inlet patches but no intestinal metaplasia is found [199, 202, 209]. *Helicobacter pylori* organisms can be identified in a subset of patients with *Helicobacter pylori* gastritis. Ectopic sebaceous glands consist of sebaceous glands, morphologically identical to dermal sebaceous glands, aberrantly located in the squamous esophageal mucosa (Fig. 5.25a, b).

Differential Diagnosis

The identification of columnar epithelium in the esophagus can raise concern for Barrett esophagus. In contrast to Barrett esophagus, which involves the distal esophagus, inlet patches usually involve the proximal esophagus. Furthermore, inlet

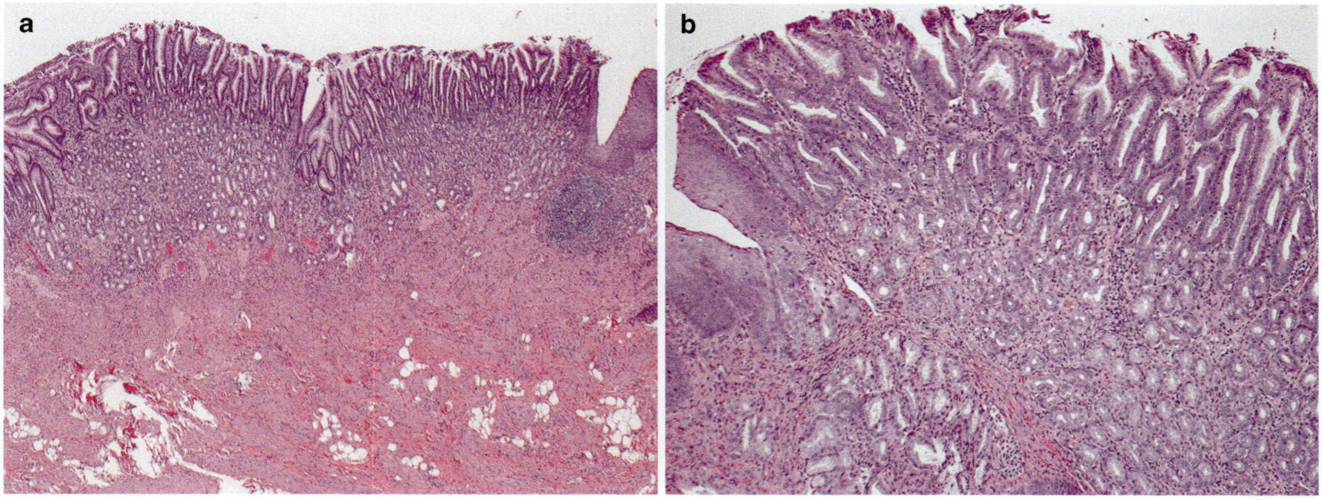

Fig. 5.24 Gastric heterotopia. Gastric heterotopia consists of an island of gastric mucosa completely separated from the stomach by normal squamous esophageal mucosa (right end of the image). This is often associated with inflammation (lymphoid aggregate, right) (**a**). Although most cases of gastric heterotopia are of fundic phenotype, this example is of antral phenotype, featuring gastric mucus glands and foveolar epithelium (**b**)

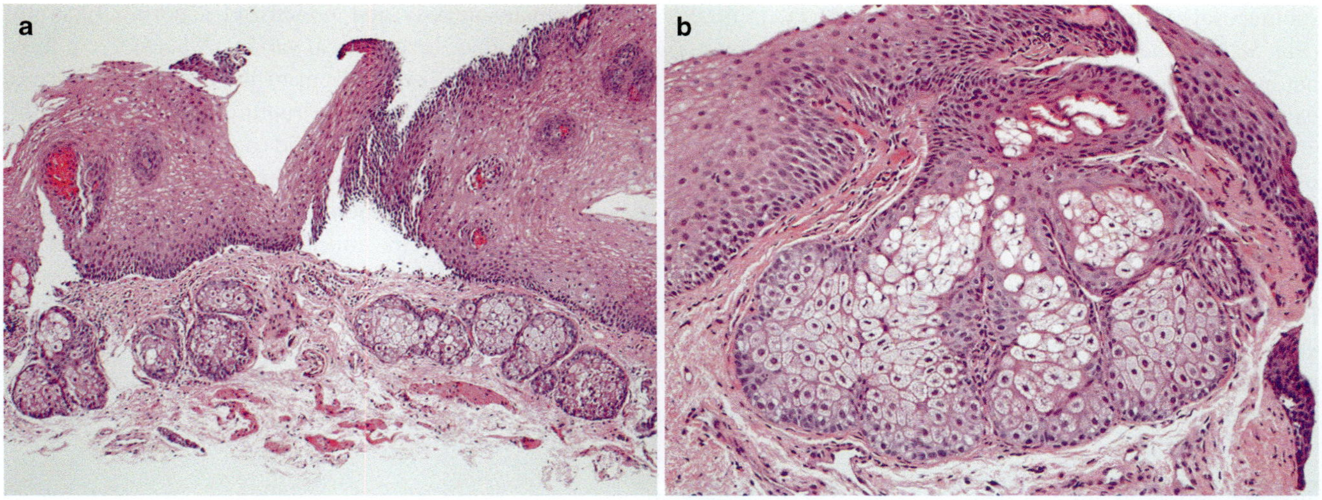

Fig. 5.25 Ectopic sebaceous glands. Ectopic sebaceous glands consist of sebaceous glands, morphologically identical to dermal sebaceous glands, aberrantly located in the squamous esophageal mucosa (**a**). The ectopic sebaceous glands are located in the lamina propria of the squamous esophageal mucosa (**b**)

patches lack the intestinal metaplasia and are separated from the stomach by normal squamous epithelium. Ectopic sebaceous glands can resemble glycogenic acanthosis endoscopically, but the two entities are easily distinguished histologically.

Miscellaneous Disorders

Acute Esophageal Necrosis

Definition

Acute esophageal necrosis, also known as black esophagus, is a unique esophageal condition characterized by mucosal friability and necrosis, causing blackening of the distal esophagus with a sharp demarcation at the gastroesophageal junction.

Clinical Features

Acute esophageal necrosis is very rare, with a reported incidence of 0.01%–0.2% in patients undergoing upper endoscopy [213–215]. The mean age at diagnosis is 68 years [214, 216]. Established risk factors include alcohol abuse (binge drinking) and duodenal ulcers [214, 217, 218]. Most patients present with upper gastrointestinal bleeding [214]. The exact pathogenesis of this disorder remains unknown, but most believe that acute esophageal necrosis is likely the result of hypoperfusion-associated ischemia [214, 217–219]. This condition can be fatal; the reported mortality rate attributed to acute esophageal necrosis is up to 50% [213, 216, 220–222]. The diagnosis is made endoscopically, based on the unique gross appearance. The treatment approach is mainly supportive [217].

Gross Findings

Endoscopically, acute esophageal necrosis is characterized by dark brown to black discoloration of the esophagus, whose mucosa appears necrotic, friable, and ulcerated (Fig. 5.26a). The lesion is identified in the mid and distal portions with a sharp demarcation at the gastroesophageal junction; the stomach is usually unremarkable [222].

Microscopic Findings

Because the endoscopic picture is very characteristic, the diagnosis is made endoscopically and no biopsy is usually obtained. Nevertheless, microscopic examination shows extensive mucosal sloughing, necrosis of residual mucosa, submucosal edema, and an acute inflammatory infiltrate (Fig. 5.26b). The inflammation is not confined to the mucosa but extends through the esophageal wall. Ischemic changes have been described in the muscularis propria, but it is usually intact. A characteristic finding is the presence of brown pigmentation in the mucosa; the pigment is positive for PAS (with and without diastase digestion) and might represent lipofuscin.

Differential Diagnosis

The endoscopic differential diagnosis includes melanosis, pseudomelanosis, coal dust deposition, corrosive esophagitis, and acanthosis nigricans [217, 219, 222]. Microscopically, distinction from these entities is generally straightforward. Histologic distinction from melanosis and pseudomelanosis is facilitated by the use of melanin and iron stains, if necessary. Melanosis shows a positive melanin stain, and pseudomelanosis can be positive for both melanin and iron stains.

Esophageal Varices

Definition

Esophageal varices are dilated and tortuous veins located in the esophageal mucosa and submucosa that bulge into the esophageal lumen as a result of portal hypertension and porto-systemic shunting.

Clinical Features

Esophageal varices usually develop in conditions that cause portal hypertension, most commonly as result of hepatic cirrhosis (particularly alcoholic cirrhosis) [223]. Portal hypertension not associated with liver cirrhosis (e.g., schistosomiasis and noncirrhotic portal hypertension) also produces esophageal varices. Varices occur most frequently in the distal 3–4 cm of the esophagus. Varices are asymptomatic unless they rupture and bleed, causing hematemesis or melena. Ruptured esophageal varices are a serious complication of portal hypertension, leading to death in 20%–30% in patients with cirrhotic portal hypertension [224]. After the initial bleeding, episodes of rebleeding are frequent. Varices are treated with sclerosis and banding techniques, portosystemic shunting, and medical management of portal hypertension [225]. In patients with end-stage cirrhosis, liver transplantation causes the varices to regress.

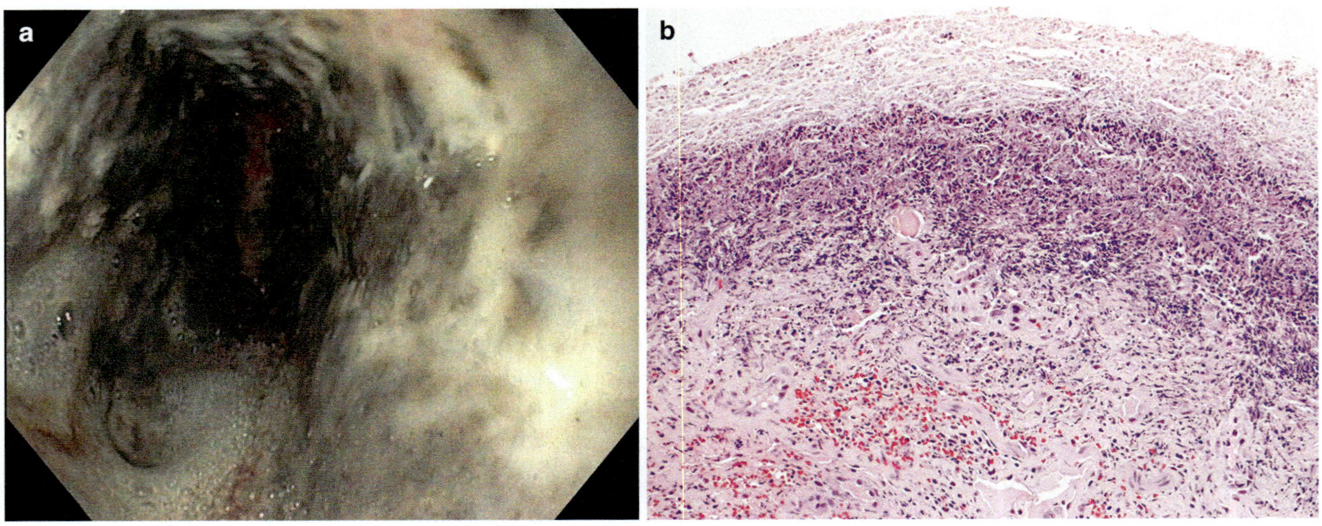

Fig. 5.26 Acute esophageal necrosis. Endoscopically, acute esophageal necrosis is characterized by the presence of friable, dark-brown to black-colored mucosa, indicating extensive mucosal necrosis (**a**). Esophageal biopsy shows extensive mucosal sloughing and necrosis, submucosal edema, and an acute inflammatory infiltrate (**b**)

Gross Findings

Endoscopically, dilated and tortuous veins are identified bulging into the lumen of the distal esophagus. Focally, fresh hemorrhage and/or thrombosis can sometimes be observed. Because varices tend to collapse upon cessation of blood flow (tissue removal), they are better appreciated endoscopically in comparison to pathologic specimens (autopsies or resections); in autopsy specimens, pinned fixation of the open esophagus can help demonstrate varices. Likewise, identification of a bleeding site in esophageal varices can also be challenging in pathology specimens.

Microscopic Findings

Histologic examination shows dilated veins in the esophageal mucosa and submucosa filled with blood. Organizing thrombosis can sometimes be identified. The overlying mucosa can also demonstrate erosion, ulceration, and associated inflammation; these features often occur after the application of therapeutic sclerosis and/or banding techniques [226, 227].

Glycogenic Acanthosis

Definition

Glycogenic acanthosis is a benign entity of unknown pathogenesis, characterized by the presence of small raised esophageal plaques usually identified endoscopically.

Clinical Features

Glycogenic acanthosis is a common endoscopic finding, probably affecting up to 25% of the general population. Despite its name, glycogenic acanthosis is not associated with skin disorders or abnormalities of glucose metabolism, and has no clear relationship to smoking, alcohol or hot liquid intake, or GERD [76, 228]. The only known clinical associations of glycogenic acanthosis are Cowden syndrome or tuberous sclerosis; both conditions can be associated with extensive glycogenic acanthosis [229]. In fact, the presence of extensive glycogenic acanthosis in association with gastrointestinal polyposis has been proposed to be pathognomonic for the diagnosis of Cowden's disease. Unless there is a coexisting disease, patients with glycogenic acanthosis are asymptomatic [230]. The etiology of glycogenic acanthosis is unknown; a possible pathogenesis could be age-related degenerative change of the squamous esophageal epithelium [231].

Gross Findings

Endoscopy shows multiple white mucosal elevations or plaques usually measuring less than 0.5 cm. The lesions are surrounded by normal mucosa and are most commonly found in the lower esophagus. The lesions can be extensive in syndrome patients, assuming a confluent conglomeration with a cobblestone mucosal pattern.

Microscopic Findings

Histologically, the squamous epithelium is focally thickened by groups of enlarged and clear cells located in the upper layers of the squamous epithelium (Fig. 5.27a). The enlarged and clear appearance of these cells is a result of abundant cytoplasmic glycogen [76, 230, 231]. The glycogen contents can sometimes be highlighted by PAS stain (Fig. 5.27b). There is no epithelial atypia or inflammation.

Differential Diagnosis

Glycogenic acanthosis lesions have a unique endoscopic appearance. Therefore, the lesions are typically recognized

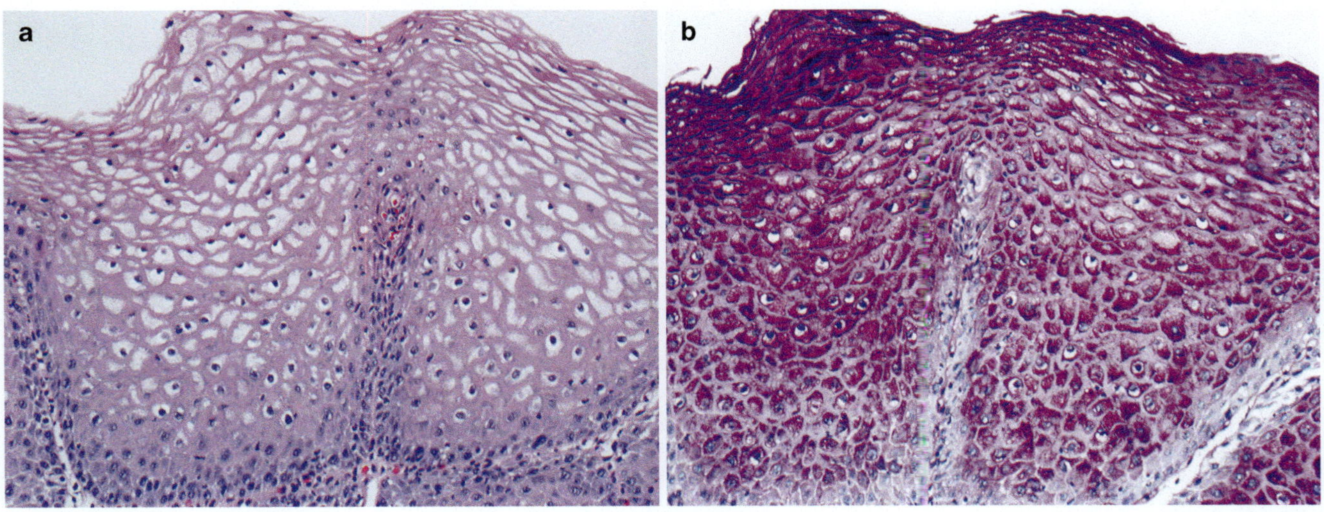

Fig. 5.27 Glycogenic acanthosis. In glycogenic acanthosis, the squamous epithelium features thickening by groups of enlarged and clear cells located in the upper layers of the squamous epithelium (**a**). PAS stain highlights the increased glycogen contents of the distended squamous cells (**b**)

endoscopically and not usually biopsied. On occasion, however, the lesions can be macroscopically confused with *Candida* plaques or leukoplakia. Biopsies of such lesions can be easily differentiated from *Candida* and leukoplakia by the absence of organisms, inflammation, and epidermoid metaplasia and by the presence of patchy epithelial thickening by groups of enlarged and clear cells located in the upper layers of the squamous epithelium, typical for glycogenic acanthosis.

Inflammatory/Hyperplastic Polyps

Definition

Inflammatory or hyperplastic polyps, also known as inflammatory esophagogastric polyp, are benign non-neoplastic polyps of the esophagus that result from an exaggerated response to mucosal injury.

Clinical Features

Although uncommon, inflammatory/hyperplastic polyps are the most common benign squamous lined polyps of the esophagus. They occur most frequently in men and have a predilection to arise in the distal esophagus near the gastroesophageal junction. Inflammatory/hyperplastic polyps are associated with GERD and Barrett esophagus [232–235]. They are not associated with risk of malignant transformation. Inflammatory/hyperplastic polyps are thought to represent an exaggerated response to mucosal injury of various types, such as GERD, healing ulcers, protracted vomiting, Crohn's disease, and sclerotherapy for varices. When these polyps arise proximal to the gastroesophageal junction, they are often associated with surgical anastomoses, pill-induced esophagitis, or infection [236]. Inflammatory/hyperplastic polyps can be treated with endoscopic mucosal resection or other methods of excision [237].

Microscopic Findings

Inflammatory/hyperplastic polyps can be lined by squamous or columnar epithelium or both. The columnar epithelial phenotype arises near the gastroesophageal junction and features hyperplastic primarily gastric-type foveolar epithelium with ulceration, edema, and lamina propria inflammation (Fig. 5.28a, b) [236]. If lined purely by squamous epithelium, the polyps usually have smooth surface and are lined by elongated and irregular tongues of squamous epithelium that extends deep into the underlying lamina propria. Because this phenotype can harbor human papillomaviruses (HPV), it is debatable whether it represents true inflammatory/hyperplastic polyps or endophytic type squamous papilloma [238]. Such polyps might still arise in association with various forms of mucosal injury such as GERD; HPV might promote epithelial growth following this initial damage [238].

Differential Diagnosis

As mentioned above, inflammatory/hyperplastic polyps lined purely by squamous epithelium can overlap with the endophytic-type squamous papilloma. The columnar phenotype can show marked epithelial atypia arising in association with significant inflammation and erosion/ulceration; these

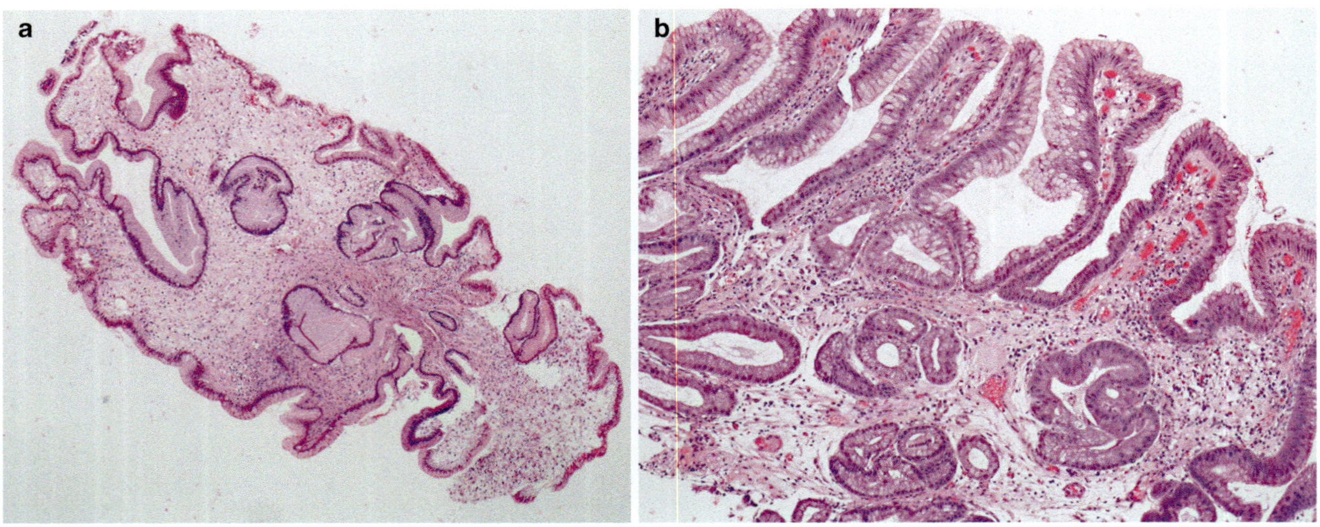

Fig. 5.28 Inflammatory/hyperplastic polyp. An esophageal hyperplastic polyp arising near the GE junction is lined by columnar gastric-type mucosa; it shows foveolar hyperplasia and mucosal edema (**a**); higher-power view shows foveolar hyperplasia, lamina propria edema, and inflammation (**b**)

changes could be mistaken for columnar epithelial dysplasia. In contrast to columnar epithelial dysplasia, however, the atypical reactive epithelium lacks architectural complexity, retains surface maturation, and tends to be most evident in areas of inflammation and erosion/ulceration. Furthermore, the atypical nuclei tend to have open chromatin and prominent nucleoli, in opposition to the hyperchromatic changes usually seen in dysplasia.

Squamous Papilloma

Definition

Esophageal squamous papillomas are benign esophageal polyps consisting of mature stratified squamous epithelium overlying lamina propria.

Clinical Features

Squamous papillomas are the most common benign tumor of the esophagus [238–240]. However, they are still rare; less than 1% of individuals develop them, but some suggest that they may be underdiagnosed [239]. Most patients are asymptomatic; the papilloma is usually an incidental finding during endoscopy. Large tumors, however, can cause dysphagia and epigastric pain. The etiology of squamous papillomas includes HPV infection (detected in up to 86% of polyps) or chronic mucosal irritation from various forms of esophagitis including GERD and Barrett esophagus [238, 240, 241]. The majority (80%–90%) of tumors is solitary, and instances of papillomatosis are rare, usually arising in children [242, 243]. Although rare cases of squamous dysplasia and even carcinoma have been reported [243, 244], squamous papillomas are benign and are not considered premalignant [238, 245]. Squamous papilloma is treated with endoscopic excision and recurrence is rare [246].

Gross Findings

Endoscopically, squamous papillomas are small (usually measuring less than 1 cm), pink to white, sessile and soft polyps. In rare instances, papillomas can be larger, measuring up to 3 cm. Most squamous papillomas involve the distal and middle esophagus. A cauliflower-like appearance is associated with the exophytic microscopic type (see below).

Microscopic Findings

Squamous papilloma have three main histologic types [238]:

1. Exophytic: This is the most common type of squamous papilloma. It most frequently arises in the distal esophagus. Microscopically (Fig. 5.29a), this type features branching finger-like papillae lined by mature thickened squamous epithelium, overlying delicate fibrovascular cores of lamina propria. HPV is frequently found in this subtype (Fig. 5.29b, c), involving up 78% of tumors [238, 247]; koilocytosis may be present.
2. Endophytic: The endophytic type of papilloma has a round, smooth surface and is lined by elongated and irregular tongues of thickened squamous epithelium showing inverted growth and extending deep into the underlying lamina propria. Some consider these tumors as a variant of inflammatory/hyperplastic polyps.
3. Spiked (verrucoid): This is the least common type of squamous papilloma. This type has a verrucous appearance, featuring a corrugated surface with acanthosis, hyperkeratosis, and a prominent granular cell layer. HPV is present in approximately 40% of cases [238].

All the abovementioned types frequently show lamina propria inflammation and vascular congestion. The squamous epithelium is acanthotic in all types and shows reactive changes and hyperplasia of the basal layer. Surface maturation is preserved.

Differential Diagnosis

The differential diagnosis includes pseudoepitheliomatous hyperplasia, squamous cell carcinoma, and verrucous carcinoma. Pseudoepitheliomatous hyperplasia is a reactive process that develops in association with mucosal ulcerations and erosions. The squamous epithelium is acanthotic and irregular and shows elongated and irregular tongues of thickened squamous epithelium. These features can mimic squamous papilloma. Pseudoepitheliomatous hyperplasia, however, does not present endoscopically as a discrete polyp, lacks true papillae and fibrovascular cores, and shows more pronounced inflammation and ulceration. Furthermore, pseudoepitheliomatous hyperplasia is negative for HPV and lacks koilocytosis.

Squamous papilloma is usually easily distinguished from squamous cell carcinoma and verrucous carcinoma. However, if a squamous papilloma is large and significantly inflamed/eroded, with associated marked epithelial atypia, it could raise consideration for carcinoma. In contrast to carcinoma, however, squamous papilloma, even in the presence of marked inflammation-associated epithelial atypia, retains surface maturation, lacks mitoses in the middle and upper thirds of the squamous epithelium, and lacks atypical mitotic figures. It also lacks the central keratinous crater characteristic of verrucous carcinoma. More importantly, squamous papilloma lacks the infiltrative growth pattern characteristic of squamous cell carcinoma. Finally, squamous papilloma, even if large, is a discrete polyp; in contrast, carcinoma forms a poorly demarcated mass that can be associated with stricture formation.

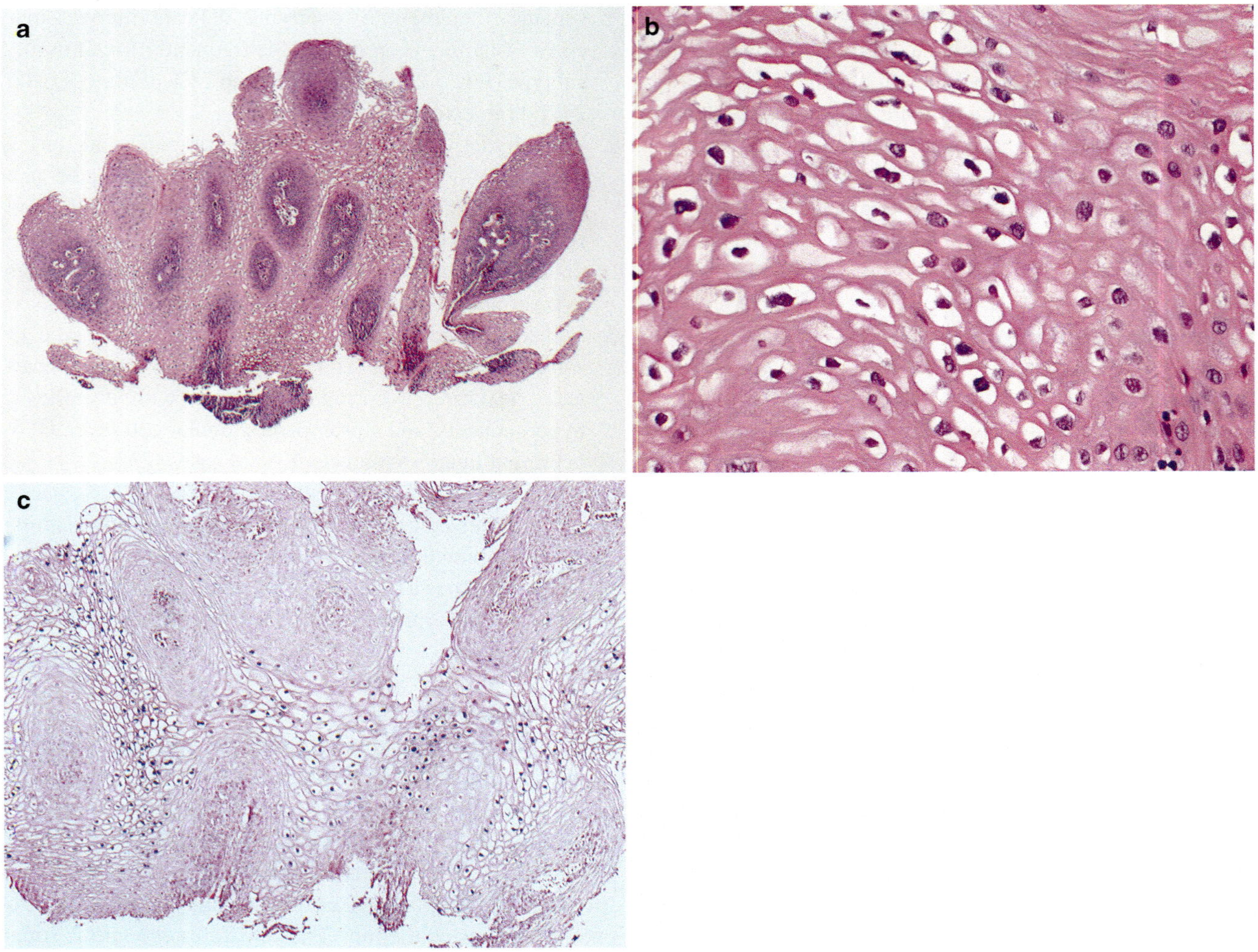

Fig. 5.29 Squamous papilloma. The exophytic type of squamous papilloma features branching finger-like papillae lined by mature squamous epithelium, overlying delicate fibrovascular cores of lamina propria (**a**). The exophytic type of squamous papilloma harbors HPV, suggested by the presence of koilocytic changes (**b**) and evidenced by positive in situ hybridization for low-risk HPV (**c**)

References

1. Abraham SC, Cruz-Correa M, Lee LA, Yardley JH, Wu TT. Alendronate-associated esophageal injury: pathologic and endoscopic features. Mod Pathol. 1999;12(12):1152–7.
2. Abraham SC, Yardley JH, Wu TT. Erosive injury to the upper gastrointestinal tract in patients receiving iron medication: an underrecognized entity. Am J Surg Pathol. 1999;23(10):1241–7.
3. Bott S, Prakash C, McCallum RW. Medication-induced esophageal injury: survey of the literature. Am J Gastroenterol. 1987;82(8):758–63.
4. Boyce HW Jr. Drug-induced esophageal damage: diseases of medical progress. Gastrointest Endosc. 1998;47(6):547–50.
5. Kikendall JW, Friedman AC, Oyewole MA, Fleischer D, Johnson LF. Pill-induced esophageal injury. Case reports and review of the medical literature. Dig Dis Sci. 1983;28(2):174–82.
6. Semble EL, Wu WC, Castell DO. Nonsteroidal antiinflammatory drugs and esophageal injury. Semin Arthritis Rheum. 1989;19(2):99–109.
7. Taha AS, Dahill S, Nakshabendi I, Lee FD, Sturrock RD, Russell RI. Oesophageal histology in long term users of non-steroidal anti-inflammatory drugs. J Clin Pathol. 1994;47(8):705–8.
8. Parfitt JR, Driman DK. Pathological effects of drugs on the gastrointestinal tract: a review. Hum Pathol. 2007;38(4):527–36. https://doi.org/10.1016/j.humpath.2007.01.014.
9. Lewis JH. Gastrointestinal injury due to medicinal agents. Am J Gastroenterol. 1986;81(9):819–34.
10. Kaye P, Abdulla K, Wood J, James P, Foley S, Ragunath K, et al. Iron-induced mucosal pathology of the upper gastrointestinal tract: a common finding in patients on oral iron therapy. Histopathology. 2008;53(3):311–7. https://doi.org/10.1111/j.1365-2559.2008.03081.x.
11. Haig A, Driman DK. Iron-induced mucosal injury to the upper gastrointestinal tract. Histopathology. 2006;48(7):808–12. https://doi.org/10.1111/j.1365-2559.2006.02448.x.
12. Abraham SC, Bhagavan BS, Lee LA, Rashid A, Wu TT. Upper gastrointestinal tract injury in patients receiving kayexalate (sodium polystyrene sulfonate) in sorbitol: clinical, endoscopic, and histopathologic findings. Am J Surg Pathol. 2001;25(5):637–44.
13. Gaduputi V, Tariq H, Ihimoyan A. A rare cause of esophagitis with crystal deposition. Can J Gastroenterol Hepatol. 2015;29(3):123–4.
14. Swanson BJ, Limketkai BN, Liu TC, Montgomery E, Nazari K, Park JY, et al. Sevelamer crystals in the gastrointestinal tract (GIT): a new entity associated with mucosal injury. Am

J Surg Pathol. 2013;37(11):1686–93. https://doi.org/10.1097/PAS.0b013e3182999d8d.
15. Stemmermann GN, Hayashi T. Colchicine intoxication. A reappraisal of its pathology based on a study of three fatal cases. Hum Pathol. 1971;2(2):321–32.
16. Iacobuzio-Donahue CA, Lee EL, Abraham SC, Yardley JH, Wu TT. Colchicine toxicity: distinct morphologic findings in gastrointestinal biopsies. Am J Surg Pathol. 2001;25(8):1067–73.
17. Daniels JA, Gibson MK, Xu L, Sun S, Canto MI, Heath E, et al. Gastrointestinal tract epithelial changes associated with taxanes: marker of drug toxicity versus effect. Am J Surg Pathol. 2008;32(3):473–7. https://doi.org/10.1097/PAS.0b013e3181582331.
18. Hruban RH, Yardley JH, Donehower RC, Boitnott JK. Taxol toxicity. Epithelial necrosis in the gastrointestinal tract associated with polymerized microtubule accumulation and mitotic arrest. Cancer. 1989;63(10):1944–50.
19. Novak JM, Collins JT, Donowitz M, Farman J, Sheahan DG, Spiro HM. Effects of radiation on the human gastrointestinal tract. J Clin Gastroenterol. 1979;1(1):9–39.
20. Trowers E, Thomas C Jr, Silverstein FE. Chemical- and radiation-induced esophageal injury. Gastrointest Endosc Clin N Am. 1994;4(4):657–75.
21. Davila M, Bresalier RS. Gastrointestinal complications of oncologic therapy. Nat Clin Pract Gastroenterol Hepatol. 2008;5(12):682–96. https://doi.org/10.1038/ncpgasthep1277.
22. Maguire PD, Sibley GS, Zhou SM, Jamieson TA, Light KL, Antoine PA, et al. Clinical and dosimetric predictors of radiation-induced esophageal toxicity. Int J Radiat Oncol Biol Phys. 1999;45(1):97–103.
23. Choy H, LaPorte K, Knill-Selby E, Mohr P, Shyr Y. Esophagitis in combined modality therapy for locally advanced non-small cell lung cancer. Semin Radiat Oncol. 1999;9(2 Suppl 1):90–6.
24. Qiao WB, Zhao YH, Zhao YB, Wang RZ. Clinical and dosimetric factors of radiation-induced esophageal injury: radiation-induced esophageal toxicity. World J Gastroenterol. 2005;11(17):2626–9.
25. O'Rourke IC, Tiver K, Bull C, Gebski V, Langlands AO. Swallowing performance after radiation therapy for carcinoma of the esophagus. Cancer. 1988;61(10):2022–6.
26. Coia LR, Myerson RJ, Tepper JE. Late effects of radiation therapy on the gastrointestinal tract. Int J Radiat Oncol Biol Phys. 1995;31(5):1213–36. https://doi.org/10.1016/0360-3016(94)00419-L.
27. Rubio CA, Sjodahl K, Lagergren J. Lymphocytic esophagitis: a histologic subset of chronic esophagitis. Am J Clin Pathol. 2006;125(3):432–7.
28. Purdy JK, Appelman HD, Golembeski CP, McKenna BJ. Lymphocytic esophagitis: a chronic or recurring pattern of esophagitis resembling allergic contact dermatitis. Am J Clin Pathol. 2008;130(4):508–13. https://doi.org/10.1309/D3PCF6D6YYMQRX9A.
29. Haque S, Genta RM. Lymphocytic oesophagitis: clinicopathological aspects of an emerging condition. Gut. 2012;61(8):1108–14. https://doi.org/10.1136/gutjnl-2011-301014.
30. Cohen S, Saxena A, Waljee AK, Piraka C, Purdy J, Appelman H, et al. Lymphocytic esophagitis: a diagnosis of increasing frequency. J Clin Gastroenterol. 2012;46(10):828–32. https://doi.org/10.1097/MCG.0b013e3182500de8.
31. Kasirye Y, John A, Rall C, Resnick J. Lymphocytic esophagitis presenting as chronic dysphagia. Clin Med Res. 2012;10(2):83–4. https://doi.org/10.3121/cmr.2011.1009.
32. Isolauri J, Markkula H. Lye ingestion and carcinoma of the esophagus. Acta Chir Scand. 1989;155(4–5):269–71.
33. de Jong AL, Macdonald R, Ein S, Forte V, Turner A. Corrosive esophagitis in children: a 30-year review. Int J Pediatr Otorhinolaryngol. 2001;57(3):203–11.
34. Garcia Diaz E, Castro Fernandez M, Romero Gomez M, Castilla Higuero L. Upper gastrointestinal tract injury caused by ingestion of caustic substances. Gastroenterol Hepatol. 2001;24(4):191–5.
35. Ein SH, Shandling B, Stephens CA. Twenty-one year experience with the pediatric gastric tube. J Pediatr Surg. 1987;22(1):77–81.
36. Friedman EM. Caustic ingestions and foreign bodies in the aerodigestive tract of children. Pediatr Clin N Am. 1989;36(6):1403–10.
37. Appelqvist P, Salmo M. Lye corrosion carcinoma of the esophagus: a review of 63 cases. Cancer. 1980;45(10):2655–8.
38. Cesar WG, Barrios MM, Maruta CW, Aoki V, Santi GG. Oesophagitis dissecans superficialis: an acute, benign phenomenon associated with pemphigus vulgaris. Clin Exp Dermatol. 2009;34(8):e614–6. https://doi.org/10.1111/j.1365-2230.2009.03308.x.
39. Carmack SW, Vemulapalli R, Spechler SJ, Genta RM. Esophagitis dissecans superficialis ("sloughing esophagitis"): a clinicopathologic study of 12 cases. Am J Surg Pathol. 2009;33(12):1789–94. https://doi.org/10.1097/PAS.0b013e3181b7ce21.
40. Hokama A, Ihama Y, Nakamoto M, Kinjo N, Kinjo F, Fujita J. Esophagitis dissecans superficialis associated with bisphosphonates. Endoscopy. 2007;39(Suppl 1):E91. https://doi.org/10.1055/s-2006-945146.
41. Hage-Nassar G, Rotterdam H, Frank D, Green PH. Esophagitis dissecans superficialis associated with celiac disease. Gastrointest Endosc. 2003;57(1):140–1. https://doi.org/10.1067/mge.2003.42.
42. Hokama A, Yamamoto Y, Taira K, Nakamura M, Kobashigawa C, Nakamoto M, et al. Esophagitis dissecans superficialis and autoimmune bullous dermatoses: a review. World J Gastrointest Endosc. 2010;2(7):252–6. https://doi.org/10.4253/wjge.v2.i7.252.
43. Purdy JK, Appelman HD, McKenna BJ. Sloughing esophagitis is associated with chronic debilitation and medications that injure the esophageal mucosa. Mod Pathol. 2012;25(5):767–75. https://doi.org/10.1038/modpathol.2011.204.
44. Beck RN. Oesophagitis dissecans superficialis. Br Med J. 1954;1(4860):501–2.
45. Ponsot P, Molas G, Scoazec JY, Ruszniewski P, Henin D, Bernades P. Chronic esophagitis dissecans: an unrecognized clinicopathologic entity? Gastrointest Endosc. 1997;45(1):38–45.
46. Stanley JR, Amagai M. Pemphigus, bullous impetigo, and the staphylococcal scalded-skin syndrome. N Engl J Med. 2006;355(17):1800–10. https://doi.org/10.1056/NEJMra061111.
47. Montgobert J, Bellaiche G, Nouts A, Ley G, Slama JL. Transmural esophageal dissection after iatrogenic perforation of esophagitis dissecans visualized by thoracic x-ray computed tomography. Gastroenterol Clin Biol. 1999;23(8–9):987–8.
48. Ramaswami G, Jain PK, Talati VR. Oesophagitis dissecans superficialis complicating repeated rigid oesophagoscopy and dilatation. J Laryngol Otol. 2007;121(1):92–3. https://doi.org/10.1017/S002221510600274X.
49. Baehr PH, McDonald GB. Esophageal infections: risk factors, presentation, diagnosis, and treatment. Gastroenterology. 1994;106(2):509–32.
50. Canalejo Castrillero E, Garcia Duran F, Cabello N, Garcia Martinez J. Herpes esophagitis in healthy adults and adolescents: report of 3 cases and review of the literature. Medicine (Baltimore). 2010;89(4):204–10. https://doi.org/10.1097/MD.0b013e3181e949ed.
51. McBane RD, Gross JB Jr. Herpes esophagitis: clinical syndrome, endoscopic appearance, and diagnosis in 23 patients. Gastrointest Endosc. 1991;37(6):600–3.
52. Buss DH, Scharyj M. Herpesvirus infection of the esophagus and other visceral organs in adults. Incidence and clinical significance. Am J Med. 1979;66(3):457–62.
53. McDonald GB, Sharma P, Hackman RC, Meyers JD, Thomas ED. Esophageal infections in immunosuppressed patients after marrow transplantation. Gastroenterology. 1985;88(5 Pt 1):1111–7.

54. Greenson JK, Beschorner WE, Boitnott JK, Yardley JH. Prominent mononuclear cell infiltrate is characteristic of herpes esophagitis. Hum Pathol. 1991;22(6):541–9.
55. Chetty R, Roskell DE. Cytomegalovirus infection in the gastrointestinal tract. J Clin Pathol. 1994;47(11):968–72.
56. Wang HW, Kuo CJ, Lin WR, Hsu CM, Ho YP, Lin CJ, et al. The clinical characteristics and manifestations of cytomegalovirus esophagitis. Dis Esophagus. 2016;29(4):392–9. https://doi.org/10.1111/dote.12340.
57. Griffiths PD, Grundy JE. The status of CMV as a human pathogen. Epidemiol Infect. 1988;100(1):1–15.
58. Bonacini M, Young T, Laine L. The causes of esophageal symptoms in human immunodeficiency virus infection. A prospective study of 110 patients. Arch Intern Med. 1991;151(8):1567–72.
59. Wilcox CM, Straub RF, Schwartz DA. Prospective endoscopic characterization of cytomegalovirus esophagitis in AIDS. Gastrointest Endosc. 1994;40(4):481–4.
60. Lemonovich TL, Watkins RR. Update on cytomegalovirus infections of the gastrointestinal system in solid organ transplant recipients. Curr Infect Dis Rep. 2012;14(1):33–40. https://doi.org/10.1007/s11908-011-0224-6.
61. Whitley RJ, Jacobson MA, Friedberg DN, Holland GN, Jabs DA, Dieterich DT, et al. Guidelines for the treatment of cytomegalovirus diseases in patients with AIDS in the era of potent antiretroviral therapy: recommendations of an international panel. International AIDS Society-USA. Arch Intern Med. 1998;158(9):957–69.
62. Greenson JK. Macrophage aggregates in cytomegalovirus esophagitis. Hum Pathol. 1997;28(3):375–8.
63. Teot LA, Ducatman BS, Geisinger KR. Cytologic diagnosis of cytomegaloviral esophagitis. A report of three acquired immunodeficiency syndrome-related cases. Acta Cytol. 1993;37(1):93–6.
64. Samonis G, Skordilis P, Maraki S, Datseris G, Toloudis P, Chatzinikolaou I, et al. Oropharyngeal candidiasis as a marker for esophageal candidiasis in patients with cancer. Clin Infect Dis. 1998;27(2):283–6.
65. Kodsi BE, Wickremesinghe C, Kozinn PJ, Iswara K, Goldberg PK. Candida esophagitis: a prospective study of 27 cases. Gastroenterology. 1976;71(5):715–9.
66. Simon MR, Houser WL, Smith KA, Long PM. Esophageal candidiasis as a complication of inhaled corticosteroids. Ann Allergy Asthma Immunol. 1997;79(4):333–8. https://doi.org/10.1016/S1081-1206(10)63024-4.
67. Larner AJ, Lendrum R. Oesophageal candidiasis after omeprazole therapy. Gut. 1992;33(6):860–1.
68. Pappas PG, Rex JH, Sobel JD, Filler SG, Dismukes WE, Walsh TJ, et al. Guidelines for treatment of candidiasis. Clin Infect Dis. 2004;38(2):161–89. https://doi.org/10.1086/380796.
69. Barbaro G, Barbarini G, Calderon W, Grisorio B, Alcini P, Di Lorenzo G. Fluconazole versus itraconazole for candida esophagitis in acquired immunodeficiency syndrome. Candida Esophagitis. Gastroenterology. 1996;111(5):1169–77.
70. Wagner C, Graninger W, Presterl E, Joukhadar C. The echinocandins: comparison of their pharmacokinetics, pharmacodynamics and clinical applications. Pharmacology. 2006;78(4):161–77. https://doi.org/10.1159/000096348.
71. Arathoon EG, Gotuzzo E, Noriega LM, Berman RS, DiNubile MJ, Sable CA. Randomized, double-blind, multicenter study of caspofungin versus amphotericin B for treatment of oropharyngeal and esophageal candidiases. Antimicrob Agents Chemother. 2002;46(2):451–7.
72. Mathieson R, Dutta SK. Candida esophagitis. Dig Dis Sci. 1983;28(4):365–70.
73. Gornig M, Emmert-Buck M, Walsh TJ. Patterns of Candida esophagitis in cancer and AIDS patients: histopathological study of 23 patients. Mycoses. 1997;40(Suppl 1):81–5.
74. Bertoni G, Sassatelli R, Nigrisoli E, Conigliaro R, Bedogni G. Ectopic sebaceous glands in the esophagus: report of three new cases and review of the literature. Am J Gastroenterol. 1994;89(10):1884–7.
75. Rywlin AM, Ortega R. Glycogenic acanthosis of the esophagus. Arch Pathol. 1970;90(5):439–43.
76. Bender MD, Allison J, Cuartas F, Montgomery C. Glycogenic acanthosis of the esophagus: a form of benign epithelial hyperplasia. Gastroenterology. 1973;65(3):373–80.
77. Maguire A, Sheahan K. Pathology of oesophagitis. Histopathology. 2012;60(6):864–79. https://doi.org/10.1111/j.1365-2559.2011.03855.x.
78. Ezzell JH Jr, Bremer J, Adamec TA. Bacterial esophagitis: an often forgotten cause of odynophagia. Am J Gastroenterol. 1990;85(3):296–8.
79. Walsh TJ, Belitsos NJ, Hamilton SR. Bacterial esophagitis in immunocompromised patients. Arch Intern Med. 1986;146(7):1345–8.
80. Forsmark CE, Wilcox CM, Darragh TM, Cello JP. Disseminated histoplasmosis in AIDS: an unusual case of esophageal involvement and gastrointestinal bleeding. Gastrointest Endosc. 1990;36(6):604–5.
81. Eng J, Sabanathan S. Tuberculosis of the esophagus. Dig Dis Sci. 1991;36(4):536–40.
82. Disease GBD, Injury I, Prevalence C. Global, regional, and national incidence, prevalence, and years lived with disability for 310 diseases and injuries, 1990–2015: a systematic analysis for the Global Burden of Disease Study 2015. Lancet. 2016;388(10053):1545–602. https://doi.org/10.1016/S0140-6736(16)31678-6.
83. Rassi A Jr, Rassi A, Marin-Neto JA. Chagas disease. Lancet. 2010;375(9723):1388–402. https://doi.org/10.1016/S0140-6736(10)60061-X.
84. Prata A. Evolution of the clinical and epidemiological knowledge about Chagas disease 90 years after its discovery. Mem Inst Oswaldo Cruz. 1999;94(Suppl 1):81–8.
85. Schmunis GA. Prevention of transfusional Trypanosoma cruzi infection in Latin America. Mem Inst Oswaldo Cruz. 1999;94(Suppl 1):93–101.
86. Rassi A Jr, Rassi A. Marcondes de Rezende J. American trypanosomiasis (Chagas disease). Infect Dis Clin N Am. 2012;26(2):275–91. https://doi.org/10.1016/j.idc.2012.03.002.
87. Teixeira AR, Hecht MM, Guimaro MC, Sousa AO, Nitz N. Pathogenesis of Chagas' disease: parasite persistence and autoimmunity. Clin Microbiol Rev. 2011;24(3):592–630. https://doi.org/10.1128/CMR.00063-10.
88. Nascimento RD, de Souza Lisboa A, Fujiwara RT, de Freitas MA, Adad SJ, Oliveira RC, et al. Characterization of enteroglial cells and denervation process in chagasic patients with and without megaesophagus. Hum Pathol. 2010;41(4):528–34. https://doi.org/10.1016/j.humpath.2009.05.018.
89. Coura JR, Borges-Pereira J. Chagas disease. What is known and what should be improved: a systemic review. Rev Soc Bras Med Trop. 2012;45(3):286–96.
90. de Oliveira RB, Troncon LE, Dantas RO, Menghelli UG. Gastrointestinal manifestations of Chagas' disease. Am J Gastroenterol. 1998;93(6):884–9. https://doi.org/10.1111/j.1572-0241.1998.270_r.x.
91. de Oliveira RB, Rezende Filho J, Dantas RO, Iazigi N. The spectrum of esophageal motor disorders in Chagas' disease. Am J Gastroenterol. 1995;90(7):1119–24.
92. Dantas RO, Godoy RA, Oliveira RB, Meneghelli UG, Troncon LE. Lower esophageal sphincter pressure in Chagas' disease. Dig Dis Sci. 1990;35(4):508–12.
93. Coura JR, Borges-Pereira J. Chronic phase of Chagas disease: why should it be treated? A comprehensive review. Mem Inst Oswaldo Cruz. 2011;106(6):641–5.

94. Coura JR. Present situation and new strategies for Chagas disease chemotherapy: a proposal. Mem Inst Oswaldo Cruz. 2009;104(4):549–54.
95. Coura JR. Current prospects of specific treatment of Chagas' disease. Bol Chil Parasitol. 1996;51(3–4):69–75.
96. Koberle F. Chagas' disease and Chagas' syndromes: the pathology of American trypanosomiasis. Adv Parasitol. 1968;6:63–116.
97. Koberle F. The causation and importance of nervous lesions in American trypanosomiasis. Bull World Health Organ. 1970;42(5):739–43.
98. Decker GA, Loftus EV Jr, Pasha TM, Tremaine WJ, Sandborn WJ. Crohn's disease of the esophagus: clinical features and outcomes. Inflamm Bowel Dis. 2001;7(2):113–9.
99. D'Haens G, Rutgeerts P, Geboes K, Vantrappen G. The natural history of esophageal Crohn's disease: three patterns of evolution. Gastrointest Endosc. 1994;40(3):296–300.
100. De Felice KM, Katzka DA, Raffals LE. Crohn's disease of the esophagus: clinical features and treatment outcomes in the biologic era. Inflamm Bowel Dis. 2015;21(9):2106–13. https://doi.org/10.1097/MIB.0000000000000469.
101. Ramaswamy K, Jacobson K, Jevon G, Israel D. Esophageal Crohn disease in children: a clinical spectrum. J Pediatr Gastroenterol Nutr. 2003;36(4):454–8.
102. Wagtmans MJ, Verspaget HW, Lamers CB, van Hogezand RA. Clinical aspects of Crohn's disease of the upper gastrointestinal tract: a comparison with distal Crohn's disease. Am J Gastroenterol. 1997;92(9):1467–71.
103. Estrada CA, Lewandowski C, Schubert TT, Dorman PJ. Esophageal involvement in secondary amyloidosis mimicking achalasia. J Clin Gastroenterol. 1990;12(4):447–50.
104. Rose S, Young MA, Reynolds JC. Gastrointestinal manifestations of scleroderma. Gastroenterol Clin N Am. 1998;27(3):563–94.
105. Lopez-Cepero Andrada JM, Jimenez Arjona J, Amaya Vidal A, Rubio Garrido J, Navas Relinque C, Soria de la Cruz MJ, et al. Pseudoachalasia and secondary amyloidosis in a patient with rheumatoid arthritis. Gastroenterol Hepatol. 2002;25(6):398–400.
106. Chua S, Dodd H, Saeed IT, Chakravarty K. Dysphagia in a patient with lupus and review of the literature. Lupus. 2002;11(5):322–4. https://doi.org/10.1191/0961203302lu195cr.
107. de Merieux P, Verity MA, Clements PJ, Paulus HE. Esophageal abnormalities and dysphagia in polymyositis and dermatomyositis. Arthritis Rheum. 1983;26(8):961–8.
108. Fitzgerald RC, Triadafilopoulos G. Esophageal manifestations of rheumatic disorders. Semin Arthritis Rheum. 1997;26(4):641–66.
109. Palma R, Freire A, Freitas J, Morbey A, Costa T, Saraiva F, et al. Esophageal motility disorders in patients with Sjogren's syndrome. Dig Dis Sci. 1994;39(4):758–61.
110. Cozzi F, Zucchetta P, Durigon N, Marzola MC, Bullo A, Favaro M, et al. Changes in esophageal peristalsis in diverse clinical forms and antibody specificity in scleroderma: a scintigraphic study in 100 cases. Reumatismo. 2003;55(2):86–92.
111. Weston S, Thumshirn M, Wiste J, Camilleri M. Clinical and upper gastrointestinal motility features in systemic sclerosis and related disorders. Am J Gastroenterol. 1998;93(7):1085–9. https://doi.org/10.1111/j.1572-0241.1998.00334.x.
112. Recht MP, Levine MS, Katzka DA, Reynolds JC, Saul SH. Barrett's esophagus in scleroderma: increased prevalence and radiographic findings. Gastrointest Radiol. 1988;13(1):1–5. https://doi.org/10.1007/BF01889012.
113. Katzka DA, Reynolds JC, Saul SH, Plotkin A, Lang CA, Ouyang A, et al. Barrett's metaplasia and adenocarcinoma of the esophagus in scleroderma. Am J Med. 1987;82(1):46–52.
114. Bargon J, Stein J, Dietrich CF, Muller U, Caspary WF, Wagner TO. Gastrointestinal complications of adult patients with cystic fibrosis. Z Gastroenterol. 1999;37(8):739–49.
115. Pauwels A, Blondeau K, Dupont LJ, Sifrim D. Mechanisms of increased gastroesophageal reflux in patients with cystic fibrosis. Am J Gastroenterol. 2012;107(9):1346–53. https://doi.org/10.1038/ajg.2012.213.
116. Dziekiewicz MA, Banaszkiewicz A, Urzykowska A, Lisowska A, Rachel M, Sands D, et al. Gastroesophageal reflux disease in children with cystic fibrosis. Adv Exp Med Biol. 2015;873:1–7. https://doi.org/10.1007/5584_2015_154.
117. Scott RB, O'Loughlin EV, Gall DG. Gastroesophageal reflux in patients with cystic fibrosis. J Pediatr. 1985;106(2):223–7.
118. Agrons GA, Corse WR, Markowitz RI, Suarez ES, Perry DR. Gastrointestinal manifestations of cystic fibrosis: radiologic-pathologic correlation. Radiographics. 1996;16(4):871–93. https://doi.org/10.1148/radiographics.16.4.8835977.
119. Hassall E, Israel DM, Davidson AG, Wong LT. Barrett's esophagus in children with cystic fibrosis: not a coincidental association. Am J Gastroenterol. 1993;88(11):1934–8.
120. Blondeau K, Pauwels A, Dupont L, Mertens V, Proesmans M, Orel R, et al. Characteristics of gastroesophageal reflux and potential risk of gastric content aspiration in children with cystic fibrosis. J Pediatr Gastroenterol Nutr. 2010;50(2):161–6. https://doi.org/10.1097/MPG.0b013e3181acae98.
121. McDonald GB, Sullivan KM, Plumley TF. Radiographic features of esophageal involvement in chronic graft-vs.-host disease. AJR Am J Roentgenol. 1984;142(3):501–6. https://doi.org/10.2214/ajr.142.3.501.
122. Trabulo D, Ferreira S, Lage P, Rego RL, Teixeira G, Pereira AD. Esophageal stenosis with sloughing esophagitis: a curious manifestation of graft-vs-host disease. World J Gastroenterol. 2015;21(30):9217–22 https://doi.org/10.3748/wjg.v21.i30.9217.
123. Nakshabendi IM, Maldonado ME, Coppola D, Mamel JJ. Esophageal cast: a manifestation of graft-versus-host disease. Dig Dis. 2000;18(2):103–5. https://doi.org/10.1159/000016962.
124. Sodhi SS, Srinivasan R, Thomas RM. Esophageal graft versus host disease. Gastrointest Endosc. 2000;52(2):235. https://doi.org/10.1067/mge.2000.107289.
125. Otero Lopez-Cubero S, Sale GE, McDonald GB. Acute graft-versus-host disease of the esophagus. Endoscopy. 1997;29(7):S35–6.
126. Minocha A, Mandanas RA, Kida M, Jazzar A. Bullous esophagitis due to chronic graft-versus-host disease. Am J Gastroenterol. 1997;92(3):529–30.
127. Shulman HM, Kleiner D, Lee SJ, Morton T, Pavletic SZ, Farmer E, et al. Histopathologic diagnosis of chronic graft-versus-host disease: National Institutes of Health consensus development project on criteria for clinical trials in chronic graft-versus-host disease: II. Pathology working group report. Biol Blood Marrow Transplant. 2006;12(1):31–47. https://doi.org/10.1016/j.bbmt.2005.10.023.
128. Lamireau T, Leaute-Labreze C, Le Bail B, Taieb A. Esophageal involvement in Stevens-Johnson syndrome. Endoscopy. 2001;33(6):550–3. https://doi.org/10.1055/s-2001-15091.
129. Wise JL, Murray JA. Esophageal manifestations of dermatologic disease. Curr Gastroenterol Rep. 2002;4(3):205–12.
130. Stewart MI, Woodley DT, Briggaman RA. Epidermolysis bullosa acquisita and associated symptomatic esophageal webs. Arch Dermatol. 1991;127(3):373–7.
131. Abraham SC, Ravich WJ, Anhalt GJ, Yardley JH, Wu TT. Esophageal lichen planus: case report and review of the literature. Am J Surg Pathol. 2000;24(12):1678–82.
132. Bobadilla J, van der Hulst RW, ten Kate FJ, Tytgat GN. Esophageal lichen planus. Gastrointest Endosc. 1999;50(2):268–71.
133. Jobard-Drobacheff C, Blanc D, Quencez E, Zultak M, Paris B, Ottignon Y, et al. Lichen planus of the oesophagus. Clin Exp Dermatol. 1988;13(1):38–41.

134. Leyva-Leon F, Wright AL, Wight RG, Harrington CI. Esophageal lichen planus presenting with dysphagia. Int J Dermatol. 1990;29(5):354–5.
135. Kirsch M. Esophageal lichen planus: a forgotten diagnosis. J Clin Gastroenterol. 1995;20(2):145–6.
136. Van Maercke P, Gunther M, Groth W, Gheorghiu T, Habermann U. Lichen ruber mucosae with esophageal involvement. Endoscopy. 1988;20(4):158–60. https://doi.org/10.1055/s-2007-1018165.
137. Chandan VS, Murray JA, Abraham SC. Esophageal lichen planus. Arch Pathol Lab Med. 2008;132(6):1026–9. https://doi.org/10.1043/1543-2165(2008)132[1026:ELP]2.0.CO;2.
138. Torzecka JD, Sysa-Jedrzejowska A, Waszczykowska E, Wozniacka A, Dziankowska-Bartkowiak B, Narbutt J. Immunopathological examination of esophagus as a useful criterion of cure in pemphigus vulgaris. J Eur Acad Dermatol Venereol. 1999;12(2):115–8.
139. Bernard P, Souyri N, Pillegand B, Bonnetblanc JM. Immunofluorescent studies of gastrointestinal tract mucosa in bullous pemphigoid. Arch Dermatol. 1986;122(2):137–8.
140. Gomi H, Akiyama M, Yakabi K, Nakamura T, Matsuo I. Oesophageal involvement in pemphigus vulgaris. Lancet. 1999;354(9192):1794. https://doi.org/10.1016/S0140-6736(99)04708-X.
141. Trattner A, Lurie R, Leiser A, David M, Hazaz B, Kadish U, et al. Esophageal involvement in pemphigus vulgaris: a clinical, histologic, and immunopathologic study. J Am Acad Dermatol. 1991;24(2 Pt 1):223–6.
142. Sharon P, Greene ML, Rachmilewitz D. Esophageal involvement in bullous pemphigoid. Gastrointest Endosc. 1978;24(3):122–3.
143. Ahmed AR, Hombal SM. Cicatricial pemphigoid. Int J Dermatol. 1986;25(2):90–6.
144. Epstein EH Jr. Molecular genetics of epidermolysis bullosa. Science. 1992;256(5058):799–804.
145. Shields HM, Shaffer K, O'Farrell RP, Travers R, Hayward JN, Becker LS, et al. Gastrointestinal manifestations of dermatologic disorders. Clin Gastroenterol Hepatol. 2007;5(9):1010–7; quiz 05–6. https://doi.org/10.1016/j.cgh.2007.05.018.
146. Travis SP, McGrath JA, Turnbull AJ, Schofield OM, Chan O, O'Connor AF, et al. Oral and gastrointestinal manifestations of epidermolysis bullosa. Lancet. 1992;340(8834–8835):1505–6.
147. Ergun GA, Lin AN, Dannenberg AJ, Carter DM. Gastrointestinal manifestations of epidermolysis bullosa. A study of 101 patients. Medicine (Baltimore). 1992;71(3):121–7.
148. Zweiban B, Cohen H, Chandrasoma P. Gastrointestinal involvement complicating Stevens-Johnson syndrome. Gastroenterology. 1986;91(2):469–74.
149. Mahe A, Keita S, Blanc L, Bobin P. Esophageal necrosis in the Stevens-Johnson syndrome. J Am Acad Dermatol. 1993;29(1):103–4.
150. Harewood GC, Murray JA, Cameron AJ. Esophageal lichen planus: the Mayo Clinic experience. Dis Esophagus. 1999;12(4):309–11.
151. Galloro G, Diamantis G, Magno L, Inzirillo M, Mignogna MC, Mignogna C, et al. Technical aspects in endoscopic biopsy of lesions in esophageal pemphigus vulgaris. Dig Liver Dis. 2007;39(4):363–7. https://doi.org/10.1016/j.dld.2006.12.008.
152. Lever WF. Pemphigus. Medicine (Baltimore). 1953;32(1):1–123.
153. Mignogna MD, Lo Muzio L, Galloro G, Satriano RA, Ruocco V, Bucci E. Oral pemphigus: clinical significance of esophageal involvement: report of eight cases. Oral Surg Oral Med Oral Pathol Oral Radiol Endod. 1997;84(2):179–84.
154. Park W, Vaezi MF. Etiology and pathogenesis of achalasia: the current understanding. Am J Gastroenterol. 2005;100(6):1404–14. https://doi.org/10.1111/j.1572-0241.2005.41775.x.
155. Spechler SJ, Castell DO. Classification of oesophageal motility abnormalities. Gut. 2001;49(1):145–51.
156. Pandolfino JE, Gawron AJ. Achalasia: a systematic review. JAMA. 2015;313(18):1841–52. https://doi.org/10.1001/jama.2015.2996.
157. Farrokhi F, Vaezi MF. Idiopathic (primary) achalasia. Orphanet J Rare Dis. 2007;2:38. https://doi.org/10.1186/1750-1172-2-38.
158. Spiess AE, Kahrilas PJ. Treating achalasia: from whalebone to laparoscope. JAMA. 1998;280(7):638–42.
159. Lake JM, Wong RK. Review article: the management of achalasia—a comparison of different treatment modalities. Aliment Pharmacol Ther. 2006;24(6):909–18. https://doi.org/10.1111/j.1365-2036.2006.03079.x.
160. Dughera L, Cassolino P, Cisaro F, Chiaverina M. Achalasia. Minerva Gastroenterol Dietol. 2008;54(3):277–85.
161. Spechler SJ, Souza RF, Rosenberg SJ, Ruben RA, Goyal RK. Heartburn in patients with achalasia. Gut. 1995;37(3):305–8.
162. Ott DJ, Richter JE, Chen YM, Wu WC, Gelfand DW, Castell DO. Esophageal radiography and manometry: correlation in 172 patients with dysphagia. AJR Am J Roentgenol. 1987;149(2):307–11. https://doi.org/10.2214/ajr.149.2.307.
163. Omura N, Kashiwagi H, Yano F, Tsuboi K, Ishibashi Y, Hoshino M, et al. Effect of laparoscopic esophagomyotomy on chest pain associated with achalasia and prediction of therapeutic outcomes. Surg Endosc. 2011;25(4):1048–53. https://doi.org/10.1007/s00464-010-1314-5.
164. Sharp KW, Khaitan L, Scholz S, Holzman MD, Richards WO. 100 consecutive minimally invasive Heller myotomies: lessons learned. Ann Surg. 2002;235(5):631–8; discussion 8–9
165. Patti MG, Pellegrini CA, Horgan S, Arcerito M, Omelanczuk P, Tamburini A, et al. Minimally invasive surgery for achalasia: an 8-year experience with 168 patients. Ann Surg. 1999;230(4):587–93; discussion 93–4
166. Triadafilopoulos G, Aaronson M, Sackel S, Burakoff R. Medical treatment of esophageal achalasia. Double-blind crossover study with oral nifedipine, verapamil, and placebo. Dig Dis Sci. 1991;36(3):260–7.
167. Clark SB, Rice TW, Tubbs RR, Richter JE, Goldblum JR. The nature of the myenteric infiltrate in achalasia: an immunohistochemical analysis. Am J Surg Pathol. 2000;24(8):1153–8.
168. Goldblum JR, Whyte RI, Orringer MB, Appelman HD. Achalasia. A morphologic study of 42 resected specimens. Am J Surg Pathol. 1994;18(4):327–37.
169. Goldblum JR, Rice TW, Richter JE. Histopathologic features in esophagomyotomy specimens from patients with achalasia. Gastroenterology. 1996;111(3):648–54.
170. Lehman MB, Clark SB, Ormsby AH, Rice TW, Richter JE, Goldblum JR. Squamous mucosal alterations in esophagectomy specimens from patients with end-stage achalasia. Am J Surg Pathol. 2001;25(11):1413–8.
171. Gockel I, Bohl JR, Doostkam S, Eckardt VF, Junginger T. Spectrum of histopathologic findings in patients with achalasia reflects different etiologies. J Gastroenterol Hepatol. 2006;21(4):727–33. https://doi.org/10.1111/j.1440-1746.2006.04250.x.
172. Kjellin AP, Ost AE, Pope CE 2nd. Histology of esophageal mucosa from patients with achalasia. Dis Esophagus. 2005;18(4):257–61. https://doi.org/10.1111/j.1442-2050.2005.00478.x.
173. Shoenut JP, Micflikier AB, Yaffe CS, Den Boer B, Teskey JM. Reflux in untreated achalasia patients. J Clin Gastroenterol. 1995;20(1):6–11.
174. Knauer CM. Mallory-Weiss syndrome. Characterization of 75 Mallory-Weiss lacerations in 528 patients with upper gastrointestinal hemorrhage. Gastroenterology. 1976;71(1):5–8.
175. Younes Z, Johnson DA. The spectrum of spontaneous and iatrogenic esophageal injury: perforations, Mallory-Weiss tears, and hematomas. J Clin Gastroenterol. 1999;29(4):306–17.
176. Caroli A, Follador R, Gobbi V, Breda P, Ricci G. Mallory-Weiss syndrome. Personal experience and review of the literature. Minerva Dietol Gastroenterol. 1989;35(1):7–12.

177. Dagradi AE, Broderick JT, Juler G, Wolinsky S, Stempien SJ. The Mallory-Weiss syndrome and lesion. A study of 30 cases. Am J Dig Dis. 1966;11(9):710–21.
178. Watts HD, Admirand WH. Mallory-Weiss syndrome. A reappraisal. JAMA. 1974;230(12):1674–5.
179. Yin A, Li Y, Jiang Y, Liu J, Luo H. Mallory-Weiss syndrome: clinical and endoscopic characteristics. Eur J Intern Med. 2012;23(4):e92–6. https://doi.org/10.1016/j.ejim.2012.02.005.
180. Parva M, Finnegan M, Keiter C, Mercogliano G, Perez CM. Mallory-Weiss tear diagnosed in the immediate postpartum period: a case report. J Obstet Gynaecol Can. 2009;31(8):740–3. https://doi.org/10.1016/S1701-2163(16)34280-3.
181. Lawrence DR, Ohri SK, Moxon RE, Townsend ER, Fountain SW. Primary esophageal repair for Boerhaave's syndrome. Ann Thorac Surg. 1999;67(3):818–20.
182. Lawrence DR, Moxon RE, Fountain SW, Ohri SK, Townsend ER. Iatrogenic oesophageal perforations: a clinical review. Ann R Coll Surg Engl. 1998;80(2):115–8.
183. Woo KM, Schneider JI. High-risk chief complaints I: chest pain—the big three. Emerg Med Clin North Am. 2009;27(4):685–712, x. https://doi.org/10.1016/j.emc.2009.07.007.
184. Vial CM, Whyte RI. Boerhaave's syndrome: diagnosis and treatment. Surg Clin North Am. 2005;85(3):515–24, ix. https://doi.org/10.1016/j.suc.2005.01.010.
185. de Lutio di Castelguidone E, Merola S, Pinto A, Raissaki M, Gagliardi N, Romano L. Esophageal injuries: spectrum of multidetector row CT findings. Eur J Radiol. 2006;59(3):344–8. https://doi.org/10.1016/j.ejrad.2006.04.027.
186. Gubbins GP, Nensey YM, Schubert TT, Batra SK. Barogenic perforation of the esophagus distal to a stricture after endoscopy. J Clin Gastroenterol. 1990;12(3):310–2.
187. de Schipper JP, Pull ter Gunne AF, Oostvogel HJ, van Laarhoven CJ. Spontaneous rupture of the oesophagus: Boerhaave's syndrome in 2008. Literature review and treatment algorithm. Dig Surg. 2009;26(1):1–6. https://doi.org/10.1159/000191283.
188. Korn O, Onate JC, Lopez R. Anatomy of the Boerhaave syndrome. Surgery. 2007;141(2):222–8. https://doi.org/10.1016/j.surg.2006.06.034.
189. Tobin RW. Esophageal rings, webs, and diverticula. J Clin Gastroenterol. 1998;27(4):285–95.
190. Atmatzidis K, Papaziogas B, Pavlidis T, Mirelis C, Papaziogas T. Plummer-Vinson syndrome. Dis Esophagus. 2003;16(2):154–7.
191. Rice TW. Esophageal diverticula: introduction. Semin Thorac Cardiovasc Surg. 1999;11(4):325.
192. Reznik SI, Rice TW, Murthy SC, Mason DP, Apperson-Hansen C, Blackstone EH. Assessment of a pathophysiology-directed treatment for symptomatic epiphrenic diverticulum. Dis Esophagus. 2007;20(4):320–7. https://doi.org/10.1111/j.1442-2050.2007.00716.x.
193. Bhattacharya S, Mahmud S, McGlinchey I, Nassar AH. Intramural pseudodiverticulosis of the esophagus. Surg Endosc. 2002;16(4):714–5. https://doi.org/10.1007/s00464-001-4234-6.
194. Bruhlmann WF, Zollikofer CL, Maranta E, Hefti ML, Bivetti J, Giger M, et al. Intramural pseudodiverticulosis of the esophagus: report of seven cases and literature review. Gastrointest Radiol. 1981;6(3):199–208.
195. Sabanathan S, Salama FD, Morgan WE. Oesophageal intramural pseudodiverticulosis. Thorax. 1985;40(11):849–57.
196. Neumann WL, Lujan GM, Genta RM. Gastric heterotopia in the proximal oesophagus ("inlet patch"): association with adenocarcinomas arising in Barrett mucosa. Dig Liver Dis. 2012;44(4):292–6. https://doi.org/10.1016/j.dld.2011.11.008.
197. Yuksel I, Uskudar O, Koklu S, Basar O, Gultuna S, Unverdi S, et al. Inlet patch: associations with endoscopic findings in the upper gastrointestinal system. Scand J Gastroenterol. 2008;43(8):910–4.
198. Weickert U, Wolf A, Schroder C, Autschbach F, Vollmer H. Frequency, histopathological findings, and clinical significance of cervical heterotopic gastric mucosa (gastric inlet patch): a prospective study in 300 patients. Dis Esophagus. 2011;24(2):63–8. https://doi.org/10.1111/j.1442-2050.2010.01091.x.
199. Tang P, McKinley MJ, Sporrer M, Kahn E. Inlet patch: prevalence, histologic type, and association with esophagitis, Barrett esophagus, and antritis. Arch Pathol Lab Med. 2004;128(4):444–7. https://doi.org/10.1043/1543-2165(2004)128<444:IPPHTA>2.0.CO;2.
200. Terada T. Heterotopic gastric mucosa of the gastrointestinal tract: a histopathologic study of 158 cases. Pathol Res Pract. 2011;207(3):148–50. https://doi.org/10.1016/j.prp.2010.12.004.
201. Borhan-Manesh F, Farnum JB. Incidence of heterotopic gastric mucosa in the upper oesophagus. Gut. 1991;32(9):968–72.
202. Jabbari M, Goresky CA, Lough J, Yaffe C, Daly D, Cote C. The inlet patch: heterotopic gastric mucosa in the upper esophagus. Gastroenterology. 1985;89(2):352–6.
203. Azar C, Jamali F, Tamim H, Abdul-Baki H, Soweid A. Prevalence of endoscopically identified heterotopic gastric mucosa in the proximal esophagus: endoscopist dependent? J Clin Gastroenterol. 2007;41(5):468–71. https://doi.org/10.1097/01.mcg.0000225519.59030.8d.
204. Sanchez-Pernaute A, Hernando F, Diez-Valladares L, Gonzalez O, Perez Aguirre E, Furio V, et al. Heterotopic gastric mucosa in the upper esophagus ("inlet patch"): a rare cause of esophageal perforation. Am J Gastroenterol. 1999;94(10):3047–50. https://doi.org/10.1111/j.1572-0241.1999.01458.x.
205. Yarborough CS, McLane RC. Stricture related to an inlet patch of the esophagus. Am J Gastroenterol. 1993;88(2):275–6.
206. Chatelain D, de Lajarte-Thirouard AS, Tiret E, Flejou JF. Adenocarcinoma of the upper esophagus arising in heterotopic gastric mucosa: common pathogenesis with Barrett's adenocarcinoma? Virchows Arch. 2002;441(4):406–11.
207. Alrawi SJ, Winston J, Tan D, Gibbs J, Loree TR, Hicks W, et al. Primary adenocarcinoma of cervical esophagus. J Exp Clin Cancer Res. 2005;24(2):325–30.
208. Gutierrez O, Akamatsu T, Cardona H, Graham DY, El-Zimaity HM. Helicobacter pylori and hetertopic gastric mucosa in the upper esophagus (the inlet patch). Am J Gastroenterol. 2003;98(6):1266–70. https://doi.org/10.1111/j.1572-0241.2003.07488.x.
209. Akbayir N, Alkim C, Erdem L, Sokmen HM, Sungun A, Basak T, et al. Heterotopic gastric mucosa in the cervical esophagus (inlet patch): endoscopic prevalence, histological and clinical characteristics. J Gastroenterol Hepatol. 2004;19(8):891–6. https://doi.org/10.1111/j.1440-1746.2004.03474.x.
210. Borhan-Manesh F, Farnum JB. Study of Helicobacter pylori colonization of patches of heterotopic gastric mucosa (HGM) at the upper esophagus. Dig Dis Sci. 1993;38(1):142–6.
211. Shah KK, DeRidder PH, Shah KK. Ectopic gastric mucosa in proximal esophagus. Its clinical significance and hormonal profile. J Clin Gastroenterol. 1986;8(5):509–13.
212. Jacobs E, Dehou MF. Heterotopic gastric mucosa in the upper esophagus: a prospective study of 33 cases and review of literature. Endoscopy. 1997;29(8):710–5. https://doi.org/10.1055/s-2007-1004294.
213. Gurvits GE, Shapsis A, Lau N, Gualtieri N, Robilotti JG. Acute esophageal necrosis: a rare syndrome. J Gastroenterol. 2007;42(1):29–38. https://doi.org/10.1007/s00535-006-1974-z.
214. Grudell AB, Mueller PS, Viggiano TR. Black esophagus: report of six cases and review of the literature, 1963–2003. Dis Esophagus. 2006;19(2):105–10. https://doi.org/10.1111/j.1442-2050.2006.00549.x.
215. Hong JW, Kim SU, Park HN, Seo JH, Lee YC, Kim H. Black esophagus associated with alcohol abuse. Gut Liver. 2008;2(2):133–5. https://doi.org/10.5009/gnl.2008.2.2.133.

216. Odelowo OO, Hassan M, Nidiry JJ, Marshalleck JJ. Acute necrotizing esophagitis: a case report. J Natl Med Assoc. 2002;94(8):735–7.
217. Endo T, Sakamoto J, Sato K, Takimoto M, Shimaya K, Mikami T, et al. Acute esophageal necrosis caused by alcohol abuse. World J Gastroenterol. 2005;11(35):5568–70.
218. Burtally A, Gregoire P. Acute esophageal necrosis and low-flow state. Can J Gastroenterol. 2007;21(4):245–7.
219. Lacy BE, Toor A, Bensen SP, Rothstein RI, Maheshwari Y. Acute esophageal necrosis: report of two cases and a review of the literature. Gastrointest Endosc. 1999;49(4 Pt 1):527–32.
220. Khan AM, Hundal R, Ramaswamy V, Korsten M, Dhuper S. Acute esophageal necrosis and liver pathology, a rare combination. World J Gastroenterol. 2004;10(16):2457–8.
221. Watermeyer GA, Shaw JM, Krige JE. Education and imaging. Gastrointestinal: acute necrotizing esophagitis. J Gastroenterol Hepatol. 2007;22(7):1162. https://doi.org/10.1111/j.1440-1746.2007.05013.x.
222. Day A, Sayegh M. Acute oesophageal necrosis: a case report and review of the literature. Int J Surg. 2010;8(1):6–14. https://doi.org/10.1016/j.ijsu.2009.09.014.
223. Luketic VA, Sanyal AJ. Esophageal varices. I. Clinical presentation, medical therapy, and endoscopic therapy. Gastroenterol Clin N Am. 2000;29(2):337–85.
224. de Franchis R, Primignani M. Natural history of portal hypertension in patients with cirrhosis. Clin Liver Dis. 2001;5(3):645–63.
225. Ashkenazi E, Kovalev Y, Zuckerman E. Evaluation and treatment of esophageal varices in the cirrhotic patient. Isr Med Assoc J. 2013;15(2):109–15.
226. Arakawa M, Kage M. Haemorrhage in the upper digestive tract due to portal hypertension: clinicopathological examinations of the foci of haemorrhage. J Gastroenterol Hepatol. 1989;4(Suppl 1):168–70.
227. Evans DM, Jones DB, Cleary BK, Smith PM. Oesophageal varices treated by sclerotherapy: a histopathological study. Gut. 1982;23(7):615–20.
228. Vadva MD, Triadafilopoulos G. Glycogenic acanthosis of the esophagus and gastroesophageal reflux. J Clin Gastroenterol. 1993;17(1):79–83.
229. Kay PS, Soetikno RM, Mindelzun R, Young HS. Diffuse esophageal glycogenic acanthosis: an endoscopic marker of Cowden's disease. Am J Gastroenterol. 1997;92(6):1038–40.
230. Glick SN, Teplick SK, Goldstein J, Stead JA, Zitomer N. Glycogenic acanthosis of the esophagus. AJR Am J Roentgenol. 1982;139(4):683–8. https://doi.org/10.2214/ajr.139.4.683.
231. Ghahremani GG, Rushovich AM. Glycogenic acanthosis of the esophagus: radiographic and pathologic features. Gastrointest Radiol. 1984;9(2):93–8.
232. Quitadamo M, Benson J. Squamous papilloma of the esophagus: a case report and review of the literature. Am J Gastroenterol. 1988;83(2):194–201.
233. Rabin MS, Bremner CG, Botha JR. The reflux gastroesophageal polyp. Am J Gastroenterol. 1980;73(5):451–2.
234. Long KB, Odze RD. Gastroesophageal junction hyperplastic (inflammatory) polyps: a clinical and pathologic study of 46 cases. Am J Surg Pathol. 2011;35(7):1038–44. https://doi.org/10.1097/PAS.0b013e3182189425.
235. Fernandez-Rodriguez CM, Badia-Figuerola N, Ruiz del Arbol L, Fernandez-Seara J, Dominguez F, Aviles-Ruiz JF. Squamous papilloma of the esophagus: report of six cases with long-term follow-up in four patients. Am J Gastroenterol. 1986;81(11):1059–62.
236. Abraham SC, Singh VK, Yardley JH, Wu TT. Hyperplastic polyps of the esophagus and esophagogastric junction: histologic and clinicopathologic findings. Am J Surg Pathol. 2001;25(9):1180–7.
237. De Ceglie A, Lapertosa G, Blanchi S, Di Muzio M, Picasso M, Filiberti R, et al. Endoscopic mucosal resection of large hyperplastic polyps in 3 patients with Barrett's esophagus. World J Gastroenterol. 2006;12(35):5699–704.
238. Odze R, Antonioli D, Shocket D, Noble-Topham S, Goldman H, Upton M. Esophageal squamous papillomas. A clinicopathologic study of 38 lesions and analysis for human papillomavirus by the polymerase chain reaction. Am J Surg Pathol. 1993;17(8):803–12.
239. Yoo SS, Lee WH, Ha J, Choi SP, Kim HJ, Kim TH, et al. The prevalence of esophageal disorders in the subjects examined for health screening. Korean J Gastroenterol. 2007;50(5):306–12.
240. Bohn OL, Navarro L, Saldivar J, Sanchez-Sosa S. Identification of human papillomavirus in esophageal squamous papillomas. World J Gastroenterol. 2008;14(46):7107–11.
241. Carr NJ, Bratthauer GL, Lichy JH, Taubenberger JK, Monihan JM, Sobin LH. Squamous cell papillomas of the esophagus: a study of 23 lesions for human papillomavirus by in situ hybridization and the polymerase chain reaction. Hum Pathol. 1994;25(5):536–40.
242. Kato H, Orito E, Yoshinouchi T, Ueda R, Koizumi T, Yoshinouchi M, et al. Regression of esophageal papillomatous polyposis caused by high-risk type human papilloma virus. J Gastroenterol. 2003;38(6):579–83.
243. Attila T, Fu A, Gopinath N, Streutker CJ, Marcon NE. Esophageal papillomatosis complicated by squamous cell carcinoma. Can J Gastroenterol. 2009;23(6):415–9.
244. Van Cutsem E, Geboes K, Vantrappen G. Malignant degeneration of esophageal squamous papilloma associated with the human papillomavirus. Gastroenterology. 1992;103(3):1119–20.
245. Carr NJ, Monihan JM, Sobin LH. Squamous cell papilloma of the esophagus: a clinicopathologic and follow-up study of 25 cases. Am J Gastroenterol. 1994;89(2):245–8.
246. Szanto I, Szentirmay Z, Banai J, Nagy P, Gonda G, Voros A, et al. Squamous papilloma of the esophagus. Clinical and pathological observations based on 172 papillomas in 155 patients. Orv Hetil. 2005;146(12):547–52.
247. Politoske EJ. Squamous papilloma of the esophagus associated with the human papillomavirus. Gastroenterology. 1992;102(2):668–73.

Part III

Non-neoplastic Diseases of the Stomach

Common Types of Gastritis

6

Michael Torbenson

Reactive Gastropathy

Definition

Reactive gastropathy, also known as chemical gastropathy, refers to gastric mucosal injury with minimal inflammation, typically caused by chemicals.

Clinical Features

There are no strong or consistent associations between clinical symptoms that lead to endoscopy and the finding of reactive gastropathy on biopsy [1]. Endoscopic findings are also nonspecific, mostly consisting of mucosal hyperemia.

Reactive gastropathy results from a variety of chemical-type injuries that irritate the gastric mucosa but do not cause significant inflammation. The most common causes are bile reflux disease (anecdotally about 35%) and use of nonsteroidal anti-inflammatory drugs (NSAIDs) (anecdotally about 50%). There are many less common causes, including other drugs and sometimes alcohol. A substantial minority of cases do not have a clearly identifiable cause. On the other hand, visual identification of bile in the stomach by endoscopy does not always correlate with histological findings of reactive gastropathy. Likewise, many patients (20–90%) with chronic NSAID use do not develop histological findings of reactive gastropathy [2, 3].

Reactive gastropathy is identified in 15–20% of endoscopic biopsy specimens, based on several large multicenter studies [1, 4]. The frequency, however, varies significantly by age, being rare in children and increasing with age. Reactive gastropathy is evenly distributed throughout the USA, in contrast to *Helicobacter pylori* (*H. pylori*) gastritis, which has strong regional associations [1]. In terms of other gastrointestinal conditions, bile reflux gastropathy is associated with an increased risk for reflux esophagitis [5], Barrett mucosa [1], and duodenitis [1], all of which are linked by bile reflux disease. The link with chronic NSAID use explains the statistical clustering of reactive gastropathy with focal active ileitis and with collagenous colitis [1].

M. Torbenson (✉)
Department of Laboratory Medicine and Pathology, Mayo Clinic, Rochester, MN, USA
e-mail: Torbenson.Michael@mayo.edu

Pathological Features

Reactive gastropathy is diagnosed when a constellation of histological findings are present. The pattern is straightforward in well-developed cases. However, there are many biopsies that show some but not all of the findings of reactive gastropathy, making them harder to classify. Some pathologists take the approach of making the diagnosis of reactive gastropathy early and often, to avoid missing any cases. Unfortunately, this approach leads to a considerable loss of specificity, with many of the diagnoses of reactive gastropathy that are made in this setting having little clinical relevance and so little clinical value. A better approach uses a higher diagnostic threshold, so that when a diagnosis is made, it has strong positive predictive value.

Reactive gastropathy is primarily an antral disease. The core injury pattern with reactive gastropathy is that of foveolar hyperplasia. In the normal antral mucosa, the glands and the pits are each about equal in thickness, but with reactive gastropathy, there is striking foveolar hyperplasia, and the pits become elongated, often developing a cork-screw appearance (Fig. 6.1). The epithelium often shows some degree of mucin depletion (Fig. 6.2). The foveolar hyperplasia is typically accompanied by smooth muscle hyperplasia, with thin vertical strands of smooth muscle within the lamina propria (Fig. 6.3). Lamina propria edema is common, as is mild vascular congestion. The body mucosa can also show reactive changes in severe cases of reactive gastropathy (Fig. 6.4). Intestinal metaplasia is rare and when present

L. Zhang et al. (eds.), *Surgical Pathology of Non-neoplastic Gastrointestinal Diseases*,
https://doi.org/10.1007/978-3-030-15573-5_6

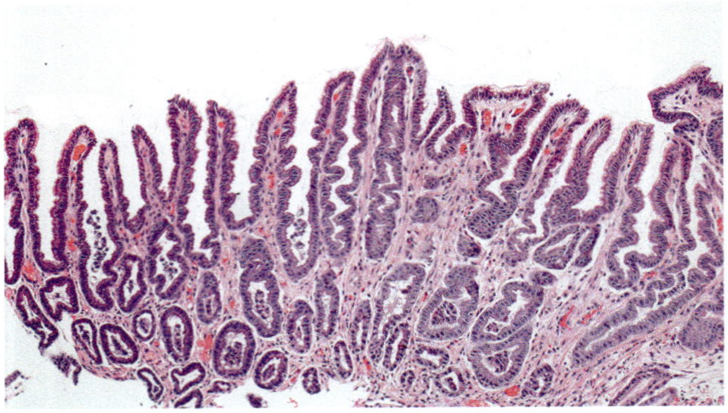

Fig. 6.1 Reactive gastropathy, antrum. Foveolar hyperplasia results from hyperplasia of the gastric pits. The antral pits have a cork-screw appearance

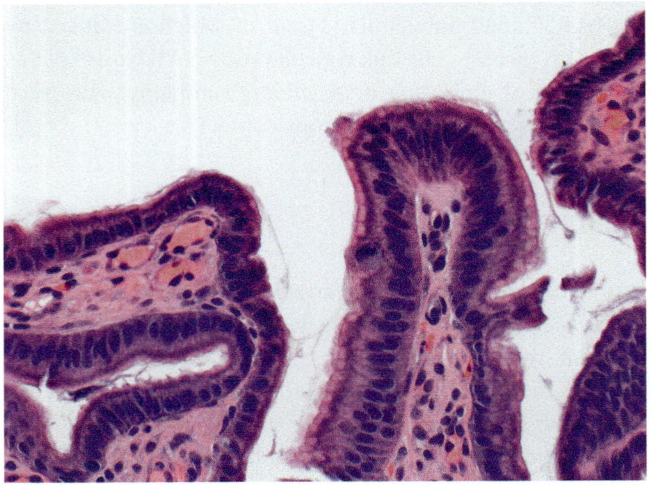

Fig. 6.2 Reactive gastropathy, antrum. The surface epithelium shows mucin depletion

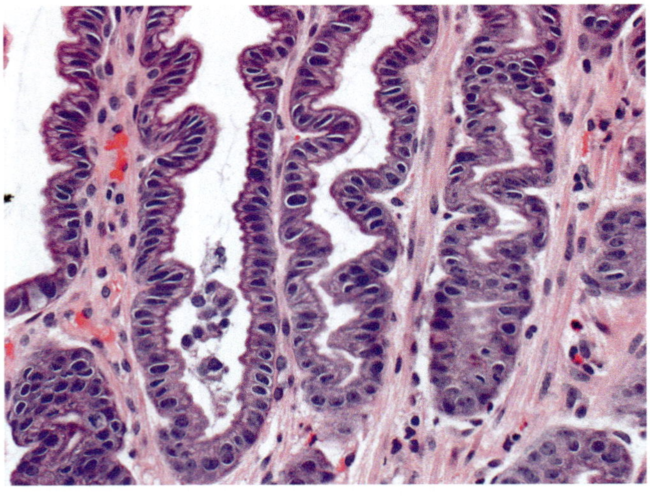

Fig. 6.3 Reactive gastropathy, antrum. There are thin vertical wisps of smooth muscle in the lamina propria

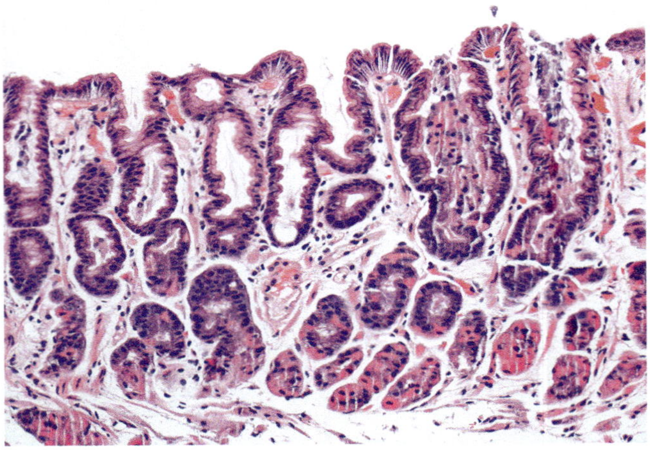

Fig. 6.4 Reactive gastropathy, body. The body mucosa also shows reactive gastropathy and severe reactive gastropathy in the antrum (not shown)

tends to be focal, in contrast to the more extensive metaplasia seen in some cases of chronic *H. pylori* gastritis.

Superficial erosions are fairly common with reactive gastropathy, but inflammation in the lamina propria is absent or sparse. When present, the sparse lamina propria inflammation shows occasional eosinophils, lymphocytes, and, in rare cases, isolated foci of acute inflammation. Less commonly, the reactive gastropathy pattern can be superimposed on chronic gastritis. In these cases, the background mucosa can show active chronic or inactive chronic gastritis.

Differential Diagnosis

Several additional disease processes may seem to be essentially similar to that of reactive gastropathy. First, biopsy findings at the edge of an antral ulcer can show essentially all of the findings of reactive gastropathy. Correlation with endoscopic findings will clarify the correct diagnosis. Second, biopsies from the pylorus can have hyperplastic changes that closely resemble reactive gastropathy, though they tend to have less mucin depletion and little or no lamina propria edema.

Acute Gastritis

The term acute gastritis is not specific for an etiology but is used to indicate gastritis with an acute clinical presentation, with symptoms that promptly resolve if the underlying condition is corrected. This term should not be confused with active gastritis, with the latter term indicating the presence of neutrophils. Essentially all causes of acute gastritis fall into one of these three categories: ischemic injury, usually from debilitating illness; caustic injury from ingestion of various industrial chemicals; and bacterial infection (also called phlegmonous or suppurative gastritis). Acute gastritis can sometimes also result from alcohol or NSAID injury.

There are several broad correlates between the etiology of acute gastritis and the endoscopic and/or gross findings [6]. Ischemic injury from debilitating illnesses often manifests as uncontrollable hemorrhage, and endoscopy shows multiple foci of hemorrhage/mucosa necrosis with a body-predominant pattern. In more severe cases, the entire stomach can be involved. In contrast, gastric injury from caustic agents tends to be antral predominant. Injury from alcohol or NSAIDs also tends to be antral predominant.

The histological findings will vary depending on the agent and the severity of injury, but non-phlegmonous causes tend to show extensive lamina propria edema, hemorrhage (Fig. 6.5), and erosion. Inflammation is generally sparse. Severe cases can also show deep ulcerations, often leading to gastric perforation. Gastric fibrosis and strictures can develop as sequelae of healed acute gastritis.

Phlegmonous gastritis results from acute bacterial infection of the stomach and typically presents with acute abdominal and intense gastric pain, vomiting, fevers, and elevated white blood cell counts. Even with prompt antibiotic therapy, the disease is often fatal. On histological examination, the inflammation is neutrophil rich and tends to be predominately submucosal in location [7, 8]. Patients may have other forms of chronic gastritis, so the mucosa can show varying degrees of chronic inflammation and metaplasia. Rare cases have presented as mass lesions [9]. The most common bacterial cause of phlegmonous gastritis is *Streptococcus*, but there are many other potential causes including *Staphylococcus*, *Pneumococcus*, *Enterobacter*, and *Escherichia coli* [7].

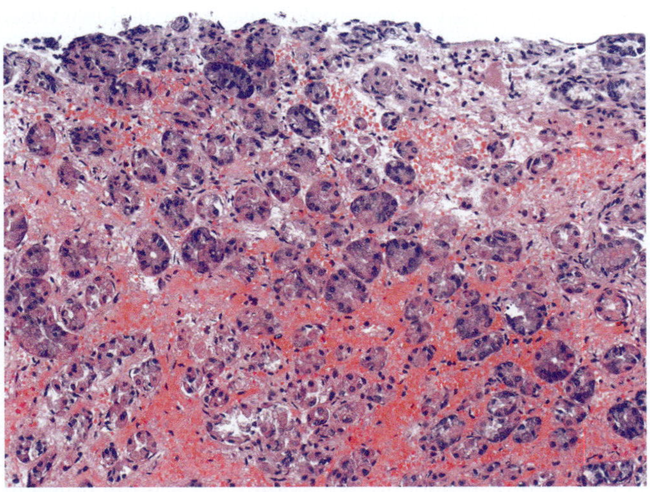

Fig. 6.5 Acute gastritis, stomach body biopsy. The lamina propria shows hemorrhage and edema, with no inflammation

Peptic Ulcer Disease

Definition

Peptic ulcer disease refers to gastric and duodenal ulcers mainly caused by *H. pylori* infection and NSAID use.

Clinical Features

Peptic ulcer disease primarily involves the duodenum and stomach but rarely can involve the esophagus or Meckel's diverticulum. *H. pylori* infection and NSAIDs/aspirin use are by far the most important clinical causes of peptic ulcer disease. Both diseases demonstrate an independent and an additive risk for peptic ulcers. To illustrate, individuals with both *H. pylori* infection and chronic use of NSAIDs have a 61-fold increase in risk for peptic ulcer disease [10]. There has been a sharp decline in the prevalence of peptic ulcer disease over the past several decades in industrialized communities, paralleling a decrease in *H. pylori* infections [11]. Recent studies suggest about 20% of peptic ulcers are not related to *H. pylori* infection or to NSAIDs/aspirin use [12]. Some of these cases are associated with high stress conditions such as major natural disasters [11].

Pathological Features

The ulcers in peptic disease show the typical changes of an ulcer (Fig. 6.6a, b), with no unique histological findings. The background mucosa often shows a reactive gastropathy pattern of injury. Gastric ulcers are much more likely to be biopsied than their duodenal counterparts, because gastric ulcers in general have a higher association with malignancy. Uncomplicated benign duodenal ulcers are generally not biopsied unless they have atypical endoscopic findings or fail to heal after therapy [13–15]. The inflammatory exudates in cases of malignant gastric ulcers are more likely to have colonies of non-Helicobacter bacteria, filamentous bacteria, and/or fungal organisms [16]. In many cases, the ulcer may not be directly sampled because the endoscopist is targeting the edge of the ulcer, which has a higher clinical value for ruling out carcinoma.

Helicobacter pylori Gastritis

Definition

Helicobacter pylori gastritis is the most common form of gastritis which refers to a primary infection of the stomach caused by *Helicobacter pylori*.

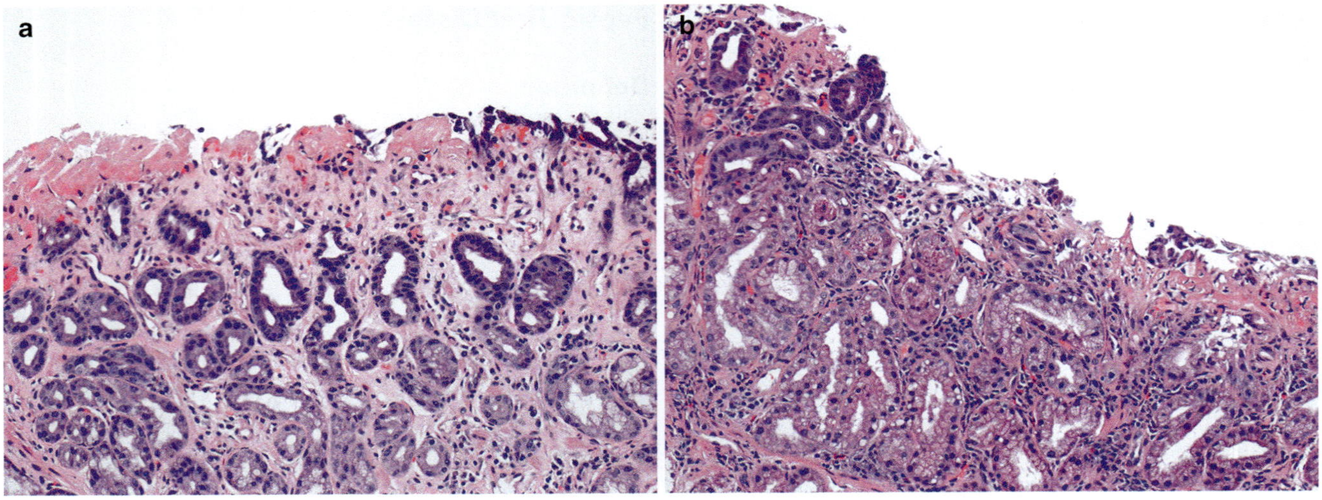

Fig. 6.6 Peptic ulcer, antral biopsy. The duodenum (**a**) and the antrum (**b**) show mucosal erosions

Clinical Features

H. pylori infection is mainly acquired during childhood to adolescence years [17]. Transmission is oral-fecal, and mother-to-child transmission appears to be the main route of infection [18, 19]. The infections are asymptomatic in both their acute and chronic phases. However, if *H. pylori* leads to peptic ulcer disease, then patients can have a wide variety of clinical symptoms, such as dyspepsia.

H. pylori gastritis is defined histologically by the presence of *H. pylori* organisms on H&E and/or special stains. The presence of organisms on histology or by culture is 100% specific for *H. pylori* infection. Of note, however, for reasons that are obscure, some pediatric guidelines do not consider histology-proven *H. pylori* gastritis to be sufficient to establish the diagnosis, requiring additional confirmation by PCR or FISH [20].

In several situations, the organisms can be absent on histology, but other tests such as the stool antigen test or the urease breath test can be positive. The most common situations are individuals who are currently on, or who recently stopped, proton pump inhibitor therapy or individuals who have recently been on antibiotics for other infections. These cases that are negative for *H. pylori* on histology but are positive by stool test or breath test are also generally considered as positive for active *H. pylori* gastritis for clinical care.

Serology for *H. pylori* infection is available but has limited clinical usefulness even when positive. IgG and/or IgA antibodies to *H. pylori* are detectable after infection and can last for years after sporadic or treatment induced clearance, but do not indicate active infection. Negative serologies, however, make active infection very unlikely [21]. Also of note, individuals with prior *H. pylori* gastritis can serorevert in time after clearing the infection, losing positive serology testing for *H. pylori*. In one study, the frequency of seroreversion was 8% [22].

The urease breath test for *H. pylori* is based on ingesting urea that has been labeled with carbon isotopes ^{13}C or ^{14}C. The *H. pylori* bacteria contain urease that breaks down the urea, releasing the carbon isotopes, which are subsequently exhaled and detected in the breath. The test is reported in some studies to have excellent sensitivity and specificity (>95%) [23], although the use of proton pump inhibitors (which are used by 15% of all adults [24] and seem to be nearly ubiquitous among patients visiting a gastroenterologist) is known to decrease the test sensitivity [25]. The stool test for bacterial antigens is another noninvasive outpatient test that has clinical value but relatively low clinical usage because of patient inconvenience and general patient disinterest in home-based fecal testing. The stool antigen test uses ELISA to detect bacterial antigens and is not influenced as strongly by the use of proton pump inhibitors.

In terms of invasive testing, the endoscopist can use a mucosal tissue fragment for the rapid urease test, which is based on the ability of bacterial urease to break down urea, with breakdown products detected by a color substrate. Tissue can also be submitted for PCR, which has high sensitivity but lower specificity, being at risk for false-positive results. All of these tests (other than serology and to some degree the stool assay) are less sensitive if patients are taking antibiotics, proton pump inhibitors, or bismuth subsalicylate (Pepto-Bismol), so testing is optimal if the patient is off these agents for several weeks prior to testing. In practice, however, this is essentially impossible to routinely implement.

Biopsy specimens can also be submitted for culture, which is not routinely available or routinely desirable but can be useful when there is concern for antibiotic-resistant *H. pylori*. Epidemiology studies suggest the problem of antibiotic-resistant organisms will likely increase in time [26].

Terminology for Histological Pattern of Injury

The Sydney Classification System for gastritis was published in 1990 in a series of six papers [27–32] and the updated Sydney Classification System in 1994 [33]. These seminal papers played a major role in standardizing the terminology used to describe histological findings in gastric injury. Gastritis was classified based on topography, morphology, and etiology. Several terms in these papers are important parts of the history of gastric pathology, but are no longer used today, because gastritis is now classified by etiology (e.g., *H. pylori* gastritis, autoimmune gastritis, etc.), with additional comments to indicate when there is metaplasia. For example, terms such as *environmental metaplastic atrophic gastritis* (*EMAG*) or *multifocal atrophic gastritis* or *type B gastritis* are no longer used for clinical care (Table 6.1).

Pathological Features

Inflammation *H. pylori* gastritis is an antral-predominant disease in most untreated cases, with active chronic gastritis involving the antrum, the transition zone, and the body to a lesser degree. This pattern was often encapsulated by the statement "one grade higher inflammation in the antrum than the body." However, the body mucosa is commonly involved when patients are taking proton pump inhibitors (a large proportion of patients today), which can shift the pattern of inflammation and organisms to more heavy involvement of the body mucosa [33].

The histological findings in untreated *H. pylori* gastritis show lymphoplasmacytic inflammation of the lamina propria, commonly with at least mild neutrophilic inflammation (Fig. 6.7). The chronic inflammation can vary in intensity from mild to marked. The inflammation often is more prominent in the superficial half of the lamina propria (Fig. 6.8). Lymphoid aggregates are also common (Fig. 6.9). Active inflammation varies in intensity but is never as striking as the chronic inflammation Active inflammation will disappear within days after successful treatment [33], while chronic inflammation can linger on, slowly abating to baseline over several years (Fig. 6.10).

Children In most cases, the histological findings in children and adults are broadly similar. However, atrophy and metaplasia are less common in children because of the relatively shorter length of infection. Some studies have also reported that the frequency and degree of active inflammation are

Table 6.1 Classification of common forms of gastritis

Disease	Topographic pattern	Older terminology
Reactive gastropathy	Antrum ≫ body	Type C gastritis
H. pylori gastritis	Antrum > or = body	Type B gastritis Environmental metaplastic atrophic gastritis (EMAG) for cases with atrophy; with less severe atrophy the term was multifocal atrophic gastritis
H. pylori-negative chronic gastritis	Antrum > body	None
Autoimmune gastritis	Body	Type A gastritis Autoimmune metaplastic atrophic gastritis (AMAG)
Autoimmune pangastritis	Antrum and body	None

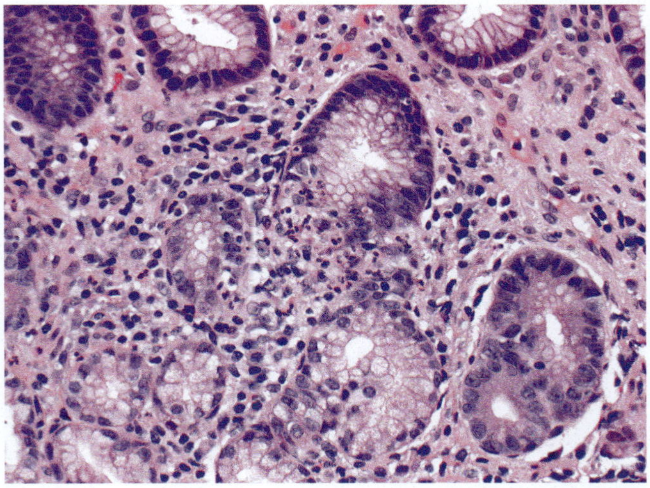

Fig. 6.7 *H. pylori* gastritis. This antral biopsy shows mild active chronic gastritis. The active inflammation is defined as neutrophils in the gastric epithelium

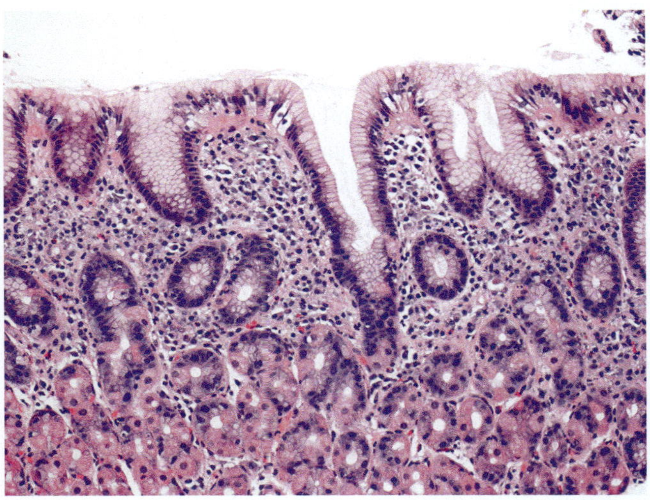

Fig. 6.8 *H. pylori* gastritis. The chronic inflammation in this body biopsy is denser in the upper half of the lamina propria

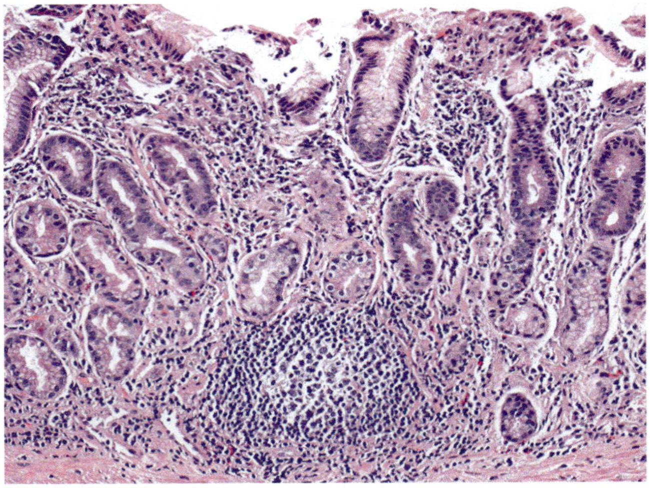

Fig. 6.9 *H. pylori* gastritis. The biopsy shows active chronic gastritis with a lymphoid aggregate

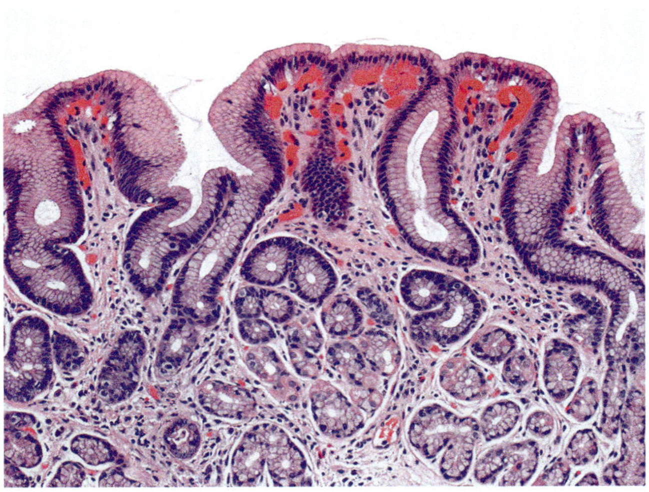

Fig. 6.10 Treated *H. pylori* gastritis. This biopsy of the gastric body was taken 1.5 years after successful treatment for *H. pylori* and shows mild chronic inflammation

lower in pediatric than adult cases, while pediatric cases have more prominent chronic inflammation [34]. The chronic inflammation can be accompanied by prominent lymphoid aggregates, leading to a distinctive nodular appearance on endoscopy [35, 36]. The presence of prominent lymphoid aggregates sometimes leads to the histological term follicular gastritis [37].

Organisms The *H. pylori* organism is shaped as a thin, straight to slightly curved rod (Figs. 6.11 and 6.12). Organisms can be rare to abundant. After partial treatment, the organisms can be round and sparse in numbers (Fig. 6.13). The organisms are mostly located in the layer of mucin that lies at the mucosa surface, but they can also be found deeper in the gastric pits. Rarely, it is reported that

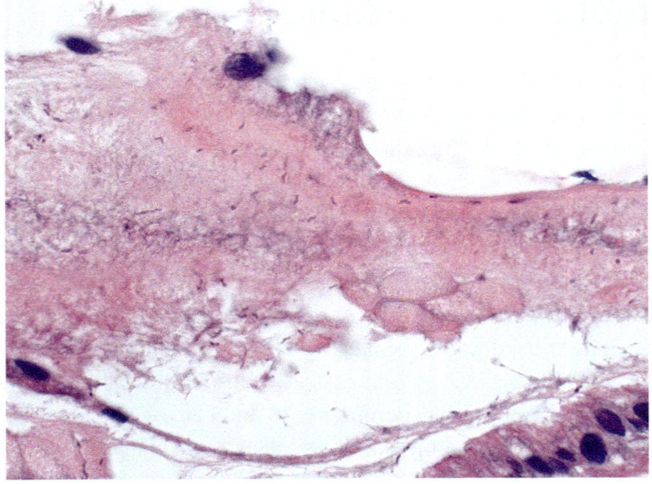

Fig. 6.11 *H. pylori* organisms, H&E. The organisms are thin rods

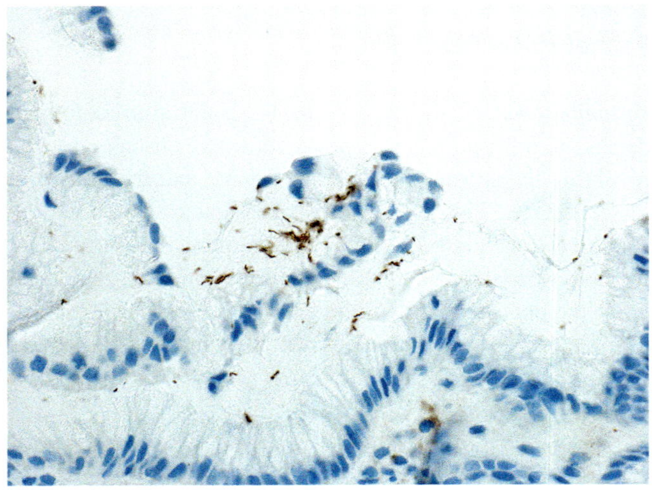

Fig. 6.12 *H. pylori* organisms, immunostain. The organisms are nicely highlighted on an immunostain

Fig. 6.13 *H. pylori* organisms, immunostain. The organisms in this case of partial treatment are present only focally and the sparse organisms are round

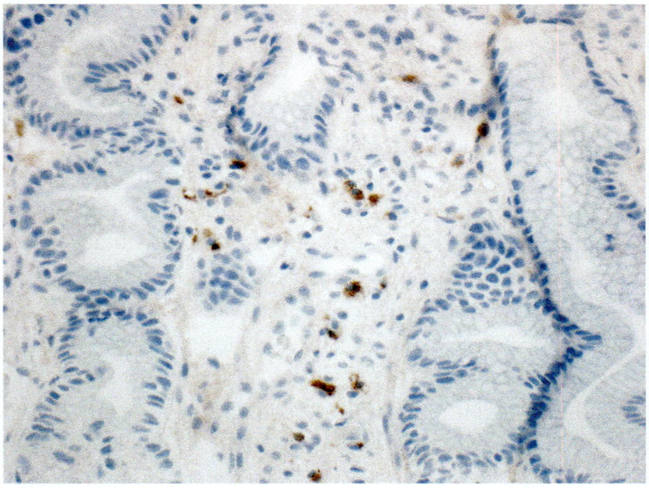

Fig. 6.14 *H. pylori* organisms, immunostain. There is nonspecific granular staining in occasional macrophages, but this should not be interpreted as *H. pylori*

organisms are also identifiable in macrophages, but often this seems to be somewhat in the eye of the beholder. Of note, immunostains often show nonspecific, irregular granular staining of macrophage cytoplasm, and this should not be interpreted as *H. pylori* infection (Fig. 6.14). Organisms are absent to rare in areas of intestinal metaplasia, so biopsies that show extensive or near-total metaplasia of the mucosa are inadequate to rule out *H. pylori* infection. Also of note, organisms tend to be sparse to absent in the reactive epithelium adjacent to an ulcer, so endoscopic sampling that is limited to the edge of the ulcer can miss organisms.

Currently, clinical care decisions are based on the presence or absence of organisms and not on their density, but some pathologists prefer to indicate their density in the pathology report, as suggested in the Sydney classification, which is fine to do as a personal/practice-based preference. For research studies, visual analog scales are available to provide semi-quantitative data [33].

Special Stains for H. pylori Histochemical and immunostains (Figs. 6.12 and 6.13) are available to help identify organisms. In the updated Sydney Classification System and in other expert reviews, reflex stains to identify *H. pylori* were either implicitly [33] or explicitly [38] endorsed in order to identify those rare cases that are *H. pylori* positive but lack the typical active chronic gastritis pattern, including cases with minimal inflammation, cases with more of a reactive gastropathy pattern, and cases with mild chronic gastritis lacking activity. For example, one study showed that 11% of *H. pylori*-positive gastric biopsies do not have the typical pattern of active chronic mucosal inflammation [39]. Reflexive staining is undoubtedly helpful in capturing these cases, but the pendulum has swung (because of cost concerns) to ordering stains for *H. pylori* in situations with a higher likelihood of positivity (Table 6.2) [21].

Table 6.2 Use of special stains to identify *H. pylori*

Biopsy findings	Degree of suspicion for *H. pylori* based on histology	Stains for *H. pylori*
Definite organism seen on H&E	Biopsy proven	Not needed (though some guidelines for the pediatric population recommend confirming studies by PCR or FISH)
Active chronic gastritis with no organisms on H&E	High	Yes
Inactive chronic gastritis with no organisms on H&E	Moderate	Yes, if moderate or marked inflammation; situation dependent with mild chronic gastritis Special situations where *H. pylori* stains are usually needed: prior *H. pylori* treatment with biopsy to assess response; MALT lymphoma; history of gastric or duodenal ulcers; high risk demographics (e.g., household members with known infection)
Antral or fundic mucosa with minimal or mild chronic inflammation, with or without focal minimal activity	Low	Generally not. Consider stain if patient is known to have positive serology or has other risk factors for *H. pylori* (such as actively infected household members)
Antral hyperplastic polyps	Low	No, unless additional finding of chronic gastritis or active chronic gastritis in background mucosa
Fundic gland polyps	Minimal	No, unless additional finding of chronic gastritis or active chronic gastritis in background mucosa
Reactive gastropathy	Minimal	No, unless additional finding of chronic gastritis
Normal antral or fundic mucosa	Absent	No

Metaplasia Metaplasia in the stomach can take the form of intestinal metaplasia (Fig. 6.15), pancreatic acinar cell metaplasia (Fig. 6.16), and pyloric metaplasia (also called pseudopyloric metaplasia) (Fig. 6.17). Intestinal and pancreatic acinar cell metaplasia can be found anywhere in the stomach, while pyloric metaplasia is recognizable in the stomach body/fundus only.

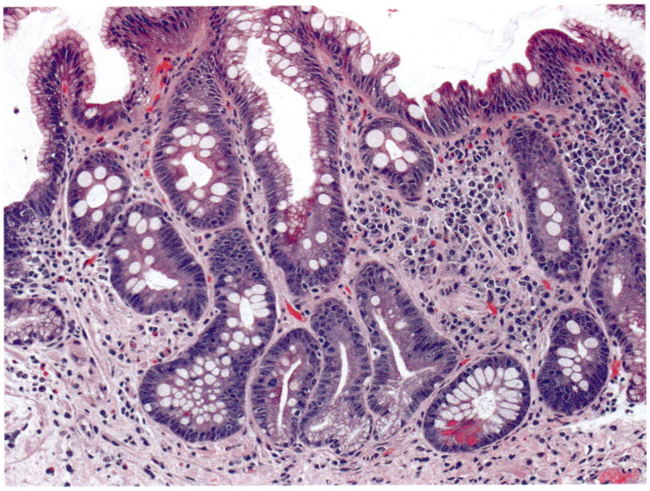

Fig. 6.15 Intestinal metaplasia. The usual gastric mucinous epithelium has been replaced by epithelium with goblet cells interspersed among absorptive-type cells

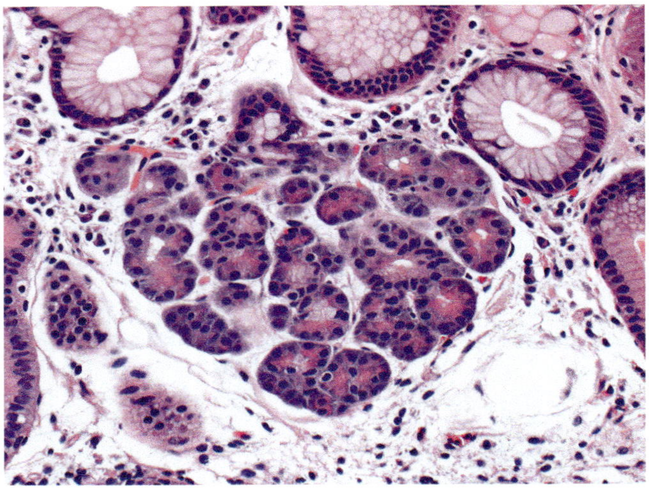

Fig. 6.16 Pancreatic acinar cell metaplasia. This pattern of metaplasia is found mostly in the stomach body and is more common in autoimmune gastritis than in *H. pylori* gastritis

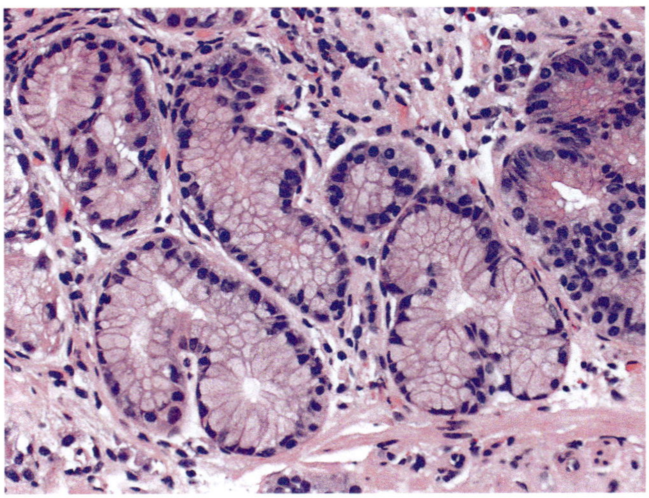

Fig. 6.17 Pseudopyloric metaplasia. The metaplastic glands resemble pylori glands. This pattern of metaplasia is more common in autoimmune gastritis than in *H. pylori* gastritis

Intestinal metaplasia can be further divided into incomplete and complete metaplasia. Incomplete metaplasia has occasional to scattered goblet cells interspersed within gastric-type cells that lack a well-defined brush border and contain neutral mucin (pink on PAS/AB stains at pH 2.5) or contain acidic sialomucins and sulfomucins (purple on PAS/AB stains at pH 2.5). In contrast, complete intestinal metaplasia has a greater number of goblet cells, which are interspersed with non-secretory absorptive-type cells that have well-formed brush borders (negative on PAS/AB stains at pH 2.5) [33]. There have been studies linking incomplete intestinal metaplasia to higher risk of dysplasia and carcinoma [40, 41], but to date the association is not sufficiently established to warrant routine subtyping of metaplasia for clinical purposes.

At the clinical care level, it is sufficient to comment on the presence or absence of intestinal metaplasia. Another useful practice is to provide a sense of how much of the biopsy is metaplastic (e.g., focal metaplasia, diffuse metaplasia, etc.). If the mucosa in the biopsy sample is entirely or nearly entirely metaplastic, then it is inadequate for excluding *H. pylori* infection. There are well-developed and validated visual analog tools to provide semi-quantitative data on the degree of metaplasia [33]. These work well and are important for research studies but are generally not used for clinical care. Sampling error is a well-understood consideration in attempting to extend the biopsy findings to the entire stomach, so it is not the role of the pathologist but the endoscopist to visualize the entire stomach and know whether the findings are targeted toward a lesion or are random samples that are intended to be representative of the stomach.

Intestinal metaplasia is a known intermediate step toward carcinoma, so biopsies with metaplasia should be carefully searched for dysplasia. Intestinal metaplasia often appears somewhat polypoid on endoscopy, especially when the background mucosa shows significant atrophy, and can be received as "biopsy of a polyp."

Atrophy Mucosal atrophy is intuitively easy to understand as thinning of the mucosa because of loss of gastric glands and is easily seen when atrophy is severe. However, this finding is not reproducibly identified in the early stages of disease, even with the use of visual analog tools. Nor is atrophy part of the modern approach to classification of gastric disease, which is instead based on etiology, with atrophy being a consequence of long-standing disease. Almost all causes of chronic injury can lead to mucosal atrophy with sufficient length and severity of disease. At a practical level, atrophy is almost always accompanied by metaplasia, so much so in fact that some pathologists use the terms essentially interchangeably for clinical care.

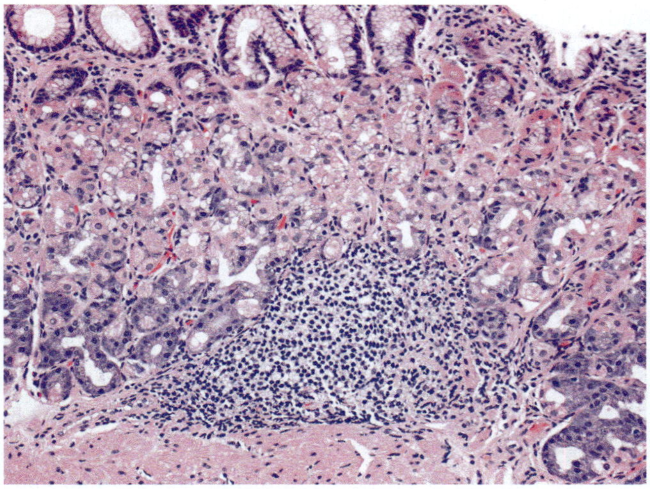

Fig. 6.18 Mild chronic gastritis with lymphoid aggregates. This pattern is sometimes classified as prior or "ex" *H. pylori* gastritis, but the specificity of this pattern for previous *H. pylori* gastritis is not clear

Prior H. pylori Infection The updated Sydney Classification System [33] and subsequent expert reviews [42] suggested that prior *H. pylori* gastritis could be recognized by finding a low-grade inactive chronic gastritis that also contained lymphoid aggregates (Fig. 6.18). This proposal is based on studies that followed the natural history of inflammation after successful treatment of *H. pylori* gastritis. However, it remains unproven that all or even most cases of minimal or mild chronic gastritis with lymphoid aggregates represent prior *H. pylori* infection.

Risk for Gastric Carcinoma and for Lymphoma Chronic *H. pylori* gastritis is strongly associated with an increased risk for mucosal associated lymphoid tissue (MALT) lymphomas. MALT lymphomas are rare, with an incidence rate in the USA of 3.8 per million people years [43], but serological studies show that 80–95% of patients with MALT lymphoma have a history of *H. pylori* exposure [44, 45]. Up to 80% of patients with stage I/II disease achieve complete regression of the lymphoma after eradication of *H. pylori* [46]. Diffuse large B-cell lymphoma (DLBCL) of the stomach can be de novo or associated with *H. pylori* infection [44]. DLBCL patients with limited disease can also achieve remission of their lymphoma by eradication of *H. pylori* in cases where the lymphoma is associated with *H. pylori* infection [47].

Chronic H. pylori infection also increases risk for gastric adenocarcinoma, through the resulting atrophy, metaplasia, and dysplasia sequence [48]. Nonetheless, gastric adenocarcinoma is rare in the Western world, despite the much higher frequency of *H. pylori* infection, and the overall odds ratio of developing gastric carcinoma is modestly elevated, at 2–3 [49].

Treatment

There are at least seven FDA-approved treatment regiments for *H. pylori*, with most involving 10–14 days of therapy [50]. Several common examples are as follows: proton pump inhibitor, amoxicillin or metronidazole, and clarithromycin (clarithromycin triple therapy); proton pump inhibitor, bismuth subsalicylate, nitroimidazole, and tetracycline (bismuth quadruple therapy). The various treatments have reported cure rates of about 90%.

Helicobacter heilmannii Gastritis

H. heilmannii gastritis is caused by a number of different organisms that are closely related and show a similar morphology on H&E and histochemical stains. There are about 30 formal species, such as *H. felix* or *H. suis* [51], but all of them are generally referred to as *H. heilmannii* when are identified solely on immunohistochemistry. In human tissue, *H. suis* is the most prevalent [51]. The prevalence is much lower than *H. pylori* gastritis, typically about 0.1% [52–54]. In rare cases, both *H. pylori* and *H. heilmannii* can be present [53].

The mucosal findings in *H. heilmannii* gastritis are largely similar to those of *H. pylori* gastritis, with antral-predominant active chronic gastritis. However, the activity and the degree of chronic inflammation tend to be lower in grade [54, 55]. Lymphoid aggregates can be present [53] and MALT lymphoma can develop [55].

The organisms are about twice as long, and distinct spirals can sometimes be discerned on higher magnification (Fig. 6.19). The organisms can be less numerous and more patchy in comparison to *H. pylori*. Both organisms are read-

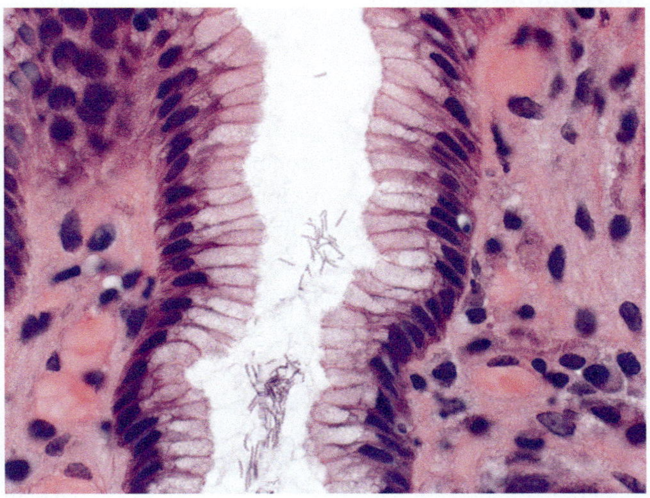

Fig. 6.19 *H. heilmannii* gastritis. The organisms are longer than typical *H. pylori* and show distinctive spirals

ily visualized on histochemical stains. Many but not all commercial antibodies to *H. pylori* will cross react with *H. heilmannii*.

Helicobacter pylori-Negative Chronic Gastritis

The criteria used to define a chronic gastritis have not been rigorously established. The updated Sydney Classification System suggested that the maximum number of mononuclear cells in the normal gastric mucosa is 2 to –5 lymphocytes, plasma cells, or macrophages per high-power field (40X objective) [33]. As an alternative approach, a normal biopsy could have clusters of no more than two to three lymphocytes or plasma cells in the superficial lamina propria [33]. These thresholds seem low and are not well validated. Despite the lack of established criteria, cases of *H. pylori*-negative chronic gastritis are not uncommon in clinical practice. One study of 1240 patients found that 10% of antral biopsies showed *H. pylori*-negative chronic gastritis [56]. A subset of these cases will also show active (neutrophilic) inflammation, and the historical adage that active chronic inflammation, outside the setting of Crohn's disease, almost always indicates *H. pylori* infection no longer matches the empirical evidence.

Some cases of *H. pylori*-negative gastritis reflect sampling effect, partial inadvertent treatment from antibiotics used for recent or concurrent infections of other organs, or *H. pylori* infections that are masked by the use of proton pump inhibitors. However, there remains a substantial proportion of cases that are unexplained with our current fund of knowledge.

Autoimmune Gastritis

Definition

Older terms for autoimmune gastritis were based on either topography or etiology plus morphology and include type A gastritis and autoimmune metaplastic atrophic gastritis (AMAG). These older terms are important for historical reasons, but the current approach is to classify disease by etiology, using the term autoimmune gastritis.

Clinical Features

Autoimmune gastritis is most commonly seen in middle-aged individuals with a median age of about 55 [57]. About 70% of cases are identified in women [57]. The prevalence has not been well established, but in a European multicenter study of surgical pathology specimens, the frequency of autoimmune gastritis was 2% [4]. On the other hand, in a population-based study from Germany, one that focused on individuals between 50 and 74 years of age, the prevalence was 19% based on serological studies [58]. The frequency of pernicious anemia (a result of late-stage autoimmune gastritis) is lower, estimated to be about 2% in those older than 60 years of age [59]. The data is mixed on whether autoimmune gastritis is specifically associated with Northern European ancestry. While most cases are found in adults, the disease is also well documented in the pediatric population [60].

Autoimmune gastritis can be asymptomatic or be associated with nonspecific complaints such as dyspepsia [57]. Common findings at presentation include fatigue and anemia. Autoimmune gastritis is associated with pernicious anemia (anemia resulting from lack of vitamin B12, leading to macrocytic, megaloblastic anemia), but this finding is now less common because of supplementation of food with vitamins, including B12. Nonetheless, one study found 54% of patients with autoimmune gastritis had pernicious anemia [57]. This same study found iron deficiency anemia at presentation in 35% of cases [57]. Patients with late-stage disease and significant B12 deficiency can also have a wide variety of neurological clinical signs and symptoms.

Patients can have serum autoantibodies to intrinsic factor and/or to parietal cells. Anti-parietal cell antibodies have a sensitivity for autoimmune gastritis of about 80%, with a specificity of about 70%. Intrinsic factor antibodies are highly specific (>95%) but less sensitive (40%). Other autoimmune conditions common in patients with autoimmune gastritis include autoimmune thyroid disease [61] and type 1 diabetes mellitus [62].

The destruction of the parietal cells by autoimmune gastritis leads to a hypochloridic gastric lumen. This triggers antral G cells to produce high levels of gastrin, as gastrin in the normal stomach increases acid production. The chronically increased gastrin levels in turn lead to proliferation of endocrine cells in the stomach body, which are called enterochromaffin-like (ECL) cells. These ECL cells can become hyperplastic and eventually form neuroendocrine tumors. As a result of these changes, patients with autoimmune gastritis typically have elevated serum levels of both gastrin and chromogranin A [63].

Pathological Features

Autoimmune gastritis is a body-predominant pattern of disease, with inflammatory destruction of the oxyntic glands leading to mucosal atrophy, metaplasia, and ECL cell hyperplasia (Figs. 6.20 and 6.21). The inflammation is predominately lymphocytic, but plasma cells can be prominent.

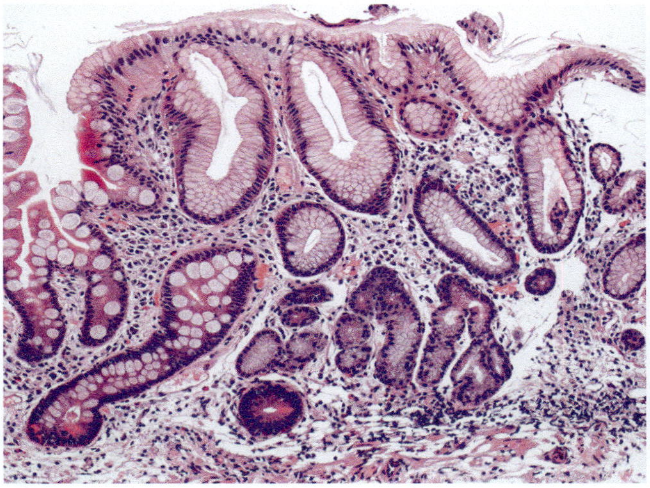

Fig. 6.20 Autoimmune gastritis. The stomach body biopsies show chronic inflammation with loss of the normal oxyntic glands and intestinal and pyloric metaplasia

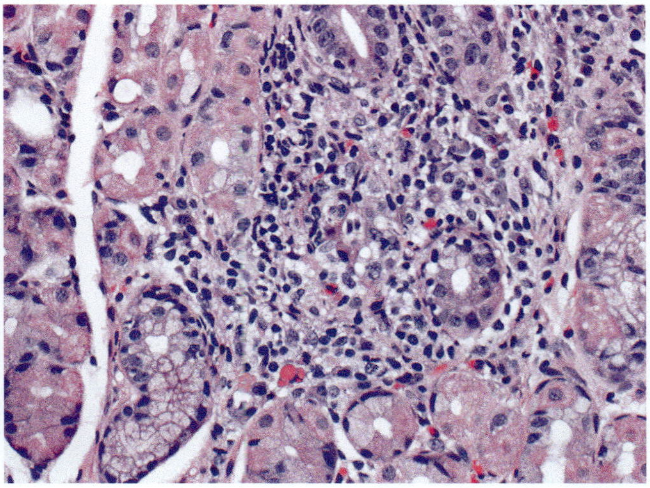

Fig. 6.22 Autoimmune gastritis, early. This biopsy from the stomach body shows oxyntic glands with lymphocytosis and injury

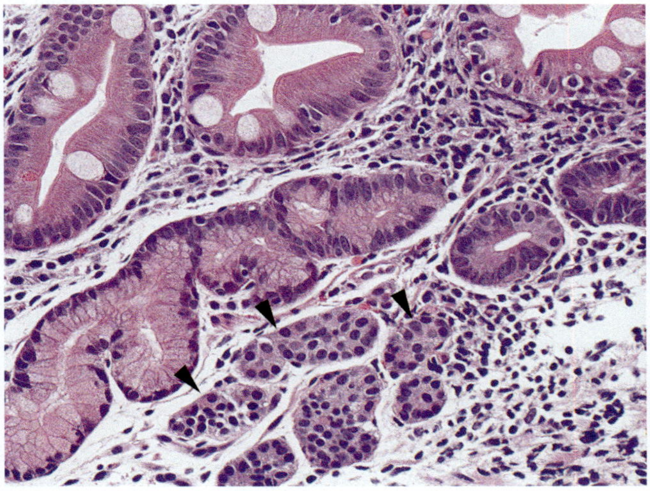

Fig. 6.21 Autoimmune gastritis, ECL cell hyperplasia. Nodules of ECL cell hyperplasia (arrowheads) are evident on H&E

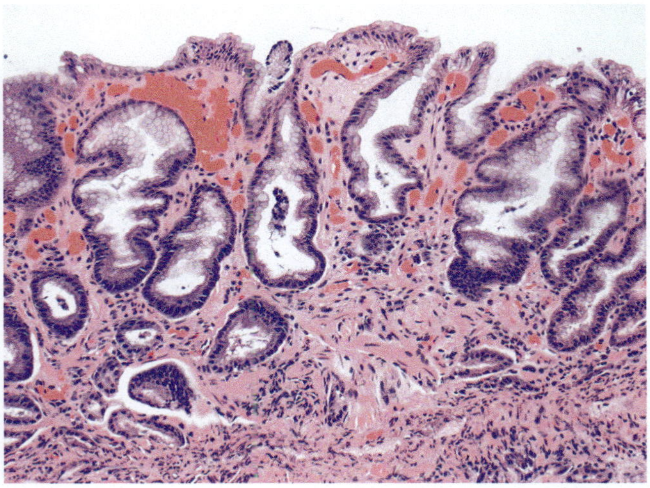

Fig. 6.23 Autoimmune gastritis, antrum. The antral biopsy showed mild nonspecific inflammation with no atrophy or metaplasia. There is mild corkscrewing of the glands, suggesting a component of reactive gastropathy

Neutrophilic inflammation is generally sparse or absent. In early disease, the atrophy and metaplasia are patchy and there can be lymphocytic inflammation of the body glands (Fig. 6.22) [64]. Metaplasia is usually pyloric or intestinal, but pancreatic acinar metaplasia is also common. Pancreatic acinar cell metaplasia is present in about 50% of all cases and is more commonly seen in autoimmune gastritis than in *H. pylori* gastritis [65]. Biopsies of the antrum (Fig. 6.23) can show mild nonspecific chronic inflammation, mild reactive gastropathy-type changes, or both.

The diagnosis of autoimmune gastritis is made by finding chronic gastritis of the body that is often accompanied by at least patchy atrophy and metaplasia. Because of the common clinical practice of either not designating the biopsy location or putting biopsies from both the antrum and the body in the same container, it is best to prove a tissue fragment of body origin by the lack of G cells. Gastrin immunostain is positive in the antrum, shows patchy staining in the antral-fundic transition zone, and is negative in the body. Of note, gastrin-positive cells can be present in intestinal metaplasia, so that the atrophic body mucosa with intestinal metaplasia may be mistakenly considered as antral mucosa. In addition, essentially all cases of autoimmune gastritis, even early ones, show at least mild ECL cell hyperplasia. ECL cell hyperplasia is defined as the presence of at least five adjacent positive cells on chromogranin or synaptophysin immunostain. There can be linear hyperplasia (Fig. 6.24) or nodular hyperplasia (Fig. 6.25). Nodular ECL cell hyperplasia can be seen on

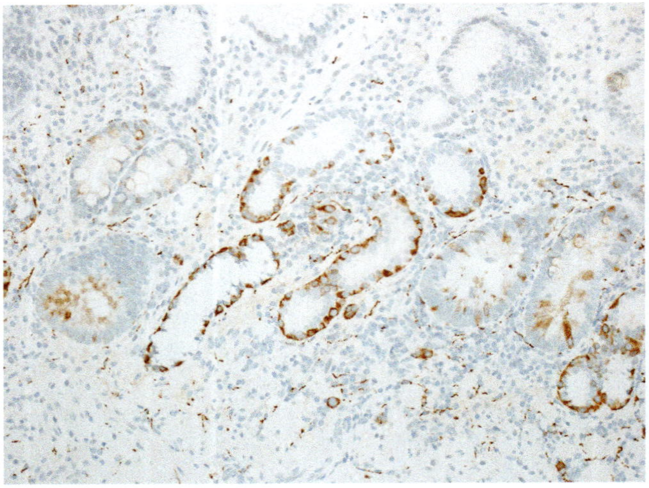

Fig. 6.24 ECL cell hyperplasia, chromogranin A immunostain. The gastric pits are lined by ECL cells that are in continuous chains of at least five cells in length

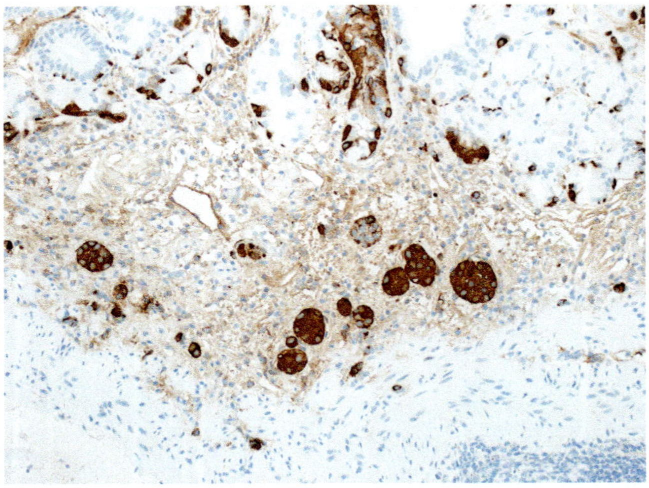

Fig. 6.25 Autoimmune gastritis, nodular ECL cell hyperplasia, chromogranin A immunostain. Distinctive nodules of ECL cells are seen

H&E, but it is best to confirm the findings with immunohistochemistry. The ECL cell hyperplasia can progress over time, leading to increasing sized neuroendocrine proliferations (Fig. 6.26) (Table 6.3). Neuroendocrine tumors are usually well differentiated, WHO grade 1 [66].

Autoimmune gastritis has been linked to both pseudopolyps and epithelial polyps. Pseudopolyps are found in the body mucosa when relatively preserved islands of mucosa appear polypoid, being juxtaposed to adjacent areas of mucosal atrophy [67]. The antral mucosa can also show hyperplastic polyps [68]. The most common epithelial polyp in autoimmune gastritis is the pyloric gland adenoma. While pyloric gland adenomas make up only 3% of all gastric polyps, 36% occur in the setting of autoimmune gastritis [69]. Tubular adenomas can also develop in cases of autoimmune gastritis [70].

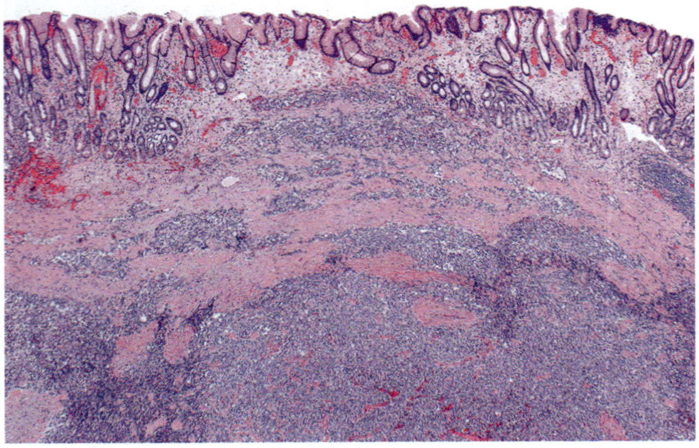

Fig. 6.26 Autoimmune gastritis, neuroendocrine tumor. A large submucosal tumor is seen

Table 6.3 Classification of ECL cell proliferations in the setting of autoimmune gastritis

Finding	Definition	Notes
Normal	Scattered positive cells	
ECL cell hyperplasia	Linear hyperplasia = at least five adjacent immunostain-positive ECL cells Nodular hyperplasia = nodule of at least five immunostain-positive ECL cells	Linear hyperplasia typically precedes nodular hyperplasia
Neuroendocrine dysplasia	Nodules of ECL cells that are between 150 and 500 μm	500 μm = 0.5 mm
Microcarcinoid	Nodules of ECL cells that are between >0.5 mm and <0.5 cm	
Neuroendocrine tumor	Nodule of ECL cells >0.5 cm	Should be graded using standard WHO approach

Autoimmune Pangastritis

Definition

This is a rare form of chronic gastritis involving both gastric antrum and body which is believed due to an autoimmune etiology.

Clinical Features

Autoimmune pangastritis can affect both children and adults. Essentially all patients have concurrent autoimmune conditions of other organs. In children and teenaged individuals, the most common association is with autoimmune enterocolitis, some of whom also have the X-linked syndrome of immune dysregulation, polyendocrinopathy, and enteropathy (IPEX) [71]. One study also reported a similar pattern of gastritis in two children with X-linked lymphoproliferative disease [72]. In adults, cases have been reported in individuals with systemic lupus, autoimmune hemolytic anemia, refractory sprue, and disabling fibromyalgia [71]. Serologies are commonly positive for ANA and other autoimmune markers. Data on the presence of anti-parietal bodies and anti-intrinsic factor is limited to one case, but they were negative [71].

Pathological Features

Autoimmune pangastritis shows marked chronic gastritis that leads to progressive atrophy and metaplasia of both the body and the antrum (Figs. 6.27, 6.28, and 6.29) [71]. The inflammation is predominately lymphoplasmacytic with patchy areas of activity.

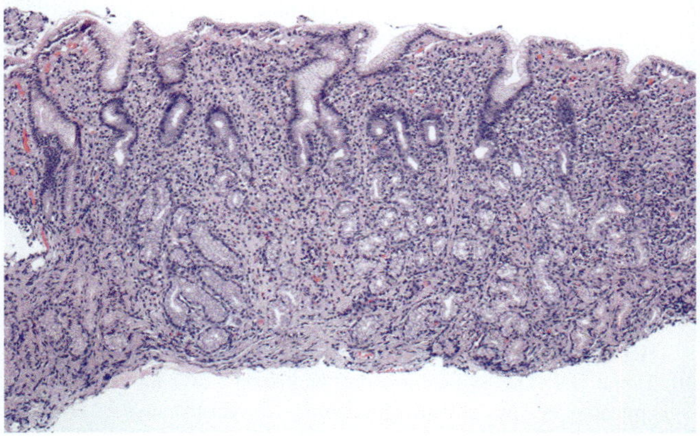

Fig. 6.27 Autoimmune pangastritis. The antral mucosa shows marked chronic inflammation

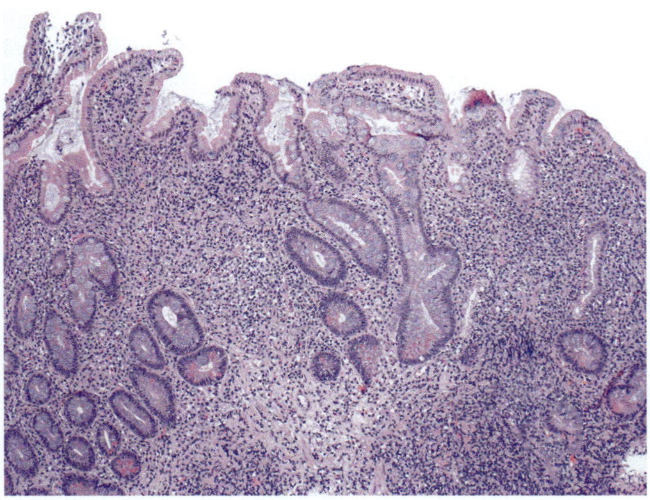

Fig. 6.28 Autoimmune pangastritis. The body shows marked chronic inflammation

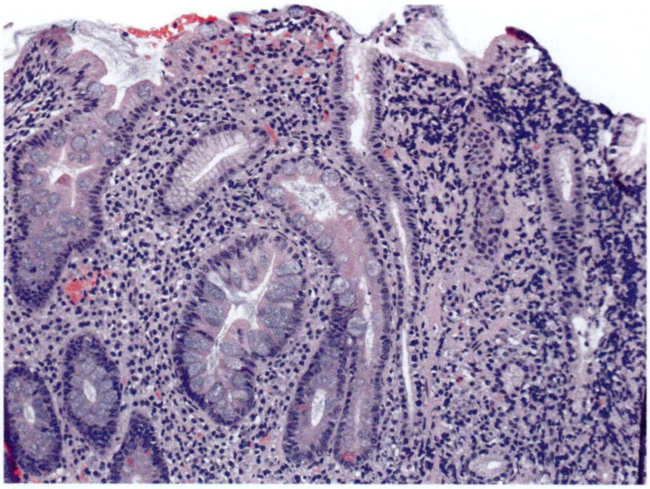

Fig. 6.29 Autoimmune pangastritis. The body shows extensive intestinal metaplasia with loss of oxyntic glands

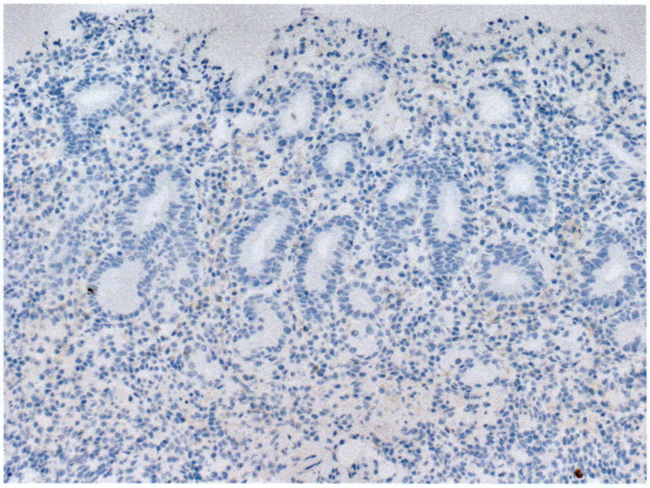

Fig. 6.30 Autoimmune pangastritis, chromogranin immunostain. There is no evidence for ECL cell hyperplasia in this body biopsy, despite extensive atrophy and metaplasia

The inflammation is equally present in the antrum and the body and fairly evenly distributed throughout the lamina propria. The mucosal atrophy and metaplasia are generally marked and diffuse. In contrast to typical autoimmune gastritis, ECL cell hyperplasia is not evident because the antral G cells that produce gastrin are also destroyed (Fig. 6.30). Low-grade dysplasia has been reported [71]. The autoimmune pangastritis pattern is distinct from typical autoimmune gastritis both because of the antral involvement and the lack of ECL cell hyperplasia.

References

1. Maguilnik I, Neumann WL, Sonnenberg A, Genta RM. Reactive gastropathy is associated with inflammatory conditions throughout the gastrointestinal tract. Aliment Pharmacol Ther. 2012;36(8):736–43. https://doi.org/10.1111/apt.12031.

2. Frezza M, Gorji N, Melato M. The histopathology of non-steroidal anti-inflammatory drug induced gastroduodenal damage: correlation with Helicobacter pylori, ulcers, and haemorrhagic events. J Clin Pathol. 2001;54(7):521–5.
3. Haber MM, Lopez I. Gastric histologic findings in patients with nonsteroidal anti-inflammatory drug-associated gastric ulcer. Mod Pathol. 1999;12(6):592–8.
4. Wolf EM, Plieschnegger W, Geppert M, Wigginghaus B, Hoss GM, Eherer A, et al. Changing prevalence patterns in endoscopic and histological diagnosis of gastritis? Data from a cross-sectional Central European multicentre study. Dig Liver Dis. 2014;46(5):412–8. https://doi.org/10.1016/j.dld.2013.12.017.
5. Nakos A, Kouklakis G, Pitiakoudis M, Zezos P, Efraimidou E, Giatromanolaki A, et al. The histological and immunohistochemical aspects of bile reflux in patients with gastroesophageal reflux disease. Gastroenterol Res Pract. 2011;2011:905872. https://doi.org/10.1155/2011/905872.
6. Srivastava A, Lauwers GY. Pathology of non-infective gastritis. Histopathology. 2007;50(1):15–29. https://doi.org/10.1111/j.1365-2559.2006.02553.x.
7. Yu QQ, Tariq A, Unger SW, Cabello-Inchausti B, Robinson MJ. Phlegmonous gastritis associated with Kaposi sarcoma: a case report and review of the literature. Arch Pathol Lab Med. 2004;128(7):801–3. https://doi.org/10.1043/1543-2165(2004)128<801:PGAWKS>2.0.CO;2.
8. O'Toole PA, Morris JA. Acute phlegmonous gastritis. Postgrad Med J. 1988;64(750):315–6.
9. Munroe CA, Chen A. Suppurative (phlegmonous) gastritis presenting as a gastric mass. Dig Dis Sci. 2010;55(1):11–3. https://doi.org/10.1007/s10620-009-0961-7.
10. Huang JQ, Sridhar S, Hunt RH. Role of Helicobacter pylori infection and non-steroidal anti-inflammatory drugs in peptic-ulcer disease: a meta-analysis. Lancet. 2002;359(9300):14–22. https://doi.org/10.1016/S0140-6736(02)07273-2.
11. Lanas A, Chan FKL. Peptic ulcer disease. Lancet. 2017;390(10094):613–24. https://doi.org/10.1016/S0140-6736(16)32404-7.
12. Charpignon C, Lesgourgues B, Pariente A, Nahon S, Pelaquier A, Gatineau-Sailliant G, et al. Peptic ulcer disease: one in five is related to neither Helicobacter pylori nor aspirin/NSAID intake. Aliment Pharmacol Ther. 2013;38(8):946–54. https://doi.org/10.1111/apt.12465.
13. Committee ASoP, Banerjee S, Cash BD, Dominitz JA, Baron TH, Anderson MA, et al. The role of endoscopy in the management of patients with peptic ulcer disease. Gastrointest Endosc. 2010;71(4):663–8. https://doi.org/10.1016/j.gie.2009.11.026.
14. Peixoto A, Silva M, Pereira P, Macedo G. Biopsies in gastrointestinal endoscopy: when and how. GE Port J Gastroenterol. 2016;23(1):19–27. https://doi.org/10.1016/j.jpge.2015.07.004.
15. Forbat LN, Walker MM, Gribble RJ, Baron JH. Lack of clinical value of biopsy of duodenal ulcer at endoscopy. Gastrointest Endosc. 1987;33(3):269–70.
16. Hissong E, Jessurun J, Yantiss RK. Findings in exudates can help distinguish benign gastric ulcers from ulcerated adenocarcinomas. Histopathology. 2018;73(2):215–9. https://doi.org/10.1111/his.13510.
17. Kalach N, Bontems P, Raymond J. Helicobacter pylori infection in children. Helicobacter. 2017;22(Suppl 1) https://doi.org/10.1111/hel.12414.
18. Mamishi S, Eshaghi H, Mahmoudi S, Bahador A, Hosseinpour Sadeghi R, Najafi M, et al. Intrafamilial transmission of Helicobacter pylori: genotyping of faecal samples. Br J Biomed Sci. 2016;73(1):38–43. https://doi.org/10.1080/09674845.2016.1150666.
19. Konno M, Yokota S, Suga T, Takahashi M, Sato K, Fujii N. Predominance of mother-to-child transmission of Helicobacter pylori infection detected by random amplified polymorphic DNA fingerprinting analysis in Japanese families. Pediatr Infect Dis J. 2008;27(11):999–1003. https://doi.org/10.1097/INF.0b013e31817d756e.
20. Jones NL, Koletzko S, Goodman K, Bontems P, Cadranel S, Casswall T, et al. Joint ESPGHAN/NASPGHAN guidelines for the management of Helicobacter pylori in children and adolescents (update 2016). J Pediatr Gastroenterol Nutr. 2017;64(6):991–1003. https://doi.org/10.1097/MPG.0000000000001594.
21. Batts KP, Ketover S, Kakar S, Krasinskas AM, Mitchell KA, Wilcox R, et al. Appropriate use of special stains for identifying Helicobacter pylori: recommendations from the Rodger C. Haggitt Gastrointestinal Pathology Society. Am J Surg Pathol. 2013;37(11):e12–22. https://doi.org/10.1097/PAS.0000000000000097.
22. Rosenstock S, Jorgensen T, Andersen L, Bonnevie O. Seroconversion and seroreversion in IgG antibodies to Helicobacter pylori: a serology based prospective cohort study. J Epidemiol Community Health. 2000;54(6):444–50.
23. Wang YK, Kuo FC, Liu CJ, Wu MC, Shih HY, Wang SS, et al. Diagnosis of Helicobacter pylori infection: current options and developments. World J Gastroenterol. 2015;21(40):11221–35. https://doi.org/10.3748/wjg.v21.i40.11221.
24. Targownik LE, Metge C, Roos L, Leung S. The prevalence of and the clinical and demographic characteristics associated with high-intensity proton pump inhibitor use. Am J Gastroenterol. 2007;102(5):942–50. https://doi.org/10.1111/j.1572-0241.2007.01106.x.
25. McColl KE. Clinical practice. Helicobacter pylori infection. N Engl J Med. 2010;362(17):1597–604. https://doi.org/10.1056/NEJMcp1001110.
26. Vilaichone RK, Quach DT, Yamaoka Y, Sugano K, Mahachai V. Prevalence and pattern of antibiotic resistant strains of Helicobacter pylori infection in ASEAN. Asian Pac J Cancer Prev. 2018;19(5):1411–3. https://doi.org/10.22034/APJCP.2018.19.5.1411.
27. Misiewicz JJ. The Sydney System: a new classification of gastritis. Introduction. J Gastroenterol Hepatol. 1991;6(3):207–8.
28. Goodwin CS. The Sydney System: microbial gastritis. J Gastroenterol Hepatol. 1991;6(3):235–7.
29. Price AB. The Sydney System: histological division. J Gastroenterol Hepatol. 1991;6(3):209–22.
30. Tytgat GN. The Sydney System: endoscopic division. Endoscopic appearances in gastritis/duodenitis. J Gastroenterol Hepatol. 1991;6(3):223–34.
31. Strickland RG. The Sydney System: auto-immune gastritis. J Gastroenterol Hepatol. 1991;6(3):238–43.
32. Sipponen P, Kekki M, Siurala M. The Sydney System: epidemiology and natural history of chronic gastritis. J Gastroenterol Hepatol. 1991;6(3):244–51.
33. Dixon MF, Genta RM, Yardley JH, Correa P. Classification and grading of gastritis. The updated Sydney System. International Workshop on the Histopathology of Gastritis, Houston 1994. Am J Surg Pathol. 1996;20(10):1161–81.
34. Yang HR. Updates on the diagnosis of Helicobacter pylori infection in children: what are the differences between adults and children? Pediatr Gastroenterol Hepatol Nutr. 2016;19(2):96–103. https://doi.org/10.5223/pghn.2016.19.2.96.
35. Yang HR, Choi HS, Paik JH, Lee HS. Endoscopic and histologic analysis of gastric mucosa-associated lymphoid tissue in children with Helicobacter pylori infection. J Pediatr Gastroenterol Nutr. 2013;57(3):298–304. https://doi.org/10.1097/MPG.0b013e318298020a.
36. Mazigh Mrad S, Abidi K, Brini I, Boukthir S, Sammoud A. Nodular gastritis: an endoscopic indicator of Helicobacter pylori infection in children. Tunis Med. 2012;90(11):789–92.
37. Mejia CR, Vera CA, Huiza-Espinoza L. Association between follicular gastritis and Helicobacter pylori in children seen at a public hospital in Peru. Rev Gastroenterol Mex. 2016;81(2):80–5. https://doi.org/10.1016/j.rgmx.2016.01.003.

38. Genta RM, Lash RH. Helicobacter pylori-negative gastritis: seek, yet ye shall not always find. Am J Surg Pathol. 2010;34(8):e25–34. https://doi.org/10.1097/PAS.0b013e3181e51067.
39. Glickman JN, Noffsinger A, Nevin DT, Ray M, Lash RH, Genta RM. Helicobacter infections with rare bacteria or minimal gastritis: expecting the unexpected. Dig Liver Dis. 2015;47(7):549–55. https://doi.org/10.1016/j.dld.2015.04.005.
40. Pittayanon R, Rerknimitr R, Klaikaew N, Sanpavat A, Chaithongrat S, Mahachai V, et al. The risk of gastric cancer in patients with gastric intestinal metaplasia in 5-year follow-up. Aliment Pharmacol Ther. 2017;46(1):40–5. https://doi.org/10.1111/apt.14082.
41. Gonzalez CA, Sanz-Anquela JM, Companioni O, Bonet C, Berdasco M, Lopez C, et al. Incomplete type of intestinal metaplasia has the highest risk to progress to gastric cancer: results of the Spanish follow-up multicenter study. J Gastroenterol Hepatol. 2016;31(5):953–8. https://doi.org/10.1111/jgh.13249.
42. Stolte M, Meining A. The updated Sydney system: classification and grading of gastritis as the basis of diagnosis and treatment. Can J Gastroenterol. 2001;15(9):591–8.
43. Khalil MO, Morton LM, Devesa SS, Check DP, Curtis RE, Weisenburger DD, et al. Incidence of marginal zone lymphoma in the United States, 2001–2009 with a focus on primary anatomic site. Br J Haematol. 2014;165(1):67–77. https://doi.org/10.1111/bjh.12730.
44. Delchier JC, Lamarque D, Levy M, Tkoub EM, Copie-Bergman C, Deforges L, et al. Helicobacter pylori and gastric lymphoma: high seroprevalence of CagA in diffuse large B-cell lymphoma but not in low-grade lymphoma of mucosa-associated lymphoid tissue type. Am J Gastroenterol. 2001;96(8):2324–8. https://doi.org/10.1111/j.1572-0241.2001.04036.x.
45. Eck M, Schmausser B, Haas R, Greiner A, Czub S, Muller-Hermelink HK. MALT-type lymphoma of the stomach is associated with Helicobacter pylori strains expressing the CagA protein. Gastroenterology. 1997;112(5):1482–6.
46. Fischbach W. Gastric MALT lymphoma—update on diagnosis and treatment. Best Pract Res Clin Gastroenterol. 2014;28(6):1069–77. https://doi.org/10.1016/j.bpg.2014.09.006.
47. Kuo SH, Yeh KH, Wu MS, Lin CW, Hsu PN, Wang HP, et al. Helicobacter pylori eradication therapy is effective in the treatment of early-stage H pylori-positive gastric diffuse large B-cell lymphomas. Blood. 2012;119(21):4838–44; quiz 5057. https://doi.org/10.1182/blood-2012-01-404194.
48. Correa P, Piazuelo MB. Helicobacter pylori infection and gastric adenocarcinoma. US Gastroenterol Hepatol Rev. 2011;7(1):59–64.
49. Pormohammad A, Ghotaslou R, Leylabadlo HE, Nasiri MJ, Dabiri H, Hashemi A. Risk of gastric cancer in association with Helicobacter pylori different virulence factors: a systematic review and meta-analysis. Microb Pathog. 2018;118:214–9. https://doi.org/10.1016/j.micpath.2018.03.004.
50. Chey WD, Leontiadis GI, Howden CW, Moss SF. ACG clinical guideline: treatment of Helicobacter pylori infection. Am J Gastroenterol. 2017;112(2):212–39. https://doi.org/10.1038/ajg.2016.563.
51. Bento-Miranda M, Figueiredo C. Helicobacter heilmannii sensu lato: an overview of the infection in humans. World J Gastroenterol. 2014;20(47):17779–87. https://doi.org/10.3748/wjg.v20.i47.17779.
52. Okiyama Y, Matsuzawa K, Hidaka E, Sano K, Akamatsu T, Ota H. Helicobacter heilmannii infection: clinical, endoscopic and histopathological features in Japanese patients. Pathol Int. 2005;55(7):398–404. https://doi.org/10.1111/j.1440-1827.2005.01844.x.
53. Ierardi E, Monno RA, Gentile A, Francavilla R, Burattini O, Marangi S, et al. Helicobacter heilmannii gastritis: a histological and immunohistochemical trait. J Clin Pathol. 2001;54(10):774–7.
54. Joo M, Kwak JE, Chang SH, Kim H, Chi JG, Kim KA, et al. Helicobacter heilmannii-associated gastritis: clinicopathologic findings and comparison with Helicobacter pylori-associated gastritis. J Korean Med Sci. 2007;22(1):63–9. https://doi.org/10.3346/jkms.2007.22.1.63.
55. Stolte M, Kroher G, Meining A, Morgner A, Bayerdorffer E, Bethke B. A comparison of Helicobacter pylori and H. heilmannii gastritis. A matched control study involving 404 patients. Scand J Gastroenterol. 1997;32(1):28–33.
56. Shiota S, Thrift AP, Green L, Shah R, Verstovsek G, Rugge M, et al. Clinical manifestations of Helicobacter pylori-negative gastritis. Clin Gastroenterol Hepatol. 2017;15(7):1037–46.e3. https://doi.org/10.1016/j.cgh.2017.01.006.
57. Carabotti M, Lahner E, Esposito G, Sacchi MC, Severi C, Annibale B. Upper gastrointestinal symptoms in autoimmune gastritis: a cross-sectional study. Medicine (Baltimore). 2017;96(1):e5784. https://doi.org/10.1097/MD.0000000000005784.
58. Zhang Y, Weck MN, Schottker B, Rothenbacher D, Brenner H. Gastric parietal cell antibodies, Helicobacter pylori infection, and chronic atrophic gastritis: evidence from a large population-based study in Germany. Cancer Epidemiol Biomark Prev. 2013;22(5):821–6. https://doi.org/10.1158/1055-9965.EPI-12-1343.
59. Andres E, Serraj K. Optimal management of pernicious anemia. J Blood Med. 2012;3:97–103. https://doi.org/10.2147/JBM.S25620.
60. Pogoriler J, Kamin D, Goldsmith JD. Pediatric non-Helicobacter pylori atrophic gastritis: a case series. Am J Surg Pathol. 2015;39(6):786–92. https://doi.org/10.1097/PAS.0000000000000378.
61. Venerito M, Radunz M, Reschke K, Reinhold D, Frauenschlager K, Jechorek D, et al. Autoimmune gastritis in autoimmune thyroid disease. Aliment Pharmacol Ther. 2015;41(7):686–93. https://doi.org/10.1111/apt.13097.
62. De Block CE, De Leeuw IH, Van Gaal LF. Autoimmune gastritis in type 1 diabetes: a clinically oriented review. J Clin Endocrinol Metab. 2008;93(2):363–71. https://doi.org/10.1210/jc.2007-2134.
63. Miceli E, Padula D, Lenti MV, Gallia A, Albertini R, Di Stefano M, et al. A laboratory score in the diagnosis of autoimmune atrophic gastritis: a prospective study. J Clin Gastroenterol. 2015;49(1):e1–5. https://doi.org/10.1097/MCG.0000000000000101.
64. Torbenson M, Abraham SC, Boitnott J, Yardley JH, Wu TT. Autoimmune gastritis: distinct histological and immunohistochemical findings before complete loss of oxyntic glands. Mod Pathol. 2002;15(2):102–9. https://doi.org/10.1038/modpathol.3880499.
65. Jhala NC, Montemor M, Jhala D, Lu L, Talley L, Haber MM, et al. Pancreatic acinar cell metaplasia in autoimmune gastritis. Arch Pathol Lab Med. 2003;127(7):854–7. https://doi.org/10.1043/1543-2165(2003)127<854:PACMIA>2.0.CO;2.
66. Lee HE, Mounajjed T, Erickson LA, Wu TT. Sporadic gastric well-differentiated neuroendocrine tumors have a higher Ki-67 proliferative index. Endocr Pathol. 2016;27(3):259–67. https://doi.org/10.1007/s12022-016-9443-6.
67. Krasinskas AM, Abraham SC, Metz DC, Furth EE. Oxyntic mucosa pseudopolyps: a presentation of atrophic autoimmune gastritis. Am J Surg Pathol. 2003;27(2):236–41.
68. Abraham SC, Singh VK, Yardley JH, Wu TT. Hyperplastic polyps of the stomach: associations with histologic patterns of gastritis and gastric atrophy. Am J Surg Pathol. 2001;25(4):500–7.
69. Vieth M, Kushima R, Borchard F, Stolte M. Pyloric gland adenoma: a clinico-pathological analysis of 90 cases. Virchows Arch. 2003;442(4):317–21. https://doi.org/10.1007/s00428-002-0750-6.
70. Chlumska A, Boudova L, Benes Z, Zamecnik M. Autoimmune gastritis. A clinicopathologic study of 25 cases. Cesk Patol. 2005;41(4):137–42.
71. Jevremovic D, Torbenson M, Murray JA, Burgart LJ, Abraham SC. Atrophic autoimmune pangastritis: a distinctive form of antral and fundic gastritis associated with systemic autoimmune disease. Am J Surg Pathol. 2006;30(11):1412–9. https://doi.org/10.1097/01.pas.0000213337.25111.37.
72. Rougemont AL, Fournet JC, Martin SR, de Saint-Basile G, Latour S, Primeau MN, et al. Chronic active gastritis in X-linked lymphoproliferative disease. Am J Surg Pathol. 2008;32(2):323–8. https://doi.org/10.1097/PAS.0b013e318141fca1.

7 Special Forms of Gastritis

Saba Yasir

Lymphocytic Gastritis

Definition

Lymphocytic gastritis (LG) is characterized by intraepithelial lymphocytosis involving the foveolar epithelium, as well as expansion of lamina propria by chronic inflammation.

Clinical Features

LG is an uncommon form of chronic gastritis. The prevalence of LG was reported to be 0.83–1.4% among adult patients with nonulcer dyspepsia, 1.63–4.5% among adult patients with chronic gastritis, and 3.7% among children undergoing upper endoscopy for symptoms of diarrhea, vomiting, and failure to thrive [1–4]. Adult patients are most commonly affected, with a peak incidence in the sixth decade of life. There is no sex predilection [3, 5]. The most common presenting symptoms are abdominal pain, dyspepsia, iron deficiency anemia, weight loss, anorexia, and severe hypoproteinemia [1, 5, 6]. Children usually present with recurrent vomiting, epigastric pain, and diarrhea [4].

Endoscopic Findings

LG is known to be associated with variable endoscopic findings. Previous studies have suggested a strong association of LG with varioliform gastritis, an uncommon form of gastritis which gives discrete endoscopic appearance to gastric mucosa when present throughout the stomach. It was reported that up to 80% of LG cases showed an endoscopic appearance of varioliform gastritis [1, 7, 8]. It was also reported that the vast majority of cases (82%) with varioliform gastritis had LG, and the presence of LG was strongly associated with diffuse or body-predominant disease compared to antrum-predominant disease [1]. The strong association between the two was not seen in subsequent studies, which reported the diagnosis of LG to be associated with varioliform gastritis in only 3.9–30% of cases [3, 9, 10]. Patients with LG can present with erythema with or without erosions. The endoscopy may be completely normal in up to 50% of patients [10]. Some studies have reported that LG can produce giant mucosal folds in gastric body, mimicking Menetrier disease [11–13].

Pathologic Features

Microscopic Findings

LG is characterized by the presence of increased intraepithelial lymphocytes, more prominent in surface and foveolar epithelium as compared to the deeper crypts (Fig. 7.1a, b). The surface layer also shows epithelial damage as well as loss of mucin. In most of the cases, intraepithelial lymphocytosis is quite prominent on lower magnification; therefore, formal count of intraepithelial lymphocytes is not required on routine basis. Typically, intraepithelial lymphocytosis ranges from 40 to 60 per 100 epithelial cells [1, 14]. The lymphocytes are small, round, and have a clear halo around the cells, likely due to a fixation artifact. Most cases also show an increase in small lymphocytes and plasma cells within the lamina propria. However, the degree of lamina propria inflammation does not correlate with the degree of intraepithelial lymphocytosis [5, 7]. Active inflammation involving surface lining epithelium and lamina propria has also been noted in a few cases. Rarely, hyperplastic/regenerative changes of the foveolar epithelium can be seen in LG (Fig. 7.1c, d). These changes may be quite prominent in cases as to mimic endoscopic and clinical manifestations of Menetrier disease.

S. Yasir (✉)
Department of Laboratory Medicine and Pathology, Mayo Clinic, Rochester, MN, USA
e-mail: Yasir.Saba@mayo.edu

L. Zhang et al. (eds.), *Surgical Pathology of Non-neoplastic Gastrointestinal Diseases*,
https://doi.org/10.1007/978-3-030-15573-5_7

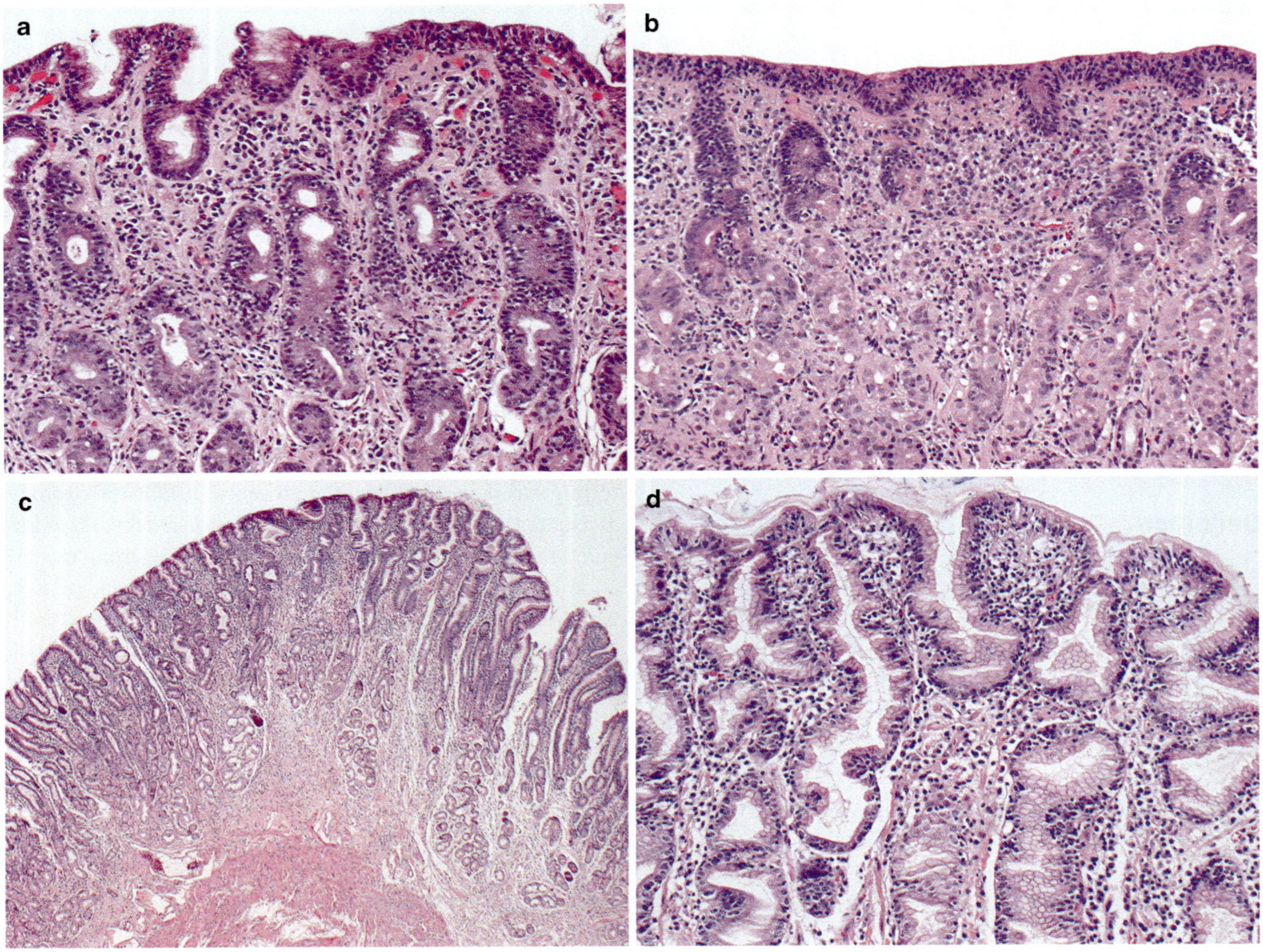

Fig. 7.1 Lymphocytic gastritis. (**a**) Prominent intraepithelial lymphocytosis in the surface and foveolar epithelium in antrum. (**b**) Prominent intraepithelial lymphocytosis in the surface and foveolar epithelium in gastric body. (**c**) Lymphocytic gastritis with marked foveolar hyperplasia. (**d**) High-power view from panel (**c**) shows prominent intraepithelial lymphocytosis

H. pylori immunohistochemical stain should be performed in all cases of LG. LG pattern of injury is seen commonly in association with *H. pylori* infection [9].

Disease Associations

Table 7.1 shows various disease entities which are commonly associated with LG. Common etiologic associations include immune-mediated diseases, infections, medications, or idiopathy. LG is known to be associated with celiac disease. The prevalence of LG has been reported to be 10–45% among patients with celiac disease [4, 9, 15–17]. In addition, about 33% of adult patients with LG have celiac disease. LG is even more strongly associated with celiac disease in pediatric population; 60–100% of cases with LG have underlying celiac disease. Therefore, any pediatric patient with LG

Table 7.1 Diseases associated with lymphocytic gastritis

Diseases
Immune-related disease
Celiac disease
Common variable immunodeficiency
Crohn's disease
Lymphocytic colitis
Infections
H. pylori gastritis
HIV infection
Neoplasia
Gastric and esophageal carcinoma
Lymphoma
Others
Varioliform gastritis
Inflammatory polyp
Idiopathic

should undergo duodenal biopsy as well as serologic workup for celiac disease. LG can also be seen in association with *H. pylori* infection. The reported prevalence of LG in patients with *H. pylori* infection ranges from 29% to 85% [3, 9, 18, 19]. In addition, approximately 4% of patients with histological diagnosis of *H. pylori*-associated chronic gastritis have the LG pattern of injury [9]. Approximately 22% of the patients with common variable immunodeficiency have been reported to be associated with LG [20]. Rarely, LG has been reported in patient with inflammatory bowel disease/Crohn's disease and concomitant lymphocytic colitis [9].

The disease severity and distribution of LG are different among the associated diseases. The intraepithelial lymphocytosis was greater in antrum than in body in majority of LG associated with celiac disease (83%, 20 of 24), but in only 19% (4 of 21) of LG associated with *H. pylori* infection. Patients with varioliform gastritis had more severe involvement of body [9].

Differential Diagnosis

Morphologic features of LG can mimic non-specific chronic gastritis if intraepithelial lymphocytosis is less prominent. In these cases, especially in pediatric population, the diagnosis of LG may be overlooked, which can further delay the diagnostic workup for an underlying disorder, such as celiac disease. In patients with LG and concomitant *H. pylori* infection, chronic inflammation of the lamina propria can be quite prominent so as to simulate mucosal-associated lymphoid tissue (MALT) lymphoma. Intraepithelial lymphocytosis is also a feature of MALT lymphoma. Distinctive features of MALT lymphoma include dense mononuclear cell infiltrate with associated lymphoepithelial lesions in the gastric crypts. On the other hand, LG is characterized by more uniform distribution of intraepithelial lymphocytes, mainly involving the surface epithelium. Immunohistochemical stain can be performed in difficult cases, as MALT lymphomas are composed of neoplastic B-cells, whereas lymphocytes in LG are of T-cell origin.

Treatment and Prognosis

The treatment for LG has not been well established. The main therapy is to control the associated disease such as celiac disease or *H. pylori* gastritis. Eradication of *H. pylori* can reach a complete and long-lasting resolution of LG in the majority of patients [21]. Some cases may spontaneously resolve. Proton pump inhibitors may also be effective on some patients with LG.

Collagenous Gastritis

Definition

Collagenous gastritis (CG) is defined by the deposition of subepithelial collagen band thicker than 10 μm and increased chronic inflammation of the lamina propria.

Clinical Features

CG is a rare disease entity with a slight female predominance. The age of the patients ranges from 9 months to 80 years [22–26]. The most common presenting complaints in patients with CG include abdominal pain, anemia, diarrhea, nausea and vomiting, and weight loss [23–28]. The clinical presentation of CG differs in pediatric and adult patients and depends on the severity of disease and the involvement of different parts of the gastrointestinal tract. The children typically present in their early teens with iron deficiency anemia due to isolated involvement of the stomach [26, 29]. Adult patients, on the other hand, have a more diffuse gastrointestinal tract involvement, being associated with collagenous colitis or collagenous sprue, and present with chronic watery diarrhea [26, 30, 31]. CG has been reported to be associated with immune-mediated and autoimmune disorders, including combined variable immunodeficiency, celiac disease, systemic lupus erythematosus, autoimmune atrophic gastritis, and medications [26, 32].

Endoscopic Findings

The characteristic endoscopic finding of CG is mucosal nodularity of the stomach [26]. The mucosal nodularity is seen in most of the cases of CG, with equal frequency in children and adults. The mucosal nodules vary in size and are distributed throughout the gastric body and antrum. The size and extent of mucosal involvement depends on the severity of inflammation. The inflammatory process in CG is uneven and heterogeneous leading to typical mucosal nodular appearance. Interestingly, the depressed areas surrounding gastric nodules are more involved with inflammation, atrophy, and collagen deposition, compared to the nodular lesions which demonstrate fewer inflammatory cells and minimal histological changes of CG. Recent studies have found that the depressed mucosa in CG showed amorphous surface structure and abnormal capillaries including blind ending and irregular caliber changes, whereas nodular mucosa demonstrate no abnormal surface structure or abnormal capillary vessels [33]. Other endoscopic findings of CG include mucosal erythema, erosions, and exudates [26]. The mucosa can be completely normal in some patients of CG.

Microscopic Findings

CG is histologically characterized by thickening of subepithelial collagen band, typically >10 μm, and accompanied by chronic inflammation of the lamina propria (Fig. 7.2a). Similar to collagenous colitis, CG has distinct collagen band with entrapment of superficial capillaries (Fig. 7.2a). Collagen layer is ragged in appearance and has irregular interface with the underlying lamina propria. Surface lining epithelium is sometimes sloughed off (Fig. 7.2a). The thickness of the collagen band varies from 10 μm to 120 μm [26, 34–37]. The collagen deposition can be heterogeneous in any particular case and depend on the location of the biopsy, and severity and duration of disease. The inflammatory infiltrate is composed of a mixed population of small lymphocytes, plasma cells, and eosinophils. The inflammatory infiltrate can also vary in intensity and composition. Some cases display distinct intraepithelial lymphocytosis, mimicking lymphocytic gastritis. Some reported cases had concurrent areas of lymphocytic gastritis [26]. Eosinophils can be a prominent component of inflammation in about half the cases (Fig. 7.2b) [32]. Atrophic changes of the gastric corpus have also been described [32].

Trichrome stain can be performed to highlight subepithelial collagen band. In most cases, collagen band is prominent on H&E staining; however, in difficult cases where collagen deposition is patchy and variable, trichrome stain would be very helpful to confirm an increase in collagen band thickness (Fig. 7.2c). Some studies have reported the use of tenascin immunohistochemical stain to highlight collagen band [32]. In cases with subtle changes of CG, tenascin immunostain can be a sensitive marker to detect subepithelial collagen layer [32].

Differential Diagnosis

Gastric mucosa with erosion and fibrin deposition can mimic CG. Mucosal fibrosis associated with autoimmune

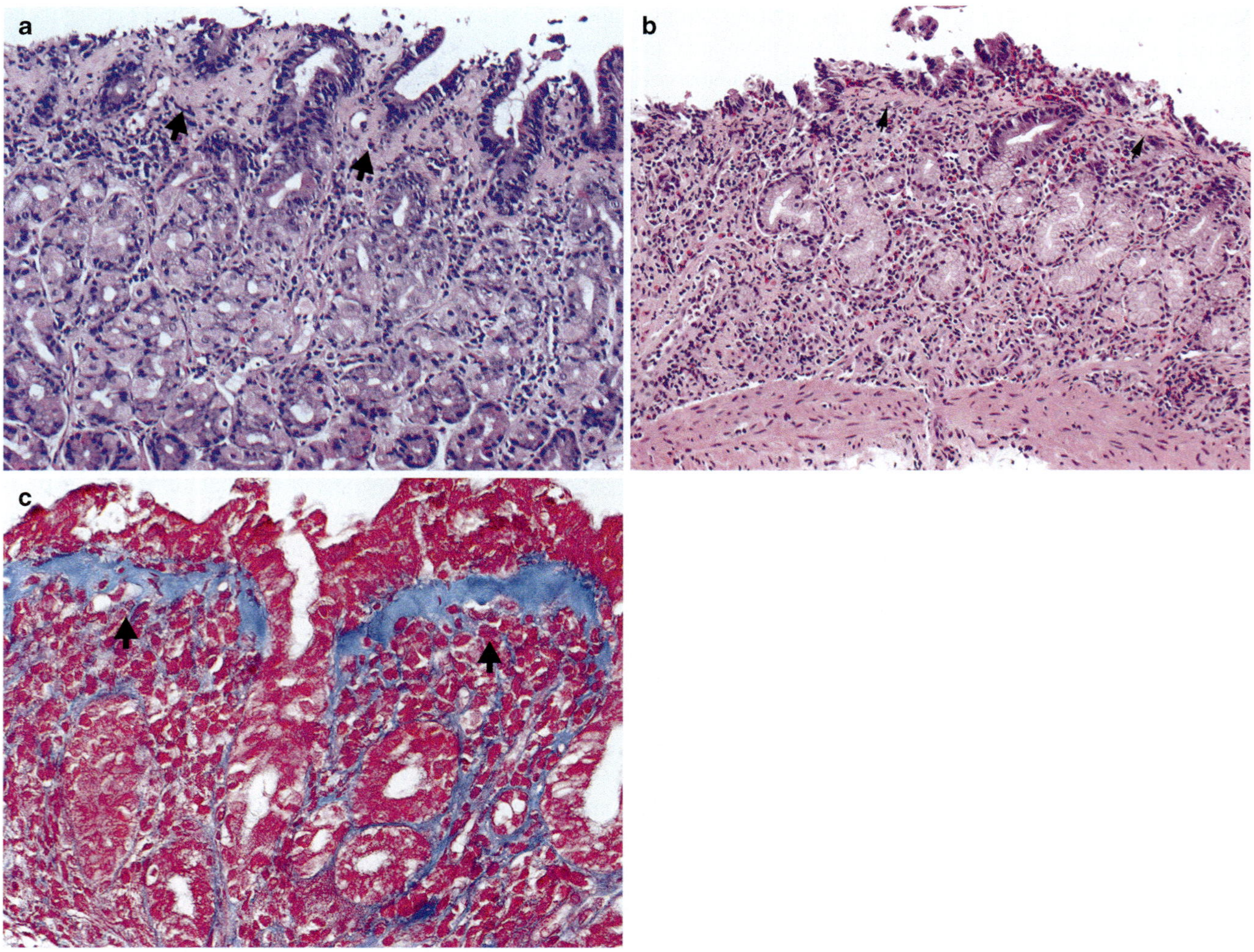

Fig. 7.2 Collagenous gastritis. (**a**) Gastric fundic mucosa with striking increase in subepithelial collagen band thickness (arrows). The collagen layer entraps the capillaries and inflammatory cells. (**b**) Antral mucosa with thickened subepithelial collagenous band (arrows) and prominent eosinophils in lamina propria. (**c**) Trichrome stain nicely highlights subepithelial collagen deposition (arrows)

gastritis, ischemia, radiation therapy, or healed ulcer resembles collagen deposition in CG. The mucosal fibrosis in the above mentioned conditions diffusely involves gastric mucosa. In contrast, the collagen deposition in CG is purely subepithelial in location. Gastric mucosal amyloidosis can also show morphologic similarities with CG. Subepithelial location of the collagen band and negative Congo red stain would lead to the right diagnosis. Sometimes, tangential sectioning of poorly oriented gastric biopsies can give a false impression of increased collagen band thickness. In these cases, other features of CG including surface epithelial damage and chronic inflammation of the lamina propria will be absent. CG with prominent eosinophilia may be confused with eosinophilic gastritis (EG), but thickened collagen band is absent in eosinophilic gastritis (EG).

Treatment and Prognosis

There is no established therapy for CG. Proton pump inhibitors, steroids, iron supplementation, and hypoallergenic diets have been tried with limited success. There are a few case reports with follow-up information of CG, but the natural course and prognosis are still unclear. In most cases, the collagen deposits remain unchanged or even thicker due to persistent inflammation [26, 33].

Eosinophilic Gastritis

Definition

Eosinophilic gastritis (EG) is defined by the presence of dense infiltration of eosinophils within gastric mucosa, gastric wall, and serosa.

Clinical Features

EG is a rare entity and usually presents as a component of eosinophilic gastroenteritis. Eosinophilic gastritis/gastroenteritis is a clinicopathological diagnosis which includes (1) clinical symptoms of gastrointestinal tract, (2) histological evidence of eosinophilic infiltration, (3) absence of eosinophilic infiltration in other organs, and (4) absence of known causes of secondary eosinophilia. Increased number of eosinophils within gastric biopsies has been reported in several conditions including parasitic infection [38], after therapy for *H. pylori* infection [39], drug reaction [40], Crohn's disease, connective tissue disorders, and hematopoietic disorders. EG affects both children and adult population with no sex predilection. Most common presenting symptoms are epigastric pain, reflux disease or dysphagia, nausea, and vomiting. Some patients present with gastric outlet obstruction [41] or as acute abdomen with perforation requiring emergency laparotomy.

Endoscopic Findings

The most common endoscopic abnormalities are mucosal erythema, erosion, gastritis, or nodularity [42]. The endoscopic mucosal appearance can be normal in some cases.

Pathologic Findings

Histological examination is critical to diagnosis. EG is characterized by a striking increase in eosinophils within the lamia propria (Fig. 7.3a). Marked infiltration of eosinophils into the epithelium is considered a pathognomonic feature of EG. The eosinophils infiltrate the surface epithelium as well as the foveolar crypts with associated epithe-

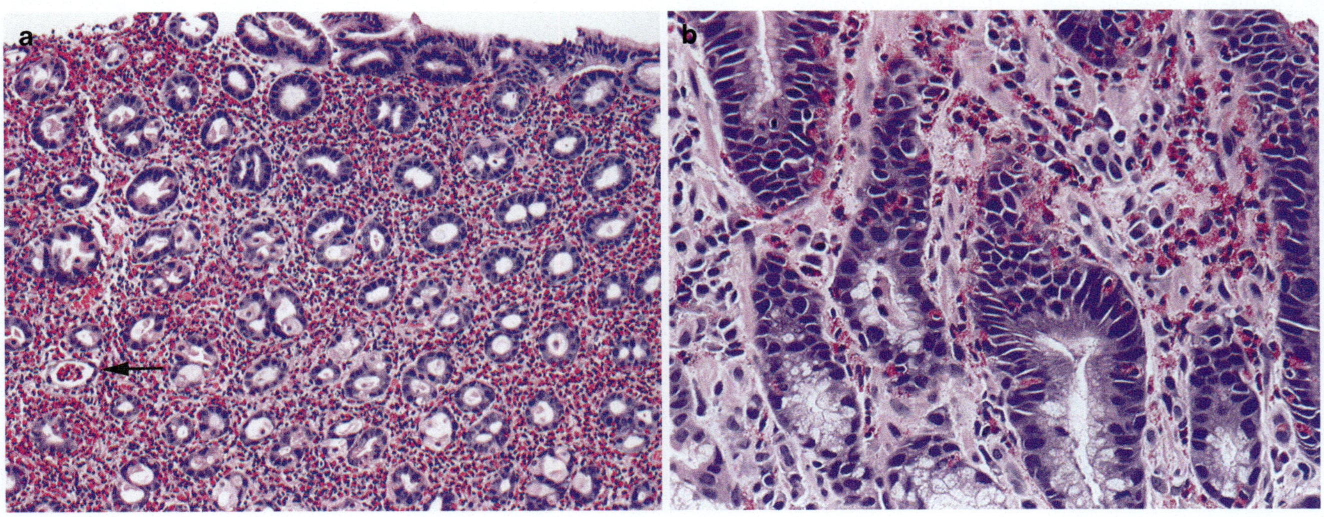

Fig. 7.3 Eosinophilic gastritis. (**a**) Marked eosinophilic infiltration into the lamia propria. Focal eosinophilic crypt abscess (arrow) is also present. (**b**) Infiltration of eosinophils into the crypt epithelium

lial damage and regenerative changes (Fig. 7.3b). Eosinophilic crypt abscesses are rarely seen (Fig. 7.3a). Some cases show diffuse sheets of eosinophilic infiltrate, whereas others show discrete clusters of eosinophils which tend to surround gastric crypts. Involvement of muscularis mucosa and submucosa is frequently seen. Studies have reported a wide range of eosinophils in patients with EG, ranging from 127/mm^2 to 2108/mm^2 [42]. A histological diagnosis of EG should be considered in biopsies with eosinophilic infiltrate >30 per high-power field in several separate high-power fields [42]. In routine clinical practice, the histological diagnosis of EG is etiologically nonspecific. In all such cases, possibility of both idiopathic and secondary EG should be entertained. *H. pylori* infection should be excluded by performing immunostain. Other secondary causes such as drugs, parasites, hypereosinophilic syndrome, and Crohn's disease can be excluded by clinical and endoscopic correlation.

Immunohistochemical stains are not routinely performed to document increased eosinophils. Immunohistochemical workup is sometimes done to exclude associated infections (e.g., H. pylori) or hematolymphoid neoplasia.

Differential Diagnosis

Histological pattern of EG raises several important clinical differentials. Certain parasitic infestations, such as *Strongyloides*, *Ascaris*, and *Anisakiasis*, elicit a striking eosinophilic tissue reaction. Identification of parasitic ova, larvae, or nematodes in tissue as well as in stool studies is essential for proper diagnosis. Drug reaction is another known etiology which needs to be excluded clinically. Some diseases can have quite prominent eosinophilic infiltrate, such as CG, Crohn's disease, Langerhans cell histiocytosis, and mast cell disease. Recognition of characteristic histological clues and pertinent immunohistochemical workup is key to proper diagnosis. Certain hematolymphoid malignancies, such as Hodgkin lymphoma, can show dense population of eosinophils. Finally, connective tissue disorders, hypereosinophilic syndromes, and vasculitis are other conditions with increased gastric eosinophils.

Treatment and Prognosis

Spontaneous remission may occur in a small subset of patients. The standard treatment strategy for EG has not been established. Treatment options may include proton pump inhibitor and *H. pylori* eradication, dietary considerations, steroids, biologic agents, and mast cells stabilizers.

Granulomatous Gastritis

Definition

Granulomatous gastritis (GG) is defined by the involvement of gastric mucosa by necrotizing or non-necrotizing granulomatous inflammation.

Clinical Features

GG is an uncommon entity comprising only 0.35% of all gastric biopsies or resection [43]. GG is a distinct histological entity, and definite diagnosis requires thorough clinical and radiologic correlation, microbiological studies, and follow-up data. GG encompasses a wide spectrum of disease entities such as Crohn's disease, infections, sarcoidosis, drug reaction, foreign body reaction, malignant neoplasms including malignant lymphomas, and rarely idiopathic GG [44]. Association of GG with *H. pylori* infection has not been well established; however, GG has been reported with coexisting *H. pylori* gastritis [43, 44].

Endoscopic Findings

The gastric mucosa can be normal in appearance or can show linear ulcers, erythema, deep mucosal ulcers, mucosal thickening, or nodularity. Findings are typically more prominent in antrum in cases with GG associated with Crohn's disease. Patients with sarcoidosis can present with gastric outlet obstruction or linitis plastic-like appearance [45].

Pathological Features

The defining histological feature of GG is the presence of mucosal and/or submucosal granulomas. The granulomas are composed of well-defined nodules of epithelioid or spindled histiocytes admixed with small lymphocytes, eosinophils, and multinucleated giant cells (Fig. 7.4a). The number, size, type, and location of granulomas vary in different patients. Granulomas can be necrotizing and non-necrotizing. Most cases of granulomatous inflammation with central necrosis or caseation are associated with mycobacterial or fungal infections.

The background gastric mucosa shows variable degree of chronic and active inflammation. In Crohn's disease, the gastric mucosa shows mild, moderate, or severe lymphoplasmacytic infiltrate within the lamina propria with cystitis or crypt abscesses (Fig. 7.4b). The distribution of disease can be from very focal, patchy, to diffuse. Atrophic mucosal changes and intestinal metaplasia are also noted in rare cases. The inter-

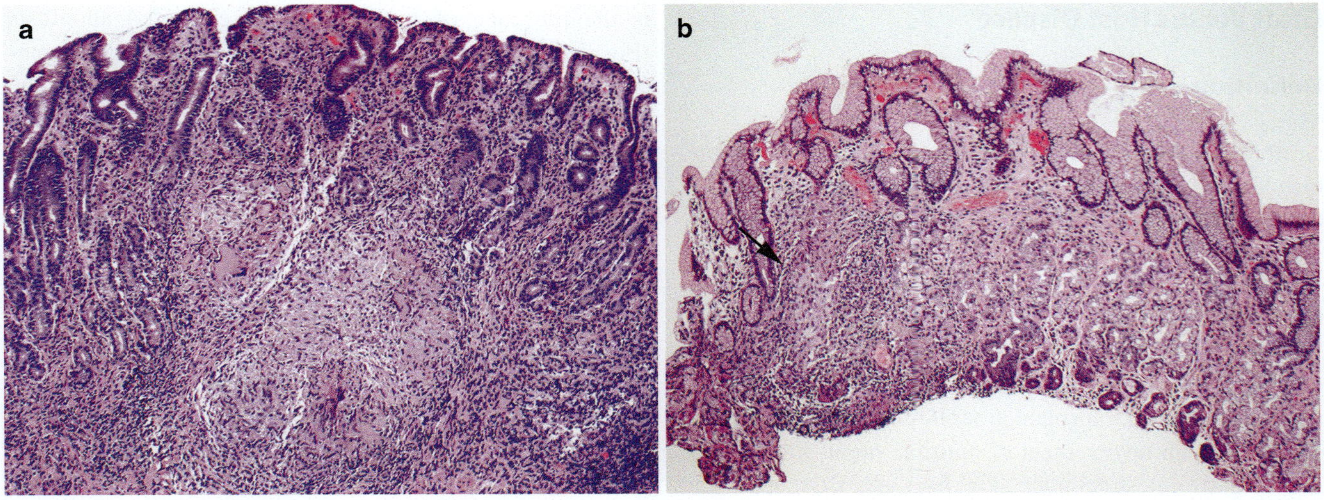

Fig. 7.4 Granulomatous gastritis. (**a**) Well-defined non-necrotizing granulomas with multinucleated giant cells are seen within the lamina propria in a patient with sarcoidosis. (**b**) Non-necrotizing granuloma (arrow) with chronic inflammation in lamina propria in Crohn's disease

vening mucosa can be completely normal. Resection specimens demonstrate additional characteristic features of Crohn's disease, including transmural inflammation and lymphoid aggregates, and neuronal hyperplasia.

Sarcoidosis is a systemic granulomatous disease that rarely involves the stomach. The granulomas typically seen in sarcoidosis are numerous, compact and coalescing, and fibrotic and are surrounded by a cuff of small lymphocytes (Fig. 7.4a). However, these histological features are not pathognomonic of sarcoidosis. Sarcoidosis is a diagnosis of exclusion, and final diagnosis is made after careful clinical and radiological correlation.

Special stains for fungal and mycobacterial organisms (Grocott's methenamine silver and acid-fast stains) should be performed in all cases of GG. In cases with diffuse and intense lymphoplasmacytic infiltrate, possibility of associated lymphoproliferative disorders should also be excluded. Immunostains for MALT lymphoma and Hodgkin's lymphoma are performed in selected cases. *H. pylori* immunostain should also be performed in cases with GG.

Differential Diagnosis

GG is a histologic diagnosis with multiple different etiologies (Table 7.2).

A large proportion of cases with GG are diagnosed with Crohn's disease, either retrospectively or prospectively. Crohn's diseases should always be considered in biopsies with active chronic gastritis and associated granulomas, although these findings are not entirely specific to Crohn's disease. Most patients with gastric Crohn's disease have concurrent ileal and colonic involvement. Therefore, correlation with colonoscopy and biopsy findings will lead to the right diagnosis. *H. pylori* stain should also be performed because about 10% of patients with Crohn's disease have concurrent *H. pylori* gastritis [43].

Table 7.2 Etiologies of granulomatous gastritis

Diseases
Infections Mycobacterial Fungal
Crohn's disease associated granulomas
Drug reaction
Malignant neoplasms Lymphoma
Sarcoidosis
Foreign-body granulomas
Idiopathic granulomatous gastritis

Idiopathic/isolated granulomatous gastritis (IGG) was initially reported by Fehimini in 1963 [46]. These cases were classified as IGG since all known causes of GG were excluded. However, the concept of IGG was challenged by several subsequent studies. Most of the cases of IGG reported so far had coexisting chronic atrophic gastritis, chronic active gastritis, or chronic gastritis with or without intestinal metaplasia [46–49] and had been linked to *H. pylori* infection. Therefore, it is preferred that a descriptive diagnosis should be rendered instead of using a terminology of IGG.

Treatment and Prognosis

The treatment and prognosis of GG rely on the underlying etiology. Therefore, following an appropriate clinical approach to determine the underlying cause is the key in managing GG.

Graft Versus Host Disease

Definition

Graft versus host disease (GVHD) is a clinical syndrome, histologically characterized by variable degree of inflammation with epithelial cell apoptosis and crypt drop out.

Clinical Features

GVHD is one of the most common complications of hematopoietic stem cell transplantation. It is considered a clinical syndrome with involvement of multiple organ sites including the gastrointestinal tract, skin, liver, etc. Both upper and lower gastrointestinal tracts are involved, with the stomach, duodenum, and colon being the most commonly biopsied sites. Most common presenting symptoms are nausea, vomiting, and diarrhea. Severe cases of GVHD may present with gastrointestinal bleeding, protein-losing enteropathy, or ileus [50].

Endoscopic Findings

Endoscopic features are variable and do not correlate well with histopathological findings. The findings range from normal mucosa to severe ulceration. The most commonly reported findings are mucosal edema, erythema, and friability [51].

Pathological Features

GVHD is a clinicopathological diagnosis. There are no validated set of histopathological criteria for acute GVHD. The most common histological feature of GVHD is the presence of increased crypt epithelial apoptosis (Fig. 7.5a). The epithelial apoptosis is seen in most regenerative parts of the mucosa, such as deeper crypts of the antrum or neck of the gastric body glands. The epithelial apoptosis is much easier to recognize when the cell is vacuolated containing karyorrhectic debris. Identification of small individual cell apoptosis in gastric biopsies is quite challenging. Other histological findings include gland dilatation with luminal debris (Fig. 7.5b), regenerative epithelial changes, gastric antral vascular ectasia-like changes, increased inflammatory infiltrate of the lamina propria with prominent eosinophils, and occasional neutrophilic infiltrate. The extent of mucosal involvement depends on the severity of the disease. The mucosal involvement can be patchy and variable in distribution. The minimal threshold for increased apoptosis is subjective. Scattered apoptotic bodies in more than one gland or one apoptotic body per biopsy piece are considered minimal required criteria for diagnosing GVHD. The final diagnosis of GVHD cannot be based on just biopsy findings. The histological findings, in an appropriate clinical and serological context, are diagnostic of GVHD. There is no universally accepted grading scheme for acute GVHD. The most commonly used grading system for gastrointestinal GVHD is for colonic GVHD which was described by Lerner [52] and modified by Sale [53]:

- Grade 1: occasional crypt apoptosis without crypt loss.
- Grade 2: crypt apoptosis with individual crypt loss.
- Grade 3: loss of two or more contiguous crypts.
- Grade 4: extensive crypt loss with mucosal denudation.

CMV and adenovirus infections can show similar histological findings. Therefore, immunohistochemical stains should be performed on every case to exclude the possibility of infections.

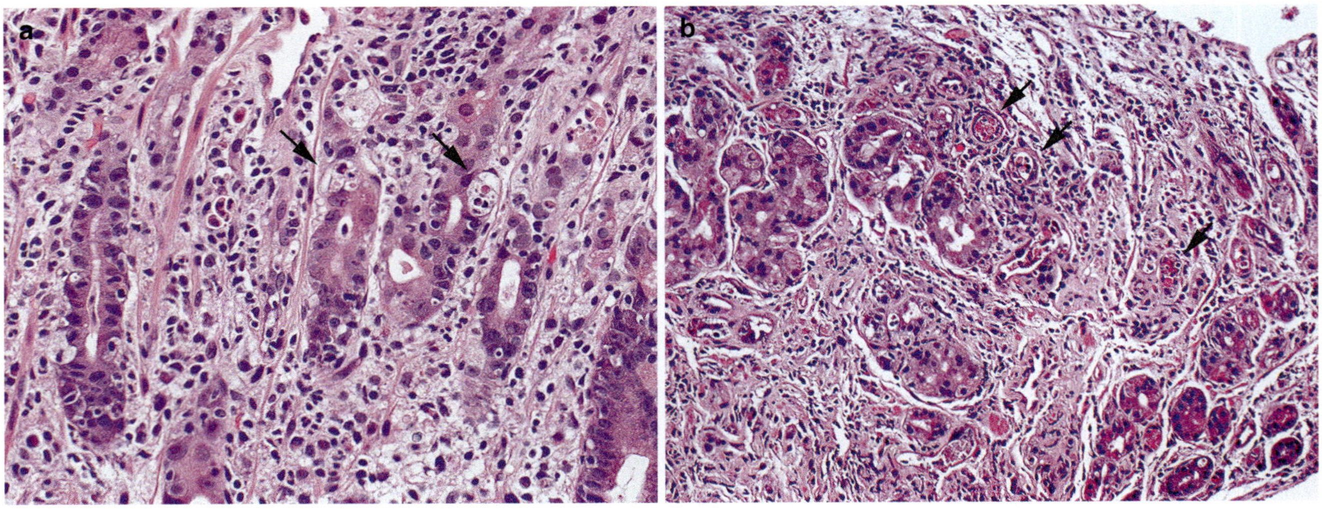

Fig. 7.5 GVHD. (**a**) Epithelial crypt apoptosis/karyorrhectic debris (arrows) is a histological hallmark of GVHD. (**b**) Crypt blunting and loss and multiple luminal debris (arrows)

Differential Diagnosis

There are several entities that histologically mimic GVHD. The most important differential diagnosis includes infections, particularly CMV, and medication-related injury, such as with mycophenolate, NSAIDs, or proton pump inhibitors. Careful search for CMV and adenovirus cytopathic effect/nuclear inclusions should be made. CMV immunostain is required on biopsies even if viral inclusions are absent on histology. Medication especially mycophenolate-related injury is another important differential diagnosis. There are no validated set of features that can reliably differentiate between the two entities. Some authors [54] have reported histological features which can differentiate between the two entities. The presence of crypt abscesses and neuroendocrine cell aggregates indicates GVHD. On the other hand, lamina propria eosinophils are more frequently present in mycophenolate-related injury than GVHD. The diagnosis of GVHD should be made with caution if the patient is on mycophenolate regimen.

Treatment and Prognosis

Immunosuppression with corticosteroids is the first-line treatment, with sustained response in <50% of patients with acute GVHD, and 40–50% with chronic GVHD. Chronic GVHD is still a major cause of morbidity and mortality, despite the treatment.

Focally Enhanced Gastritis

Definition

Focally enhanced gastritis (FEG) is defined by the presence of small collections of small lymphocytes, histiocytes, and neutrophils surrounding some foveolar epithelium or gastric glands.

Clinical Features

FEG has historically been described as a marker of inflammatory bowel disease. FEG was commonly seen in Crohn's disease patients with a prevalence ranging from 43% to 76% [55–59]. The specificity of FEG for Crohn's disease was challenged later on as FEG was seen in 10–24% of ulcerative colitis patients and 2–19% of non-inflammatory bowel disease patients [56, 59–61]. In pediatric population, the presence of FEG has been reported to be more predictive of inflammatory bowel disease compared with adult population [62].

Endoscopic Findings

The endoscopic mucosal appearance of FEG can be erythematous, nodular, polypoid, thickened, or edematous. The mucosa can be normal as well.

Pathological Features

FEG is not a common diagnosis in clinical practice. The gastric biopsy shows discrete focus/foci of localized inflammation (Fig. 7.6a). The inflammatory focus is composed of a mixture of small lymphocytes, histiocytes, and plasma cells. Neutrophils and eosinophils can be seen in some cases (Fig. 7.6b). The inflammation surrounds the individual gastric gland or small group of glands. There is glandular injury with infiltration of lymphocytes and associated aggregates of histiocytes or ill-defined granulomas. *H. pylori* immunostain can be performed to rule out *H. pylori*-associated gastritis.

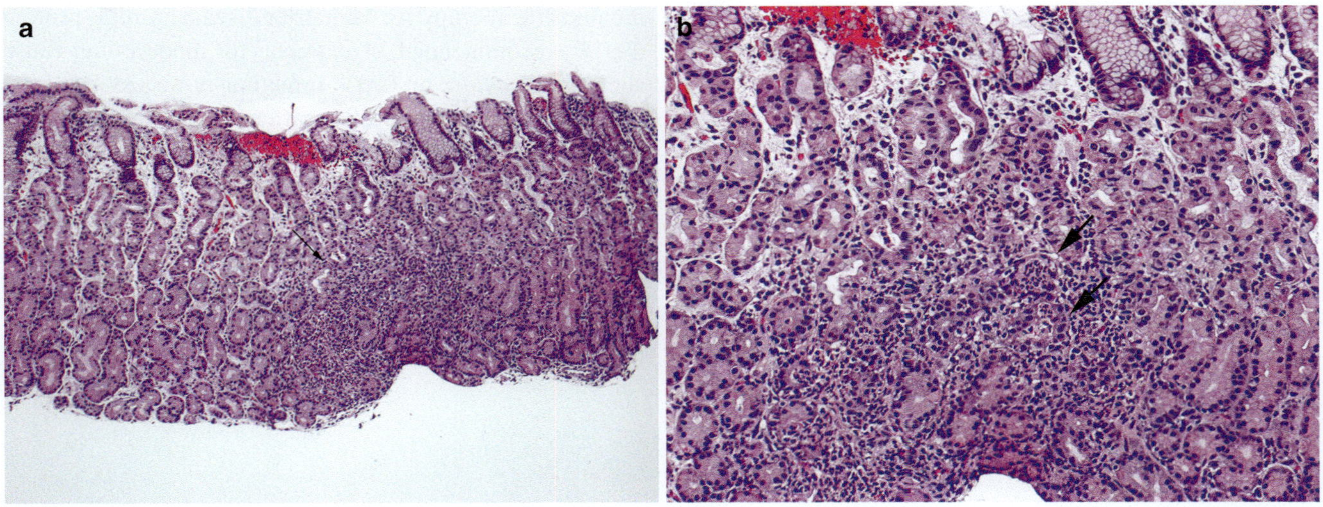

Fig. 7.6 Focally enhanced gastritis. (**a**) A small discrete focus containing group of glands surrounded by inflammatory infiltrate (arrow). Adjacent gastric mucosa is uninvolved. (**b**) The inflammatory infiltrate is composed of small lymphocytes, a few plasma cells, neutrophils (arrows), and rare eosinophils

Differential Diagnosis

FEG is a morphologic pattern of mucosal injury that can mimic other forms of chronic gastritis, e.g., *H. pylori*-associated chronic gastritis or sometimes granulomatous gastritis.

Treatment and Prognosis

To rule out *H. pylori* infection is necessary and may require proton pump inhibitors and *H. pylori* eradication. Given its potential relationship with inflammatory bowel disease, correlation with pathological findings in other sites of gastrointestinal tracts and other clinical features is necessary in determining whether it is an incidental finding or is associated with inflammatory bowel disease.

Hypertrophic Gastropathy

Menetrier Disease

Definition

Menetrier Disease is a rare protein-losing gastropathy which is characterized by giant mucosal hypertrophy of the gastric body and fundus.

Clinical Features

Menetrier disease is a rare acquired disorder, and its pathogenesis is not fully understood. The most common presenting complaints include nausea, vomiting, diarrhea, abdominal pain, weight loss, malnutrition, and peripheral edema due to hypoalbuminemia. Patients typically present with insidious onset and progressive symptoms and have an increased risk of gastric cancer [63, 64]. Children can present with self-limited disease and can be associated with CMV infection [65]. Menetrier disease has also been reported in patients with autoimmune diseases such as inflammatory bowel disease, sclerosing cholangitis, and ankylosing spondylitis [66, 67].

Endoscopic and Gross Findings

The characteristics endoscopic finding is marked thickening and hypertrophy of gastric mucosal folds (Fig. 7.7a). These endoscopic findings are not entirely specific to Menetrier disease. Other conditions including Zollinger-Ellison syndrome, gastric lymphoma, signet ring cell adenocarcinoma, gastric polyps, etc. can show similar endoscopic picture.

Pathological Features

Grossly, the mucosa has polypoid and spongy appearance which mimic cerebral convolutions (Fig. 7.7b). The gastric body and fundus is typically involved with relative sparing of the gastric antrum (Fig. 7.7b, c).

The histological features are striking, which include marked hyperplasia, elongation, and tortuosity of the gastric foveolar epithelium (Fig. 7.7d). The oxyntic glands are usually replaced by mucous glands, which are often cystically dilated (Fig. 7.7e). The lamina propria shows variable degree of edema and inflammatory infiltrate.

Differential Diagnosis

There is a wide spectrum of disease that can mimic Menetrier disease both endoscopically and histologically (Table 7.3). In contrast to Menetrier disease, Zollinger-Ellison syndrome has marked hyperplasia of the parietal cells and is not associated with foveolar hyperplasia and protein loss. Hypertrophic lymphocytic gastritis involves gastric fundus and body with sparing of antrum but shows striking increase in intraepithelial lymphocytes. Hypertrophic hypersecretory gastropathy shows hyperplasia of all the glandular components. There is no protein loss and gastrin level is normal. Hyperplastic polyps usually involve gastric antrum. The mucosa is edematous and hyperplastic foveolar epithelium often shows prominent regenerative changes and surface erosions. Cronkite-Canada syndrome may mimic Menetrier disease both clinically and endoscopically. However, Cronkite-Canada syndrome tends to involve the entire gastrointestinal tract with lamina propria edema, gland architectural distortion, and inflammation in the intervening non-polypoid gastric mucosa, while Menetrier disease is always limited to the proximal stomach with no endoscopic and histological evidence of disease in antrum and duodenum.

Treatment and Prognosis

Cetuximab, a monoclonal antibody against EGFR, now is the first-line therapy for Menetrier disease. A high-protein diet is recommended. Treatment for underlying cause such as *H. pylori* or CMV infection is necessary. Total gastrectomy is indicated for patients with severe disease despite cetuximab treatment. The prognosis is variable. Resolution may occur spontaneously or after treating underlying *H. pylori* or CMV infection. It was estimated that 2–15% of individuals with Menetrier disease may develop stomach cancer in their lifetime [63, 64], and annual or biannual endoscopic surveillance has been recommended [68].

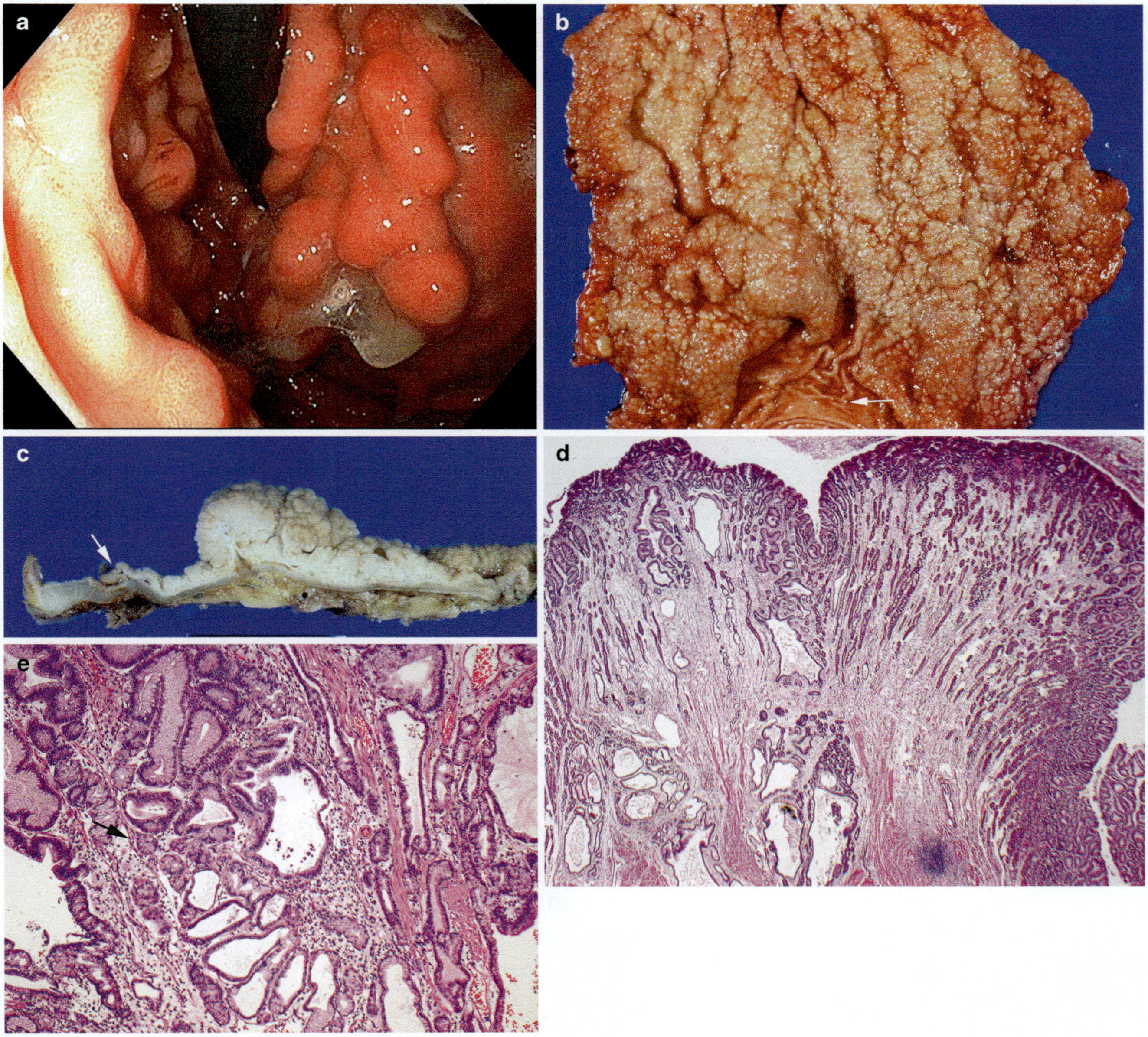

Fig. 7.7 Menetrier Disease. (**a**) Endoscopic appearance of Menetrier disease with markedly thickened and polypoid mucosal folds. (**b**) Gastrectomy specimen. The disease typically involves gastric fundus and body and spares gastric antrum (arrow). Mucosal appearance mimics cerebral convolutions. (**c**) Cross section of a surgical specimen shows marked mucosal thickening and polypoid appearance involving body and fundus and spare antrum (arrow). (**d**) The foveolar epithelium shows marked elongation and hyperplasia and glandular dilatation. There is loss of gastric oxyntic glands. (**e**) Residual parietal cells (arrow) in background of marked foveolar hyperplasia

Zollinger-Ellison Syndrome

Definition

Zollinger-Ellison Syndrome (ZES) is characterized by gastrinomas causing hypergastrinemia, increased acid production, and peptic ulcer disease.

Clinical Features

ZES is a rare condition which is caused by increased gastric secretion from duodenal and pancreatic gastrinomas. The annual incidence of gastrinoma is 0.5–2 per million populations [69, 70]. Most gastrinomas are sporadic, but approximately 30% of gastrinomas are associated with multiple endocrine neo-

Table 7.3 Differential diagnosis of Menetrier disease

Diseases
Zollinger-Ellison Syndrome
Hypertrophic lymphocytic gastritis
Hypertrophic hypersecretory gastropathy
Chronic *H. pylori* gastritis or CMV infection
Gastric polyps Hyperplastic polyps Cronkhite-Canada Syndrome Juvenile polyposis Cowden syndrome
Gastric malignancy Diffuse gastric carcinoma Lymphoma
Gastric adenocarcinoma and proximal polyposis of the stomach (GAPPS)

plasia type 1 (MEN 1) [71]. The most common presenting symptoms are abdominal pain and chronic diarrhea. Other symptoms include weight loss and gastrointestinal bleeding.

Endoscopic Findings

There is massive hypertrophy of the gastric rugal folds which involves fundus and body of the stomach.

Pathological Features

Grossly, the gastric folds are thickened (Fig. 7.8a). There is striking increase in thickness of oxyntic mucosa (Fig. 7.8b). The parietal cells show marked hyperplasia and hypertrophy, and extend up to foveolar neck (Fig. 7.8b, c). These histological changes are secondary to marked increase in gastrin

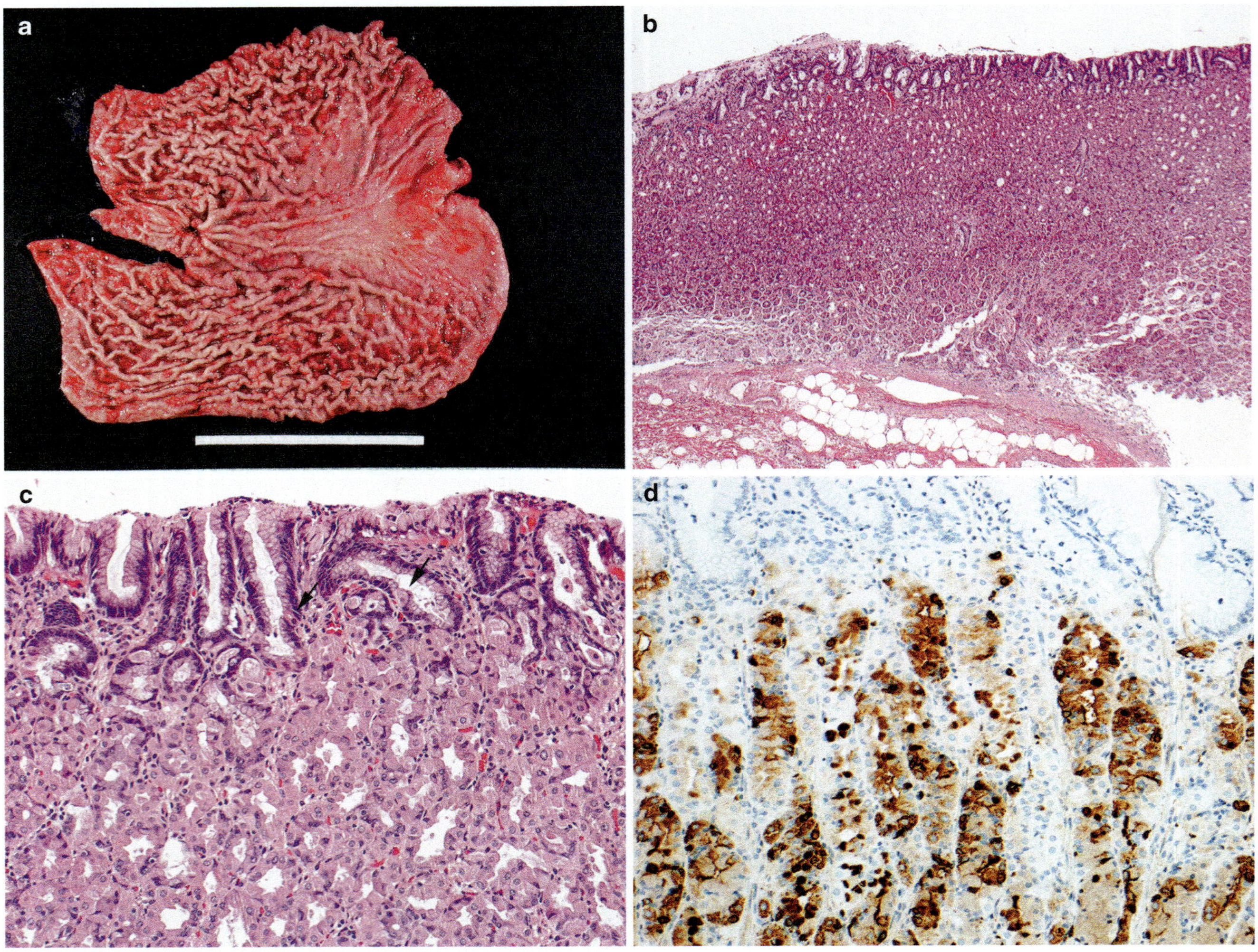

Fig. 7.8 Zollinger-Ellison Syndrome. (**a**) Gastrectomy specimen shows hypertrophy of the gastric rugal folds. (**b**) There is marked thickening of the gastric oxyntic mucosa. (**c**) The parietal cells show hyperplasia and reach up to the neck of foveolar epithelium (arrows). (**d**) Chromogranin stain highlights ECL hyperplasia, mainly linear pattern

levels. Another effect of hypergastrinemia is endocrine cell (ECL) hyperplasia of the gastric fundus and body (Fig. 7.8d). The ECL hyperplasia can be linear and/or nodular. Gastric neuroendocrine tumors have been reported in ZES associated with MEN type 1.

Gastrin immunostain is used to confirm the diagnosis of duodenal or pancreatic gastrinomas. Chromogranin immunostain can highlight ECL hyperplasia and gastric neuroendocrine tumors.

Differential Diagnosis

Menetrier disease is characterized by gastric rugal hypertrophy, protein losing gastropathy, and hypochlorhydria. In contrast to ZES, Menetrier disease shows massive foveolar hyperplasia and loss of oxyntic glands. Autoimmune gastritis is also characterized by hypergastrinemia. In contrast to ZES, autoimmune gastritis shows loss/atrophy of the oxyntic mucosa and has hypochlorhydria.

Treatment and Prognosis

Medical therapy is the mainstream in managing ZES and the goal is to limit the clinical manifestations and complications of peptic ulcer disease. Surgical resection of sporadic gastrinomas with no metastasis is curative. Metastatic gastrinoma is the main cause of morbidity and mortality in patients with ZES, but current treatment modalities are still of limited benefit.

References

1. Haot J, et al. Lymphocytic gastritis—prospective study of its relationship with varioliform gastritis. Gut. 1990;31(3):282–5.
2. Jaskiewicz K, et al. Lymphocytic gastritis in nonulcer dyspepsia. Dig Dis Sci. 1991;36(8):1079–83.
3. Dixon MF, et al. Lymphocytic gastritis—relationship to Campylobacter pylori infection. J Pathol. 1988;154(2):125–32.
4. De Giacomo C, et al. Lymphocytic gastritis: a positive relationship with celiac disease. J Pediatr. 1994;124(1):57–62.
5. Hayat M, et al. The pattern of involvement of the gastric mucosa in lymphocytic gastritis is predictive of the presence of duodenal pathology. J Clin Pathol. 1999;52(11):815–9.
6. Crampton JR, et al. Chronic lymphocytic gastritis and protein losing gastropathy. Gut. 1989;30(Spec No):71–4.
7. Haot J, et al. Lymphocytic gastritis: a newly described entity: a retrospective endoscopic and histological study. Gut. 1988;29(9):1258–64.
8. Haot J, et al. Lymphocytic gastritis versus varioliform gastritis. A historical series revisited. J Pathol. 1989;158(1):19–22.
9. Wu TT, Hamilton SR. Lymphocytic gastritis: association with etiology and topology. Am J Surg Pathol. 1999;23(2):153–8.
10. Lynch DA, et al. Lymphocytic gastritis and associated small bowel disease: a diffuse lymphocytic gastroenteropathy? J Clin Pathol. 1995;48(10):939–45.
11. Wolfsen HC, Carpenter HA, Talley NJ. Menetrier's disease: a form of hypertrophic gastropathy or gastritis? Gastroenterology. 1993;104(5):1310–9.
12. Mosnier JF, et al. Hypertrophic gastropathy with gastric adenocarcinoma: Menetrier's disease and lymphocytic gastritis? Gut. 1991;32(12):1565–7.
13. Haot J, et al. Menetrier's disease with lymphocytic gastritis: an unusual association with possible pathogenic implications. Hum Pathol. 1991;22(4):379–86.
14. Oberhuber G, et al. High proportion of granzyme B-positive (activated) intraepithelial and lamina propria lymphocytes in lymphocytic gastritis. Am J Surg Pathol. 1998;22(4):450–8.
15. Feeley KM, et al. Lymphocytic gastritis and coeliac disease: evidence of a positive association. J Clin Pathol. 1998;51(3):207–10.
16. Wolber R, et al. Lymphocytic gastritis in patients with celiac sprue or spruelike intestinal disease. Gastroenterology. 1990;98(2):310–5.
17. Karttunen T, Niemela S. Lymphocytic gastritis and coeliac disease. J Clin Pathol. 1990;43(5):436–7.
18. Hayat M, et al. Effects of Helicobacter pylori eradication on the natural history of lymphocytic gastritis. Gut. 1999;45(4):495–8.
19. Niemela S, et al. Ten year follow up study of lymphocytic gastritis: further evidence on Helicobacter pylori as a cause of lymphocytic gastritis and corpus gastritis. J Clin Pathol. 1995;48(12):1111–6.
20. Daniels JA, et al. Gastrointestinal tract pathology in patients with common variable immunodeficiency (CVID): a clinicopathologic study and review. Am J Surg Pathol. 2007;31(12):1800–12.
21. Madisch A, et al. Healing of lymphocytic gastritis after Helicobacter pylori eradication therapy—a randomized, double-blind, placebo-controlled multicentre trial. Aliment Pharmacol Ther. 2006;23(4):473–9.
22. Rustagi T, Rai M, Scholes JV. Collagenous gastroduodenitis. J Clin Gastroenterol. 2011;45(9):794–9.
23. Gopal P, McKenna BJ. The collagenous gastroenteritides: similarities and differences. Arch Pathol Lab Med. 2010;134(10):1485–9.
24. Brain O, et al. Collagenous gastritis: reports and systematic review. Eur J Gastroenterol Hepatol. 2009;21(12):1419–24.
25. Colletti RB, Trainer TD. Collagenous gastritis. Gastroenterology. 1989;97(6):1552–5.
26. Leung ST, et al. Collagenous gastritis: histopathologic features and association with other gastrointestinal diseases. Am J Surg Pathol. 2009;33(5):788–98.
27. Hijaz NM, et al. Clinical outcome of pediatric collagenous gastritis: case series and review of literature. World J Gastroenterol. 2013;19(9):1478–84.
28. Maguire AA, et al. Collagenous sprue: a clinicopathologic study of 12 cases. Am J Surg Pathol. 2009;33(10):1440–9.
29. Lagorce-Pages C, et al. Collagenous gastritis: a report of six cases. Am J Surg Pathol. 2001;25(9):1174–9.
30. Stancu M, et al. Collagenous gastritis associated with lymphocytic gastritis and celiac disease. Arch Pathol Lab Med. 2001;125(12):1579–84.
31. Vesoulis Z, et al. Collagenous gastritis: a case report, morphologic evaluation, and review. Mod Pathol. 2000;13(5):591–6.
32. Arnason T, et al. Collagenous gastritis: a morphologic and immunohistochemical study of 40 patients. Mod Pathol. 2015;28(4):533–44.
33. Kamimura K, et al Collagenous gastritis: review. World J Gastrointest Endosc. 2015;7(3):265–73.

34. Cote JF, et al. Collagenous gastritis revealed by severe anemia in a child. Hum Pathol. 1998;29(8):883–6.
35. Kajino Y, et al. Collagenous gastritis in a young Japanese woman. Pathol Int. 2003;53(3):174–8.
36. Park S, et al. Collagenous gastritis in a Korean child: a case report. J Korean Med Sci. 2005;20(1):146–9.
37. Soeda A, et al. Collagenous gastroduodenitis coexisting repeated Dieulafoy ulcer: a case report and review of collagenous gastritis and gastroduodenitis without colonic involvement. Clin J Gastroenterol. 2014;7(5):402–9.
38. Muraoka A, et al. Acute gastric anisakiasis: 28 cases during the last 10 years. Dig Dis Sci. 1996;41(12):2362–5.
39. Genta RM, Lew GM, Graham DY. Changes in the gastric mucosa following eradication of Helicobacter pylori. Mod Pathol. 1993;6(3):281–9.
40. Pusztaszeri MP, Genta RM, Cryer BL. Drug-induced injury in the gastrointestinal tract: clinical and pathologic considerations. Nat Clin Pract Gastroenterol Hepatol. 2007;4(8):442–53.
41. Katiyar R, et al. Primary eosinophilic gastritis in a child with gastric outlet obstruction. J Gastrointest Surg. 2016;20(6):1270–1.
42. Lwin T, Melton SD, Genta RM. Eosinophilic gastritis: histopathological characterization and quantification of the normal gastric eosinophil content. Mod Pathol. 2011;24(4):556–63.
43. Shapiro JL, Goldblum JR, Petras RE. A clinicopathologic study of 42 patients with granulomatous gastritis. Is there really an "idiopathic" granulomatous gastritis? Am J Surg Pathol. 1996;20(4):462–70.
44. Ectors NL, et al. Granulomatous gastritis: a morphological and diagnostic approach. Histopathology. 1993;23(1):55–61.
45. Tokala H, Polsani K, Kalavakunta JK. Gastric sarcoidosis: a rare clinical presentation. Case Rep Gastrointest Med. 2013;2013:260704.
46. Fahimi HD, et al. Isolated granulomatous gastritis: its relationship to disseminated sarcoidosis and regional enteritis. Gastroenterology. 1963;45:161–75.
47. Tukiainen H, et al. Granulomatous gastritis as a diagnostic problem between sarcoidosis and other granulomatous disorders. Sarcoidosis. 1988;5(1):66–7.
48. Weinstock JV. Idiopathic isolated granulomatous gastritis: spontaneous resolution without surgical intervention. Dig Dis Sci. 1980;25(3):233–5.
49. Woolf IL, et al. Granulomatous gastritis, iron deficiency, vitamin B12 malabsorption and immunoglobulin deficiency. Postgrad Med J. 1976;52(607):303–5.
50. Deeg HJ, Antin JH. The clinical spectrum of acute graft-versus-host disease. Semin Hematol. 2006;43(1):24–31.
51. Khan K, et al. Diagnostic endoscopy in children after hematopoietic stem cell transplantation. Gastrointest Endosc. 2006;64(3):379–85; quiz 389–92
52. Lerner KG, et al. Histopathology of graft-vs.-host reaction (GvHR) in human recipients of marrow from HL-A-matched sibling donors. Transplant Proc. 1974;6(4):367–71.
53. Sale GE, et al. Gastrointestinal graft-versus-host disease in man. A clinicopathologic study of the rectal biopsy. Am J Surg Pathol. 1979;3(4):291–9.
54. Star KV, et al. Histologic features in colon biopsies can discriminate mycophenolate from GVHD-induced colitis. Am J Surg Pathol. 2013;37(9):1319–28.
55. Kundhal PS, et al. Gastral antral biopsy in the differentiation of pediatric colitides. Am J Gastroenterol. 2003;98(3):557–61.
56. Meining A, et al. Focal inflammatory infiltrations in gastric biopsy specimens are suggestive of Crohn's disease. Crohn's Disease Study Group, Germany. Scand J Gastroenterol. 1997;32(8):813–8.
57. Oberhuber G, et al. Focally enhanced gastritis: a frequent type of gastritis in patients with Crohn's disease. Gastroenterology. 1997;112(3):698–706.
58. Oberhuber G, Hirsch M, Stolte M. High incidence of upper gastrointestinal tract involvement in Crohn's disease. Virchows Arch. 1998;432(1):49–52.
59. Parente F, et al. Focal gastric inflammatory infiltrates in inflammatory bowel diseases: prevalence, immunohistochemical characteristics, and diagnostic role. Am J Gastroenterol. 2000;95(3):705–11.
60. Hummel TZ, et al. Additional value of upper GI tract endoscopy in the diagnostic assessment of childhood IBD. J Pediatr Gastroenterol Nutr. 2012;54(6):753–7.
61. Sharif F, et al. Focally enhanced gastritis in children with Crohn's disease and ulcerative colitis. Am J Gastroenterol. 2002;97(6):1415–20.
62. McHugh JB, Gopal P, Greenson JK. The clinical significance of focally enhanced gastritis in children. Am J Surg Pathol. 2013;37(2):295–9.
63. Coffey RJ, et al. Menetrier disease and gastrointestinal stromal tumors: hyperproliferative disorders of the stomach. J Clin Invest. 2007;117(1):70–80.
64. Scharschmidt BF. The natural history of hypertrophic gastrophy (Menetrier's disease). Report of a case with 16 year follow-up and review of 120 cases from the literature. Am J Med. 1977;63(4):644–52.
65. Eisenstat DD, et al. Acute cytomegalovirus infection in a child with Menetrier's disease. Gastroenterology. 1995;109(2):592–5.
66. Fiske WH, et al. Efficacy of cetuximab in the treatment of Menetrier's disease. Sci Transl Med. 2009;1(8):8ra18.
67. Hatemi I, et al. Menetrier's disease coexisting with ulcerative colitis and sclerosing cholangitis. Dig Liver Dis. 2008;40(1):78–9.
68. Nalle SC, Turner JR. Menetrier's disease therapy: rebooting mucosal signaling. Sci Transl Med. 2009;1(8):8ps10.
69. Kulke MH, et al. NANETS treatment guidelines: well-differentiated neuroendocrine tumors of the stomach and pancreas. Pancreas. 2010;39(6):735–52.
70. Metz DC, Jensen RT. Gastrointestinal neuroendocrine tumors: pancreatic endocrine tumors. Gastroenterology. 2008;135(5):1469–92.
71. Norton JA. Neuroendocrine tumors of the pancreas and duodenum. Curr Probl Surg. 1994;31(2):77–156.

Drugs-Induced Injury, Infections, Vascular, Congenital, and Miscellaneous Disorders

8

Vishal S. Chandan

Drug-Induced Injury

Medication-associated gastric injuries have been known for decades. The first report on aspirin-associated gastric injury was published in 1938 [1]. In the recent years, the number of different drug-associated gastric injuries has significantly increased. Some of the injury patterns are nonspecific but generate a differential diagnosis which could be narrowed to a specific drug by incorporating the clinical history and patient's medication list. However, specific patterns of injury can also be seen which are typically associated with a particular drug. A surgical pathologist's familiarity with the general and specific patterns of drug-induced injury to the stomach can be an invaluable tool to pathologic interpretation. Recognition and reporting of drug-induced injury by pathologists can alert clinicians to this under-recognized condition that can usually be easily corrected.

Iron Pill-Associated Gastric Injury

Oral iron medication is commonly used to treat and prevent iron deficiency anemia. Ferrous sulfate is the most common iron medication associated with gastric injury. Iron overdose can cause severe corrosive injury to the stomach and result in ulceration and hemorrhagic necrosis which can even lead to gastric perforation in severe cases [2, 3]. However, a small subset of patients can also develop localized gastric mucosal injury from iron tablet ingestion at the therapeutic level due to impaction of iron material [4, 5]. Iron pill-associated gastric injury can cause various endoscopic abnormalities such as erythema, erosion, ulceration, subepithelial hemorrhages, flat black dots, and even dark brown appearance of gastric mucosa. Rarely, iron-induced gastric ulceration can also mimic gastric carcinoma both radiologically and endoscopically [6]. The pathogenesis of mucosal injury related to therapeutic iron medication is not well understood. However, it is most likely a combined effect of dysmotility or preexisting mucosal damage and prolonged contact of trapped iron pill material.

Identification of iron deposition in the gastric mucosa is usually straightforward. Iron pill material shows a characteristic brown crystalline and clumpy fibrillary material which is refractile but not polarizable (Fig. 8.1a). This material represents oxidized inorganic iron and is generally extracellular. Most of the time, this brown crystalline material is luminal, seen adjacent to the surface epithelium and admixed with luminal inflammatory exudate (Fig. 8.1b). It can be also seen deposited within the lamina propria, either covered by intact epithelium or adjacent to superficial erosions or even within granulation tissue. A small subset of cases may show iron-containing thrombi in mucosal blood vessels or iron deposition within mucosal vessel walls.

The adjacent gastric mucosa can show reactive foveolar hyperplasia with mucin depletion and elongated tortuous gastric pits (Fig. 8.2). The gastric epithelium can show marked epithelial atypia with prominent nucleoli, retained mucosal architecture, low nuclear to cytoplasmic ratio, and lack of nuclear hyperchromasia and should be differentiated from dysplasia.

Hemosiderin deposition can also be frequently seen within the surface epithelium and/or the gastric glands. On an iron stain, the crystalline iron pill material can be easily distinguished from hemosiderin pigment, despite positive staining for both on the iron stain (Fig. 8.3).

Proton Pump Inhibitors

Proton pump inhibitors (PPIs) are very commonly used for treatment of reflux esophagitis and gastric peptic ulcer dis-

V. S. Chandan (✉)
Department of Pathology, University of California – Irvine, Irvine, CA, USA
e-mail: vchandan@uci.edu

L. Zhang et al. (eds.), *Surgical Pathology of Non-neoplastic Gastrointestinal Diseases*, https://doi.org/10.1007/978-3-030-15573-5_8

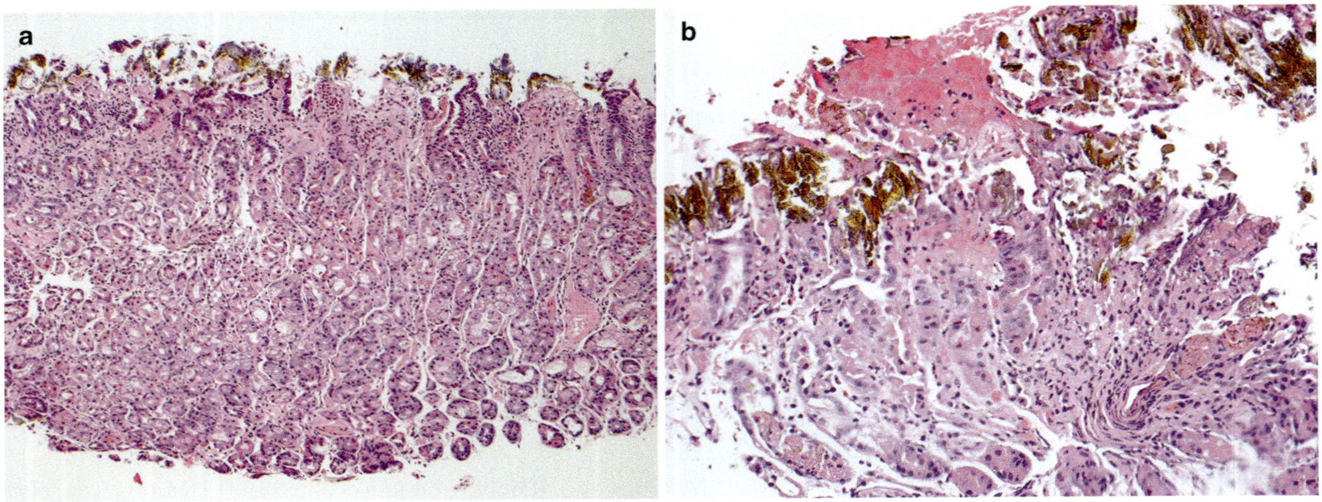

Fig. 8.1 Iron pill-associated gastric injury. Brown crystalline and clumpy fibrillary iron pill material encrusted on the surface epithelium with erosive injury (**a**). Refractile iron pill material is admixed with luminal inflammatory exudate (**b**)

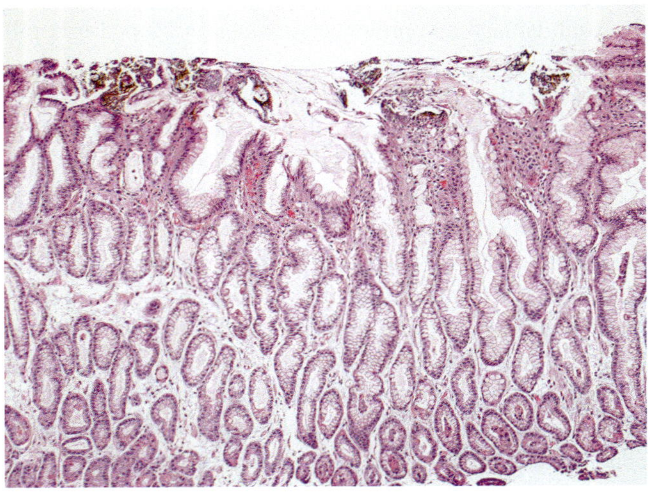

Fig. 8.2 Reactive epithelial changes in iron pill-associated injury. Gastric mucosa shows reactive foveolar hyperplasia and elongated tortuous gastric pits

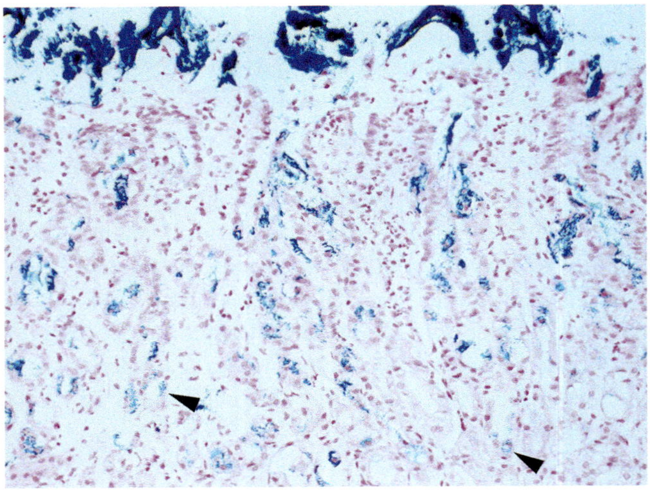

Fig. 8.3 The crystalline iron pill material is positive on the iron stain. There is also iron deposition within the crypt lumen and occasional within the gastric epithelial cells (arrowheads)

ease. These medications are freely available over the counter and are very effective in reducing gastric acidity. However, there is some concern about their long-term usage leading to gastric polyps, atrophic gastritis, and even gastric endocrine cell hyperplasia.

A subset of patients develop gastric parietal cell hyperplasia within the body, characterized by enlarged and increased parietal cells protruding into the gastric glands and even imparting a serrated appearance to the glandular lumen (Fig. 8.4). The obstruction of the acid flow by the hypertrophic parietal cells presumably leads to fundic gland cysts and fundic gland polyps. Several studies have confirmed prolonged use of PPIs with development of fundic gland polyps [7–9]. A study has also shown disappearance of the fundic gland polyps with discontinuation of PPIs and recurrence with resumed use of PPIs, further supporting the relationship between PPIs and fundic gland polyps [10]. However, some authors disputed this association [11, 12].

Long-term PPI usage has also been associated with two- to fourfold increase in serum gastrin levels in some patients [13–16]. Similarly, due to increased gastrin levels, endocrine cell hyperplasia has also been seen in some patients on long-term PPI usage [16–18]. However, no increased risk of gastric neuroendocrine tumors has been reported with long-term PPI usage. PPI usage among *H. pylori*-infected patients has also been associated with aggravation of gastritis and atrophy of gastric corpus [13, 17–21]. Hence, there has been suggestion about patients being tested for *H. pylori* before long-term PPI therapy [19].

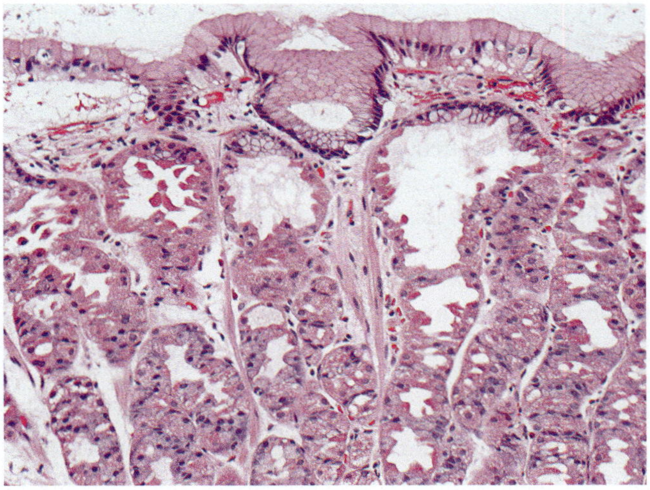

Fig. 8.4 Proton pump inhibitors' effects. Enlarged and increased parietal cells protruding into the gastric glands with a serrated appearance to the glandular lumen in body and fundus

OsmoPrep-Associated Gastritis

OsmoPrep is a tablet form of osmotic laxative sometimes used for bowel preparation as a colon preparatory agent. It is usually used in patients who cannot tolerate the large chalky fluid which constitutes the more commonly prescribed liquid sodium phosphate agent. The active ingredient is sodium phosphate and has been associated with risk of acute phosphate nephrotoxicity.

In a recent study, a subset of patients who were prescribed OsmoPrep showed purple to black inorganic deposits in the superficial lamina propria of the stomach [22]. The deposits varied in size (<100 m) and showed irregular contour with the appearance of crushed pill fragments. The gastric mucosa showed features of reactive gastropathy with marked reactive epithelial changes, including mucin loss and nuclear hyperchromasia. No erosions or ulcers were seen. However, in some cases congestion and mild edema were seen adjacent to these deposits. The differential for these deposits included iron pill material and mucosal calcinosis. However, these OsmoPrep deposits were positive on von Kossa stain but negative on alizarin red (a calcium chelating dye) arguing against mucosal calcinosis. The deposits were also negative on Perl's iron stain.

Mycophenolate Mofetil

Mycophenolate mofetil (MMF) is an immunosuppressant used in solid organ and bone marrow as well as stem cell transplant patients to prevent allograft rejection and graft versus host disease (GVHD), respectively. It is also used to treat some autoimmune and inflammatory diseases such as psoriasis, lupus nephritis, and myasthenia gravis. The histological hallmark of MMF-associated injury is increased apoptosis, characterized by condensation and fragmentation of blue nuclear and pink cytoplasmic material with an empty space surrounding the degenerated cell components. Gastric biopsies can show a range of histological changes varying from severe reactive gastropathy, Crohn's-like features including granulomatous inflammation, to nonspecific changes [23, 24]. A small subset of patients can also show ballooning degeneration of the parietal cells characterized by enlarged parietal cell to more than twice its normal size and clearing of the cytoplasm [24].

Medications Associated with Mitotic Arrest (Colchicine and Taxol)

Colchicine is an alkaloid used for treatment of gout and other medical conditions including immune/rheumatologic disorders. Colchicine exhibits antimitotic activity due to its ability to bind to tubulin and preventing the polymerization of tubulin into microtubules. Patients with renal and/or hepatic failure may develop colchicine toxicity. The most noticeable feature of colchicine toxicity is mitotic arrest in metaphase with absent mitotic spindles and bizarre chromatin patterns, especially ring mitosis (Fig. 8.5) [25, 26]. The mucous neck region of the stomach usually shows the prominent mitosis with colchicine toxicity. The gastric foveolar epithelium may also show enlarged hyperchromatic nuclei with loss of polarity and epithelial stratification. Increased apoptosis may also be seen. It is important for the pathologists to recognize the epithelial atypia to be related to colchicine toxicity in order to avoid confusion with high-grade

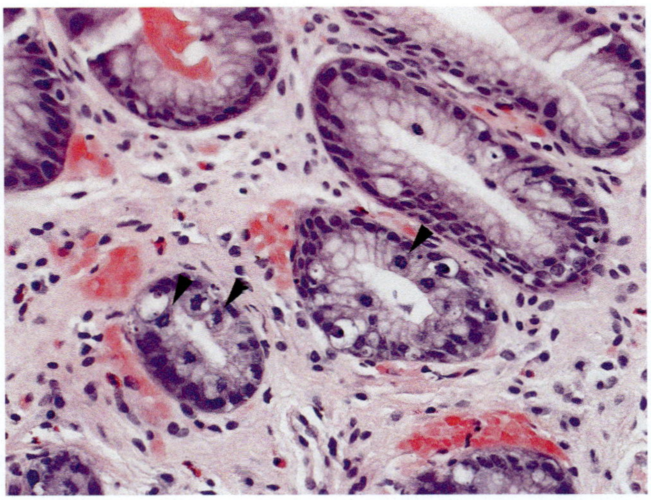

Fig. 8.5 Colchicine toxicity. Gastric biopsy from a chronic renal failure patients taking colchicine shows mitotic arrest in metaphase (ring mitosis, arrowheads) and increased apoptosis

dysplasia. These changes are not seen in patients taking colchicine who do not have clinical evidence of toxicity. Hence when these changes are identified by the pathologists, it is important to reconcile with the patient's medication list, since if colchicine is the offending agent, then the patient is probably toxic. Of note, even therapeutic doses of colchicine may rarely cause ring mitosis, especially in colorectal polyps [27]. The histological findings of colchicine toxicity regress on cessation of the drug.

Taxol (paclitaxel) is a chemotherapy drug used to treat malignancies of lung, esophagus, and breast. Taxol binds to the microtubules of the mitotic spindle causing metaphase arrest. Like colchicine, Taxol causes increased and arrested mitotic activity including ring mitosis [25, 28]. The mitotic figures are predominantly seen in the proliferative zone of the gastric mucosa. Taxol effects are histologically identical to those of colchicine toxicity and morphologically indistinguishable. However, the histological features of Taxol effect can be seen in any patient undergoing chemotherapy with this drug, and unlike colchicine, mitotic arrest and ring mitosis after Taxol administration do not indicate Taxol toxicity. Rarely, patients with telomere-mediated disorders may also show ring mitosis and apoptosis [29].

Nonsteroidal Anti-inflammatory Drugs (NSAIDs)

NSAIDs are widely used for their analgesic and anti-inflammatory effects. They prevent prostaglandin synthesis by inhibiting cyclooxygenase-1 (COX-1) and cyclooxygenase-2 (COX-2). The decreased prostaglandin synthesis results in mucosal ischemia and decreased mucosal integrity within the gastrointestinal tract due to decreased production of mucosal protectants. Within the stomach, three major histologic types of gastric injuries are noted: acute hemorrhagic gastritis (described in detail in Chap. 6), ulcers, and reactive gastropathy (described in detail in Chap. 6) [30, 31]. NSAID-related erosions frequently develop in the gastric body, whereas NSAIDs ulcers are often large, multiple, and painless and develop in the antrum [32, 33].

Chemotherapy and Radiation-Associated Changes

Chemotherapeutic agents, such as 5-fluoro-2-deoxuridin (FUDR) and mitomycin C when used for hepatic arterial infusion chemotherapy, have been associated with erosions and ulcers within the distal stomach [34, 35]. In some patients, chemotherapy-related gastric ulcers may show marked epithelial atypia that can be mistaken for gastric dysplasia or even early carcinoma [36, 37]. These changes can be distinguished from "true" dysplasia by its patchy distribution, absence of a mass lesion, surface maturation, lack of intestinal metaplasia, lack of infiltrative pattern, open nuclear chromatin with prominent nucleoli, retained nuclear polarity, lack of atypical mitosis, and cytoplasmic eosinophilia and/or vacuolization [38].

Yttrium-90 microspheres injected for selective internal radiation can be associated with gastric ulceration and presence of black microspheres within the mucosal capillaries [39, 40]. This occurs when the Yttrium-90-labeled microspheres accidentally enter the arteries supplying the stomach, causing unintended radiation damage. The stomach shows lamina propria hyalinization, atypical stromal and endothelial cells, as well as damaged ectatic vessels (Fig. 8.6a). The microspheres are basophilic and uniform and measure about 30–40 m in diameter (Fig. 8.6b) [40, 41].

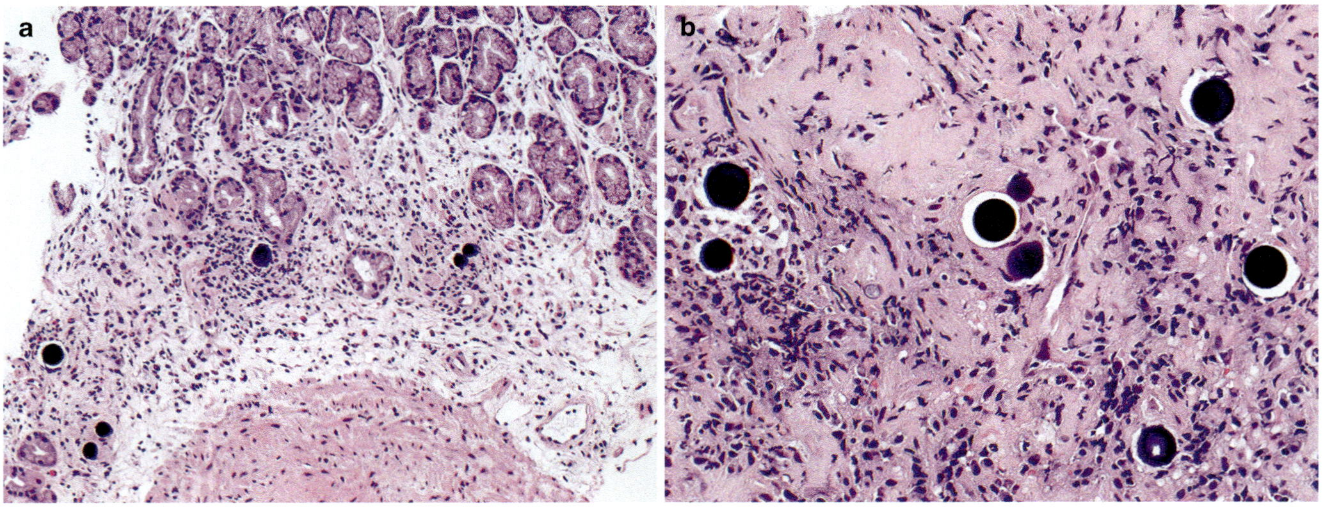

Fig. 8.6 Yttrium-90-induced gastric mucosal injury. The stomach shows lamina propria hyalinization and basophilic, uniform Yttrium-90 microspheres within lamina propria (**a**) and granulation tissue (**b**)

Resins (Kayexalate-Sorbitol, Cholestyramine, Colesevelam, Colestipol, and Sevelamer)

Resins are nonabsorbable medications which act as platforms for ion exchange in the gastrointestinal tract. The commonly used resins include Kayexalate (sodium polystyrene sulfonate), sevelamer, and bile acid sequestrants (BAS).

Kayexalate-sorbitol enemas are used for treatment of hyperkalemia in patients with renal insufficiency. Kayexalate is a cation exchange resin that picks up excess potassium ions in exchange for sodium ions within the large intestine. The resin and excess potassium ions are then excreted in the stool. Sorbitol is a laxative agent which is administered with Kayexalate, as it can cause constipation and bezoar formation. However, as a result of vascular shunting due to osmotic load, a subset of patients with uremia can develop gastrointestinal tract ischemia and even necrosis [42–44]. There is also some suggestion that Kayexalate can itself directly inflict mucosal injury [43]. Within the stomach, hemorrhagic gastritis, serpiginous ulcers, and erosions have been described to be related to Kayexalate-sorbitol (Fig. 8.7a) [42, 44, 45]. Kayexalate crystals are rhomboid or triangular in shape and deeply basophilic on hematoxylin and eosin (H&E) stain (Fig. 8.7b). They also can be highlighted on PAS-D (the crystals are magenta color), Diff-Quik, and acid-fast stains (the crystals are black). They exhibit a distinctive internal mosaic pattern that resembles fish scales [42]. These crystals are refractile but do not polarize. The crystals remain attached to the intact mucosa or can be seen admixed with the inflammatory exudates in cases with ulcers or erosions.

Cholestyramine is a bile acid sequestrant which is clinically used in treatment of hyperlipidemia. Cholestyramine crystals are irregularly shaped and have a near black to deep red to bright orange color on H&E stain depending on the tissue thickness and stain variability [46–48]. They also lack the fish-scale pattern of Kayexalate and appear to have a smooth glassy texture (Fig. 8.8). Large cholestyramine crystals may occasionally show irregular cracking lines but still would lack the geometric fish scale pattern. They appear dull yellow on acid-fast stain and variable gray or hot pink on PAS-D stain [48, 49]. Cholestyramine is probably not directly harmful to the gastrointestinal tract mucosa, but it can potentiate preexisting lesions, thereby increasing the risk of bleeding [49]. However, in the stomach, it has been associated with superficial erosions to ulcerations [50].

Colesevelam and colestipol are also bile acid sequestrants that are used to treat diarrhea, hypercholesteremia, and dyslipidemia. They probably lack the ability to cause significant

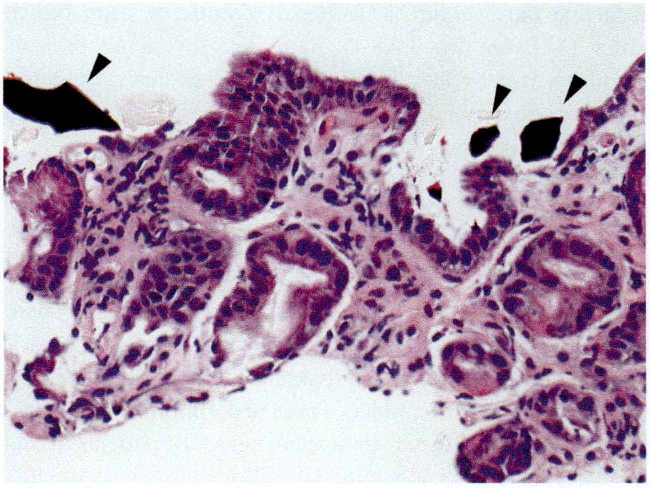

Fig. 8.8 Cholestyramine crystals. Cholestyramine crystals (arrowheads) are irregularly shaped and have a near black to deep-red to bright orange color with smooth glassy texture and no fish scale on H&E stain

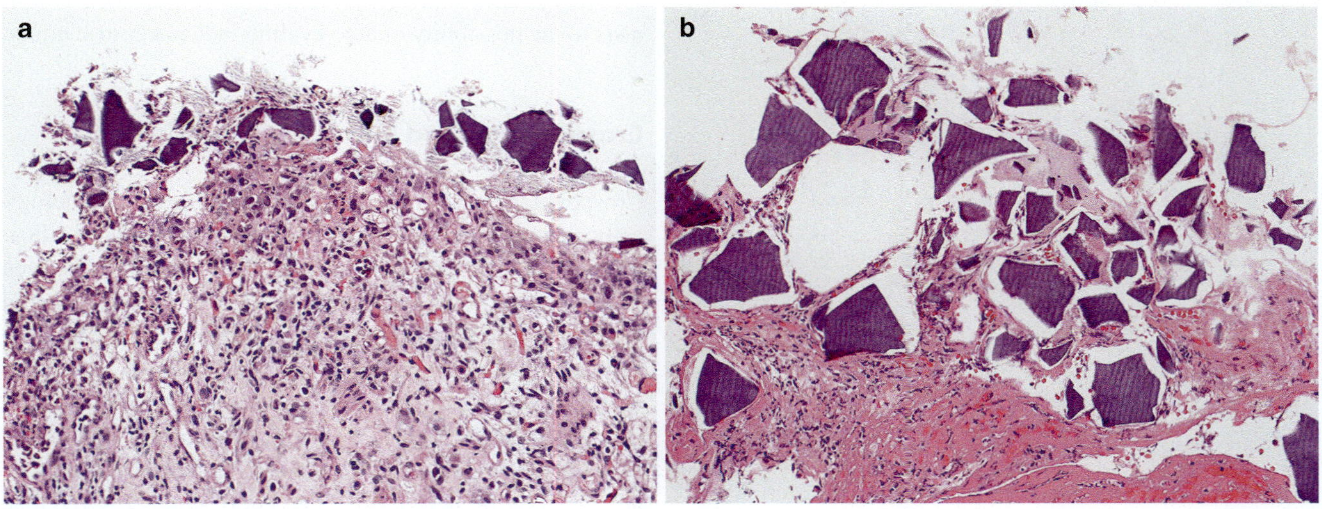

Fig. 8.7 Kayexalate-sorbitol-associated gastric injury. Kayexalate crystals present in gastric ulcer (a). Kayexalate crystals are rhomboid or triangular in shape and deeply basophilic with mosaic pattern that resembles fish scales on H&E stain (b)

direct mucosal injury to the gastrointestinal tract [48]. However, crystals can be seen occasionally within stomach biopsies. Morphologically the crystals of colesvelam and colestipol are identical to cholestyramine crystals and cannot be distinguished from one another.

Sevelamer carbonate is another anion exchange resin which is a phosphate binder. It is used in patients with chronic renal failure to treat hyperphosphatemia. It has been associated with gastric mucosal injury, but its exact etiological role remains unclear as it may just be an innocent bystander [47]. On the H&E stain the crystals of sevelamer appear broad, curved, and irregularly spaced (Fig. 8.9). Like Kayexalate, they also show fish-scale pattern. However, they also show a characteristic two-toned color imparted by bright pink linear accentuations with a rusty yellow background. Some crystals embedded in an area of ulcer, necrosis, or ischemia may acquire a deep eosinophilic or rusty brown color [47]. On the PAS-D stain, the sevelamer crystals acquire a violet color. These crystals are exclusively identified in patients with chronic kidney disease, and this is an important clue toward their diagnosis.

Lanthanum

Lanthanum carbonate (Fosrenol) is used in patients with chronic renal failure for treatment of hyperphosphatemia. It is a rare alkaline earth metal that binds with phosphate in the gastrointestinal tract and has a poor absorption from the gastrointestinal tract. However, a small subset of patients taking this drug develops lanthanum deposition within mucosal histiocytes (Fig. 8.10a–c) [51–53]. Small foreign body granulomas may also be seen [54]. The histiocytes show a fine to coarse granular material that varies in color from brown, gray, to violet. These histiocytes may stain positive with Prussian blue and toluidine blue in some cases. Lanthanum can be identified in the histiocytes by electron microscopy, but the diagnosis is usually confirmed by correlation with the clinical history. There are some reports suggesting that this accumulation reverses after stopping lanthanum, but in rare cases, the deposits are seen even years after the discontinuation of lanthanum [55, 56].

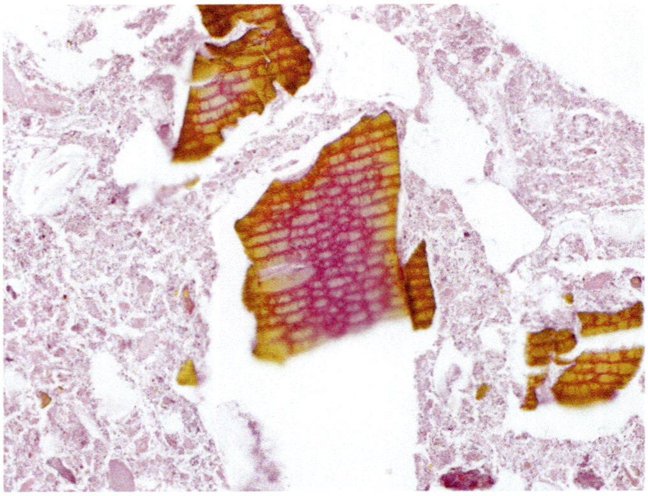

Fig. 8.9 Sevelamer crystals. Sevelamer crystals have broad, curved, and irregularly spaced fish-scale pattern and a characteristic two-toned color imparted by bright pink linear accentuations with a rusty yellow background on the H&E stain

Olmesartan

Angiotensin II receptor antagonists such as olmesartan (Benicar) are commonly used for treatment of hypertension. A subset of patients taking olmesartan may show lymphocytic gastritis (Fig. 8.11), collagenous gastritis, or chronic gastritis [57].

Tetracycline/Doxycycline

Doxycycline is an oral tetracycline antibiotic. Recently, there have been reports of doxycycline causing superficial gastric mucosal necrosis with a peculiar form of vascular degeneration [58, 59]. Endoscopy showed white to yellow plaque-like lesions or non-bleeding ulcers. Histologically, the superficial mucosal necrosis was characterized by hyperplastic foveolar cells, inflamed lamina propria, and sloughing of the superficial epithelial cells. They also show vascular degeneration of the capillaries characterized by eosinophilic necrosis of the vessel wall creating a ringlike deeply eosinophilic granular structure, sometimes even creating a halo effect due to separation from the surrounding tissue. These vessels often show intraluminal neutrophils and microthrombi [58]. This pattern of injury is unique and its presence should alert the pathologists to the possibility of doxycycline-induced gastric injury.

Crospovidone and Microcrystalline Cellulose

Crospovidone and microcrystalline cellulose are biologically inert pharmaceutical fillers incorporated into medications to facilitate drug delivery. They can sometimes be seen in stomach biopsies. Awareness of their morphology would be helpful for the pathologists to differentiate them from parasites, calcifications, and other medications associated with mucosal injuries. In a recent study by Shaddy et al., the overall filler incidence in gastric biopsies was about 3% [60]. Their presence outside the luminal bowel may be an indicator of perforation. On H&E stain crospovidone appears non-birefringent, coral, or sponge shaped with pink core and purple coat and measures 0.4–1.5 mm in diameter

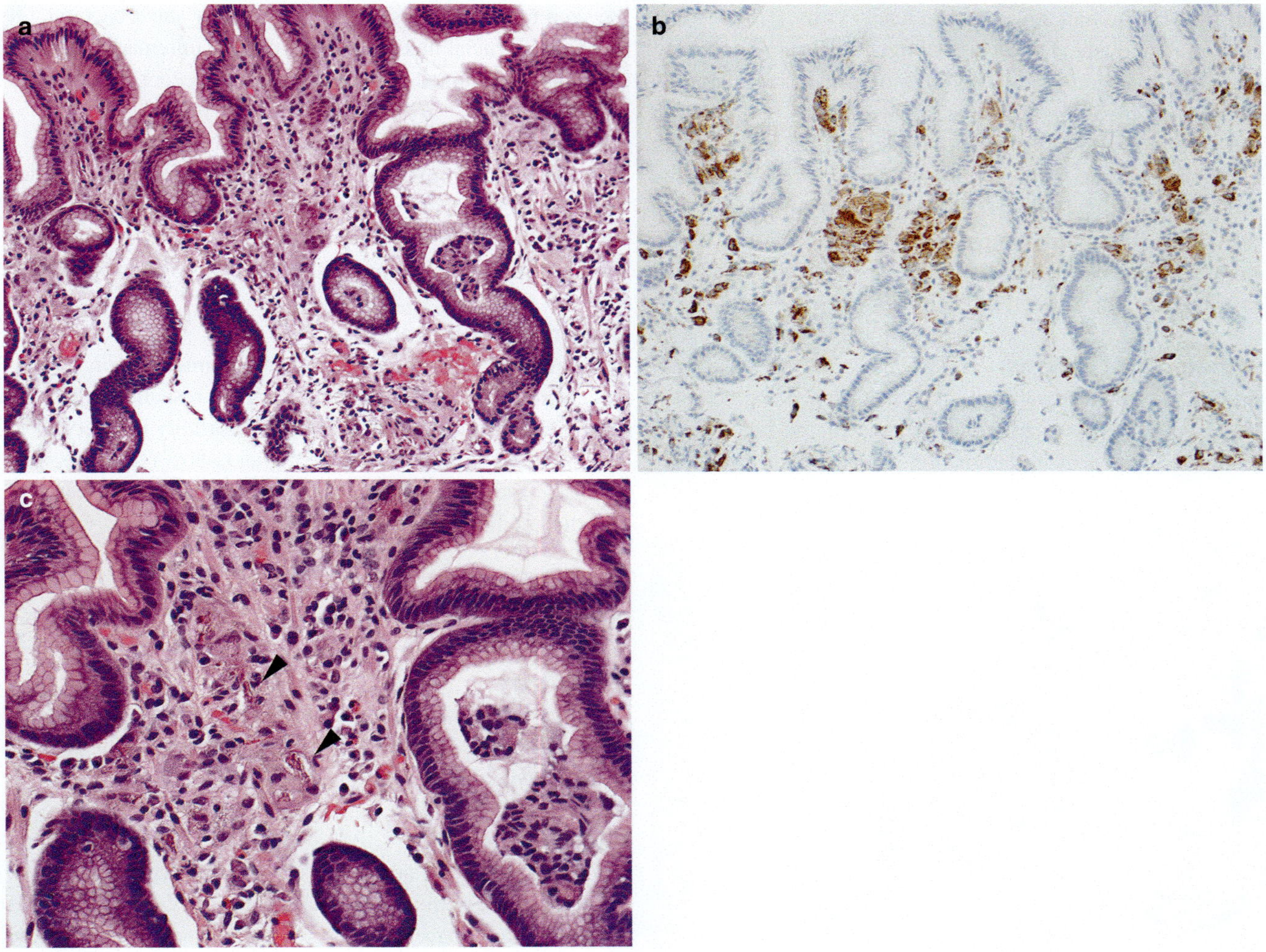

Fig. 8.10 Lanthanum deposition. Antral mucosal biopsy from a chronic renal failure patient receiving lanthanum carbonate for hyperphosphatemia shows histiocytic aggregates within lamina propria (**a**). The histiocytes within the lamina propria are positive for CD68 by immunohistochemical stain (**b**). There are cytoplasmic coarse inclusion-like brownish materials with irregular branching (arrowheads) present within the histiocytes (**c**)

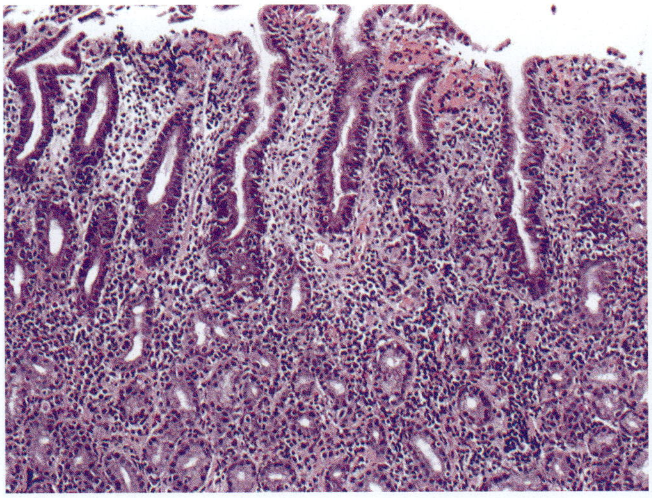

Fig. 8.11 Olmesartan-associated gastric injury. Lymphocytic gastritis pattern in a patient with olmesartan-associated enteropathy

(Fig. 8.12). Microcrystalline cellulose on H&E stain appears transparent with a rod or matchstick shape (Fig. 8.13a) and is brightly birefringent under polarized light (Fig. 8.13b) [60].

Infections

Phlegmonous (Suppurative) Gastritis

Definition

Phlegmonous gastritis is a rare form of rapidly progressive suppurative bacterial infection that affects the stomach. Its hallmarks are necrosis and gangrene.

Clinical Features

Patients usually have an underlying condition, such as immunocompromised status or debilitating condition such as malignancy, human immunodeficiency virus (HIV) infection, or alcoholism. The exact pathogenesis is not known but is often caused by a variety of bacteria including *Staphylococcus*, *Streptococcus*, *Enterococcus*, *Escherichia coli*, *Proteus*, and *Clostridium* species [61–63]. Presenting symptoms include fever, abdominal pain, nausea, vomiting, and hematemesis [61]. Computed tomography (CT) scan may show diffuse thickening of the gastric wall with intramural low density. Endoscopy may show ulcers, thickened gastric folds, mass effect, or necrotic material.

Pathological Features

Grossly the stomach wall may appear thickened and necrotic. Microscopy shows suppurative necrosis of the mucosa and submucosa with acute inflammation. Transmural necrosis may be seen in severe cases. A Gram stain may show bacteria. Of note, a superficial mucosal biopsy may be unremarkable if the findings are confined to the submucosa or deeper structures.

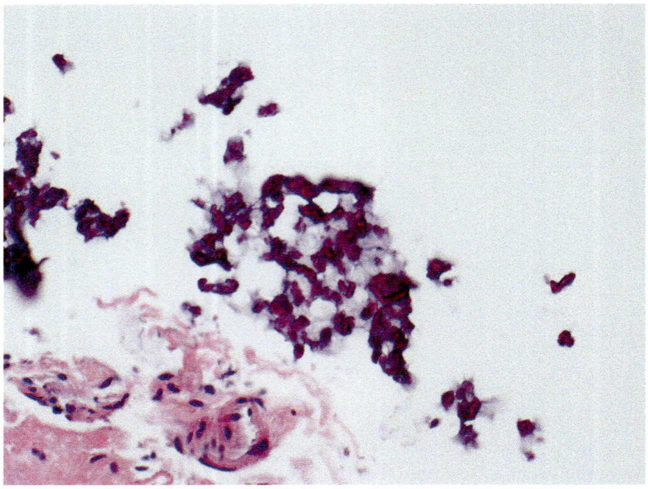

Fig. 8.12 Crospovidone. This filler material appears non-birefringent, coral, or sponge shaped with pink core and purple coat on H&E stain

Differential Diagnosis

Differential diagnosis includes gastric lymphoma, gastrointestinal stromal tumor, linitis plastic, and superinfected malignancy. These conditions can be differentiated by careful histological review and use of special stains as needed.

Treatment and Prognosis

Treatment includes medical and surgical intervention. Broad-spectrum antibiotics are useful. Surgical resection is also an option and may offer better survival. Mortality is low (~10%) for localized disease but can be higher (>50%) for cases with diffuse gastric involvement. Early diagnosis and treatment are the key for improved survival [61, 62].

Sarcina ventriculi

Definition

Sarcina ventriculi is a Gram-positive anaerobic coccus that can be identified within the stomach, especially in patients with delayed gastric emptying.

Clinical Features

It occurs mainly in adults but can also be seen in children, more commonly in females than males [64]. More than half of the patients have a history of gastric outlet obstruction, gastroparesis, and/or gastrointestinal surgery. It has also been associated with gastric perforation and emphysematous gastritis [65, 66]. Most patients present with abdominal pain, nausea, and vomiting. In some patients, it may just be an

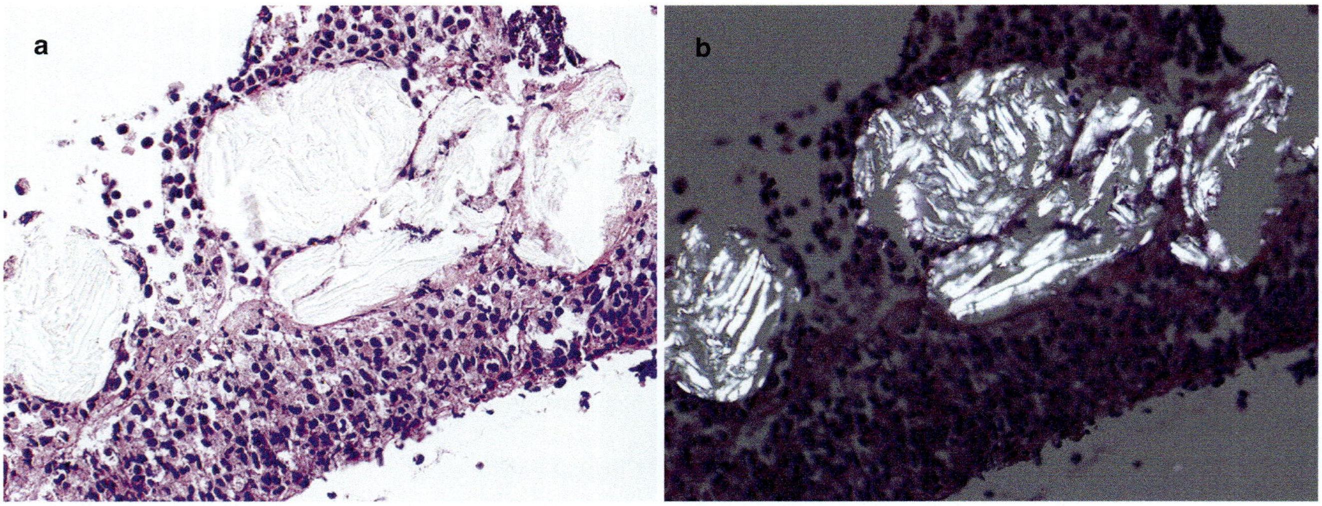

Fig. 8.13 Microcrystalline cellulose. This filler material appears transparent with a rod or matchstick shape in background of inflammatory exudates on H&E stain (**a**) and is brightly birefringent under polarized light (**b**)

incidental finding and the patient may be asymptomatic [67]. Endoscopy may show gastric bezoar, retained food residue, erosions, and ulcerations [64].

Pathological Features

The organisms are not invasive and generally seen near the mucosal surface in the gastric mucin. On H&E stain, *Sarcina ventriculi* appear as basophilic cuboid-shaped organisms measuring 1.8–3 m and arranged in tetrad packet arrangement (Fig. 8.14a). There may be flattening of the cell walls in areas of contact with adjacent organism and it may even be refractile in nature [64]. On Gram stain, the organisms are strongly positive. The organism can also be confirmed by molecular methods using polymerase chain reaction (PCR) and sequencing of the 16S ribosomal RNA gene and pyruvate decarboxylase gene. The adjacent gastric mucosa is usually unremarkable, but, in some cases, it may show diffuse hemorrhagic gastritis with ulceration (Fig. 8.14b) [68]. The exact mechanism of mucosal injury caused by *Sarcina* is not entirely clear. There has been a suggestion that it may simply be a bystander in an underlying disease process. The organism has also been reported in feces of healthy people, especially those on vegetarian diet [69]. It can also be found in the soil and air [70]. However, identification of Sarcina in gastric biopsies is important for surgical pathologists due to its strong association with gastric stasis and rare cases of life-threatening emphysematous gastritis. Its presence in a gastric biopsy should raise a consideration for gastric outlet obstruction and delayed gastric emptying.

Differential Diagnosis

The main differential is *Micrococcus* species, a Gram-positive coccus that occurs in tetrads or packets. However, the *Micrococcus* is considerably smaller measuring 0.5 m and unlike *Sarcina* species, the *Micrococcus* species tend to form tightly packed clusters [68]. In addition, the *Micrococcus* bacterium is aerobic and catalase positive and does not form spores, while *Sarcina ventriculi* is anaerobic, catalase negative, and spore forming [71]. *Staphylococcus* species can also be in the differential, and they are also Gram-positive. However, *Staphylococcus* bacteria are smaller in size, measuring around 1 m in diameter, and arranged in grape-like clusters, rather than a tetrad pattern.

Treatment and Prognosis

There is no standard regimen for treatment. Antibiotics such as metronidazole are successful in eradication of the organism. There is also suggestion to omit treatment if the patient is healthy and asymptomatic, as the organism can occur commensally [64].

Syphilis Gastritis

Definition

It is a gastric infection caused by spirochete *Treponema pallidum*, which is mostly a sexually transmitted disease.

Clinical Features

Median age is 39 years, more common in males and black race [72]. Epigastric or abdominal pain is the most common presenting symptom, followed by vomiting and weight loss. Only a small subset of patients may have a history of syphilis but many of them may have prior or concurrent clinical manifestations of the disease. Majority of cases have positive serological tests for syphilis (Venereal Disease Research Laboratory (VDRL), Rapid Plasma Reagin (RPR), and/or Kolmer). Endoscopy may show gastric ulceration, erosion, nodular mucosa, thickened folds, or rarely even a mass lesion [72].

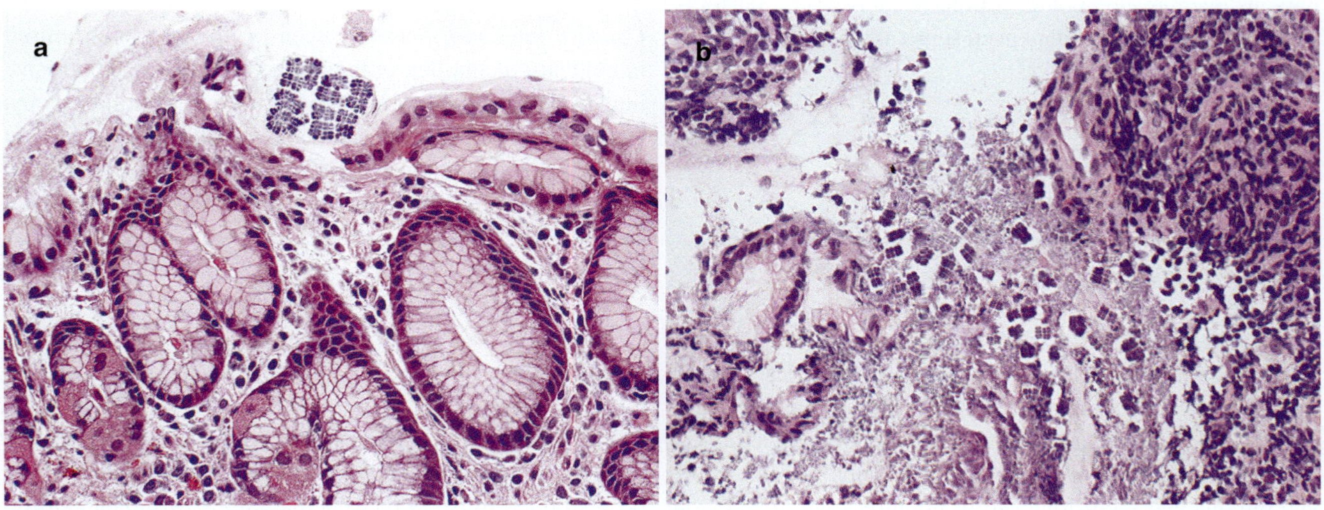

Fig. 8.14 *Sarcina ventriculi*. Basophilic, cuboid-shaped organisms in tetrad packet arrangement on luminal surface of gastric mucosa with mild chronic inflammation (**a**) and in foci of ulceration with inflammatory exudates (**b**)

Pathological Features

Microscopy shows gastritis with a prominent plasma cell infiltrate, admixed lymphocytes, and varying number of neutrophils. The dense plasmacytic infiltrate may show a perivascular distribution. Vasculitis is seen in the form of proliferative endoarteritis; however, endophlebitis may also be seen in occasional cases. Rare cases may also show atrophic gastritis [72]. *T. pallidum* immunostain can be used to highlight the organisms and confirm the diagnosis. Silver stains such as Warthin-Starry can also be useful in detecting the organisms, but it can be difficult to read and is also not highly sensitive [73]. Immunofluorescence microscopy and PCR testing is also available [74]. *Treponema pallidum* is a Gram-negative spirochete measuring 8–15 m in length and 0.1–0.2 m in diameter. The organisms are usually present in the lamina propria and between the glandular epithelial cells.

Differential Diagnosis

Helicobacter pylori and *Helicobacter heilmannii* enter the differential as they share some morphological similarity with *Treponema pallidum*. *Helicobacter pylori* are much smaller and measure 1–3 m in length and 0.5–1 m in diameter. *Helicobacter heilmannii* is longer and wider than *Helicobacter pylori* but shorter and plumper than *Treponema pallidum* with 4–6 helical turns giving a corkscrew-like appearance [75, 76]. Immunostains for *Helicobacter pylori* and *Treponema pallidum* can be useful in their distinction. The *Treponema* immunostain has recently been reported to show crossed reactivity with *Helicobacter heilmannii* [77].

Treatment and Prognosis

Antibiotics like penicillin usually resolve the infection. The clinical symptoms usually disappear in a week and the endoscopy findings return to normal in about 10 days. Rare patients may develop complications such as gastric perforation or obstruction and may need surgical resection.

Viral Infections

Cytomegalovirus (CMV)

Cytomegalovirus (CMV) gastritis is usually seen in immunocompromised patients, such as those with malignancies, HIV infection, and post-transplant or on steroids [78]. Symptoms include fever and abdominal pain. Endoscopy may show erythema, erosions, and ulceration. Rare cases may show hypertrophic gastritis resembling Menetrier's disease [79]. Histopathology shows characteristically enlarged endothelial, stromal, or rarely epithelial cells with an owl's eye intranuclear inclusions and/or granular basophilic cytoplasmic inclusions (Fig. 8.15). CMV immunostain can be used to confirm the diagnosis.

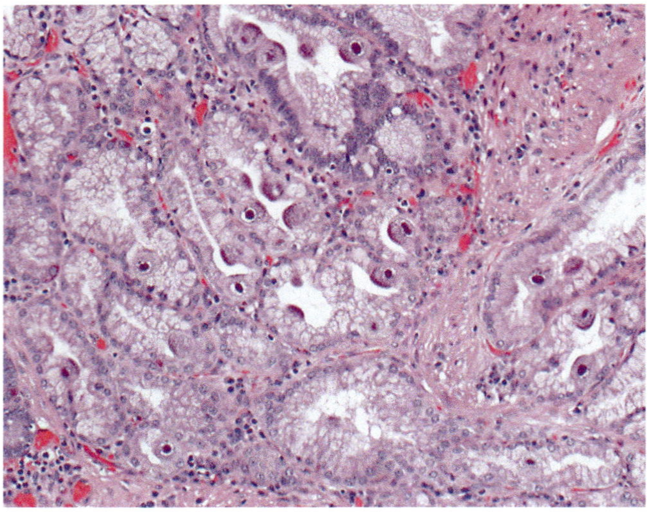

Fig. 8.15 CMV gastritis. Antral mucosa with multiple owl's eye intranuclear inclusions and granular basophilic cytoplasmic inclusions within epithelial cells

Herpesvirus (HSV)

Gastric infection by herpesvirus (HSV) and varicella zoster virus (VZV) is rare but can be seen in immunosuppressed patients [80, 81]. The epithelial cells typically show ground glass nuclei and eosinophilic inclusion surrounded by a clear halo, demonstrating margination, multinucleation, and molding.

Epstein-Barr Virus (EBV)

Rare cases of Epstein-Barr virus (EBV) gastritis (Fig 8.16a, b) have been reported with associated prominent lymphoid hyperplasia simulating a lymphoma [82, 83].

Fungal Infections

Candida infection is usually seen in immunocompromised individuals, alcoholics, or those who have ingested corrosive liquids. Mucosa shows erosions or ulcers. On microscopy, yeasts and pseudohyphae can be identified using silver stain or PAS-D stain. Large gastric ulcers with cancer can also show fungal contamination by *Candida* [84]. A rare fatal case of invasive mucormycosis associated with emphysematous gastritis has also been reported [85].

Parasites

Gastric infection by parasites is rare. However, *Schistosoma ova* can be seen within the stomach [86]. Cryptosporidiosis has been reported in AIDS patients, presenting as subtotal gastric obstruction due to stricturing [87, 88]. Gastric invasive anisakiasis has also been reported after consumption of fish [89].

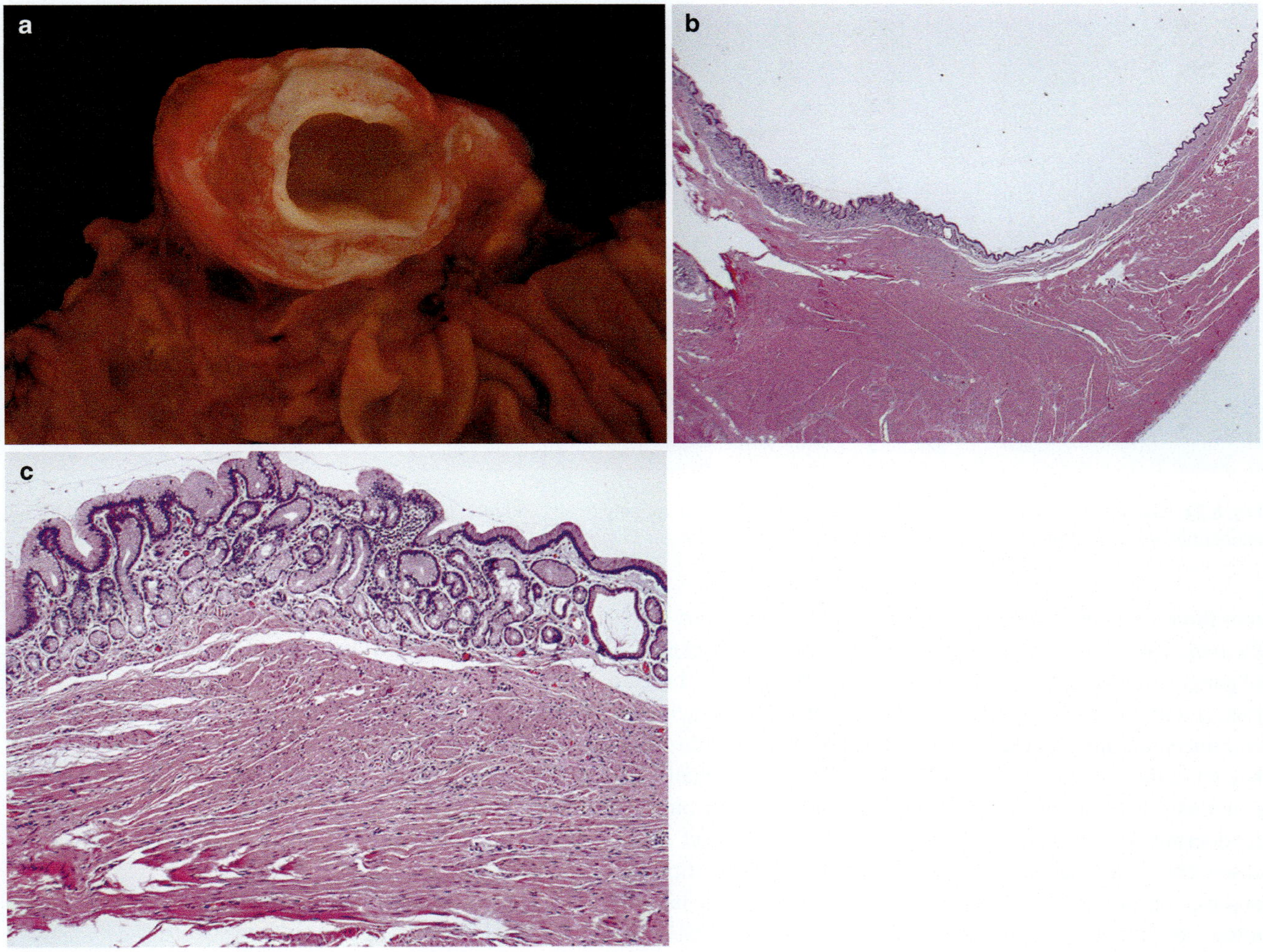

Fig. 8.20 Gastric duplication cyst. The duplication cyst is adhered to the pancreas (**a**). Muscular propria is present within the cyst wall (**b**), and the lining epithelium shows normal gastric epithelium (**c**)

tomic, functional, and vascular connection with the original organ.

Clinical Features

In general, pancreatic heterotopia is a relatively infrequent lesion, with an autopsy frequency ranging between 0.6% and 13% [132, 133]. Stomach is the most frequent site of pancreatic heterotopia. It can be associated with other congenital anomalies such as gastrointestinal atresia and duplication. The exact pathogenesis of this lesion is unknown. It is believed to arise during embryonic development of the gastrointestinal tract. During embryogenesis, if one or more evaginations from developing pancreas remain entrapped, then it may be carried away from the remainder of the gland by the developing gastrointestinal tract and may give rise to heterotopic pancreas. The other theory proposes pancreatic metaplasia of endodermal tissues that end up in the submucosa during embryonic life. Majority of the patients remain asymptomatic and the lesion is found incidentally during endoscopy, surgery, or autopsy. A small subset of patients may present with abdominal pain, bleeding, nausea, and vomiting [134].

Pathological Features

Grossly it appears as a single, well-circumscribed, solid, or cystic tan mass within the submucosa. Endoscopically the lesion may appear as a mucosal polyp with central umbilication and normal-appearing overlying mucosa. Occasionally, it may also be seen within the muscularis propria or serosa. It varies in size from 0.2 cm to 6 cm. Rare cases can be multiple or pedunculated. Histologically, it contains a mixture of tissues that may be found in the normal pancreas. Most consists primarily of ducts and surrounding simple mucin-producing glands. Special stains are usually not needed but trypsin immunostain can be used to confirm the presence of pancreatic acini. Cytokeratin 7 immunostain has also been shown to facilitate recognition of pancreatic heterotopia in gastric biopsies [135]. Ectopic pancreas can be classified

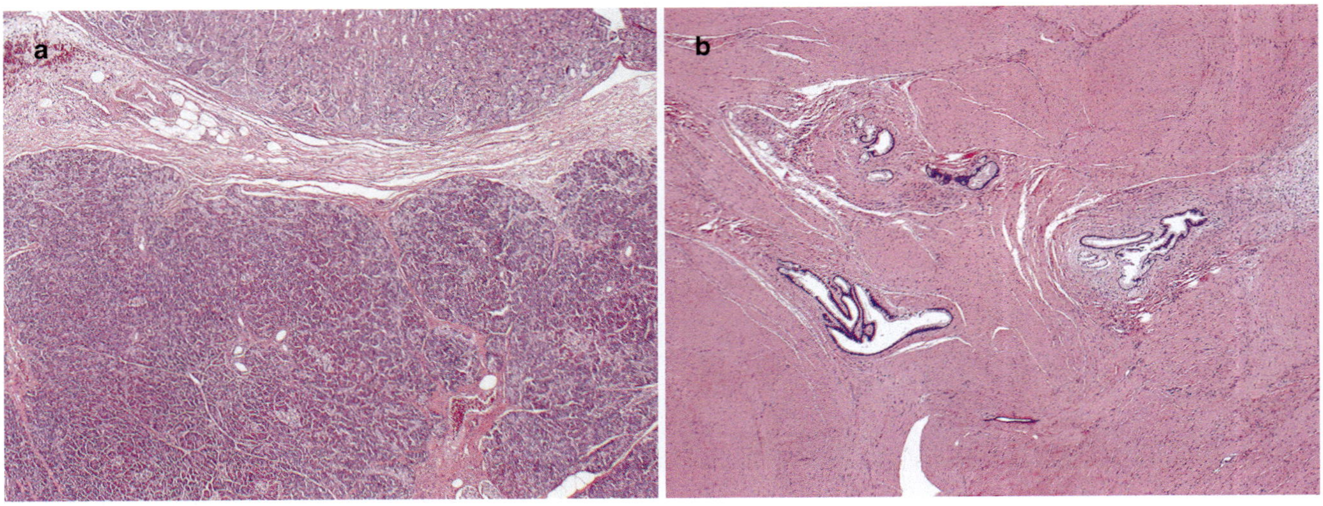

Fig. 8.21 Gastric pancreatic heterotopia. Pancreatic heterotopia comprising of all cell types, including exocrine cells, endocrine cells, and ductal epithelium present within gastric submucosa (**a**). Pancreatic heterotopia composed of ducts only in muscularis propria of stomach (**b**)

into three types according to Heinrich based on the types of the pancreatic cells present: type I with all three components of pancreatic tissues (acini, ducts, and islet cells) (Fig. 8.21a); type II with exocrine components of pancreatic tissues (acini and ducts, but no islet cells); and type III with mainly ducts but no acini or islet cells (Fig. 8.21b) [136]. Occasionally, pancreatic heterotopia can be composed of islet cells only (endocrine heterotopia) (Fig. 8.22a, b) [137]. A subset of cases can show secondary changes such as pancreatitis, abscess formation, fibrosis, or fat necrosis, distorting the histology of the heterotopic tissue. Rarely, endocrine and/or glandular neoplasms as well as pancreatic cysts can also develop within pancreatic heterotopia [138, 139].

Differential Diagnosis

If only pancreatic acinar cells are present, especially in the gastroesophageal junction region, then it may represent pancreatic acinar metaplasia [140]. Cases of autoimmune atrophic gastritis can also show pancreatic acinar metaplasia in the stomach [141]. Purely endocrine heterotopic pancreas may mimic a well-differentiated neuroendocrine tumor (Fig. 8.22a, b). Both show monomorphic neuroendocrine cells arranged in small nests or microtubules. However, the scattered nature of the lesion, small size of the nests, and absence of stromal reaction argue against a neuroendocrine tumor and favor an endocrine pancreatic heterotopia. Immunostains may also help in making this distinction as cases of endocrine pancreatic heterotopia would show majority of cells expressing insulin (Fig. 8.22c), mostly in the center of the nodules, with fewer peripheral cells showing somatostatin (Fig. 8.22d) and glucagon (Fig. 8.22e) positivity [142].

Treatment and Prognosis

Asymptomatic cases do not need treatment unless complications develop. Localized surgical resection is usually the treatment of choice.

Congenital Pyloric Stenosis

Definition

Congenital pyloric stenosis is defined as narrowing of the stomach due to abnormal thickening of the pylorus resulting in gastric outlet obstruction.

Clinical Features

Congenital pyloric stenosis is the most common cause of gastric outlet obstruction and surgical cause of vomiting in infants. Incidence ranges from 1 to 6 per 1000 live births [143, 144]. Commonly occurs in whites, first-born child, and males. Congenital pyloric stenosis can be associated with other anomalies like esophageal atresia, intestinal malrotation, and urinary tract defects [145]. The etiology remains unknown but probably is multifactorial involving genetic predisposition and perinatal as well as environmental factors [146]. However, it has been associated with several chromosomal aneuploidy syndromes such as deletion 11q, duplica-

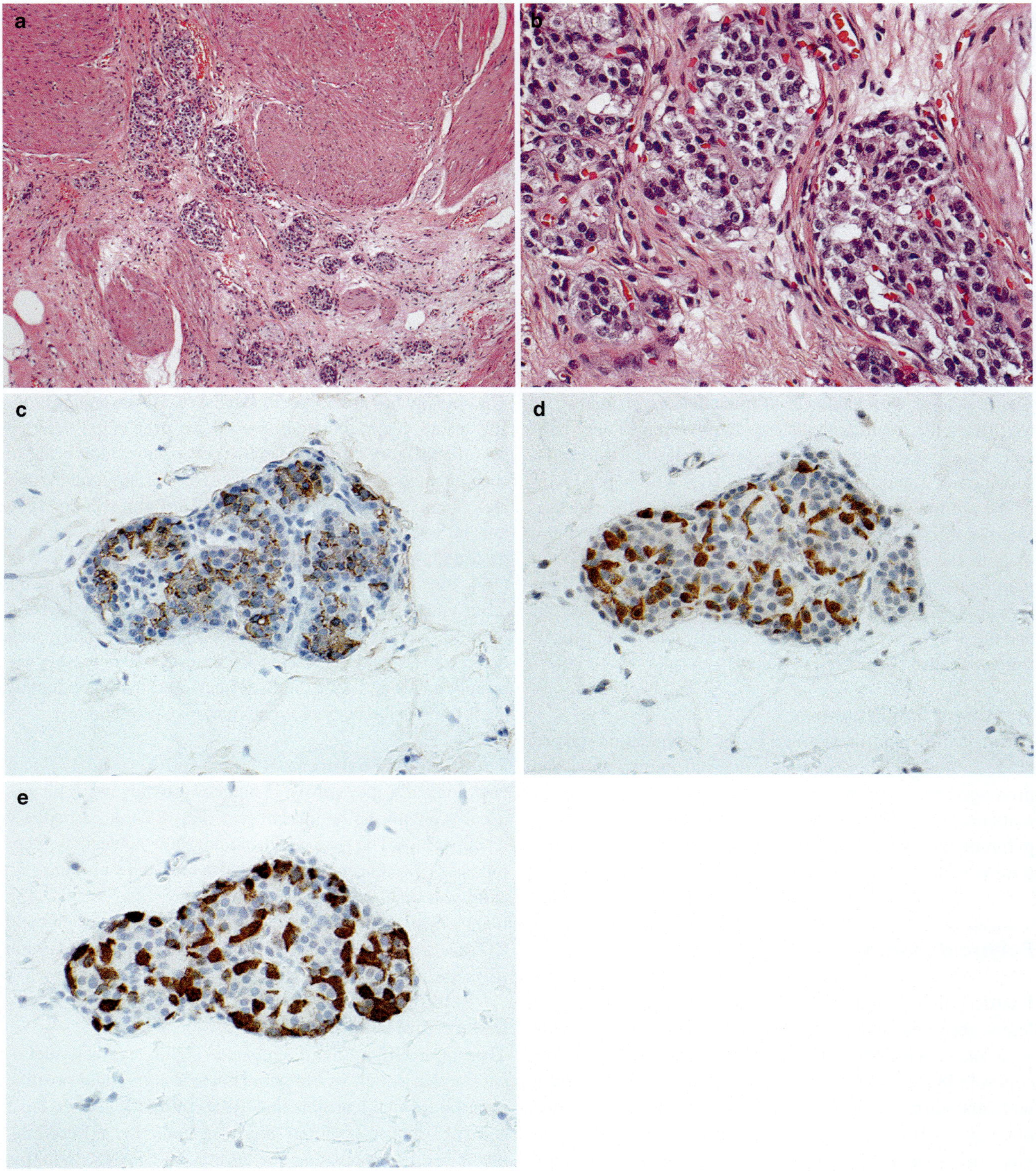

Fig. 8.22 Gastric pancreatic endocrine heterotopia. Pancreatic heterotopia comprising islet cells only in muscularis propria of stomach (**a**). The neuroendocrine cells arranged in small nests and absence of stromal reaction (**b**) and the majority of cells, mostly in the center of the nodules expressing insulin (**c**), with fewer peripheral cells expressing somatostatin (**d**) and glucagon (**e**) by immunostains

tion 14q, duplication 9q, trisomy 18, and trisomy 21 [147]. Formula feeding and azithromycin have also been associated with increased risk of developing hypertrophic pyloric stenosis [148, 149]. Clustering of cases has been seen within families [147]. Patients typically present with progressive projectile nonbilious vomiting between the second and eighth weeks of life [150, 151]. If untreated, the infant may develop hypochloremic and hypokalemic metabolic alkalosis. The clinical diagnosis can be made by feeling the thickened pylorus as an olive-shaped mass in the mid-epigastrium and observing the gastric peristaltic waves. Abdominal ultrasound can confirm the diagnosis [152, 153].

Pathological Features

The characteristic finding on gross is concentrically enlarged gastric pylorus with thickness of more than 1 cm and two to four times its usual length. The pylorus becomes very hard due to the hypertrophy of the muscle and elastic tissue in the submucosa. The proximal stomach dilates with hypertrophy of the antrum and gastric outlet obstruction at the pylorus. Microscopically, there will be hyperplasia and hypertrophy of both the circular and longitudinal muscle fibers of the muscularis propria. The vessels in the submucosa may appear dilated. The nerve fibers may be reduced or absent and the ganglion cells may also disappear. Interstitial cells of Cajal may also be reduced in number [154].

Treatment and Prognosis

Extramucosal pyloromyotomy is the treatment of choice [155, 156]. Age below 2 weeks, delayed presentation, and prolonged preoperative hospital stay are predictors of poor outcome [157]. However, majority of the infants undergoing pyloromyotomy have an excellent prognosis with no long-term sequelae.

Polypoid Lesions

Gastric polyp is any lesion that protrudes into the gastric lumen above the mucosal surface. They are identified mostly as an incidental finding during about 1–6% of upper endoscopies [158–160]. A small subset of large polys may present with abdominal pain, bleeding, anemia, or gastric outlet obstruction [161]. The endoscopic appearance of gastric polyps is not specific for a particular subtype and hence histopathological examination is necessary for their accurate pathological diagnosis. The role of the pathologists is to identify a specific subtype of gastric polyp as it may have prognostic implications with a central goal of identifying whether the polyp is dysplastic or not. Many subtypes of gastric polyps arise in a background of chronic gastritis or association with polyposis syndromes. Hence, accurate identification of a particular subtype of gastric polyp may provide useful clues about its etiology as well as abnormalities in the background gastric mucosa.

Gastric Xanthoma

Definition

Gastric xanthoma is composed of benign aggregate of foamy lipid-laden histiocytes. It is also known as gastric xanthelasma or gastric lipid islands.

Clinical Features

Reported incidence varies between 1% and 6% in non-operated stomachs, most commonly seen in the stomach but can also be seen in small bowel, colon, and esophagus [162]. The etiology has not yet been established. However, it is probably a response to initial localized destruction of cells caused by inflammatory and degenerative changes, which leads to accumulation of cholesterol or fat [163]. Gastric xanthomas are commonly seen in patients after Billroth resection. They may be associated with hyperlipidemia, *H. pylori* infection, or gastric dysplasia; however, the evidence is not consistent [164–166]. It is usually an incidental finding as most patients are asymptomatic. On endoscopy, they appear as single or multiple, yellow to white plaques that are typically well demarcated, round to flat and vary from 1 to 10 mm. They are usually antral and near the lesser curvature but occasionally are located in the body or fundus and may be multiple.

Pathological Features

Histologically, they consist of numerous foamy macrophages usually within the lamina propria (Fig. 8.23a), particularly its upper half. The foamy cells do not show nuclear atypia or mitosis. The adjacent gastric mucosa may show chronic gastritis, intestinal metaplasia, or even atrophic gastritis. The foamy histiocytes are positive for CD68 (Fig. 8.23b) and CD163, and are negative for mucicarmine and cytokeratin (Fig. 8.23c).

Differential Diagnosis

The major differential diagnosis is signet ring cell adenocarcinoma, which would show nuclear atypia and positive staining for mucicarmine and cytokeratin. Metastatic clear cell renal cell carcinoma may also enter the differential, but it would be positive for keratin and PAX8. Whipple disease and *Mycobacterium avium*-intracellulare are rare infections of the stomach that also enter into consideration, and they can be evaluated by special stains (PAS-D and acid-fast bacilli).

Treatment and Prognosis

No treatment or follow-up is needed. However, recent studies have shown a high prevalence rate of gastric xanthoma in

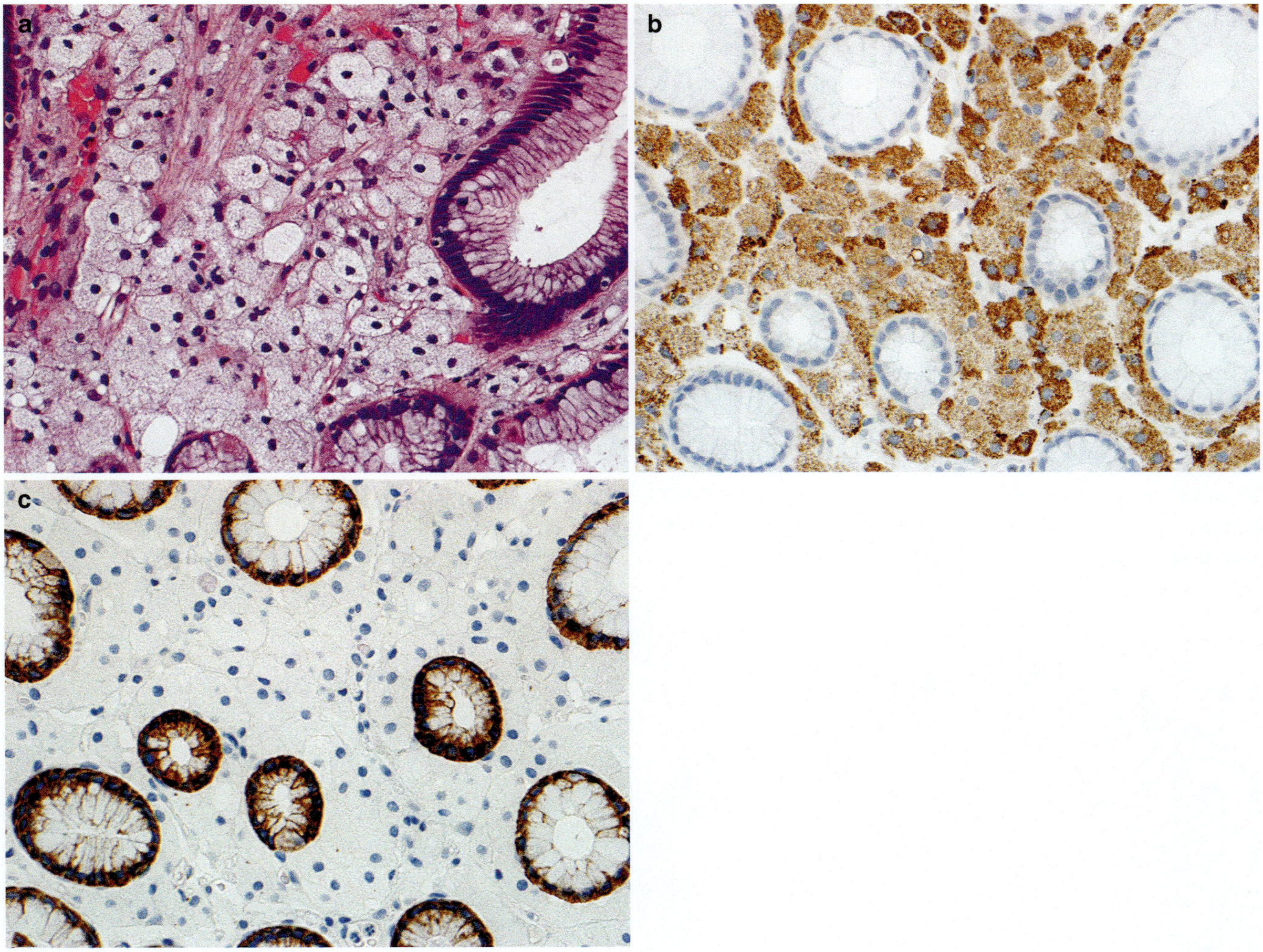

Fig. 8.23 Gastric xanthoma. Numerous foamy histiocytes within the lamina propria of gastric mucosa (**a**). The foamy histiocytes are positive for CD68 (**b**) and are negative for cytokeratin (**c**) by immunostains

gastric cancer cases with its presence as a predictive marker for metachronous and synchronous gastric cancer [167, 168].

Hyperplastic Polyp

Definition

Hyperplastic polyp is a benign polyp lined by gastric foveolar epithelium composed of elongated and distorted gastric pits with an inflamed and edematous stroma. It is also known as regenerative polyp and hyperplasiogenous polyp.

Clinical Features

It is the second most common type (about 15%) of gastric polyp after fundic gland polyp in the western populations [158, 161]. It can be found at any age but commonly seen in adults with a mean age range of 65–75 years. They are usually asymptomatic, most commonly seen in the gastric antrum, but can be seen throughout the stomach [169]. They can be single or multiple and range in size from a few millimeters to a few centimeters with a majority being less than 2 cm. They tend to arise in response to a variety of mucosal injuries and are strongly associated with chronic gastritis related to *H. pylori*, chemical, or autoimmune gastritis [169, 170]; hence evaluation of the background gastric mucosa is important in cases of hyperplastic polyps due to clinical consequences. Multiple hyperplastic polyps can be found in Menetrier's disease. Solid organ transplant has also been reported as a risk factor for development of hyperplastic polyps [171, 172]. Endoscopically, hyperplastic polyps may show superficial ulceration and a broad pedicle.

Pathological Features

Histologically, hyperplastic polyps are composed of elongated and dilated gastric pits with an edematous inflamed lamina propria and lined by reactive foveolar epithelium (Figs. 8.24a, b). A rich vasculature is common. The surface may be eroded or ulcerated with prominent reactive atypia within the foveolar epithelium (Fig. 8.24c). Pyloric-type glands and foci of intestinal metaplasia may be seen (Fig. 8.24d). Wisps of smooth muscle originating from the muscularis mucosa may be seen in larger polyps.

Differential Diagnosis

Polypoid foveolar hyperplasia is considered a precursor of gastric hyperplastic polyp by some and measures less than 1 cm. It differs slightly from hyperplastic polyp with absence of cystically dilated gastric pits and normal or only slightly swollen lamina propria and mild inflammatory component. Considering the concept of a continuum between these two entities, a definitive distinction may be not important [173].

Gastric mucosal prolapse polyp can show varying degree of elongation and cystic dilatation of the pit region (Fig. 8.25). However, it contains thick-walled vessels and prominent bundles of arborizing smooth muscle. The glandular component is usually compact with back to back glands [173].

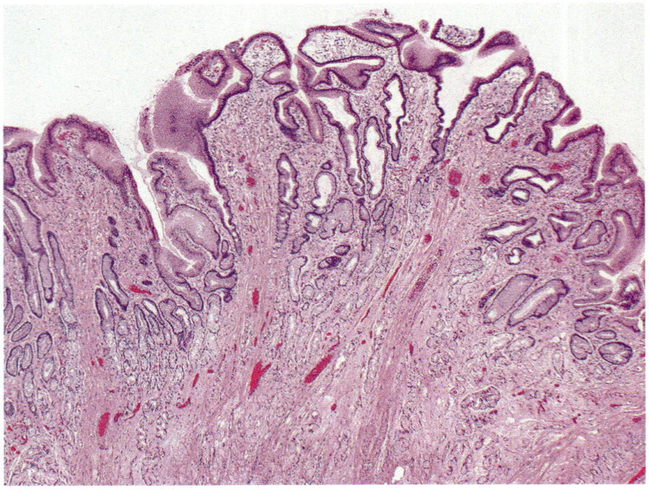

Fig. 8.25 Mucosal prolapse polyp. Antral mucosa with elongation and cystic dilatation of the pit region and prominent bundles of smooth muscle in lamina propria

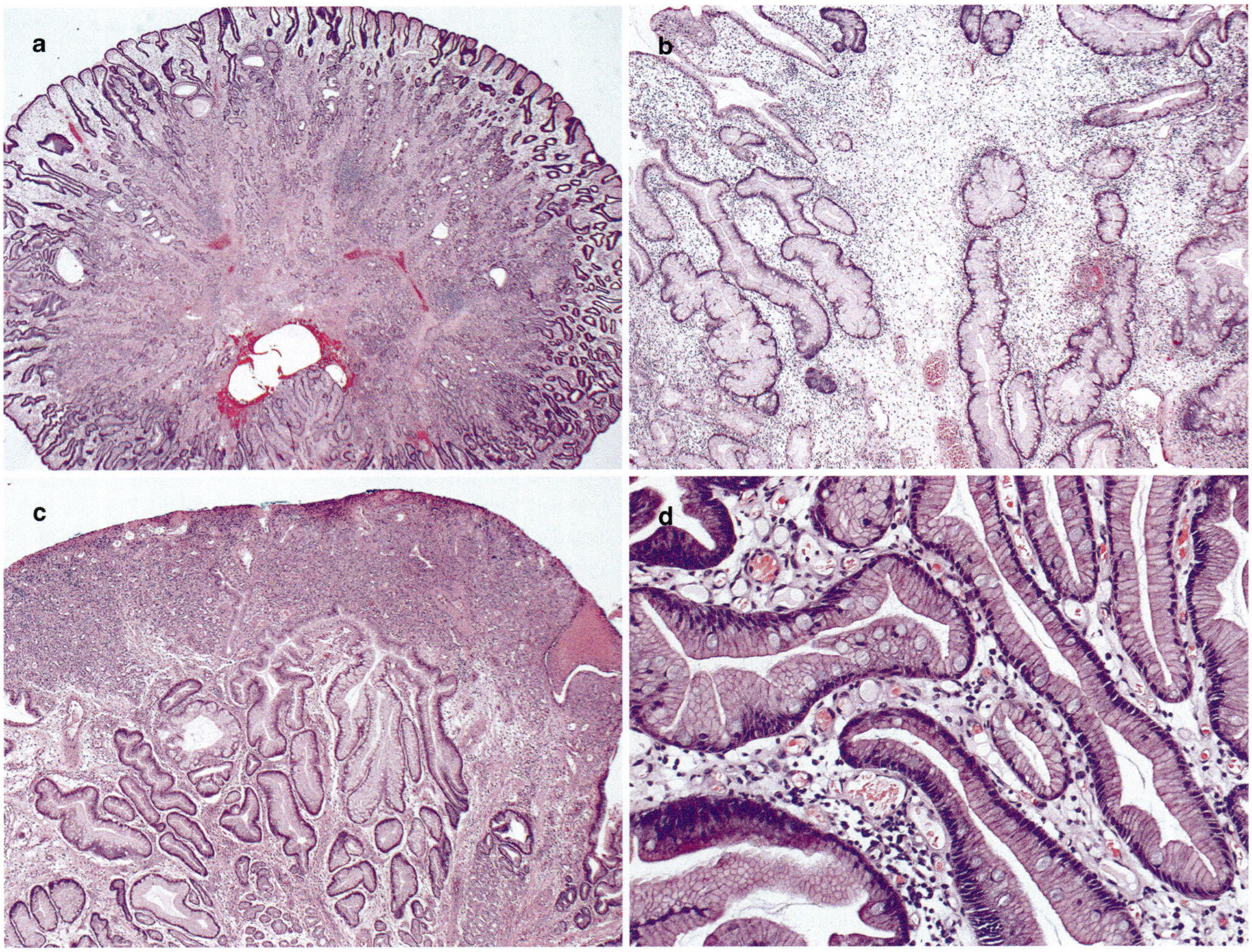

Fig. 8.24 Hyperplastic polyp. Gastric hyperplastic polyp is composed of elongated and dilated gastric pits (**a**) with an edematous inflamed lamina propria (**b**), erosion and granulation tissue in lamina propria (**c**), and foci of intestinal metaplasia (**d**)

Patients with Menetrier's disease can have multiple hyperplastic polyps. However, Menetrier's disease is usually limited to the gastric body and fundus. It shows prominent foveolar hyperplasia with lesser degree of inflammation. There is absence of intervening normal gastric mucosa between the polyps.

Morphological differentiation of hyperplastic polyps from hamartomatous polyps seen in Cronkhite-Canada syndrome and juvenile polyposis can be very difficult as they share significant morphologic overlap. Communication with the clinical colleagues to see if the patient has other features to support a particular syndrome is usually helpful in such situations to establish a correct diagnosis. However, a useful distinguishing feature of Cronkhite-Canada syndrome is the presence of inflammatory and edematous changes in the non-polypoid areas similar to those seen in the polypoid areas. In contrast, the inflammatory changes in juvenile polyposis are limited to the polypoid areas only with intervening normal mucosa.

Circumscribed foci of pseudosignet ring cell changes can occur in a small subset of hyperplastic polyps related to gland degeneration from torsion or ischemic injury and results in epithelial sloughing, and the epithelial cells assume a signet ring-like appearance (Fig. 8.26). The distinction from signet ring cell adenocarcinoma can be made by appreciating the lack of usual high-grade cytologic atypia and absence of infiltrative growth pattern within these sloughed epithelial cells showing pseudosignet ring cell change as well as ischemic/degenerative changes within the surrounding mucosa. E-cadherin and Ki-67 immunostain as well as reticulin stain may be useful adjuncts in such situations. E-cadherin is usually positive in the sloughed pseudosignet ring cells while it would be negative in signet ring cell adenocarcinoma. Reticulin stain would highlight the confinement of the pseudosignet ring cells within the gland basement membrane and the absence of an infiltrative pattern. The Ki-67 labeling in pseudosignet ring cells would be low (<2% staining), while the Ki-67 labeling would be increased in signet ring cell adenocarcinoma [174].

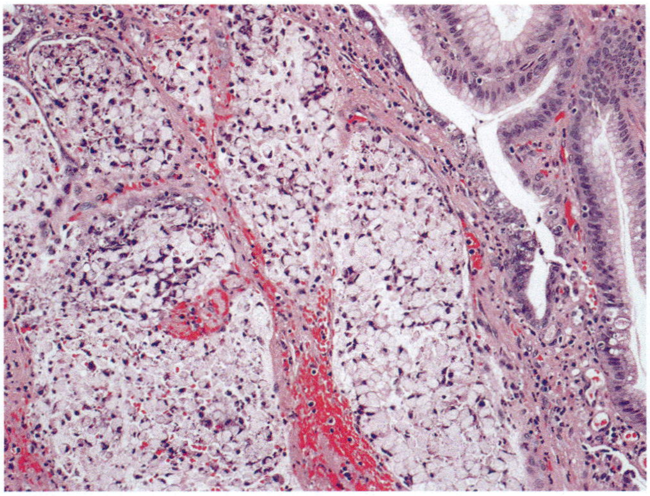

Fig. 8.26 Gastric hyperplastic polyp with pseudosignet ring cell changes. Circumscribed foci of epithelial sloughing assuming a signet ringlike appearance related to gland degeneration from torsion or ischemic injury in a gastric hyperplastic polyp

Treatment and Prognosis

Up to 80% of hyperplastic polyps have been reported to regress after eradication of *H. pylori* before endoscopic removal [175, 176]. Hence, testing for *H. pylori* infection and its eradication are important in patients with hyperplastic polyps. They rarely undergo neoplastic change, and dysplasia in hyperplastic polyps is rare, ranging from 1.5% to 4%. It is more common in polyps measuring >2 cm [169, 177–179]. Adenocarcinoma is even rarer with a reported range of up to 2%. However, hyperplastic polyps are associated with an increased risk of synchronous cancer occurring elsewhere in the gastric mucosa [180]. Hence, endoscopic and microscopic assessment of the surrounding gastric mucosa is important. There is controversy regarding whether they should be simply biopsied or whether they should be entirely removed by polypectomy. Some recommend performing polypectomy for all small polyps and periodic biopsy of larger hyperplastic polyps that are too big for polypectomy. Others recommend polypectomy for only large hyperplastic polyps as they have the highest risk for neoplastic change.

Peutz-Jeghers Polyp

Definition

Peutz-Jeghers polyp is a hamartomatous polyp arising in patients with Peutz-Jeghers syndrome (PJS).

Clinical Features

PJS is an autosomal dominant syndrome caused by a germline mutation of the *LKB1/STK11* gene. WHO criteria for clinical diagnosis of PJSs are: (1) detection of three or more histologically confirmed Peutz-Jeghers polyps; or (2) the presence of any number of Peutz-Jeghers polyps in a patient with a family history of the syndrome; or (3) detection of characteristic, prominent mucocutaneous pigmentation in the patient with a family history of the syndrome; or (4) detection of any number of Peutz-Jeghers polyps in a patient with prominent mucocutaneous pigmentation [181]. Patients with PJS have gastrointestinal polyposis, perioral pigmentation, and overtime cancer risk of >80% by the age 70 years [182, 183]. About 25% of patients with PJS develop gastric polyps [184].

Pathological Features

The polyps usually vary in size between 0.1 cm and 5 cm and they are often sessile. The gastric polyps commonly arise in the antrum. Microscopically, they are composed of promi-

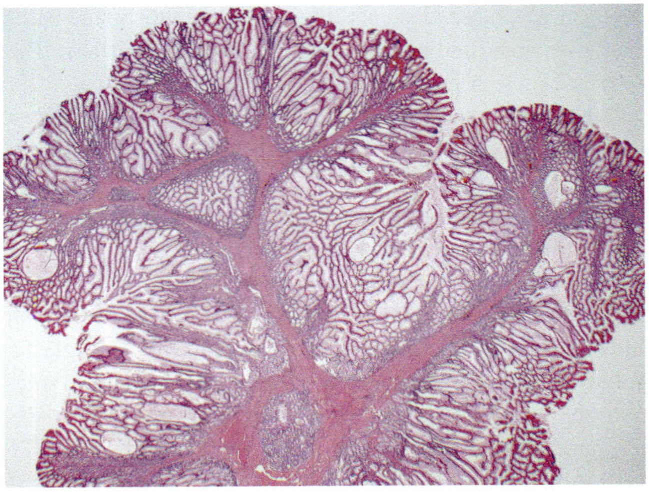

Fig. 8.27 Peutz-Jeghers polyp. A hamartomatous polyp composed of prominent, dilated, or branching mucin-filled gastric pits lined by foveolar epithelium and variable number of deep glands. Some arborizing smooth muscle bundles are present in this gastric Peutz-Jeghers polyp

nent dilated or branching mucin-filled gastric pits lined by foveolar epithelium and variable number of deep glands (Fig. 8.27). The surfaces of polyps may be superficially eroded and acutely inflamed. They usually lack an arborizing architecture with prominent bands of smooth muscle as seen in small bowel or colonic Peutz-Jeghers polyps; however, a subset of them may show some degree of smooth muscle proliferation. The background gastric mucosa is usually unremarkable. A subset of large polyps may show displaced benign glands and mucinous cysts within the submucosa, muscularis propria, or even the serosa. The benign histologic appearance of the epithelium differentiates these areas from invasive adenocarcinoma.

Differential Diagnosis

Gastric Peutz-Jeghers polyps are often difficult to distinguish from gastric hyperplastic polyps and juvenile polyps [185]. They are best distinguished by correlation with the clinical history and other features that characterize each syndrome to establish the correct diagnosis. A subset of large gastric hyperplastic polyps may develop prominent smooth muscle bundles within the polyp due to mucosal prolapse. Therefore, the identification of prominent smooth muscle bundles is also not diagnostic of Peutz-Jeghers polyps in the stomach. Hence, one should be cautious in making a new diagnosis of Peutz-Jeghers syndrome while evaluating gastric polyps in isolation of the clinical context.

Treatment and Prognosis

These patients are at an increased risk for a variety of extraintestinal and gastrointestinal malignancies including gastric, small bowel, and colorectal cancers. Patients with PJS have a 29% lifetime risk of gastric cancer [186, 187]. Dysplasia in gastric Peutz-Jeghers polyp is rare. It has been proposed that Peutz-Jeghers polyps are not malignant precursors but in fact just an epiphenomenon to cancer prone condition [188]. The gastric mucosa of PJS patients has yet not been studied for pre-tumor progression [189]. Surveillance guidelines for PJS patients recommend upper gastrointestinal endoscopy and colonoscopy be done first at the age of 8 years. If polyps are found, it should be repeated every 3 years. If no polyps are found, then a second baseline examination should be done at the age of 18 years and then every 3 years, or earlier if symptoms occur [182]. It has also been suggested that gastric Peutz-Jeghers polyps larger than 1 cm should be resected endoscopically, and patients should receive annual surveillance [170].

Juvenile Polyp

Definition

Juvenile polyp is a hamartomatous polyp arising in patients with juvenile polyposis syndrome (JPS).

Clinical Features

JPS is an autosomal dominant syndrome and is the most common of the hamartomatous polyposis syndromes. Synonyms for this syndrome include generalized juvenile polyposis, juvenile polyposis of infancy, and gastric juvenile polyposis. It is caused by mutations of the *SMAD4* gene (also called the *MADH4* gene) or the *BMPR1A* gene in 20% and 25% of patients, respectively [190–192]. *SMAD4* mutation is associated with the greatest risk factor for upper-gastrointestinal tract involvement, as more than 80% of patients with a germline *SMAD4* mutation will have extra-colonic involvement [193, 194]. The early childhood presentation has been associated with *ENG* germline mutations [195]. Majority of the patients have a family history of JPS; however, about 25% of newly diagnosed cases represent new or de novo mutations and hence they are sporadic [196]. WHO criteria for the clinical diagnosis of JPS include: (1) more than three to five juvenile polyps of the large bowel; or (2) multiple juvenile polyps throughout the gastrointestinal tract; or (3) any number of juvenile polyps with a family history of JPS [197]. JPS patients develop hamartomatous polyps in the colon, the stomach, and less commonly in the small bowel. More than 80% of JPS patients have lesions in the stomach. Most develop polyps before the age of 20 years; hence, the diagnosis can be made much later in life in late adulthood (the word "juvenile" signifies the type of polyp and not the age of diagnosis or onset of the polyp). The clinical manifestations can vary in severity, as a subset of patients developing only a few polyps, whereas others have extensive polyposis, presenting with diarrhea or malabsorption.

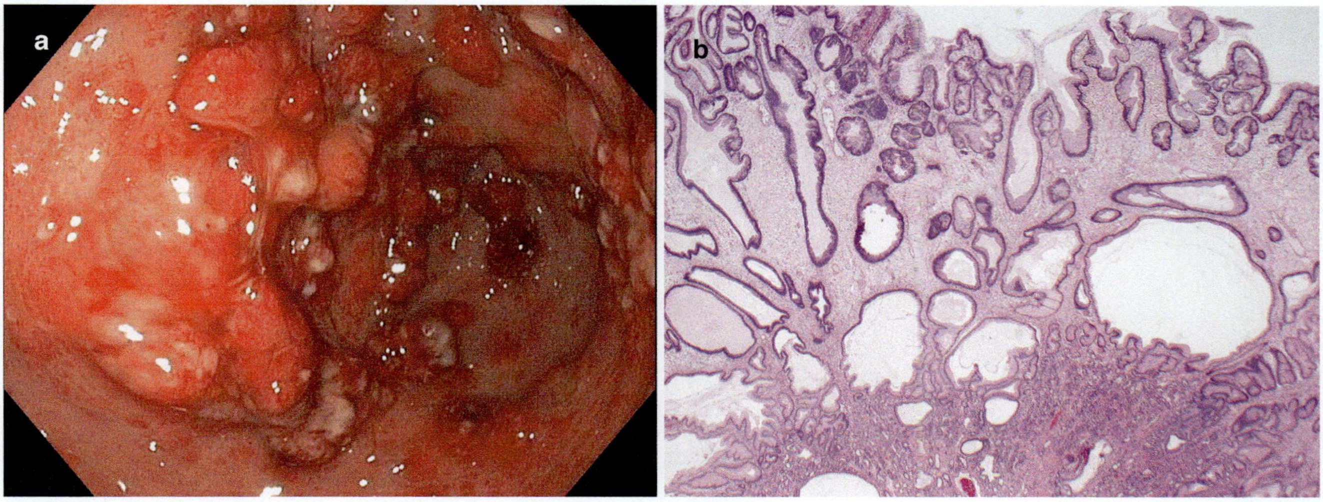

Fig. 8.28 Juvenile polyposis syndrome. Multiple polyps in stomach affecting the antrum, body, and fundus in a patient with juvenile polyposis syndrome on upper endoscopy (**a**). The polyp shows abundant distorted and mucus-filled dilated gastric glands with prominent edema in lamina propria (**b**)

Pathological Features

Grossly juvenile polyps are usually multiple polyps ranging from 0.1 cm to 5 cm affecting the antrum and extending to the fundus/body (Fig. 8.28a). They usually have spherical shape with a smooth surface. The larger polyps can be multilobated or may show a villiform architecture. Microscopically, they show abundant distorted and mucus-filled dilated gastric glands with excess of lamina propria showing edema and inflammatory cells (Fig. 8.28b). The stroma/epithelium ratio is abnormally greater than normal. Smooth muscle is rarely seen within the lamina propria. Dysplasia can be found in 15% of gastric juvenile polyps [198]. A subset of patients with JPS may develop massive gastric juvenile polyposis showing total or near-total carpeting of the gastric mucosa by innumerable polyps, ranging from a few millimeters to 10 cm [199, 200].

Differential Diagnosis

Gastric juvenile polyps share resemblance with hyperplastic polyps or other hamartomatous gastric polyps such as PJS, Cronkhite-Canada syndrome, and Cowden syndrome [185]; hence, they are difficult to almost impossible to differentiate on morphology alone. One clue may be the abnormal intervening mucosa seen in Cronkhite-Canada syndrome polyps but not in JPS. The polyps in JPS are usually more extensive and densely distributed, and they also have more abundant inflamed stroma and less foveolar hyperplasia than hyperplastic polyps.

JPS polyps should be distinguished from sporadic juvenile polyps unassociated with a syndrome, which are typically single incidental lesions in the antrum, with a prevalence of about 2% of the pediatric and adult population. In contrast, JPS gastric polyps are typically multiple with involvement of both gastric antrum and body. There are no morphological features that can help separate syndromic from non-syndromic polyps.

Treatment and Prognosis

Patients with JPS have a 20% risk of developing gastric carcinoma [201]. Upper gastrointestinal endoscopy is recommended between the age of 12 and 15 years, and it should be repeated annually if polyps are found and every 1–3 years if no polyps are found [182].

Cronkhite-Canada Syndrome

Definition

Cronkhite-Canada syndrome is a rare non-congenital protein-losing enteropathy characterized by diffuse gastrointestinal tract polyposis and ectodermal changes such as alopecia and nail dystrophy.

Clinical Features

Majority of the patients manifest in middle to late adulthood, and >80% of patients are over 50 years at the time of diagnosis with a mean age at presentation of 59 years. Abdominal pain, diarrhea, and weight loss are the common presenting symptoms. Patients may also present with protein-losing enteropathy and peripheral edema due to malabsorption. Almost all patients also show ectodermal manifestations such as alopecia (of the body and scalp), nail dystrophy, and skin hyperpigmentation. Its exact cause is unknown but an autoimmune etiology has been suggested [202].

Pathological Features

The polyposis in Cronkhite-Canada syndrome involves the entire gastrointestinal tract except the esophagus [203, 204]. The polyps range in size from a few millimeters to 1.5 cm. The polyps may involve the entire stomach (Fig. 8.29a).

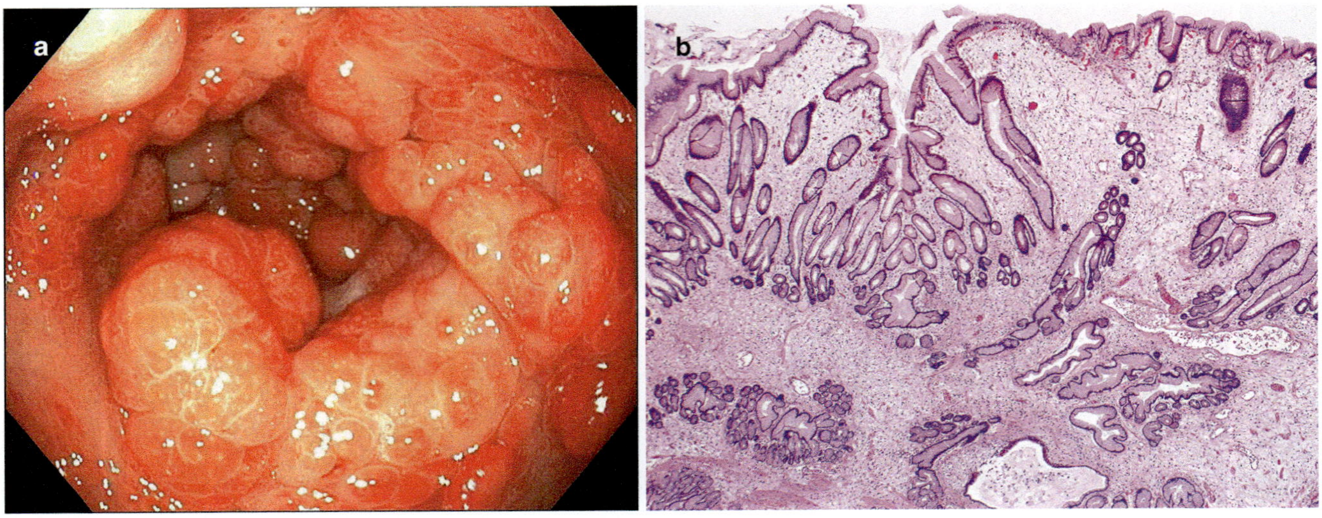

Fig. 8.29 Cronkhite-Canada syndrome. Numerous polypoid lesions present in the entire stomach on upper endoscopy in a patient with Cronkhite-Canada syndrome (**a**). The polyps have a hamartomatous appearance with cystically dilated gastric glands and edematous lamina propria (**b**)

Occasionally, there may be selective sparing of the stomach [204]. Microscopically, the Cronkhite-Canada syndrome polyps have a hamartomatous appearance. They show cystically dilated gastric glands and edematous lamina propria with mild mononuclear inflammation (Fig. 8.29b). Oxyntic, chief, Paneth, and endocrine cells are usually inconspicuous. A prominent mast cell, eosinophils, or IgG4 positive plasma cell infiltrate may be seen [203, 205–207]. The most important microscopic finding that distinguishes Cronkhite-Canada syndrome from other polyposis syndromes is the presence of lamina propria edema, gland/crypt architectural distortion, and inflammation in the intervening endoscopically/macroscopically normal-appearing non-polypoid gastric mucosa.

Differential Diagnosis

Gastric Cronkhite-Canada syndrome polyps share resemblance with hyperplastic polyps or other hamartomatous gastric polyps such as PJS, JPS, and Cowden syndrome [202]. Hence, they are very difficult to differentiate on morphology alone. One clue may be the abnormal intervening mucosa seen in Cronkhite-Canada syndrome polyps but not in others.

An infiltrative or infectious etiology may also be in the differential especially if endoscopy shows a diffusely thickened or atrophic appearance rather than a polypoid mucosa. Careful histopathological evaluation will easily exclude neoplasia as well as infection and confirm the characteristic architectural distortion and lamina propria changes of Cronkhite-Canada syndrome. Special stains for infectious etiology can also be helpful.

Menetrier's disease can also present as polypoid gastric mucosa on endoscopy, and Cronkhite-Canada syndrome is clinically associated with peripheral edema, diarrhea, and protein-losing enteropathy. However, the hyperplastic changes on microscopy are virtually always limited to the proximal stomach with an endoscopically and histologically unremarkable antral mucosa. Moreover, the duodenal mucosa would also be normal in Menetrier's disease [208].

Treatment and Prognosis

Cronkhite-Canada syndrome polyps are considered nonneoplastic with controversial malignant potential. However, carcinomas of the stomach have been described in patients with Cronkhite-Canada syndrome [209–211]. Due to its rarity, it is debatable if the patients with Cronkhite-Canada syndrome are truly at risk for gastrointestinal cancers. Variety of treatment approaches such as nutritional support, antibiotics, immune suppression, and surgery have been tried, often in different combinations and they have had variable success [202]. Less than 5% of patients have a complete remission and the overall outcome remains poor [212]. The 5-year disease-related mortality is reported as high as 55% and is most frequently related to gastrointestinal hemorrhage, infection, malnutrition, or congestive heart failure [204, 213].

Cowden Syndrome

Definition

Cowden syndrome is a rare autosomal dominant condition characterized by multiple hamartomatous lesions. It is included in the spectrum of *PTEN* hamartoma tumor syndromes. Recent studies have shown a prevalence of 25–35% for *PTEN* mutations in Cowden syndrome patients [214–216].

Clinical Features

It is characterized by pathognomonic mucocutaneous lesions (facial trichilemmoma, acral keratoses, papillomatous papules, and mucosal lesions), increased cancer risk (breast, thyroid, endometrial, colorectal, kidney, and melanoma), benign hamartomatous overgrowth of tissues (including gastrointestinal polyposis), and macrocephaly. Gastrointestinal polyposis involving the entire gastrointestinal tract is a common manifestation in patients with Cowden syndrome. Almost all patients with Cowden syndrome have gastric polyps. Most of the patients with Cowden syndrome manifest the phenotype by the second decade. Consensus-based diagnostic criteria for Cowden syndrome has been established by the International Cowden Consortium [217, 218].

Pathological Features

Gastric polyps are usually numerous and range in size from 0.1 cm to 2 cm (Fig. 8.30a). Microscopically, the polyps are hyperplastic or hamartomatous (Fig. 8.30b) as seen in other polyposis syndromes such as Cronkhite-Canada syndrome and JPS. Dysplasia is extremely rare.

Differential Diagnosis

Gastric polyps in Cowden syndrome share resemblance with hyperplastic polyps or other hamartomatous gastric polyps such as PJS, JPS, and Cronkhite-Canada syndrome. Hence, they are very difficult to differentiate on morphology alone.

Treatment and Prognosis

It is unclear if patients with Cowden syndrome have an increased risk for gastric cancer. However, there are a few reported cases of gastric cancer in patients with Cowden syndrome [219, 220]. Endoscopic upper gastrointestinal tract surveillance is recommended in patients with Cowden syndrome every 2–3 years starting at 15 years of age [182].

Miscellaneous Disorders

Pancreatic Acinar Metaplasia

Definition

Pancreatic acinar metaplasia (PAM) is defined as nests or lobules of pancreatic acinar tissue composed of cells with coarse apical eosinophilic granules with or without mucous cells. Synonyms include pancreatic cell metaplasia and pancreatic metaplasia.

Clinical Features

Usually an incidental finding that can be seen in children and adults with no gender preference. It is may represent a congenital rest or a type of metaplasia [140, 221–225]. Studies have shown PAM in up to 11% of investigated subjects [140, 141, 221]. It is commonly seen in the gastric cardia and antrum without any significant association with inflammation, atrophy, or intestinal metaplasia. However, PAM in the gastric body has been associated with autoimmune atrophic gastritis [141]. A study has also shown PAM located above the gastroesophageal junction to be associated with *H. pylori* gastritis and gastroesophageal reflux [226].

Pathological Features

On H&E-stained sections, PAM appears as pancreatic acinar-like cells with abundant cytoplasm that is eosinophilic and granular in the apical and middle portions and basophilic in the basal area (Fig. 8.31). The nuclei are basally situated, small,

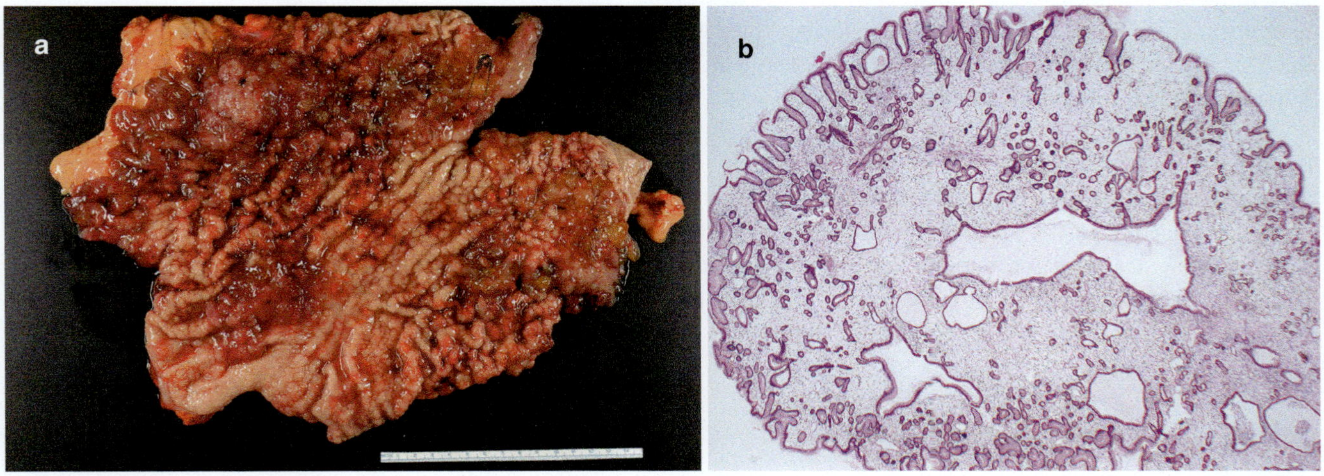

Fig. 8.30 Cowden syndrome. A gastrectomy specimen shows numerous polyps in the antrum, body, and fundus in a patient with Cowden syndrome (**a**). The polyps have hyperplastic or hamartomatous appearance similar to the histological features of juvenile polyp or Cronkhite-Canada syndrome (**b**)

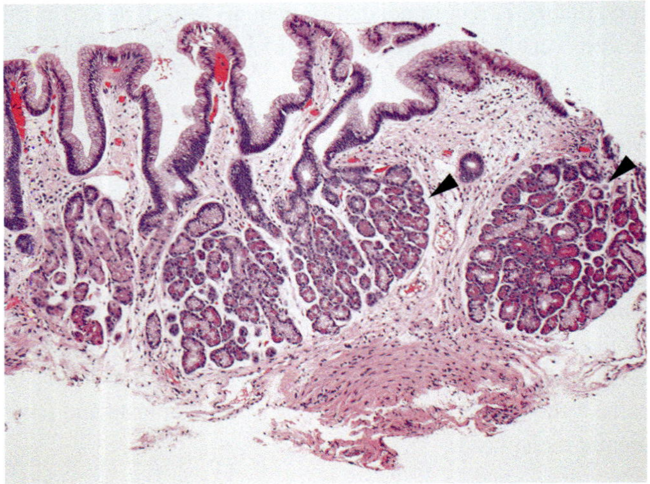

Fig. 8.31 Pancreatic acinar metaplasia. A few foci of well-circumscribed pancreatic acinar cells (arrowheads) present in a biopsy from gastric cardia with mild chronic inflammation in lamina propria

round, and uniform with inconspicuous nucleoli. Mucous cells may be intermingled with acinar-like cells within the lobules or could line tubules or small cystic spaces. The foci of PAM may be in continuity with the adjacent gastric glands or may be separated from them by smooth muscle or fibrous tissue. Immunohistochemically, PAM is positive for pancreatic lipase, amylase, and trypsinogen [140, 221]. However, immunostains are usually not required for diagnosis. Rare cells in PAM may be positive for chromogranin, synaptophysin, or gastrin.

Differential Diagnosis

Pancreatic heterotopia is differentiated from PAM by presence of ductal elements and/or well-defined islets. Paneth cells may also come in the differential, but the presence of large refractile granules within Paneth cells helps to distinguish them from PAM in which the zymogen granules are much smaller and eosinophilic. Immunostains for trypsin or lipase may be helpful in difficult cases.

Treatment and Prognosis

No treatment is needed as it is an incidental finding. However, its presence in adult gastric mucosa from the body or fundus should raise a suspicion for autoimmune atrophic gastritis especially if there is presence of associated chronic inflammation and/or atrophy of the oxyntic glands.

Gastritis Cystica Polyposa or Profunda

Definition

Gastritis cystica polyposa is a rare pseudotumor of the stomach characterized by benign growth of deep gastric glands through the muscularis mucosa into the submucosa or beyond. A polypoid lesion is known as polyposa, and when it is predominantly inverted, forming a submucosal lesion or mass, it is referred to as profunda.

Clinical Features

Gastritis cystica polyposa is usually seen in adults in the 5th or 6th decades of life. Patients may remain asymptomatic or present with abdominal pain, gastrointestinal bleed, and rarely gastric outlet obstruction. Endoscopy may show a nodular mucosa. It is commonly seen in patients who have undergone gastric surgery such as gastroenterostomy [227–229]. However, it can also be seen in non-operated stomachs [230–232]. Chronic inflammation, gastric surgery, and ischemia are considered to be the most important factors in its pathogenesis [233]. Epithelial displacement and implantation into the submucosa or beyond occurs following mucosal ulceration, herniation, iatrogenic mucosal defect (due to surgery, biopsy or polypectomy), or microdiverticula. Standard endoscopic biopsy is usually less helpful in making the diagnosis as it seldom offers information about the submucosa. In many cases, the preoperative diagnosis of this entity can be challenging and the patient may have to undergo gastric resection for definitive diagnosis.

Pathological Features

Histology shows dilated glands extending through the muscularis mucosa into the submucosa, muscularis propria, and even into the serosa (Fig. 8.32). These glands are lined by bland foveolar epithelium with absence of nuclear atypia or mitotic activity. The glands are surrounded by a rim of normal lamina propria and absence of desmoplastic stromal reaction. The surrounding stroma may be edematous with varying degrees of mixed inflammation, hemosiderin deposition, and fibrosis. The overlying gastric mucosa may show active chronic inflammation, ulceration, glandular atrophy, or intestinal metaplasia.

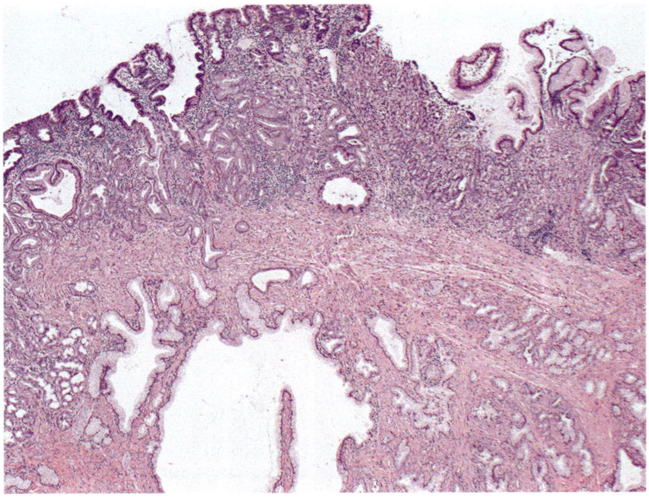

Fig. 8.32 Gastritis cystica profunda. Dilated gastric glands with absence of nuclear atypia extend through the muscularis mucosa into the submucosa. The glands present in the submucosa are surrounded by a rim of normal lamina propria and are without desmoplastic stromal reaction

Differential Diagnosis

Invasive well-differentiated adenocarcinoma is the main differential, and its distinction can be challenging [234]. However, careful attention to the absence of invasive growth pattern, lack of cytologic atypia, absence of desmoplastic stromal reaction, presence of lamina propria around the glands, and history of prior surgical procedure helps in distinguishing invasive adenocarcinoma from gastritis cystica polyposa or profunda (Table 8.2). Endometriosis may also come in the differential, but the presence of endometrial stroma and its positivity for estrogen receptor immunostain can help in making this distinction.

Treatment and Prognosis

Localized surgical excision including endoscopic submucosal dissection and endoscopic mucosal resection are usually curative [231]. However, recurrence can be rarely seen after surgical resection [235]. There has been a suggestion that gastritis cystica profunda/polyposa may be a precancerous condition, but this is controversial and not universally accepted [236–238]. However, there are rare cases of gastritis cystica profunda/polyposa reported in association with gastric adenocarcinoma in unoperated stomach [239, 240].

Table 8.2 Differences between gastritis cystica profunda/polyposa and invasive adenocarcinoma

Features	Gastritis cystica profunda/polyposa	Invasive adenocarcinoma
Overlying dysplastic epithelium	Absent	Present
Rim of lamina propria around the glands	Present	Absent
Desmoplastic stromal reaction around the glands	Absent	Present
Mitosis	Absent to rare	Present
Contour of glands	Smooth, regular, and lobular	Irregular and distorted
Cytologic atypia	Absent	Present

Mucosal Calcinosis

Definition

Gastric mucosal calcinosis is defined as deposition of calcium salts within the gastric mucosa.

Clinical Features

Gastric mucosal calcinosis is typically seen in adults with a female predominance. Usually asymptomatic but occasional patients can present with dyspepsia, nausea, vomiting, and epigastric pain. Most examples are detected at autopsy or due to the use of bone-seeking radiopharmaceuticals such as technetium-99 m methylene diphosphate. In routine practice, gastric calcifications are rare and seen in less than 0.1% of gastric biopsies [241]. However, up to 33% of gastric biopsies in transplant patients and up to 60% of chronically uremic, dialyzed patients can have calcinosis in their gastric biopsies [242, 243]. Gastric mucosal calcinosis has been associated with a number of etiological conditions such as hypercalcemia and/or hyperphosphatemia (related to chronic renal disease, uremia, dialysis, and secondary hyperparathyroidism), antacids, sucralfate, citrate-containing blood products, and organ transplantation [241]. Endoscopy may show 1–5 mm white flat plaques or nodules in the gastric fundus, body, and/or antrum [244, 245]. Rarely, it may appear as a large ulcerative lesion mimicking malignancy [246].

Pathological Features

Histological findings include amorphous irregular basophilic deposits in the lamina propria usually just below the epithelium or foveolar tips (Fig. 8.33a). These deposits may

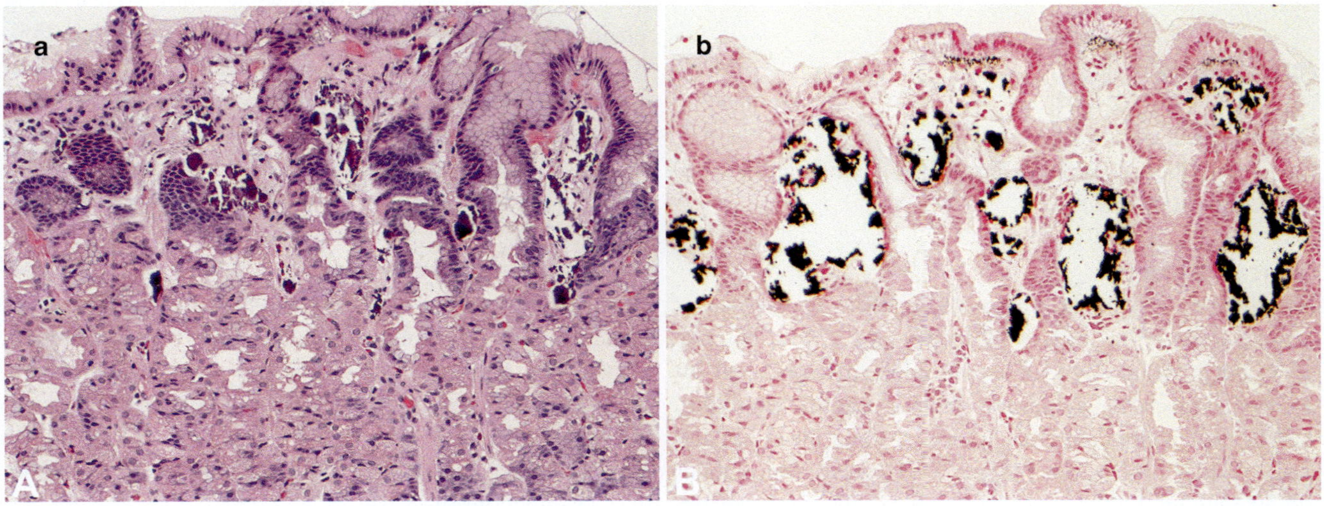

Fig. 8.33 Mucosal calcinosis. Amorphous irregular basophilic deposits in the lamina propria below the gastric surface epithelium or foveolar tips (**a**). These deposits are positive on Von Kossa stain (**b**)

also be found in the deeper lamina propria or muscularis mucosa. The deposits may be slightly refractile but do not polarize. Von Kossa (Fig. 8.33b) and alizarin red stains are positive. There is no predilection for any particular part of the stomach as they can be found in the fundus, body, and/or antrum. In severe cases, the calcinosis may also be seen in the submucosal vessels with associated luminal stenosis. In majority of cases, the background gastric mucosa may be unremarkable (metastatic calcification). However, about 30% of cases may show some background changes such as inflammation, edema, ulceration, atrophy, and foveolar hyperplasia (dystrophic calcification). There is no significant association between gastric mucosal calcinosis and *H. pylori*.

Differential Diagnosis

Kayexalate crystals may come in the differential but are rhomboid or triangular in shape, deeply basophilic on H&E stain, and exhibit a distinctive internal mosaic pattern that resembles fish scales [42]. Schistosomal eggs and strongyloides worm can undergo calcification and be in the differential. However, identification of parasitic structures within the areas of calcifications and presence of eosinophils and Charcot-Leyden crystals can help make the differentiation. OsmoPrep deposits can mimic mucosal deposits, but they are purple to black in color. They are also positive on von Kossa stain but negative with alizarin red helping to make the distinction [22].

Treatment and Prognosis

The presence of mucosal calcinosis in gastric biopsies should be reported as its presence serves as a marker for the presence of metastatic calcifications in organs such as the heart, where it may be fatal [243]. Some cases of mucosal calcification are reversible with normalization of the biochemical parameters [241].

Amyloidosis

Definition

Gastric amyloidosis is defined as deposition of amyloid protein within the stomach.

Clinical Features

In patients with systemic amyloidosis, gastric involvement is seen in around 8% of cases by biopsy and 12% at autopsy [247] and is commonly seen in male adults in the 6th and 7th decades. Presenting symptoms include nausea, vomiting, weight loss, abdominal pain, gastrointestinal bleeding, and gastric outlet obstruction [248–252]. However, only about 1% of patients with gastric amyloidosis are symptomatic. Endoscopy may show varying appearances including thickened gastric folds, loss of rugal folds, ulcers, hematomas, granular mucosa, gastroparesis, nodular appearance, mass lesion, and plaque-like lesions [247, 253]. Up to a third of patients may show unremarkable gastric mucosa suggesting that a gastric biopsy is essential for diagnosis of gastric amyloidosis [249].

Pathological Features

Histologically, amyloid deposits appear pale eosinophilic and acellular on H&E stain (Fig. 8.34a). Congo red stain is positive exhibiting an apple green birefringence (Fig. 8.34b, c). Amyloid deposition can be seen within the body/fundus and/or antrum. Muscularis mucosae is the most common location for amyloid deposition, followed by the lamina propria, and submucosa [249]. The blood vessels also commonly show amyloid deposition. The surrounding gastric mucosa may show changes of reactive gastropathy, gastritis, intestinal metaplasia, and *H. pylori* infection. A recent series on gastric amyloidosis showed AL (amyloid light chain) type to be the most common subtype of amyloid involving the stomach, followed by the ATTR (transthyretin amyloidosis), AA (acquired amyloidosis), and AApo A1 (Apolipoprotein A1 amyloidosis) types [249].

Differential Diagnosis

Differential diagnosis includes extracellular deposits that can mimic amyloidosis on H&E stain such as collagen deposits, light chain deposition disease, and elastosis (Fig. 8.35a). Collagen fibers tend to be brighter and more eosinophilic than amyloid on H&E stain. Trichrome stain will show strong positivity for collagen, in comparison amyloid tends to be negative or very weakly positive. Congo red stain can also help, as collagen is not congophilic. Under polarizing light, the collagen does not show the apple green birefringence but shows a silvery white birefringence. Light chain deposition disease is rare in the stomach [254, 255]. They will be negative on Congo red stain. The monoclonal light chains are usually kappa light chain restricted. Elastosis will be negative on Congo red stain. Acid orcein-Giemsa and Verhoeff-van Gieson stains (Fig. 8.35b) can be used to highlight the elastic fibers.

Treatment and Prognosis

The treatment and prognosis of amyloidosis depends on the underlying disease. Hence, accurate subtyping of amyloid deposits by mass spectrometry is important for therapeutic purposes and prognosis. In AL amyloidosis, treatment focuses on the underlying plasma cell dyscrasia. While in AA amyloidosis, cure is aimed at the underlying inflammatory or infectious disorder.

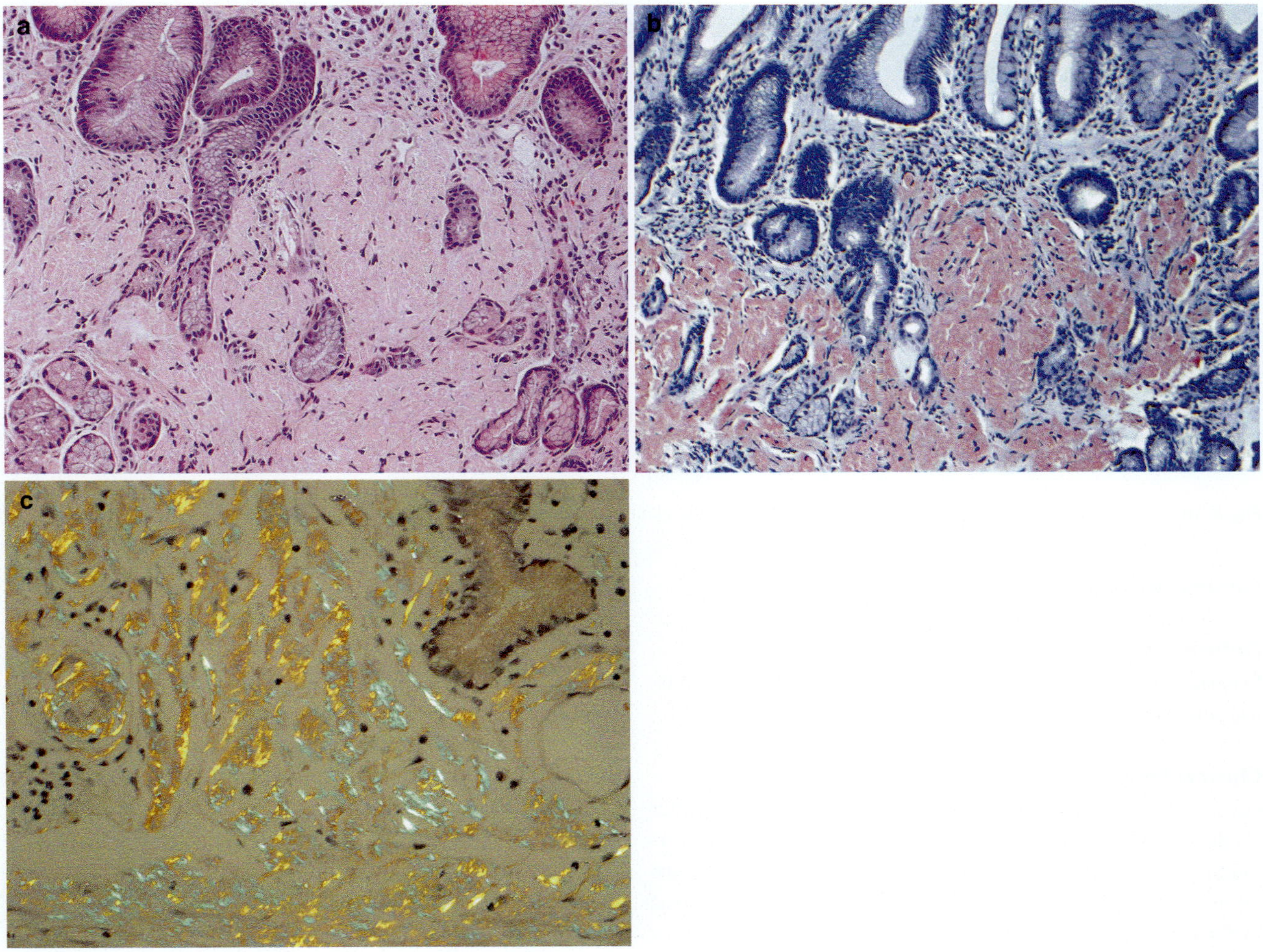

Fig. 8.34 Gastric amyloidosis. Pale eosinophilic and acellular amyloid deposits within lamina propria on H&E stain (**a**). The amyloid deposits are positive on Congo red stain (**b**) and show an apple green birefringence under polarized light (**c**)

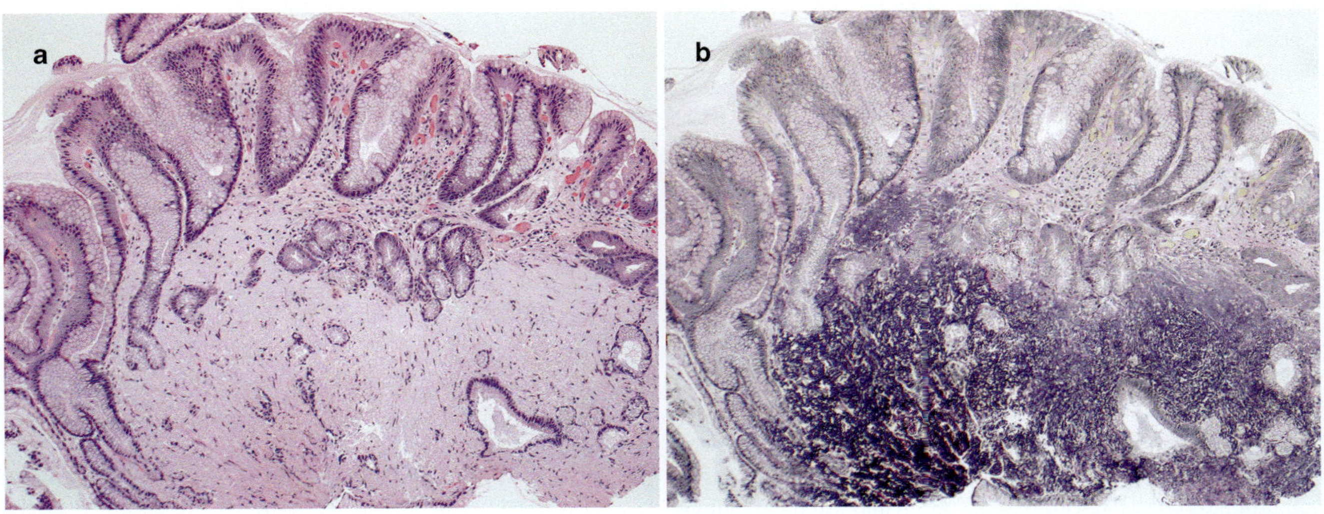

Fig. 8.35 Elastosis. Gastric antral biopsy with pale pink eosinophilic amorphous deposition within the lamina propria on H&E stain (**a**). The pale pink eosinophilic amorphous depositions are elastic fibers and positive on Verhoeff-van Gieson stain (**b**)

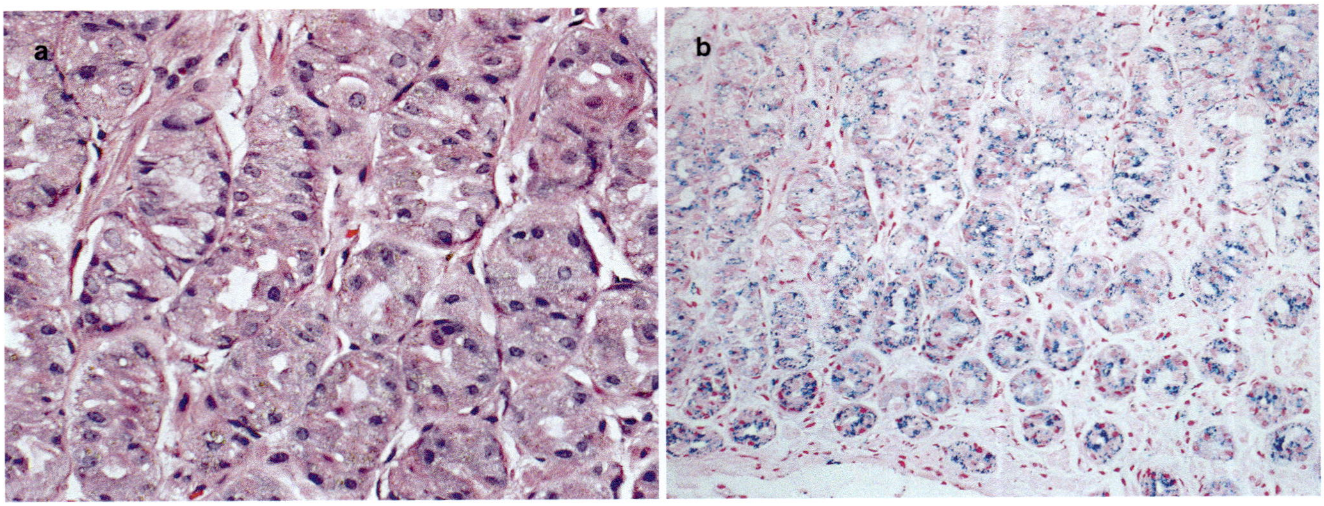

Fig. 8.36 Gastric siderosis. Brownish iron deposition in the fundic glandular epithelium (**a**) and is positive on Prussian blue stain (**b**)

Gastric Siderosis

Definition

Gastric siderosis is defined as iron deposition within the gastric mucosa.

Clinical Features

Gastric siderosis is typically seen in adults with no gender predominance and is usually seen in patients with iron overload/hemochromatosis, heavy alcohol abusers, or patients taking iron medications. One study showed gastric siderosis in 50–69% of gastric biopsies from patients with hemochromatosis or alcoholics [256]. However, overall it is an uncommon condition with a prevalence of 3.6% in gastric biopsies [257]. This condition is usually asymptomatic and the patients may present with symptoms related to the underlying disorder. Laboratory tests can show an elevated ferritin. Endoscopy may show speckled areas of brown pigmentation within the stomach [258].

Pathological Features

Iron deposits appear as brown granules that are consistent with hemosiderin. Sometimes it may form large coarse clumps with a fibrillary appearance. Three patterns of gastric siderosis have been described. [257]. First and the most common pattern shows predominant iron deposition in the stromal cells and macrophages, and it is most likely a result of gastric inflammation or prior trauma or hemorrhage. The second pattern shows predominantly extracellular iron deposition with associated mild gastritis and reactive gastropathy. This pattern is associated with oral iron medication use. The third pattern shows predominant iron deposition in the antral and fundic glandular epithelium and may be associated with systemic iron overload/hemochromatosis (Fig.8.36a). Prussian blue (iron) stain can highlight the iron in cases of gastric siderosis (Fig. 8.36b).

Differential Diagnosis

Iron pill-associated gastritis may come in the differential. However, iron pill material shows a characteristic brown crystalline and clumpy fibrillary material which is refractile (Fig. 8.1). Most of the time, this brown crystalline material is luminal, seen adjacent to the surface epithelium and admixed with luminal inflammatory exudate. The adjacent gastric mucosa can show reactive foveolar hyperplasia with mucin depletion and elongated tortuous gastric pits. On an iron stain, the crystalline iron pill material can be easily distinguished from hemosiderin pigment, despite positive staining for both on the iron stain.

Treatment and Prognosis

Treatment depends on the underlying disorder. When gastric siderosis is identified, it should be an indication for further workup to rule out iron overload/hemochromatosis and portal hypertension within the patient.

References

1. Douthwaite AH, Lintott GAM. Gastroscopic observation of the effect of aspirin and certain other substances of the stomach. Lancet. 1938;232(6013):1225. https://doi.org/10.1016/S0140-6736(00)78970-7.
2. Banner W Jr, Tong TG. Iron poisoning. Pediatr Clin N Am. 1986;33(2):393–409.
3. McGuigan MA. Acute iron poisoning. Pediatr Ann. 1996;25(1):33–8.
4. Eckstein RP, Symons P. Iron tablets cause histopathologically distinctive lesions in mucosal biopsies of the stomach and esophagus. Pathology. 1996;28(2):142–5.
5. Abraham SC, Yardley JH, Wu TT. Erosive injury to the upper gastrointestinal tract in patients receiving iron medication: an underrecognized entity. Am J Surg Pathol. 1999;23(10):1241–7.
6. Smith IM, Bryson G, Glen P. Iron-induced gastric ulceration with radiological and endoscopic appearance of carcinoma. BMJ Case Reports. 2015;2015 https://doi.org/10.1136/bcr-2015-211997.

7. Jalving M, Koornstra JJ, Wesseling J, Boezen HM, De Jong S, Kleibeuker JH. Increased risk of fundic gland polyps during long-term proton pump inhibitor therapy. Aliment Pharmacol Ther. 2006;24(9):1341–8. https://doi.org/10.1111/j.1365-2036.2006.03127.x.
8. Ally MR, Veerappan GR, Maydonovitch CL, Duncan TJ, Perry JL, Osgard EM, et al. Chronic proton pump inhibitor therapy associated with increased development of fundic gland polyps. Dig Dis Sci. 2009;54(12):2617–22. https://doi.org/10.1007/s10620-009-0993-z.
9. Zelter A, Fernández JL, Bilder C, Rodríguez P, Wonaga A, Dorado F, et al. Fundic gland polyps and association with proton pump inhibitor intake: a prospective study in 1,780 endoscopies. Dig Dis Sci. 2011;56(6):1743–8. https://doi.org/10.1007/s10620-010-1493-x.
10. Choudhry U, Boyce HW Jr, Coppola D. Proton pump inhibitor-associated gastric polyps: a retrospective analysis of their frequency, and endoscopic, histologic, and ultrastructural characteristics. Am J Clin Pathol. 1998;110(5):615–21.
11. Declich P, Ambrosiani L, Bellone S, Tavani E, Prada A, Bortoli A, et al. Fundic gland polyps under omeprazole treatment [1] (multiple letters). Am J Clin Pathol. 1999;112(4):576–7.
12. Declich P, Tavani E, Porcellati M, Bellone S, Grassini R. Long-term omeprazole treatment and fundic gland polyps: a very authoritative proof against a link? [7]. Am J Gastroenterol. 2001;96(5):1650.
13. Berstad AE, Hatlebakk JG, Maartmann-Moe H, Berstad A, Brandtzaeg P. Helicobacter pylori gastritis and epithelial cell proliferation in patients with reflux oesophagitis after treatment with lansoprazole. Gut. 1997;41(6):740–7.
14. Klinkenberg-Knol EC, Festen HPM, Jansen JBMJ, Lamers CBHW, Nelis F, Snel P, et al. Long-term treatment with omeprazole for refractory reflux esophagitis: efficacy and safety. Ann Intern Med. 1994;121(3):161–7.
15. McCloy RF, Arnold R, Bardhan KD, Cattan D, Klinkenberg-Knol E, Maton PN, et al. Pathophysiological effects of long-term acid suppression in man. Dig Dis Sci. 1995;40(2 Supplement):96S–120S. https://doi.org/10.1007/BF02214874.
16. Lamberts R, Creutzfeldt W, Strüber HG, Brunner G, Solcia E. Long-term omeprazole therapy in peptic ulcer disease: gastrin, endocrine cell growth, and gastritis. Gastroenterology. 1993;104(5):1356–70.
17. Lamberts R, Brunner G, Solcia E. Effects of very long (up to 10 years) proton pump blockade on human gastric mucosa. Digestion. 2001;64(4):205–13. https://doi.org/10.1159/000048863.
18. Kuipers EJ, Lundell L, Klinkenberg-Knol EC, Havu N, Festen HPM, Liedman B, et al. Atrophic gastritis and helicobacter pylori infection in patients with reflux esophagitis treated with omeprazole or fundoplication. N Engl J Med. 1996;334(16):1018–22. https://doi.org/10.1056/NEJM199604183341603.
19. Kuipers EJ, Uyterlinde AM, Pena AS, Hazenberg HJA, Bloemena E, Lindeman J, et al. Increase of helicobacter pylori-associated corpus gastritis during acid suppressive therapy: implications for long-term safety. Am J Gastroenterol. 1995;90(9):1401–6.
20. Meining A, Kiel G, Stolte M. Changes in helicobacter pylori-induced gastritis in the antrum and corpus during and after 12 months of treatment with ranitidine and lansoprazole in patients with duodenal ulcer disease. Aliment Pharmacol Ther. 1998;12(8):735–40. https://doi.org/10.1046/j.1365-2036.1998.00370.x.
21. Kuipers EJ, Lee A, Klinkenberg-Knol EC, Meuwissen SGM. The development of atrophic gastritis—helicobacter pylori and the effects of acid suppressive therapy. Aliment Pharmacol Ther. 1995;9(4):331–40. https://doi.org/10.1111/j.1365-2036.1995.tb00391.x.
22. Matsukuma K, Gui D, Olson KA, Tejaswi S, Clayton EF, Thai A. OsmoPrep-associated gastritis. Am J Surg Pathol. 2016;40(11):1550–6. https://doi.org/10.1097/PAS.0000000000000706.
23. Parfitt JR, Jayakumar S, Driman DK. Mycophenolate Mofetil-related gastrointestinal mucosal injury: variable injury patterns, including graft-versus-host disease-like changes. Am J Surg Pathol. 2008;32(9):1367–72. https://doi.org/10.1097/PAS.0b013e31816bf3fe.
24. Nguyen T, Park JY, Scudiere JR, Montgomery E. Mycophenolic acid (cellcept and myofortic) induced injury of the upper gi tract. Am J Surg Pathol. 2009;33(9):1355–63. https://doi.org/10.1097/PAS.0b013e3181a755bd.
25. Iacobuzio-Donahue CA, Lee EL, Abraham SC, Yardley JH, Wu TT. Colchicine toxicity: distinct morphologic findings in gastrointestinal biopsies. Am J Surg Pathol. 2001;25(8):1067–73. https://doi.org/10.1097/00000478-200108000-00012.
26. Al-Daraji WI, Al-Mahmoud RM, Ilyas M. Gastric changes following colchicine therapy in patients with FMF. Dig Dis Sci. 2008;53(8):2079–82. https://doi.org/10.1007/s10620-007-0132-7.
27. Torbenson M, Montgomery EA, Iacobuzio-Donahue C, Yardley JH, Wu TT, Abraham SC. Colchicine effect in a colonic hyperplastic polyp: a lesion mimicking serrated adenoma. Arch Pathol Lab Med. 2002;126(5):615–7.
28. Daniels JA, Gibson MK, Xu L, Sun S, Canto MI, Heath E, et al. Gastrointestinal tract epithelial changes associated with taxanes: marker of drug toxicity versus effect. Am J Surg Pathol. 2008;32(3):473–7. https://doi.org/10.1097/PAS.0b013e3181582331.
29. Jonassaint NL, Guo N, Califano JA, Montgomery EA, Armanios M. The gastrointestinal manifestations of telomere-mediated disease. Aging Cell. 2013;12(2):319–23. https://doi.org/10.1111/acel.12041.
30. Taha AS. Histopathological aspects of mucosal injury related to non-steroidal anti-inflammatory drugs. Ital J Gastroenterol. 1996;28(SUPPL. 4):12–5.
31. Quinn CM, Bjarnason I, Price AB. Gastritis in patients on non-steroidal anti-inflammatory drugs. Histopathology. 1993;23(4):341–8. https://doi.org/10.1111/j.1365-2559.1993.tb01217.x.
32. Hirschowitz BI, Lanas A. Atypical and aggressive upper gastrointestinal ulceration associated with aspirin abuse. J Clin Gastroenterol. 2002;34(5):523–8. https://doi.org/10.1097/00004836-200205000-00008.
33. Sung JJY, Russell RI, Yeomans N, Chan FKL, Chen SL, Fock KM, et al. Non-steroidal anti-inflammatory drug toxicity in the upper gastrointestinal tract. J Gastroenterol Hepatol. 2000;15(SUPPL. OCTOBER):G58–68. https://doi.org/10.1046/j.1440-1746.2000.02267.x.
34. Jewell LD, Fields AL, Murray CJW, Thomson ABR. Erosive gastroduodenitis with marked epithelial atypia after hepatic arterial infusion chemotherapy. Am J Gastroenterol. 1985;80(6):421–4. https://doi.org/10.1111/j.1572-0241.1985.tb02136.x.
35. Wells JJ, Nostrant TT, Wilson JAP, Gyves JW. Gastroduodenal ulcerations in patients receiving selective hepatic artery infusion chemotherapy. Am J Gastroenterol. 1985;80(6):425–9. https://doi.org/10.1111/j.1572-0241.1985.tb02137.x.
36. Weidner N, Smith JG, LaVanway JM. Peptic ulceration with marked epithelial atypia following hepatic arterial infusion chemotherapy. A lesion initially misinterpreted as carcinoma. Am J Surg Pathol. 1983;7(3):261–8.
37. Petras RE, Hart WR, Bukowski RM. Gastric epithelial atypia associated with hepatic arterial infusion chemotherapy. Its distinction from early gastric carcinoma. Cancer. 1985;56(4):745–50. https://doi.org/10.1002/1097-0142(19850815)56:4<745::AID-CNCR2820560408>3.0.CO;2-Q.
38. Brien TP, Farraye FA Odze RD. Gastric dysplasia-like epithelial atypia associated with chemoradiotherapy for esophageal cancer: a clinicopathologic and immunohistochemical study of 15 cases. Mod Pathol. 2001;14(5):389–96. https://doi.org/10.1038/modpathol.3880323.

39. Lim LC, Gibbs P, Yip D, Shapiro JD, Dowling R, Smith D, et al. A prospective evaluation of treatment with selective internal radiation therapy (SIR-spheres) in patients with unresectable liver metastases from colorectal cancer previously treated with 5-FU based chemotherapy. BMC Cancer. 2005;5 https://doi.org/10.1186/1471-2407-5-132.
40. Ogawa F, Mino-Kenudson M, Shimizu M, Ligato S, Lauwers GY. Gastroduodenitis associated with yttrium 90-microsphere selective internal radiation: an iatrogenic complication in need of recognition. Arch Pathol Lab Med. 2008;132(11):1734–8. https://doi.org/10.1043/1543-2165-132.11.1734.
41. Crowder CD, Grabowski C, Inampudi S, Sielaff T, Sherman CA, Batts KP. Selective internal radiation therapy-induced extrahepatic injury an emerging cause of iatrogenic organ damage. Am J Surg Pathol. 2009;33(7):963–75. https://doi.org/10.1097/PAS.0b013e31817ed787.
42. Abraham SC, Bhagavan BS, Lee LA, Rashid A, Wu TT. Upper gastrointestinal tract injury in patients receiving Kayexalate (sodium polystyrene sulfonate) in sorbitol: clinical, endoscopic, and histopathologic findings. Am J Surg Pathol. 2001; 25(5):637–44. https://doi.org/10.1097/00000478-200105000-00011.
43. Harel Z, Harel S, Shah PS, Wald R, Perl J, Bell CM. Gastrointestinal adverse events with sodium polystyrene sulfonate (Kayexalate) use: a systematic review. Am J Med. 2013;126(3):264 .e9–e.e24. https://doi.org/10.1016/j.amjmed.2012.08.016.
44. Rashid A, Hamilton SR. Necrosis of the gastrointestinal tract in uremic patients as a result of sodium polystyrene sulfonate (kayexalate) in sorbitol: an underrecognized condition. Am J Surg Pathol. 1997;21(1):60–9. https://doi.org/10.1097/00000478-199701000-00007.
45. Roy-Chaudhury P, Meisels IS, Freedman S, Steinman TI, Steer M. Combined gastric and ileocecal toxicity (serpiginous ulcers) after oral Kayexalate in sorbital therapy. Am J Kidney Dis. 1997;30(1):120–2. https://doi.org/10.1016/S0272-6386(97)90574-6.
46. Chen Z, Scudiere JR, Montgomery E. Medication-induced upper gastrointestinal tract injury. J Clin Pathol. 2009;62(2):113–9. https://doi.org/10.1136/jcp.2008.058263.
47. Swanson BJ, Limketkai BN, Liu TC, Montgomery E, Nazari K, Park JY, et al. Sevelamer crystals in the gastrointestinal tract (GIT): a new entity associated with mucosal injury. Am J Surg Pathol. 2013;37(11):1686–93. https://doi.org/10.1097/PAS.0b013e3182999d8d.
48. Arnold MA, Swanson BJ, Crowder CD, Frankel WL, Lam-Himlin D, Singhi AD, et al. Colesevelam and colestipol: novel medication resins in the gastrointestinal tract. Am J Surg Pathol. 2014;38(11):1530–7. https://doi.org/10.1097/PAS.0000000000000260.
49. Vieth M, Montgomery E. Medication-associated gastrointestinal tract injury. Virchows Arch. 2017;470(3):245–66. https://doi.org/10.1007/s00428-017-2077-3.
50. Seminerio J, McGrath K, Arnold CA, Voltaggio L, Singhi AD. Medication-associated lesions of the GI tract. Gastrointest Endosc. 2014;79(1):140–50. https://doi.org/10.1016/j.gie.2013.08.027.
51. Goto K, Ogawa K. Lanthanum deposition is frequently observed in the gastric mucosa of dialysis patients with lanthanum carbonate therapy: a clinicopathologic study of 13 cases, including 1 case of lanthanum granuloma in the colon and 2 nongranulomatous gastric cases. Int J Surg Pathol. 2016;24(1):89–92. https://doi.org/10.1177/1066896915613434.
52. Rothenberg ME, Araya H, Longacre TA, Pasricha PJ. Lanthanum-induced gastrointestinal histiocytosis. ACG Case Rep J. 2015;2:187–9.
53. Yasunaga C, Haratake J, Ohtani A. Specific accumulation of lanthanum carbonate in the gastric mucosal histiocytes in a dialysis patient. Ther Apher Dial. 2015;19(6):622–4. https://doi.org/10.1111/1744-9987.12325.
54. Yabuki K, Shiba E, Harada H, Uchihashi K, Matsuyama A, Haratake J, et al. Lanthanum deposition in the gastrointestinal mucosa and regional lymph nodes in dialysis patients: analysis of surgically excised specimens and review of the literature. Pathol Res Pract. 2016;212(10):919–26. https://doi.org/10.1016/j.prp.2016.07.017.
55. Hoda RS, Sanyal S, Abraham JL, Everett JM, Hundemer GL, Yee E, et al. Lanthanum deposition from oral lanthanum carbonate in the upper gastrointestinal tract. Histopathology. 2017;70(7):1072–8. https://doi.org/10.1111/his.13178.
56. Davis RL, Abraham JL. Lanthanum deposition in a dialysis patient. Nephrol Dial Transplant. 2009;24(10):3247–50. https://doi.org/10.1093/ndt/gfp364.
57. Rubio-Tapia A, Herman ML, Ludvigsson JF, Kelly DG, Mangan TF, Wu TT, et al. Severe spruelike enteropathy associated with olmesartan. Mayo Clin Proc. 2012;87(8):732–8. https://doi.org/10.1016/j.mayocp.2012.06.003.
58. Shih AR, Lauwers GY, Mattia A, Schaefer EA, Misdraji J. Vascular injury characterizes doxycycline-induced upper gastrointestinal tract mucosal injury. Am J Surg Pathol. 2017;41(3):374–81. https://doi.org/10.1097/PAS.0000000000000792.
59. Xiao SY, Zhao L, Hart J, Semrad CE. Doxycycline-induced gastric and esophageal mucosal injuries with vascular degeneration. Am J Surg Pathol. 2013;37(7):1115–6. https://doi.org/10.1097/PAS.0b013e31828f5b3a.
60. Shaddy SM, Arnold MA, Shilo K, Frankel WL, Harzman AE, Stanich PP, et al. Crospovidone and microcrystalline cellulose. Am J Surg Pathol. 2017;41(4):564–9. https://doi.org/10.1097/PAS.0000000000000790.
61. Rada-Palomino A, Muñoz-Duyos A, Pérez-Romero N, Vargas-Pierola H, Puértolas-Rico N, Ruiz-Campos L, et al. Phlegmonous gastritis: a rare entity as a differential diagnostic of an acute abdomen. Description of a case and a bibliographic review. Revista Espanola de Enfermedades Digestivas. 2014;106(6):418–24.
62. Kim GY, Ward J, Henessey B, Peji J, Godell C, Desta H, et al. Phlegmonous gastritis: case report and review. Gastrointest Endosc. 2005;61(1):168–74. https://doi.org/10.1016/S0016-5107(04)02217-5.
63. Guo J, Young SK, Lorenzo CR, Lee CM, Kanel GC, Brynes RK, et al. Phlegmonous gastritis in a patient with myeloid sarcoma: a case report. Appl Immunohistochem Mol Morphol. 2009;17(5):458–62. https://doi.org/10.1097/PAI.0b013e31819f86e2.
64. Al Rasheed MR, Senseng CG. Sarcina ventriculi : review of the literature. Arch Pathol Lab Med. 2016;140(12):1441–5. https://doi.org/10.5858/arpa.2016-0028-RS.
65. Laass MW, Pargac N, Fischer R, Bernhardt H, Knoke M, Henker J. Emphysematous gastritis caused by Sarcina ventriculi. Gastrointest Endosc. 2010;72(5):1101–3. https://doi.org/10.1016/j.gie.2010.02.021.
66. Tolentino LF, Kallichanda N, Javier B, Yoshimori R, French SW. A case report of gastric perforation and peritonitis associated with opportunistic infection by Sarcina ventriculi. Lab Med. 2003;34(7):535–7. https://doi.org/10.1309/CDFF-04HE-9FHD-QPAN.
67. Haroon Al Rasheed MR, Kim GJ, Senseng C. A rare case of Sarcina ventriculi of the stomach in an asymptomatic patient. Int J Surg Pathol. 2016;24(2):142–5.
68. Lam-Himlin D, Tsiatis AC, Montgomery E, Pai RK, Brown JA, Razavi M, et al. Sarcina organisms in the gastrointestinal tract: a clinicopathologic and molecular study. Am J Surg Pathol. 2011;35(11):1700–5. https://doi.org/10.1097/PAS.0b013e31822911e6.
69. Crowther JS. Sarcina ventriculi in human faeces. J Med Microbiol. 1971;4(3):343–50.

70. Lowe SE, Pankratz HS, Zeikus JG. Influence of pH extremes on sporulation and ultrastructure of Sarcina ventriculi. J Bacteriol. 1989;171(7):3775–81.
71. Canale-Parola E. Biology of the sugar-fermenting Sarcinae. Bacteriol Rev. 1970;34(1):82–97.
72. Mylona EE, Baraboutis IG, Papastamopoulos V, Tsagalou EP, Vryonis E, Samarkos M, et al. Gastric syphilis: a systematic review of published cases of the last 50 years. Sex Transm Dis. 2010;37(3):177–83. https://doi.org/10.1097/OLQ.0b013e3181c0d51f.
73. Martín-Ezquerra G, Fernandez-Casado A, Barco D, Jucglà A, Juanpere-Rodero N, Manresa JM, et al. Treponema pallidum distribution patterns in mucocutaneous lesions of primary and secondary syphilis: an immunohistochemical and ultrastructural study. Hum Pathol. 2009;40(5):624–30. https://doi.org/10.1016/j.humpath.2008.10.017.
74. Chen CY, Chi KH, George RW, Cox DL, Srivastava A, Rui Silva M, et al. Diagnosis of gastric syphilis by direct immunofluorescence staining and real-time PCR testing. J Clin Microbiol. 2006;44(9):3452–6. https://doi.org/10.1128/JCM.00721-06.
75. Neafie RC, Marty AM. Unusual infections in humans. Clin Microbiol Rev. 1993;6(1):34–56.
76. Rank EL, Goldenberg SA, Hasson J, Cartun RW, Grey N. Treponema pallidum and helicobacter pylori recovered in a case of chronic active gastritis. Am J Clin Pathol. 1992;97(1):116–20.
77. Fernandez-Flores A, Garcia Varona A. Anti-Treponema antibody also stains helicobacter heilmannii. Appl Immunohistochem Mol Morphol. 2016;24(3):e20–1. https://doi.org/10.1097/PAI.0000000000000266.
78. Hinnant KL, Rotterdam HZ, Bell ET, Tapper ML. Cytomegalovirus infection of the alimentary tract: a clinicopathological correlation. Am J Gastroenterol. 1986;81(10):944–50.
79. Xiao SY, Hart J. Marked gastric foveolar hyperplasia associated with active cytomegalovirus infection. Am J Gastroenterol. 2001;96(1):223–6. https://doi.org/10.1111/j.1572-0241.2001.03480.x.
80. Nohr EW, Itani DM, Andrews CN, Kelly MM. Varicella-zoster virus gastritis: case report and review of the literature. Int J Surg Pathol. 2017;25(5):449–52. https://doi.org/10.1177/1066896917696751.
81. Rivera-Vaquerizo PA, Gomez-Garrido J, Vicente-Gutierrez M, Blasco-Colmenarejo M, Mayor-Lopez J, Perez-Flores R. Varicella zoster gastritis 3 years after bone marrow transplantation for treatment of acute leukemia. Gastrointest Endosc. 2001;53(7):809–10.
82. Chen ZM, Shah R, Zuckerman GR, Wang HL. Epstein-Barr virus gastritis: an underrecognized form of severe gastritis simulating gastric lymphoma. Am J Surg Pathol. 2007;31(9):1446–51. https://doi.org/10.1097/PAS.0b013e318050072f.
83. Kitayama Y, Honda S, Sugimura H. Epstein-Barr virus-related gastric pseudolymphoma in infectious mononucleosis. Gastrointest Endosc. 2000;52(2):290–1. https://doi.org/10.1067/mge.2000.107715.
84. Loffeld RJ, Loffeld BC, Arends JW, Flendrig JA, van Spreeuwel JP. Fungal colonization of gastric ulcers. Am J Gastroenterol. 1988;83(7):730–3.
85. Cherney CL, Chutuape A, Fikrig MK. Fatal invasive gastric mucormycosis occurring with emphysematous gastritis: case report and literature review. Am J Gastroenterol. 1999;94(1):252–6. https://doi.org/10.1111/j.1572-0241.1999.00809.x.
86. Mohamed AE, Ghandour ZM, Al-Karawi MA, Yasawy MI, Sammak B. Gastrointestinal parasites presentations and histological diagnosis from endoscopic biopsies and surgical specimens. Saudi Med J. 2000;21(7):629–34.
87. Forester G, Sidhom O, Nahass R, Andavolu R. AIDS-associated cryptosporidiosis with gastric stricture and a therapeutic response to paromomycin. Am J Gastroenterol. 1994;89(7):1096–8.
88. Garone MA, Winston BJ, Lewis JH. Cryptosporidiosis of the stomach. Am J Gastroenterol. 1986;81(6):465–70.
89. Sohn WM, Na BK, Kim TH, Park TJ. Anisakiasis: report of 15 gastric cases caused by Anisakis type I larvae and a brief review of Korean Anisakiasis cases. Korean J Parasitol. 2015;53(4):465–70. https://doi.org/10.3347/kjp.2015.53.4.465.
90. Rider JA, Klotz AP, Kirsner JB. Gastritis with veno-capillary ectasia as a source of massive gastric hemorrhage. Gastroenterology. 1953;24(1):118–23. https://doi.org/10.1016/S0016-5085(53)80070-3.
91. Jabbari M, Cherry R, Lough JO, Daly DS, Kinnear DG, Goresky CA. Gastric antral vascular ectasia: the watermelon stomach. Gastroenterology. 1984;87(5):1165–70. https://doi.org/10.1016/S0016-5085(84)80080-3.
92. Dulai GS, Jensen DM, Kovacs TOG, Gralnek IM, Jutabha R. Endoscopic treatment outcomes in watermelon stomach patients with and without portal hypertension. Endoscopy. 2004;36(1):68–72. https://doi.org/10.1055/s-2004-814112.
93. Charneau J, Petit R, Cales P, Dauver A, Boyer J. Antral motility in patients with cirrhosis with or without gastric antral vascular ectasia. Gut. 1995;37(4):488–92.
94. Quintero E, Pique JM, Bombi JA, Bordas JM, Sentis J, Elena M, et al. Gastric mucosal vascular ectasias causing bleeding in cirrhosis. A distinct entity associated with hypergastrinemia and low serum levels of pepsinogen I. Gastroenterology. 1987;93(5):1054–61.
95. Gostout CJ, Viggiano TR, Ahlquist DA, Wang KK, Larson MV, Balm R. The clinical and endoscopic spectrum of the watermelon stomach. J Clin Gastroenterol. 1992;15(3):256–63.
96. Ward EM, Raimondo M, Rosser BG, Wallace MB, Dickson RD. Prevalence and natural history of gastric antral vascular ectasia in patients undergoing orthotopic liver transplantation. J Clin Gastroenterol. 2004;38(10):898–900. https://doi.org/10.1097/00004836-200411000-00013.
97. Tobin RW, Hackman RC, Kimmey MB, Durtschi B, Hayashi A, Malik R, et al. Bleeding from gastric antral vascular ectasia in marrow transplant patients. Gastrointest Endosc. 1996;44(3):223–9. https://doi.org/10.1016/S0016-5107(96)70155-4.
98. Smith E, Tekola B, Patrie J, Cornella S, Caldwell S. Clinical characterization of gastric antral vascular ectasia: a potential manifestation of the metabolic syndrome. Am J Med. 2016;129(12):1329 e19–23. https://doi.org/10.1016/j.amjmed.2016.07.007.
99. Hudson C, Fontenot E, Landreneau S. Gastric antral vascular ectasia presenting as a polypoid mass in a patient with cirrhosis. Gastrointest Endosc. 2017; https://doi.org/10.1016/j.gie.2017.08.002.
100. Selinger CP, Ang YS. Gastric antral vascular ectasia (GAVE): an update on clinical presentation, pathophysiology and treatment. Digestion. 2008;77(2):131–7. https://doi.org/10.1159/000124339.
101. James Sarfeh I, Tarnawski A. Portal hypertensive gastritis. Gastroenterology. 1984;86(3):592. https://doi.org/10.1016/S0016-5085(84)80052-9.
102. Sarin SK, Sreenivas DV, Lahoti D, Saraya A. Factors influencing development of portal hypertensive gastropathy in patients with portal hypertension. Gastroenterology. 1992;102(3):994–9.
103. Parikh SS, Desai SB, Prabhu SR, Trivedi MH, Shankaran K, Bhukhanwala FA, et al. Congestive Gastropathy: factors influencing development, endoscopic features, helicobacter pylori infection, and microvessel changes. Am J Gastroenterol. 1994;89(7):1036–42. https://doi.org/10.1111/j.1572-0241.1994.tb03219.x.
104. Primignani M, Carpinelli L, Preatoni P, Battaglia G, Carta A, Prada A, et al. Natural history of portal hypertensive gastropathy in patients with liver cirrhosis. Gastroenterology. 2000;119(1):181–7. https://doi.org/10.1053/gast.2000.8555.

105. Thuluvath PJ, Yoo HY. Portal hypertensive gastropathy. Am J Gastroenterol. 2002;97(12):2973–8. https://doi.org/10.1016/S0002-9270(02)05511-9.
106. Sogaard KK, Astrup LB, Vilstrup H, Gronbaek H. Portal vein thrombosis; risk factors, clinical presentation and treatment. BMC Gastroenterol. 2007;7 https://doi.org/10.1186/1471-230X-7-34.
107. Kamath PS, Lacerda M, Ahlquist DA, McKusick MA, Andrews JC, Nagorney DA. Gastric mucosal responses to intrahepatic portosystemic shunting in patients with cirrhosis. Gastroenterology. 2000;118(5):905–11. https://doi.org/10.1016/S0016-5085(00)70176-4.
108. Cubillas R, Rockey DC. Portal hypertensive gastropathy: a review. Liver Int. 2010;30(8):1094–102. https://doi.org/10.1111/j.1478-3231.2010.02286.x.
109. Ohta M, Yamaguchi S, Gotoh N, Tomikawa M. Pathogenesis of portal hypertensive gastropathy: a clinical and experimental review. Surgery. 2002;131(1):S165–S70. https://doi.org/10.1067/msy.2002.119499.
110. Ohta M, Higashi MHH, Ueno K, Tomikawa M, Kishihara F, Kawanaka H, et al. Portal and gastric mucosal hemodynamics in cirrhotic patients with portal-hypertensive gastropathy. Hepatology. 1994;20(6):1432–6. https://doi.org/10.1002/hep.1840200609.
111. Massoni F, Ricci L, Pelosi M, Ricci S. The portal hypertensive Gastropathy: a case and review of literature. J Clin Diagn Res. 2016;10(6):HD01–2. https://doi.org/10.7860/JCDR/2016/14489.7942.
112. McCormack TT, Sims J, Eyre-Brook I, Kennedy H, Goepel J, Johnson AG, et al. Gastric lesions in portal hypertension: inflammatory gastritis or congestive gastropathy? Gut. 1985;26(11):1226–32. https://doi.org/10.1136/gut.26.11.1226.
113. Han S, Chaudhary N, Wassef W. Portal hypertensive gastropathy and gastric antral vascular ectasia. Curr Opin Gastroenterol. 2015;31(6):506–12. https://doi.org/10.1097/MOG.0000000000000214.
114. Chaer RA, Helton WS. Dieulafoy's disease. J Am Coll Surg. 2003;196(2):290–6. https://doi.org/10.1016/S1072-7515(02)01801-X.
115. Nguyen DC, Jackson CS. The Dieulafoy's lesion: an update on evaluation, diagnosis, and management. J Clin Gastroenterol. 2015;49(7):541–9. https://doi.org/10.1097/MCG.0000000000000321.
116. Baxter M, Aly EH. Dieulafoy's lesion: current trends in diagnosis and management. Ann R Coll Surg Engl. 2010;92(7):548–54. https://doi.org/10.1308/003588410X12699663905311.
117. Marangoni G, Cresswell AB, Faraj W, Shaikh H, Bowles MJ. An uncommon cause of life-threatening gastrointestinal bleeding: 2 synchronous Dieulafoy lesions. J Pediatr Surg. 2009;44(2):441–3. https://doi.org/10.1016/j.jpedsurg.2008.09.033.
118. Juler GL, Labitzke HG, Lamb R, Allen R. The pathogenesis of Dieulafoy's gastric erosion. Am J Gastroenterol. 1984;79(3):195–200. https://doi.org/10.1111/j.1572-0241.1984.tb05118.x.
119. Miko TL, Thomázy VA. The caliber persistent artery of the stomach: a unifying approach to gastric aneurysm, Dieulafoy's lesion, and submucosal arterial malformation. Hum Pathol. 1988;19(8):914–21. https://doi.org/10.1016/S0046-8177(88)80006-6.
120. Stark ME, Gostout CJ, Balm RK. Clinical features and endoscopic management of Dieulafoy's disease. Gastrointest Endosc. 1992;38(5):545–50. https://doi.org/10.1016/S0016-5107(92)70513-6.
121. Senger JL, Kanthan R. The evolution of Dieulafoy's lesion since 1897: then and now-a journey through the Lens of a pediatric lesion with literature review. Gastroenterol Res Pract. 2012;2012:432517. https://doi.org/10.1155/2012/432517.
122. Chung IK, Kim EJ, Lee MS, Kim HS, Park SH, Lee MH, et al. Bleeding Dieulafoy's lesions and the choice of endoscopic method: comparing the hemostatic efficacy of mechanical and injection methods. Gastrointest Endosc. 2000;52(6):721–4. https://doi.org/10.1067/mge.2000.108040.
123. Matsui S, Kamisako T, Kudo M, Inoue R. Endoscopic band ligation for control of nonvariceal upper GI hemorrhage: comparison with bipolar electrocoagulation. Gastrointest Endosc. 2002;55(2):214–8. https://doi.org/10.1067/mge.2002.121337.
124. Park CH, Sohn YH, Lee WS, Joo YE, Choi SK, Rew JS, et al. The usefulness of endoscopic hemoclipping for bleeding Dieulafoy lesions. Endoscopy. 2003;35(5):388–92. https://doi.org/10.1055/s-2003-38780.
125. Park CH, Joo YE, Kim HS, Choi SK, Rew JS, Kim SJ. A prospective, randomized trial of endoscopic band ligation versus endoscopic hemoclip placement for bleeding gastric Dieulafoy's lesions. Endoscopy. 2004;36(8):677–81. https://doi.org/10.1055/s-2004-825661.
126. Khoury T, Rivera L. Foregut duplication cysts: a report of two cases with emphasis on embryogenesis. World J Gastroenterol. 2011;17(1):130–4. https://doi.org/10.3748/wjg.v17.i1.130.
127. Sharma S, Nezakatgoo N, Sreenivasan P, Vanatta J, Jabbour N. Foregut cystic developmental malformation: new taxonomy and classification—unifying embryopathological concepts. Indian J Pathol Microbiol. 2009;52(4):461–72. https://doi.org/10.4103/0377-4929.56119.
128. Horne G, Ming-Lum C, Kirkpatrick AW, Parker RL. High-grade neuroendocrine carcinoma arising in a gastric duplication cyst: a case report with literature review. Int J Surg Pathol. 2007;15(2):187–91. https://doi.org/10.1177/1066896906295777.
129. Rowling JT. Some observations on gastric cysts. Br J Surg. 1959;46(199):441–5.
130. Holcomb Iii GW, Gheissari A, O'Neill JA Jr, Shorter NA, Bishop HC. Surgical management of alimentary tract duplications. Ann Surg. 1989;209(2):167–74.
131. Kuraoka K, Nakayama H, Kagawa T, Ichikawa T, Yasui W. Adenocarcinoma arising from a gastric duplication cyst with invasion to the stomach: a case report with literature review. J Clin Pathol. 2004;57(4):428–31. https://doi.org/10.1136/jcp.2003.013946.
132. Dolan RV, Remine WH, Dockerty MB. The fate of heterotopic pancreatic tissue: a study of 212 cases. Arch Surg. 1974;109(6):762–5. https://doi.org/10.1001/archsurg.1974.01360060032010.
133. Martinez NS, Morlock CG, Dockerty MB, Waugh JM, Weber HM. Heterotopic pancreatic tissue involving the stomach. Ann Surg. 1958;147(1):1–12.
134. Chen HL, Chang WH, Shih SC, Bair MJ, Lin SC. Changing pattern of ectopic pancreas: 22 years of experience in a medical center. J Formos Med Assoc. 2008;107(12):932–6. https://doi.org/10.1016/S0929-6646(09)60016-4.
135. Lindtner RA, Schreiber F, Langner C. Cytokeratin 7 immunostaining facilitates recognition of pancreatic heterotopia in gastric biopsies. Pathol Int. 2007;57(8):548–50. https://doi.org/10.1111/j.1440-1827.2007.02138.x.
136. Distler M, Ruckert F, Aust D, Saeger HD, Grutzmann R. Pancreatic heterotopia of the duodenum: anatomic anomaly or clinical challenge? J Gastrointest Surg. 2011;15(4):631–6. https://doi.org/10.1007/s11605-011-1420-2.
137. Gaspar Fuentes A, Campos Tarrech JM, Fernández Burgui JL, Castells Tejón E, Ruíz Rossello J, Gómez Pérez J, et al. Pancreatic ectopias. Revista Espanola de las Enfermedades del Aparato Digestivo. 1973;39(3):255–68.
138. Osanai M, Miyokawa N, Tamaki T, Yonekawa M, Kawamura A, Sawada N. Adenocarcinoma arising in gastric heterotopic pancreas: clinicopathological and immunohistochemical study with

genetic analysis of a case. Pathol Int. 2001;51(7):549–54. https://doi.org/10.1046/j.1440–1827.2001.01240.x.
139. Chetty R, Weinreb I. Gastric neuroendocrine carcinoma arising from heterotopic pancreatic tissue. J Clin Pathol. 2004;57(3):314–7. https://doi.org/10.1136/jcp.2003.013557.
140. Wang HH, Zeroogian JM, Spechler SJ, Goyal RK, Antonioli DA. Prevalence and significance of pancreatic acinar metaplasia at the gastroesophageal junction. Am J Surg Pathol. 1996;20(12):1507–10.
141. Jhala NC, Montemor M, Jhala D, Lu L, Talley L, Haber MM, et al. Pancreatic acinar cell metaplasia in autoimmune gastritis. Arch Pathol Lab Med. 2003;127(7):854–7. https://doi.org/10.1043/1543–2165(2003)127<854:PACMIA>2.0.CO;2.
142. Hammock L, Jorda M. Gastric endocrine pancreatic heterotopia: report of a case with histologic and immunohistochemical findings and review of the literature. Arch Pathol Lab Med. 2002;126(4):464–7.
143. To T, Wajja A, Wales PW, Langer JC. Population demographic indicators associated with incidence of pyloric stenosis. Arch Pediatr Adolesc Med. 2005;159(6):520–5. https://doi.org/10.1001/archpedi.159.6.520.
144. Mullassery D, Perry D, Goyal A, Jesudason EC, Losty PD. Surgical practice for infantile hypertrophic pyloric stenosis in the United Kingdom and Ireland-a survey of members of the British Association of Paediatric Surgeons. J Pediatr Surg. 2008;43(6):1227–9. https://doi.org/10.1016/j.jpedsurg.2007.12.075.
145. Applegate MS, Druschel CM. The epidemiology of infantile hypertrophic pyloric stenosis in New York state: 1983 to 1990. Arch Pediatr Adolesc Med. 1995;149(10):1123–9. https://doi.org/10.1001/archpedi.1995.02170230077011.
146. Zhu J, Zhu T, Lin Z, Qu Y, Mu D. Perinatal risk factors for infantile hypertrophic pyloric stenosis: a meta-analysis. J Pediatr Surg. 2017;52(9):1389–97. https://doi.org/10.1016/j.jpedsurg.2017.02.017.
147. Peeters B, Benninga MA, Hennekam RC. Infantile hypertrophic pyloric stenosis—genetics and syndromes. Nat Rev Gastroenterol Hepatol. 2012;9(11):646–60. https://doi.org/10.1038/nrgastro.2012.133.
148. Wayne C, Hung JH, Chan E, Sedgwick I, Bass J, Nasr A. Formula-feeding and hypertrophic pyloric stenosis: is there an association? A case-control study. J Pediatr Surg. 2016;51(5):779–82. https://doi.org/10.1016/j.jpedsurg.2016.02.021.
149. Eberly MD, Eide MB, Thompson JL, Nylund CM. Azithromycin in early infancy and pyloric stenosis. Pediatrics. 2015;135(3):483–8. https://doi.org/10.1542/peds.2014–2026.
150. Poon TS, Zhang AL, Cartmill T, Cass DT. Changing patterns of diagnosis and treatment of infantile hypertrophic pyloric stenosis: a clinical audit of 303 patients. J Pediatr Surg. 1996;31(12):1611–5.
151. Panteli C. New insights into the pathogenesis of infantile pyloric stenosis. Pediatr Surg Int. 2009;25(12):1043–52. https://doi.org/10.1007/s00383-009–2484-x.
152. Taylor ND, Cass DT, Holland AJA. Infantile hypertrophic pyloric stenosis: has anything changed? J Paediatr Child Health. 2013;49(1):33–7. https://doi.org/10.1111/jpc.12027.
153. Hernanz-Schulman M. Infantile hypertrophic pyloric stenosis. Radiology. 2003;227(2):319–31. https://doi.org/10.1148/radiol.2272011329.
154. Rolle U, Piaseczna-Piotrowska A, Puri P. Interstitial cells of Cajal in the normal gut and in intestinal motility disorders of childhood. Pediatr Surg Int. 2007;23(12):1139–52. https://doi.org/10.1007/s00383–007–2022–7.
155. Aspelund G, Langer JC. Current management of hypertrophic pyloric stenosis. Semin Pediatr Surg. 2007;16(1):27–33. https://doi.org/10.1053/j.sempedsurg.2006.10.004.
156. Perger L, Fuchs JR, Komidar L, Mooney DP. Impact of surgical approach on outcome in 622 consecutive pyloromyotomies at a pediatric teaching institution. J Pediatr Surg. 2009;44(11):2119–25. https://doi.org/10.1016/j.jpedsurg.2009.02.067.
157. Chalya PL, Manyama M, Kayange NM, Mabula JB, Massenga A. Infantile hypertrophic pyloric stenosis at a tertiary care hospital in Tanzania: a surgical experience with 102 patients over a 5-year period. BMC Res Notes. 2015;8:690. https://doi.org/10.1186/s13104–015–1660–4.
158. Carmack SW, Genta RM, Schuler CM, Saboorian MH. The current spectrum of gastric polyps: a 1-year national study of over 120,000 patients. Am J Gastroenterol. 2009;104(6):1524–32. https://doi.org/10.1038/ajg.2009.139.
159. Cao H, Wang B, Zhang Z, Zhang H, Qu R. Distribution trends of gastric polyps: an endoscopy database analysis of 24121 northern Chinese patients. J Gastroenterol Hepatol. 2012;27(7):1175–80. https://doi.org/10.1111/j.1440–1746.2012.07116.x.
160. Archimandritis A, Spiliadis C, Tzivras M, Vamvakousis B, Davaris P, Manika Z, et al. Gastric epithelial polyps: a retrospective endoscopic study of 12974 symptomatic patients. Ital J Gastroenterol. 1996;28(7):387–90.
161. Islam RS, Patel NC, Lam-Himlin D, Nguyen CC. Gastric polyps: a review of clinical, endoscopic, and histopathologic features and management decisions. Gastroenterol Hepatol. 2013;9(10):640–51.
162. Gencosmanoglu R, Sen-Oran E, Kurtkaya-Yapicier O, Tozun N. Xanthelasmas of the upper gastrointestinal tract. J Gastroenterol. 2004;39(3):215–9. https://doi.org/10.1007/s00535–003–1288–3.
163. Chandan VS, Wang W, Landas SK. Gastric lipid islands. Arch Pathol Lab Med. 2004;128(8):937–8. https://doi.org/10.1043/1543–2165(2004)128<937:GLI>2.0.CO;2.
164. Hori S, Tsutsumi Y. Helicobacter pylori infection in gastric xanthomas: Immunohistochemical analysis of 145 lesions. Pathol Int. 1996;46(8):589–93.
165. Isomoto H, Mizuta Y, Inoue K, Matsuo T, Hayakawa T, Miyazaki M, et al. A close relationship between helicobacter pylori infection and gastric xanthoma. Scand J Gastroenterol. 1999;34(4):346–52. https://doi.org/10.1080/003655299750026344.
166. Yi SY. Dyslipidemia and H pylori in gastric xanthomatosis. World J Gastroenterol. 2007;13(34):4598–601.
167. Shibukawa N, Ouchi S, Wakamatsu S, Wakahara Y, Kaneko A. Gastric xanthoma is a predictive marker for metachronous and synchronous gastric cancer. World J Gastrointest Oncol. 2017;9(8):327–32. https://doi.org/10.4251/wjgo.v9.i8.327.
168. Kitamura S, Muguruma N, Okamoto K, Tanahashi T, Fukuya A, Tanaka K, et al. Clinicopathological assessment of gastric xanthoma as potential predictive marker of gastric Cancer. Digestion. 2017;96(4):199–206. https://doi.org/10.1159/000481346.
169. Abraham SC, Singh VK, Yardley JH, Wu TT. Hyperplastic polyps of the stomach: associations with histologic patterns of gastritis and gastric atrophy. Am J Surg Pathol. 2001;25(4):500–7. https://doi.org/10.1097/00000478–200104000–00010.
170. Goddard AF, Badreldin R, Pritchard DM, Walker MM, Warren B. The management of gastric polyps. Gut. 2010;59(9):1270–6. https://doi.org/10.1136/gut.2009.182089.
171. Amaro R, Neff GW, Karnam US, Tzakis AG, Raskin JB. Acquired hyperplastic gastric polyps in solid organ transplant patients. Am J Gastroenterol. 2002;97(9):2220–4. https://doi.org/10.1016/S0002–9270(02)04332–0.
172. Jewell KD, Toweill DL, Swanson PE, Upton MP, Yeh MM. Gastric hyperplastic polyps in post transplant patients: a clinicopathologic study. Mod Pathol. 2008;21(9):1108–12. https://doi.org/10.1038/modpathol.2008.87.
173. Gonzalez-Obeso E, Fujita H, Deshpande V, Ogawa F, Lisovsky M, Genevay M, et al. Gastric hyperplastic polyps: a heterogeneous clinicopathologic group including a distinct subset best categorized

as mucosal prolapse polyp. Am J Surg Pathol. 2011;35(5):670–7. https://doi.org/10.1097/PAS.0b013e3182127d2b.
174. Boncher J, Bronner M, Goldblum JR, Liu X. Reticulin staining clarifies florid benign signet ring cell change with mitotic activity in a penetrating gastric ulcer. Am J Surg Pathol. 2011;35(5):762–6. https://doi.org/10.1097/PAS.0b013e318213f833.
175. Ohkusa T, Takashimizu I, Fujiki K, Suzuki S, Shimoi K, Horiuchi T, et al. Disappearance of hyperplastic polyps in the stomach after eradication of helicobacter pylori: a randomized, controlled trial. Ann Intern Med. 1998;129(9):712–5.
176. Ljubičić N, Banić M, Kujundžić M, Antić Z, Vrkljan M, Kovačević I, et al. The effect of eradicating helicobacter pylori infection on the course of adenomatous and hyperplastic gastric polyps. Eur J Gastroenterol Hepatol. 1999;11(7):727–30.
177. Daibo M, Itabashi M, Hirota T. Malignant transformation of gastric hyperplastic polyps. Am J Gastroenterol. 1987;82(10):1016–25.
178. Han AR, Sung CO, Kim KM, Park CK, Min BH, Lee JH, et al. The clinicopathological features of gastric hyperplastic polyps with neoplastic transformations: a suggestion of indication for endoscopic polypectomy. Gut Liver. 2009;3(4):271–5. https://doi.org/10.5009/gnl.2009.3.4.271.
179. Hattori T. Morphological range of hyperplastic polyps and carcinomas arising in hyperplastic polyps of the stomach. J Clin Pathol. 1985;38(6):622–30.
180. Dirschmid K, Platz-Baudin C, Stolte M. Why is the hyperplastic polyp a marker for the precancerous condition of the gastric mucosa? Virchows Arch. 2006;448(1):80–4. https://doi.org/10.1007/s00428–005–0068–2.
181. Offerhaus GJA, Billaud M, Gruber SB. Peutz-Jehgers syndrome. Tumours of the Digestive System. Editors Bosman FT, Carneiro F, Hruban RH and Theise ND, IARC, Lyon, 2010:166–70.
182. Syngal S, Brand RE, Church JM, Giardiello FM, Hampel HL, Burt RW. ACG clinical guideline: genetic testing and management of hereditary gastrointestinal cancer syndromes. Am J Gastroenterol. 2015;110(2):223–62. https://doi.org/10.1038/ajg.2014.435.
183. Brosens LAA, van Hattem WA, Jansen M, de Leng WWJ, Giardiello FM, Offerhaus GJA. Gastrointestinal polyposis syndromes. Curr Mol Med. 2007;7(1):29–46. https://doi.org/10.2174/156652407779940404.
184. McGarrity TJ, Kulin HE, Zaino RJ. Peutz-Jeghers syndrome. Am J Gastroenterol. 2000;95(3):596–604. https://doi.org/10.1016/S0002–9270(99)00890–4.
185. Lam-Himlin D, Park JY, Cornish TC, Shi C, Montgomery E. Morphologic characterization of syndromic gastric polyps. Am J Surg Pathol. 2010;34(11):1656–62. https://doi.org/10.1097/PAS.0b013e3181f2b1f1.
186. Van Lier MGF, Westerman AM, Wagner A, Looman CWN, Wilson JHP, De Rooij FWM, et al. High cancer risk and increased mortality in patients with Peutz—Jeghers syndrome. Gut. 2011;60(2):141–7. https://doi.org/10.1136/gut.2010.223750.
187. Giardiello FM, Brensinger JD, Tersmette AC, Goodman SN, Petersen GM, Booker SV, et al. Very high risk of cancer in familial Peutz-Jeghers syndrome. Gastroenterology. 2000;119(6):1447–53. https://doi.org/10.1053/gast.2000.20228.
188. Jansen M, De Leng WWJ, Baas AF, Myoshi H, Mathus-Vliegen L, Taketo MM, et al. Mucosal prolapse in the pathogenesis of Peutz-Jeghers polyposis. Gut. 2006;55(1):1–5. https://doi.org/10.1136/gut.2005.069062.
189. Langeveld D, Jansen M, De Boer DV, Van Sprundel M, Brosens LAA, Morsink FH, et al. Aberrant intestinal stem cell lineage dynamics in Peutz-Jeghers syndrome and familial adenomatous polyposis consistent with protracted clonal evolution in the crypt. Gut. 2012;61(6):839–46. https://doi.org/10.1136/gutjnl-2011–300622.
190. Howe JR, Roth S, Ringold JC, Summers RW, Järvinen HJ, Sistonen P, et al. Mutations in the SMAD4/DPC4 gene in juvenile polyposis. Science. 1998;280(5366):1086–8. https://doi.org/10.1126/science.280.5366.1086.
191. Howe JR, Ringold JC, Summers RW, Mitros FA, Nishimura DY, Stone EM. A gene for familial juvenile polyposis maps to chromosome 18q21.1. Am J Hum Genet. 1998;62(5):1129–36. https://doi.org/10.1086/301840.
192. Howe JR, Bair JL, Sayed MG, Anderson ME, Mitros FA, Petersen GM, et al. Germline mutations of the gene encoding bone morphogenetic protein receptor 1A in juvenile polyposis. Nat Genet. 2001;28(2):184–7. https://doi.org/10.1038/88919.
193. Aretz S, Stienen D, Uhlhaas S, Stolte M, Entius MM, Loff S, et al. High proportion of large genomic deletions and a genotype-phenotype update in 80 unrelated families with juvenile polyposis syndrome. J Med Genet. 2007;44(11):702–9. https://doi.org/10.1136/jmg.2007.052506.
194. Sayed MG, Ahmed AF, Ringold JR, Anderson ME, Bair JL, Mitros FA, et al. Germline SMAD4 or BMPR1A mutations and phenotype of juvenile polyposis. Ann Surg Oncol. 2002;9(9):901–6.
195. Sweet K, Willis J, Zhou XP, Gallione C, Sawada T, Alhopuro P, et al. Molecular classification of patients with unexplained hamartomatous and hyperplastic polyposis. J Am Med Assoc. 2005;294(19):2465–73. https://doi.org/10.1001/jama.294.19.2465.
196. Schreibman IR, Baker M, Amos C, McGarrity TJ. The hamartomatous polyposis syndromes: a clinical and molecular review. Am J Gastroenterol. 2005;100(2):476–90. https://doi.org/10.1111/j.1572–0241.2005.40237.x.
197. Offerhaus GJA, Howe JR. Juvenile polyposis. WHO Classification of Tumours of the Digestive System 2010:166–7.
198. Ma C, Giardiello FM, Montgomery EA. Upper tract juvenile polyps in juvenile polyposis patients: dysplasia and malignancy are associated with foveolar, intestinal, and pyloric differentiation. Am J Surg Pathol. 2014;38(12):1618–26.
199. Gonzalez RS, Adsay V, Graham RP, Shroff SG, Feely MM, Drage MG, et al. Massive gastric juvenile-type polyposis: a clinicopathological analysis of 22 cases. Histopathology. 2017;70(6):918–28. https://doi.org/10.1111/his.13149.
200. Lawless ME, Toweill DL, Jewell KD, Jain D, Lamps L, Krasinskas AM, et al. Massive gastric juvenile polyposis: a clinicopathologic study using SMAD4 immunohistochemistry. Am J Clin Pathol. 2017;147(4):390. https://doi.org/10.1093/ajcp/aqx015.
201. Howe JR, Mitros FA, Summers RW. The risk of gastrointestinal carcinoma in familial juvenile polyposis. Ann Surg Oncol. 1998;5(8):751–6.
202. Slavik T, Montgomery EA. Cronkhite-Canada syndrome six decades on: the many faces of an enigmatic disease. J Clin Pathol. 2014;67(10):891–7. https://doi.org/10.1136/jclinpath-2014–202488.
203. Ward EM, Wolfsen HC. Review article: the non-inherited gastrointestinal polyposis syndromes. Aliment Pharmacol Ther. 2002;16(3):333–42. https://doi.org/10.1046/j.1365–2036.2002.01172.x.
204. Daniel ES, Ludwig SL, Lewin KJ, Ruprecht RM, Rajacich GM, Schwabe AD. The cronkhite-Canada syndrome: an analysis of clinical and pathologic features and therapy in 55 patients. Medicine (United States). 1982;61(5):293–309.
205. Riegert-Johnson DL, Osborn N, Smyrk T, Boardman LA. Cronkhite-Canada syndrome hamartomatous polyps are infiltrated with IgG4 plasma cells [1]. Digestion. 2007;75(2–3):96–7. https://doi.org/10.1159/000102963.
206. Sweetser S, Ahlquist DA, Osborn NK, Sanderson SO, Smyrk TC, Chari ST, et al. Clinicopathologic features and treatment outcomes in Cronkhite-Canada syndrome: support for autoimmunity. Dig Dis Sci. 2012;57(2):496–502. https://doi.org/10.1007/s10620–011–1874–9.

207. Burke AP, Sobin LH. The pathology of Cronkhite-Canada polyps. A comparison to juvenile polyposis. Am J Surg Pathol. 1989;13(11):940–6. https://doi.org/10.1097/00000478-198911000-00004.
208. Wolfsen HC, Carpenter HA, Talley NJ. Menetrier's disease: a form of hypertrophic gastropathy or gastritis? Gastroenterology. 1993;104(5):1310–9. https://doi.org/10.1016/0016-5085(93)90339-E.
209. Isobe T, Kobayashi T, Hashimoto K, Kizaki J, Miyagi M, Aoyagi K, et al. Cronkhite-Canada syndrome complicated with multiple gastric cancers and multiple colon adenomas. Am J Case Rep. 2013;14:120–8. https://doi.org/10.12659/AJCR.889083.
210. Egawa T, Kubota T, Otani Y, Kurihara N, Abe S, Kimata M, et al. Surgically treated Cronkhite-Canada syndrome associated with gastric cancer. Gastric Cancer. 2000;3(3):156–60.
211. Watanabe T, Kudo M, Shirane H, Kashida H, Tomita S, Orino A, et al. Cronkhite-Canada syndrome associated with triple gastric cancers: a case report. Gastrointest Endosc. 1999;50(5):688–91.
212. Chadalavada R, Brown DK, Walker AN, Sedghi S. Cronkhite-Canada syndrome: sustained remission after corticosteroid treatment. Am J Gastroenterol. 2003;98(6):1444–6. https://doi.org/10.1111/j.1572-0241.2003.07509.x.
213. Goto A. Cronkhite-Canada syndrome: epidemiological study of 110 cases reported in Japan. Archiv fur Japanische Chirurgie. 1995;64(1):3–14.
214. Pilarski R, Stephens JA, Noss R, Fisher JL, Prior TW. Predicting PTEN mutations: an evaluation of cowden syndrome and Bannayan-Riley-Ruvalcaba syndrome clinical features. J Med Genet. 2011;48(8):505–12. https://doi.org/10.1136/jmg.2011.088807.
215. Pilarski R, Burt R, Kohlman W, Pho L, Shannon KM, Swisher E. Cowden syndrome and the PTEN hamartoma tumor syndrome: systematic review and revised diagnostic criteria. J Natl Cancer Inst. 2013;105(21):1607–16. https://doi.org/10.1093/jnci/djt277.
216. Ngeow J, Sesock K, Eng C. Clinical implications for Germline PTEN Spectrum disorders. Endocrinol Metab Clin N Am. 2017;46(2):503–17. https://doi.org/10.1016/j.ecl.2017.01.013.
217. Eng C. Will the real Cowden syndrome please stand up: revised diagnostic criteria. J Med Genet. 2000;37(11):828–30.
218. Pilarski R, Eng C. Will the real Cowden syndrome please stand up (again)? Expanding mutational and clinical spectra of the PTEN hamartoma tumour syndrome. J Med Genet. 2004;41(5):323–6.
219. Al-Thihli K, Palma L, Marcus V, Cesari M, Kushner YB, Barkun A, et al. A case of Cowden's syndrome presenting with gastric carcinomas and gastrointestinal polyposis. Nat Clin Pract Gastroenterol Hepatol. 2009;6(3):184–9. https://doi.org/10.1038/ncpgasthep1359.
220. Hamby LS, Lee EY, Schwartz RW. Parathyroid adenoma and gatric carcinoma as manifestations of cowden's disease. Surgery. 1995;118(1):115–7. https://doi.org/10.1016/S0039-6060(05)80018-2.
221. Doglioni C, Laurino L, Dei Tos AP, De Boni M, Franzin G, Braidotti P, et al. Pancreatic (acinar) metaplasia of the gastric mucosa: histology, ultrastructure, immunocytochemistry, and clinicopathologic correlations of 101 cases. Am J Surg Pathol. 1993;17(11):1134–43. https://doi.org/10.1097/00000478-199311000-00006.
222. Krishnamurthy S, Dayal Y. Pancreatic metaplasia in Barrett's esophagus: an immunohistochemical study. Am J Surg Pathol. 1995;19(10):1172–80.
223. Integlia MJ. Pancreatic metaplasia of the gastric mucosa in pediatric patients. Am J Gastroenterol. 1997;92(9):1553–6.
224. Krishnamurthy S, Integlia MJ, Grand RJ, Dayal Y. Pancreatic acinar cell clusters in pediatric gastric mucosa. Am J Surg Pathol. 1998;22(1):100–5. https://doi.org/10.1097/00000478-199801000-00013.
225. Jhala N, Jhala D, West B, Atkinson BF, Haber MH. Pancreatic (acinar cell) metaplasia or early pancreatic heterotopia? Am J Clin Pathol. 1994;101:385
226. Johansson J, Hakansson HO, Mellblom L, Kempas A, Kjellen G, Brudin L, et al. Pancreatic acinar metaplasia in the distal oesophagus and the gastric cardia: prevalence, predictors and relation to GORD. J Gastroenterol. 2010;45(3):291–9. https://doi.org/10.1007/s00535-009-0161-4.
227. Littler ER, Gleibermann E. Gastritis cystica polyposa. (Gastric mucosal prolapse at gastroenterostomy site, with cystic and infiltrative epithelial hyperplasia). Cancer. 1972;29(1):205–9. https://doi.org/10.1002/1097-0142(197201)29:1<205::AID-CNCR2820290130>3.0.CO;2-J.
228. Qizilbash AH. Gastritis cystica and carcinoma arising in old gastrojejunostomy stoma. Can Med Assoc J. 1975;112(12):1432–3.
229. Tomizuka T, Mazaki T, Mado K, Henmi A, Ishii Y, Masuda H, et al. A case of gastritis cystica profunda. Surgery. 2008;143(3):449–50. https://doi.org/10.1016/j.surg.2007.02.009.
230. Béchade D, Desramé J, Algayres JP. Gastritis cystica profunda in a patient with no history of gastric surgery. Endoscopy. 2007;39(Suppl 1):E80–1. https://doi.org/10.1055/s-2006-945070.
231. Xu G, Peng C, Li X, Zhang W, Lv Y, Ling T, et al. Endoscopic resection of gastritis cystica profunda: preliminary experience with 34 patients from a single center in China. Gastrointest Endosc. 2015;81(6):1493–8. https://doi.org/10.1016/j.gie.2014.11.017.
232. Yu XF, Guo LW, Chen ST, Teng LS. Gastritis cystica profunda in a previously unoperated stomach: a case report. World J Gastroenterol. 2015;21(12):3759–62. https://doi.org/10.3748/wjg.v21.i12.3759.
233. Franzin G, Novelli P. Gastritis cystica profunda. Histopathology. 1981;5(5):535–47. https://doi.org/10.1111/j.1365-2559.1981.tb01817.x.
234. Odze RD, Greenson J, Lauwers G, Goldblum J. Gastritis cystica profunda versus invasive adenocarcinoma. Am J Surg Pathol. 2012;36(2):316. https://doi.org/10.1097/PAS.0b013e31823edb3b.
235. Wang L, Yan H, Cao DC, Huo L, Huo HZ, Wang B, et al. Gastritis cystica profunda recurrence after surgical resection: 2-year follow-up. World J Surg Oncol. 2014;12(1) https://doi.org/10.1186/1477-7819-12-133.
236. Fonde EC, Rodning CB. Gastritis cystica profunda. Am J Gastroenterol. 1986;81(6):459–64. https://doi.org/10.1111/j.1572-0241.1986.tb01523.x.
237. Franzin G, Musola R, Zamboni G, Manfrini C. Gastritis cystica polyposa: a possible precancerous lesion. Tumori. 1985;71(1):13–8.
238. Choi MG, Jeong JY, Kim KM, Bae JM, Noh JH, Sohn TS, et al. Clinical significance of gastritis cystica profunda and its association with Epstein-Barr virus in gastric cancer. Cancer. 2012;118(21):5227–33. https://doi.org/10.1002/cncr.27541.
239. Park CH, Park JM, Jung CK, Kim DB, Kang SH, Lee SW, et al. Early gastric cancer associated with gastritis cystica polyposa in the unoperated stomach treated by endoscopic submucosal dissection. Gastrointest Endosc. 2009;69(6):e47–50. https://doi.org/10.1016/j.gie.2008.10.020.
240. Deery S, Yates R, Hata J, Shi C, Parikh AA. Gastric adenocarcinoma associated with gastritis cystica profunda in an unoperated stomach. Am Surg. 2012;78(8):E379–E80.
241. Gorospe M, Fadare O. Gastric mucosal calcinosis: clinicopathologic considerations. Adv Anat Pathol. 2007;14(3):224–8. https://doi.org/10.1097/PAP.0b013e31805048ea.
242. Greenson JK, Trinidad SB, Pfeil SA, Brainard JA, McBride PT, Colijn HO, et al. Gastric mucosal calcinosis: calcified aluminum phosphate deposits secondary to aluminum-containing antacids or sucralfate therapy in organ transplant

patients. Am J Surg Pathol. 1993;17(1):45–50. https://doi.org/10.1097/00000478-199301000-00005.
243. Kuzela DC, Huffer WE, Conger JD, Winter SD, Hammond WS. Soft tissue calcification in chronic dialysis patients. Am J Pathol. 1977;86(2):403–24.
244. Ou Tim L, Hurwitz S, Tuch P. The endoscopic diagnosis of gastric calcification. J Clin Gastroenterol. 1982;4(3):213–5.
245. Saab S, Venkataramani A, Behling CA, Savides TJ. Gastric mucosal calcinosis in a patient with dyspepsia. J Clin Gastroenterol. 1996;22(2):156–7. https://doi.org/10.1097/00004836-199603000-00020.
246. Nayak HK, Mohindra S, Iqbal S, Saraswat VA, Agarwal V, Pande G. Gastric mucosal calcinosis mimicking malignancy. Am J Gastroenterol. 2016;111(10):1380. https://doi.org/10.1038/ajg.2016.274.
247. Ebert EC, Nagar M. Gastrointestinal manifestations of amyloidosis. Am J Gastroenterol. 2008;103(3):776–87. https://doi.org/10.1111/j.1572-0241.2007.01669.x.
248. Menke DM, Kyle RA, Fleming CR, Wolfe JT III, Kurtin PJ, Oldenburg WA. Symptomatic gastric amyloidosis in patients with primary systemic amyloidosis. Mayo Clin Proc. 1993;68(8):763–7. https://doi.org/10.1016/S0025-6196(12)60634-X.
249. Said SM, Grogg KL, Smyrk TC. Gastric amyloidosis: clinicopathological correlations in 79 cases from a single institution. Human Pathology. 2015;46(4):491–8. Original contribution. https://doi.org/10.1016/j.humpath.2014.12.009.
250. Seon CS, Park YS, Jung YM, Choi JH, Son BK, Ahn SB, et al. Gastric outlet obstruction due to gastric amyloidosis mimicking malignancy in a patient with ankylosing spondylitis. Clin Endosc. 2013;46(6):651–5. https://doi.org/10.5946/ce.2013.46.6.651.
251. Khan Z, Darr U, Renno A, Tiwari A, Sofi A, Nawras A. Massive upper and lower GI bleed from simultaneous primary (AL) amyloidosis of the stomach and transverse colon in a patient with multiple myeloma. Case Rep Gastroenterol. 2017;11(3):625–31. https://doi.org/10.1159/000480073.
252. Rivera R, Kaul V, DeCross A, Whitney-Miller C. Primary gastric amyloidosis presenting as an isolated gastric mass. Gastrointest Endosc. 2012;76(1):186–7. https://doi.org/10.1016/j.gie.2012.02.059.
253. Tada S, Lida M, Iwashita A, Matsui T, Fuchigami T, Yamamoto T, et al. Endoscopic and biopsy findings of the upper digestive tract in patients with amyloidosis. Gastrointest Endosc. 1990;36(1):10–4. https://doi.org/10.1016/S0016-5107(90)70913-3.
254. Jimenez-Zepeda VH, Vajpeyi R, John R, Trudel S. Light chain deposition disease affecting the gastrointestinal tract in the setting of post-living donor kidney transplantation. Int J Hematol. 2012;96(1):125–31. https://doi.org/10.1007/s12185-012-1090-1.
255. Kwon JH, Jeong SH, Kim JW, Bang SM, Kim H, Kim YH, et al. Case report: a case of light chain deposition disease involving liver and stomach with chronic hepatitis C virus infection and hepatocellular carcinoma. J Med Virol. 2011;83(5):810–4. https://doi.org/10.1002/jmv.22050.
256. Conte D, Velio P, Brunelli L, Mandelli C, Cesana M, Ferrario L, et al. Stainable Iron in gastric and duodenal mucosa of primary hemochromatosis patients and alcoholics. Am J Gastroenterol. 1987;82(3):237–40. https://doi.org/10.1111/j.1572-0241.1987.tb05298.x.
257. Marginean EC, Bennick M, Cyczk J, Robert ME, Jain D. Gastric siderosis: patterns and significance. Am J Surg Pathol. 2006;30(4):514–20. https://doi.org/10.1097/00000478-200604000-00013.
258. Antunes AG, Cadilla J, Guerreiro H. Gastric siderosis as a cause of dyspepsia. BMJ Case Rep. 2016;2016 https://doi.org/10.1136/bcr-2016-216862.

Part IV

Non-neoplastic Diseases of the Duodenum

9 Malabsorption and Malnutrition Disorders

Tsung-Teh Wu

Celiac Disease

Definition

Celiac disease is a common immune-mediated and genetically predisposed chronic malabsorptive disorder caused by intolerance to gluten. It is also known as celiac sprue, nontropical sprue, gluten-induced enteropathy, or gluten-sensitive enteropathy [1–4].

Clinical Features

Epidemiology Celiac disease can occur at any age and is approximately twice more common in women than in men [5]. The prevalence of celiac disease varies geographically and has increased in the past decades due to improved detection and awareness of disease. In Western and US population, the prevalence is around 1% [6–8]. The prevalence is even higher in patients at risk: up to 20% in first-degree relatives of celiac disease, 3–6% in type I diabetes, up to 15% in patients with iron deficiency anemia, and 1–3% in patients with osteoporosis [9]. Patients with Down's syndrome, Turner's syndrome, William's syndrome, and sarcoidosis also have increased risk of celiac disease [10–13].

Pathogenesis Ingestion of gluten is the prerequisite for the development of celiac disease, and environmental factors such as large-dose gluten exposure without ongoing breastfeeding, gastrointestinal infections, drugs, interferon α[alpha], and surgery may increase the risk or trigger the development of celiac disease [14, 15]. Celiac disease has a strong association with HLA-DQ heterodimers DQ2 and DQ8; HLA-DQ2 present in 95% and HLA-DQ8 in 5% of patients with celiac disease [16, 17]. Negative test for both HLA-DQ types makes diagnosis of celiac disease very unlikely [18]. The pathogenesis involves a T-cell-mediated immune response to gluten presented by HLA-DQ2 and HLA-DQ8 molecules. The gliadin peptides modified and deaminated by the tissue transglutaminase 2 (TG2) can bind with much higher affinity to HLA-DQ2 and HLA-DQ8 molecules and activate CD4-positive T cell in lamina propria, resulting in a cascade of inflammatory response, mucosal remodeling, and villous atrophy [19]. Untreated celiac disease patients typically have a high titer of antibody to tissue transglutaminase (IgA-TG2) and deaminated gliadin peptides [20–22].

Clinical Presentations Malabsorption with diarrhea, steatorrhea, weight loss, and failure to thrive are the classical presentations of celiac disease. Newly diagnosed celiac disease can also be asymptomatic or present with other symptoms such as anemia, vague abdominal pain, neuropathy, ataxia, depression, short stature, osteoporosis, and liver disease [23]. Iron deficiency anemia is a common manifestation of celiac disease and can occur in 33% of adult celiac disease patients [24]. Vitamin deficiency such as vitamin B12 deficiency can occur in 12–41% and low serum folate level in 35–49% of celiac disease patients [25]. Bone disease from malabsorption of calcium and/or vitamin D causing osteopenia, osteoporosis, or osteomalacia is frequent in celiac disease [26].

Endoscopic Findings Mucosal fold loss, scalloping, mosaic pattern, nodularity, fissuring, and prominent submucosal vascularity are the main endoscopic features of celiac disease (Fig. 9.1) [27, 28]. The endoscopic pattern differs between children and adults, and the mosaic pattern is commonly found in children. Video capsule endoscopy, double-balloon endoscopy, and chromoendoscopy can also be used to make diagnosis of celiac disease.

The pattern of villous atrophy is typical, with diffuse involvement of distal duodenum and proximal jejunum, but

T.-T. Wu (✉)
Department of Laboratory and Medical Pathology, Mayo Clinic, Rochester, MN, USA
e-mail: Wu.TsungTeh@mayo.edu

L. Zhang et al. (eds.), *Surgical Pathology of Non-neoplastic Gastrointestinal Diseases*,
https://doi.org/10.1007/978-3-030-15573-5_9

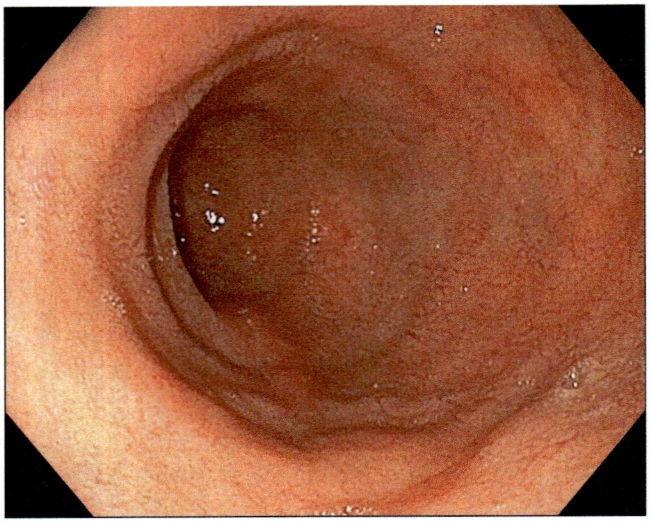

Fig. 9.1 Endoscopic features of celiac disease. The duodenum shows loss of normal duodenal folds with scalloping and mosaic pattern

villous atrophy can also be patchy and present in 9–19% of celiac disease [29–32]. Celiac disease with only isolated duodenal bulb involvement (ultrashort celiac disease) can occur in 9–13% of patients [33–36]. Inclusion of biopsy from duodenal bulb can increase the diagnostic yield of celiac disease. Multiple duodenal biopsies including at least four biopsies from distal duodenum and one or two from the duodenal bulb (either the 9- or 12-o'clock position) are recommended for diagnosing celiac disease [37].

Laboratory Findings Serological tests for celiac disease include endomysial antibody (EMA), IgA anti-transglutaminase antibodies (IgA TTG), IgG anti-transglutaminase antibodies (IgG TTG), and deaminated antigliadin antibodies (DGP, either IgA or IgG isotype). The serological tests for celiac disease should be performed with patients on gluten-contaminating diet. IgA TTG is the preferred single test for the detection of celiac disease in individuals over 2 years old with both sensitivity and specificity about 95% as recommended in the current American Gastroenterological Association (AGA) guideline [37]. For screening children younger than 2 years of age, the IgA TTG should be combined with IgA and IgG DGP. Of note, IgA deficiency is present in 2–3% of patients with celiac disease and is more common than in general population (1 in 400–800) [38]. Total IgA should be measured with IgG DGP in patients suspected with celiac disease and IgA deficiency [37].

A diagnosis of celiac disease should be based on the positive serology, history, endoscopic findings, and histological finding of villous atrophy on duodenal biopsy [37]. IgA TTG can be negative in 5–16% of patients with biopsy-confirmed celiac disease [21, 39]. Serological tests for celiac disease can be negative, particularly when patients are on gluten-free diets. A negative test for HLA-DQ2 and HLA-DQ8 can be used to exclude celiac disease in patients with equivocal duodenal biopsy or individuals following a gluten-free diet [40].

The requirement of duodenal biopsy for confirming the diagnosis of celiac disease has been challenging in the pediatric population. In 2012, the European Society for Paediatric Gastroenterology, Hepatology, and Nutrition (ESPGHAN) proposed that it may be possible to avoid any biopsy in children who meet the following criteria: characteristic symptoms of celiac disease, IgA TTG levels >10x the upper limit of normal, confirmed by detection of EMA and positive HLA-DQ2/DQ8 [41]. Using this criteria, >50% of children and adolescents with celiac disease can be diagnosed without duodenal biopsy; however, biopsy still is required for confirming the diagnosis for celiac disease in adults [42]. Duodenal biopsy can also be used to differentiate celiac disease from other causes of malabsorptive disorders.

Pathological Features

A well-orientated duodenal biopsy is required to determine the villous height-to-crypt depth (Vh:Cd) ratio for the evaluation of villous atrophy. The normal duodenal mucosa should have a Vh:Cd ratio >3 and scattered intraepithelial lymphocytes (IELs) (<25 per 100 enterocytes) with so-called decrescendo pattern which are more prominent along the lateral edge of villi decreasing from the base toward the tip of villi (Fig. 9.2). The characteristic histological features of celiac disease include villous atrophy, crypt hyperplasia, chronic inflammation in lamina propria, and increased IELs [43]. Increased IELs in celiac disease are present at the tip of villi or even distribution along

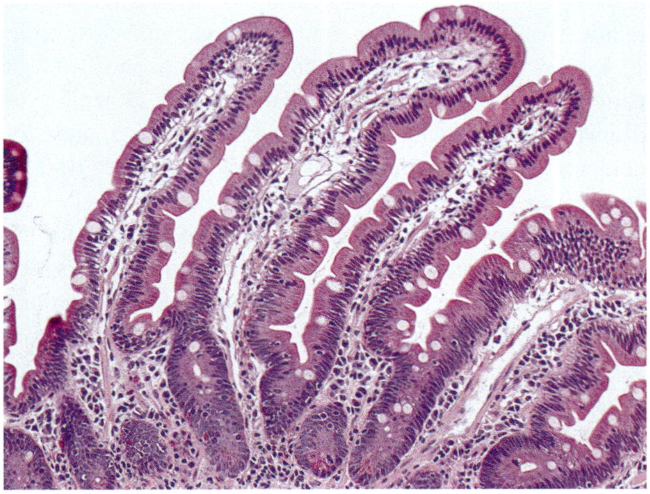

Fig. 9.2 Normal duodenal mucosa. The villous height-to-crypt depth (Vh:Cd) ratio is >3 with scattered intraepithelial lymphocytes (IELs) <25 per 100 enterocytes, which are more prominent along the lateral edge of villi decreasing from base toward tip of villi (decrescendo pattern)

the length of villi [44]. The IEL count should be assessed on H&E section and can be counted in 20 villous-tip enterocytes in five villi or 50 enterocytes in two villi [8, 45]. The characteristic histological features primarily affect proximal small bowel including duodenum and proximal jejunum, but rarely celiac disease can also affect terminal ileum. The pathological changes present in the terminal ileum are predominantly IELs with >25/100 epithelial cells present in 17–60% of cases, and villous atrophy is only rarely present [46–48].

The grading scheme to classify the histological spectrum of celiac disease was first introduced by Marsh in 1992 [49] and later modified by Oberhuber in 1999 [50]. The Marsh-Oberhuber grading scheme describes four different types of small bowel injury based on the degree of villous atrophy, absence or presence of crypt hyperplasia, and presence of IELs >40 per 100 enterocytes (Table 9.1). Type 1 is the infiltrative type with normal Vh:Cd ratio >3 and increased IELs (Fig. 9.3a–c). Type 2 is the infiltrative-hyperplastic type with

Table 9.1 Histological classification of celiac diseases

Marsh–Oberhuber	Histologic features	Corazza-Villanancci
Type 1	Normal Vh:Cd ratio, increased IELs[a]	Grade A
Type 2	Normal Vh:Cd ratio, crypt hyperplasia, increased IELs	Grade A
Type 3a	Mild villous atrophy, increased IELs	Grade B1
Type 3b	Subtotal villous atrophy, increased IELs	Grade B1
Type 3c	Total villous atrophy, increased IELs	Grade B2
Type 4[b]	Flat mucosa, normal IELs	

[a]Increased IELs is defined as >40 per 100 enterocytes determined from biopsies taken from distal small bowel by Crosby capsule, where the IELs are greater in number in the Marsh-Oberhuber classification as compared to >25 per 100 enterocytes in the Corazza-Villanacci classification determined from endoscopic biopsy from duodenum

[b]Marsh-Oberhuber Type 4 was deleted in Corazza-Villanacci classification

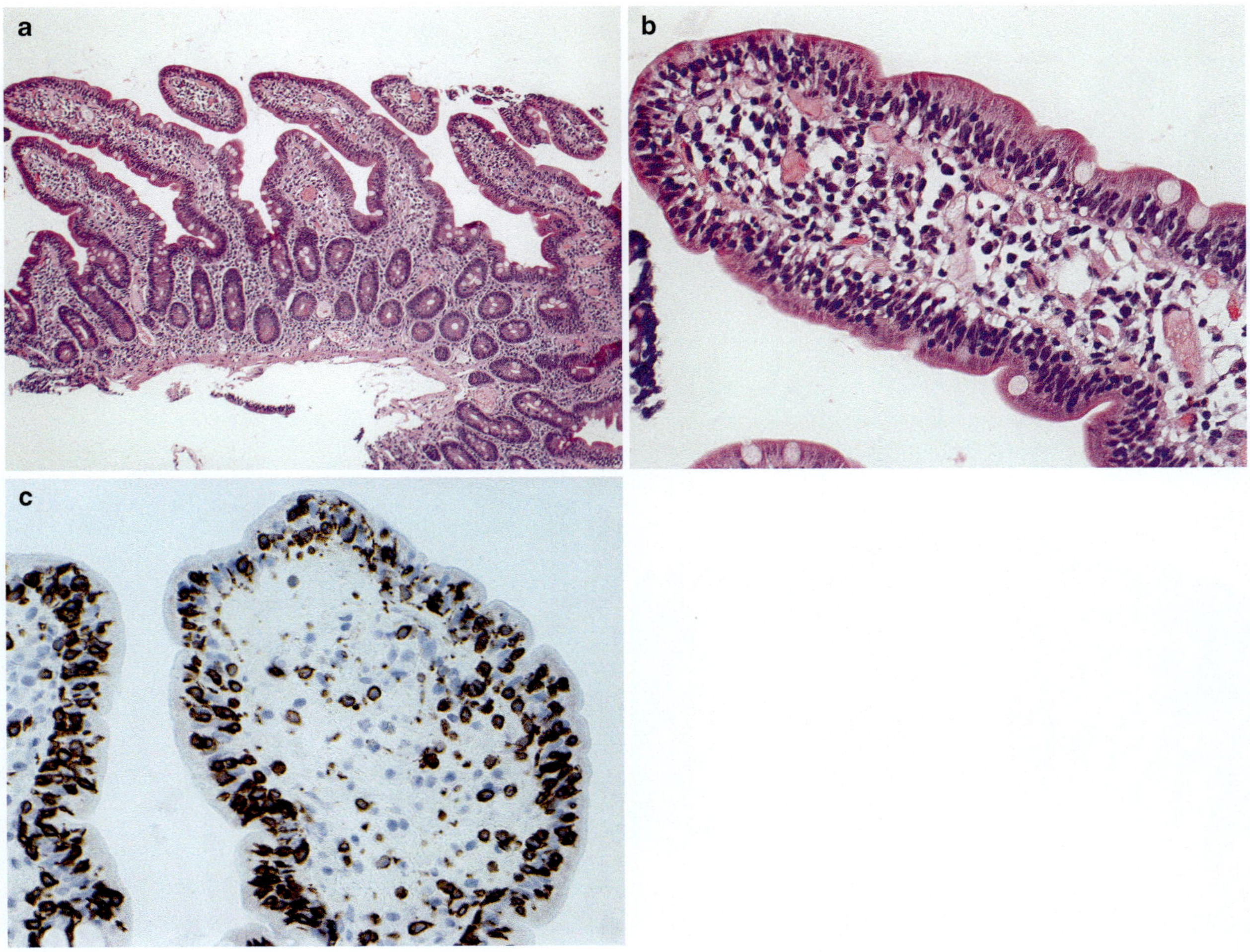

Fig. 9.3 Celiac disease with increased intraepithelial lymphocytes but normal villous architecture. (**a**) The duodenal biopsy shows normal Vh:Cd ratio and increased intraepithelial lymphocytes along the entire length of the villi on low-power view. (**b**) A high-power view of the tip of duodenal villi reveals prominent intraepithelial lymphocytosis. (**c**) A CD3 immunohistochemical stain highlights the presence of intraepithelial lymphocytosis

normal Vh:Cd ratio >3, crypt hyperplasia, and increased IELs. This is a very rare pattern and seen in experimental conditions and in patients with dermatitis herpetiformis. Type 3 is the destructive type with presence of villous atrophy and increased IELs and can be further subdivided into type 3a (mild villous atrophy, Vh:Cd ratio between 1 and 3), type 3b (subtotal villous atrophy, Vh:Cd ratio >0 but <1), and type 3c (total villous atrophy, Vh:Cd = 0) based on the degree of villous atrophy (Fig. 9.4a–d). Type 4 is the atrophic type with flat mucosa, only a few crypts identified, and near-normal IELs. This is a very rare pattern and is usually seen in patients with refractory sprue, ulcerative jejunoileitis, and enteropathy-associated T-cell lymphoma. There is significant interobserver variation in using Marsh-Oberhuber grading scheme. A simplified grading scheme was proposed by Corazza and Villanacci in 2005 [51] and divided the mucosal lesions into two grades (Grade A and B). Grade A is non-atrophic lesion with increased IELs >25 per 100 enterocytes (equivalent to Marsh-Oberhuber Types 1 and 2), and Grade B is atrophic lesion with increased IELs >25 per 100 enterocytes (B1 equivalent to Marsh-Oberhuber Types 3a and 3b, and B2 equivalent to Marsh-Oberhuber type 3c) (Table 9.1). Increased IELs defined as >40 per 100 enterocytes were originally determined from biopsies taken from distal small bowel by Crosby capsule in the Marsh-Oberhuber classification which is higher than the >25 per 100 enterocytes used in the Corazza-Villanacci classification determined from endoscopic biopsy from duodenum.

Colonic lymphocytosis can present in 30% of colonic biopsies from celiac disease patients [52]. Microscopic colitis (75–80% lymphocytic colitis and 20–25% collagenous colitis) is present in 4% of patients with celiac disease, a

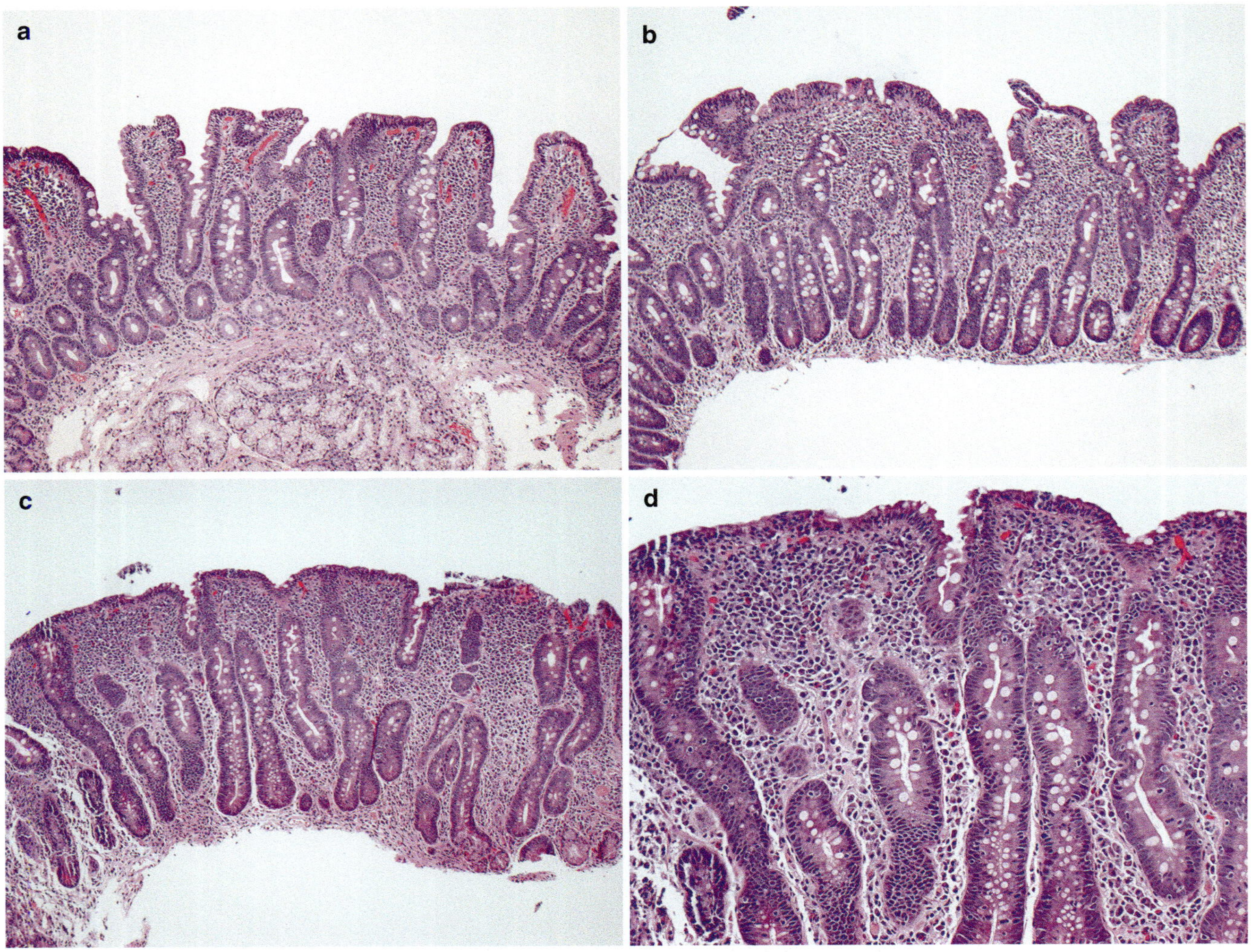

Fig. 9.4 Celiac disease with villous atrophy and increased intraepithelial lymphocytes (IELs). (**a**) Duodenal biopsy from celiac disease shows mild villous atrophy with a Vh:Cd ratio >1 but less than 3 and IELs. (**b**) Celiac disease with subtotal villous atrophy (Vh:Cd ratio <1) and IELs. (**c**) Celiac disease with total villous atrophy with IELs. (**d**) The duodenal biopsy in celiac disease shows marked increased chronic inflammatory cells composed of predominantly plasma cells in the lamina propria and crypt hyperplasia. The surface columnar epithelia show reactive epithelial changes with the presence of prominent intraepithelial lymphocytes

50–70-fold increase as compared to general population [53, 54]. Microscopic colitis is commonly present after the diagnosis of celiac disease [53]. On the other hand, celiac disease is also frequently diagnosed in 15% of patients with microscopic colitis [55] and in 13% of patients with collagenous colitis [56]. Lymphocytic gastritis is also found in 36–42% of pediatric celiac disease patients [57, 58] and in one-third of celiac disease patients [59].

Differential Diagnosis

Duodenal intraepithelial lymphocytosis and villous atrophy are not unique for celiac disease and can be seen in a variety of other conditions (Table 9.2). Lymphocytic duodenitis can be present in 3.8% of population negative for celiac serology [8] and seen in association with infections such as *Helicobacter pylori* and *Giardia* infection, tropical sprue, drugs such as nonsteroidal anti-inflammatory drugs (NSAIDs), IgA deficiency, common variable immunodeficiency (CVID), and inflammatory bowel disease such as Crohn's disease [3, 60, 61]. The distribution of IELs of the decrescendo pattern with IELs more prominent at the crypt and lower part of the villi is not typical for celiac disease. The distribution pattern of IELs in celiac disease without villous atrophy can be continuous with even distribution along the villi or in the tip of villi [44]; however, these distribution patterns of IELs are not unique to celiac disease without villous atrophy and can also be seen in IELs with normal villous architecture associated with other conditions described in Table 9.2 [60, 62–64].

Villous atrophy can also be seen in infections, drugs such as Olmesartan, food hypersensitivity, immune disorders, lymphoma, and nutritional deficiency disorders [37, 65, 66]. Acute inflammation such as cryptitis and crypt abscess (Fig. 9.5) is not a main histological feature of celiac disease, but it can present in 53% of newly diagnosed celiac disease and cannot be used as a pathological feature to exclude celiac disease [47, 67]. Gastric mucinous metaplasia commonly seen in peptic-type duodenitis can also present in celiac disease (Fig. 9.6).

Table 9.2 Histological differential diagnosis of celiac disease

Increased ILEs and normal villous architecture	Villous atrophy ± increased IELs
Dermatitis herpetiformis	Dermatitis herpetiformis
Helicobacter pylori gastritis	Tropical sprue
Bacterial overgrowth syndrome	Bacterial overgrowth syndrome
Nonsteroidal anti-inflammatory drugs (NSAIDs)	Autoimmune enteropathy
Olmesartan	Olmesartan
Crohn's disease	Crohn's disease
Infections (*Giardia*, *Cryptosporidium*, viral, etc.)	Collagenous sprue
Food hypersensitivity (Cow's milk, soy, etc.)	Refractory sprue
Peptic duodenitis	Eosinophilic enteritis
Common variable immunodeficiency (CVID)	CVID
IgA deficiency	Whipple's disease
Systemic autoimmune disease (rheumatoid arthritis, SLE, Hashimoto thyroiditis, etc.)	Lymphoma Mycobacterial infection Microvillous inclusion disease Tufting enteropathy Chemotherapy Nutritional deficiency

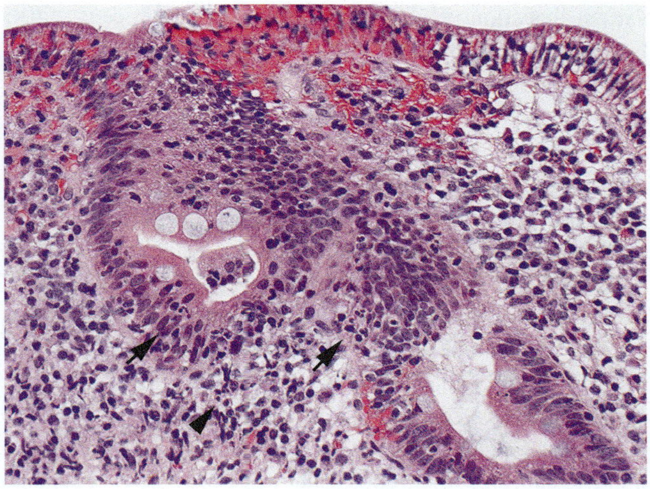

Fig. 9.5 Celiac disease with acute inflammation. A duodenal biopsy from patient with celiac disease demonstrates villous atrophy, IELs, increased chronic inflammatory cells in lamina propria and presence of acute inflammation within the lamina propria (arrowhead) and cryptitis (arrows)

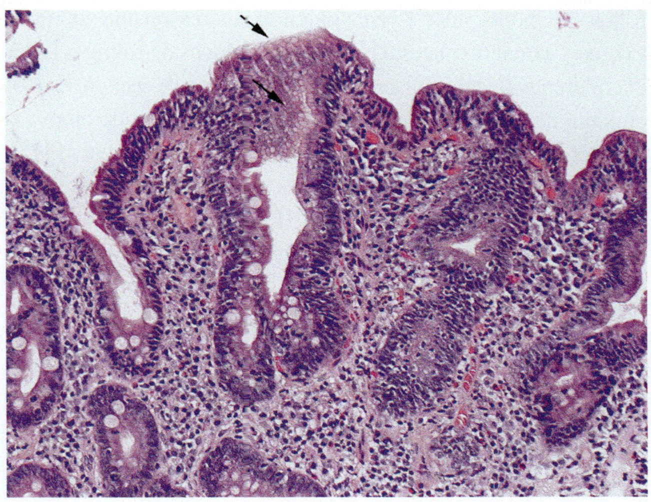

Fig. 9.6 Celiac disease with gastric mucinous metaplasia. A duodenal biopsy from patient with celiac disease demonstrates villous atrophy, IELs, increased chronic inflammatory cells in lamina propria, and presence of gastric mucinous metaplasia (arrow) seen in peptic-type injury

In the presence of negative celiac serology and negative HLA-DQ2 and HLA-DQ8, pathologists should promptly consider nonceliac entities which can mimic celiac disease when duodenal biopsy shows increased IELs and villous atrophy [68].

Treatment and Prognosis

Patients with celiac disease require lifelong adherence to a gluten-free diet (GFD). Currently, there are no medications that can be reliably used to prevent small bowel mucosal injury caused by gluten exposure in celiac disease patients [37, 69]. Nonresponsive celiac disease with persistent symptoms occurs in 4–30% patients after initiation of GFD, and inadvertent ingestion of gluten is the most common cause [70]. Food intolerance, small intestinal bacterial overgrowth, pancreatic insufficiency, irritable bowel syndrome, and refractory celiac disease (RCD) can also be the cause of non-responsive celiac disease [70–72]. Celiac serologic titers decrease soon after initiation of GFD and can be negative or normal after being on GFD for 2 years [73]. Persistent elevation of celiac serology is seen in celiac disease patients with ongoing small mucosal injury on GFD, but is not a sensitive marker for predicting presence of mucosal atrophy [74]. Ongoing mucosal atrophy can also be seen in celiac disease patients with normal or negative celiac serology on GFD [74, 75].

Histological recovery is slow and delayed in adult celiac disease on GFD as compared to symptomatic and serological improvement [75, 76]. In adult celiac disease, 57–76% of patients can achieve mucosal healing on GFD, and neither symptoms nor serology is reliable to predict ongoing small bowel injury on GFD [74, 75, 77, 78]. Complete mucosal healing with normal duodenal histology is seen in 34% at 2 years and 66% at 5 years with the median time of 3 years in celiac disease patients on GFD [75]. A follow-up biopsy after 2 years on GFD is a reasonable approach to access extent of mucosal healing [37]. Mucosal healing is faster in children with celiac disease on GFD and can be seen in 95% of children 2 years after following GFD [77]. A follow-up biopsy is not recommended routinely in children with celiac disease [37].

RCD is uncommon in patients with celiac disease [72, 79, 80], and patients with type II RCD is associated with increased mortality and can progress to enteropathy-associated T-cell lymphoma [79]. Patients with celiac disease have increased risk of non-Hodgkin lymphoma and small intestinal adenocarcinoma [81–83] and increased risk of death due to cardiovascular diseases, pulmonary diseases, and cancer [84].

Refractory Celiac Disease

Definition

Refractory celiac disease (RCD), also known as refractory sprue, is defined by persistent or recurrent malabsorptive symptoms and presence of small intestinal villous atrophy despite strict adherence to GFD for more than 12 months in the absence of other causes of nonresponsive treated celiac disease and overt lymphoma [65, 70, 72, 85]. The majority of RCD patients are diagnosed due to development of new symptoms and recurrence of diarrhea after initial response to GFD for years (secondary RCD). Primary RCD occur in a subset of RCD patients who never have response to GFD [65]. RCD is subdivided into type I and type II. Type I RCD has increased IELs with normal T-cell phenotype, and type II RCD has aberrant T-cell phenotype or monoclonal population T cells [65].

Clinical Features

Epidemiology RCD is uncommon and affects 0.7–1.5% of patients with celiac disease [72, 86]. RCD is two to three times more common in women than in men [79, 80]. Type I RCD is more common than type II RCD in the USA [72].

Pathogenesis Type I RCD is histologically similar to active celiac disease and could represent an increased sensitivity to gluten or delayed response to withdrawal of gluten. Viral infection such as *Rotavirus* or hepatitis B may play a role in developing RCD [87]. RCD has different mucosal effector cytokine profile as compared to active celiac disease. IL-15, TNF-α*[alpha]*, IL-6, and IL-17A are upregulated in RCD [87, 88]; and high Smad7 is associated with defective TGF-beta1 signaling, causing sustained inflammatory cytokine production in RCD [89]. Cytogenetic alteration such as partial trisomy 1q22–44 is frequently observed in type II RCD, and this gain of 1q can also be seen in 16% of enteropathy-associated T-cell lymphoma [90].

Clinical Presentations Persistent malabsorptive symptoms such as diarrhea, abdominal pain, and weight loss are the most common symptoms. Anemia, fatigue, malaise, multiple vitamin deficiencies, thrombotic events, and co-existing autoimmune disorders are also frequent in patients with RCD [65, 91, 92].

Endoscopic and Image Findings Macroscopic features of villous atrophy and ulcerations are frequently seen in RCD. Large ulceration (>1 cm) or ulcerative jejunitis is common in patients with type II RCD [79, 80]. Mesenteric lymphadenopathy and nonspecific small intestinal abnormalities such as bowel wall thickening are present in up to 50% of patients with RCD [79].

Laboratory Findings Positive celiac serology is present in 19–30% of patients with RCD despite on strict GFD [79, 80]. HLA-DQ2 is present in 98% of RCD patients, and the remaining cases almost all have HLA-DQ8. Chronic elevation of transaminase is present in 50% of RCD patients [80].

Pathological Features

Histological features of RCD are similar to active celiac disease. The differentiation between type I and type II RCD is based on the detection of abnormal intraepithelial lymphocyte phenotype by different methods including immunohistochemistry, flow cytometry, and molecular analysis of T-cell receptor clonality [65, 93, 94]. Normal duodenal intraepithelial lymphocytes have normal surface makers and are CD3+, CD7+, CD8+, and TCR+. Type I RCD has polyclonal IELs and normal T-cell phenotype (Fig. 9.7a–c). Type II RCD has abnormal intraepithelial T cells showing loss of normal surface CD3, CD8, and TCR with preservation of cytoplasmic CD3 (CD3ε), and presence of TCR chain (γ and δ) clonal rearrangement by PCR. Immunohistochemistry with combination of CD3 and CD8 is more commonly used than flow cytometry for detection of abnormal IEL phenotype. Typical type II RCD shows CD3ε+/CD8-phenotype by immunohistochemistry (Fig. 9.8a–c). Type II RCD can rarely present with normal CD3+/CD8+ phenotype but with monoclonal TCR gene rearrangement by PCR [95]. Detection of TCR clonal rearrangement by PCR is required to confirm the presence of clonal IELs and should be used along with CD3 and CD8 immunohistochemistry for evaluation of patients with RCD [65].

Differential Diagnosis

T-cell lymphoma including small intestinal CD4+ or CD8+ T-cell lymphoma and enteropathy-associated T-cell lymphoma should be differentiated from RCD. In RCD, the histological features are similar to active celiac disease, and no morphological features of lymphoproliferative disease are present. Small intestinal CD4+ or CD8+ lymphoproliferative disorder is a heterogeneous and indolent lymphoma with prolonged survival which can also clinically and morphologically mimic celiac disease [96–99]. Duodenal atrophy, intraepithelial lymphocytic infiltrates predominantly involving crypts rather

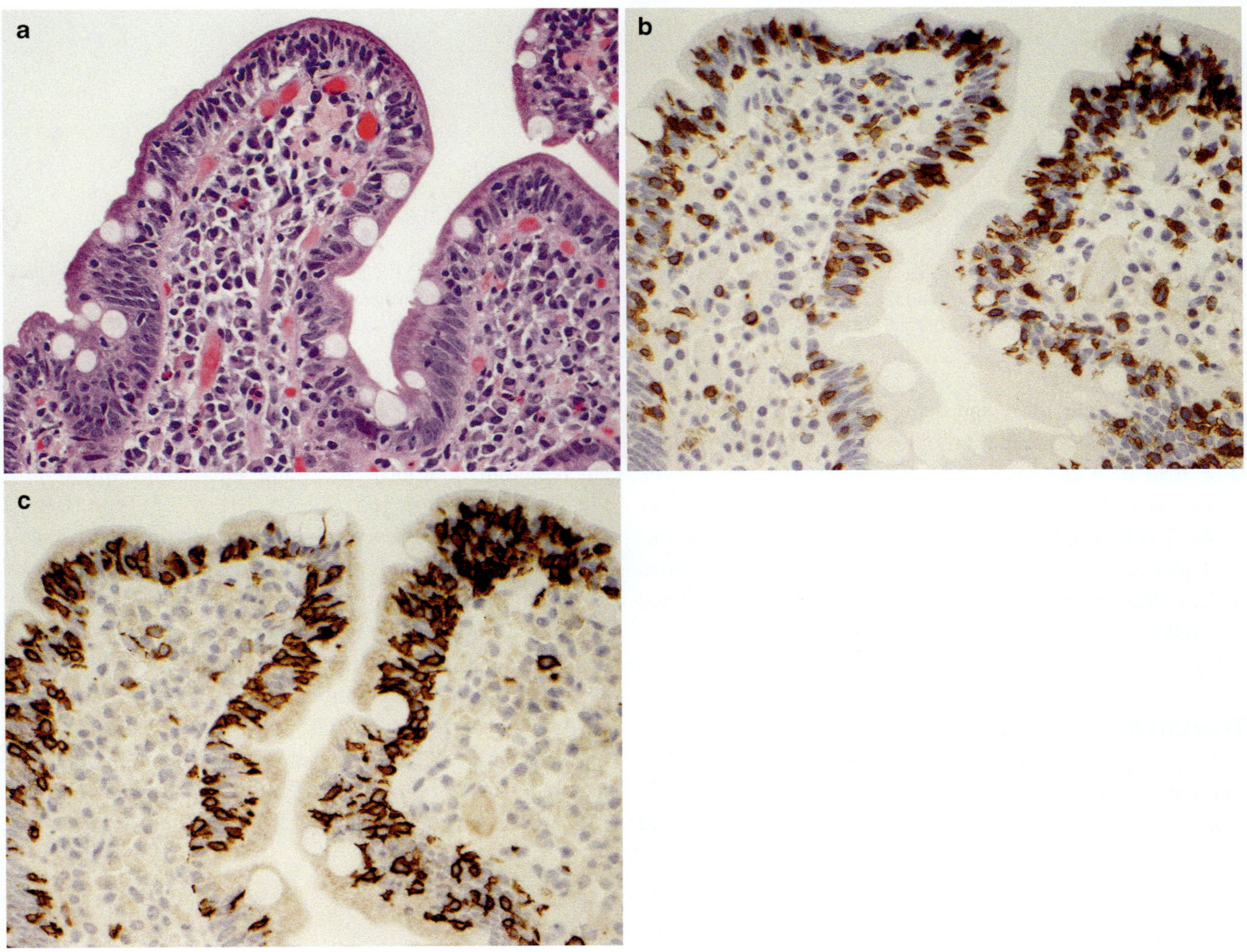

Fig. 9.7 Type I refractory celiac disease. (**a**) A duodenal biopsy from type I RCD shows villous atrophy and IELs. The IELs have normal T-cell phenotype and express both CD3 (**b**) and CD8 (**c**) by immunohistochemical stains

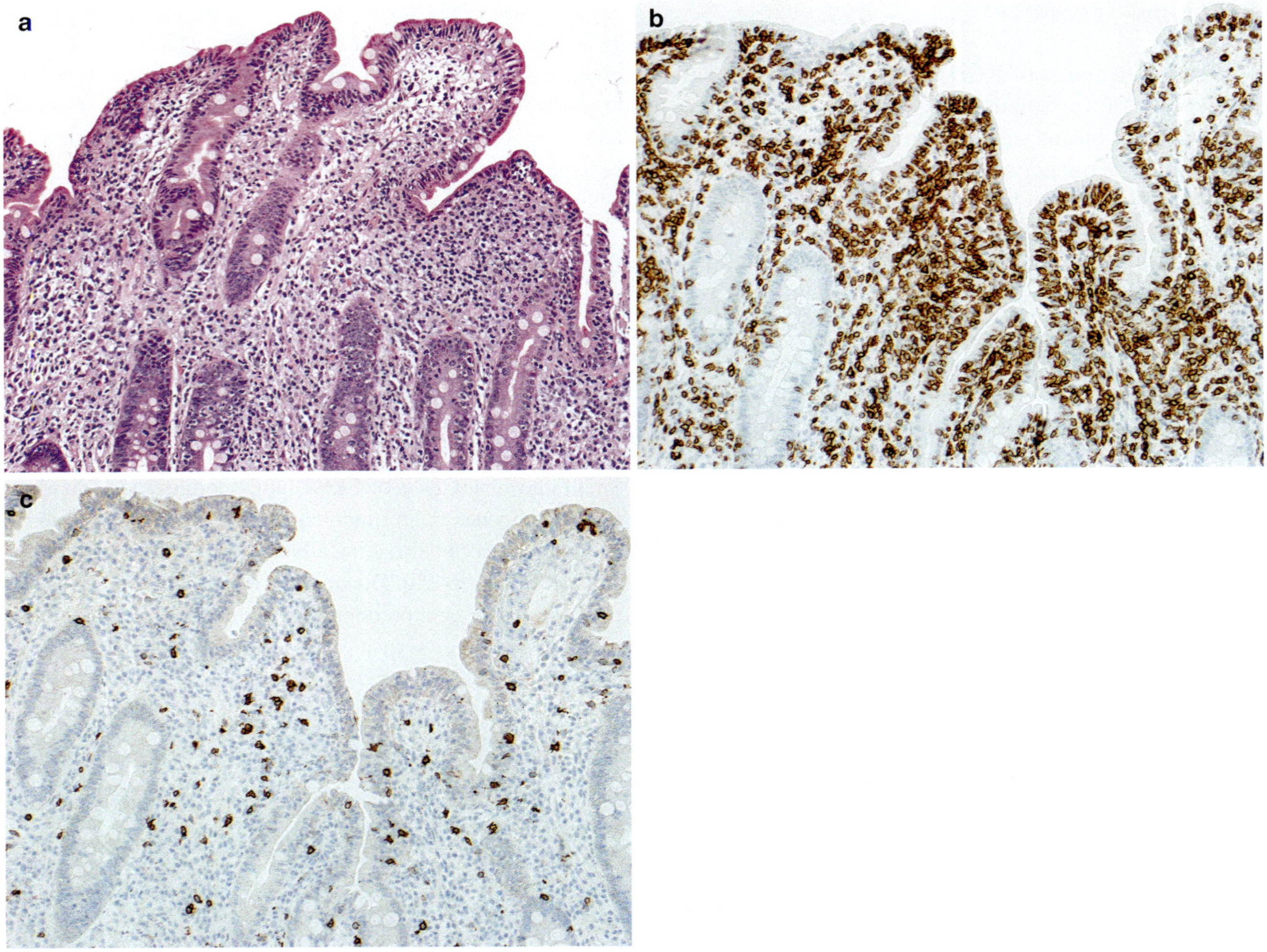

Fig. 9.8 Type II refractory celiac disease. (**a**) A duodenal biopsy from Type II RCD shows villous atrophy and IELs. The IELs have abnormal intraepithelial T cells with loss of normal surface CD3 with preservation of cytoplasmic CD3 (CD3ε) (**b**), and loss of normal CD8 expression (**c**) by immunohistochemical stains

than surface epithelium, and dense infiltrates of small-sized CD3+ T-lymphocytes that are CD4+/CD8– or CD8+/CD4– (Fig. 9.9a–e) with clonal TCR gene rearrangement are the characteristic histological features of small intestinal CD4+ or CD8+ T-cell lymphoma. These are in contrast to the prominent plasma cells, but not T-lymphocytes present in celiac disease. Recurrent *STAT3-JAK2* fusions have been identified in small intestinal CD4+ lymphoproliferative disorder [100].

Treatment and Prognosis

There is no standard treatment for RCD patients [37, 69, 87]. The general approach is elimination of gluten exposure and symptomatic control. Prednisone, budesonide, or a combination of prednisone and azathioprine is effective for clinical symptomatic improvement and mucosal healing in most type I RCD patients [65, 79, 80, 101, 102]. Type II RCD patients have more severe symptoms and signs than type I RCD and are less likely to respond to therapy. There are no treatments with proven efficacy for type II RCD. A variety of immunosuppressive agents including systemic steroids, enteric-coated budesonide, azathioprine, methotrexate, cyclosporine, anti-TNF antibodies, and cladribine have been used to treat type II RCD [37].

Low serum albumin and anemia are frequent findings and may indicate poor prognosis [79, 101]. The prognosis of type I RCD is much better than type II RCD. The 5-year survival

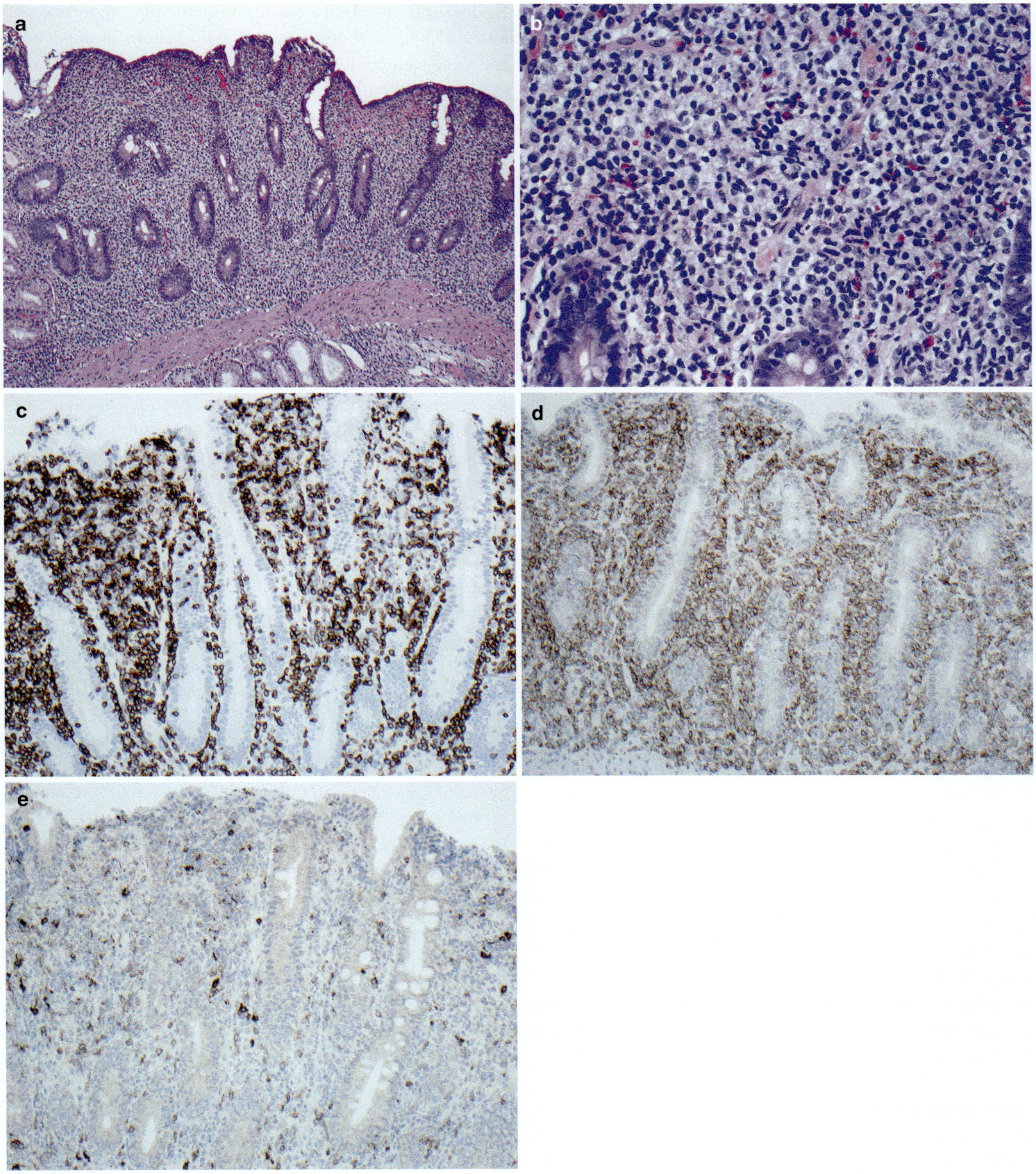

Fig. 9.9 Small intestinal CD4+ lymphoproliferative disorder can mimic refractory sprue. (**a**) A duodenal biopsy shows total villous atrophy and IELs. (**b**) The lamina propria is expanded by a monotonous infiltrate of small-sized mononuclear cells but no plasma cells on high-power view The mononuclear cell infiltrates in lamina propria are CD3+ T-lymphocytes (**c**) and are positive for CD4 (**d**) but negative for CD8 (**e**) by immunohistochemical stains

rate is 40–58% for patients with type II RCD [79, 80, 101]. The poor prognosis is largely due to frequent (33–52%) progression to overt enteropathy-associated T-cell lymphoma in type II RCD patients [80, 103].

Collagenous Sprue

Definition

Collagenous sprue (CS) is characterized by chronic diarrhea and malabsorption with presence of severe villous atrophy and subepithelial collagen deposition in small bowel mucosa [104–107].

Clinical Features

Epidemiology CS is a rare type of small bowel enteropathy. Collagenous sprue was first described by Schein in 1947 [108] and histologically confirmed in 1970 [109]. CS has been previously recognized as refractory sprue or unclassified sprue, and approximately 50% of the refractory sprue patients developed collagenous sprue during follow-up [110].

Pathogenesis The pathogenesis and etiology of CS are unknown. Associated immune-mediated disorders are present in 70% of CS, and celiac disease is the most frequent [106]. Other associated diseases include autoimmune enteropathy, hypogammaglobulinemia, hypothyroidism, microscopic colitis, and increased IgG4-positive plasma cells [106, 111]. Environmental factors and drugs such NSAIDs and olmesartan can be the contributing factors for CS [66]. Increased collagen synthesis with inadequate fibrolysis appears to contribute to the broad collagen band deposition in CS. The prominent subepithelial collagen deposition is due to increased expression of main fibrogenic genes: procollagen I and tissue inhibitor of MMP-1(TIMP-1) by myofibroblastic cells and unaltered fibrolytic matrix metalloproteinases (MMPs) [112].

Clinical Presentations CS is more common in women than in men with a 2:1 female-to-male ratio and typically affects middle-aged to elderly women [104–106]. CS accounts for 30–50% of the refractory sprue cases [110, 113]. Severe diarrhea and weight loss are the most common presentations for CS [106]. Approximately one-third of CS patients are associated with celiac disease [104, 106], and this association is even higher (89%) in the study by Vakiani [105]. Collagenous colitis, lymphocytic colitis, collagenous gastritis, and lymphocytic gastritis are frequently present in patients with CS [104–106].

Endoscopic Findings Mucosal nodularity, reduction of mucosal fold, scalloping, and mosaic pattern in duodenum and upper jejunum commonly seen in celiac disease can be seen in CS as well.

Pathological Features

Villous atrophy (total or subtotal) with subepithelial collagen deposition is the key histological feature of CS (Fig. 9.10a). The normal thickness of basement in small bowel is <1.5 μm, and mild thickening of basement or fibrosis up to 5 μm can be seen more than half of active celiac disease without clinical significance [105, 114]. In CS, the collagen band can be of variable thickness, and there is no consensus regarding the minimal thickness of the collagen band for the diagnosis of CS. The minimal thickness of the collagen band required for the diagnosis of CS varies between 5 and 12 μm among different studies [105, 107, 110]. Similar to the collagenous colitis, the broadened subepithelial collagen band extends into the lamina propria with irregular and jagged border. Entrapped capillaries and stromal and inflammatory cells are present in CS (Fig. 9.10a). Trichrome stain can be used to confirm the presence of thickened subepithelial collagen band (Fig. 9.10b). The collagen deposition can be diffuse or patchy [106]. The subepithelial collagen deposition is frequently accompanied with surface epithelial injury, and epithelial detachment can be seen in 66–100% of CS. Increased IELs are present in 25–70% of CS (Fig. 9.10c) [104–106]. Increased chronic inflammatory cells including lymphocytes, plasma cells, and occasionally eosinophils are present in the lamina propria. Increased IgG4-positive plasma cells in lamina propria can be present in 23% of CS [111]. Acute inflammation can be present in surface epithelium and crypts in 40–50% of small bowel biopsies from CS [105, 106].

The degree of mucosal abnormality seen in biopsy does not correlate with the patients' clinical symptoms, but the overall length of involved small bowel correlates with the severity of clinical presentation [115]. Clonal T cell by TCR gene rearrangement PCR can be detected in CS associated with type II refractory sprue [105] and in five of six CS cases tested [104].

Differential Diagnosis

Thickening of the basement membrane due to tangential sectioning of the duodenal mucosa can mimic thickening of the subepithelial collagen band, and deeper H&E sections with better oriented small bowel mucosa or trichrome stain can be used to resolve this issue. Increased lamina propria fibrosis associated with erosion or ulceration needs to be differentiated from subepithelial collagen deposition in CS. Fibrosis associated with erosion and ulceration is not limited to the

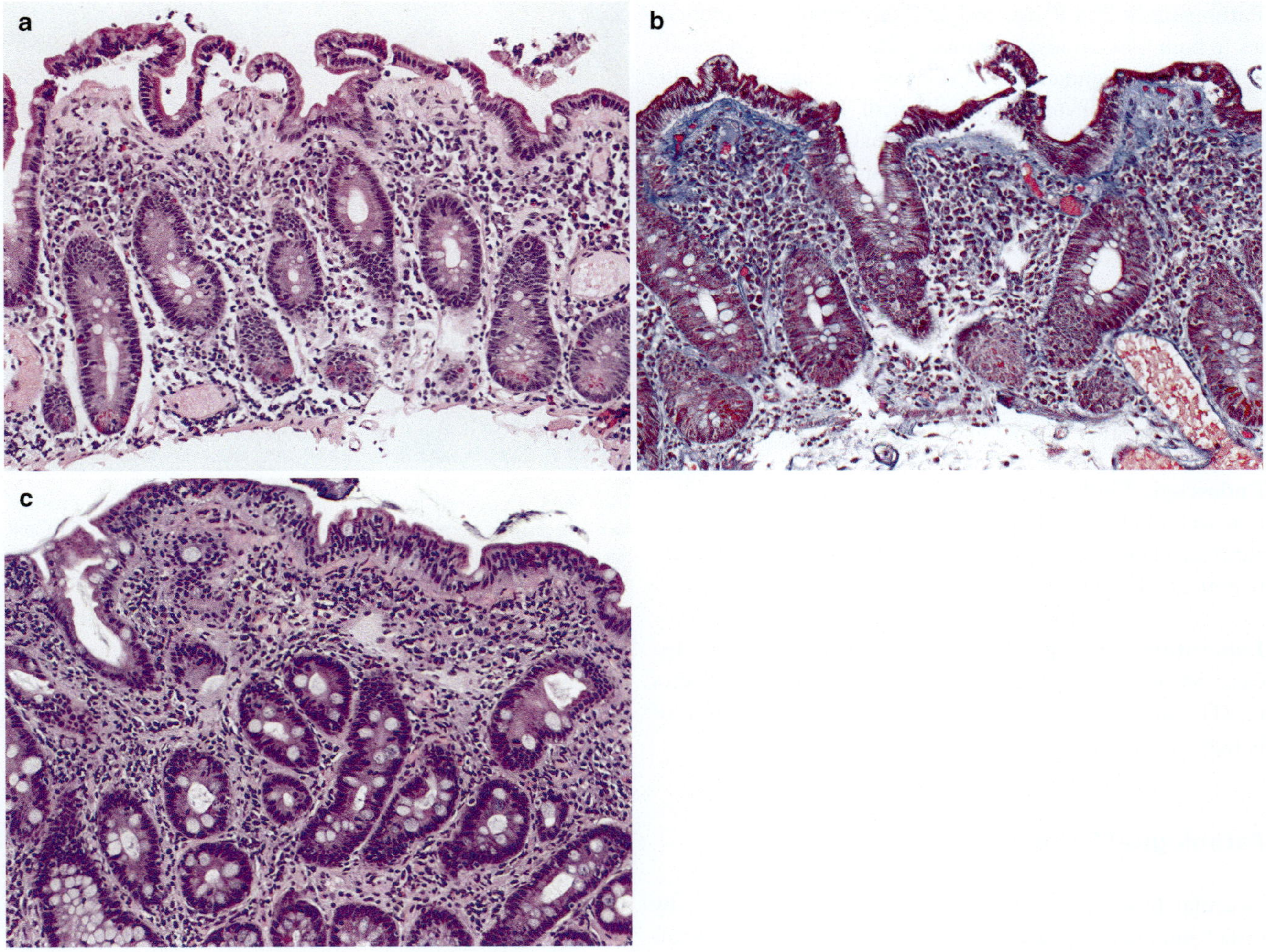

Fig. 9.10 Collagenous sprue. (**a**) Duodenal biopsy shows total villous atrophy with subepithelial collagenous band deposition. The broadened subepithelial collagen deposition extends into the lamina propria with irregular and jagged border, entrapped capillaries, and stromal and inflammatory cells. (**b**) Trichrome stain confirms the presence of thickening subepithelial collagenous band deposition. (**c**) An example of increased intraepithelial lymphocytes present in collagenous sprue

subepithelial location and typically involves a wide area of lamina propria. Amyloid deposits in particular when present as subepithelial deposition can mimic CS, and a Congo red stain can be used to confirm the diagnosis of amyloid deposits.

Treatment and Prognosis

The prognosis of CS was thought to be poor with high morbidity due to severe malnutrition and mortality, but recent studies have shown that good clinical outcomes could be achieved in up to 80% of CS patients with GFD and immunosuppressive treatment [105, 106]. Patients with CS do not develop lymphoma, but they can occasionally die from complications of malnutrition [104–106]. Perforation of small bowel is a rare complication of CS [116].

Dermatitis Herpetiformis

Definition

Dermatitis herpetiformis (DH) is the cutaneous manifestation of gluten-sensitive enteropathy precipitated by exposure to gluten diet, characterized by the deposition of granular IgA in the papillary dermis and subclinical small bowel villous atrophy or intraepithelial lymphocytosis [117, 118].

Clinical Features

Epidemiology DH can appear at any ages and is more common in middle-aged adults with a slightly male predominance. DH is relatively common in northern Europe with a prevalence of 30–75 per 100,000 and rare in Asia [118].

Pathogenesis In patients with DH, circulating IgA antibodies to both tissue transglutaminase (TG2) and a high-avidity epidermal transglutaminase (TG3) are present. The pathogenesis of DH involves deposition of IgA-TG3 antibody and TG3 immunocomplex in the dermal-epidermal junction with subsequent activation of TG3 by stretching, pressure, or other factors and results in inflammatory response influx into the papillary dermis [118, 119].

Clinical Presentations DH is a blistering, itching skin rash typically on the elbows, knees, and buttocks. Patients with DH are mostly asymptomatic and rarely present with abrupt and severe gastrointestinal symptoms or signs of malabsorption that are typically seen in celiac disease [118, 120].

Endoscopic Findings Features of celiac disease, including mucosal fold loss, scalloping, mosaic pattern, nodularity, fissuring, and prominent submucosal vascularity can be present in patients with DH but with a lesser degree.

Laboratory Findings Similar to patients with celiac disease, HLA DQ2 is present in 95–100%, and IgA antibodies to TG3 and TG2 (IgA TTG) are present in up to 95% of patients with DH [118, 121].

Pathological Features

Granular IgA deposits at the dermal-epidermal junction by direct immunofluorescence on the skin biopsy from unaffected skin close to an active lesion is required for the diagnosis of DH. In the biopsies from small bowel, villous atrophy is present in 70–75% of patients, and the remaining 25–30% of patients have intraepithelial lymphocytosis (Fig. 9.11) [118, 122–124]. The degree of villous atrophy is less severe in DH than in celiac disease [124].

Differential Diagnosis

Duodenal intraepithelial lymphocytosis and villous atrophy are not unique for DH and can be seen in celiac disease and a variety of other conditions (Table 9.2).

Treatment and Prognosis

A lifelong GFD is the treatment choice for both skin rash and small bowel enteropathy for patients with DH. It takes several weeks to months for the skin rash to respond to the GFD, and dapsone is used with GFD to treat the skin lesions [118]. The prognosis of DH on GFD is excellent [125], and only a small subset (1.7%) of patients of DH may have active rash

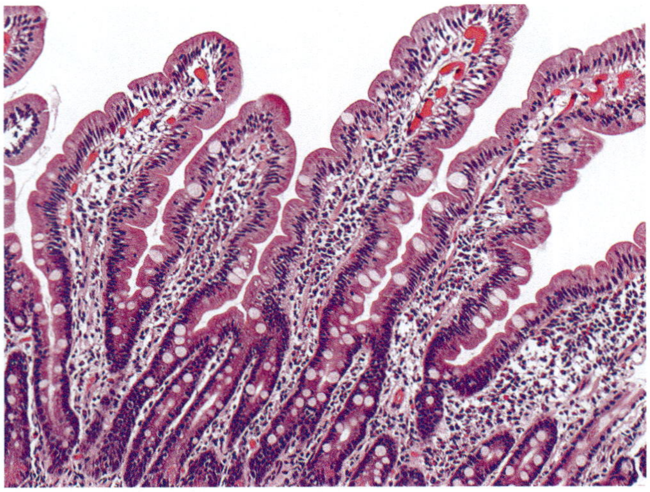

Fig. 9.11 Dermatitis herpetiformis. Duodenal biopsy from a patient with dermatitis herpetiformis shows normal villous architecture and increased intraepithelial lymphocytes

but recovered small bowel mucosa although on strict GFD [118]. The risk of non-Hodgkin's lymphoma is increased up to ten times in patients with DH, but GFD for more than 5 years appears to be protective [126–128].

IgA Deficiency

Definition

IgA deficiency is characterized by absent or decreased serum IgA level of <7 mg/ml in individuals older than 4 years in the presence of normal levels of both IgG and IgM and exclusion of other causes of hypogammaglobulinemia and T-cell defect as well as normal IgG antibody response to all vaccinations [129, 130].

Clinical Features

Epidemiology Selective IgA deficiency is the most common primary antibody deficiency [129] with a prevalence of 1:600 in general population in the Western world [131]. The prevalence varies in different ethnicities, ranging from 1:143 to 1:965 in Caucasian populations, but it is less frequent among Asians [130, 132]. IgA deficiency is present in 2–3% of celiac disease patients, an approximately 10–15-fold increased frequency as compared to general population [133, 134].

Pathogenesis IgA is the most abundant antibody isotype produced in the body and is the second most common isotype in serum following IgG. IgA has circulating monomeric form and secretary dimeric form in the intestinal tract [135]. In the intestinal tract, Peyer's patches, isolated lymphoid follicles, and lamina propria can be the site of local IgA production by T-cell-dependent or T-cell-independent mechanisms [129]. Bacteria endogenous to the intestinal tract are coated with secretary IgA, causing limited epithelial adherence and penetration; therefore, the bacteria are confined to the mucosal surface [136]. Patients with IgA deficiency has a maturation defect in B-cells to produce IgA [137], and this can be due to intrinsic B-cell defect, T-cell abnormalities, and abnormality in cytokine network [129, 130, 135]. Secretary IgM production is increased as a compensatory mechanism in most IgA-deficient patients [138]. IgA deficiency is a heterogeneous group of genetic abnormalities composed of variable chromosomal abnormalities, cytogenetic defects, and monogenic mutations [130]. Mutations in the *TNFRSF13B* gene encoding transmembrane activator and calcium-modulator and cyclophilin ligand interactor (TACI), which has a role in the isotype switching in B cells, have been found in a subset of IgA deficiency and common variable immunodeficiency (CVID) patients [139, 140]. A shared cytotoxic T lymphocyte-associated protein-4-inducible co-stimulator risk locus (CTLA4-ICOS) has been defined in celiac disease, IgA deficiency, and CVID [141].

Clinical Presentations Most (85–90%) of the individuals with IgA deficiency are asymptomatic. Some patients with IgA deficiency can develop recurrent sinopulmonary infections, gastrointestinal infections, autoimmune disorders, allergies, and malignancy [129, 130]. Recurrent sinopulmonary infection is the most common disease, occurring in 40–90% of symptomatic patients with IgA deficiency. Autoimmune disorders can occur in 5–30% patients with IgA deficiency [142–144]. The common autoimmune disorders in patients with IgA deficiency are idiopathic thrombocytopenic purpura, Graves' disease, autoimmune hemolytic anemia, type I diabetes mellitus, rheumatoid arthritis, systemic lupus erythematosus, and celiac disease [145]. The rate of gastrointestinal disorders in IgA deficiency is not high; giardiasis, malabsorption, celiac disease, lactose intolerance, ulcerative colitis, Crohn's disease, pernicious anemia, nodular lymphoid hyperplasia, and colonic adenocarcinoma have been reported [146–151]. Allergic diseases such as allergic rhinitis, conjunctivitis, urticarial, eczema, food allergy, and asthma are common presentations in 40% patients with IgA deficiency. Approximately 25% of patients with IgA deficiency are identified during evaluation of allergic diseases [152]. A severe anaphylactoid transfusion reaction can rarely be seen in patients with IgA deficiency.

Laboratory Findings Serum IgA level is <7 mg/ml with normal IgG and IgM levels. Screening for celiac disease in IgA-deficient patients should use IgG DGP instead of IgA TTG [37].

Pathological Features

Increased IELs without villous atrophy (Fig. 9.12a) is the most common histological feature in duodenal biopsy from patients with IgA deficiency [153]. Villous atrophy, increased IELs, and increased chronic inflammation in lamina propria can be seen in patients with IgA deficiency

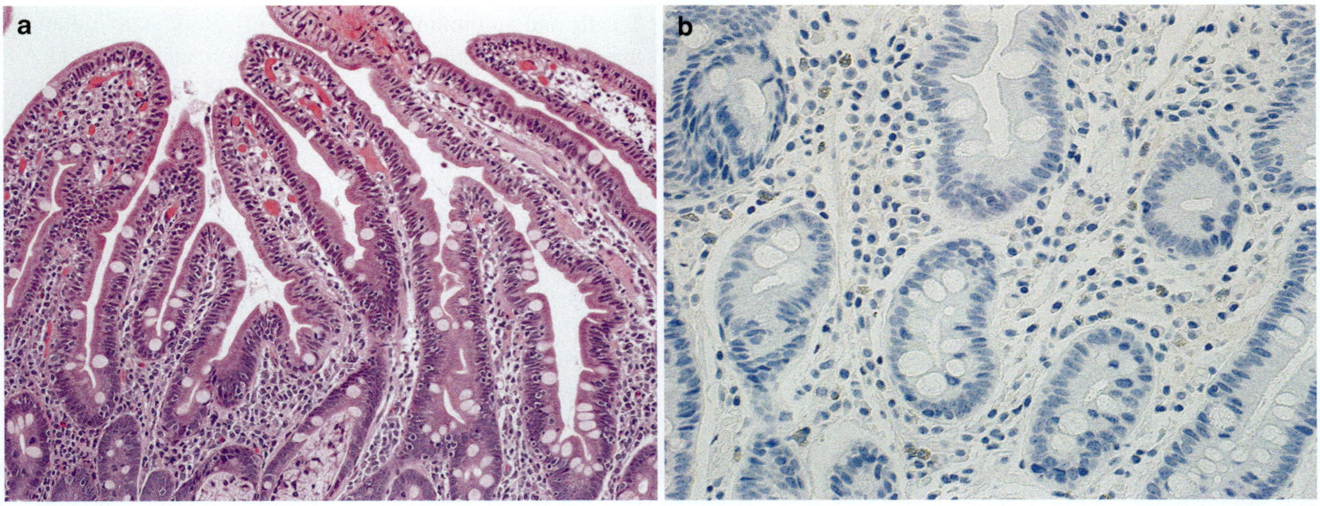

Fig. 9.12 IgA deficiency. (**a**) A duodenal biopsy from IgA deficiency patient shows presence of increased intraepithelial lymphocytes but normal villous architectures. (**b**) The plasma cells present within lamina propria are negative for IgA by immunohistochemical stain. (**c**) IgM-positive plasma cells in lamina propria are increased by immunohistochemical stain

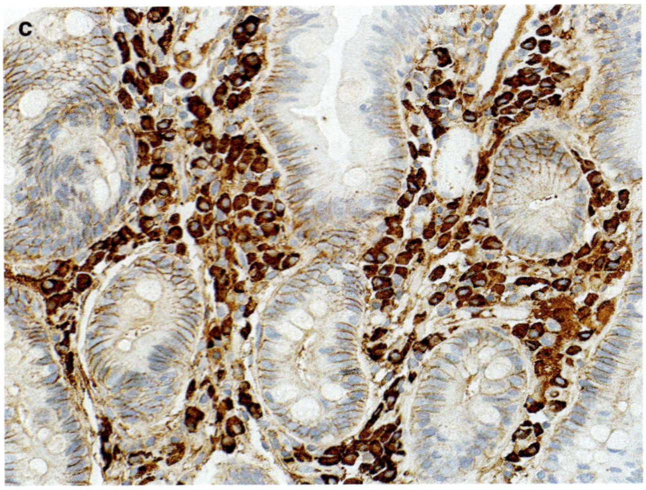

Fig. 9.12 (continued)

and celiac disease. The plasma cells are present within the lamina propria, and these plasma cells are negative for IgA (Fig. 9.12b) by immunohistochemical stain and the IgM-positive plasma cells are increased (Fig. 9.12c). Giardia infection [146] and nodular lymphoid hyperplasia [154, 155] can be present in duodenal biopsy from IgA-deficient patients (Fig. 9.13a, b).

Differential Diagnosis

Lymphocytic duodenitis can occur in a variety of diseases (Table 9.2), and identification of decreased or absent IgA-positive plasma cells in lamina propria with decreased serum IgA level is required to confirm the diagnosis of IgA deficiency. Nodular lymphoid hyperplasia is not specific for IgA deficiency and can also occur in CVID, lymphoproliferative disorders, and immunodeficiency.

Treatment and Prognosis

In asymptomatic patients with IgA deficiency, no treatment is needed except for the awareness of potential anaphylactic transfusion reaction. In symptomatic IgA-deficient patients, the treatments are individualized and targeted at the associated disorders. The prognosis depends on the associated disorders and is good in patients without associated disorders. IgA deficiency and CVID can occur in the same families, and it is also known that IgA deficiency may progress to CVID [156, 157]. The incidence of cancer in patients with IgA deficiency is not increased [158], and there are sporadic case reports of lymphoid and gastrointestinal malignancy [159, 160].

Autoimmune Enteropathy

Definition

Autoimmune enteropathy (AIE) is characterized by severe and protracted diarrhea, lack of response to exclusion diet, small intestinal villous atrophy, and presence of circulating autoantibodies or evidence of predisposition to autoimmune disease [161–164].

Clinical Features

Epidemiology AIE is a rare cause of intractable diarrhea which was first described by Walker-Smith in a 15-month-old child [165] and is primarily a pediatric disease affecting infants within the first 6 months of life. The estimated incidence is <1 in 10,000 infants and is the most frequent diagnosis in up to 25–29% of children with intractable diarrhea [163, 166, 167]. AIE can also affect adults [162, 168, 169].

Pathogenesis The underlying pathogenesis of AIE is not well understood but appears to result from dysregulation of intestinal immune function. There are two syndromic forms of AIE: IPEX (immunodysregulation, polyendocrinopathy, enteropathy, and X-linked syndrome) and APECED (autoimmune phenomenon, polyendocrinopathy, candidiasis, and ectodermal dystrophy) [170, 171]. IPEX is an X-linked recessive disorder and typically presents in infancy with AIE, insulin-dependent diabetes mellitus, and cutaneous manifestation of eczema, atopic dermatitis, and alopecia. IPEX is caused by loss-of-function mutations in Forkhead box 3 p3 (FOXP3), a transcriptional regulator critical for the normal development and function of regulatory T cells. Loss of FOXP3 activity leads to hyperactivation of immune cells by CD4+ effector T cells and autoimmune disease [172]. Rare gene mutations that affect the regulation of T-cell function, including CTLA4, CD25, STSAT1, STAT3, STAT5B, and ITCH, can have IPEX-like phenotype [173]. APECED, also known as autoimmune polyglandular syndrome type 1 (APS 1), is an autosomal recessive disease present in early childhood and adolescence and is characterized by malabsorption, diarrhea, adrenal gland insufficiency, and hypoparathyrodism. APECED is caused by loss-of-function mutations in the autoimmune regulator (AIRE) gene, which encodes a transcription factor (autoimmune regulator protein) regulating the expression of self-antigens in the thymus, presented by HLA molecules to maturing T cells. Defects in AIRE lead to the development of T cells that recognize self-antigens, resulting in autoimmune diseases [174]. Circulating autoantibodies to goblet cells or enterocytes and aberrant expression of HLA class II molecules by enterocytes are often detected in AIE patients [161, 162, 175].

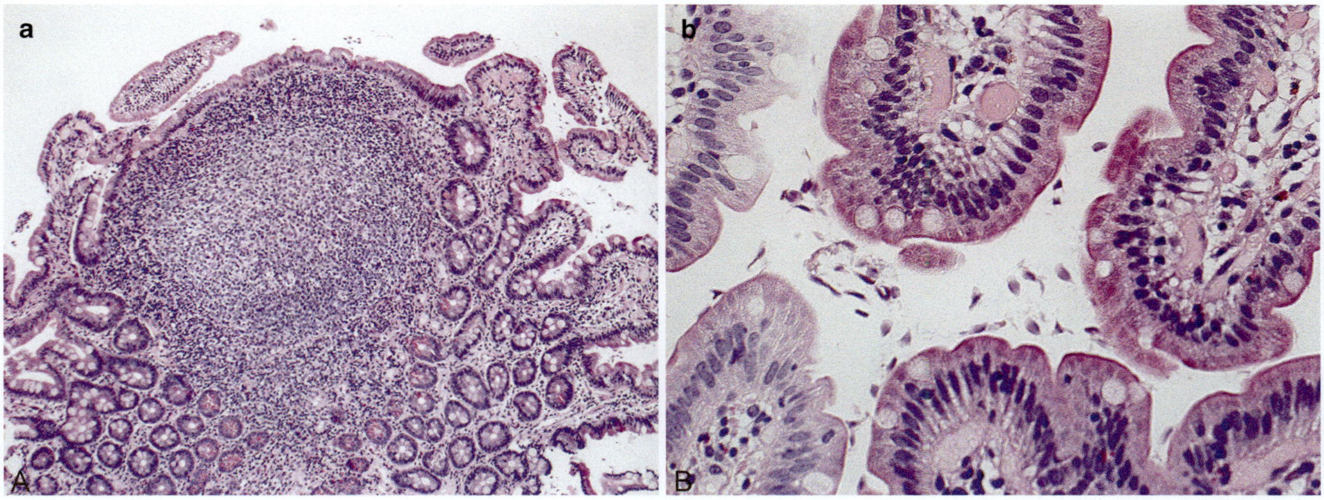

Fig. 9.13 Nodular lymphoid hyperplasia and Giardia infection in IgA deficiency. (**a**) A duodenal biopsy from IgA-deficiency patients shows presence of nodular lymphoid hyperplasia and Giardia infection without presence of acute inflammation. (**b**) Luminal pear-shaped Giardia parasites are demonstrated on high-power view

Clinical Presentations AIE in pediatric patients typically present within weeks or first 6 months of life with severe and life-threatening diarrhea requiring parental nutrition [163, 173]. The intestinal malabsorption leads to slow growth and low body weight. Local and systemic infections are common due to loss of skin and gut barriers, poor nutrition, and immunosuppressive therapies. The manifestation of pediatric AIE can be isolated to gastrointestinal tract or be part of systemic primary immunodeficiency disorders such as IPEX and APECED [171, 173]. Adult AIE presents with malabsorption, chronic diarrhea, and severe weight loss and is often initially being suspected to have gluten-sensitive enteropathy but not responsive to GFD [162, 163]. AIE is associated with other autoimmune diseases including type I diabetes mellitus, rheumatoid arthritis, autoimmune hepatitis, autoimmune thyroiditis, and CVID [162, 169]. AIE has been reported in patients with thymoma [162, 176, 177]. Multisystem extraintestinal manifestations including endocrine, pulmonary, renal, liver, hematologic, and musculoskeletal system involvement can occur in AIE [163, 164].

Endoscopic Findings In adult AIE, gross abnormalities with scalloping, fissuring, mosaic pattern, and villous atrophy can be seen in 53% of duodenum by esophagogastroduodenoscopy and in 71% of proximal small bowel by capsular enteroscopy [162].

Laboratory Findings Antienterocyte antibodies are present in 64–80% of AIE patients and antigoblet cell antibodies in 43% of patients [162, 169, 171]. The presence of autoantibodies to goblet cells or enterocytes is not specific for AIE and can be seen in other diseases and should be considered in conjunction with clinical manifestation and histological findings for the diagnosis of AIE. Antienterocyte antibodies can be seen in HIV infection, and antigoblet cell antibodies can be present in inflammatory bowel disease, celiac disease, and allergic enteropathy [164, 173]. Other autoantibodies including antinuclear antibody, antismooth muscle antibody, antiparietal cell antibody, and antibody against villin can also be present [164].

Pathological Features

Villous atrophy, increased chronic inflammatory infiltrates composed of plasma cells and lymphocytes in lamina propria, lymphocytic infiltrates in deeper crypts, increased crypt apoptotic bodies, IELs, and absence of goblet cells and/or Paneth cells can be present in AIE [162, 171]. The histological features can be grouped into four histological patterns: (1) active chronic duodenitis/enteritis, (2) celiac disease-like, (3) graft-versus-host-disease-like, and (4) mixed/no prominent pattern [169]. Active chronic duodenitis/enteritis characterized by moderate to severe villous atrophy, expansion of lamina propria by mononuclear inflammatory cells, and scattered acute inflammation such as cryptitis or crypt abscess is the most common histological pattern and occurs in 52% of adult and pediatric AIE (Fig. 9.14a) [169]. Celiac disease-like pattern with villous atrophy, crypt hyperplasia, and surface IELs (Fig. 9.14b) is the second most common pattern present in 21% of adult and pediatric AIE [169]. Prominent crypt epithelial cell apoptosis with villous atrophy and relative absence of inflammation, a histological pattern similar to graft-versus-host disease (Fig. 9.14c),

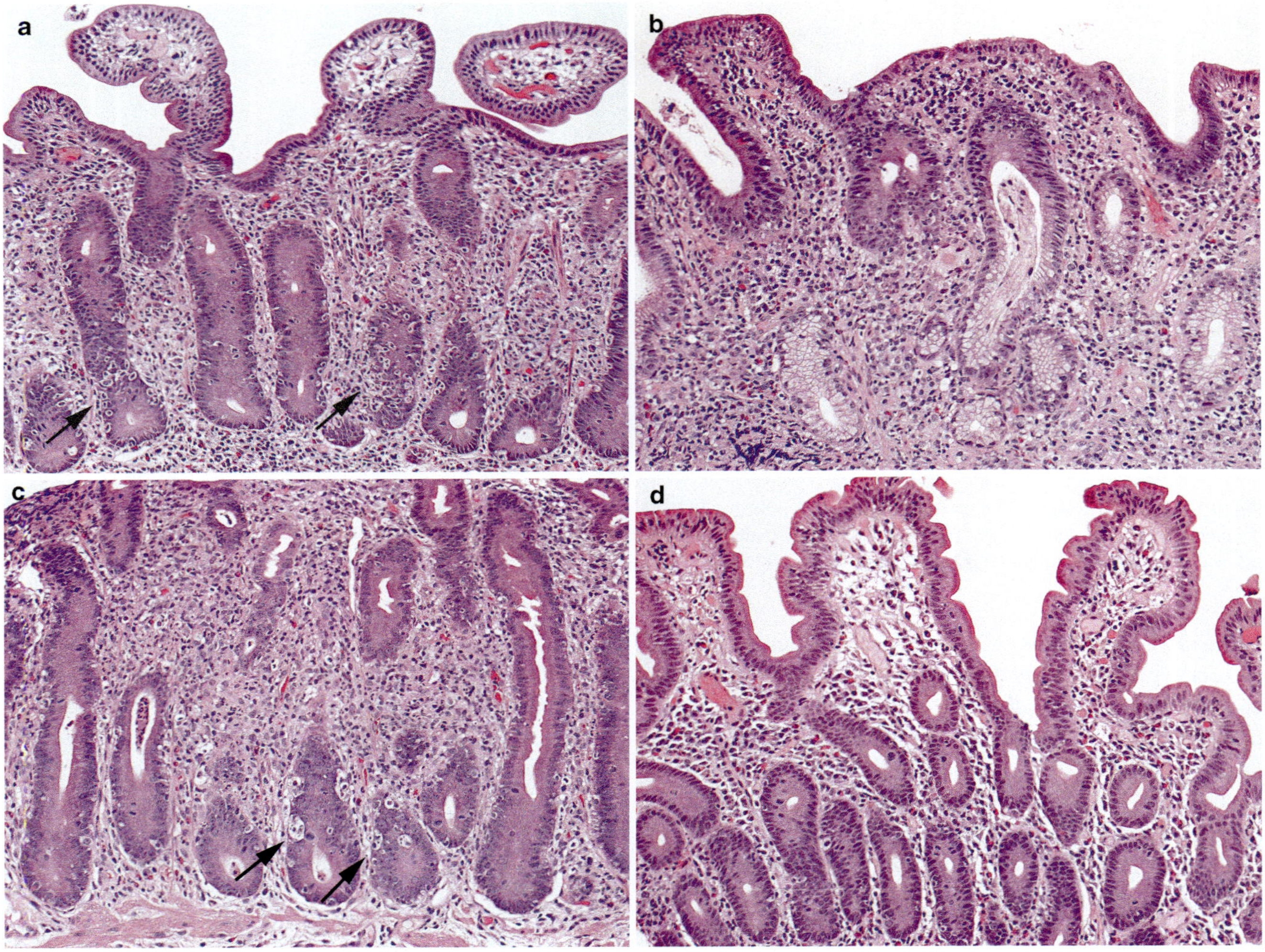

Fig. 9.14 Histological patterns in autoimmune enteropathy. (**a**) Active chronic duodenitis/enteritis pattern. Duodenal biopsy shows moderate to severe villous atrophy, expansion of lamina propria by mononuclear inflammatory cells and acute inflammation with cryptitis (arrows). (**b**) Celiac disease-like pattern with villous atrophy, crypt hyperplasia, and increased surface intraepithelial lymphocytes. (**c**) Graft-versus-host disease-like pattern with prominent crypt epithelial cell apoptosis (arrows), villous atrophy, and mild acute inflammation. (**d**) Duodenal biopsy shows the absence of goblet cells and Paneth cells

is present in 17% of adult and pediatric AIE [169] and is commonly (75%) seen in AIE in patients with IPEX [170]. The mixed/no predominant pattern characterized by villous atrophy, mononuclear cell infiltrate in lamina propria, and increased crypt apoptosis, but the histological features are not sufficient for the three abovementioned histological patterns, is present in 13% of AIE. Histological features seen in duodenum are also present in ileum [169]. Absence of goblet cells and/or Paneth cells (Fig. 9.14d) can present in 8–60% of pediatric and adult AIE [162, 169, 171, 173].

In AIE, mucosal abnormalities do not only involve small intestine. In the majority of the patients, at least one other gastrointestinal location demonstrates evidence of mucosal injury, with stomach (71–86%) being the most commonly affected site, followed by colon (50–64%) and esophagus (28–69%) [169, 171, 173]. Chronic gastritis is the most common pattern of gastric mucosal change, and active chronic gastritis, lymphocytic gastritis, and autoimmune atrophic gastritis-like pattern have also been described in patients with AIE. Active chronic inflammation is present in 32–50% of colonic biopsy from AIE patients, and lymphocytic colitis, increased crypt apoptosis, and absence of goblet cells can also occur [169, 171]. In patients with esophagus involvement, reactive epithelial changes are the most common features, and eosinophilic infiltrates in the squamous mucosa can present in 22% of patients with AIE [169, 171].

Differential Diagnosis

The main differential diagnoses for AIE include celiac disease, refractory sprue, inflammatory bowel disease, graft-versus-host disease, and drug-associated injury due to the nonspecific histological features seen in AIE. Celiac disease can be differentiated from AIE by the presence of positive celiac serology and clinical response to GFD. Inflammatory bowel disease, either Crohn's disease or ulcerative colitis, involving duodenum can present as active chronic duodenitis/enteritis pattern and the known history of inflammatory bowel disease is the key to differentiate from AIE. Drug-associated small bowel injury seen in immunomodulatory drugs such as anti-CTLA-4 (ipilimumab), anti-PD-1/PD-L1 (nivolumab and pembrolizumab) and idelalisib (a phosphoinositide 3-kinase inhibitor) can present as active chronic duodenitis/enteritis pattern mimicking AIE [178–180]. CMV and HIV infection and drugs such as NSAIDs and mycophenolate mofetil can also present with graft-versus-host-like pattern and need to be differentiated from AIE.

Treatment and Prognosis

Patients with AIE often require total parental nutrition and systemic steroids. Immunosuppressive agents such as azathioprine, methotrexate, mycophenolate mofetil, tacrolimus, cyclosporine, infliximab, and rituximan have been used in AIE refractory to steroid with varying successes [164, 173]. Most of the pediatric AIE with IPEX patients receive hematopoietic stem cell transplants [169, 181]. The prognosis typically depends on the severity of symptoms and the underlying etiologies. Histological improvement (partial or complete response) is seen in 73–93% of patients following therapy, although it is not always correlated with clinical findings [162, 169, 171]. Death due to diarrhea refractory to immunosuppressive therapy in both adults and children has been reported [162, 169, 171].

Olmesartan-Associated Enteropathy

Definition

Olmesartan is an angiotensin II receptor blocker (ARB) used for the treatment of hypertension. Severe enteropathy with chronic diarrhea and weight loss can be associated with olmesartan, and clinical and histological improvement of enteropathy occurs after suspension of olmesartan [66, 182, 183].

Clinical Features

Epidemiology Olmesartan-associated enteropathy is a rare disease, and the prevalence among the olmesartan users has not been determined [182, 183]. Olmesartan-associated enteropathy is the second most common (26%) etiology next to seronegative celiac disease (28%) for villous atrophy in patients with negative celiac serology [184].

Pathogenesis The mechanisms of olmesartan-associated enteropathy are unknown. Cell-mediated inflammatory immunity injury has been suggested because of the long delay between the initiation of olmesartan therapy and development of enteropathy. ARBs have been suggested to have inhibitory effects on TGFβ[beta] action which is important in the maintenance of gut immune homeostasis [66]. Olmesartan-associated enteropathy shares a similar immunopathogenetic pathway with increased CD8+ cells and overexpression of IL-15 by epithelial cells in duodenum seen in celiac disease [185] Enteropathy associated with ARBs other than olmesartan has rarely been reported in patients taking irbesartan, valsartan, and telmisartan [182, 186, 187].

Clinical Presentations Olmesartan-associated enteropathy affects both men and women and mostly affects older patients in their seventh to eighth decades of life [66, 182, 188]. Chronic diarrhea and weight loss are the most common presentations, and other common symptoms include nausea, vomiting, abdominal pain, bloating, and fatigue [66, 189]. The clinical symptoms occur months or years after the olmesartan therapy [183]. The clinical symptoms can be severe which require hospitalization in 64% of patients [66].

Endoscopic Findings Endoscopic features of olmesartan-associated enteropathy have not been well characterized, but can show mucosal nodularity, villous atrophy, and ulceration [189].

Laboratory Findings HLA DQ2/DQ8 is frequently present in 43–92% of patients with olmesartan-associated enteropathy, and celiac serology is typically negative [66, 183]. Normocytic anemia, hypoalbuminemia, electrolyte abnormalities, zinc deficiency, and small bowel bacterial overgrowth can also occur [66]. Antienterocyte antibody and antigoblet cell antibody can rarely be detected in patients with olmesartan-associated enteropathy [66, 190].

Pathological Features

Olmesartan-associated enteropathy has a spectrum of histological features including celiac sprue-like, collagenous sprue, autoimmune enteropathy-like, and graft-versus-host disease-like patterns [66, 183, 190]. Villous atrophy (total or partial) is the most common finding seen in 95% of duodenal biopsies, followed by intraepithelial lymphocytosis in 70%, chronic inflammation in lamina propria, and thickening subepithelial collagen band (collagenous sprue) in 30% (Fig. 9.15) [183]. Acute inflammation is also common in 73% of duodenal biopsy [66]. Increased crypt apoptosis and paucity of goblet cells can occasionally present in duodenal biopsies [183, 190]. No aberrant T-cell phenotypes have been detected within the intraepithelial lymphocytes in olmesartan-associated enteropathy [66, 182, 190]. Sprue-like histological features such as villous atrophy and crypt hyperplasia tend to be more frequently present in patients with abdominal pain and taking olmesartan as compared with other ARBs [191].

Colon and stomach can also be involved by olmesartan-associated enteropathy. Lymphocytic or collagenous colitis is present in 19–100% of patients with olmesartan-associated enteropathy [183]. Colonic crypt apoptosis, acute inflammation, and active chronic inflammation have been also reported [66, 183]. Lymphocytic or collagenous gastritis is present in 14–100% of patients with olmesartan-associated enteropathy [183]. Active chronic gastritis can also occur [66].

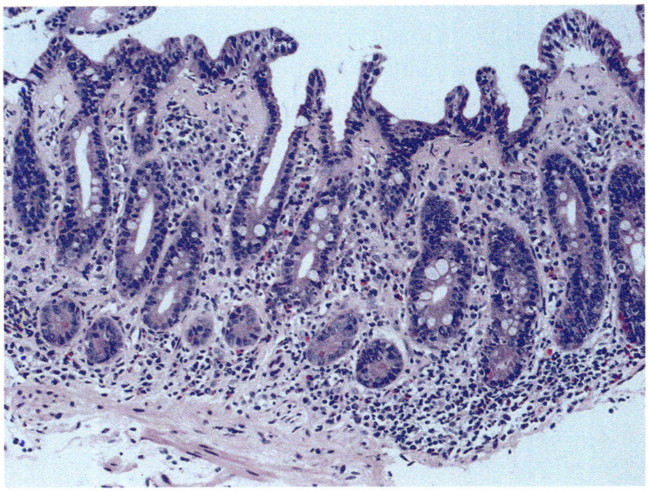

Fig. 9.15 Olmesartan-associated enteropathy. Duodenal biopsy shows presence of collagenous sprue with villous atrophy, increased chronic inflammation in lamina propria, and thickening of subepithelial collagenous band

Differential Diagnosis

The histological features present in olmesartan-associated enteropathy are not unique and cannot be used to separate from other diseases such as celiac disease, tropical sprue, CS, AIE, other medication-associated injuries, inflammatory bowel disease, and graft-versus-host disease (Table 9.2) [183, 188]. Most of the olmesartan-associated enteropathy has been diagnosed as unclassified sprue, CS, or AIE before this entity was described in 2012 [66, 182]. Correlation with medication history and clinical remission after stopping olmesartan are the keys to differentiate olmesartan-associated enteropathy from the abovementioned diseases. Positive celiac serology is present in celiac disease but not in olmesartan-associated enteropathy. Patients with AIE are accompanied by other autoimmune diseases and/or positive antienterocyte or anti-goblet cell antibodies.

Treatment and Prognosis

The prognosis is excellent. The clinical resolution of enteropathy symptoms and histological recovery of villous atrophy are present in the majority (up to 100%) of patients after drug cessation (Fig. 9.16a, b) [66, 182, 183, 189]. Rare cases can have persistent diarrhea despite discontinuation of olmesartan and require anti-TNFα[alpha] therapy [190].

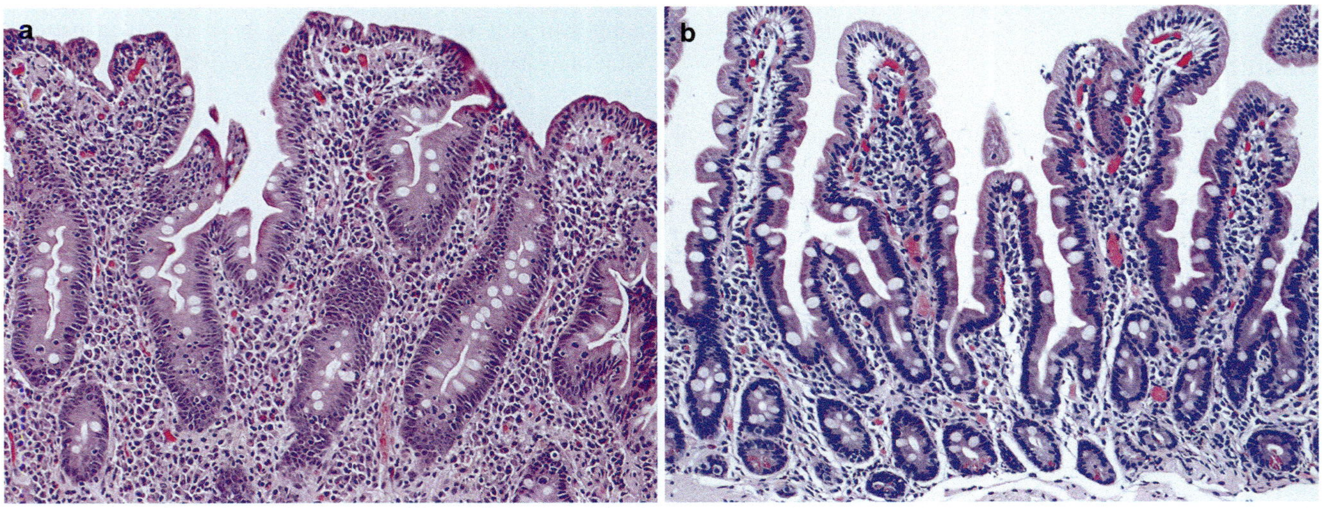

Fig. 9.16 Histological recovery of villous atrophy after drug cessation in Olmesartan-associated enteropathy. (**a**) Duodenal biopsy shows villous atrophy, increased chronic inflammation in lamina propria and increased intraepithelial lymphocytes similar to celiac disease in a patient on olmesartan. (**b**) The duodenal biopsy returned to normal villous architecture and no evidence of increased intraepithelial lymphocytes after cessation of olmesartan and was put on gluten challenge

Tropical Sprue

Definition

Tropical sprue is an acquired chronic inflammatory disease with intestinal malabsorption syndrome that affects residents and tourists of tropical regions including India, South East of Asia, West Africa, Central America, and Northern South America [192, 193].

Clinical Features

Pathogenesis The precise pathogenesis of tropical sprue remains unknown, but infectious etiology has been suggested because of epidemics particularly in rural areas with poor sanitation, and it is also known as "postinfective tropical malabsorption" [194, 195]. A contamination of small intestine by aerobic enteric bacteria including *Escherichia coli*, *Klebsiella pneumoniae*, and *Enterobacter cloacae* has been identified in patients with tropical sprue, but no specific causal agent has been found [194–196]. The orocecal transit time is prolonged in patients with tropical sprue [195]. There is increased frequency of HLA Aw19 and Aw31 in Puerto Rican patients [197, 198].

Clinical Presentations The typical symptoms in patients with tropical sprue are chronic non-bloody diarrhea, steatorrhea, weight loss, bloating, and abdominal cramps. In severe cases, vitamin A deficiency can lead to night blindness, and vitamin B12 and folate malabsorption can cause macrocytic anemia and neurological symptoms [198, 199].

Pathological Features

The pathological features seen in tropical sprue include increased IELs, villous atrophy, and increased chronic inflammatory cells in lamina propria [199, 200]. These histological features are present in the entire small bowel including duodenum, jejunum, and ileum (Fig. 9.17a, b). Marked

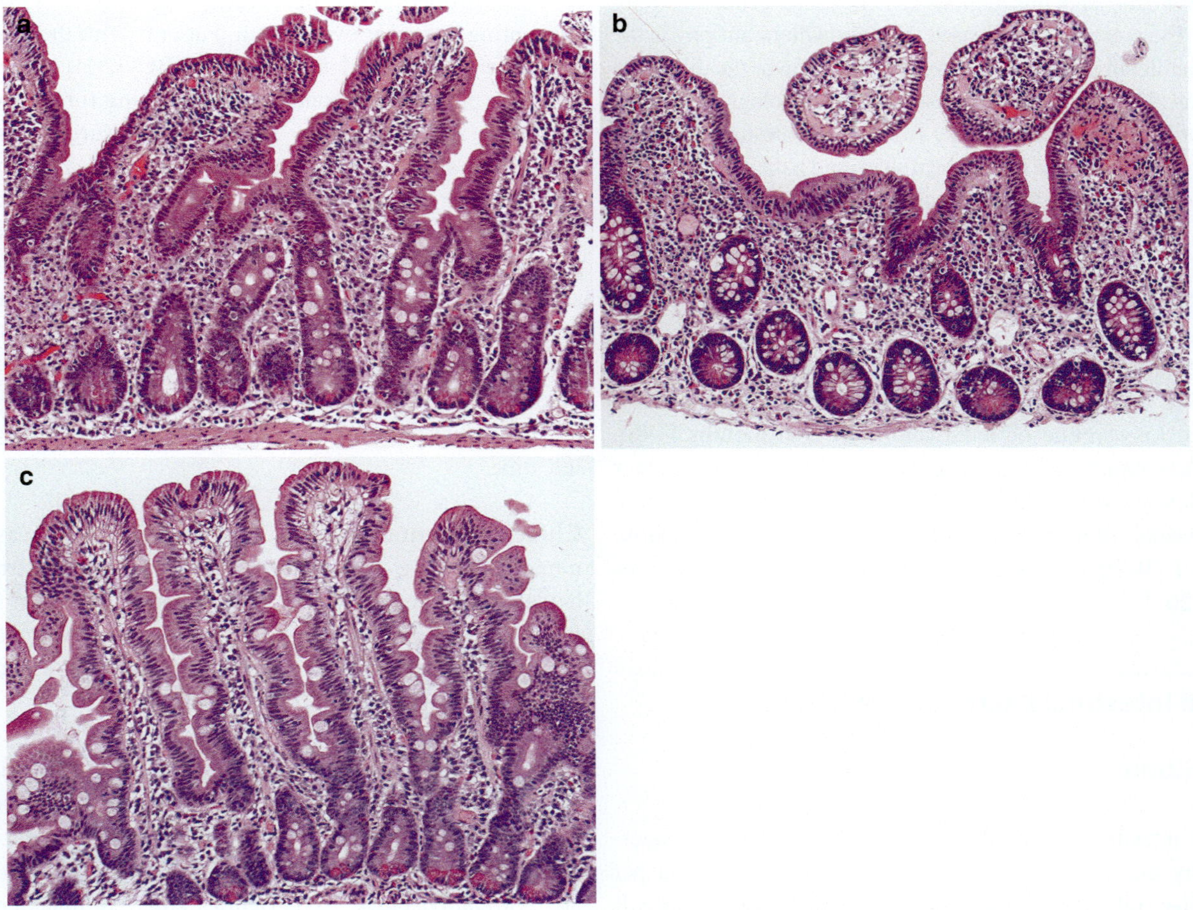

Fig. 9.17 (**a**) Tropical sprue. Duodenal biopsy shows villous atrophy and increased chronic inflammatory cells in lamina propria and increased intraepithelial lymphocytes. (**b**) Biopsy from terminal ileum demonstrates similar histological features. (**c**) Duodenal mucosa shows normal villous architecture and no evidence of increased intraepithelial lymphocytes after antibiotic doxycycline treatment

IELs and increased eosinophilic infiltrates in lamina propria are present in all duodenal biopsies from patients with tropical sprue, and increased IELs without villous atrophy can be seen in 25% of tropical sprue [199]. Gastric mucinous metaplasia can be seen in duodenal mucosa. The degree of IELs is higher in the villi without tip accentuation as compared to crypt. Acute inflammation such as intraepithelial neutrophilic infiltrates is not present in tropical sprue. The degree of villous atrophy tends to be more severe in the biopsy from terminal ileum than in duodenum, and the degree of IELs is similar between terminal ileum and duodenum [199]. Mild IELs can be present in 43% of colonic biopsies [199], and lymphocytic colitis can rarely present in patients with tropical sprue [201].

Differential Diagnosis

The main histological differential diagnoses for tropical sprue are celiac disease, small intestinal bacterial overgrowth syndrome (SIBO), and the other disease entities described in Table 9.2. Patients with tropical sprue typically have a travel history to the endemic regions and negative celiac serology [202]. The presence of increased IELs and villous atrophy in the terminal ileum as well as duodenum would favor the diagnosis of tropical sprue over celiac disease. The histological features present in the duodenal biopsy from small intestinal bacterial overgrowth syndrome tend to be milder, and patients with SIBO have underlying risk factors for motility disorders and stasis.

Treatment and Prognosis

Treatment for tropical sprue includes a combination of vitamin B12 and folate supplement and administration of antibiotics doxycycline or tetracycline for 3–6 months [196]. Travelers returning to nontropical regions generally recover completely with clinical improvement evident within 2–6 weeks after treatment (Fig. 9.17c); however, relapse rates of 20–50% are seen in patients from endemic regions [199, 203].

Small Intestinal Bacterial Overgrowth

Definition

Small intestinal bacterial overgrowth (SIBO) is characterized by the presence of increased number of bacteria per milliliter (mL) (>10^5 colony-forming units [CFU]) and colonization of gram-negative aerobic and anaerobic bacteria that are normally restricted to the colon or less frequently from oropharyngeal flora in the small intestine, associated with a spectrum of clinical symptoms including diarrhea, abdominal pain, weight loss, bloating, nausea, vomiting, and malabsorption [204, 205].

Clinical Features

Epidemiology SIBO is a common cause of chronic diarrhea [206]. The prevalence of SIBO in the general population is unknown and has been reported to be in 2.5–22% based on small studies and different diagnostic methods [204]. The prevalence of SIBO in patients with predisposed conditions varies, with 50% in liver cirrhosis, 96% in Crohn's disease with small bowel stricture, 38% in pediatric population living in an urban slum, 26% in disabled older adults, and 30–85% in patients with irritable bowel syndrome [204, 207].

Pathogenesis The pathogenesis of SIBO involves alterations of the endogenous defense mechanisms including gastric acid secretion, intestinal motility, intact ileo-cecal valve, intestinal immunoglobulin secretion, and bacteriostatic properties of pancreatic and bile secretion for preventing bacterial overgrowth. Patients with these alterations are predisposed to develop SIBO [204]. The most common predisposed conditions accounting for 90% of the SIBO are altered anatomy from previous surgery such as blind loop syndrome and stricture, impaired gut motility, and chronic pancreatitis. Other predisposing conditions include achlorhydria, immunodeficiency syndromes, celiac disease, Crohn's disease, short gut syndrome, liver cirrhosis, scleroderma, autonomic neuropathy in diabetes mellitus, radiation enteropathy, and fibromyalgia [204, 205]. In some patients, more than one predisposing factor can be involved. Bacterial overgrowth can produce various toxic agents with systemic effects and causing injury to the small intestine.

Clinical Presentations Patients with SIBO may be asymptomatic or have clinical symptoms resembling irritable bowel syndromes with nonspecific symptoms such as bloating, flatulence, abdominal pain, and diarrhea. Weight loss, steatorrhea, malnutrition, and vitamin deficiency occur in more severe cases of SIBO [204, 207].

Laboratory Findings The gold standard for the diagnosis of SIBO is the aspiration of small bowel fluid microbial culture with growth of at least 10^5 CFU/mL in duodenal or jejunal fluids [204, 207]. The main bacteria identified are *Streptococcus, Escherichia coli, Staphylococcus, Micrococcus,* and *Klebsiella* for micro-aerophilic bacteria and *Bacteroides, Lactobacillus,* and *Clostridium* for anaerobic bacteria [208]. There are other noninvasive hydrogen breath tests for the diagnosis of SIBO. The glucose hydrogen breath test is highly specific but with low sensitivity, and the early-peak criteria in the lactulose hydrogen test is highly nonspecific [209].

Pathological Features

Villous atrophy, increased IELs, increased chronic inflammatory infiltrates in lamina propria, and focal acute inflammation have been described in small bowel biopsy from patients with SIBO (Fig. 9.18a, b) [207, 210, 211]. In a large histological evaluation of 67 patients with SIBO, 52% of the duodenal biopsies have normal histology; and villous atrophy is only present in 24% and IELs in 22% of duodenal biopsies [207]. Increased IgA-positive plasma cells in lamina propria and increased CD8+ IELs have also been shown in SIBO [212].

Differential Diagnosis

Villous atrophy and increased IELs can be present in the SIBO and need to be considered among the differential diagnoses listed in Table 9.2. However, histologically unremarkable duodenal biopsies can be present in more than half of the patients with diagnosis of SIBO; and a normal duodenal biopsy does not exclude the diagnosis of SIBO.

Treatment and Prognosis

Therapy for SIBO is individualized and should include treatment of underlying disease, nutritional and vitamin support, and selective antibiotics targeting the type of the isolated bacteria on the cultures. The prognosis of SIBO is determined mainly on the underlying disease causing SIBO. The relapse rate of SIBO after successful treatment is high (44%) in 9 months after successful treatment with rifaximin [213].

Lipid Malabsorption Disorders

The transport of alimentary fat occurs predominantly in the small intestine. The absorption of fat starts with hydrolysis of lipids by pancreatic lipase, phospholipase A2, and cholesterol esterase, followed by emulsification into mixed micelles by bile salt and enters the enterocytes via passive diffusion. Within the enterocytes, the lipolytic products are re-esterified by various enzymes into glycoprotein in the endoplasmic reticulum. Synthesis of apo B-48 and its interaction with microsomal triglyceride transfer protein (MTP) is essential for pre-chylomicron assembly. The formation of pre-chylomicron is critical for the transport of nascent lipoprotein into Golgi mediated by Sar1b GTPase. The maturation of pre-chylomicron into chylomicron occurs in Golgi and released into the intestinal lymph through exocytosis [214].

Fat malabsorption disorders commonly occur in patients with severe liver disease, chronic pancreatitis, cystic fibrosis, and extensive small bowel resection in Crohn's disease due to loss of enterohepatic circulation of bile acids. Abetalipoproteinemia, hypobetalipoproteinemia, and chylomicron retention disease (Anderson disease) are the congenital intestinal lipid metabolic disorders involving defects in lipid transport within the enterocytes. These congenital lipid

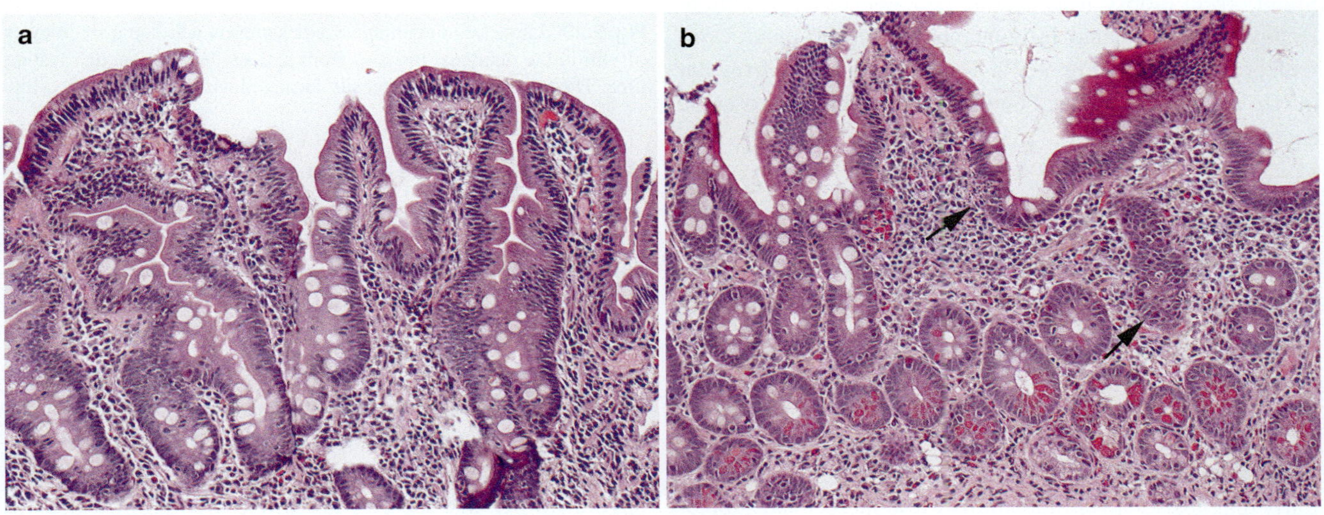

Fig. 9.18 Small intestinal bacterial overgrowth. (**a**) Duodenal biopsy shows villous atrophy, increased chronic inflammatory infiltrates in lamina propria, and increased intraepithelial lymphocytes similar to celiac disease in small intestinal bacterial overgrowth. (**b**) Focal acute inflammation with cryptitis (arrows) is present in the duodenal biopsy from a patient with small intestinal bacterial overgrowth

metabolic disorders are uncommon and share similar clinical characteristics including failure to thrive in childhood, fat malabsorption, low serum lipid levels, neurological and visual disorders due to malabsorption of fat-soluble vitamins and accumulation of fat vacuoles within the enterocytes.

Abetalipoproteinemia

Definition

Abetalipoproteinemia is a rare autosomal recessive disorder with an estimated incidence of less than one per million [215]. Abetalipoproteinemia is caused by deficiency of MTP due to loss-of-function mutations in the *MTTP* gene on chromosome 4q22–24 [216, 217]. MTP protein is expressed in the endoplasmic reticulum of enterocytes (duodenum and proximal jejunum) and hepatocytes and plays a key role in proper folding of apo B and assembly of apo B-containing lipoproteins. Absence of MTP leads to premature degradation of nascent apo B and prevents pre-chylomicron formation [218].

Clinical Features

Patients with abetalipoproteinemia can have multisystem manifestations and present with diarrhea, steatorrhea, acanthocytosis, low serum cholesterol and apo-B, and failure to thrive. Diarrhea and fat malabsorption usually occur within few months of life; however, there is clinical heterogeneity of disease, and symptoms and signs may occur in older individuals. Deficiency of fat-soluble vitamins A and E can cause neurological symptoms and retinitis pigmentosa [214]. Hepatic steatosis with elevated serum transaminase and hepatomegaly has been frequently reported, and cirrhosis can also occur [219, 220].

Pathological Features

Small bowel biopsy from fasting patients typically demonstrates multivacuolated fat contents within the enterocytes with preserved villi (Fig. 9.19). The fat vacuoles are irregular in size and not membrane bound under electron microscopic examination [221].

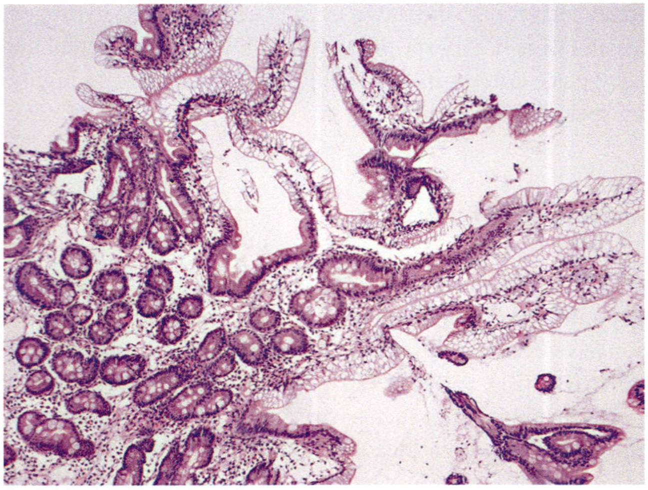

Fig. 9.19 Abetalipoproteinemia. Small bowel biopsy from a fasting patient shows multivacuolated fat contents within the enterocytes with preserved villi

Differential Diagnosis

Large fat-containing vacuoles can be present within the enterocytes of villi in the duodenal biopsies from patients without enough fasting time. The distribution of fat vacuoles is typically localized within the tip of the villi (Fig. 9.20) and is in contrast to the diffuse distribution of fat vacuoles along the entire villi seen in patients with abetalipoproteinemia.

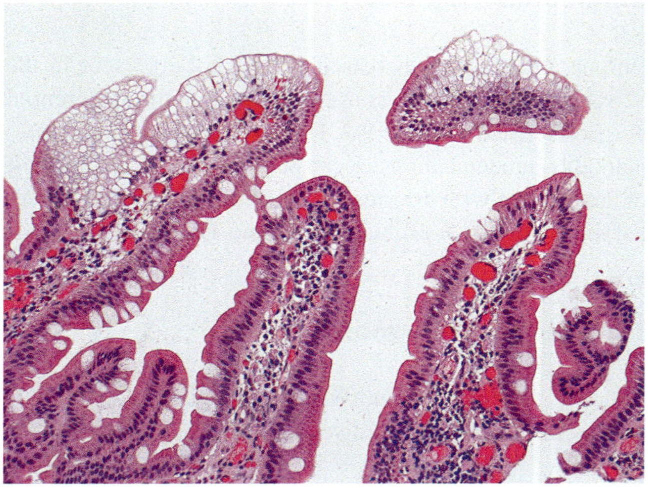

Fig. 9.20 Large fat-containing vacuoles present within the enterocytes of villi in the duodenal biopsies from patients without enough fasting time. The fat vacuoles are typically localized within the tip of the villi

Treatment and Prognosis

Early diagnosis with combination of low-fat diet and supplementation of essential fatty acids and fat-soluble vitamins helps to prevent the severe sequels of abetalipoproteinemia [214, 222].

Hypobetalipoproteinemia

Familial hypobetalipoproteinemia is an autosomal dominant disorder characterized by molecular defects in the *APOB* gene on chromosome 2p23–24 which interferes with the translation of full-length Apo B mRNA, resulting in truncated Apo B protein [223, 224]. Homozygous familial hypobetalipoproteinemia patients have clinical manifestation and histological phenotype indistinguishable from abetalipoproteinemia, and heterozygous patients have a milder disease and are often asymptomatic. Mild elevation of transaminase and hepatic steatosis are the main clinical manifestations of heterozygous familial hypobetalipoproteinemia [225, 226]. Cirrhosis and hepa-

Pathogenesis The pathogenesis of PIL is not clear. Lymphatic obstruction and mutations in genes such as vascular endothelial growth factor receptor 3, forkhead transcriptional factor (*FOXC2*), prospero-related homeobox-transcription factor (*PROX1*), and *SOX18* that involve in the lymphogenesis are the proposed possible pathogenesis for PIL [323, 324]. Mutation of the *CCBE1* gene encoding collagen and calcium-binding EGF-domain-1, responsible for the intestinal lymphangiectasia, has been identified in 23% of patients with Hennekam syndrome [332]. Intestinal lymphangiectasia is responsible for the leaking lymph into the intestinal lumen and leading to lymphopenia and hypoalbuminemia.

Clinical Presentations PIL occurs primarily in children, and the majority of the cases are diagnosed at or before 3 years of age but can also be seen in adults [323, 324]. Approximately 90% of PIL cases are sporadic and the rest are familial [331]. Pitting edema in variable degree, usually symmetrical involving lower limb, is the main clinical presentation with other common presentations including chylous ascites, pleural effusion, and pericarditis. Moderate diarrhea is the main digestive symptom, and malabsorptive syndrome can present in elder patients. Other rare clinical associations include abdominal mass, mechanical ileus, iron deficiency anemia, celiac disease, osteomalacia, and lymphedema [323, 324].

Endoscopic Findings Endoscopy reveals diffusely elongated, circumferential, and polypoid mucosa covered by whitish enlarged villi with snowflake appearance overlying intestinal mucosa (Fig. 9.27a) [324, 333].

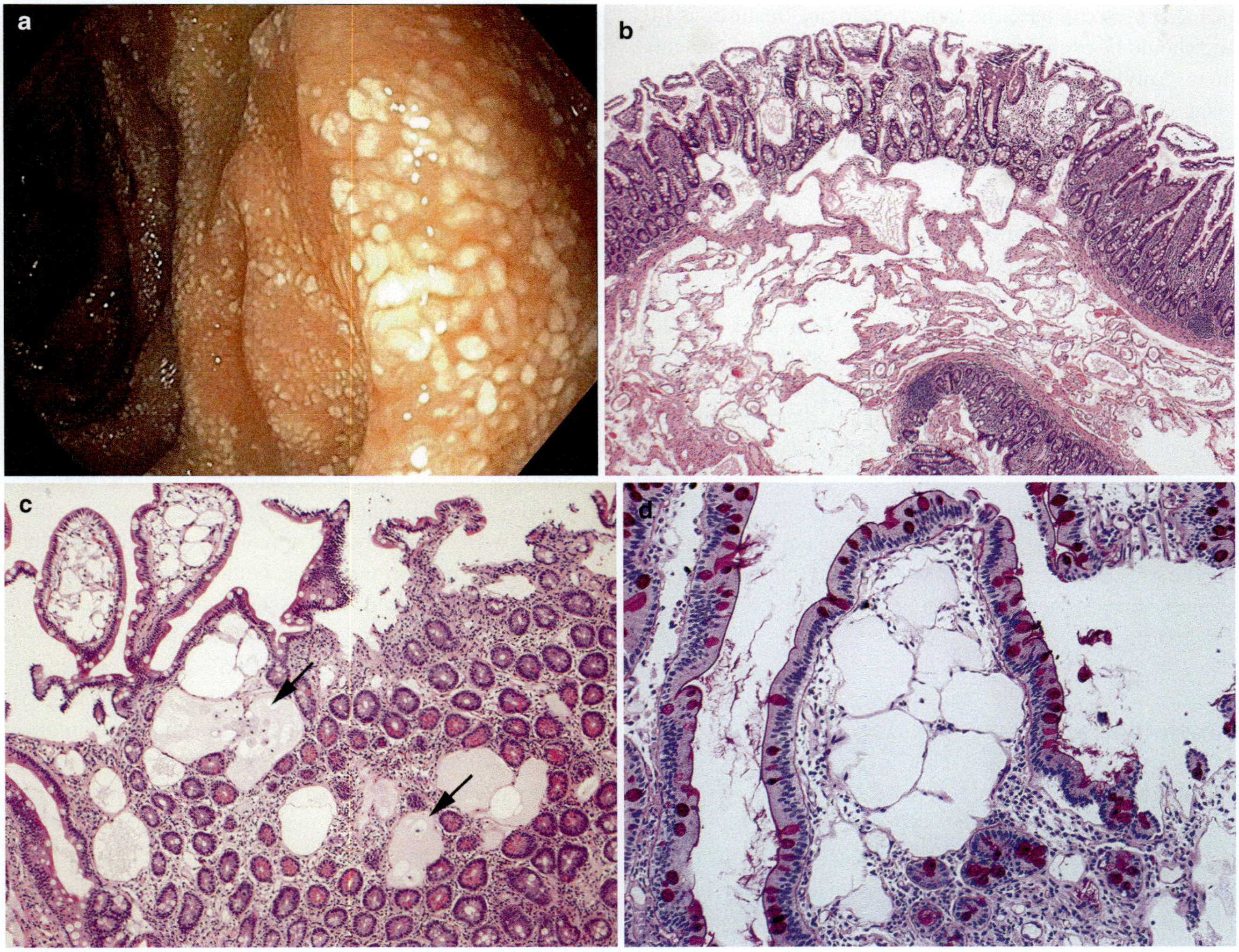

Fig. 9.27 Lymphangiectasia. (**a**) Endoscopic examination reveals snowflake appearance. (**b**) Dilated lymphatic vessels are diffusely present in the mucosa and submucosa with increased chronic inflammatory cells and plasma cells in lamina propria in duodenal biopsy. (**c**) There are scattered foamy histiocytes (arrows) mixed with clear lymph fluids within the dilated lymphatic vessels. (**d**) The lymph fluids are negative for PAS-D stain

Pathological Features

The diagnosis of PIL is based on the characteristic finding on double-balloon enteroscopy with confirmation by histological examination of the corresponding biopsy specimens [324]. Dilated lymphatic vessels are diffusely present in the mucosa and submucosa, with polyclonal plasma cells in the small bowel biopsy (Fig. 9.27b) and serosa in the resected small bowel [324]. There are scattered foamy histiocytes mixed with clear lymph fluids within the dilated lymphatic vessels (Fig. 9.27c). The lymph fluids are negative for PAS-D stain (Fig. 9.27d). The villous height is generally unaltered, and villous atrophy in small bowel has only rarely been described [334].

Differential Diagnosis

Functional intestinal lymphangiectasia and secondary lymphangiectasia can have the same histological features as PIL and should be excluded by correlation with clinical presentations. Amyloid deposits and WM can mimic lymphangiectasia. Congo red stain and IgM immunohistochemical stain can be used to differentiate between these entities.

Treatment and Prognosis

PIL is a chronic debilitating disorder. Diet rich in protein and low-fat with medium-chain triglyceride supplementation is the principal and effective treatment. In most patients, dietary treatment is permanently needed for the PIL [324]. Medium-chain triglyceride is directly absorbed in portal venous circulation and can prevent intestinal lacteal overloading. In patients not responding to dietary treatment, octreotide, antiplasmin, tranexamic acid, vitamin D supplementation, and surgical resection of segmental or localized intestinal lymphangiectasia can be used [324]. Serous effusions such as pleural and pericardial effusion can occur and can be life-threatening [323]. Malignant lymphoma is a late complication, occurring 19–45 years after the diagnosis of PIL [335].

Amyloidosis

Definition

Amyloidosis is characterized by extracellular deposition of Congo red histochemical stain-positive abnormal β[beta]-pleated fibrillar proteins and can affect any organ system.

Clinical Features

Clinical Presentations More than 25 different proteins of amyloid have been identified [336]. Amyloidosis can be systemic and localized. The most common type of amyloidosis is the systemic immunoglobulin light chain amyloidosis (AL) secondary to plasma cell dyscrasia with an incidence of nine cases per million person-years [337]. Other types of amyloidosis include serum amyloid A protein (AA) associated with infections, inflammatory or neoplastic disorders, leukocyte chemotactic factor 2 (ALECT2), β[beta]2-microglobulin (Aβ[beta]2 M), and familial forms including transthyretin (ATTR), fibrinogen A α[alpha]-chain (AFib), apolipoprotein AI (AApo AI), apolipoprotein AII (AApo AII), apolipoprotein AIV (AApo AIV), lysozyme (ALys), gelsolin (AGel), and cystatin (ACys) [338]. Gastrointestinal involvement by amyloidosis is common, and small bowel is the most commonly affected site, followed by stomach and colon, and esophagus is the least commonly involved [336, 339]. Systemic AL amyloidosis has the most common gastrointestinal involvement and can be identified in 80% of the biopsies from stomach and rectum [337]. Senile amyloidosis is found in 10–36% of patients over 80 years old, and gastrointestinal tract involvement is present in 41–44%, mainly in the colon and small bowel [340]. Hereditary lysozyme amyloidosis (ALys) is an autosomal dominant disorder with gastrointestinal symptoms, sicca syndrome, renal dysfunction, hepatic rupture, and lymphadenopathy [341]. Amyloid deposits are present in the liver in all the patients and in GI tract in the majority of ALys patients [341]. Gastrointestinal symptoms are frequent in patients with familial amyloidotic polyneuropathy [342]. Gastrointestinal tract involvement is present in approximately one-third of Aβ[beta]2M amyloidosis patients, in particular in patients on hemodialysis for more than 10 years [343].

Small bowel is the most affected site for systemic amyloidosis [344]. The clinical manifestations in amyloidosis with small bowel involvement include diarrhea, steatorrhea, protein loss, hemorrhage, obstruction, ischemia, perforation, intussusception, pneumatosis intestinalis, constipation, and pseudo-obstruction [336, 340]. Malabsorption is found in 8.5% of AL amyloidosis patients and 2.3% of AA amyloidosis patients [345], and malabsorption syndrome can be the main presentation for AL amyloidosis [346]. Steatorrhea is present in up to 98% of patients with familial amyloidotic polyneuropathy [342]. Small bowel involvement has been reported in four (three with diarrhea and weight loss and one with small intestinal perforation) of 16 patients with ALys amyloidosis [341]. Small intestinal amyloidosis can present as localized lesion [347] and can rarely be associated with gastrointestinal lymphoma [348].

Endoscopic and Imaging Findings The endoscopic features include fine granular appearance, erosions, mucosal friability, thickening of the valvulae conniventes, and multiple polypoid protrusions in amyloidosis involving small bowel

[349]. The fine granular appearance is more common in AA amyloidosis, whereas the multiple polypoid protrusions and thickening of the valvulae conniventes are more common in AL amyloidosis [350]. The most common radiological finding in small bowel amyloidosis is ischemic manifestation and edema secondary to amyloid deposition on vascular structure and symmetrical thickening of folds and "jejunalization" of ileum [351].

Pathological Features

Amyloidosis in small bowel biopsy shows eosinophilic amorphous material deposition that is positive for Congo red stain with apple green birefringence under polarized light (Fig. 9.28). Amyloid deposits can be found in lamina propria, muscularis mucosae, and submucosal vascular wall in the biopsy specimens. AL and AA amyloidosis can have different amyloid deposition patterns in the small bowel. AA amyloidosis is predominantly present in the lamina propria, while the AL amyloidosis is present in the mucosa, submucosa, and muscularis propria [349]. The amyloid deposits can be around the submucosal nerves in familial amyloidotic polyneuropathy [352]. All the different types of amyloid deposits within the gastrointestinal tract have similar histological features and need to be subtyped. The globular amyloid deposits seen in ALECT2 are only identified in the liver but have not been seen in gastrointestinal tract [353]. Immunohistochemical stains are useful for typing AA, AApoAI, Alys, ALac, and ATTR; however, classification for AL and rare hereditary amyloidosis by immunohistochemical stains can be challenging and sometimes impossible [354]. Amyloid subtyping can be performed by laser microdissection followed by tandem mass spectrometry and is currently the preferred method for subtyping amyloid [338, 355].

Differential Diagnosis

WM and elastofibromatous changes of the intestine are the main differential diagnosis for intestinal amyloidosis. WM is negative for Congo red stain but is positive for IgM immunohistochemical stain. The elastosis present in elastofibromatous change has fine granular and fibrillar amorphous appearance with a fibrous component involving muscularis mucosae and submucosa [356, 357]. Elastofibromatosis change is positive for elastin (VVG) stain (see Fig. 8.35 in Chap. 8) but is negative for Congo red stain.

Treatment and Prognosis

There is no specific treatment for the complications arising from amyloidosis involving the gastrointestinal tract. Treating the underlying cause of amyloidosis and supportive treatment can help to relieve the associated gastrointestinal symptoms [336].

Food Allergy and Protein Intolerance

The most common food allergens include milk, egg, peanut, tree nuts, wheat, crustacean shellfish, and soy. Immunological reactions to dietary proteins can be classified as IgE mediated (immediate gastrointestinal hypersensitivity and oral allergic

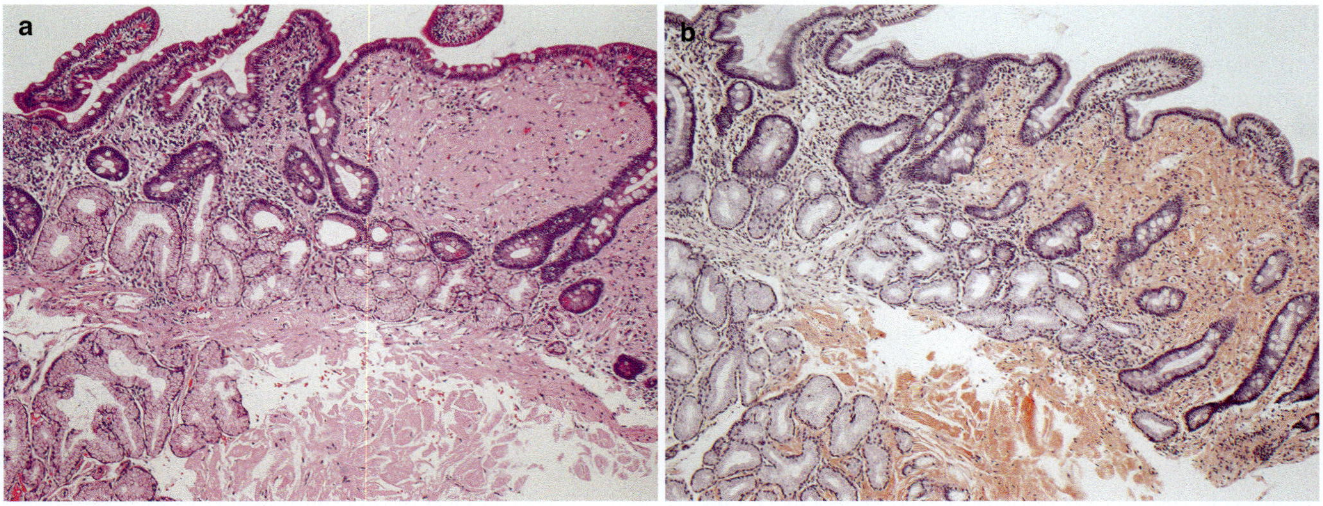

Fig. 9.28 Amyloid deposit in duodenum. (**a**) Duodenal biopsy shows eosinophilic amorphous material deposition in lamina propria, muscularis mucosae, and submucosa in a patient with AL amyloidosis. (**b**) These eosinophilic amorphous material depositions are positive for Congo red stain with apple green birefringence under polarized light

reaction), mixed (allergic eosinophilic esophagitis, gastritis, and gastroenteritis), and non-IgE mediated [358, 359]. The non-IgE-mediated food allergy presents in a subacute or chronic nature and more commonly affects gastrointestinal tract only, which includes three main clinical entities: food protein-induced enterocolitis (FPIES), food protein-induced proctocolitis, and food protein-induced enteropathy. FPIES occurs in infants and is mostly due to response to cow's milk, soy, and rice [359–361]. Profuse vomiting, diarrhea, and melena typically present within the first month of life in FPIES. With elimination of offending food, most of the children become tolerant of the offending food by the age of 3. Food protein-induced proctocolitis is a benign condition that tends to occur exclusively in breastfed infants in response to food allergens ingested by the mother and appearing in the breast milk. Food protein-induced proctocolitis usually resolves in 6 months to 2 years even without treatment [362]. Food protein-induced enteropathy occurs in infants with chronic diarrhea, steatorrhea, malabsorption, and poor weight gain within the first month of life due to response to cow's milk, soy, and less frequently chicken, rice, and fish [359].

Cow's Milk and Soy Protein Intolerance

Cow's milk protein-sensitive enteropathy (CMSE) is characterized by persistent diarrhea and malabsorption in infants and occasionally in school-age children due to intolerance of cow's milk [363, 364]. The clinical symptoms improve on cow's milk-free diet and relapse after re-exposure to cow's milk protein. CMSE is a non-IgE-mediated gastrointestinal food-allergic disorder. Infants intolerant to cow's milk protein are often intolerant to other proteins including soy protein [365]. Soy protein intolerance can also present in infants with persistent diarrhea, colitis, and flat intestinal mucosa [366, 367].

Partial villous atrophy, mild IELs, and increased chronic inflammatory cells including plasma cells and eosinophils in lamina propria are the histological features present in the jejunal biopsies from infants with cow's milk intolerance [363, 368–372]. The small bowel mucosa returns to normal architecture after 3–13 months on milk-free diet [368]. Lymphonodular hyperplasia of duodenal bulb is the typical endoscopic finding in older children with CMSE [364]. Microscopically, there are lymphoid follicles but no evidence of villous atrophy in duodenal biopsy [364].

Treatment for CMSE is the elimination of cow's milk and all foods based on cow's milk with substitution of formula free of cow's milk and extensively hydrolyzed formula or amino acid formula [373]. This dietary treatment is temporary and return to normal diet between 1 and 4 years of age is possible in the majority of infants [374, 375].

Kwashiorkor Disease (Protein-Calorie Malnutrition)

Definition

Kwashiorkor disease (KD) is a type of protein-calorie malnutrition occurring in infants or children in the setting of insufficient protein intake in the presence of sufficient calorie intake and is characterized by edema, protuberant belly, "bull-dog" face, dermatitis and thinning of hair, weight loss, failure to thrive, irritability, and lethargy [376].

Clinical Features

Epidemiology KD is most often seen in children from developing countries or areas of famine and is endemic in Africa [376]. KD is extremely rare in developed countries and is mainly due to nutritional ignorance and deliberate deviation to a protein-deficient diet because of a perceived intolerance to formula or milk [377, 378].

Pathogenesis The pathogenesis of KD is not clear, but inadequate dietary protein in the presence of sufficient calorie intake is the commonly accepted theory. Expression of enterocyte heparin sulfate proteoglycan (HSPG) and sulfated glycosaminoglycan (GAG) are marked decreased in both epithelium and lamina propria in the duodenum may precipitate protein-losing enteropathy to cause edema [379].

Clinical Presentations Early symptoms of KD are nonspecific and include irritability, fatigue and lethargy, growth failure, loss of muscle mass, edema, diarrhea, and decreased immunity occurring after protein deprivation continues. Affected children have a large protuberant belly due to ascites secondary to hypoalbuminemia and grossly enlarged liver because of fatty infiltration, characteristic "bull-dog" eye, dermatitis with exfoliative or flaky paint in appearance, and thinning of hair [378]. KD can rarely occur in adult secondary to Roux-en-Y gastric bypass surgery [380].

Pathological Features

Jejunal or duodenal biopsies from patients with KD reveal partial or subtotal villous atrophy, increased IELs, and increased chronic inflammatory cells including plasma cells, lymphocytes, and eosinophils in lamina propria [381, 382]. Small bowel mucosa remains abnormal even after 12 months of treatment but can show normal architecture 4–10 years after treatment of KD [382, 383].

disease. Clin Gastroenterol Hepatol. 2007;5(4):445–50. https://doi.org/10.1016/j.cgh.2006.12.006.

71. Abdulkarim AS, Burgart LJ, See J, Murray JA. Etiology of non-responsive celiac disease: results of a systematic approach. Am J Gastroenterol. 2002;97(8):2016–21. https://doi.org/10.1111/j.1572–0241.2002.05917.x.
72. Roshan B, Leffler DA, Jamma S, Dennis M, Sheth S, Falchuk K, et al. The incidence and clinical spectrum of refractory celiac disease in a north american referral center. Am J Gastroenterol. 2011;106(5):923–8. https://doi.org/10.1038/ajg.2011.104.
73. Nachman F, Sugai E, Vazquez H, Gonzalez A, Andrenacci P, Niveloni S, et al. Serological tests for celiac disease as indicators of long-term compliance with the gluten-free diet. Eur J Gastroenterol Hepatol. 2011;23(6):473–80. https://doi.org/10.1097/MEG.0b013e328346e0f1.
74. Silvester JA, Kurada S, Szwajcer A, Kelly CP, Leffler DA, Duerksen DR. Tests for serum transglutaminase and endomysial antibodies do not detect most patients with celiac disease and persistent villous atrophy on gluten-free diets: a meta-analysis. Gastroenterology. 2017;153(3):689–701.e1. https://doi.org/10.1053/j.gastro.2017.05.015.
75. Rubio-Tapia A, Rahim MW, See JA, Lahr BD, Wu TT, Murray JA. Mucosal recovery and mortality in adults with celiac disease after treatment with a gluten-free diet. Am J Gastroenterol. 2010;105(6):1412–20. https://doi.org/10.1038/ajg.2010.10.
76. Lanzini A, Lanzarotto F, Villanacci V, Mora A, Bertolazzi S, Turini D, et al. Complete recovery of intestinal mucosa occurs very rarely in adult coeliac patients despite adherence to gluten-free diet. Aliment Pharmacol Ther. 2009;29(12):1299–308. https://doi.org/10.1111/j.1365–2036.2009.03992.x.
77. Wahab PJ, Meijer JW, Mulder CJ. Histologic follow-up of people with celiac disease on a gluten-free diet: slow and incomplete recovery. Am J Clin Pathol. 2002;118(3):459–63. https://doi.org/10.1309/evxt-851x-whlc-rlx9.
78. Kaukinen K, Peraaho M, Lindfors K, Partanen J, Woolley N, Pikkarainen P, et al. Persistent small bowel mucosal villous atrophy without symptoms in coeliac disease. Aliment Pharmacol Ther. 2007;25(10):1237–45. https://doi.org/10.1111/j.1365–2036.2007.03311.x.
79. Rubio-Tapia A, Kelly DG, Lahr BD, Dogan A, Wu TT, Murray JA. Clinical staging and survival in refractory celiac disease: a single center experience. Gastroenterology. 2009;136(1):99–107; quiz 352–3. https://doi.org/10.1053/j.gastro.2008.10.013.
80. Malamut G, Afchain P, Verkarre V, Lecomte T, Amiot A, Damotte D, et al. Presentation and long-term follow-up of refractory celiac disease: comparison of type I with type II. Gastroenterology. 2009;136(1):81–90. https://doi.org/10.1053/j.gastro.2008.09.069.
81. Leslie LA, Lebwohl B, Neugut AI, Gregory Mears J, Bhagat G, Green PH. Incidence of lymphoproliferative disorders in patients with celiac disease. Am J Hematol. 2012;87(8):754–9. https://doi.org/10.1002/ajh.23237.
82. Olen O, Askling J, Ludvigsson JF, Hildebrand H, Ekbom A, Smedby KE. Coeliac disease characteristics, compliance to a gluten free diet and risk of lymphoma by subtype. Dig Liver Dis. 2011;43(11):862–8. https://doi.org/10.1016/j.dld.2011.07.012.
83. Elfstrom P, Granath F, Ye W, Ludvigsson JF. Low risk of gastrointestinal cancer among patients with celiac disease, inflammation, or latent celiac disease. Clin Gastroenterol Hepatol. 2012;10(1):30–6. https://doi.org/10.1016/j.cgh.2011.06.029.
84. Ludvigsson JF, Montgomery SM, Ekbom A, Brandt L, Granath F. Small-intestinal histopathology and mortality risk in celiac disease. JAMA. 2009;302(11):1171–8. https://doi.org/10.1001/jama.2009.1320.
85. Biagi F, Corazza GR. Defining gluten refractory enteropathy. Eur J Gastroenterol Hepatol. 2001;13(5):561–5.
86. West J. Celiac disease and its complications: a time traveller's perspective. Gastroenterology. 2009;136(1):32–4. https://doi.org/10.1053/j.gastro.2008.11.026.
87. Malamut G, Cellier C. Refractory coeliac disease. Curr Opin Oncol. 2013;25(5):445–51. https://doi.org/10.1097/01.cco.0000432526.47228.b6.
88. Caruso R, Marafini I, Sedda S, Del Vecchio Blanco G, Giuffrida P, MacDonald TT, et al. Analysis of the cytokine profile in the duodenal mucosa of refractory coeliac disease patients. Clin Sci (Lond). 2014;126(6):451–8. https://doi.org/10.1042/cs20130478.
89. Sedda S, De Simone V, Marafini I, Bevivino G, Izzo R, Paoluzi OA, et al. High Smad7 sustains inflammatory cytokine response in refractory coeliac disease. Immunology. 2017;150(3):356–63. https://doi.org/10.1111/imm.12690.
90. Verkarre V, Romana SP, Cellier C, Asnafi V, Mention JJ, Barbe U, et al. Recurrent partial trisomy 1q22-q44 in clonal intraepithelial lymphocytes in refractory celiac sprue. Gastroenterology. 2003;125(1):40–6.
91. Daum S, Cellier C, Mulder CJ. Refractory coeliac disease. Best Pract Res Clin Gastroenterol. 2005;19(3):413–24. https://doi.org/10.1016/j.bpg.2005.02.001.
92. Daum S, Ipczynski R, Schumann M, Wahnschaffe U, Zeitz M, Ullrich R. High rates of complications and substantial mortality in both types of refractory sprue. Eur J Gastroenterol Hepatol. 2009;21(1):66–70. https://doi.org/10.1097/MEG.0b013e328307c20c.
93. Patey-Mariaud De Serre N, Cellier C, Jabri B, Delabesse E, Verkarre V, Roche B, et al. Distinction between coeliac disease and refractory sprue: a simple immunohistochemical method. Histopathology. 2000;37(1):70–7.
94. Verbeek WH, Goerres MS, von Blomberg BM, Oudejans JJ, Scholten PE, Hadithi M, et al. Flow cytometric determination of aberrant intra-epithelial lymphocytes predicts T-cell lymphoma development more accurately than T-cell clonality analysis in Refractory Celiac Disease. Clin Immunol. 2008;126(1):48–56. https://doi.org/10.1016/j.clim.2007.09.002.
95. de Mascarel A, Belleannee G, Stanislas S, Merlio C, Parrens M, Laharie D, et al. Mucosal intraepithelial T-lymphocytes in refractory celiac disease: a neoplastic population with a variable CD8 phenotype. Am J Surg Pathol. 2008;32(5):744–51. https://doi.org/10.1097/PAS.0b013e318159b478.
96. Zivny J, Banner BF, Agrawal S, Pihan G, Barnard GF. CD4+ T-cell lymphoproliferative disorder of the gut clinically mimicking celiac sprue. Dig Dis Sci. 2004;49(4):551–5.
97. Matnani R, Ganapathi KA, Lewis SK, Green PH, Alobeid B, Bhagat G. Indolent T- and NK-cell lymphoproliferative disorders of the gastrointestinal tract: a review and update. Hematol Oncol. 2017;35(1):3–16. https://doi.org/10.1002/hon.2317.
98. Margolskee E, Jobanputra V, Lewis SK, Alobeid B, Green PH, Bhagat G. Indolent small intestinal CD4+ T-cell lymphoma is a distinct entity with unique biologic and clinical features. PLoS One. 2013;8(7):e68343. https://doi.org/10.1371/journal.pone.0068343.
99. Malamut G, Meresse B, Kaltenbach S, Derrieux C, Verkarre V, Macintyre E, et al. Small intestinal CD4+ T-cell lymphoma is a heterogenous entity with common pathology features. Clin Gastroenterol Hepatol. 2014;12(4):599–608.e1. https://doi.org/10.1016/j.cgh.2013.11.028.
100. Sharma A, Oishi N, Boddicker RL, Hu G, Benson HK, Ketterling RP, et al. Recurrent STAT3-JAK2 fusions in indolent T-cell lymphoproliferative disorder of the gastrointestinal tract. Blood. 2018;131(20):2262–6. https://doi.org/10.1182/blood-2018–01–830968.
101. Al-Toma A, Verbeek WH, Hadithi M, von Blomberg BM, Mulder CJ. Survival in refractory coeliac disease and enteropathy-associated T-cell lymphoma: retrospective evaluation of single-centre

experience. Gut. 2007;56(10):1373–8. https://doi.org/10.1136/gut.2006.114512.
102. Brar P, Lee S, Lewis S, Egbuna I, Bhagat G, Green PH. Budesonide in the treatment of refractory celiac disease. Am J Gastroenterol. 2007;102(10):2265–9. https://doi.org/10.1111/j.1572-0241.2007.01380.x.
103. Al-Toma A, Goerres MS, Meijer JW, von Blomberg BM, Wahab PJ, Kerckhaert JA, et al. Cladribine therapy in refractory celiac disease with aberrant T cells. Clin Gastroenterol Hepatol. 2006;4(11):1322–7; quiz 00. https://doi.org/10.1016/j.cgh.2006.07.007.
104. Maguire AA, Greenson JK, Lauwers GY, Ginsburg RE, Williams GT, Brown IS, et al. Collagenous sprue: a clinicopathologic study of 12 cases. Am J Surg Pathol. 2009;33(10):1440–9. https://doi.org/10.1097/PAS.0b013e3181ae2545.
105. Vakiani E, Arguelles-Grande C, Mansukhani MM, Lewis SK, Rotterdam H, Green PH, et al. Collagenous sprue is not always associated with dismal outcomes: a clinicopathological study of 19 patients. Mod Pathol. 2010;23(1):12–26. https://doi.org/10.1038/modpathol.2009.151.
106. Rubio-Tapia A, Talley NJ, Gurudu SR, Wu TT, Murray JA. Gluten-free diet and steroid treatment are effective therapy for most patients with collagenous sprue. Clin Gastroenterol Hepatol. 2010;8(4):344–9.e3. https://doi.org/10.1016/j.cgh.2009.12.023.
107. Zhao X, Johnson RL. Collagenous sprue: a rare, severe small-bowel malabsorptive disorder. Arch Pathol Lab Med. 2011;135(6):803–9. https://doi.org/10.1043/2010-0028-rs.1.
108. Schein J. Syndrome on non tropical sprue with hitherto undescribed lesions of the intestine. Gastroenterology. 1947;8(4):438–60.
109. Weinstein WM, Saunders DR, Tytgat GN, Rubin CE. Collagenous sprue—an unrecognized type of malabsorption. N Engl J Med. 1970;283(24):1297–301. https://doi.org/10.1056/nejm197012102832401.
110. Robert ME, Ament ME, Weinstein WM. The histologic spectrum and clinical outcome of refractory and unclassified sprue. Am J Surg Pathol. 2000;24(5):676–87.
111. Schoolmeester JK, Jenkins SM, Murray JA, Wu TT, Chandan VS. Increased immunoglobulin G4-positive plasma cells in collagenous sprue. Hum Pathol. 2013;44(8):1624–9. https://doi.org/10.1016/j.humpath.2013.01.013.
112. Daum S, Foss HD, Schuppan D, Riecken EO, Zeitz M, Ullrich R. Synthesis of collagen I in collagenous sprue. Clin Gastroenterol Hepatol. 2006;4(10):1232–6. https://doi.org/10.1016/j.cgh.2006.07.003.
113. Cellier C, Delabesse E, Helmer C, Patey N, Matuchansky C, Jabri B, et al. Refractory sprue, coeliac disease, and enteropathy-associated T-cell lymphoma. French Coeliac Disease Study Group. Lancet. 2000;356(9225):203–8.
114. Bossart R, Henry K, Doe WF, Booth CC. Proceedings: collagenous basement membrane thickening in jejunal biopsies from patients with adult coeliac disease. Gut. 1974;15(4):338.
115. Robert ME. Gluten sensitive enteropathy and other causes of small intestinal lymphocytosis. Semin Diagn Pathol. 2005;22(4):284–94.
116. Freeman HJ, Webber DL. Free perforation of the small intestine in collagenous sprue. World J Gastroenterol. 2009;15(35):4446–8.
117. Leonard J, Haffenden G, Tucker W, Unsworth J, Swain F, McMinn R, et al. Gluten challenge in dermatitis herpetiformis. N Engl J Med. 1983;308(14):816–9. https://doi.org/10.1056/nejm198304073081406.
118. Reunala T, Salmi TT, Hervonen K. Dermatitis herpetiformis: pathognomonic transglutaminase IgA deposits in the skin and excellent prognosis on a gluten-free diet. Acta Derm Venereol. 2015;95(8):917–22. https://doi.org/10.2340/00015555-2162.
119. Sardy M, Karpati S, Merkl B, Paulsson M, Smyth N. Epidermal transglutaminase (TGase 3) is the autoantigen of dermatitis herpetiformis. J Exp Med. 2002;195(6):747–57.
120. Karpati S. Dermatitis herpetiformis. Clin Dermatol. 2012;30(1):56–9. https://doi.org/10.1016/j.clindermatol.2011.03.010.
121. Rose C, Armbruster FP, Ruppert J, Igl BW, Zillikens D, Shimanovich I. Autoantibodies against epidermal transglutaminase are a sensitive diagnostic marker in patients with dermatitis herpetiformis on a normal or gluten-free diet. J Am Acad Dermatol. 2009;61(1):39–43. https://doi.org/10.1016/j.jaad.2008.12.037.
122. van de Staak WJ, van Tongeren JH. Dermatitis herpetiformis and pathological changes of the mucous membrane of the small intestine. Dermatologica. 1970;140(4):231–41.
123. Brow JR, Parker F, Weinstein WM, Rubin CE. The small intestinal mucosa in dermatitis herpetiformis. I. Severity and distribution of the small intestinal lesion and associated malabsorption. Gastroenterology. 1971;60(3):355–61.
124. Collin P, Salmi TT, Hervonen K, Kaukinen K, Reunala T. Dermatitis herpetiformis: a cutaneous manifestation of coeliac disease. Ann Med. 2017;49(1):23–31. https://doi.org/10.1080/07853890.2016.1222450.
125. Hervonen K, Alakoski A, Salmi TT, Helakorpi S, Kautiainen H, Kaukinen K, et al. Reduced mortality in dermatitis herpetiformis: a population-based study of 476 patients. Br J Dermatol. 2012;167(6):1331–7. https://doi.org/10.1111/j.1365-2133.2012.11105.x.
126. Lewis HM, Renaula TL, Garioch JJ, Leonard JN, Fry JS, Collin P, et al. Protective effect of gluten-free diet against development of lymphoma in dermatitis herpetiformis. Br J Dermatol. 1996;135(3):363–7.
127. Hervonen K, Vornanen M, Kautiainen H, Collin P, Reunala T. Lymphoma in patients with dermatitis herpetiformis and their first-degree relatives. Br J Dermatol. 2005;152(1):82–6. https://doi.org/10.1111/j.1365-2133.2005.06345.x.
128. Grainge MJ, West J, Solaymani-Dodaran M, Card TR, Logan RF. The long-term risk of malignancy following a diagnosis of coeliac disease or dermatitis herpetiformis: a cohort study. Aliment Pharmacol Ther. 2012;35(6):730–9. https://doi.org/10.1111/j.1365-2036.2012.04998.x.
129. Yel L. Selective IgA deficiency. J Clin Immunol. 2010;30(1):10–6. https://doi.org/10.1007/s10875-009-9357-x.
130. Yazdani R, Azizi G, Abolhassani H, Aghamohammadi A. Selective IgA deficiency: epidemiology, pathogenesis, clinical phenotype, diagnosis, prognosis and management. Scand J Immunol. 2017;85(1):3–12. https://doi.org/10.1111/sji.12499.
131. Burrows PD, Cooper MD. IgA deficiency. Adv Immunol. 1997;65:245–76.
132. Abolhassani H, Gharib B, Shahinpour S, Masoom SN, Havaei A, Mirminachi B, et al. Autoimmunity in patients with selective IgA deficiency. J Investig Allergol Clin Immunol. 2015;25(2):112–9.
133. Cataldo F, Marino V, Ventura A, Bottaro G, Corazza GR. Prevalence and clinical features of selective immunoglobulin A deficiency in coeliac disease: an Italian multicentre study. Italian Society of Paediatric Gastroenterology and Hepatology (SIGEP) and "Club del Tenue" Working Groups on Coeliac Disease. Gut. 1998;42(3):362–5.
134. Chow MA, Lebwohl B, Reilly NR, Green PH. Immunoglobulin A deficiency in celiac disease. J Clin Gastroenterol. 2012;46(10):850–4. https://doi.org/10.1097/MCG.0b013e31824b2277.
135. Woof JM, Kerr MA. The function of immunoglobulin A in immunity. J Pathol. 2006;208(2):270–82. https://doi.org/10.1002/path.1877.
136. Macpherson AJ, Geuking MB, McCoy KD. Immune responses that adapt the intestinal mucosa to commensal intestinal bacteria. Immunology. 2005;115(2):153–62. https://doi.org/10.1111/j.1365-2567.2005.02159.x.

137. Wang Z, Yunis D, Irigoyen M, Kitchens B, Bottaro A, Alt FW, et al. Discordance between IgA switching at the DNA level and IgA expression at the mRNA level in IgA-deficient patients. Clin Immunol. 1999;91(3):263–70. https://doi.org/10.1006/clim.1999.4702.
138. Brandtzaeg P, Karlsson G, Hansson G, Petruson B, Bjorkander J, Hanson LA. The clinical condition of IgA-deficient patients is related to the proportion of IgD- and IgM-producing cells in their nasal mucosa. Clin Exp Immunol. 1987;67(3):626–36.
139. Castigli E, Wilson SA, Garibyan L, Rachid R, Bonilla F, Schneider L, et al. TACI is mutant in common variable immunodeficiency and IgA deficiency. Nat Genet. 2005;37(8):829–34. https://doi.org/10.1038/ng1601.
140. Rachid R, Castigli E, Geha RS, Bonilla FA. TACI mutation in common variable immunodeficiency and IgA deficiency. Curr Allergy Asthma Rep. 2006;6(5):357–62.
141. Haimila K, Einarsdottir E, de Kauwe A, Koskinen LL, Pan-Hammarstrom Q, Kaartinen T, et al. The shared CTLA4-ICOS risk locus in celiac disease, IgA deficiency and common variable immunodeficiency. Genes Immun. 2009;10(2):151–61. https://doi.org/10.1038/gene.2008.89.
142. Jacob CM, Pastorino AC, Fahl K, Carneiro-Sampaio M, Monteiro RC. Autoimmunity in IgA deficiency: revisiting the role of IgA as a silent housekeeper. J Clin Immunol. 2008;28(Suppl 1):S56–61. https://doi.org/10.1007/s10875–007–9163–2.
143. Singh K, Chang C, Gershwin ME. IgA deficiency and autoimmunity. Autoimmun Rev. 2014;13(2):163–77. https://doi.org/10.1016/j.autrev.2013.10.005.
144. Yazdani R, Latif A, Tabassomi F, Abolhassani H, Azizi G, Rezaei N, et al. Clinical phenotype classification for selective immunoglobulin A deficiency. Expert Rev Clin Immunol. 2015;11(11):1245–54. https://doi.org/10.1586/1744666x.2015.1081565.
145. Wang N, Shen N, Vyse TJ, Anand V, Gunnarson I, Sturfelt G, et al. Selective IgA deficiency in autoimmune diseases. Mol Med. 2011;17(11–12):1383–96. https://doi.org/10.2119/molmed.2011.00195.
146. Zinneman HH, Kaplan AP. The association of giardiasis with reduced intestinal secretory immunoglobulin A. Am J Dig Dis. 1972;17(9):793–7.
147. Meini A, Pillan NM, Villanacci V, Monafo V, Ugazio AG, Plebani A. Prevalence and diagnosis of celiac disease in IgA-deficient children. Ann Allergy Asthma Immunol. 1996;77(4):333–6. https://doi.org/10.1016/s1081–1206(10)63329–7.
148. Brandtzaeg P. Update on mucosal immunoglobulin A in gastrointestinal disease. Curr Opin Gastroenterol. 2010;26(6):554–63. https://doi.org/10.1097/MOG.0b013e32833dccf8.
149. Iizuka M, Itou H, Sato M, Yukawa M, Shirasaka T, Chiba M, et al. Crohn's disease associated with selective immunoglobulin a deficiency. J Gastroenterol Hepatol. 2001;16(8):951–2.
150. Asada Y, Isomoto H, Shikuwa S, Wen CY, Fukuda E, Miyazato M, et al. Development of ulcerative colitis during the course of rheumatoid arthritis: association with selective IgA deficiency. World J Gastroenterol. 2006;12(32):5240–3.
151. Lai Ping So A, Mayer L. Gastrointestinal manifestations of primary immunodeficiency disorders. Semin Gastrointest Dis. 1997;8(1):22–32.
152. Cunningham-Rundles C. Physiology of IgA and IgA deficiency. J Clin Immunol. 2001;21(5):303–9.
153. Klemola T. Immunohistochemical findings in the intestine of IgA-deficient persons: number of intraepithelial T lymphocytes is increased. J Pediatr Gastroenterol Nutr. 1988;7(4):537–43.
154. Piascik M, Rydzewska G, Pawlik M, Milewski J, Furmanek MI, Wronska E, et al. Diffuse nodular lymphoid hyperplasia of the gastrointestinal tract in patient with selective immunoglobulin A deficiency and sarcoid-like syndrome—case report. Adv Med Sci. 2007;52:296–300.
155. Joo M, Shim SH, Chang SH, Kim H, Chi JG, Kim NH. Nodular lymphoid hyperplasia and histologic changes mimicking celiac disease, collagenous sprue, and lymphocytic colitis in a patient with selective IgA deficiency. Pathol Res Pract. 2009;205(12):876–80. https://doi.org/10.1016/j.prp.2009.02.005.
156. Hammarstrom L, Vorechovsky I, Webster D. Selective IgA deficiency (SIgAD) and common variable immunodeficiency (CVID). Clin Exp Immunol. 2000;120(2):225–31.
157. Aghamohammadi A, Mohammadi J, Parvaneh N, Rezaei N, Moin M, Espanol T, et al. Progression of selective IgA deficiency to common variable immunodeficiency. Int Arch Allergy Immunol. 2008;147(2):87–92. https://doi.org/10.1159/000135694.
158. Mellemkjaer L, Hammarstrom L, Andersen V, Yuen J, Heilmann C, Barington T, et al. Cancer risk among patients with IgA deficiency or common variable immunodeficiency and their relatives: a combined Danish and Swedish study. Clin Exp Immunol. 2002;130(3):495–500.
159. Mir-Madjlessi SH, Vafai M, Khademi J, Kamalian N. Coexisting primary malignant lymphoma and adenocarcinoma of the large intestine in an IgA-deficient boy. Dis Colon Rectum. 1984;27(12):822–4.
160. Kersey JH, Shapiro RS, Filipovich AH. Relationship of immunodeficiency to lymphoid malignancy. Pediatr Infect Dis J. 1988;7(5 Suppl):S10–2.
161. Unsworth DJ, Walker-Smith JA. Autoimmunity in diarrhoeal disease. J Pediatr Gastroenterol Nutr. 1985;4(3):375–80.
162. Akram S, Murray JA, Pardi DS, Alexander GL, Schaffner JA, Russo PA, et al. Adult autoimmune enteropathy: Mayo Clinic Rochester experience. Clin Gastroenterol Hepatol. 2007;5(11):1282–90; quiz 45. https://doi.org/10.1016/j.cgh.2007.05.013.
163. Montalto M, D'Onofrio F, Santoro L, Gallo A, Gasbarrini A, Gasbarrini G. Autoimmune enteropathy in children and adults. Scand J Gastroenterol. 2009;44(9):1029–36. https://doi.org/10.1080/00365520902783691.
164. Gentile NM, Murray JA, Pardi DS. Autoimmune enteropathy: a review and update of clinical management. Curr Gastroenterol Rep. 2012;14(5):380–5. https://doi.org/10.1007/s11894–012–0276–2.
165. Walker-Smith JA, Unsworth DJ, Hutchins P, Phillips AD, Holborow EJ. Autoantibodies against gut epithelium in child with small-intestinal enteropathy. Lancet. 1982;1(8271):566–7.
166. Catassi C, Fabiani E, Spagnuolo MI, Barera G, Guarino A. Severe and protracted diarrhea: results of the 3-year SIGEP multicenter survey. Working Group of the Italian Society of Pediatric Gastroenterology and Hepatology (SIGEP). J Pediatr Gastroenterol Nutr. 1999;29(1):63–8.
167. Goulet OJ, Brousse N, Canioni D, Walker-Smith JA, Schmitz J, Phillips AD. Syndrome of intractable diarrhoea with persistent villous atrophy in early childhood: a clinicopathological survey of 47 cases. J Pediatr Gastroenterol Nutr. 1998;26(2):151–61.
168. Corazza GR, Biagi F, Volta U, Andreani ML, De Franceschi L, Gasbarrini G. Autoimmune enteropathy and villous atrophy in adults. Lancet. 1997;350(9071):106–9. https://doi.org/10.1016/s0140–6736(97)01042–8.
169. Masia R, Peyton S, Lauwers GY, Brown I. Gastrointestinal biopsy findings of autoimmune enteropathy: a review of 25 cases. Am J Surg Pathol. 2014;38(10):1319–29. https://doi.org/10.1097/pas.0000000000000317.
170. Patey-Mariaud de Serre N, Canioni D, Ganousse S, Rieux-Laucat F, Goulet O, Ruemmele F, et al. Digestive histopathological presentation of IPEX syndrome. Mod Pathol. 2009;22(1):95–102. https://doi.org/10.1038/modpathol.2008.161.
171. Singhi AD, Goyal A, Davison JM, Regueiro MD, Roche RL, Ranganathan S. Pediatric autoimmune enteropathy: an entity frequently associated with immunodeficiency disorders. Mod Pathol. 2014;27(4):543–53. https://doi.org/10.1038/modpathol.2013.150.

172. Ruemmele FM, Moes N, de Serre NP, Rieux-Laucat F, Goulet O. Clinical and molecular aspects of autoimmune enteropathy and immune dysregulation, polyendocrinopathy autoimmune enteropathy X-linked syndrome. Curr Opin Gastroenterol. 2008;24(6):742–8. https://doi.org/10.1097/MOG.0b013e32830c9022.
173. Umetsu SE, Brown I, Langner C, Lauwers GY. Autoimmune enteropathies. Virchows Arch. 2017; https://doi.org/10.1007/s00428-017-2243-7.
174. Kisand K, Peterson P. Autoimmune polyendocrinopathy candidiasis ectodermal dystrophy. J Clin Immunol. 2015;35(5):463–78. https://doi.org/10.1007/s10875-015-0176-y.
175. Mirakian R, Hill S, Richardson A, Milla PJ, Walker-Smith JA, Bottazzo GF. HLA product expression and lymphocyte subpopulations in jejunum biopsies of children with idiopathic protracted diarrhoea and enterocyte autoantibodies. J Autoimmun. 1988;1(3):263–77.
176. Mais DD, Mulhall BP, Adolphson KR, Yamamoto K. Thymoma-associated autoimmune enteropathy. A report of two cases. Am J Clin Pathol. 1999;112(6):810–5.
177. Elwing JE, Clouse RE. Adult-onset autoimmune enteropathy in the setting of thymoma successfully treated with infliximab. Dig Dis Sci. 2005;50(5):928–32.
178. Oble DA, Mino-Kenudson M, Goldsmith J, Hodi FS, Seliem RM, Dranoff G, et al. Alpha-CTLA-4 mAb-associated panenteritis: a histologic and immunohistochemical analysis. Am J Surg Pathol. 2008;32(8):1130–7. https://doi.org/10.1097/PAS.0b013e31817150e3.
179. Gonzalez RS, Salaria SN, Bohannon CD, Huber AR, Feely MM, Shi C. PD-1 inhibitor gastroenterocolitis: case series and appraisal of 'immunomodulatory gastroenterocolitis'. Histopathology. 2017;70(4):558–67. https://doi.org/10.1111/his.13118.
180. Louie CY, DiMaio MA, Matsukuma KE, Coutre SE, Berry GJ, Longacre TA. Idelalisib-associated enterocolitis: clinicopathologic features and distinction from other enterocolitides. Am J Surg Pathol. 2015;39(12):1653–60. https://doi.org/10.1097/pas.0000000000000525.
181. Moes N, Rieux-Laucat F, Begue B, Verdier J, Neven B, Patey N, et al. Reduced expression of FOXP3 and regulatory T-cell function in severe forms of early-onset autoimmune enteropathy. Gastroenterology. 2010;139(3):770–8. https://doi.org/10.1053/j.gastro.2010.06.006.
182. Marthey L, Cadiot G, Seksik P, Pouderoux P, Lacroute J, Skinazi F, et al. Olmesartan-associated enteropathy: results of a national survey. Aliment Pharmacol Ther. 2014;40(9):1103–9. https://doi.org/10.1111/apt.12937.
183. Burbure N, Lebwohl B, Arguelles-Grande C, Green PH, Bhagat G, Lagana S. Olmesartan-associated sprue-like enteropathy: a systematic review with emphasis on histopathology. Hum Pathol. 2016;50:127–34. https://doi.org/10.1016/j.humpath.2015.12.001.
184. DeGaetani M, Tennyson CA, Lebwohl B, Lewis SK, Abu Daya H, Arguelles-Grande C, et al. Villous atrophy and negative celiac serology: a diagnostic and therapeutic dilemma. Am J Gastroenterol. 2013;108(5):647–53. https://doi.org/10.1038/ajg.2013.45.
185. Marietta EV, Nadeau AM, Cartee AK, Singh I, Rishi A, Choung RS, et al. Immunopathogenesis of olmesartan-associated enteropathy. Aliment Pharmacol Ther. 2015;42(11–12):1303–14. https://doi.org/10.1111/apt.13413.
186. Mandavdhare HS, Sharma V, Prasad KK, Kumar A, Rathi M, Rana SS. Telmisartan-induced sprue-like enteropathy: a case report and a review of patients using non-olmesartan angiotensin receptor blockers. Intest Res. 2017;15(3):419–21. https://doi.org/10.5217/ir.2017.15.3.419.
187. Zanelli M, Negro A, Santi R, Bisagni A, Ragazzi M, Ascani S, et al. Letter: sprue-like enteropathy associated with angiotensin II receptor blockers other than olmesartan. Aliment Pharmacol Ther. 2017;46(4):471–3. https://doi.org/10.1111/apt.14176.
188. Choi EY, McKenna BJ. Olmesartan-associated enteropathy: a review of clinical and histologic findings. Arch Pathol Lab Med. 2015;139(10):1242–7. https://doi.org/10.5858/arpa.2015-0204-RA.
189. Ianiro G, Bibbo S, Montalto M, Ricci R, Gasbarrini A, Cammarota G. Systematic review: sprue-like enteropathy associated with olmesartan. Aliment Pharmacol Ther. 2014;40(1):16–23. https://doi.org/10.1111/apt.12780.
190. Scialom S, Malamut G, Meresse B, Guegan N, Brousse N, Verkarre V, et al. Gastrointestinal disorder associated with olmesartan mimics autoimmune enteropathy. PLoS One. 2015;10(6):e0125024. https://doi.org/10.1371/journal.pone.0125024.
191. Lagana SM, Braunstein ED, Arguelles-Grande C, Bhagat G, Green PH, Lebwohl B. Sprue-like histology in patients with abdominal pain taking olmesartan compared with other angiotensin receptor blockers. J Clin Pathol. 2015;68(1):29–32. https://doi.org/10.1136/jclinpath-2014-202615.
192. Mathan VI. Tropical sprue. Springer Semin Immunopathol. 1990;12(2–3):231–7.
193. Nath SK. Tropical sprue. Curr Gastroenterol Rep. 2005;7(5):343–9.
194. Cook GC. Aetiology and pathogenesis of postinfective tropical malabsorption (tropical sprue). Lancet. 1984;1(8379):721–3.
195. Ghoshal UC, Ghoshal U, Ayyagari A, Ranjan P, Krishnani N, Misra A, et al. Tropical sprue is associated with contamination of small bowel with aerobic bacteria and reversible prolongation of orocecal transit time. J Gastroenterol Hepatol. 2003;18(5):540–7.
196. Walker MM. What is tropical sprue? J Gastroenterol Hepatol. 2003;18(8):887–90.
197. Haghighi P, Wolf PL. Tropical sprue and subclinical enteropathy: a vision for the nineties. Crit Rev Clin Lab Sci. 1997;34(4):313–41. https://doi.org/10.3109/10408369708998096.
198. Batheja MJ, Leighton J, Azueta A, Heigh R. The face of tropical sprue in 2010. Case Rep Gastroenterol. 2010;4(2):168–72. https://doi.org/10.1159/000314231.
199. Brown IS, Bettington A, Bettington M, Rosty C. Tropical sprue: revisiting an underrecognized disease. Am J Surg Pathol. 2014;38(5):666–72. https://doi.org/10.1097/pas.0000000000000153.
200. Swanson VL, Thomassen RW. Pathology of the jejunal mucosa in tropical sprue. Am J Pathol. 1965;46:511–51.
201. Puri AS, Khan EM, Kumar M, Pandey R, Choudhuri G. Association of lymphocytic (microscopic) colitis with tropical sprue. J Gastroenterol Hepatol. 1994;9(1):105–7.
202. Langenberg MC, Wismans PJ, van Genderen PJ. Distinguishing tropical sprue from celiac disease in returning travellers with chronic diarrhoea: a diagnostic challenge? Travel Med Infect Dis. 2014;12(4):401–5. https://doi.org/10.1016/j.tmaid.2014.05.001.
203. Rickles FR, Klipstein FA, Tomasini J, Corcino JJ, Maldonado N. Long-term follow-up of antibiotic-treated tropical sprue. Ann Intern Med. 1972;76(2):203–10.
204. Bures J, Cyrany J, Kohoutova D, Forstl M, Rejchrt S, Kvetina J, et al. Small intestinal bacterial overgrowth syndrome. World J Gastroenterol. 2010;16(24):2978–90.
205. Rezaie A, Pimentel M, Rao SS. How to test and treat small intestinal bacterial overgrowth: an evidence-based approach. Curr Gastroenterol Rep. 2016;18(2):8. https://doi.org/10.1007/s11894-015-0482-9.
206. Teo M, Chung S, Chitti L, Tran C, Kritas S, Butler R, et al. Small bowel bacterial overgrowth is a common cause of chronic diarrhea. J Gastroenterol Hepatol. 2004;19(8):904–9. https://doi.org/10.1111/j.1440-1746.2004.03376.x.
207. Lappinga PJ, Abraham SC, Murray JA, Vetter EA, Patel R, Wu TT. Small intestinal bacterial overgrowth: histopathologic features and clinical correlates in an underrecognized

entity. Arch Pathol Lab Med. 2010;134(2):264–70. https://doi.org/10.1043/1543-2165-134.2.264.
208. Bouhnik Y, Alain S, Attar A, Flourie B, Raskine L, Sanson-Le Pors MJ, et al. Bacterial populations contaminating the upper gut in patients with small intestinal bacterial overgrowth syndrome. Am J Gastroenterol. 1999;94(5):1327–31. https://doi.org/10.1111/j.1572-0241.1999.01016.x.
209. Ghoshal UC, Shukla R, Ghoshal U. Small intestinal bacterial overgrowth and irritable bowel syndrome: a bridge between functional organic dichotomy. Gut Liver. 2017;11(2):196–208. https://doi.org/10.5009/gnl16126.
210. Ament ME, Shimoda SS, Saunders DR, Rubin CE. Pathogenesis of steatorrhea in three cases of small intestinal stasis syndrome. Gastroenterology. 1972;63(5):728–47.
211. Haboubi NY, Lee GS, Montgomery RD. Duodenal mucosal morphometry of elderly patients with small intestinal bacterial overgrowth: response to antibiotic treatment. Age Ageing. 1991;20(1):29–32.
212. Riordan SM, McIver CJ, Wakefield D, Duncombe VM, Bolin TD, Thomas MC. Luminal antigliadin antibodies in small intestinal bacterial overgrowth. Am J Gastroenterol. 1997;92(8):1335–8.
213. Lauritano EC, Gabrielli M, Scarpellini E, Lupascu A, Novi M, Sottili S, et al. Small intestinal bacterial overgrowth recurrence after antibiotic therapy. Am J Gastroenterol. 2008;103(8):2031–5.
214. Levy E. Insights from human congenital disorders of intestinal lipid metabolism. J Lipid Res. 2015;56(5):945–62. https://doi.org/10.1194/jlr.R052415.
215. Burnett JR, Bell DA, Hooper AJ, Hegele RA. Clinical utility gene card for: Abetalipoproteinaemia—Update 2014. Eur J Hum Genet. 2015;23(6) https://doi.org/10.1038/ejhg.2014.224.
216. Wetterau JR, Aggerbeck LP, Bouma ME, Eisenberg C, Munck A, Hermier M, et al. Absence of microsomal triglyceride transfer protein in individuals with abetalipoproteinemia. Science (New York, NY). 1992;258(5084):999–1001.
217. Shoulders CC, Brett DJ, Bayliss JD, Narcisi TM, Jarmuz A, Grantham TT, et al. Abetalipoproteinemia is caused by defects of the gene encoding the 97 kDa subunit of a microsomal triglyceride transfer protein. Hum Mol Genet. 1993;2(12):2109–16.
218. Berriot-Varoqueaux N, Aggerbeck LP, Samson-Bouma M, Wetterau JR. The role of the microsomal triglygeride transfer protein in abetalipoproteinemia. Annu Rev Nutr. 2000;20:663–97. https://doi.org/10.1146/annurev.nutr.20.1.663.
219. Collins JC, Scheinberg IH, Giblin DR, Sternlieb I. Hepatic peroxisomal abnormalities in abetalipoproteinemia. Gastroenterology. 1989;97(3):766–70.
220. Avigan MI, Ishak KG, Gregg RE, Hoofnagle JH. Morphologic features of the liver in abetalipoproteinemia. Hepatology. 1984;4(6):1223–6.
221. Sidler AK, Huston BM, Thomas DB. Pathological case of the month. Abetalipoproteinemia (Bassen-Kornzweig syndrome). Arch Pediatr Adolesc Med. 1997;151(12):1265–6.
222. Lee J, Hegele RA. Abetalipoproteinemia and homozygous hypobetalipoproteinemia: a framework for diagnosis and management. J Inherit Metab Dis. 2014;37(3):333–9. https://doi.org/10.1007/s10545-013-9665-4.
223. Burnett JR, Zhong S, Jiang ZG, Hooper AJ, Fisher EA, McLeod RS, et al. Missense mutations in APOB within the betaalpha1 domain of human APOB-100 result in impaired secretion of ApoB and ApoB-containing lipoproteins in familial hypobetalipoproteinemia. J Biol Chem. 2007;282(33):24270–83. https://doi.org/10.1074/jbc.M702442200.
224. Vongsuvanh R, Hooper AJ, Coakley JC, Macdessi JS, O'Loughlin EV, Burnett JR, et al. Novel mutations in abetalipoproteinaemia and homozygous familial hypobetalipoproteinaemia. J Inherit Metab Dis. 2007;30(6):990. https://doi.org/10.1007/s10545-007-0693-9.
225. Tarugi P, Lonardo A, Ballarini G, Grisendi A, Pulvirenti M, Bagni A, et al. Fatty liver in heterozygous hypobetalipoproteinemia caused by a novel truncated form of apolipoprotein B. Gastroenterology. 1996;111(4):1125–33.
226. Schonfeld G, Patterson BW, Yablonskiy DA, Tanoli TS, Averna M, Elias N, et al. Fatty liver in familial hypobetalipoproteinemia: triglyceride assembly into VLDL particles is affected by the extent of hepatic steatosis. J Lipid Res. 2003;44(3):470–8. https://doi.org/10.1194/jlr.M200342-JLR200.
227. Lonardo A, Tarugi P, Ballarini G, Bagni A. Familial heterozygous hypobetalipoproteinemia, extrahepatic primary malignancy, and hepatocellular carcinoma. Dig Dis Sci. 1998;43(11):2489–92.
228. Bonnefont-Rousselot D, Condat B, Sassolas A, Chebel S, Bittar R, Federspiel MC, et al. Cryptogenic cirrhosis in a patient with familial hypocholesterolemia due to a new truncated form of apolipoprotein B. Eur J Gastroenterol Hepatol. 2009;21(1):104–8. https://doi.org/10.1097/MEG.0b013e3282ffd9f8.
229. Cefalu AB, Pirruccello JP, Noto D, Gabriel S, Valenti V, Gupta N, et al. A novel APOB mutation identified by exome sequencing cosegregates with steatosis, liver cancer, and hypocholesterolemia. Arterioscler Thromb Vasc Biol. 2013;33(8):2021–5. https://doi.org/10.1161/atvbaha.112.301101.
230. Jones B, Jones EL, Bonney SA, Patel HN, Mensenkamp AR, Eichenbaum-Voline S, et al. Mutations in a Sar1 GTPase of COPII vesicles are associated with lipid absorption disorders. Nat Genet. 2003;34(1):29–31. https://doi.org/10.1038/ng1145.
231. Silvain M, Bligny D, Aparicio T, Laforet P, Grodet A, Peretti N, et al. Anderson's disease (chylomicron retention disease): a new mutation in the SARA2 gene associated with muscular and cardiac abnormalities. Clin Genet. 2008;74(6):546–52. https://doi.org/10.1111/j.1399-0004.2008.01069.x.
232. Boldrini R, Biselli R, Bosman C. Chylomicron retention disease—the role of ultrastructural examination in differential diagnosis. Pathol Res Pract. 2001;197(11):753–7. https://doi.org/10.1078/0344-0338-00154.
233. Peretti N, Sassolas A, Roy CC, Deslandres C, Charcosset M, Castagnetti J, et al. Guidelines for the diagnosis and management of chylomicron retention disease based on a review of the literature and the experience of two centers. Orphanet J Rare Dis. 2010;5:24. https://doi.org/10.1186/1750-1172-5-24.
234. Avery GB, Villavicencio O, Lilly JR, Randolph JG. Intractable diarrhea in early infancy. Pediatrics. 1968;41(4):712–22.
235. Reifen RM, Cutz E, Griffiths AM, Ngan BY, Sherman PM. Tufting enteropathy: a newly recognized clinicopathological entity associated with refractory diarrhea in infants. J Pediatr Gastroenterol Nutr. 1994;18(3):379–85.
236. Sivagnanam M, Mueller JL, Lee H, Chen Z, Nelson SF, Turner D, et al. Identification of EpCAM as the gene for congenital tufting enteropathy. Gastroenterology. 2008;135(2):429–37. https://doi.org/10.1053/j.gastro.2008.05.036.
237. Goulet O, Salomon J, Ruemmele F, de Serres NP, Brousse N. Intestinal epithelial dysplasia (tufting enteropathy). Orphanet J Rare Dis. 2007;2:20. https://doi.org/10.1186/1750-1172-2-20.
238. Patey N, Scoazec JY, Cuenod-Jabri B, Canioni D, Kedinger M, Goulet O, et al. Distribution of cell adhesion molecules in infants with intestinal epithelial dysplasia (tufting enteropathy). Gastroenterology. 1997;113(3):833–43.
239. Guerra E, Lattanzio R, La Sorda R, Dini F, Tiboni GM, Piantelli M, et al. mTrop1/Epcam knockout mice develop congenital tufting enteropathy through dysregulation of intestinal E-cadherin/beta-catenin. PLoS One. 2012;7(11):e49302. https://doi.org/10.1371/journal.pone.0049302.

240. Mueller JL, McGeough MD, Pena CA, Sivagnanam M. Functional consequences of EpCam mutation in mice and men. Am J Physiol Gastrointest Liver Physiol. 2014;306(4):G278–88. https://doi.org/10.1152/ajpgi.00286.2013.
241. Salomon J, Goulet O, Canioni D, Brousse N, Lemale J, Tounian P, et al. Genetic characterization of congenital tufting enteropathy: epcam associated phenotype and involvement of SPINT2 in the syndromic form. Hum Genet. 2014;133(3):299–310. https://doi.org/10.1007/s00439-013-1380-6.
242. Abely M, Hankard GF, Hugot JP, Cezard JP, Peuchmaur M, Navarro J. Intractable infant diarrhea with epithelial dysplasia associated with polymalformation. J Pediatr Gastroenterol Nutr. 1998;27(3):348–52.
243. Bird LM, Sivagnanam M, Taylor S, Newbury RO. A new syndrome of tufting enteropathy and choanal atresia, with ophthalmologic, hematologic and hair abnormalities. Clin Dysmorphol. 2007;16(4):211–21. https://doi.org/10.1097/MCD.0b013e328274264b.
244. Roche O, Putterman M, Salomon J, Lacaille F, Brousse N, Goulet O, et al. Superficial punctate keratitis and conjunctival erosions associated with congenital tufting enteropathy. Am J Ophthalmol. 2010;150(1):116–21.e1. https://doi.org/10.1016/j.ajo.2010.01.034.
245. Ranganathan S, Schmitt LA, Sindhi R. Tufting enteropathy revisited: the utility of MOC31 (EpCAM) immunohistochemistry in diagnosis. Am J Surg Pathol. 2014;38(2):265–72. https://doi.org/10.1097/pas.0000000000000106.
246. Treetipsatit J, Hazard FK. Features of gastric and colonic mucosa in congenital enteropathies: a study in histology and immunohistochemistry. Am J Surg Pathol. 2014;38(12):1697–706. https://doi.org/10.1097/pas.0000000000000287.
247. Martin BA, Kerner JA, Hazard FK, Longacre TA. Evaluation of intestinal biopsies for pediatric enteropathy: a proposed immunohistochemical panel approach. Am J Surg Pathol. 2014;38(10):1387–95. https://doi.org/10.1097/pas.0000000000000314.
248. Davidson GP, Cutz E, Hamilton JR, Gall DG. Familial enteropathy: a syndrome of protracted diarrhea from birth, failure to thrive, and hypoplastic villus atrophy. Gastroenterology. 1978;75(5):783–90.
249. Ruemmele FM, Schmitz J, Goulet O. Microvillous inclusion disease (microvillous atrophy). Orphanet J Rare Dis. 2006;1:22. https://doi.org/10.1186/1750-1172-1-22.
250. Vogel GF, Hess MW, Pfaller K, Huber LA, Janecke AR, Muller T. Towards understanding microvillus inclusion disease. Mol Cell Pediatr. 2016;3(1):3. https://doi.org/10.1186/s40348-016-0031-0.
251. Muller T, Hess MW, Schiefermeier N, Pfaller K, Ebner HL, Heinz-Erian P, et al. MYO5B mutations cause microvillus inclusion disease and disrupt epithelial cell polarity. Nat Genet. 2008;40(10):1163–5. https://doi.org/10.1038/ng.225.
252. Wiegerinck CL, Janecke AR, Schneeberger K, Vogel GF, van Haaften-Visser DY, Escher JC, et al. Loss of syntaxin 3 causes variant microvillus inclusion disease. Gastroenterology. 2014;147(1):65–8.e10. https://doi.org/10.1053/j.gastro.2014.04.002.
253. Pohl JF, Shub MD, Trevelline EE, Ingebo K, Silber G, Rayhorn N, et al. A cluster of microvillous inclusion disease in the Navajo population. J Pediatr. 1999;134(1):103–6.
254. Canani RB, Castaldo G, Bacchetta R, Martin MG, Goulet O. Congenital diarrhoeal disorders: advances in this evolving web of inherited enteropathies. Nat Rev Gastroenterol Hepatol. 2015;12(5):293–302. https://doi.org/10.1038/nrgastro.2015.44.
255. Overeem AW, Posovszky C, Rings EH, Giepmans BN, van ISC. The role of enterocyte defects in the pathogenesis of congenital diarrheal disorders. Dis Model Mech. 2016;9(1):1–12. https://doi.org/10.1242/dmm.022269.
256. Knowles BC, Roland JT, Krishnan M, Tyska MJ, Lapierre LA, Dickman PS, et al. Myosin Vb uncoupling from RAB8A and RAB11A elicits microvillus inclusion disease. J Clin Invest. 2014;124(7):2947–62. https://doi.org/10.1172/jci71651.
257. Kravtsov DV, Ahsan MK, Kumari V, van Ijzendoorn SC, Reyes-Mugica M, Kumar A, et al. Identification of intestinal ion transport defects in microvillus inclusion disease. Am J Physiol Gastrointest Liver Physiol. 2016;311(1):G142–55. https://doi.org/10.1152/ajpgi.00041.2016.
258. Stepensky P, Bartram J, Barth TF, Lehmberg K, Walther P, Amann K, et al. Persistent defective membrane trafficking in epithelial cells of patients with familial hemophagocytic lymphohistiocytosis type 5 due to STXBP2/MUNC18-2 mutations. Pediatr Blood Cancer. 2013;60(7):1215–22. https://doi.org/10.1002/pbc.24475.
259. Girard M, Lacaille F, Verkarre V, Mategot R, Feldmann G, Grodet A, et al. MYO5B and bile salt export pump contribute to cholestatic liver disorder in microvillous inclusion disease. Hepatology. 2014;60(1):301–10. https://doi.org/10.1002/hep.26974.
260. Perry A, Bensallah H, Martinez-Vinson C, Berrebi D, Arbeille B, Salomon J, et al. Microvillous atrophy: atypical presentations. J Pediatr Gastroenterol Nutr. 2014;59(6):779–85. https://doi.org/10.1097/mpg.0000000000000526.
261. Phillips AD, Jenkins P, Raafat F, Walker-Smith JA. Congenital microvillous atrophy: specific diagnostic features. Arch Dis Child. 1985;60(2):135–40.
262. Raafat F, Green NJ, Nathavitharana KA, Booth IW. Intestinal microvillous dystrophy: a variant of microvillous inclusion disease or a new entity? Hum Pathol. 1994;25(11):1243–8.
263. Al-Daraji WI, Zelger B, Zelger B, Hussein MR. Microvillous inclusion disease: a clinicopathologic study of 17 cases from the UK. Ultrastruct Pathol. 2010;34(6):327–32. https://doi.org/10.3109/01913123.2010.500447.
264. Groisman GM, Ben-Izhak O, Schwersenz A, Berant M, Fyfe B. The value of polyclonal carcinoembryonic antigen immunostaining in the diagnosis of microvillous inclusion disease. Hum Pathol. 1993;24(11):1232–7.
265. Groisman GM, Amar M, Livne E. CD10: a valuable tool for the light microscopic diagnosis of microvillous inclusion disease (familial microvillous atrophy). Am J Surg Pathol. 2002;26(7):902–7.
266. Talmon G, Holzapfel M, DiMaio DJ, Muirhead D. Rab11 is a useful tool for the diagnosis of microvillous inclusion disease. Int J Surg Pathol. 2012;20(3):252–6. https://doi.org/10.1177/1066896911430959.
267. Iancu TC, Mahajnah M, Manov I, Shaoul R. Microvillous inclusion disease: ultrastructural variability. Ultrastruct Pathol. 2007;31(3):173–88. https://doi.org/10.1080/01913120701350712.
268. Halac U, Lacaille F, Joly F, Hugot JP, Talbotec C, Colomb V, et al. Microvillous inclusion disease: how to improve the prognosis of a severe congenital enterocyte disorder. J Pediatr Gastroenterol Nutr. 2011;52(4):460–5. https://doi.org/10.1097/MPG.0b013e3181fb4559.
269. Wang J, Cortina G, Wu SV, Tran R, Cho JH, Tsai MJ, et al. Mutant neurogenin-3 in congenital malabsorptive diarrhea. N Engl J Med. 2006;355(3):270–80. https://doi.org/10.1056/NEJMoa054288.
270. Cortina G, Smart CN, Farmer DG, Bhuta S, Treem WR, Hill ID, et al. Enteroendocrine cell dysgenesis and malabsorption, a histopathologic and immunohistochemical characterization. Hum Pathol. 2007;38(4):570–80. https://doi.org/10.1016/j.humpath.2006.10.014.
271. Ohsie S, Gerney G, Gui D, Kahana D, Martin MG, Cortina G. A paucity of colonic enteroendocrine and/or enterochromaffin cells characterizes a subset of patients with chronic unexplained diarrhea/malabsorption. Hum Pathol. 2009;40(7):1006–14. https://doi.org/10.1016/j.humpath.2008.12.016.

272. Al Khalidi H, Kandel G, Streutker CJ. Enteropathy with loss of enteroendocrine and paneth cells in a patient with immune dysregulation: a case of adult autoimmune enteropathy. Hum Pathol. 2006;37(3):373–6.
273. Goulet O, Vinson C, Roquelaure B, Brousse N, Bodemer C, Cezard JP. Syndromic (phenotypic) diarrhea in early infancy. Orphanet J Rare Dis. 2008;3:6. https://doi.org/10.1186/1750–1172–3-6.
274. Hartley JL, Zachos NC, Dawood B, Donowitz M, Forman J, Pollitt RJ, et al. Mutations in TTC37 cause trichohepatoenteric syndrome (phenotypic diarrhea of infancy). Gastroenterology. 2010;138(7):2388–98, 98.e1–2. https://doi.org/10.1053/j.gastro.2010.02.010.
275. Fabre A, Bourgeois P, Coste ME, Roman C, Barlogis V, Badens C. Management of syndromic diarrhea/tricho-hepato-enteric syndrome: a review of the literature. Intractable Rare Dis Res. 2017;6(3):152–7. https://doi.org/10.5582/irdr.2017.01040.
276. Fabre A, Martinez-Vinson C, Goulet O, Badens C. Syndromic diarrhea/Tricho-hepato-enteric syndrome. Orphanet J Rare Dis. 2013;8:5. https://doi.org/10.1186/1750–1172–8-5.
277. Muller T, Rasool I, Heinz-Erian P, Mildenberger E, Hulstrunk C, Muller A, et al. Congenital secretory diarrhoea caused by activating germline mutations in GUCY2C. Gut. 2016;65(8):1306–13. https://doi.org/10.1136/gutjnl-2015–309441.
278. Janecke AR, Heinz-Erian P, Yin J, Petersen BS, Franke A, Lechner S, et al. Reduced sodium/proton exchanger NHE3 activity causes congenital sodium diarrhea. Hum Mol Genet. 2015;24(23):6614–23. https://doi.org/10.1093/hmg/ddv367.
279. Holmberg C, Perheentupa J. Congenital Na+ diarrhea: a new type of secretory diarrhea. J Pediatr. 1985;106(1):56–61.
280. Booth IW, Stange G, Murer H, Fenton TR, Milla PJ. Defective jejunal brush-border Na+/H+ exchange: a cause of congenital secretory diarrhoea. Lancet. 1985;1(8437):1066–9.
281. Heinz-Erian P, Muller T, Krabichler B, Schranz M, Becker C, Ruschendorf F, et al. Mutations in SPINT2 cause a syndromic form of congenital sodium diarrhea. Am J Hum Genet. 2009;84(2):188–96. https://doi.org/10.1016/j.ajhg.2009.01.004.
282. Sivagnanam M, Janecke AR, Muller T, Heinz-Erian P, Taylor S, Bird LM. Case of syndromic tufting enteropathy harbors SPINT2 mutation seen in congenital sodium diarrhea. Clin Dysmorphol. 2010;19(1):48. https://doi.org/10.1097/MCD.0b013e328331de38.
283. Posovszky C. Congenital intestinal diarrhoeal diseases: a diagnostic and therapeutic challenge. Best Pract Res Clin Gastroenterol. 2016;30(2):187–211. https://doi.org/10.1016/j.bpg.2016.03.004.
284. Norio R, Perheentupa J, Launiala K, Hallman N. Congenital chloride diarrhea, an autosomal recessive disease. Genetic study of 14 Finnish and 12 other families. Clin Genet. 1971;2(3):182–92.
285. Hoglund P, Auranen M, Socha J, Popinska K, Nazer H, Rajaram U, et al. Genetic background of congenital chloride diarrhea in high-incidence populations: Finland, Poland, and Saudi Arabia and Kuwait. Am J Hum Genet. 1998;63(3):760–8. https://doi.org/10.1086/301998.
286. Wedenoja S, Pekansaari E, Hoglund P, Makela S, Holmberg C, Kere J. Update on SLC26A3 mutations in congenital chloride diarrhea. Hum Mutat. 2011;32(7):715–22. https://doi.org/10.1002/humu.21498.
287. Hihnala S, Hoglund P, Lammi L, Kokkonen J, Ormala T, Holmberg C. Long-term clinical outcome in patients with congenital chloride diarrhea. J Pediatr Gastroenterol Nutr. 2006;42(4):369–75. https://doi.org/10.1097/01.mpg.0000214161.37574.9a.
288. Carmel R. Biomarkers of cobalamin (vitamin B-12) status in the epidemiologic setting: a critical overview of context, applications, and performance characteristics of cobalamin, methylmalonic acid, and holotranscobalamin II. Am J Clin Nutr. 2011;94(1):348s–58s. https://doi.org/10.3945/ajcn.111.013441.
289. Battat R, Kopylov U, Szilagyi A, Saxena A, Rosenblatt DS, Warner M, et al. Vitamin B12 deficiency in inflammatory bowel disease: prevalence, risk factors, evaluation, and management. Inflamm Bowel Dis. 2014;20(6):1120–8. https://doi.org/10.1097/mib.0000000000000024.
290. Ward MG, Kariyawasam VC, Mogan SB, Patel KV, Pantelidou M, Sobczynska-Malefora A, et al. Prevalence and risk factors for functional vitamin B12 deficiency in patients with Crohn's Disease. Inflamm Bowel Dis. 2015;21(12):2839–47. https://doi.org/10.1097/mib.0000000000000559.
291. Abd-el-Gawa G, Abrahamsson K, Norlen L, Hjalmas K, Hanson E. Vitamin B12 and folate after 5–12 years of continent ileal urostomy (Kock reservoir) in children and adolescents. Eur Urol. 2002;41(2):199–205.
292. Foroozan P, Trier JS. Mucosa of the small intestine in pernicious anemia. N Engl J Med. 1967;277(11):553–9. https://doi.org/10.1056/nejm196709142771101.
293. Pena AS, Truelove SC, Callender ST, Whitehead R. Mucosal abnormalities and disaccharidases in pernicious anemia. Gut. 1970;11(12):1066.
294. Dawson DW. Partial villous atrophy in nutritional megaloblastic anaemia corrected by folic acid therapy. J Clin Pathol. 1971;24(2):131–5.
295. Bianchi A, Chipman DW, Dreskin A, Rosensweig NS. Nutritional folic acid deficiency with megaloblastic changes in the small-bowel epithelium. N Engl J Med. 1970;282(15):859–61. https://doi.org/10.1056/nejm197004092821510.
296. Hermos JA, Adams WH, Liu YK, Sullivan LW, Trier JS. Mucosa of the small intestine in folate-deficient alcoholics. Ann Intern Med. 1972;76(6):957–65.
297. Lizarraga A, Cuerda C, Junca E, Breton I, Camblor M, Velasco C, et al. Atrophy of the intestinal villi in a post-gastrectomy patient with severe iron deficiency anemia. Nutr Hosp. 2009;24(5):618–21.
298. Kambe T, Fukue K, Ishida R, Miyazaki S. Overview of inherited zinc deficiency in infants and children. J Nutr Sci Vitaminol. 2015;61(Suppl):S44–6. https://doi.org/10.3177/jnsv.61.S44.
299. Shah KN, Yan AC. Acquired zinc deficiency acrodermatitis associated with nephrotic syndrome. Pediatr Dermatol. 2008;25(1):56–9. https://doi.org/10.1111/j.1525–1470.2007.00583.x.
300. McClain C, Soutor C, Zieve L. Zinc deficiency: a complication of Crohn's disease. Gastroenterology. 1980;78(2):272–9.
301. Krasovec M, Frenk E. Acrodermatitis enteropathica secondary to Crohn's disease. Dermatology. 1996;193(4):361–3.
302. Kasana S, Din J, Maret W. Genetic causes and gene-nutrient interactions in mammalian zinc deficiencies: acrodermatitis enteropathica and transient neonatal zinc deficiency as examples. J Trace Elem Med Biol. 2015;29:47–62. https://doi.org/10.1016/j.jtemb.2014.10.003.
303. Wang K, Zhou B, Kuo YM, Zemansky J, Gitschier J. A novel member of a zinc transporter family is defective in acrodermatitis enteropathica. Am J Hum Genet. 2002;71(1):66–73. https://doi.org/10.1086/341125.
304. Kury S, Dreno B, Bezieau S, Giraudet S, Kharfi M, Kamoun R, et al. Identification of SLC39A4, a gene involved in acrodermatitis enteropathica. Nat Genet. 2002;31(3):239–40. https://doi.org/10.1038/ng913.
305. Maverakis E, Fung MA, Lynch PJ, Draznin M, Michael DJ, Ruben B, et al. Acrodermatitis enteropathica and an overview of zinc metabolism. J Am Acad Dermatol. 2007;56(1):116–24. https://doi.org/10.1016/j.jaad.2006.08.015.
306. Braun OH, Heilmann K, Pauli W, Rossner JA, Bergmann KE. Acrodermatitis enteropathica: recent findings concerning clinical features, pathogenesis, diagnosis and therapy. Eur J Pediatr. 1976;121(4):247–61.
307. Lombeck I, von Bassewitz DB, Becker K, Tinschmann P, Kastner H. Ultrastructural findings in acrodermatitis enteropathica. Pediatr Res. 1974;8(2):82–8. https://doi.org/10.1203/00006450–197402000–00003.

308. Kelly R, Davidson GP, Townley RR, Campbell PE. Reversible intestinal mucosal abnormality in acrodermatitis enteropathica. Arch Dis Child. 1976;51(3):219–22.
309. Chowanadisai W, Lonnerdal B, Kelleher SL. Identification of a mutation in SLC30A2 (ZnT-2) in women with low milk zinc concentration that results in transient neonatal zinc deficiency. J Biol Chem. 2006;281(51):39699–707. https://doi.org/10.1074/jbc.M605821200.
310. Owen RG, Treon SP, Al-Katib A, Fonseca R, Greipp PR, McMaster ML, et al. Clinicopathological definition of Waldenstrom's macroglobulinemia: consensus panel recommendations from the Second International Workshop on Waldenstrom's Macroglobulinemia. Semin Oncol. 2003;30(2):110–5. https://doi.org/10.1053/sonc.2003.50082.
311. Gertz MA. Waldenstrom macroglobulinemia: 2017 update on diagnosis, risk stratification, and management. Am J Hematol. 2017;92(2):209–17. https://doi.org/10.1002/ajh.24557.
312. Wang H, Chen Y, Li F, Delasalle K, Wang J, Alexanian R, et al. Temporal and geographic variations of Waldenstrom macroglobulinemia incidence: a large population-based study. Cancer. 2012;118(15):3793–800. https://doi.org/10.1002/cncr.26627.
313. Treon SP, Xu L, Yang G, Zhou Y, Liu X, Cao Y, et al. MYD88 L265P somatic mutation in Waldenstrom's macroglobulinemia. N Engl J Med. 2012;367(9):826–33. https://doi.org/10.1056/NEJMoa1200710.
314. Kapoor P, Paludo J, Ansell SM. Waldenstrom macroglobulinemia: familial predisposition and the role of genomics in prognosis and treatment selection. Curr Treat Options in Oncol. 2016;17(3):16. https://doi.org/10.1007/s11864–016–0391–7.
315. Hunter ZR, Xu L, Yang G, Zhou Y, Liu X, Cao Y, et al. The genomic landscape of Waldenstrom macroglobulinemia is characterized by highly recurring MYD88 and WHIM-like CXCR4 mutations, and small somatic deletions associated with B-cell lymphomagenesis. Blood. 2014;123(11):1637–46. https://doi.org/10.1182/blood-2013–09–525808.
316. Bedine MS, Yardley JH, Elliott HL, Banwell JG, Hendrix TR. Intestinal involvement in Waldenstrom's macroglobulinemia. Gastroenterology. 1973;65(2):308–15.
317. Veloso FT, Fraga J, Saleiro JV. Macroglobulinemia and small intestinal disease. A case report with review of the literature. J Clin Gastroenterol. 1988;10(5):546–50.
318. Pruzanski W, Warren RE, Goldie JH, Katz A. Malabsorption syndrome with infiltration of the intestinal wall by extracellular monoclonal macroglobulin. Am J Med. 1973;54(6):811–8.
319. Harris M, Burton IE, Scarffe JH. Macroglobulinaemia and intestinal lymphangiectasia: a rare association. J Clin Pathol. 1983;36(1):30–6.
320. Case records of the Massachusetts General Hospital. Weekly clinicopathological exercises. Case 3–1990. A 66-year-old woman with Waldenstrom's macroglobulinemia, diarrhea, anemia, and persistent gastrointestinal bleeding. N Engl J Med. 1990;322(3):183–92. https://doi.org/10.1056/nejm199001183220308.
321. Pratz KW, Dingli D, Smyrk TC, Lust JA. Intestinal lymphangiectasia with protein-losing enteropathy in Waldenstrom macroglobulinemia. Medicine. 2007;86(4):210–4. https://doi.org/10.1097/MD.0b013e31812e5242.
322. Gertz MA, Kyle RA, Noel P. Primary systemic amyloidosis: a rare complication of immunoglobulin M monoclonal gammopathies and Waldenstrom's macroglobulinemia. J Clin Oncol. 1993;11(5):914–20. https://doi.org/10.1200/jco.1993.11.5.914.
323. Vignes S, Bellanger J. Primary intestinal lymphangiectasia (Waldmann's disease). Orphanet J Rare Dis. 2008;3:5. https://doi.org/10.1186/1750–1172–3-5.
324. Ingle SB, Hinge Ingle CR. Primary intestinal lymphangiectasia: minireview. World J Clin Cases. 2014;2(10):528–33. https://doi.org/10.12998/wjcc.v2.i10.528.
325. Femppel J, Lux G, Kaduk B, Roesch W. Functional lymphangiectasia of the duodenal mucosa. Endoscopy. 1978;10(1):44–6. https://doi.org/10.1055/s-0028–1098260.
326. Patel AS, DeRidder PH. Endoscopic appearance and significance of functional lymphangiectasia of the duodenal mucosa. Gastrointest Endosc. 1990;36(4):376–8.
327. Kim JH, Bak YT, Kim JS, Seol SY, Shin BK, Kim HK. Clinical significance of duodenal lymphangiectasia incidentally found during routine upper gastrointestinal endoscopy. Endoscopy. 2009;41(6):510–5. https://doi.org/10.1055/s-0029–1214611.
328. Bellutti M, Monkemuller K, Fry LC, Dombrowski F, Malfertheiner P. Characterization of yellow plaques found in the small bowel during double-balloon enteroscopy. Endoscopy. 2007;39(12):1059–63. https://doi.org/10.1055/s-2007–966824.
329. Macdonald J, Porter V, Scott NW, McNamara D. Small bowel lymphangiectasia and angiodysplasia: a positive association; novel clinical marker or shared pathophysiology? J Clin Gastroenterol. 2010;44(9):610–4. https://doi.org/10.1097/MCG.0b013e3181dd9c3f.
330. Waldmann TA, Steinfeld JL, Dutcher TF, Davidson JD, Gordon RS Jr. The role of the gastrointestinal system in "idiopathic hypoproteinemia". Gastroenterology. 1961;41:197–207.
331. Alshikho MJ, Talas JM, Noureldine SI, Zazou S, Addas A, Kurabi H, et al. Intestinal lymphangiectasia: insights on management and literature review. Am J Case Rep. 2016;17:512–22.
332. Alders M, Hogan BM, Gjini E, Salehi F, Al-Gazali L, Hennekam EA, et al. Mutations in CCBE1 cause generalized lymph vessel dysplasia in humans. Nat Genet. 2009;41(12):1272–4. https://doi.org/10.1038/ng.484.
333. Oh TG, Chung JW, Kim HM, Han SJ, Lee JS, Park JY, et al. Primary intestinal lymphangiectasia diagnosed by capsule endoscopy and double balloon enteroscopy. World J Gastrointest Endosc. 2011;3(11):235–40. https://doi.org/10.4253/wjge.v3.i11.235.
334. Parfitt AM. Familial neonatal hypoproteinaemia with exudative enteropathy and intestinal lymphangiectasis. Arch Dis Child. 1966;41(215):54–62.
335. Wen J, Tang Q, Wu J, Wang Y, Cai W. Primary intestinal lymphangiectasia: four case reports and a review of the literature. Dig Dis Sci. 2010;55(12):3466–72. https://doi.org/10.1007/s10620–010–1161–1.
336. Syed U, Ching Companioni RA, Alkhawam H, Walfish A. Amyloidosis of the gastrointestinal tract and the liver: clinical context, diagnosis and management. Eur J Gastroenterol Hepatol. 2016;28(10):1109–21. https://doi.org/10.1097/meg.0000000000000695.
337. Desport E, Bridoux F, Sirac C, Delbes S, Bender S, Fernandez B, et al. Al amyloidosis. Orphanet J Rare Dis. 2012;7:54. https://doi.org/10.1186/1750–1172–7-54.
338. Said SM, Grogg KL, Smyrk TC. Gastric amyloidosis: clinicopathological correlations in 79 cases from a single institution. Hum Pathol. 2015;46(4):491–8. https://doi.org/10.1016/j.humpath.2014.12.009.
339. Tada S, Iida M, Iwashita A, Matsui T, Fuchigami T, Yamamoto T, et al. Endoscopic and biopsy findings of the upper digestive tract in patients with amyloidosis. Gastrointest Endosc. 1990;36(1):10–4.
340. Ebert EC, Nagar M. Gastrointestinal manifestations of amyloidosis. Am J Gastroenterol. 2008;103(3):776–87. https://doi.org/10.1111/j.1572–0241.2007.01669.x.
341. Sattianayagam PT, Gibbs SD, Rowczenio D, Pinney JH, Wechalekar AD, Gilbertson JA, et al. Hereditary lysozyme amyloidosis—phenotypic heterogeneity and the role of solid organ transplantation. J Intern Med. 2012;272(1):36–44. https://doi.org/10.1111/j.1365–2796.2011.02470.x.
342. Steen L, Ek B. Familial amyloidosis with polyneuropathy. A long-term follow-up of 21 patients with special reference to gastrointestinal symptoms. Acta Med Scand. 1983;214(5):387–97.

343. Jimenez RE, Price DA, Pinkus GS, Owen WF Jr, Lazarus JM, Kay J, et al. Development of gastrointestinal beta2-microglobulin amyloidosis correlates with time on dialysis. Am J Surg Pathol. 1998;22(6):729–35.
344. Gilat T, Spiro HM. Amyloidosis and the gut. Am J Dig Dis. 1968;13(7):619–33.
345. Herskovic T, Bartholomew LG, Green PA. Amyloidosis and Malabsorption Syndrome. Arch Intern Med. 1964;114:629–33.
346. Hayman SR, Lacy MQ, Kyle RA, Gertz MA. Primary systemic amyloidosis: a cause of malabsorption syndrome. Am J Med. 2001;111(7):535–40.
347. Peny MO, Debongnie JC, Haot J, Van Gossum A. Localized amyloid tumor in small bowel. Dig Dis Sci. 2000;45(9):1850–3.
348. Goteri G, Ranaldi R, Pileri SA, Bearzi I. Localized amyloidosis and gastrointestinal lymphoma: a rare association. Histopathology. 1998;32(4):348–55.
349. Tada S, Iida M, Yao T, Kawakubo K, Yao T, Okada M, et al. Endoscopic features in amyloidosis of the small intestine: clinical and morphologic differences between chemical types of amyloid protein. Gastrointest Endosc. 1994;40(1):45–50.
350. Tada S, Iida M, Yao T, Kawakubo K, Yao T, Fuchigami T, et al. Gastrointestinal amyloidosis: radiologic features by chemical types. Radiology. 1994;190(1):37–42. https://doi.org/10.1148/radiology.190.1.8259424.
351. Kim SH, Han JK, Lee KH, Won HJ, Kim KW, Kim JS, et al. Abdominal amyloidosis: spectrum of radiological findings. Clin Radiol. 2003;58(8):610–20.
352. Yoshimatsu S, Ando Y, Terazaki H, Sakashita N, Tada S, Yamashita T, et al. Endoscopic and pathological manifestations of the gastrointestinal tract in familial amyloidotic polyneuropathy type I (Met30). J Intern Med. 1998;243(1):65–72.
353. Chandan VS, Shah SS, Lam-Himlin DM, Petris GD, Mereuta OM, Dogan A, et al. Globular hepatic amyloid is highly sensitive and specific for LECT2 amyloidosis. Am J Surg Pathol. 2015;39(4):558–64. https://doi.org/10.1097/pas.0000000000000373.
354. Kebbel A, Rocken C. Immunohistochemical classification of amyloid in surgical pathology revisited. Am J Surg Pathol. 2006;30(6):673–83.
355. Vrana JA, Gamez JD, Madden BJ, Theis JD, Bergen HR 3rd, Dogan A. Classification of amyloidosis by laser microdissection and mass spectrometry-based proteomic analysis in clinical biopsy specimens. Blood. 2009;114(24):4957–9. https://doi.org/10.1182/blood-2009–07–230722.
356. Hobbs CM, Burch DM, Sobin LH. Elastosis and elastofibromatous change in the gastrointestinal tract: a clinicopathologic study of 13 cases and a review of the literature. Am J Clin Pathol. 2004;122(2):232–7. https://doi.org/10.1309/lbgt-cg1q-cd96-m3nf.
357. Ishida M, Iwai M, Kagotani A, Iwamoto N, Okabe H. Elastofibromatous change of the intestine: report of four lesions from three patients with review of the literature. Int J Clin Exp Pathol. 2014;7(5):2291–7.
358. Caubet JC, Nowak-Wegrzyn A. Current understanding of the immune mechanisms of food protein-induced enterocolitis syndrome. Expert Rev Clin Immunol. 2011;7(3):317–27. https://doi.org/10.1586/eci.11.13.
359. Turnbull JL, Adams HN, Gorard DA. Review article: the diagnosis and management of food allergy and food intolerances. Aliment Pharmacol Ther. 2015;41(1):3–25. https://doi.org/10.1111/apt.12984.
360. Mehr S, Kakakios A, Frith K, Kemp AS. Food protein-induced enterocolitis syndrome: 16-year experience. Pediatrics. 2009;123(3):e459–64. https://doi.org/10.1542/peds.2008–2029.
361. Katz Y, Goldberg MR, Rajuan N, Cohen A, Leshno M. The prevalence and natural course of food protein-induced enterocolitis syndrome to cow's milk: a large-scale, prospective population-based study. J Allergy Clin Immunol. 2011;127(3):647–53. e1–3. https://doi.org/10.1016/j.jaci.2010.12.1105.
362. Guandalini S, Newland C. Differentiating food allergies from food intolerances. Curr Gastroenterol Rep. 2011;13(5):426–34. https://doi.org/10.1007/s11894–011–0215–7.
363. Iyngkaran N, Robinson MJ, Prathap K, Sumithran E, Yadav M. Cows' milk protein-sensitive enteropathy. Combined clinical and histological criteria for diagnosis. Arch Dis Child. 1978;53(1):20–6.
364. Kokkonen J, Haapalahti M, Laurila K, Karttunen TJ, Maki M. Cow's milk protein-sensitive enteropathy at school age. J Pediatr. 2001;139(6):797–803. https://doi.org/10.1067/mpd.2001.118882.
365. Iyngkaran N, Yadav M, Boey CG, Kamath KR, Lam KL. Causative effect of cow's milk protein and soy protein on progressive small bowel mucosal damage. J Gastroenterol Hepatol. 1989;4(2):127–36.
366. Halpin TC, Byrne WJ, Ament ME. Colitis, persistent diarrhea, and soy protein intolerance. J Pediatr. 1977;91(3):404–7.
367. Ament ME, Rubin CE. Soy protein—another cause of the flat intestinal lesion. Gastroenterology. 1972;62(2):227–34.
368. Fontaine JL, Navarro J. Small intestinal biopsy in cows milk protein allergy in infancy. Arch Dis Child. 1975;50(5):357–62.
369. Kuitunen P, Visakorpi JK, Savilahti E, Pelkonen P. Malabsorption syndrome with cow's milk intolerance. Clinical findings and course in 54 cases. Arch Dis Child. 1975;50(5):351–6.
370. Rosekrans PC, Meijer CJ, Cornelisse CJ, van der Wal AM, Lindeman J. Use of morphometry and immunohistochemistry of small intestinal biopsy specimens in the diagnosis of food allergy. J Clin Pathol. 1980;33(2):125–30.
371. Phillips AD, Rice SJ, France NE, Walker-Smith JA. Small intestinal intraepithelial lymphocyte levels in cow's milk protein intolerance. Gut. 1979;20(6):509–12.
372. Walker-Smith J, Harrison M, Kilby A, Phillips A, France N. Cows' milk-sensitive enteropathy. Arch Dis Child. 1978;53(5):375–80.
373. Vandenplas Y, Koletzko S, Isolauri E, Hill D, Oranje AP, Brueton M, et al. Guidelines for the diagnosis and management of cow's milk protein allergy in infants. Arch Dis Child. 2007;92(10):902–8. https://doi.org/10.1136/adc.2006.110999.
374. Walker-Smith JA. Cow milk-sensitive enteropathy: predisposing factors and treatment. J Pediatr. 1992;121(5 Pt 2):S111–5.
375. Schrander JJ, Oudsen S, Forget PP, Kuijten RH. Follow up study of cow's milk protein intolerant infants. Eur J Pediatr. 1992;151(10):783–5.
376. Williams CD. Kwashiorkor. J Am Med Assoc. 1953;153(14):1280–5.
377. Liu T, Howard RM, Mancini AJ, Weston WL, Paller AS, Drolet BA, et al. Kwashiorkor in the United States: fad diets, perceived and true milk allergy, and nutritional ignorance. Arch Dermatol. 2001;137(5):630–6.
378. Tierney EP, Sage RJ, Shwayder T. Kwashiorkor from a severe dietary restriction in an 8-month infant in suburban Detroit, Michigan: case report and review of the literature. Int J Dermatol. 2010;49(5):500–6. https://doi.org/10.1111/j.1365–4632.2010.04253.x.
379. Amadi B, Fagbemi AO, Kelly P, Mwiya M, Torrente F, Salvestrini C, et al. Reduced production of sulfated glycosaminoglycans occurs in Zambian children with kwashiorkor but not marasmus. Am J Clin Nutr. 2009;89(2):592–600. https://doi.org/10.3945/ajcn.2008.27092.
380. William JH, Tapper EB, Yee EU, Robson SC. Secondary kwashiorkor: a rare complication of gastric bypass surgery. Am J Med. 2015;128(5):e1–2. https://doi.org/10.1016/j.amjmed.2014.12.002.
381. Stanfield JP, Hutt MS, Tunnicliffe R. Intestinal biopsy in kwashiorkor. Lancet. 1965;2(7411):519–23.
382. Shiner M, Redmond AO, Hansen JD. The jejunal mucosa in protein-energy malnutrition. A clinical, histological, and ultrastructural study. Exp Mol Pathol. 1973;19(1):61–78.

383. Cook GC, Lee FD. The jejunum after kwashiorkor. Lancet. 1966;2(7476):1263–7.
384. Waterlow JC. Intensive nursing care of kwashiorkor in Malawi. Acta Paediatr. 2000;89(2):138–40.
385. Schulzke JD, Troger H, Amasheh M. Disorders of intestinal secretion and absorption. Best Pract Res Clin Gastroenterol. 2009;23(3):395–406. https://doi.org/10.1016/j.bpg.2009.04.005.
386. Kuokkanen M, Kokkonen J, Enattah NS, Ylisaukko-Oja T, Komu H, Varilo T, et al. Mutations in the translated region of the lactase gene (LCT) underlie congenital lactase deficiency. Am J Hum Genet. 2006;78(2):339–44. https://doi.org/10.1086/500053.
387. Diekmann L, Pfeiffer K, Naim HY. Congenital lactose intolerance is triggered by severe mutations on both alleles of the lactase gene. BMC Gastroenterol. 2015;15:36. https://doi.org/10.1186/s12876-015-0261-y.
388. Ritz V, Alfalah M, Zimmer KP, Schmitz J, Jacob R, Naim HY. Congenital sucrase-isomaltase deficiency because of an accumulation of the mutant enzyme in the endoplasmic reticulum. Gastroenterology. 2003;125(6):1678–85.
389. Sander P, Alfalah M, Keiser M, Korponay-Szabo I, Kovacs JB, Leeb T, et al. Novel mutations in the human sucrase-isomaltase gene (SI) that cause congenital carbohydrate malabsorption. Hum Mutat. 2006;27(1):119. https://doi.org/10.1002/humu.9392.
390. Gericke B, Amiri M, Scott CR, Naim HY. Molecular pathogenicity of novel sucrase-isomaltase mutations found in congenital sucrase-isomaltase deficiency patients. Biochim Biophys Acta. 2017;1863(3):817–26. https://doi.org/10.1016/j.bbadis.2016.12.017.
391. Nichols BL, Avery SE, Karnsakul W, Jahoor F, Sen P, Swallow DM, et al. Congenital maltase-glucoamylase deficiency associated with lactase and sucrase deficiencies. J Pediatr Gastroenterol Nutr. 2002;35(4):573–9.
392. Wright EM, Turk E, Martin MG. Molecular basis for glucose-galactose malabsorption. Cell Biochem Biophys. 2002;36(2–3):115–21. https://doi.org/10.1385/cbb:36:2-3:115.
393. Santer R, Groth S, Kinner M, Dombrowski A, Berry GT, Brodehl J, et al. The mutation spectrum of the facilitative glucose transporter gene SLC2A2 (GLUT2) in patients with Fanconi-Bickel syndrome. Hum Genet. 2002;110(1):21–9. https://doi.org/10.1007/s00439-001-0638-6.
394. Gibson PR, Newnham E, Barrett JS, Shepherd SJ, Muir JG. Review article: fructose malabsorption and the bigger picture. Aliment Pharmacol Ther. 2007;25(4):349–63. https://doi.org/10.1111/j.1365-2036.2006.03186.x.
395. Johnston I, Nolan J, Pattni SS, Walters JR. New insights into bile acid malabsorption. Curr Gastroenterol Rep. 2011;13(5):418–25. https://doi.org/10.1007/s11894-011-0219-3.
396. Wilcox C, Turner J, Green J. Systematic review: the management of chronic diarrhoea due to bile acid malabsorption. Aliment Pharmacol Ther. 2014;39(9):923–39. https://doi.org/10.1111/apt.12684.
397. Fromm H, Malavolti M. Bile acid-induced diarrhoea. Clin Gastroenterol. 1986;15(3):567–82.
398. Vitek L. Bile acid malabsorption in inflammatory bowel disease. Inflamm Bowel Dis. 2015;21(2):476–83. https://doi.org/10.1097/mib.0000000000000193.
399. Gracie DJ, Kane JS, Mumtaz S, Scarsbrook AF, Chowdhury FU, Ford AC. Prevalence of, and predictors of, bile acid malabsorption in outpatients with chronic diarrhea. Neurogastroenterol Motil. 2012;24(11):983–e538. https://doi.org/10.1111/j.1365-2982.2012.01953.x.
400. Oelkers P, Kirby LC, Heubi JE, Dawson PA. Primary bile acid malabsorption caused by mutations in the ileal sodium-dependent bile acid transporter gene (SLC10A2). J Clin Invest. 1997;99(8):1880–7. https://doi.org/10.1172/jci119355.
401. Walters JR, Tasleem AM, Omer OS, Brydon WG, Dew T, le Roux CW. A new mechanism for bile acid diarrhea: defective feedback inhibition of bile acid biosynthesis. Clin Gastroenterol Hepatol. 2009;7(11):1189–94. https://doi.org/10.1016/j.cgh.2009.04.024.

Other Inflammatory Disorders of Duodenum

10

Tsung-Teh Wu

Chronic Duodenitis

Definition

Chronic duodenitis is characterized by mucosal edema, increased plasma cells and lymphocytic infiltrates in lamina propria, fibrosis of lamina propria, mild epithelial injury, and reactive changes of surface epithelium. Villous atrophy with neutrophilic infiltrates of surface epithelium and lamina propria are present in active chronic duodenitis [1, 2].

Clinical Features

Epidemiology Chronic duodenitis is the most common and accounts for 60% of benign duodenal lesions in adults [3], and it is present in 5% of children who have undergone endoscopy [4].

Clinical presentations The most common clinical symptom is epigastric pain. Chronic duodenitis occurs in a variety of clinical settings including *Helicobacter pylori* (*H. pylori*) infection, drugs such as nonsteroidal anti-inflammatory drugs (NSAIDs), and chronic renal failure. Chronic duodenitis is present in 90% of duodenal biopsies from patients with NSAID use, the majority of them with mild to moderate chronic duodenitis, and only 7% with severe chronic duodenitis [5]. Active chronic duodenitis is not common in chronic NSAID uses [6]. Twelve to seventy-one percent of patients with chronic renal failure can present with chronic and active chronic duodenitis [7, 8], and 34% of them may have nodular duodenitis [9]. Chronic duodenitis can also be present in 12% of normal healthy individuals [1, 10].

Endoscopic findings Endoscopic appearance of chronic duodenitis is characterized by erythema, erosions, and subepithelial hemorrhages. There is no good correlation between the endoscopic duodenitis and histologically proven chronic duodenitis. Histologically absent or minimal inflammation is present in approximately 73% of endoscopically apparent duodenitis; therefore, diagnosis of chronic duodenitis requires histological confirmation [11].

Pathological Features

Increased mononuclear cell infiltrate including plasma cells and lymphocytes in lamina propria with mucosal edema and epithelial injury is a histological feature for chronic duodenitis (Fig. 10.1a) [1, 12]. Active chronic duodenitis shows the presence of neutrophilic infiltrate in epithelium and lamina propria with marked epithelial injury. In severe active chronic duodenitis, erosion and ulceration can be present (Fig. 10.1b). Villus atrophy and mucosal thickening due to fibrosis with increased chronic inflammatory infiltrates or lymphoid aggregate in lamina propria are present in the nodular duodenitis [9].

Differential Diagnosis

Normal duodenal mucosa contains a variable number of inflammatory cells including plasma cells and lymphocytes in the lamina propria and, in particular without the presence of mucosal edema and epithelial injury, should not be overdiagnosed as mild chronic duodenitis. Peptic duodenitis can have similar degree of inflammatory infiltrates and epithelial injury, and it can be differentiated from chronic duodenitis by the presence of gastric mucinous metaplasia.

T.-T. Wu (✉)
Department of Laboratory Medicine and Pathology, Mayo Clinic, Rochester, MN, USA
e-mail: Wu.TsungTeh@mayo.edu

L. Zhang et al. (eds.), *Surgical Pathology of Non-neoplastic Gastrointestinal Diseases*,
https://doi.org/10.1007/978-3-030-15573-5_10

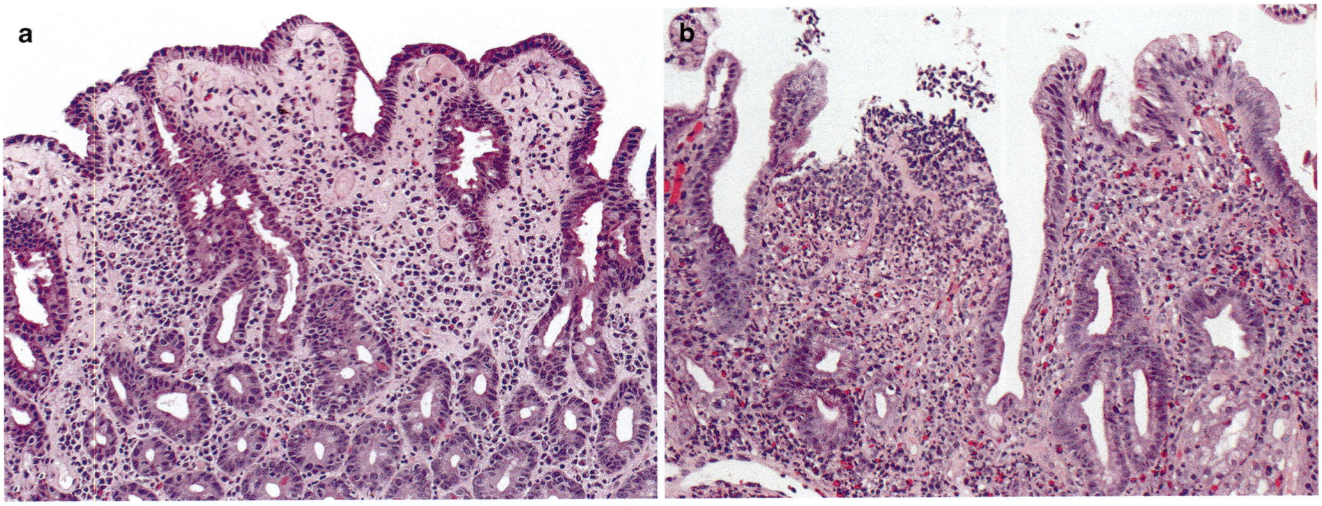

Fig. 10.1 Chronic duodenitis. (**a**) Duodenal biopsy shows increased mononuclear cell infiltrate including plasma cells and lymphocytes in lamina propria with mucosal edema, villous atrophy, and epithelial injury. (**b**) Acute inflammation and erosion are in severe active chronic duodenitis

Peptic Duodenitis

Definition

Peptic duodenitis was first described in 1962 by R. Crismer and was used to describe the presence of gastric mucinous metaplasia in duodenal mucosa whether associated with *H. pylori* infection or not [13]. Peptic duodenitis is characterized by irregular and shortening villi with edema and increased mononuclear cell infiltrates in lamina propria, superficial epithelial damage with gastric mucinous metaplasia, neutrophilic infiltrates of epithelium, and erosions [14].

Clinical Features

Epidemiology Gastric mucinous metaplasia in duodenum is present in 34–66% of adult patients with dyspepsia and in 7% of children who have undergone endoscopy [15, 16]. Peptic duodenitis with or without active inflammation is present in 7% of endoscopic duodenal biopsies [13]. *H. pylori* gastritis is associated with more than 90% of peptic duodenal ulcers [17–19]. Gastric mucinous metaplasia in duodenal mucosa can also occur in *H. pylori*-negative patients with increased acid production and hypergastrinemia. Extensive gastric mucinous metaplasia and peptic duodenitis are present in patients with Zollinger-Ellison syndrome [20].

Pathogenesis Gastric mucinous metaplasia in duodenum is more commonly present in adults than in children and is more common in males than in females [21]. The presence of gastric mucinous metaplasia in duodenum is associated with low fasting gastric pH, but not alcohol, smoking, or NSAIDs consumption. The extent of gastric mucinous metaplasia is associated with active chronic duodenitis and *H. pylori* gastritis [21, 22]. Gastric mucinous metaplasia is present in 34% of adults and 42% of children with *H. pylori* infection [23, 24]. Acid production is altered by *H. pylori* infection particularly in the antral-predominant gastritis in which the acid production is increased [22]. The high acid load in the duodenum causes gastric mucinous metaplasia in duodenal villi probably by cells migrating from Brunner's gland ducts [16]. The distribution of gastric mucinous metaplasia is patchy and more prominent in the duodenal bulb, and it is only present in the second part of the duodenum in severe cases [16]. The extent of gastric mucinous metaplasia is associated with the degree of duodenal and antral inflammation and density of *H. pylori* in antrum [23, 25]. Duodenal ulceration can be caused by a sequential effect of *H. pylori* infection in gastric antrum with increased acid secretion, peptic duodenitis, and *H. pylori* colonization on the foci with gastric mucinous metaplasia, reduced bicarbonate secretion, and mucosal damage [21, 22, 26]. There is an association with duodenal ulcers and *cagA*-positive *H. pylori* [22]; patients with duodenal ulcer have a 20-fold higher density of *H. pylori* and a higher prevalence of cagA-positive *H. pylori* strain [27].

Clinical presentations Abdominal pain, duodenal and jejunal ulcers, gastrointestinal hemorrhage, and diarrhea are the common presentations for patients with Zollinger-Ellison syndrome [28].

Pathological Features

Increased mononuclear cell infiltrates in lamina propria, gastric mucinous metaplasia, increased intramucosal Brunner's

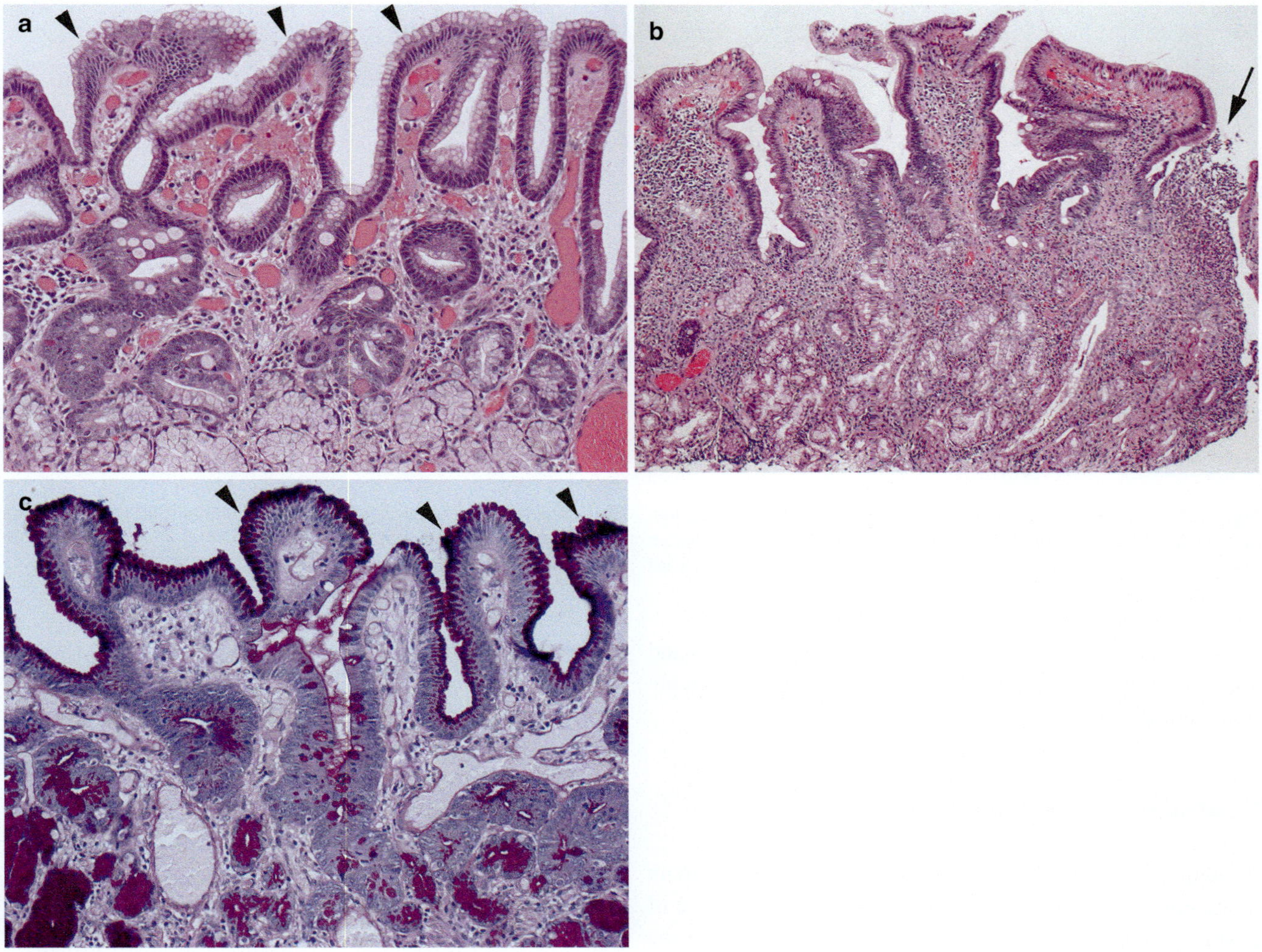

Fig. 10.2 Peptic duodenitis. (**a**) Chronic peptic duodenitis shows increased mononuclear cell infiltrates in lamina propria, gastric mucinous metaplasia (arrowheads), increased intramucosal Brunner's glands, and villous atrophy in duodenal biopsy. (**b**) Acute inflammation with neutrophilic infiltrates in epithelium and lamina propria and erosion (arrow) are present in active peptic duodenitis. (**c**) Gastric mucinous metaplasia (arrowheads) is characterized by the presence of gastric mucinous cells containing neutral mucin positive for PAS stain

glands, villous atrophy, and neutrophilic infiltrates in epithelium and lamina propria are the main features for peptic duodenitis (Fig. 10.2a, b). Gastric mucinous metaplasia is characterized by the presence of gastric mucinous cells containing apical neutral mucin in duodenal intestinal-type epithelium and can be demonstrated by a periodic acid-Schiff (PAS) stain (Fig. 10.2c). There is also a suggestion that peptic duodenitis without active inflammation should be classified as peptic duodenopathy [13]. Peptic duodenitis is more commonly present in the duodenal bulb than in second part of duodenum [14]. *H. pylori* are detected in 68% of active peptic duodenitis (Fig. 10.3a, b), more frequently than in peptic duodenitis without active inflammation which is only about 16% [13]. Increased intraepithelial lymphocytes (IELs) in the duodenum can be present in peptic duodenitis associated with *H. pylori* infection [29]. *H. pylori* infection is present in 58% of gastric mucinous metaplasia, and in 57% of diffuse nodular duodenitis [30]. Significantly decreased or complete regression of gastric mucinous metaplasia could be achieved in 54% of patients 6 months after eradication of *H. pylori*, but it had no influence on the macroscopic appearance of diffuse nodular duodenitis [30].

Differential Diagnosis

Gastric mucinous metaplasia and intramucosal Brunner's glands can be present in 64% and 96% of duodenal bulb and in 4% and 34% of second portion of duodenum in healthy individuals [1]. Gastric mucinous metaplasia in duodenum is a non-specific response to injury and inflammation and can be present in conditions other than peptic duodenitis such as in Crohn's disease and celiac disease [22]. Gastric heterotopia can be distinguished from gastric mucinous

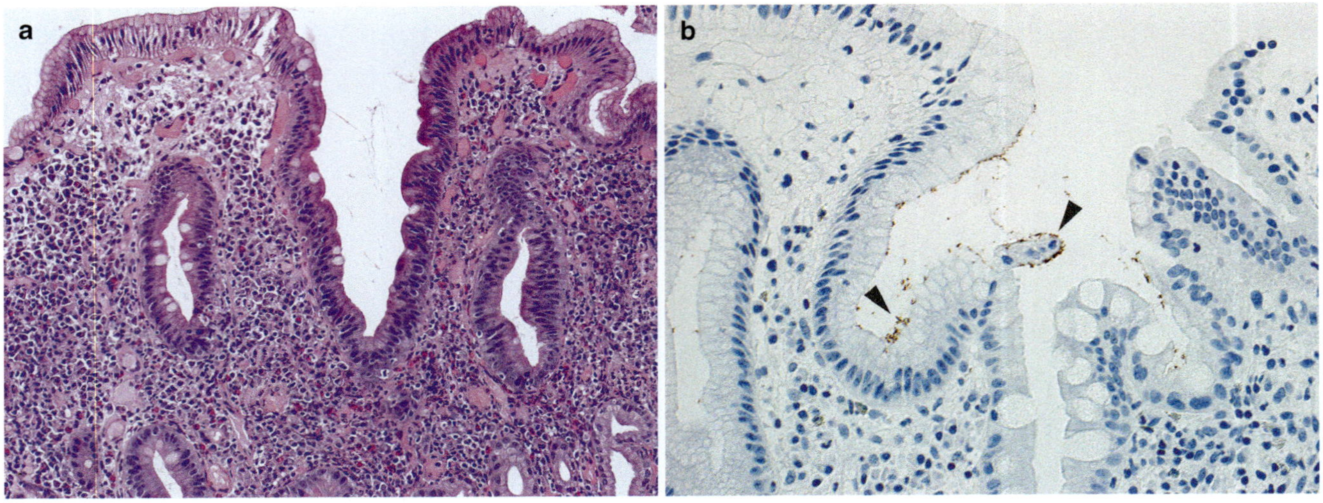

Fig. 10.3 Active peptic duodenitis with Helicobacter pylori infection. (**a**) Duodenal biopsy from a patient with active chronic Helicobacter pylori gastritis shows active peptic duodenitis. (**b**) Numerous Helicobacter pylori (arrowheads) within the luminal surface adjacent to the foci of gastric mucinous metaplasia are identified by immunohistochemical stain

metaplasia by the presence of parietal and/or chief cells and absence of increased mononuclear cell infiltrates and acute inflammation [13].

Treatment and Prognosis

Eradiation of *H. Pylori* and acid suppression are the main treatments. Acid suppression can result in 43% reduction of gastric mucinous metaplasia, but there is no effect on the degree of inflammation. Eradication of *H. pylori* can cause 42% reduction in gastric mucinous metaplasia and improvement of inflammation [25]. However, other studies showed that gastric mucinous metaplasia could persist after eradication of *H. pylori* infection [16, 31].

Lymphocytic Duodenitis

Definition

Lymphocytic duodenitis or enteritis is a histological diagnosis caused by a heterogeneous group of diseases including gluten-mediated and non-gluten-related diseases, characterized by duodenal or small bowel mucosa with normal villous architecture and increased IELs (>25 per 100 epithelial cells) [32–36]. Lymphocytic duodenitis or enteritis has also been described as microscopic enteritis, although increased IELs are not required for the diagnosis of microscopic enteritis [36, 37].

Clinical Features

Epidemiology Lymphocytic duodenitis is not an uncommon diagnosis on the duodenal biopsy in both adults and pediatric population, and the prevalence of lymphocytic duodenitis ranges from 1.3% to 10.9% [38–42]. The prevalence has increased threefold from 3% to 10.9% in a 10-year period from 2000 to 2010, mostly due to conditions other than celiac disease [41].

The most common associated etiologies for lymphocytic duodenitis or enteritis are celiac disease (9–21%), NSAIDs (8–21%), *H. pylori* infection (6–14%), irritable bowel syndrome (9–20%), inflammatory bowel disease (IBD; both Crohn's disease and ulcerative colitis—UC, 2–12%), autoimmune conditions (4–14%), and bacterial overgrowth syndrome (3–5%) [35, 36]. Lymphocytic duodenitis or enteritis can also be associated with non-celiac gluten enteropathy; dermatitis herpetiformis; wheat allergy; food or protein allergy; autoimmune enteropathy; autoimmune disorders such as rheumatoid arthritis, autoimmune thyroiditis, and psoriasis; infections such as giardia and cryptosporidium; tropical sprue; drugs such as olmesartan and idelalisib; lymphoproliferative disorders including both T-cell and B-cell lymphomas; immunodeficiency disorders such as IgA deficiency and common variable immunodeficiency (CVID), and graft-versus-host disease (GVHD) [32, 33, 35, 36, 43]. In 4–43% of the patients with diagnosis of lymphocytic duodenitis or enteritis, the underlying etiology cannot be identified [35, 36], and most of the patients are diagnosed with celiac disease or irritable bowel syndrome during the subsequent follow-up [44].

Pathogenesis Increased IEL in lymphocytic duodenitis or enteritis is a manifestation of immune response of intestinal mucosa between human host and microorganism and nonself antigens. The IELs are CD3+ and CD8+ and act as modulating cells as antigen-presenting cells for gluten, other antigens, bacteria, food, and drugs [36].

Clinical presentations The clinical presentations of lymphocytic duodenitis or enteritis vary and are associated with underlying etiology. Diarrhea, weight loss, abdominal pain, anemia, nausea, vomiting, and abdominal bloating are the most common presenting symptoms [39]. Iron, folate, vitamin B12, and vitamin D deficiency can also occur. Dyspepsia or epigastric pain can be associated with *H. pylori* infection. Recurrent infections are commonly seen in immunodeficiency. Rhinitis, asthma, and urticaria are associated with allergic disease [36].

Pathological Features

Intraepithelial lymphocytosis with normal small bowel villous architecture is the key pathologic feature for lymphocytic duodenitis or enteritis (Fig. 10.4a). The histological features are similar to the Marsh grade I in celiac disease. The distribution pattern of IELs in celiac disease-associated lymphocytic duodenitis can be continuous with even distribution along the villi or in the tip of villi [45]; however, these distribution patterns of IELs are not unique to celiac disease and can also be seen in lymphocytic duodenitis associated with inflammatory bowel disease, *H. pylori*, and other non-gluten-related etiologies [29, 39, 46]. In lymphocytic duodenitis associated with infections such giardia and cryptosporidium, the diagnostic parasites can be identified in the duodenal biopsy (Fig. 10.4b). Plasma cells are typically absent in lymphocytic duodenitis associated with CVID, and the plasma cells are negative for IgA by immunostain in IgA deficiency. Lymphocytic duodenitis is present in 44% of duodenal biopsy from patients with *H. pylori* gastritis [29].

Differential Diagnosis

Lymphocytic duodenitis or enteritis is a histological diagnosis, and determination of the associated underlying etiology typically requires clinical correlation. In lymphocytic duodenitis or enteritis associated with celiac disease, patients should have positive celiac serology and characteristic human leukocyte antigen (HLA) genotype. In patients with non-celiac gluten sensitivity who has negative IgA anti-transglutaminase antibodies (TTG), the clinical presentation is same as celiac disease, but the onset occurs shortly after gluten exposure which is in contrast to the celiac disease which usually occurs weeks later [47, 48]. The prevalence of non-celiac gluten sensitivity has been reported up to 6% in general population and is more common than celiac disease [35, 49].

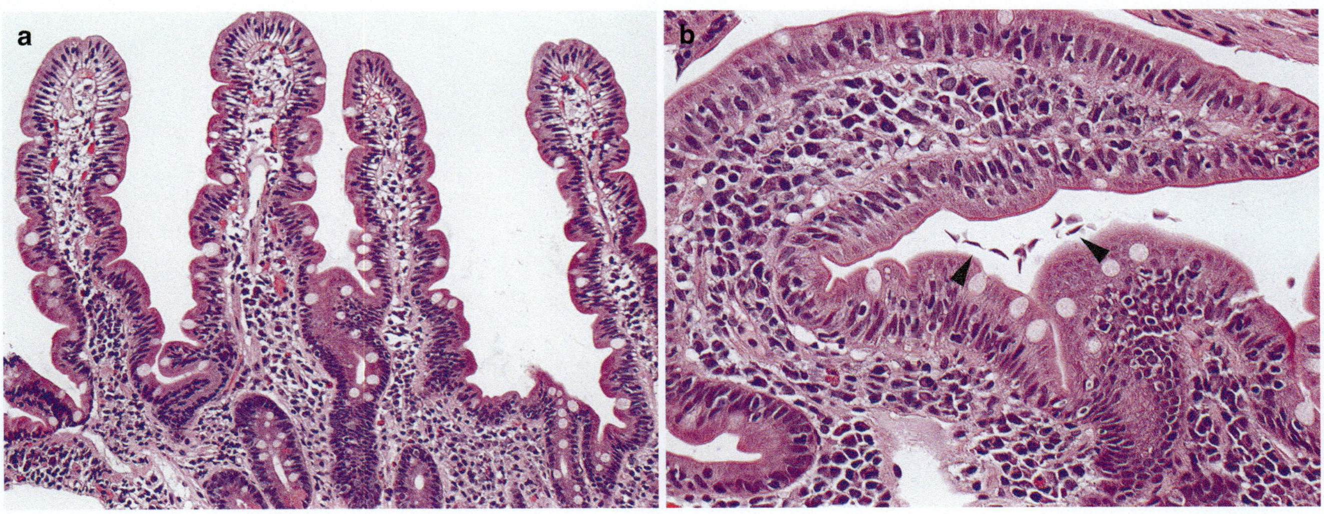

Fig. 10.4 Lymphocytic duodenitis. (**a**) Duodenal biopsy from a patient with active chronic Helicobacter pylori gastritis shows increased intraepithelial lymphocytes and normal villous architecture. (**b**) Lymphocytic duodenitis is present in a patient with giardia infection (arrowheads)

Treatment and Prognosis

The treatment of lymphocytic duodenitis or enteritis depends on the underlying associated etiologies.

Duodenal Involvement of Inflammatory Bowel Disease

Definition

Duodenitis with active and/or chronic inflammation present in patients with inflammatory bowel disease (Crohn's disease or UC) after excluding other etiologies that can cause duodenitis.

Clinical Features

Epidemiology Duodenal Crohn's disease occurs in 0.5–4% of Crohn's disease patients [50–52]. Duodenitis is found in 13% of inflammatory bowel disease patients, 26–28% of Crohn's disease patients, and 3% of UC patients. It is more frequent in children than adult IBD patients [53, 54]. In children, duodenitis has been reported in 31–33% of Crohn's disease and 3–23% of UC [55–57]. On the other hand, Crohn's disease or UC is also the common etiology for the duodenitis (13% and 3%, respectively) [4]. In children, active inflammation in stomach and duodenal bulb is more frequently seen in patients with refractory UC not responsive to medical therapy than in non-refractory UC patients [58].

Clinical presentations Upper abdominal pain, gastroduodenal obstruction, weight loss, and occasional gastrointestinal bleeding are the most common presentations for Crohn's disease involving duodenum [59]. Isolated Crohn's disease confined in the gastroduodenum is extremely rare and accounts less than 0.07% of all Crohn's disease patients [52, 60]. Gastroduodenal fistulas can occur in ileocolonic Crohn's disease or primary duodenal Crohn's disease [61, 62].

Endoscopic findings Nodularity in the descending part of the duodenum is prominent in Crohn's disease and UC. The endoscopic abnormalities in duodenum are more prominent in UC patients with pancolitis than in patients with left-sided/proctitis [63]. Granularity, nodularity, thickening mucosal folds, aphthoid ulcers, and ulcers on mucosal folds with notched appearance are present in pediatric patients with Crohn's disease [59, 64, 65].

Pathological Features

The common histological features of IBD involving duodenum are the presence of chronic duodenitis pattern with lymphoplasmacytosis in lamina propria either focal, patchy, or diffuse, villous atrophy, gastric mucinous metaplasia, and active inflammation (Fig. 10.5a, b) [66, 67]. Noncaseating granulomas are present in 3–11% of duodenal biopsies from patients with Crohn's disease (Fig. 10.5c) [66–68]. Duodenal biopsy with increased IELs and normal villous architecture (lymphocytic duodenitis) can also be seen in both Crohn's disease and UC patients (Fig. 10.5d) [35, 46, 69].

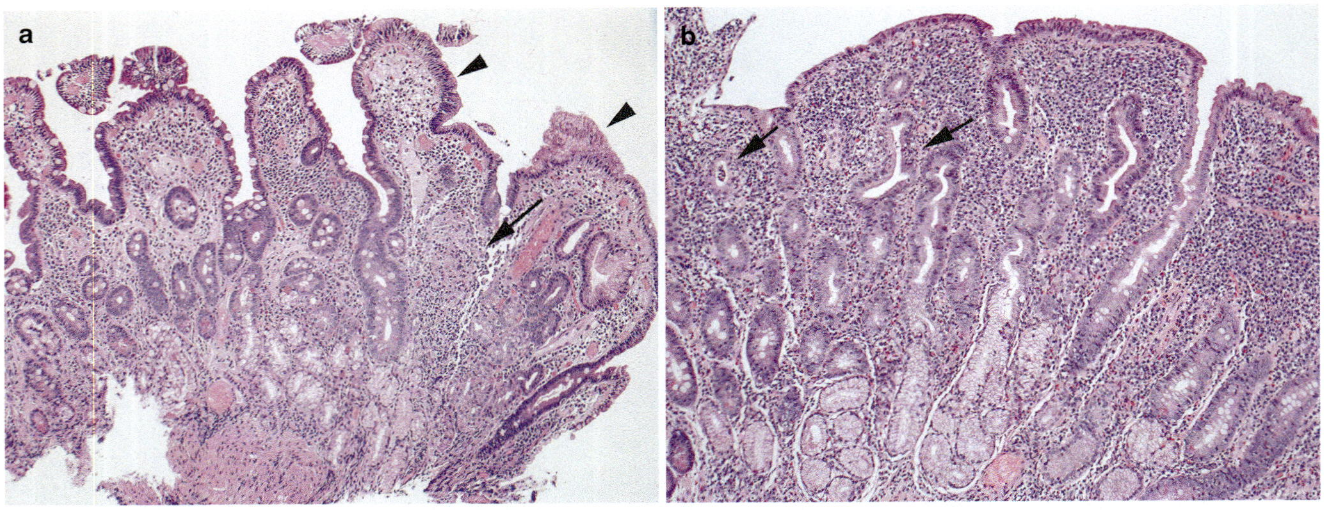

Fig. 10.5 Crohn's disease with duodenal involvement. (**a**) Duodenal biopsy shows chronic duodenitis pattern with lymphoplasmacytic infiltrates in lamina propria, villous atrophy, gastric mucinous metaplasia (arrowheads), and a small focus noncaseating granuloma (arrow) in a patient with Crohn's disease. (**b**) Active inflammation with cryptitis and crypt abscess and marked lymphoplasmacytic infiltrates in lamina propria in duodenal biopsy from another patient with Crohn's disease. (**c**) Multiple noncaseating granulomas are present in duodenal biopsy from Crohn's disease patient. (**d**) Duodenal biopsy shows increased intraepithelial lymphocytes with normal villous architecture (lymphocytic duodenitis) in Crohn's disease

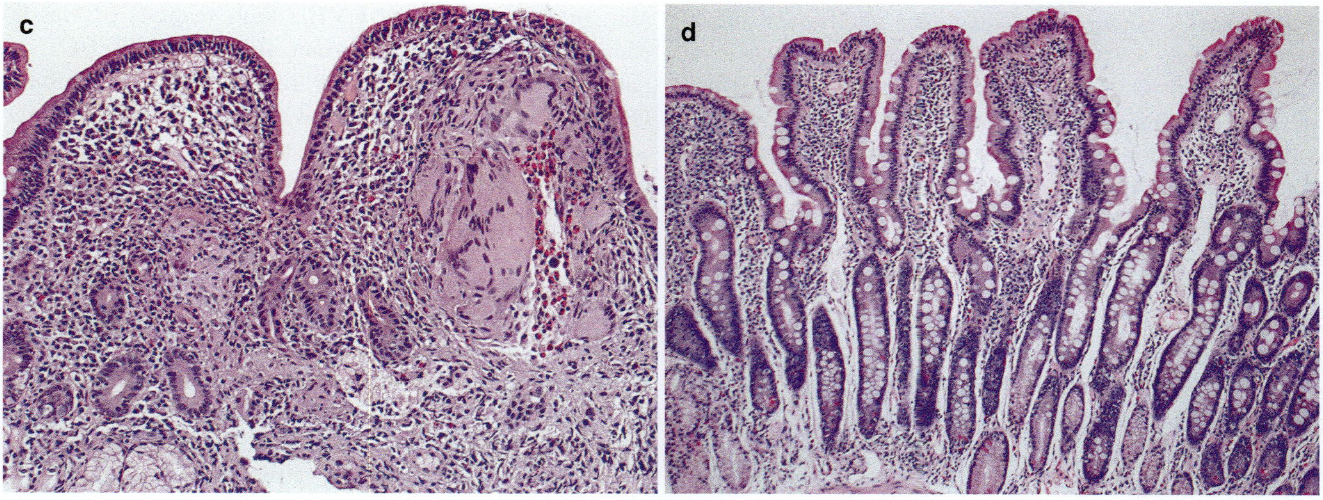

Fig. 10.5 (continued)

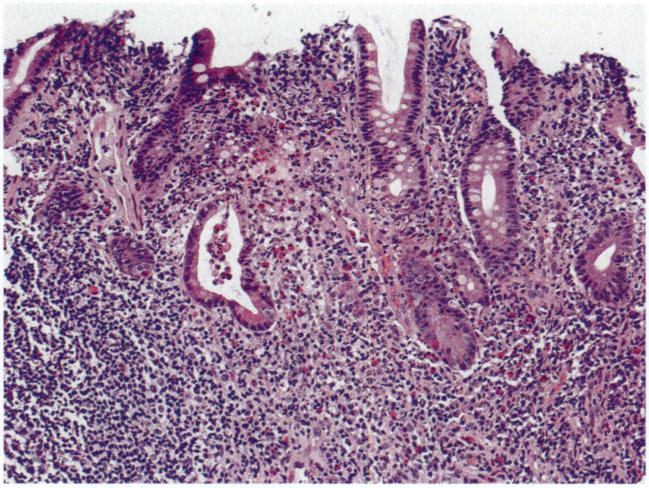

Fig. 10.6 Ulcerative colitis with duodenal involvement. Duodenal biopsy shows active chronic duodenitis with villous atrophy, diffuse lymphoplasmacytic infiltrate in lamina propria, cryptitis, and crypt abscess in a patient with ulcerative colitis

Diffuse active chronic duodenitis with villous atrophy, diffuse plasmacytosis in lamina propria, and patchy cryptitis (Fig. 10.6) have been described in 10% (4 of 40) of UC patients, and all four UC patients had pouchitis with previous colectomy [70]. Diffuse ulcerative panenteritis involving the small bowel [71, 72] and in a patient with refractory UC after colectomy with fetal outcome has been also reported [73]. Granulomatous inflammation and/or multinucleated giant cells present near glandular destruction can also present in the duodenum in pediatric UC patients [74].

Differential Diagnosis

Duodenal involvement in inflammatory bowel disease can manifest as histological patterns of active chronic duodenitis, peptic duodenitis, and lymphocytic duodenitis. Awareness of the clinical diagnosis of inflammatory bowel disease and excluding other etiologies such as infections, nutritional disorders, and medications such as NSAIDs that can cause these histological features will prompt the correct diagnosis. Crohn's disease is favored when noncaseating granulomas are present in the duodenal biopsy, and infectious etiologies have been ruled out by negative Gomori methenamine silver (GMS) and acid-fast bacteria (AFB) stains and other tests [69]. Sarcoidosis can involve duodenum and should be differentiated from duodenal Crohn's disease [75, 76].

Treatment and Prognosis

Proton pump inhibitors with steroid are the first-line treatment for active gastroduodenal Crohn's disease [65]. Gastroduodenal strictures can be treated with balloon dilatation, but duodenal fistulas need surgical closure of fistula tracts [61, 62]. Refractory gastroduodenal Crohn's disease may require surgical treatment [52].

Sarcoidosis

Sarcoidosis is a systemic granulomatous disorder of unknown etiology characterized by the formation of noncaseating granulomas in involved organs [77, 78]. Sarcoidosis affects predominantly young and middle-aged adults. The prevalence is about 4.7–64 in 100,000, and the incidence of sarcoidosis is 1–35.5 in 100,000 per year [78]. The lifetime incidence of sarcoidosis is higher in women (1.3%) than in men (1%) and higher in blacks (2.4%) than in Caucasians (0.8%) [79, 80]. Lung and lymphatic systems are the most common sites affected followed by the eyes, skin, and liver, but, virtually, every organ can be involved in sarcoidosis.

Gastrointestinal tract involvement in sarcoidosis is rare and has been reported in 0.1–1.6% of cases [81, 82]. Stomach is the most common site involved in sarcoidosis, but the entire digestive tract can also be affected [76, 83]. The common gastrointestinal symptoms are abdominal pain, weight loss, nausea/vomiting, diarrhea, and bleeding [76].

Small bowel sarcoidosis is the least common form of gastrointestinal tract sarcoidosis [76], and it can be an isolated disease or as part of disseminated gastrointestinal tract sarcoidosis [84–86]. The clinical symptoms with small bowel sarcoidosis include diarrhea, malabsorption, protein-losing enteropathy, epigastric pain, and hemorrhage [87, 88]. Nutritional deficiency, including folate and vitamin B12 [89], and duodenal obstruction [90, 91] with mass formation [75] have been reported in small bowel sarcoidosis. The pathological features of small bowel or duodenal sarcoidosis are the presence of noncaseating granulomas and partial villous atrophy [89, 92]. Multinucleated giant cells with calcium oxalate crystals and Schaumann bodies can also be seen within the noncaseating granulomas. Small bowel sarcoidosis can clinically and pathologically mimic Crohn's disease [85, 89]. Patients with Crohn's disease are not associated with elevated serum angiotensin-converting enzyme (ACE) level. The noncaseating granulomas in small bowel sarcoidosis tend to be limited in mucosa than in submucosa; in contrast, fistula tract, active chronic inflammation, and architectural distortion are commonly seen in Crohn's disease.

Graft-Versus-Host Disease

Definition

Graft-versus-host disease (GVHD) is a common complication of allogeneic hematopoietic stem cell transplantation (HCT) and can occur occasionally in autologous HCT and solid organ transplants. GVHD frequently involves the skin, gastrointestinal tract, liver, and rarely lung [93–95]. GVHD is a clinical syndrome and requires correlation with clinical, laboratory, and histopathologic findings for diagnosis [96]. GVHD can be subdivided into acute and chronic GVHDs. Acute GVHD includes (1) classic acute GVHD occurring within 100 days post HCT in patients not meeting criteria for diagnosis of chronic GVHD and (2) persistent, recurrent, or late-onset acute GVHD with features of classic acute GVHD occurring beyond 100 days post HCT in patients not meeting criteria for diagnosis of chronic GVHD. Chronic GVHD includes (1) classic chronic GVHD without features of characteristic of acute GVHD and (2) an overlap syndrome where features of acute and chronic GVHDs appear together [96].

Clinical Features

Epidemiology Acute GVHD is common (35–80%) in HCT patients [97]. The incidence of acute GVHD is around 20–50% in HLA-matched sibling HCT and is higher (60–80%) in HLA-mismatched HCT [98]. The gastrointestinal tract is the second most commonly involved organ in acute GVHD that can occur in 50–81% of patients with acute GVHD [99–101]. Acute GVHD has been described in 10% of patients after autologous HCT and is typically manifested as skin rash [94], and the incidence of gastrointestinal tract involvement by GVHD ranges from 4–13% [102, 103]. The incidence of chronic GVHD is around 30–70% in allogeneic HCT patients [96]. The estimated incidence of GVHD after solid organ transplants is 5% in small bowel transplant, 12% in multivisceral transplant, and 1–2% in liver transplant [95, 104].

Pathogenesis GVHD is a T-cell-mediated disease when the grafted donor lymphocytes encounter a foreign environment and result in activation and proliferation of inflammatory cells targeting host antigens [97, 105]. The development of acute GVHD can be conceptualized into three sequential phases [97]. Phase 1: Activation of the antigen-presenting cells (APCs) by the underlying disease and HCT conditioning regimen. "Danger" signals including proinflammatory cytokines such as TNF-α and chemokines, increased expression of adhesion molecules, major histocompatibility complex (MHC) antigens, and costimulatory molecules on host APCs are produced by damaged host tissue [105]. Phase 2: Donor T-cell activation in response to host APCs. In mouse model, CD4+ cells induce acute GVHD to MHC class II differences, and CD8+ cells induce acute GVHD to MHC class I differences. In HLA-identical HCT, both CD4+ and CD8+ cells respond to minor histocompatibility antigens and cause acute GVHD. The T-cell activations result in multiple intracellular biochemical cascades and produce excessive amount of Th1 cytokines (IFN-γ, IL-2, and TNF-α). Phase 3: Cellular and inflammatory effector phase. This phase involves both cellular effectors (cytotoxic T lymphocytes and NK cells) and soluble inflammatory mediators (TNF-α, IL-1, INF-α, and nitric oxide); both cellular effectors and inflammatory mediators synergize and amplify inflammation and tissue destruction.

Clinical presentations Nausea, vomiting, watery diarrhea, loss of appetite, bloody or mucoid stool, and abdominal pain are the common gastrointestinal manifestations of acute GVHD occurring within the first 100 days post HCT [106]. The gastrointestinal manifestations in chronic GVHD include esophageal web, proximal strictures or ring, dysphagia, anorexia, nausea, vomiting, diarrhea, weight loss, and failure to thrive [96]. The presence of esophageal web, stricture, or concentric rings documented by endoscopic or imaging study remains the only uniformly accepted diagnostic features for chronic GVHD within the gastrointestinal tract [96]. There is no difference in incidence, histological severity, and treatment response of gastrointestinal tract GVHD between allogeneic bone marrow transplantation and peripheral blood stem cell transplantation [93]. The major clinical presentations of GVHD after solid organ transplant are skin rash (100%), followed by cytopenia (16%), diarrhea (11%), and fever (5%) [95, 107].

Cytomegalovirus (CMV) and adenoviral infections can occur in allogeneic HCT patients. The incidence of CMV disease has decreased in allogeneic HCT patients after the initiation of CMV antiviral prophylaxis with acyclovir. The most important risk factors for CMV disease in allogeneic HCT patients are the serologic status of the donor and recipient. Approximately 30% of CMV-seronegative recipients who received transplant from CMV-seropositive donors develop primary CMV disease. CMV-seronegative recipients who received transplant from CMV-seronegative donors have a very low risk of primary CMV disease [108]. Patients who received alemtuzumab, an anti-CD52 monoclonal antibody that can result in CD41 and CD81 lymphopenia up to 9 months after administration, have the highest rate of CMV infection as compared to patients not receiving alemtuzumab [108, 109]. In autologous HCT, CMV infection develops in approximately 40% of patients, although CMV disease is rare after autologous HCT [108]. CMV gastroenteritis occurs in 16–25% of GVHD patients especially in HLA-mismatched transplants after allogeneic HCT [110, 111].

Adenoviral infection occurs in 3–41% of HCT patients, and it is higher in pediatric patients (31%) than in adults (14%), with 33–40% of adenovirus-positive patients having adenoviral disease [112–117]. Adenoviral infection occurs in 2–12% of autologous HCT patients [114]. The incidence of gastrointestinal tract adenoviral infection in allogeneic HCT patients is 10% [113]. Gastrointestinal symptoms of enteritis with diarrhea are the most frequent manifestations of adenoviral infection in children [115].

Endoscopic findings There is no correlation between clinical, endoscopic, and histological diagnosis of GVHD [102, 118]. The most common duodenal findings are redness, erosion, and ulceration [119]. There is no consensus regarding whether upper or lower gastrointestinal tract is the better biopsy site for diagnosing GVHD in gastrointestinal tract [93, 101, 118]. GVHD in gastrointestinal tract can involve both upper and lower gastrointestinal tracts (75–83%), and it can frequently have heterogeneous involvement of lower gastrointestinal tract only (6%) or upper gastrointestinal tract only (11–19%) due to site-specific variability in severity and partial response to treatment [93, 100, 120]. The highest diagnostic yield occurs when endoscopic visible injury or erythematous regions of both upper and lower gastrointestinal tracts are biopsied [121].

Pathological Features

The characteristic histologic features for acute GVHD are crypt apoptosis, crypt or glandular destruction, and mucosal denudation (Fig. 10.7a) [102, 118, 122]. Apoptotic bodies can appear as exploding crypts, hyperchromatic karyorrhectic nuclear debris within a large clear zone, small shrunken cells with eosinophilic cytoplasm, and a condensed nucleus (Fig. 10.7a) [118, 123]. Apoptotic debris limited to the superficial epithelium and lamina propria is a non-specific finding and cannot be used for diagnosis of acute GVHD. The minimal histological criteria for diagnosing acute GVHD in gastrointestinal tract remain controversial [118]. The proposed >6 apoptotic bodies/10 consecutive crypts criteria is similar to that used for acute cellular rejection in small bowel transplant. Although specific, it is too insensitive (59.4%) for acute GVHD [106, 124]. Using the >1–2 apoptotic bodies per biopsy piece (on average) increases sensitivity but with loss of some specificity [125, 126]. Acute GVHD in gastrointestinal tract can be graded as described in colon by Lerner et al. and Sale modification [123, 127]:

- Grade1: crypt apoptosis without crypt loss
- Grade 2: crypt apoptosis with individual crypt loss
- Grade 3: crypt apoptosis with loss of two or more contiguous crypts
- Grade 4: extensive crypt loss with mucosal denudation/ulceration (Fig. 10 7b)

This histological grading scheme is not currently recommended in routine practice by the National Institute of Health (NIH) consensus GVHD pathology working group [118]. Although eosinophils and acute inflammation are not the characteristic features of acute GVHD, eosinophils and acute inflammation with the presence of crypt apoptosis have been described in acute GVHD and cannot be used to exclude acute GVHD [102, 128].

There are no specific histological features of chronic GVHD in the gastrointestinal tract on endoscopic biopsies [102]. The characteristic features of chronic GVHD in

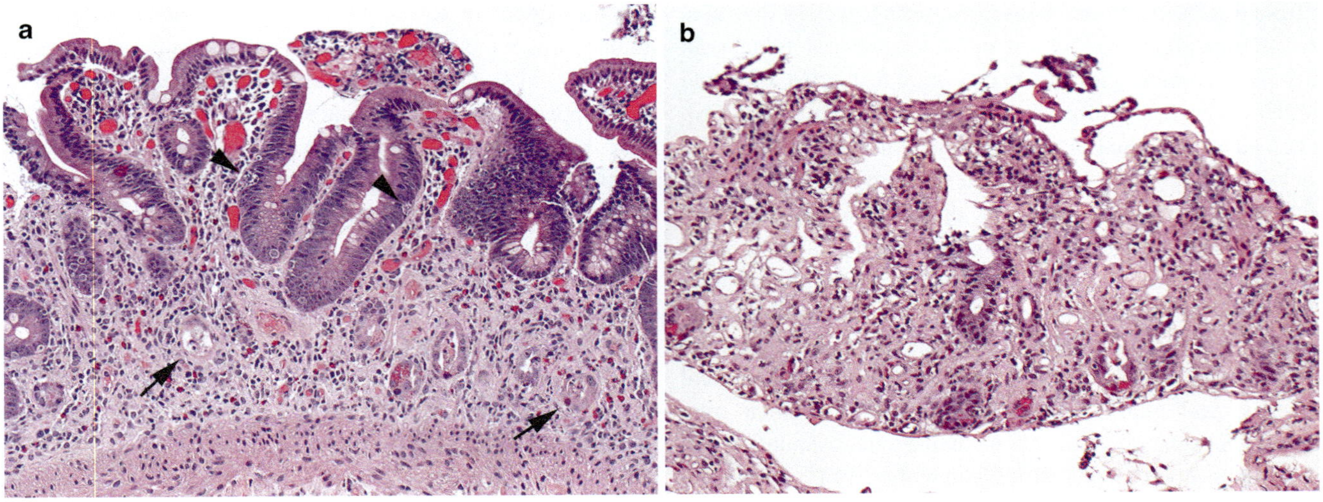

Fig. 10.7 Graft-versus-host disease. (**a**) Duodenal biopsy shows graft-versus-host disease with crypt apoptosis (arrowheads) and crypt destruction (arrows) in a patient with allogeneic bone marrow transplant. (**b**) Extensive crypt loss with mucosal denudation and ulceration in severe graft-versus-host disease

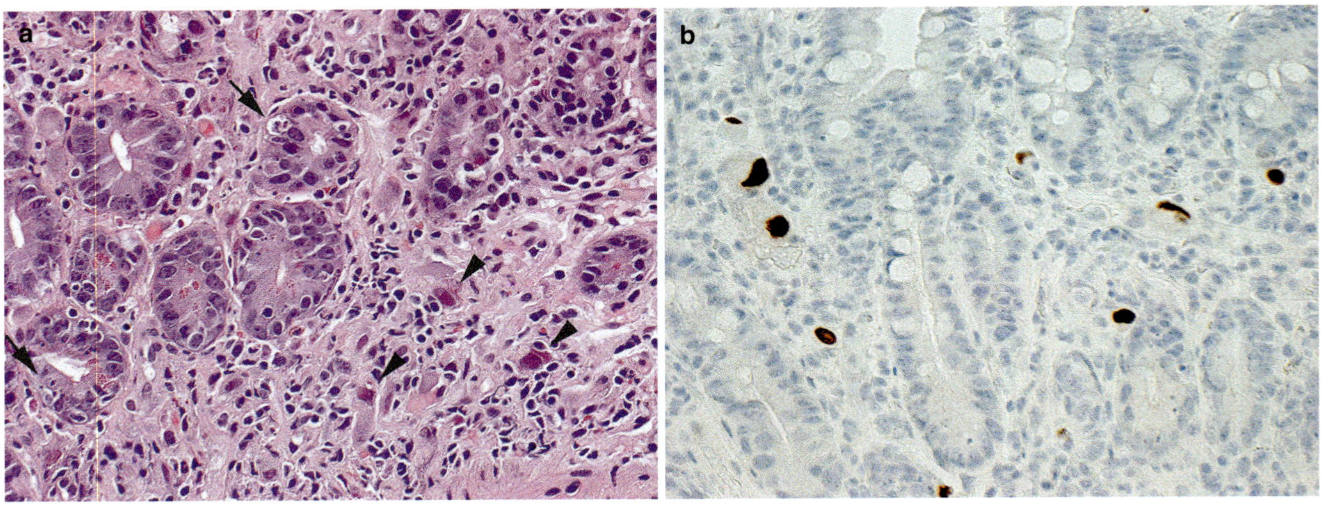

Fig. 10.8 CMV infection after bone marrow transplant. (**a**) Duodenal biopsy shows crypt apoptosis (arrows) and multiple CMV viral inclusions (arrowheads) with both nuclear and cytoplasmic inclusions in the stromal cells in a patient with allogeneic bone marrow transplant. (**b**) CMV infection is confirmed by immunohistochemical stain

gastrointestinal tracts such as submucosal or subserosal fibrosis and hyalinization of submucosal venules cannot be assessed on endoscopic biopsies [93, 122]. Mucosal fibrosis, crypt distortion, mononuclear infiltrates in lamina propria, Paneth cell metaplasia in the colon, and ulceration can be present in chronic GVHD, but they are not specific [93, 102, 129].

Differential Diagnosis

The cytoreductive conditioning therapy used before HCT can cause severe gastrointestinal tract mucosal injury, and these effects can last up to 3 weeks [93]. The presence of crypt apoptotic bodies is not unique for acute GVHD and can also be seen in infections (CMV, adenovirus, and cryptosporidium) and drug-induced gastrointestinal tract injury (mycophenolate mofetil, NSAIDs, and proton pump inhibitors). Proton pump inhibitor-associated apoptosis is mild and typically in gastric antrum [130]. CMV (Fig. 10.8a, b) and adenoviral (Fig. 10.9a, b) infections can be detected by using immunohistochemistry stains [131]. CD123 expression by immunohistochemical stain is significantly increased in colonic acute GVHD but not in CMV colitis and can be helpful in differentiating between acute GVHD and CMV infection [132]. GVHD-like histological feature is one of the histological patterns seen in mycophenolate mofetil-induced gastrointestinal tract injuries [133, 134] and needs to be differentiated from acute GVHD. The presence of increased

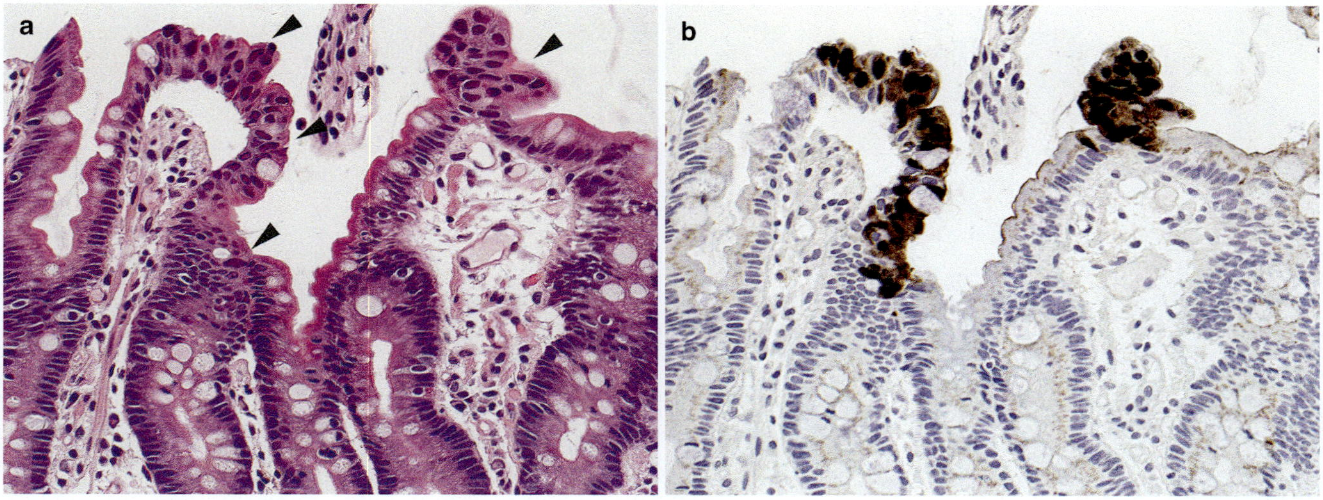

Fig. 10.9 Adenoviral infection after bone marrow transplant. (**a**) Duodenal biopsy shows numerous adenoviral inclusions with enlarged smudge nuclei (arrowheads) within the enterocytes in a patient with allogeneic bone marrow transplant. (**b**) Adenoviral infection is confirmed by immunohistochemical stain

eosinophils in the lamina propria and epithelium, and loss of neuroendocrine cell nests which are preserved in acute GVHD, would favor mycophenolate mofetil-induced gastrointestinal tract injury [135].

Treatment and Prognosis

Systemic corticosteroids are the treatment of GVHD [98]. Chronic GVHD is one of the major causes of late transplant-related mortality [96]. The mortality rate is high (30–75%) in GVHD occurring in solid organ transplants [95, 107, 136].

Eosinophilic Duodenitis/Enteritis

Eosinophilic gastroenteritis (EG) is a rare and heterogeneous disorder defined by three criteria: (1) the presence of gastrointestinal symptoms, (2) biopsies showing eosinophilic infiltrates of one or more areas of the gastrointestinal tract or characteristic radiological findings with peripheral eosinophilia, and (3) no evidence of parasitic or extraintestinal disease [137]. The commonest sites of the EG are stomach and proximal small intestine [138]. Eosinophilic duodenitis/enteritis is one of the manifestations of EG [139].

EG can affect any age group, however, most commonly between 30s and 40s years of age with a slightly male predominance [140]. The estimated prevalence of EG in the United States is between 2.5 and 30 per 100,000 individuals [140–142]. Peripheral eosinophilia is common (75–83%) but not universal in patients with EG [143–145].

EG can be classified into three different patterns by Klein classification based on the disease distribution: (1) predominantly mucosal pattern, (2) predominantly muscular pattern, and (3) predominantly subserosal pattern [146]. The anatomic locations of eosinophilic infiltrates and the depth of gastrointestinal involvement determine the clinical symptoms [138, 147]. The predominantly mucosal pattern is the most common (44–58%) form of EG, characterized by mucosal and submucosal involvement (Fig. 10.10a), and the common clinical presentations include abdominal pain, nausea, vomiting, diarrhea, bleeding, anemia, protein-losing enteropathy, malabsorption, and weight loss. The predominantly muscular pattern is the second commonest (30–39%) form of EG, characterized by muscular layer involvement, and patients can present with bowel thickening and obstructive symptoms most commonly affecting stomach and duodenum. The predominantly subserosal pattern is the rarest (12%) form of EG, characterized by eosinophilic infiltrate that permeates all layers of digestive wall and reaches the serosa (Fig. 10.10b) with the presence of eosinophilic ascites and dramatic response to steroid treatment [137, 140, 143, 144].

The range of normal number of eosinophils in the duodenum and small bowel has not been well established, and the number varies in different geographic regions with potential seasonal variation [140, 148]. There is no universal accepted criteria, and the most accepted definition of eosinophilic duodenitis/enteritis is an eosinophilic count of >20–25/ high power field (HPF) in at least one sample [149, 150]. The distribution patterns of eosinophils in the mucosa are also important clues for diagnosis of eosinophilic duodenitis/enteritis. The presence of prominent eosinophils within the crypts (intraepithelial eosinophils or eosinophilic crypt

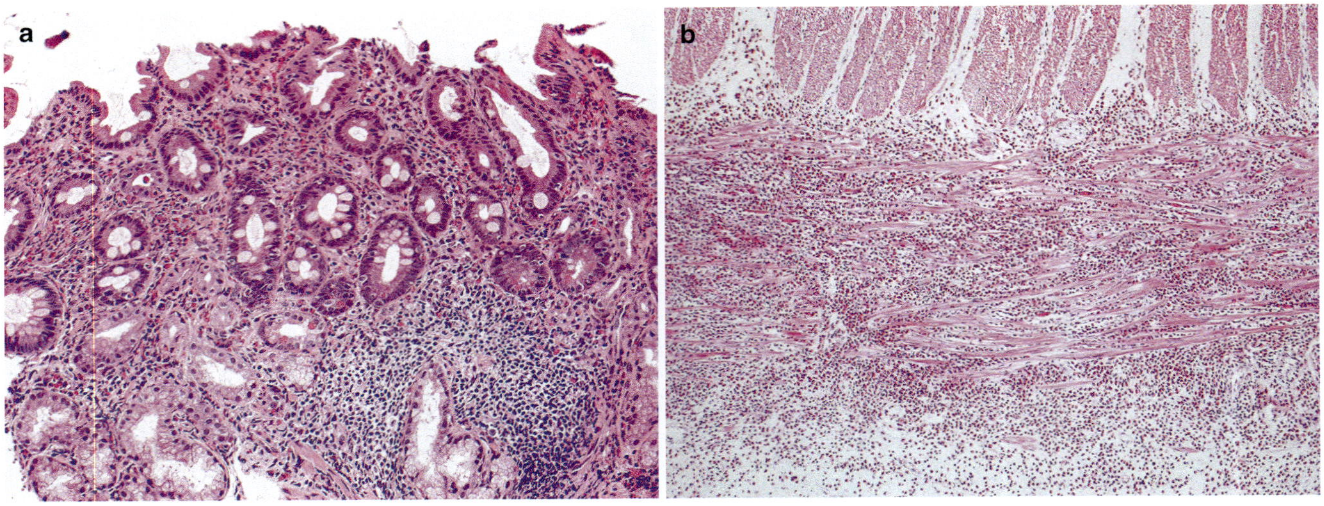

Fig. 10.10 Eosinophilic enteritis. (**a**) Eosinophilic enteritis with predominantly mucosal pattern. Duodenal biopsy shows prominent eosinophils within the crypts (intraepithelial eosinophils) and clustering of eosinophils in lamina propria. (**b**) Eosinophilic enteritis with predominantly serosal pattern. Extensive eosinophilic infiltrates are present within the muscularis propria and subserosa in resected small bowel

abscesses), clustering of eosinophils in lamina propria, and eosinophils in the muscularis mucosae is abnormal, and the diagnosis of eosinophilic duodenitis/enteritis should be suspected irrespective of the eosinophilic counts [151]. The eosinophilic infiltrates can be patchy in EG and can be missed in biopsies due to sampling issue.

EG needs to be differentiated from secondary eosinophilic gastroenteritis due to hypereosinophilic syndrome and protein hypersensitivity enteropathy. Increased eosinophilic infiltrate in gastrointestinal tract can also be present in inflammatory bowel disease; celiac disease; infections such as *H. pylori*, tuberculosis, fungal, and parasitic infections; connective tissue disorder (scleroderma); vasculitis (polyarteritis nodosa and Churg-Strauss syndrome); systemic mastocytosis; GVHD; drug reaction; food allergy; and malignancy such as lymphoma or leukemia [152]. Systemic corticosteroid is the mainstay treatment for EG if dietary treatment is not feasible or fails to achieve improvement [140, 147].

Common Variable Immunodeficiency

Definition

Common variable immunodeficiency (CVID) is characterized by hypogammaglobulinemia, with marked decrease in levels of IgG, IgA, and/or IgM, defective antibody responses to vaccines, and recurrent infections mostly in the respiratory and gastrointestinal tracts, after excluding other known primary or secondary causes of hypogammaglobulinemia [153, 154].

Clinical Features

Epidemiology CVID is the most common symptomatic form of primary immunodeficiency deficiency. The age of onset is variable, and the peak incidence is in childhood and in the second and third decades of life [154]. The prevalence of CVID is estimated between 1/50,000 and 1/10,000 in Caucasians, and it is rare in Asian and African populations [154, 155]. Most of the CVID cases occur sporadically, and familial occurrence mostly with autosomal dominant inheritance is reported in 5–25% of patients [154, 155].

Pathogenesis CVID is a heterogeneous disease with considerable phenotypical and genetic heterogeneity. With the advances in next-generation sequencing technologies, it is believed that CVID is a polygenetic or multifactorial disorder. Monogenic mutations have been identified in only 2–10% of CVID patients [156, 157]. Multiple genes have been implicated for the monogenic CVID including *ICOS*, *TNFRSF13B* (TACI), *TNFRSF13C* (BAFF-R), *TNFSF12* (TWEAK), *CD19*, *CD81*, *CR2* (CD21), *MS4A1* (CD20), *TNFRSF7* (CD27), *IL21*, *IL21R*, *LRBA*, *CTLA4*, *PRKCD*, *PLCG2*, *NFκB1*, *NFκB2*, *PIK3CD*, *PIK3R1*, *VAV1*, *RAC2*, *BLK*, *IKZF1*, and *IRF2BP2* [156, 158–160].

A subset (9%) of CVID patients can present with severe T-cell defect as late-onset combined immune deficiency (LOCID) defined by the occurrence of opportunistic infection and/or a CD4+ T-cell count $<200 \times 10^6$ cells/L [161]. Patients with LOCID have a higher prevalence of splenomegaly, granulomas, gastrointestinal disease, and lymphoma as compared to CVID patients [161].

The pathogenesis of intestinal lesions in CVID patients remains unclear. The absence of plasma cells in lamina propria of gastrointestinal tract is suggestive of the role of local defect in secretory antibodies [162]. The mononuclear cells in lamina propria produce significantly more T-helper (Th) 1 cytokeratin, IL-12 and IFNγ, which is similar to Crohn's disease [163].

Clinical presentations The most common initial clinical symptom is sinopulmonary infections [164]. Autoimmunity, granulomatous disorders (8–22%), and lymphoproliferative disorders are also common in patients with CVID [165–167]. Gastrointestinal symptoms ranging from dyspepsia, bloating, and abdominal pain to chronic diarrhea are present in up to 50–82% of CVID patients [162, 164, 168–172]. The gastrointestinal symptoms can be due to infectious or noninfectious etiologies. Acute and chronic infectious diarrhea is the most common gastrointestinal symptom in CVID [164, 173]. Giardia, salmonella, and campylobacter are the common infections in CVID patients and are more frequent in patients with undetectable serum IgA level [164]. Norovirus has also been increasingly noted in CVID patients with enteropathy [174, 175]. Noninfectious enteropathy is present in 10–50% of CVID patients and may resemble other gastrointestinal diseases such as celiac disease, Crohn's disease, and UC [162, 173]. Chronic diarrhea is the most frequent symptom occurring in up to 92%, followed by dyspepsia (66%), anemia (56%), malabsorption (54%), and abdominal pain (52%) in CVID patients with gastrointestinal symptoms [162]. Chronic diarrhea in CVID patients is associated with lymphoid hyperplasia, villous atrophy, granulomas, and inflammatory bowel disease-like lesions [164]. Inflammatory bowel disease-like disorders are present in 6–10% of CVID patients [163, 176].

Endoscopic findings Gastrointestinal endoscopic abnormalities are present in 83% of CVID patients undergoing screening endoscopy with colitis and gastritis being the most common manifestations [177]. Endoscopic abnormalities are present in stomach in 77% of CVID patients with gastrointestinal symptoms, including erythematous (27%), atrophic (27%), follicular (13%), and ulcerative (10%) gastritis [162]. Duodenal macroscopic abnormalities are present in 68% of CVID patients with gastrointestinal symptoms, including nodular lymphoid hyperplasia in 44%, disappearance of duodenal folds and mosaic pattern in 22%, and ulcerative duodenitis in 2% [162]. Endoscopic inflammation, nodular lymphoid hyperplasia, or ulcer are present in colon in 26%, 31%, and 14% of CVID patients with gastrointestinal symptoms [162].

Pathological Features

Pathological abnormalities can be present in the entire gastrointestinal tracts. Prominent intraepithelial lymphocytosis is present in 50% (5 of 10), acute inflammation with candida infection in 40% (4 of 10), and prominent apoptosis in 10% (1 of 10) of the esophagus in CVID patients [178]. In the stomach, paucity of plasma cells in lamina propria is present in 66%; lymphoid aggregates in 61%; increased apoptosis, mononuclear cell infiltrate, and occasional glandular or crypt dropouts resembling GVHD in 33–40%; lymphocytic gastritis in 22%; acute inflammation with accompanied CMV, *H. pylori*, and cryptosporidium infections in 44%; and granulomas in 6% of CVID patients [178, 179]. In the colon, lymphoid aggregates are present in 81%; paucity of plasma cells in lamina propria in 63%; increased apoptosis, mononuclear cell infiltrate, and occasional glandular or crypt dropouts resembling GVHD in 50%; lymphocytic colitis in 38–70%; acute inflammation in 88%; crypt distortion in 43%; and granulomas in 19% of CVID patients [168, 178, 179].

In the duodenum and small bowel, paucity of plasma cells in lamina propria (Fig. 10.11a) is present in 62–71%; increased apoptosis, mononuclear infiltrate, and occasional glandular or crypt dropouts resembling GVHD (Fig. 10.11b) in 21–40%; increased IELs in 30–63%; villous atrophy in 30–52%; IELs with villous atrophy resembling celiac disease (Fig. 10.11c) in 30–52%; prominent lymphoid aggregates in 10–49%; acute inflammation in 32–35%; granulomas (Fig. 10.11d) in 11%; collagenous sprue in 5%; and autoimmune enteropathy (Fig. 10.11e) in 5% of CVID patients [162, 168, 171, 172, 178–180]. IELs and villous atrophy (partial more frequently than severe) are even more frequently present in 76% (31 of 41) and 51% (21 of 41) of CVID patients with gastrointestinal symptoms [162]. Giardia, CMV, and cryptosporidium infection can be identified in up to 30% of duodenal biopsies from CVID patients [162, 178, 179]. One patient with prominent foamy macrophages without PAS-positive bacilli resembling Whipple's disease has also been described [179].

Differential Diagnosis

Acute GVHD and celiac disease are the main differential diagnoses for duodenal manifestation of CVID. Prominent apoptosis with presence of plasma cells in lamina propria and history of bone marrow or solid organ transplant are present in patients with diagnosis of acute GVHD. Villous atrophy with IELs and absence of lamina propria plasma

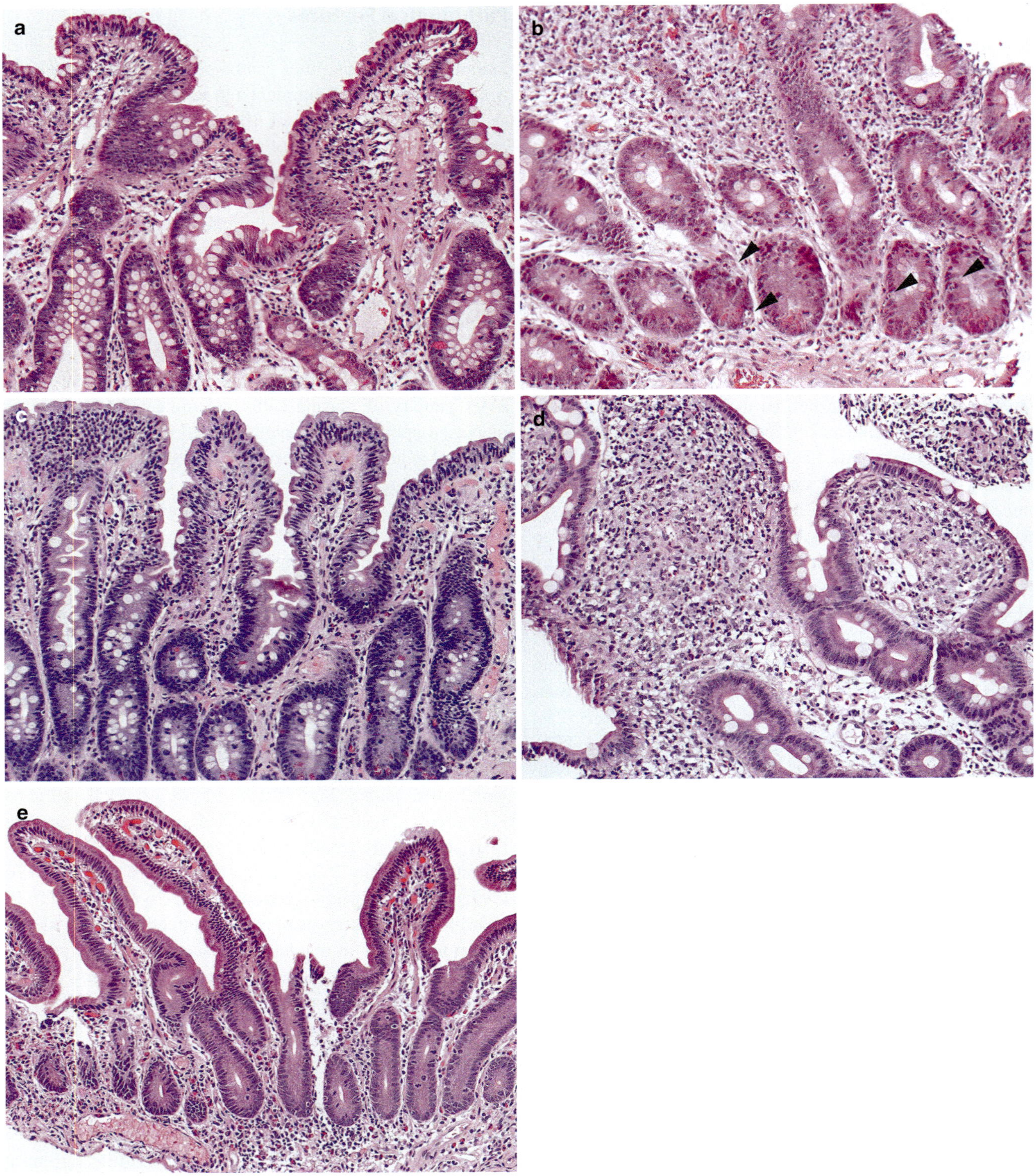

Fig. 10.11 Histological features in common variable immunodeficiency. (**a**) Duodenal biopsy shows paucity of plasma cells and chronic inflammatory cells in lamina propria. (**b**) Increased apoptosis (arrowheads) and mononuclear cell infiltrate resembling GVHD. (**c**) Increased intraepithelial lymphocytes with villous atrophy resembling celiac disease. (**d**) Noncaseating granulomas resembling Crohn's disease. (**e**) Absence of goblet cells and Paneth cells, features resembling autoimmune enteropathy

cells with presence of apoptosis, prominent lymphoid aggregates, and clinically no response of chronic diarrhea on gluten-free diet are supportive of the diagnosis of CVID [181].

Treatment and Prognosis

The standard treatment for CVID is periodic intravenous immunoglobulin (IVIg) therapy [169, 182]. IVIg therapy is not effective in reducing gastrointestinal symptoms in particular chronic diarrhea and malabsorption. Steroid treatment can significantly reduce the symptoms of chronic diarrhea and malabsorption [162]. CVID patients have a tenfold increased risk for gastric adenocarcinoma [183], and lymphoma can develop in 2–10% of CVID patients [153, 166] arising in the setting of nodular lymphoid hyperplasia [162, 184].

X-Linked Agammaglobulinemia

Definition

X-linked agammaglobulinemia (XLA) is a primary immunodeficiency disorder characterized by marked reduced level of B lymphocytes, hypogammaglobulinemia of all immunoglobulin isotypes, and recurrent sinopulmonary infections due to deficient development of B lymphocytes caused by mutations in the gene of Bruton's tyrosine kinase (*BTK*) [185–188].

Clinical Features

Epidemiology XLA accounts for 6–11% of primary immunodeficiency. The incidence of XLA varies in different countries and has been reported between 1/100,000 and 1/20,000,000 live births [189].

Pathogenesis XLA is caused by mutations in the *BTK* gene on chromosome Xq21.3-Xq22 and accounts for 85% of congenital agammaglobulinemia [186, 187]. The mutations in *BTK* gene are highly heterogeneous, and no single mutation accounts for more than 3% of XLA patients [190]. The *BTK* gene encodes a cytoplasmic non-receptor protein tyrosine kinase that belongs to the Tec kinase family and plays a fundamental role in B-cell receptor signaling pathway and B-cell development. Defect in B-cell receptor signaling pathway results in the absence of mature B cells in the peripheral blood [191]. There is no correlation between the distinct genotypes and clinical phenotypes [192], but specific mutations such as amino acid substitution occurring at conserved but not invariant sites in *BTK* gene are associated with milder disease [193, 194].

Clinical presentations XLA typically manifests in young boys within the first 2 years of life after depletion of maternal antibodies with recurrent bacterial and enteroviral infections [195].

Gastrointestinal manifestations occur in 35% of XLA patients and are less common in XLA as compared to other antibody deficiency syndromes, mainly due to T-cell dysfunctions which drive the intestinal disorders present in other immunodeficiency syndromes [196, 197]. Chronic diarrhea is the most common gastrointestinal symptoms in 21%, followed by abdominal pain in 17% and inflammatory bowel disease or Crohn's disease in 4–10% of XLA patients [189, 197–199]. Gastrointestinal tract infections occur in 35% of XLA patients [198]. Infectious diarrhea is most commonly due to *Giardia lamblia*, *Salmonella*, *Campylobacter*, and *Cryptosporidium* [189, 196]. Enteroviral infections due to coxsackievirus and echovirus can occur in the gut and cause severe neurological defects [196, 200].

Pathological Features

Recurrent fissuring ulceration of small bowel resembling Crohn's disease has been reported in patients with XLA [179, 200, 201]. In contrast to typical Crohn's disease, no granulomas and plasma cells are identified in XLA [179].

Treatment and Prognosis

The main treatment is intravenous or subcutaneous gamma globulin infusion. Rare cases of gastric adenocarcinoma and colorectal adenocarcinomas have been reported in patients with XLA [202–204].

Autosomal Recessive Agammaglobulinemia

Autosomal-recessive agammaglobulinemia (ARA) accounts for 15% of congenital agammaglobulinemia [190]. The incidence of ARA is very low (about 1/2,000,000 births) [205]. ARA is associated with mutations in several genes including immunoglobulin heavy constant Mu (*IGHM*), *CD79A*, *CD79B*, *IGLL1*, *BLNK*, *LRRC8A*, and *PIK3R1* [190, 205]. Mutations in the IGHM gene located at chromosome 14q32.2 consist of 20–30% of patients with ARA [206, 207]. Patients with ARA present at a younger age and have more severe complications as compared to XLA patients [190, 205, 207]. This clinical presentation is partially explained by mutations in the *BTK* gene resulting in a partial blockage of B-cell development, and almost all patients with XLA do have a small number of B cells and some IgG in the peripheral blood, in contrast to the defect in the IGHM which results in complete block of B-cell development [207].

X-Linked Hyper-IgM Syndrome

Definition

X-linked hyper-IgM syndrome (XHIGM) is an uncommon primary immunodeficiency disorder characterized by recurrent infections; normal or elevated level of IgM and reduced levels of IgG, IgA, and IgE; and variable defects in antigen-induced proliferative response and T-lymphocytes and macrophage effector function [208]. T-lymphocyte numbers are usually normal, and B-cell numbers are normal or slightly reduced.

Clinical Features

Epidemiology The incidence of XHIGM is approximately 1/1,030,000 live births [209].

Pathogenesis XHIGM is the most common (70%) subtype of hyper-IgM syndromes [210]. XHIGM is caused by defects in the CD40 ligand/CD40 signaling pathways or NF-κB essential modulator (NEMO), resulting in impairment of immunoglobulin isotype switching in B cells [211]. CD40L is encoded by *CD40L* gene located at chromosome Xq26.3-Xq27.1 and is mainly expressed on activated mature T cells [212–215]. CD40 is the receptor for CD40L and is expressed on B cells, monocytes/macrophages, dendritic cells, endothelial cells, and epithelial cells. CD40-CD40L interactions affect both cellular and humoral immunity, by providing a costimulatory signal for T-cell activation, and can lead to B-cell proliferation and immunoglobulin class switching [211]. Hyper-IgM syndromes can also be caused by autosomal recessive disease due to mutations in *CD40*, *AICDA* (activation-induced cytidine deaminase), and *UNG* (uracil-DNA glycosylase) [210] and autosomal dominant disease with gain-of-function mutations in *PIK3CD* (phosphoinositide 3-kinase catalytic delta component) [216].

Clinical presentations A majority (more than 90%) of the XHIMG patients are diagnosed by 4 years of age [209]. The most common clinical manifestations are pneumonia (81%), upper respiratory infections (49%), and recurrent/protracted diarrhea (32–50%) [196, 209, 216]. Gastrointestinal manifestations include oral ulcer, gingivitis, and rectal ulcer, which are most likely secondary to neutropenia [217]. Infectious diarrhea is commonly due to *Cryptosporidium*, *Giardia*, *Salmonella*, and *Entamoeba histolytica* [196, 217]. Nodular lymphoid hyperplasia can also involve gastrointestinal tract [196].

Treatment and Prognosis

The treatment for XHIGM is replacement of immunoglobulin with antibiotics for infectious complications [216]. HCT along or with liver transplant has been used to treat XHIMG patients [196, 209, 216]. There are rare reports of hepatocellular carcinoma, cholangiocarcinoma, and neuroendocrine tumors or carcinomas occurring in liver, pancreas, and gastrointestinal tract in XHIMG patients [209, 218, 219].

Severe Combined Immunodeficiency

Definition

Severe combined immunodeficiency (SCID) is a heterogeneous group of inherited disorders characterized by severe dysfunctions of T and B cells derived from thymus and bone marrow and affecting both cellular and humoral adaptive immunity [220].

Clinical Features

Epidemiology The incidence of SCID is 1 in 40,000–75,000 live births, and it is most frequently observed in the first few months of life with the median age at diagnosis of 4–7 months with severe recurrent bacterial or viral infections, sepsis, failure to thrive, and eczematoid rashes [220–223].

Pathogenesis X-linked SCID due to mutations in the interleukin-2 receptor γ (*IL2RG*) located on chromosome Xq13.1 is the most common form of SCID and accounts for 40–50% of all SCID cases [220]. Typical SCIDs are defined by the absence or severe reduction of T cells ($CD3^+ < 300$ μL), absence or severe reduction (<10% of the lower limit) of a proliferative response to phytohemagglutinin, or a maternal lymphocyte engraftment [224]. Typical SCIDs can be due to five mechanisms:

1. Reticular dygenesis due to apoptosis of hematopoietic progenitor cells, an autosomal recessive syndrome due to mutations in adenylate kinase 2 (*AK2*)
2. Premature apoptosis of lymphocyte progenitors caused by products of purine metabolism due to mutations in

adenosine deaminase (*ADA*), accounting for 10–20% cases of SCID
3. Defective cytokine-dependent signaling in T cells and NK progenitor cells due to mutations in *IL2RG, interleukin-7 receptor α* (*IL7RA*), and *Janus kinase 3* (*JAK3*)
4. Defective generation of antigen-specific T-cell and B-cell receptors due to mutations in *V(D)J recombination activating gene 1* (*RAG1*), *RAG2*, *DNA cross-link repair 1C* (*DCLRE1C*), *DNA ligase 4* (*LIG4*), and *NHEJ factor 1* (*NHEJ1*), accounting for 30% of cases of SCID
5. Defective signaling from the pre-T-cell receptor (TCR) and TCR due to defects in the CD45, CD3δ, CD3ε, and CD3ζ subunits of the pre-TCR-TCR complexes and accounting for 2% of cases of SCID [223]

In addition to the typical SCIDs, hypomorphic mutations in the *RAG1*, *RAG2*, *DCLRE1C*, and *LIG4* genes can cause Omenn syndrome and leaky SCID [225–227]. Omenn syndrome is characterized by early and severe inflammatory symptoms including generalized erythroderma, diarrhea, hepatosplenomegaly, lymphadenopathy with hypereosinophilia, and increased IgE levels, and T-cell counts can be normal or even increased [226, 228]. Leaky SCIDs are a milder form of SCID and can also be caused by mutations in *ADA*, *IL7RA*, *IL2RG*, and *JAK3* [226].

Nude SCID is a rare autosomal recessive disorder due to loss-of-function mutations in the *FOXN1* gene, characterized by the absence of thymus, alopecia universalis, and nail dystrophy [220, 229]. Autosomal recessive familial multiple gastrointestinal atresias have been reported to be associated with SCID [230, 231], but a recent study suggested that immune defect may not be the primary cause for the intestinal atresias [232].

Clinical presentations Failure to thrive, diarrhea, and susceptibility to opportunistic organisms such as *Pneumocystis jiroveci* are the common presentations. SCID patients can develop severe systemic fatal disease when inadvertently given live vaccines [223]. Maternal engraftments of lymphocytes can cause GVHD most commonly in skin and liver in 16% of SCID patients [233, 234]. SCID patients have increased susceptibility to fungal infections in gastrointestinal tract and the most common ones are *Candida* and *Aspergillus* [196, 235]. Gastroesophageal reflux disease can also occur in 21% of patients with SCID [236].

Treatment and Prognosis

SCID can be successfully treated with allogeneic transplantation of hematopoietic stem cells [223]. Gene therapy and enzyme replacement therapy can be used in selected forms of SCID [237, 238].

Wiskott-Aldrich Syndrome

Wiskott-Aldrich syndrome (WAS) is a rare X-linked primary immunodeficiency disorder characterized by immunodeficiency, microthrombocytopenia, severe eczema, recurrent infections, and increased incidence of autoimmunity and malignancy [239–241]. WAS is caused by mutations in the *WAS* gene encoding the WAS protein located on chromosome Xp11.22-p11.23 [242]. WAS protein is exclusively expressed in hematopoietic cells, a key regulator of actin polymerization in hematopoietic cells, and is involved in signaling, cell locomotion, and immune synapse formation [239, 241].

The estimated incidence of symptomatic WAS is 1 in 1000,000 [239, 243]. Mutations in the *WAS* gene have various effects on the level of WAS protein and correlate with the severity of the disease and further classify WAS into classic WAS, X-linked thrombocytopenia (XLT), intermittent X-linked thrombocytopenia (IXLT), and X-linked neutropenia (XLN) [239, 241, 244]. Classic WAS and XLT often present at birth with petechiae, bruise, and bloody diarrhea. Thrombocytopenia and small platelet size, infections, bacterial pneumonia, and skin infections are the most common symptoms. Patients with XLT often have fewer problems of eczema and infections and can be misdiagnosed as idiopathic thrombocytopenia [244]. Patients with XLN are also affected at birth, but they do not have similar symptoms of classic WAS and XLT [239].

Autoimmune disorders frequently develop in 40–70% of WAS patients with most of the cases the onset age is less than 2 years [240]. Autoimmune hemolytic anemia, thrombocytopenia, and neutropenia are the most common autoimmune diseases followed by vasculitis, renal disease, and Henoch-Schönlein-like purpura [239, 240, 245]. Inflammatory bowel disease resembling UC has been reported in up to 9% of patients with WAS, and WAS should be considered in the differential diagnosis for early-onset inflammatory bowel disease [196, 245–247]. Malignancies, mainly lymphoma (often Epstein-Barr virus-positive), leukemia, and myelodysplasia, can occur in 10–20% of patients with WAS [239, 240]. HCT is the curative therapy for WAS [243].

References

1. Kreuning J, Bosman FT, Kuiper G, Wal AM, Lindeman J. Gastric and duodenal mucosa in 'healthy' individuals. An endoscopic and histopathological study of 50 volunteers. J Clin Pathol. 1978;31(1):69–77.
2. Jenkins D, Goodall A, Gillet FR, Scott BB. Defining duodenitis: quantitative histological study of mucosal responses and their correlations. J Clin Pathol. 1985;38(10):1119–26.
3. Terada T. Pathologic observations of the duodenum in 615 consecutive duodenal specimens: I. benign lesions. Int J Clin Exp Pathol. 2012;5(1):46–51.

4. Alper A, Hardee S, Rojas-Velasquez D, Escalera S, Morotti RA, Pashankar DS. Prevalence and clinical, endoscopic, and pathological features of duodenitis in children. J Pediatr Gastroenterol Nutr. 2016;62(2):314–6. https://doi.org/10.1097/mpg.0000000000000942.
5. Moghal N, Jafarey NA. A histological study of the effects of non-steroidal anti-inflammatory drugs (NSAIDs) on the gastric and duodenal mucosa. J Pak Med Assoc. 1989;39(11):287–90.
6. Taha AS. Histopathological aspects of mucosal injury related to non-steroidal anti-inflammatory drugs. Ital J Gastroenterol. 1996;28(Suppl 4):12–5.
7. Wee A, Kang JY, Ho MS, Choong HL, Wu AY, Sutherland IH. Gastroduodenal mucosa in uraemia: endoscopic and histological correlation and prevalence of helicobacter-like organisms. Gut. 1990;31(10):1093–6.
8. Misra V, Misra SP, Shukla SK, Jaiswal PK, Agarwal R, Tondon S. Endoscopic and histological changes in upper gastrointestinal tract of patients with chronic renal failure. Indian J Pathol Microbiol. 2004;47(2):170–3.
9. Zukerman GR, Mills BA, Koehler RE, Siegel A, Harter HR, DeSchryver-Kecskemeti K. Nodular duodenitis. Pathologic and clinical characteristics in patients with end-stage renal disease. Dig Dis Sci. 1983;28(11):1018–24.
10. Kreuning J, vd Wal AM, Kuiper G, Lindeman J. Chronic nonspecific duodenitis. A multiple biopsy study of the duodenal bulb in health and disease. Scand J Gastroenterol Suppl. 1989;167:16–20.
11. Lewis S, Stableforth W, Awasthi R, Awasthi A, Pitts N, Ottaway J, et al. An examination of the relationship between the endoscopic appearance of duodenitis and the histological findings in patients with epigastric pain. Int J Clin Exp Pathol. 2012;5(6):581–7.
12. Whitehead R, Roca M, Meikle DD, Skinner J, Truelove SC. The histological classification of duodenitis in fibreoptic biopsy specimens. Digestion. 1975;13(3):129–36.
13. Genta RM, Kinsey RS, Singhal A, Suterwala S. Gastric foveolar metaplasia and gastric heterotopia in the duodenum: no evidence of an etiologic role for Helicobacter pylori. Hum Pathol. 2010;41(11):1593–600. https://doi.org/10.1016/j.humpath.2010.04.010.
14. Leonard N, Feighery CF, Hourihane DO. Peptic duodenitis—does it exist in the second part of the duodenum? J Clin Pathol. 1997;50(1):54–8.
15. Frierson HF Jr, Caldwell SH, Marshall BJ. Duodenal bulb biopsy findings for patients with non-ulcer dyspepsia with or without Campylobacter pylori gastritis. Mod Pathol. 1990;3(3):271–6.
16. Walker MM, Dixon MF. Gastric metaplasia: its role in duodenal ulceration. Aliment Pharmacol Ther. 1996;10(Suppl 1):119–28.
17. Marshall BJ, Goodwin CS, Warren JR, Murray R, Blincow ED, Blackbourn SJ, et al. Prospective double-blind trial of duodenal ulcer relapse after eradication of Campylobacter pylori. Lancet (London, England). 1988;2(8626–8627):1437–42.
18. Blaser MJ. Gastric Campylobacter-like organisms, gastritis, and peptic ulcer disease. Gastroenterology. 1987;93(2):371–83.
19. Graham DY. Campylobacter pylori and peptic ulcer disease. Gastroenterology. 1989;96(2 Pt 2 Suppl):615–25.
20. Parrish JA, Rawlins DC. Intestinal mucosa in the Zollinger-Ellison syndrome. Gut. 1965;6(3):286–9.
21. Wyatt JI, Rathbone BJ, Sobala GM, Shallcross T, Heatley RV, Axon AT, et al. Gastric epithelium in the duodenum: its association with Helicobacter pylori and inflammation. J Clin Pathol. 1990;43(12):981–6.
22. Walker MM, Crabtree JE. Helicobacter pylori infection and the pathogenesis of duodenal ulceration. Ann N Y Acad Sci. 1998;859:96–111.
23. Wyatt JI, Rathbone BJ, Dixon MF, Heatley RV. Campylobacter pyloridis and acid induced gastric metaplasia in the pathogenesis of duodenitis. J Clin Pathol. 1987;40(8):841–8.
24. Shabib SM, Cutz E, Drumm B, Sherman PM. Association of gastric metaplasia and duodenitis with Helicobacter pylori infection in children. Am J Clin Pathol. 1994;102(2):188–91.
25. Khulusi S, Badve S, Patel P, Lloyd R, Marrero JM, Finlayson C, et al. Pathogenesis of gastric metaplasia of the human duodenum: role of Helicobacter pylori, gastric acid, and ulceration. Gastroenterology. 1996;110(2):452–8.
26. Wyatt JI. Histopathology of gastroduodenal inflammation: the impact of Helicobacter pylori. Histopathology. 1995;26(1):1–15.
27. Hamlet A, Thoreson AC, Nilsson O, Svennerholm AM, Olbe L. Duodenal Helicobacter pylori infection differs in cagA genotype between asymptomatic subjects and patients with duodenal ulcers. Gastroenterology. 1999;116(2):259–68.
28. Ellison EH, Wilson SD. The Zollinger-Ellison syndrome: reappraisal and evaluation of 260 registered cases. Ann Surg. 1964;160:512–30.
29. Memeo L, Jhang J, Hibshoosh H, Green PH, Rotterdam H, Bhagat G. Duodenal intraepithelial lymphocytosis with normal villous architecture: common occurrence in *H. pylori* gastritis. Mod Pathol. 2005;18(8):1134–44. https://doi.org/10.1038/modpathol.3800404.
30. Li XB, Ge ZZ, Chen XY, Liu WZ. Duodenal gastric metaplasia and Helicobacter pylori infection in patients with diffuse nodular duodenitis. Braz J Med Biol Res. 2007;40(7):897–902.
31. Noach LA, Rolf TM, Bosma NB, Schwartz MP, Oosting J, Rauws EA, et al. Gastric metaplasia and Helicobacter pylori infection. Gut. 1993;34(11):1510–4.
32. Brown I, Mino-Kenudson M, Deshpande V, Lauwers GY. Intraepithelial lymphocytosis in architecturally preserved proximal small intestinal mucosa: an increasing diagnostic problem with a wide differential diagnosis. Arch Pathol Lab Med. 2006;130(7):1020–5. https://doi.org/10.1043/1543–2165(2006)130[1020:iliapp]2.0.co;2.
33. Hammer ST, Greenson JK. The clinical significance of duodenal lymphocytosis with normal villus architecture. Arch Pathol Lab Med. 2013;137(9):1216–9. https://doi.org/10.5858/arpa.2013–0261-RA.
34. Vande Voort JL, Murray JA, Lahr BD, Van Dyke CT, Kroning CM, Moore SB, et al. Lymphocytic duodenosis and the spectrum of celiac disease. Am J Gastroenterol. 2009;104(1):142–8. https://doi.org/10.1038/ajg.2008.7.
35. Lauwers GY, Fasano A, Brown IS. Duodenal lymphocytosis with no or minimal enteropathy: much ado about nothing? Mod Pathol. 2015;28(Suppl 1):S22–9. https://doi.org/10.1038/modpathol.2014.135.
36. Ierardi E, Losurdo G, Iannone A, Piscitelli D, Amoruso A, Barone M, et al. Lymphocytic duodenitis or microscopic enteritis and gluten-related conditions: what needs to be explored? Ann Gastroenterol. 2017;30(4):380–92. https://doi.org/10.20524/aog.2017.0165.
37. Rostami K, Aldulaimi D, Holmes G, Johnson MW, Robert M, Srivastava A, et al. Microscopic enteritis: Bucharest consensus. World J Gastroenterol. 2015;21(9):2593–604. https://doi.org/10.3748/wjg.v21.i9.2593.
38. Mahadeva S, Wyatt JI, Howdle PD. Is a raised intraepithelial lymphocyte count with normal duodenal villous architecture clinically relevant? J Clin Pathol. 2002;55(6):424–8.
39. Kakar S, Nehra V, Murray JA, Dayharsh GA, Burgart LJ. Significance of intraepithelial lymphocytosis in small bowel biopsy samples with normal mucosal architecture. Am J Gastroenterol. 2003;98(9):2027–33. https://doi.org/10.1111/j.1572–0241.2003.07631.x.
40. Shmidt E, Smyrk TC, Faubion WA, Oxentenko AS. Duodenal intraepithelial lymphocytosis with normal villous architecture in pediatric patients: Mayo Clinic experience, 2000–2009. J Pediatr

Gastroenterol Nutr. 2013;56(1):51–5. https://doi.org/10.1097/MPG.0b013e318267c353.
41. Shmidt E, Smyrk TC, Boswell CL, Enders FT, Oxentenko AS. Increasing duodenal intraepithelial lymphocytosis found at upper endoscopy: time trends and associations. Gastrointest Endosc. 2014;80(1):105–11. https://doi.org/10.1016/j.gie.2014.01.008.
42. Galli G, Purchiaroni F, Lahner E, Sacchi MC, Pilozzi E, Corleto VD, et al. Time trend occurrence of duodenal intraepithelial lymphocytosis and celiac disease in an open access endoscopic population. United European Gastroenterol J. 2017;5(6):811–8. https://doi.org/10.1177/2050640616680971.
43. Sergi C, Shen F, Bouma G. Intraepithelial lymphocytes, scores, mimickers and challenges in diagnosing gluten-sensitive enteropathy (celiac disease). World J Gastroenterol. 2017;23(4):573–89. https://doi.org/10.3748/wjg.v23.i4.573.
44. Losurdo G, Piscitelli D, Giangaspero A, Principi M, Buffelli F, Giorgio F, et al. Evolution of nonspecific duodenal lymphocytosis over 2 years of follow-up. World J Gastroenterol. 2015;21(24):7545–52. https://doi.org/10.3748/wjg.v21.i24.7545.
45. Goldstein NS, Underhill J. Morphologic features suggestive of gluten sensitivity in architecturally normal duodenal biopsy specimens. Am J Clin Pathol. 2001;116(1):63–71. https://doi.org/10.1309/5prj-cm0u-6kld-6kcm.
46. Patterson ER, Shmidt E, Oxentenko AS, Enders FT, Smyrk TC. Normal villous architecture with increased intraepithelial lymphocytes: a duodenal manifestation of Crohn disease. Am J Clin Pathol. 2015;143(3):445–50. https://doi.org/10.1309/ajcpbkqnd4shvx9q.
47. Fasano A, Sapone A, Zevallos V, Schuppan D. Nonceliac gluten sensitivity. Gastroenterology. 2015;148(6):1195–204. https://doi.org/10.1053/j.gastro.2014.12.049.
48. Volta U, Caio G, Karunaratne TB, Alaedini A, De Giorgio R. Non-coeliac gluten/wheat sensitivity: advances in knowledge and relevant questions. Expert Rev Gastroenterol Hepatol. 2017;11(1):9–18. https://doi.org/10.1080/17474124.2017.1260003.
49. Aziz I, Lewis NR, Hadjivassiliou M, Winfield SN, Rugg N, Kelsall A, et al. A UK study assessing the population prevalence of self-reported gluten sensitivity and referral characteristics to secondary care. Eur J Gastroenterol Hepatol. 2014;26(1):33–9. https://doi.org/10.1097/01.meg.0000435546.87251.f7.
50. Wise L, Kyriakos M, McCown A, Ballinger WF. Crohn's disease of the duodenum. A report and analysis of eleven new cases. Am J Surg. 1971;121(2):184–94.
51. Nugent FW, Roy MA. Duodenal Crohn's disease: an analysis of 89 cases. Am J Gastroenterol. 1989;84(3):249–54.
52. Ingle SB, Adgaonkar BD, Jamadar NP, Siddiqui S, Hinge CR. Crohn's disease with gastroduodenal involvement: diagnostic approach. World J Clin Cases. 2015;3(6):479–83. https://doi.org/10.12998/wjcc.v3.i6.479.
53. Sonnenberg A, Melton SD, Genta RM. Frequent occurrence of gastritis and duodenitis in patients with inflammatory bowel disease. Inflamm Bowel Dis. 2011;17(1):39–44. https://doi.org/10.1002/ibd.21356.
54. Diaz L, Hernandez-Oquet RE, Deshpande AR, Moshiree B. Upper gastrointestinal involvement in Crohn disease: histopathologic and endoscopic findings. South Med J. 2015;108(11):695–700. https://doi.org/10.14423/smj.0000000000000373.
55. Ruuska T, Vaajalahti P, Arajarvi P, Maki M. Prospective evaluation of upper gastrointestinal mucosal lesions in children with ulcerative colitis and Crohn's disease. J Pediatr Gastroenterol Nutr. 1994;19(2):181–6.
56. Tobin JM, Sinha B, Ramani P, Saleh AR, Murphy MS. Upper gastrointestinal mucosal disease in pediatric Crohn disease and ulcerative colitis: a blinded, controlled study. J Pediatr Gastroenterol Nutr. 2001;32(4):443–8.
57. Hummel TZ, ten Kate FJ, Reitsma JB, Benninga MA, Kindermann A. Additional value of upper GI tract endoscopy in the diagnostic assessment of childhood IBD. J Pediatr Gastroenterol Nutr. 2012;54(6):753–7. https://doi.org/10.1097/MPG.0b013e318243e3e3.
58. Sullivan KJ, Wei M, Chernetsova E, Hallani S, de Nanassy J, Benchimol EI, et al. Value of upper endoscopic biopsies in predicting medical refractoriness in pediatric patients with ulcerative colitis. Hum Pathol. 2017;66:167–76. https://doi.org/10.1016/j.humpath.2017.06.006.
59. Nugent FW, Richmond M, Park SK. Crohn's disease of the duodenum. Gut. 1977;18(2):115–20.
60. Song DJ, Whang IS, Choi HW, Jeong CY, Jung SH. Crohn's disease confined to the duodenum: a case report. World J Clin Cases. 2016;4(6):146–50. https://doi.org/10.12998/wjcc.v4.i6.146.
61. Yamamoto T, Bain IM, Connolly AB, Keighley MR. Gastroduodenal fistulas in Crohn's disease: clinical features and management. Dis Colon Rectum. 1998;41(10):1287–92.
62. Uchino M, Ikeuchi H, Matsuoka H, Matsumoto T, Takesue Y, Tomita N. Clinical features and management of duodenal fistula in patients with Crohn's disease. Hepatogastroenterology. 2012;59(113):171–4. https://doi.org/10.5754/hge10205.
63. Honma J, Mitomi H, Murakami K, Igarashi M, Saigenji K, Toyama K. Nodular duodenitis involving CD8+ cell infiltration in patients with ulcerative colitis. Hepatogastroenterology. 2001;48(42):1604–10.
64. Cameron DJ. Upper and lower gastrointestinal endoscopy in children and adolescents with Crohn's disease: a prospective study. J Gastroenterol Hepatol. 1991;6(4):355–8.
65. Laube R, Liu K, Schifter M, Yang JL, Suen MK, Leong RW. Oral and upper gastrointestinal Crohn's disease. J Gastroenterol Hepatol. 2018;33(2):355–64. https://doi.org/10.1111/jgh.13866.
66. Hardee S, Alper A, Pashankar DS, Morotti RA. Histopathology of duodenal mucosal lesions in pediatric patients with inflammatory bowel disease: statistical analysis to identify distinctive features. Pediatr Dev Pathol. 2014;17(6):450–4. https://doi.org/10.2350/14-07-1529-oa.1.
67. Brown IS, Miller GC, Bettington ML, Rosty C. Histopathological findings of extra-ileal manifestations at initial diagnosis of Crohn's disease-related ileitis. Virchows Arch. 2016;469(5):515–22. https://doi.org/10.1007/s00428-016-2009-7.
68. Sakuraba A, Iwao Y, Matsuoka K, Naganuma M, Ogata H, Kanai T, et al. Endoscopic and pathologic changes of the upper gastrointestinal tract in Crohn's disease. Biomed Res Int. 2014;2014:610767. https://doi.org/10.1155/2014/610767.
69. Wright CL, Riddell RH. Histology of the stomach and duodenum in Crohn's disease. Am J Surg Pathol. 1998;22(4):383–90.
70. Lin J, McKenna BJ, Appelman HD. Morphologic findings in upper gastrointestinal biopsies of patients with ulcerative colitis: a controlled study. Am J Surg Pathol. 2010;34(11):1672–7. https://doi.org/10.1097/PAS.0b013e3181f3de93.
71. Rubenstein J, Sherif A, Appelman H, Chey WD. Ulcerative colitis associated enteritis: is ulcerative colitis always confined to the colon? J Clin Gastroenterol. 2004;38(1):46–51.
72. Corporaal S, Karrenbeld A, van der Linde K, Voskuil JH, Kleibeuker JH, Dijkstra G. Diffuse enteritis after colectomy for ulcerative colitis: two case reports and review of the literature. Eur J Gastroenterol Hepatol. 2009;21(6):710–5. https://doi.org/10.1097/MEG.0b013e32831bc400.
73. Annese V, Caruso N, Bisceglia M, Lombardi G, Clemente R, Modola G, et al. Fatal ulcerative panenteritis following colectomy in a patient with ulcerative colitis. Dig Dis Sci. 1999;44(6):1189–95.

74. Queliza K, Ihekweazu FD, Schady D, Jensen C, Kellermayer R. Granulomatous upper gastrointestinal inflammation in pediatric ulcerative colitis. J Pediatr Gastroenterol Nutr. 2017. https://doi.org/10.1097/mpg.0000000000001771.
75. Tsujino T, Ito Y, Yoshida H, Ikushima S, Takemura T, Nakata R, et al. Duodenal mass in a patient with weight loss and liver dysfunction. Duodenal and liver sarcoidosis. Gut. 2011;60(12):1659–60, 77. https://doi.org/10.1136/gut.2010.212365.
76. Ghrenassia E, Mekinian A, Chapelon-Albric C, Levy P, Cosnes J, Seve P, et al. Digestive-tract sarcoidosis: French nationwide case-control study of 25 cases. Medicine. 2016;95(29):e4279. https://doi.org/10.1097/md.0000000000004279.
77. Baughman RP, Lower EE, du Bois RM. Sarcoidosis. Lancet (London, England). 2003;361(9363):1111–8. https://doi.org/10.1016/s0140–6736(03)12888–7.
78. Valeyre D, Prasse A, Nunes H, Uzunhan Y, Brillet PY, Muller-Quernheim J. Sarcoidosis. Lancet (London, England). 2014;383(9923):1155–67. https://doi.org/10.1016/s0140–6736(13)60680–7.
79. Hillerdal G, Nou E, Osterman K, Schmekel B. Sarcoidosis: epidemiology and prognosis. A 15-year European study. Am Rev Respir Dis. 1984;130(1):29–32. https://doi.org/10.1164/arrd.1984.130.1.29.
80. Nunes H, Bouvry D, Soler P, Valeyre D. Sarcoidosis. Orphanet J Rare Dis. 2007;2:46. https://doi.org/10.1186/1750–1172–2-46.
81. Morimoto T, Azuma A, Abe S, Usuki J, Kudoh S, Sugisaki K, et al. Epidemiology of sarcoidosis in Japan. Eur Respir J. 2008;31(2):372–9. https://doi.org/10.1183/09031936.00075307.
82. Farman J, Ramirez G, Rybak B, Lebwohl O, Semrad C, Rotterdam H. Gastric sarcoidosis. Abdom Imaging. 1997;22(3):248–52.
83. Vahid B, Spodik M, Braun KN, Ghazi LJ, Esmaili A. Sarcoidosis of gastrointestinal tract: a rare disease. Dig Dis Sci. 2007;52(12):3316–20. https://doi.org/10.1007/s10620–006–9448-y.
84. Sprague R, Harper P, McClain S, Trainer T, Beeken W. Disseminated gastrointestinal sarcoidosis. Case report and review of the literature. Gastroenterology. 1984;87(2):421–5.
85. Bulger K, O'Riordan M, Purdy S, O'Brien M, Lennon J. Gastrointestinal sarcoidosis resembling Crohn's disease. Am J Gastroenterol. 1988;83(12):1415–7.
86. Rauf A, Davis P, Levendoglu H. Sarcoidosis of the small intestine. Am J Gastroenterol. 1988;83(2):187–9.
87. Lindgren A, Engstrom CP, Nilsson O, Abrahamsson H. Protein-losing enteropathy in an unusual form of sarcoidosis. Eur J Gastroenterol Hepatol. 1995;7(10):1005–7.
88. Popovic OS, Brkic S, Bojic P, Kenic V, Jojic N, Djuric V, et al. Sarcoidosis and protein losing enteropathy. Gastroenterology. 1980;78(1):119–25.
89. MacRury SM, McQuaker G, Morton R, Hume R. Sarcoidosis: association with small bowel disease and folate deficiency. J Clin Pathol. 1992;45(9):823–5.
90. Stampfl DA, Grimm IS, Barbot DJ, Rosato FE, Gordon SJ. Sarcoidosis causing duodenal obstruction. Case report and review of gastrointestinal manifestations. Dig Dis Sci. 1990;35(4):526–32.
91. Noel JM, Katona IM, Pineiro-Carrero VM. Sarcoidosis resulting in duodenal obstruction in an adolescent. J Pediatr Gastroenterol Nutr. 1997;24(5):594–8.
92. Esmadi M, Ahmad DS, Odum B, Diaz-Arias A, Hammad H. Sarcoidosis: an extremely rare cause of granulomatous enterocolitis. J Gastrointestin Liver Dis. 2012;21(4):423–5.
93. Kambham N, Higgins JP, Sundram U, Troxell ML. Hematopoietic stem cell transplantation: graft versus host disease and pathology of gastrointestinal tract, liver, and lung. Adv Anat Pathol. 2014;21(5):301–20. https://doi.org/10.1097/pap.0000000000000032.
94. Holmberg L, Kikuchi K, Gooley TA, Adams KM, Hockenbery DM, Flowers ME, et al. Gastrointestinal graft-versus-host disease in recipients of autologous hematopoietic stem cells: incidence, risk factors, and outcome. Biol Blood Marrow Transplant. 2006;12(2):226–34. https://doi.org/10.1016/j.bbmt.2005.10.011.
95. Zhang Y, Ruiz P. Solid organ transplant-associated acute graft-versus-host disease. Arch Pathol Lab Med. 2010;134(8):1220–4. https://doi.org/10.1043/2008–0679-rs.1.
96. Jagasia MH, Greinix HT, Arora M, Williams KM, Wolff D, Cowen EW, et al. National Institutes of Health consensus development project on criteria for clinical trials in chronic graft-versus-host disease: I. The 2014 diagnosis and staging working group report. Biol Blood Marrow Transplant. 2015;21(3):389–401.e1. https://doi.org/10.1016/j.bbmt.2014.12.001.
97. Ferrara JL, Levine JE, Reddy P, Holler E. Graft-versus-host disease. Lancet (London, England). 2009;373(9674):1550–61. https://doi.org/10.1016/s0140–6736(09)60237–3.
98. Ross WA, Couriel D. Colonic graft-versus-host disease. Curr Opin Gastroenterol. 2005;21(1):64–9.
99. Przepiorka D, Smith TL, Folloder J, Khouri I, Ueno NT, Mehra R, et al. Risk factors for acute graft-versus-host disease after allogeneic blood stem cell transplantation. Blood. 1999;94(4):1465–70.
100. Aslanian H, Chander B, Robert M, Cooper D, Proctor D, Seropian S, et al. Prospective evaluation of acute graft-versus-host disease. Dig Dis Sci. 2012;57(3):720–5. https://doi.org/10.1007/s10620–011–1938-x.
101. Ross WA, Ghosh S, Dekovich AA, Liu S, Ayers GD, Cleary KR, et al. Endoscopic biopsy diagnosis of acute gastrointestinal graft-versus-host disease: rectosigmoid biopsies are more sensitive than upper gastrointestinal biopsies. Am J Gastroenterol. 2008;103(4):982–9. https://doi.org/10.1111/j.1572–0241.2007.01639.x.
102. Washington K, Jagasia M. Pathology of graft-versus-host disease in the gastrointestinal tract. Hum Pathol. 2009;40(7):909–17. https://doi.org/10.1016/j.humpath.2009.04.001.
103. Cogbill CH, Drobyski WR, Komorowski RA. Gastrointestinal pathology of autologous graft-versus-host disease following hematopoietic stem cell transplantation: a clinicopathological study of 17 cases. Mod Pathol. 2011;24(1):117–25. https://doi.org/10.1038/modpathol.2010.163.
104. Wu G, Selvaggi G, Nishida S, Moon J, Island E, Ruiz P, et al. Graft-versus-host disease after intestinal and multivisceral transplantation. Transplantation. 2011;91(2):219–24. https://doi.org/10.1097/TP.0b013e3181ff86ec.
105. Choi SW, Levine JE, Ferrara JL. Pathogenesis and management of graft-versus-host disease. Immunol Allergy Clin North Am. 2010;30(1):75–101. https://doi.org/10.1016/j.iac.2009.10.001.
106. Gomez AJ, Arai S, Higgins JP, Kambham N. Clinicopathologic threshold of acute colorectal graft-versus-host disease. Arch Pathol Lab Med. 2016;140(6):570–7. https://doi.org/10.5858/arpa.2015–0187-OA.
107. Assi MA, Pulido JS, Peters SG, McCannel CA, Razonable RR. Graft-vs.-host disease in lung and other solid organ transplant recipients. Clin Transplant. 2007;21(1):1–6. https://doi.org/10.1111/j.1399–0012.2006.00573.x.
108. Ljungman P, Hakki M, Boeckh M. Cytomegalovirus in hematopoietic stem cell transplant recipients. Hematol Oncol Clin North Am. 2011;25(1):151–69. https://doi.org/10.1016/j.hoc.2010.11.011.
109. Park SH, Choi SM, Lee DG, Choi JH, Yoo JH, Kim SH, et al. Infectious complications associated with alemtuzumab use for allogeneic hematopoietic stem cell transplantation: comparison with anti-thymocyte globulin. Transpl Infect Dis. 2009;11(5):413–23. https://doi.org/10.1111/j.1399–3062.2009.00414.x.
110. Cho BS, Yahng SA, Kim JH, Yoon JH, Shin SH, Lee SE, et al. Impact of cytomegalovirus gastrointestinal disease on the clinical outcomes in patients with gastrointestinal graft-versus-host disease

in the era of preemptive therapy. Ann Hematol. 2013;92(4):497–504. https://doi.org/10.1007/s00277-012-1632-x.
111. Bhutani D, Dyson G, Manasa R, Deol A, Ratanatharathorn V, Ayash L, et al. Incidence, risk factors, and outcome of cytomegalovirus viremia and gastroenteritis in patients with gastrointestinal graft-versus-host disease. Biol Blood Marrow Transplant. 2015;21(1):159–64. https://doi.org/10.1016/j.bbmt.2014.10.004.
112. Flomenberg P, Babbitt J, Drobyski WR, Ash RC, Carrigan DR, Sedmak GV, et al. Increasing incidence of adenovirus disease in bone marrow transplant recipients. J Infect Dis. 1994;169(4):775–81.
113. Runde V, Ross S, Trenschel R, Lagemann E, Basu O, Renzing-Kohler K, et al. Adenoviral infection after allogeneic stem cell transplantation (SCT): report on 130 patients from a single SCT unit involved in a prospective multi center surveillance study. Bone Marrow Transplant. 2001;28(1):51–7. https://doi.org/10.1038/sj.bmt.1703083.
114. Suparno C, Milligan DW, Moss PA, Mautner V. Adenovirus infections in stem cell transplant recipients: recent developments in understanding of pathogenesis, diagnosis and management. Leuk Lymphoma. 2004;45(5):873–85. https://doi.org/10.1080/10428190310001628176.
115. Feuchtinger T, Lang P, Handgretinger R. Adenovirus infection after allogeneic stem cell transplantation. Leuk Lymphoma. 2007;48(2):244–55. https://doi.org/10.1080/10428190600881157.
116. Kampmann B, Cubitt D, Walls T, Naik P, Depala M, Samarasinghe S, et al. Improved outcome for children with disseminated adenoviral infection following allogeneic stem cell transplantation. Br J Haematol. 2005;130(4):595–603. https://doi.org/10.1111/j.1365-2141.2005.05649.x.
117. Yilmaz M, Chemaly RF, Han XY, Thall PF, Fox PS, Tarrand JJ, et al. Adenoviral infections in adult allogeneic hematopoietic SCT recipients: a single center experience. Bone Marrow Transplant. 2013;48(9):1218–23. https://doi.org/10.1038/bmt.2013.33.
118. Shulman HM, Cardona DM, Greenson JK, Hingorani S, Horn T, Huber E, et al. NIH Consensus development project on criteria for clinical trials in chronic graft-versus-host disease: II. The 2014 pathology working group report. Biol Blood Marrow Transplant. 2015;21(4):589–603. https://doi.org/10.1016/j.bbmt.2014.12.031.
119. Nomura K, Iizuka T, Kaji D, Yamamoto H, Kuribayashi Y, Kimura R, et al. Clinicopathological features of patients with acute graft-versus-host disease of the upper digestive tract. J Gastroenterol Hepatol. 2014;29(11):1867–72. https://doi.org/10.1111/jgh.12651.
120. Ma C, Maluf HM, Liu TC. Acute graft-versus-host disease is more prevalent and severe in the lower than the upper gastrointestinal tract. Hum Pathol. 2015;46(10):1480–7. https://doi.org/10.1016/j.humpath.2015.06.005.
121. Thompson B, Salzman D, Steinhauer J, Lazenby AJ, Wilcox CM. Prospective endoscopic evaluation for gastrointestinal graft-versus-host disease: determination of the best diagnostic approach. Bone Marrow Transplant. 2006;38(5):371–6. https://doi.org/10.1038/sj.bmt.1705453.
122. Snover DC. Graft-versus-host disease of the gastrointestinal tract. Am J Surg Pathol. 1990;14(Suppl 1):101–8.
123. Sale GE, Shulman HM, McDonald GB, Thomas ED. Gastrointestinal graft-versus-host disease in man. A clinicopathologic study of the rectal biopsy. Am J Surg Pathol. 1979;3(4):291–9.
124. Lin J, Fan R, Zhao Z, Cummings OW, Chen S. Is the presence of 6 or fewer crypt apoptotic bodies sufficient for diagnosis of graft versus host disease? A decade of experience at a single institution. Am J Surg Pathol. 2013;37(4):539–47. https://doi.org/10.1097/PAS.0b013e318272c62a.
125. Shulman HM, Kleiner D, Lee SJ, Morton T, Pavletic SZ, Farmer E, et al. Histopathologic diagnosis of chronic graft-versus-host disease: National Institutes of Health consensus development project on criteria for clinical trials in chronic graft-versus-host disease: II. Pathology working group report. Biol Blood Marrow Transplant. 2006;12(1):31–47. https://doi.org/10.1016/j.bbmt.2005.10.023.
126. Nguyen CV, Kastenberg DM, Choudhary C, Katz LC, DiMarino A, Palazzo JP. Is single-cell apoptosis sufficient for the diagnosis of graft-versus-host disease in the colon? Dig Dis Sci. 2008;53(3):747–56. https://doi.org/10.1007/s10620-007-9904-3.
127. Lerner KG, Kao GF, Storb R, Buckner CD, Clift RA, Thomas ED. Histopathology of graft-vs.-host reaction (GvHR) in human recipients of marrow from HL-A-matched sibling donors. Transplant Proc. 1974;6(4):367–71.
128. Wong NA. Gastrointestinal pathology in transplant patients. Histopathology. 2015;66(4):467–79. https://doi.org/10.1111/his.12542.
129. Akpek G, Chinratanalab W, Lee LA, Torbenson M, Hallick JP, Anders V, et al. Gastrointestinal involvement in chronic graft-versus-host disease: a clinicopathologic study. Biol Blood Marrow Transplant. 2003;9(1):46–51. https://doi.org/10.1053/bbmt.2003.49999.
130. Welch DC, Wirth PS, Goldenring JR, Ness E, Jagasia M, Washington K. Gastric graft-versus-host disease revisited: does proton pump inhibitor therapy affect endoscopic gastric biopsy interpretation? Am J Surg Pathol. 2006;30(4):444–9.
131. Weidner AS, Panarelli NC, Rennert H, Jessurun J, Yantiss RK. Immunohistochemistry improves the detection of adenovirus in gastrointestinal biopsy specimens from hematopoietic stem cell transplant recipients. Am J Clin Pathol. 2016;146(5):627–31. https://doi.org/10.1093/ajcp/aqw179.
132. Lin J, Chen S, Zhao Z, Cummings OW, Fan R. CD123 is a useful immunohistochemical marker to facilitate diagnosis of acute graft-versus-host disease in colon. Hum Pathol. 2013;44(10):2075–80. https://doi.org/10.1016/j.humpath.2013.02.023.
133. Parfitt JR, Jayakumar S, Driman DK. Mycophenolate mofetil-related gastrointestinal mucosal injury: variable injury patterns, including graft-versus-host disease-like changes. Am J Surg Pathol. 2008;32(9):1367–72.
134. Nguyen T, Park JY, Scudiere JR, Montgomery E. Mycophenolic acid (cellcept and myofortic) induced injury of the upper GI tract. Am J Surg Pathol. 2009;33(9):1355–63. https://doi.org/10.1097/PAS.0b013e3181a755bd.
135. Star KV, Ho VT, Wang HH, Odze RD. Histologic features in colon biopsies can discriminate mycophenolate from GVHD-induced colitis. Am J Surg Pathol. 2013;37(9):1319–28. https://doi.org/10.1097/PAS.0b013e31829ab1ef.
136. Shin CR, Nathan J, Alonso M, Yazigi N, Kocoshis S, Tiao G, et al. Incidence of acute and chronic graft-versus-host disease and donor T-cell chimerism after small bowel or combined organ transplantation. J Pediatr Surg. 2011;46(9):1732–8. https://doi.org/10.1016/j.jpedsurg.2011.04.016.
137. Talley NJ, Shorter RG, Phillips SF, Zinsmeister AR. Eosinophilic gastroenteritis: a clinicopathological study of patients with disease of the mucosa, muscle layer, and subserosal tissues. Gut. 1990;31(1):54–8.
138. Ingle SB, Hinge Ingle CR. Eosinophilic gastroenteritis: an unusual type of gastroenteritis. World J Gastroenterol. 2013;19(31):5061–6. https://doi.org/10.3748/wjg.v19.i31.5061.
139. Reed C, Woosley JT, Dellon ES. Clinical characteristics, treatment outcomes, and resource utilization in children and adults with eosinophilic gastroenteritis. Dig Liver Dis. 2015;47(3):197–201. https://doi.org/10.1016/j.dld.2014.11.009.

140. Zhang M, Li Y. Eosinophilic gastroenteritis: a state-of-the-art review. J Gastroenterol Hepatol. 2017;32(1):64–72. https://doi.org/10.1111/jgh.13463.
141. Mansoor E, Saleh MA, Cooper GS. Prevalence of eosinophilic gastroenteritis and colitis in a population-based study, from 2012 to 2017. Clin Gastroenterol Hepatol. 2017;15(11):1733–41. https://doi.org/10.1016/j.cgh.2017.05.050.
142. Jensen ET, Martin CF, Kappelman MD, Dellon ES. Prevalence of eosinophilic gastritis, gastroenteritis, and colitis: estimates from a national administrative database. J Pediatr Gastroenterol Nutr. 2016;62(1):36–42. https://doi.org/10.1097/mpg.0000000000000865.
143. Yan BM, Shaffer EA. Primary eosinophilic disorders of the gastrointestinal tract. Gut. 2009;58(5):721–32. https://doi.org/10.1136/gut.2008.165894.
144. Pineton de Chambrun G, Gonzalez F, Canva JY, Gonzalez S, Houssin L, Desreumaux P, et al. Natural history of eosinophilic gastroenteritis. Clin Gastroenterol Hepatol. 2011;9(11):950–6.e1. https://doi.org/10.1016/j.cgh.2011.07.017.
145. Zhang L, Duan L, Ding S, Lu J, Jin Z, Cui R, et al. Eosinophilic gastroenteritis: clinical manifestations and morphological characteristics, a retrospective study of 42 patients. Scand J Gastroenterol. 2011;46(9):1074–80. https://doi.org/10.3109/00365521.2011.579998.
146. Klein NC, Hargrove RL, Sleisenger MH, Jeffries GH. Eosinophilic gastroenteritis. Medicine. 1970;49(4):299–319.
147. Prussin C. Eosinophilic gastroenteritis and related eosinophilic disorders. Gastroenterol Clin North Am. 2014;43(2):317–27. https://doi.org/10.1016/j.gtc.2014.02.013.
148. Conner JR, Kirsch R. The pathology and causes of tissue eosinophilia in the gastrointestinal tract. Histopathology. 2017;71(2):177–99. https://doi.org/10.1111/his.13228.
149. McCarthy AJ, Sheahan K. Classification of eosinophilic disorders of the small and large intestine. Virchows Arch. 2017. https://doi.org/10.1007/s00428–017–2249–1.
150. Alhmoud T, Hanson JA, Parasher G. Eosinophilic gastroenteritis: an underdiagnosed condition. Dig Dis Sci. 2016;61(9):2585–92. https://doi.org/10.1007/s10620–016–4203–5.
151. Yantiss RK. Eosinophils in the GI tract: how many is too many and what do they mean? Mod Pathol. 2015;28(Suppl 1):S7–21. https://doi.org/10.1038/modpathol.2014.132.
152. Hurrell JM, Genta RM, Melton SD. Histopathologic diagnosis of eosinophilic conditions in the gastrointestinal tract. Adv Anat Pathol. 2011;18(5):335–48. https://doi.org/10.1097/PAP.0b013e318229bfe2.
153. Gathmann B, Grimbacher B, Beaute J, Dudoit Y, Mahlaoui N, Fischer A, et al. The European internet-based patient and research database for primary immunodeficiencies: results 2006–2008. Clin Exp Immunol. 2009;157(Suppl 1):3–11. https://doi.org/10.1111/j.1365–2249.2009.03954.x.
154. Bonilla FA, Barlan I, Chapel H, Costa-Carvalho BT, Cunningham-Rundles C, de la Morena MT, et al. International Consensus Document (ICON): common variable immunodeficiency disorders. J Allergy Clin Immunol Pract. 2016;4(1):38–59. https://doi.org/10.1016/j.jaip.2015.07.025.
155. Hammarstrom L, Vorechovsky I, Webster D. Selective IgA deficiency (SIgAD) and common variable immunodeficiency (CVID). Clin Exp Immunol. 2000;120(2):225–31.
156. Bogaert DJ, Dullaers M, Lambrecht BN, Vermaelen KY, De Baere E, Haerynck F. Genes associated with common variable immunodeficiency: one diagnosis to rule them all? J Med Genet. 2016;53(9):575–90. https://doi.org/10.1136/jmedgenet-2015–103690.
157. Kienzler AK, Hargreaves CE, Patel SY. The role of genomics in common variable immunodeficiency disorders. Clin Exp Immunol. 2017;188(3):326–32. https://doi.org/10.1111/cei.12947.
158. Grimbacher B, Hutloff A, Schlesier M, Glocker E, Warnatz K, Drager R, et al. Homozygous loss of ICOS is associated with adult-onset common variable immunodeficiency. Nat Immunol. 2003;4(3):261–8. https://doi.org/10.1038/ni902.
159. Castigli E, Wilson SA, Garibyan L, Rachid R, Bonilla F, Schneider L, et al. TACI is mutant in common variable immunodeficiency and IgA deficiency. Nat Genet. 2005;37(8):829–34. https://doi.org/10.1038/ng1601.
160. Salzer U, Chapel HM, Webster AD, Pan-Hammarstrom Q, Schmitt-Graeff A, Schlesier M, et al. Mutations in TNFRSF13B encoding TACI are associated with common variable immunodeficiency in humans. Nat Genet. 2005;37(8):820–8. https://doi.org/10.1038/ng1600.
161. Malphettes M, Gerard L, Carmagnat M, Mouillot G, Vince N, Boutboul D, et al. Late-onset combined immune deficiency: a subset of common variable immunodeficiency with severe T cell defect. Clin Infect Dis. 2009;49(9):1329–38. https://doi.org/10.1086/606059.
162. Malamut G, Verkarre V, Suarez F, Viallard JF, Lascaux AS, Cosnes J, et al. The enteropathy associated with common variable immunodeficiency: the delineated frontiers with celiac disease. Am J Gastroenterol. 2010;105(10):2262–75. https://doi.org/10.1038/ajg.2010.214.
163. Mannon PJ, Fuss IJ, Dill S, Friend J, Groden C, Hornung R, et al. Excess IL-12 but not IL-23 accompanies the inflammatory bowel disease associated with common variable immunodeficiency. Gastroenterology. 2006;131(3):748–56. https://doi.org/10.1053/j.gastro.2006.06.022.
164. Oksenhendler E, Gerard L, Fieschi C, Malphettes M, Mouillot G, Jaussaud R, et al. Infections in 252 patients with common variable immunodeficiency. Clin Infect Dis. 2008;46(10):1547–54. https://doi.org/10.1086/587669.
165. Ardeniz O, Cunningham-Rundles C. Granulomatous disease in common variable immunodeficiency. Clin Immunol (Orlando, FL). 2009;133(2):198–207. https://doi.org/10.1016/j.clim.2009.05.001.
166. Cunningham-Rundles C. The many faces of common variable immunodeficiency. Hematology Am Soc Hematol Educ Program. 2012;2012:301–5. https://doi.org/10.1182/asheducation-2012.1.301.
167. Boursiquot JN, Gerard L, Malphettes M, Fieschi C, Galicier L, Boutboul D, et al. Granulomatous disease in CVID: retrospective analysis of clinical characteristics and treatment efficacy in a cohort of 59 patients. J Clin Immunol. 2013;33(1):84–95. https://doi.org/10.1007/s10875–012–9778–9.
168. Teahon K, Webster AD, Price AB, Weston J, Bjarnason I. Studies on the enteropathy associated with primary hypogammaglobulinaemia. Gut. 1994;35(9):1244–9.
169. Cunningham-Rundles C, Bodian C. Common variable immunodeficiency: clinical and immunological features of 248 patients. Clin Immunol (Orlando, FL). 1999;92(1):34–48. https://doi.org/10.1006/clim.1999.4725.
170. Khodadad A, Aghamohammadi A, Parvaneh N, Rezaei N, Mahjoob F, Bashashati M, et al. Gastrointestinal manifestations in patients with common variable immunodeficiency. Dig Dis Sci. 2007;52(11):2977–83. https://doi.org/10.1007/s10620–006–9736–6.
171. Jorgensen SF, Reims HM, Frydenlund D, Holm K, Paulsen V, Michelsen AE, et al. A cross-sectional study of the prevalence of gastrointestinal symptoms and pathology in patients with common variable immunodeficiency. Am J Gastroenterol. 2016;111(10):1467–75. https://doi.org/10.1038/ajg.2016.329.
172. Lougaris V, Ravelli A, Villanacci V, Salemme M, Soresina A, Fuoti M, et al. Gastrointestinal pathologic abnormalities in pediatric- and adult-onset common variable immunodeficiency. Dig Dis Sci. 2015;60(8):2384–9. https://doi.org/10.1007/s10620–015–3638–4.

173. Uzzan M, Ko HM, Mehandru S, Cunningham-Rundles C. Gastrointestinal disorders associated with common variable immune deficiency (CVID) and chronic granulomatous disease (CGD). Curr Gastroenterol Rep. 2016;18(4):17. https://doi.org/10.1007/s11894-016-0491-3.
174. Woodward JM, Gkrania-Klotsas E, Cordero-Ng AY, Aravinthan A, Bandoh BN, Liu H, et al. The role of chronic norovirus infection in the enteropathy associated with common variable immunodeficiency. Am J Gastroenterol. 2015;110(2):320–7. https://doi.org/10.1038/ajg.2014.432.
175. Woodward J, Gkrania-Klotsas E, Kumararatne D. Chronic norovirus infection and common variable immunodeficiency. Clin Exp Immunol. 2017;188(3):363–70. https://doi.org/10.1111/cei.12884.
176. Agarwal S, Smereka P, Harpaz N, Cunningham-Rundles C, Mayer L. Characterization of immunologic defects in patients with common variable immunodeficiency (CVID) with intestinal disease. Inflamm Bowel Dis. 2011;17(1):251–9. https://doi.org/10.1002/ibd.21376.
177. Maarschalk-Ellerbroek LJ, Oldenburg B, Mombers IM, Hoepelman AI, Brosens LA, Offerhaus GJ, et al. Outcome of screening endoscopy in common variable immunodeficiency disorder and X-linked agammaglobulinemia. Endoscopy. 2013;45(4):320–3. https://doi.org/10.1055/s-0032-1326078.
178. Daniels JA, Lederman HM, Maitra A, Montgomery EA. Gastrointestinal tract pathology in patients with common variable immunodeficiency (CVID): a clinicopathologic study and review. Am J Surg Pathol. 2007;31(12):1800–12. https://doi.org/10.1097/PAS.0b013e3180cab60c.
179. Washington K, Stenzel TT, Buckley RH, Gottfried MR. Gastrointestinal pathology in patients with common variable immunodeficiency and X-linked agammaglobulinemia. Am J Surg Pathol. 1996;20(10):1240–52.
180. Luzi G, Zullo A, Iebba F, Rinaldi V, Sanchez Mete L, Muscaritoli M, et al. Duodenal pathology and clinical-immunological implications in common variable immunodeficiency patients. Am J Gastroenterol. 2003;98(1):118–21. https://doi.org/10.1111/j.1572-0241.2003.07159.x.
181. Biagi F, Bianchi PI, Zilli A, Marchese A, Luinetti O, Lougaris V, et al. The significance of duodenal mucosal atrophy in patients with common variable immunodeficiency: a clinical and histopathologic study. Am J Clin Pathol. 2012;138(2):185–9. https://doi.org/10.1309/ajcpeiilh2c0wfye.
182. Quinti I, Soresina A, Guerra A, Rondelli R, Spadaro G, Agostini C, et al. Effectiveness of immunoglobulin replacement therapy on clinical outcome in patients with primary antibody deficiencies: results from a multicenter prospective cohort study. J Clin Immunol. 2011;31(3):315–22. https://doi.org/10.1007/s10875-011-9511-0.
183. Dhalla F, da Silva SP, Lucas M, Travis S, Chapel H. Review of gastric cancer risk factors in patients with common variable immunodeficiency disorders, resulting in a proposal for a surveillance programme. Clin Exp Immunol. 2011;165(1):1–7. https://doi.org/10.1111/j.1365-2249.2011.04384.x.
184. Gangemi S, Allegra A, Musolino C. Lymphoproliferative disease and cancer among patients with common variable immunodeficiency. Leuk Res. 2015;39(4):389–96. https://doi.org/10.1016/j.leukres.2015.02.002.
185. Bruton OC. Agammaglobulinemia. Pediatrics. 1952;9(6):722–8.
186. Vetrie D, Vorechovsky I, Sideras P, Holland J, Davies A, Flinter F, et al. The gene involved in X-linked agammaglobulinaemia is a member of the src family of protein-tyrosine kinases. Nature. 1993;361(6409):226–33. https://doi.org/10.1038/361226a0.
187. Tsukada S, Saffran DC, Rawlings DJ, Parolini O, Allen RC, Klisak I, et al. Deficient expression of a B cell cytoplasmic tyrosine kinase in human X-linked agammaglobulinemia. Cell. 1993;72(2):279–90.
188. Conley ME, Rohrer J, Minegishi Y. X-linked agammaglobulinemia. Clin Rev Allergy Immunol. 2000;19(2):183–204. https://doi.org/10.1385/criai:19:2:183.
189. Winkelstein JA, Marino MC, Lederman HM, Jones SM, Sullivan K, Burks AW, et al. X-linked agammaglobulinemia: report on a United States registry of 201 patients. Medicine. 2006;85(4):193–202. https://doi.org/10.1097/01.md.0000229482.27398.ad.
190. Conley ME, Broides A, Hernandez-Trujillo V, Howard V, Kanegane H, Miyawaki T, et al. Genetic analysis of patients with defects in early B-cell development. Immunol Rev. 2005;203:216–34. https://doi.org/10.1111/j.0105-2896.2005.00233.x.
191. Ponader S, Burger JA. Bruton's tyrosine kinase: from X-linked agammaglobulinemia toward targeted therapy for B-cell malignancies. J Clin Oncol. 2014;32(17):1830–9. https://doi.org/10.1200/jco.2013.53.1046.
192. Holinski-Feder E, Weiss M, Brandau O, Jedele KB, Nore B, Backesjo CM, et al. Mutation screening of the BTK gene in 56 families with X-linked agammaglobulinemia (XLA): 47 unique mutations without correlation to clinical course. Pediatrics. 1998;101(2):276–84.
193. Broides A, Yang W, Conley ME. Genotype/phenotype correlations in X-linked agammaglobulinemia. Clin Immunol (Orlando, FL). 2006;118(2–3):195–200. https://doi.org/10.1016/j.clim.2005.10.007.
194. Lopez-Granados E, Perez de Diego R, Ferreira Cerdan A, Fontan Casariego G, Garcia Rodriguez MC. A genotype-phenotype correlation study in a group of 54 patients with X-linked agammaglobulinemia. J Allergy Clin Immunol. 2005;116(3):690–7. https://doi.org/10.1016/j.jaci.2005.04.043.
195. Bearden D, Collett M, Quan PL, Costa-Carvalho BT, Sullivan KE. Enteroviruses in X-linked agammaglobulinemia: update on epidemiology and therapy. J Allergy Clin Immunol Pract. 2016;4(6):1059–65. https://doi.org/10.1016/j.jaip.2015.12.015.
196. Agarwal S, Mayer L. Diagnosis and treatment of gastrointestinal disorders in patients with primary immunodeficiency. Clin Gastroenterol Hepatol. 2013;11(9):1050–63. https://doi.org/10.1016/j.cgh.2013.02.024.
197. Barmettler S, Otani IM, Minhas J, Abraham RS, Chang Y, Dorsey MJ, et al. Gastrointestinal manifestations in X-linked agammaglobulinemia. J Clin Immunol. 2017;37(3):287–94. https://doi.org/10.1007/s10875-017-0374-x.
198. Lederman HM, Winkelstein JA. X-linked agammaglobulinemia: an analysis of 96 patients. Medicine. 1985;64(3):145–56.
199. Hernandez-Trujillo VP, Scalchunes C, Cunningham-Rundles C, Ochs HD, Bonilla FA, Paris K, et al. Autoimmunity and inflammation in X-linked agammaglobulinemia. J Clin Immunol. 2014;34(6):627–32. https://doi.org/10.1007/s10875-014-0056-x.
200. Cellier C, Foray S, Hermine O. Regional enteritis associated with enterovirus in a patient with X-linked agammaglobulinemia. N Engl J Med. 2000;342(21):1611–2. https://doi.org/10.1056/nejm200005253422113.
201. Abramowsky CR, Sorensen RU. Regional enteritis-like enteropathy in a patient with agammaglobulinemia: histologic and immunocytologic studies. Hum Pathol. 1988;19(4):483–6.
202. van der Meer JW, Weening RS, Schellekens PT, van Munster IP, Nagengast FM. Colorectal cancer in patients with X-linked agammaglobulinaemia. Lancet (London, England). 1993;341(8858):1439–40.
203. Bachmeyer C, Monge M, Cazier A, Le Deist F, de Saint Basile G, Durandy A, et al. Gastric adenocarcinoma in a patient with X-linked agammaglobulinaemia. Eur J Gastroenterol Hepatol. 2000;12(9):1033–5.
204. Staines Boone AT, Torres Martinez MG, Lopez Herrera G, de Leija Portilla JO, Espinosa Padilla SE, Espinosa Rosales FJ, et al.

Gastric adenocarcinoma in the context of X-linked agammaglobulinemia: case report and review of the literature. J Clin Immunol. 2014;34(2):134–7. https://doi.org/10.1007/s10875-013-9971-5.
205. Silva P, Justicia A, Regueiro A, Farina S, Couselo JM, Loidi L. Autosomal recessive agammaglobulinemia due to defect in μ heavy chain caused by a novel mutation in the IGHM gene. Genes Immun. 2017;18(3):197–9. https://doi.org/10.1038/gene.2017.14.
206. Yel L, Minegishi Y, Coustan-Smith E, Buckley RH, Trubel H, Pachman LM, et al. Mutations in the mu heavy-chain gene in patients with agammaglobulinemia. N Engl J Med. 1996;335(20): 1486–93. https://doi.org/10.1056/nejm199611143352003.
207. Lopez Granados E, Porpiglia AS, Hogan MB, Matamoros N, Krasovec S, Pignata C, et al. Clinical and molecular analysis of patients with defects in micro heavy chain gene. J Clin Invest. 2002;110(7):1029–35. https://doi.org/10.1172/jci15658.
208. Notarangelo LD, Duse M, Ugazio AG. Immunodeficiency with hyper-IgM (HIM). Immunodefic Rev. 1992;3(2):101–21.
209. Winkelstein JA, Marino MC, Ochs H, Fuleihan R, Scholl PR, Geha R, et al. The X-linked hyper-IgM syndrome: clinical and immunologic features of 79 patients. Medicine. 2003;82(6):373–84. https://doi.org/10.1097/01.md.0000100046.06009.b0.
210. Davies EG, Thrasher AJ. Update on the hyper immunoglobulin M syndromes. Br J Haematol. 2010;149(2):167–80. https://doi.org/10.1111/j.1365-2141.2010.08077.x.
211. Qamar N, Fuleihan RL. The hyper IgM syndromes. Clin Rev Allergy Immunol. 2014;46(2):120–30. https://doi.org/10.1007/s12016-013-8378-7.
212. Allen RC, Armitage RJ, Conley ME, Rosenblatt H, Jenkins NA, Copeland NG, et al. CD40 ligand gene defects responsible for X-linked hyper-IgM syndrome. Science (New York, NY). 1993;259(5097):990–3.
213. Aruffo A, Farrington M, Hollenbaugh D, Li X, Milatovich A, Nonoyama S, et al. The CD40 ligand, gp39, is defective in activated T cells from patients with X-linked hyper-IgM syndrome. Cell. 1993;72(2):291–300.
214. DiSanto JP, Bonnefoy JY, Gauchat JF, Fischer A, de Saint Basile G. CD40 ligand mutations in x-linked immunodeficiency with hyper-IgM. Nature. 1993;361(6412):541–3. https://doi.org/10.1038/361541a0.
215. Korthauer U, Graf D, Mages HW, Briere F, Padayachee M, Malcolm S, et al. Defective expression of T-cell CD40 ligand causes X-linked immunodeficiency with hyper-IgM. Nature. 1993;361(6412):539–41. https://doi.org/10.1038/361539a0.
216. Leven EA, Maffucci P, Ochs HD, Scholl PR, Buckley RH, Fuleihan RL, et al. Hyper IgM syndrome: a report from the USIDNET registry. J Clin Immunol. 2016;36(5):490–501. https://doi.org/10.1007/s10875-016-0291-4.
217. Levy J, Espanol-Boren T, Thomas C, Fischer A, Tovo P, Bordigoni P, et al. Clinical spectrum of X-linked hyper-IgM syndrome. J Pediatr. 1997;131(1 Pt 1):47–54.
218. Hayward AR, Levy J, Facchetti F, Notarangelo L, Ochs HD, Etzioni A, et al. Cholangiopathy and tumors of the pancreas, liver, and biliary tree in boys with X-linked immunodeficiency with hyper-IgM. J Immunol. 1997;158(2):977–83.
219. Erdos M, Garami M, Rakoczi E, Zalatnai A, Steinbach D, Baumann U, et al. Neuroendocrine carcinoma associated with X-linked hyper-immunoglobulin M syndrome: report of four cases and review of the literature. Clin Immunol (Orlando, FL). 2008;129(3):455–61. https://doi.org/10.1016/j.clim.2008.08.005.
220. Cirillo E, Giardino G, Gallo V, D'Assante R, Grasso F, Romano R, et al. Severe combined immunodeficiency—an update. Ann N Y Acad Sci. 2015;1356:90–106. https://doi.org/10.1111/nyas.12849.
221. Agarwal S, Mayer L. Gastrointestinal manifestations in primary immune disorders. Inflamm Bowel Dis. 2010;16(4):703–11. https://doi.org/10.1002/ibd.21040.
222. Cossu F. Genetics of SCID. Ital J Pediatr. 2010;36:76. https://doi.org/10.1186/1824-7288-36-76.
223. Fischer A, Notarangelo LD, Neven B, Cavazzana M, Puck JM. Severe combined immunodeficiencies and related disorders. Nat Rev Dis Primers. 2015;1:15061. https://doi.org/10.1038/nrdp.2015.61.
224. Shearer WT, Dunn E, Notarangelo LD, Dvorak CC, Puck JM, Logan BR, et al. Establishing diagnostic criteria for severe combined immunodeficiency disease (SCID), leaky SCID, and Omenn syndrome: the Primary Immune Deficiency Treatment Consortium experience. J Allergy Clin Immunol. 2014;133(4):1092–8. https://doi.org/10.1016/j.jaci.2013.09.044.
225. Honig M, Schwarz K. Omenn syndrome: a lack of tolerance on the background of deficient lymphocyte development and maturation. Curr Opin Rheumatol. 2006;18(4):383–8. https://doi.org/10.1097/01.bor.0000231907.50290.6f.
226. Felgentreff K, Perez-Becker R, Speckmann C, Schwarz K, Kalwak K, Markelj G, et al. Clinical and immunological manifestations of patients with atypical severe combined immunodeficiency. Clin Immunol (Orlando, FL). 2011;141(1):73–82. https://doi.org/10.1016/j.clim.2011.05.007.
227. Humblet-Baron S, Schonefeldt S, Garcia-Perez JE, Baron F, Pasciuto E, Liston A. Cytotoxic T-lymphocyte-associated protein 4-Ig effectively controls immune activation and inflammatory disease in a novel murine model of leaky severe combined immunodeficiency. J Allergy Clin Immunol. 2017;140(5):1394–403.e8. https://doi.org/10.1016/j.jaci.2016.12.968.
228. Omenn GS. Familial reticuloendotheliosis with eosinophilia. N Engl J Med. 1965;273:427–32. https://doi.org/10.1056/nejm196508192730806.
229. Rota IA, Dhalla F. FOXN1 deficient nude severe combined immunodeficiency. Orphanet J Rare Dis. 2017;12(1):6. https://doi.org/10.1186/s13023-016-0557-1.
230. Moreno LA, Gottrand F, Turck D, Manouvrier-Hanu S, Mazingue F, Morisot C, et al. Severe combined immunodeficiency syndrome associated with autosomal recessive familial multiple gastrointestinal atresias: study of a family. Am J Med Genet. 1990;37(1):143–6. https://doi.org/10.1002/ajmg.1320370133.
231. Rothenberg ME, White FV, Chilmonczyk B, Chatila T. A syndrome involving immunodeficiency and multiple intestinal atresias. Immunodeficiency. 1995;5(3):171–8.
232. Cole C, Freitas A, Clifton MS, Durham MM. Hereditary multiple intestinal atresias: 2 new cases and review of the literature. J Pediatr Surg. 2010;45(4):E21–4. https://doi.org/10.1016/j.jpedsurg.2010.01.017.
233. Snover DC, Filipovich AH, Ramsay NK, Weisdorf SA, Kersey JH. Graft-versus-host-disease-like histopathological findings in pre-bone-marrow transplantation biopsies of patients with severe T cell deficiency. Transplantation. 1985;39(1):95–7.
234. Muller SM, Ege M, Pottharst A, Schulz AS, Schwarz K, Friedrich W. Transplacentally acquired maternal T lymphocytes in severe combined immunodeficiency: a study of 121 patients. Blood. 2001;98(6):1847–51.
235. Antachopoulos C. Invasive fungal infections in congenital immunodeficiencies. Clin Microbiol Infect. 2010;16(9):1335–42. https://doi.org/10.1111/j.1469-0691.2010.03289.x.
236. Boeck A, Buckley RH, Schiff RI. Gastroesophageal reflux and severe combined immunodeficiency. J Allergy Clin Immunol. 1997;99(3):420–4.
237. Sponzilli I, Notarangelo LD. Severe combined immunodeficiency (SCID): from molecular basis to clinical management. Acta Biomed. 2011;82(1):5–13.
238. Thrasher AJ, Williams DA. Evolving gene therapy in primary immunodeficiency. Mol Ther. 2017;25(5):1132–41. https://doi.org/10.1016/j.ymthe.2017.03.018.

239. Ochs HD, Filipovich AH, Veys P, Cowan MJ, Kapoor N. Wiskott-Aldrich syndrome: diagnosis, clinical and laboratory manifestations, and treatment. Biol Blood Marrow Transplant. 2009;15(1 Suppl):84–90. https://doi.org/10.1016/j.bbmt.2008.10.007.
240. Ariga T. Wiskott-Aldrich syndrome; an x-linked primary immunodeficiency disease with unique and characteristic features. Allergol Int. 2012;61(2):183–9. https://doi.org/10.2332/allergolint.11-RAI-0412.
241. Massaad MJ, Ramesh N, Geha RS. Wiskott-Aldrich syndrome: a comprehensive review. Ann N Y Acad Sci. 2013;1285:26–43. https://doi.org/10.1111/nyas.12049.
242. Derry JM, Ochs HD, Francke U. Isolation of a novel gene mutated in Wiskott-Aldrich syndrome. Cell. 1994;78(4):635–44.
243. Ozsahin H, Cavazzana-Calvo M, Notarangelo LD, Schulz A, Thrasher AJ, Mazzolari E, et al. Long-term outcome following hematopoietic stem-cell transplantation in Wiskott-Aldrich syndrome: collaborative study of the European Society for Immunodeficiencies and European Group for Blood and Marrow Transplantation. Blood. 2008;111(1):439–45. https://doi.org/10.1182/blood-2007-03-076679.
244. Notarangelo LD, Miao CH, Ochs HD. Wiskott-Aldrich syndrome. Curr Opin Hematol. 2008;15(1):30–6. https://doi.org/10.1097/MOH.0b013e3282f30448.
245. Dupuis-Girod S, Medioni J, Haddad E, Quartier P, Cavazzana-Calvo M, Le Deist F, et al. Autoimmunity in Wiskott-Aldrich syndrome: risk factors, clinical features, and outcome in a single-center cohort of 55 patients. Pediatrics. 2003;111(5 Pt 1):e622–7.
246. Cannioto Z, Berti I, Martelossi S, Bruno I, Giurici N, Crovella S, et al. IBD and IBD mimicking enterocolitis in children younger than 2 years of age. Eur J Pediatr. 2009;168(2):149–55. https://doi.org/10.1007/s00431-008-0721-2.
247. Folwaczny C, Ruelfs C, Walther J, Konig A, Emmerich B. Ulcerative colitis in a patient with Wiskott-Aldrich syndrome. Endoscopy. 2002;34(10):840–1. https://doi.org/10.1055/s-2002-34272.

Infectious Disorders of the Duodenum and Small Bowel

11

Audrey N. Schuetz

Introduction

Infectious disorders of the small bowel are common worldwide. Most small bowel infections lead to diarrhea and are self-limited. Such infections usually do not require further investigation to identify an infectious etiology. Occasionally, small intestinal infections are chronic in their course either due to the immunocompromised status of the host or due to the nature of disease caused by the infectious agent itself. In this chapter, we will review the pathology of the infectious agents which cause disease of the small bowel. The histopathologic appearances of infectious entities which may lead the clinician to perform a diagnostic procedure via duodenal or small intestinal biopsies will be reviewed. A variety of viral, bacterial, fungal, and parasitic agents which cause small bowel disorders will be covered. Clinical features which will be discussed include the epidemiology, pathogenesis, and clinical presentation. When applicable, endoscopic appearance of the lesions will be described. Laboratory and radiologic ancillary approaches to diagnosis, including molecular techniques, will be mentioned. Finally, histopathologic appearance of the lesions, clinical and pathologic differential diagnosis, treatment, and prognosis will conclude each section. Infectious agents which cause intestinal diseases more commonly in other parts of the gastrointestinal tract are covered in other chapters of this book.

Viral Diseases

Adenovirus

Definition

Adenoviruses comprise a group of DNA viruses capable of infecting a variety of cell types throughout the body. Most frequently associated with upper respiratory tract infections and pneumonia, adenoviruses can also cause gastrointestinal disease. Although adenoviruses are potentially pathogenic in immunocompetent and immunocompromised persons, the majority of intestinal biopsies obtained for assessment of gastrointestinal tract originate from immunocompromised persons.

Clinical Features

Worldwide in distribution, adenoviruses cause disease throughout the year. Over 60 adenovirus serotypes capable of infecting humans have been identified, with certain serotypes showing predilections for causing infection in certain body sites [1]. Transmission occurs via aerosolized droplets, the fecal-oral route, or by fomites. Viral particles can survive on environmental surfaces for long periods of time. Most individuals have serologic evidence of prior adenoviral infection in childhood.

Adenoviruses may cause gastroenteritis, diarrhea, and intussusception as well as diseases outside of the gastrointestinal tract. Disease in immunocompetent patients is usually mild and self-limited. Enteritis due to adenovirus has been described in small bowel transplant and allogeneic stem cell transplant recipients, and disease may be severe in immunocompromised persons [2, 3]. Intussusception associated with adenoviral infection is likely due to lymphoid hyperplasia. Other adenovirus disease presentations include hepatitis, hemorrhagic cystitis, nephritis, acute respiratory disease, pharyngitis, pneumonia, keratoconjunctivitis, encephalitis, and myocarditis.

Besides histopathology, ancillary diagnostic methods include culture and molecular assays. Viral culture of fresh tissue allows identification of the organism which produces a characteristic cytopathologic effect upon infecting the host cells within 3–5 days of culture; the cytopathologic effect is described as a cluster of grapes in cell culture. Due to the length of time required for a diagnosis by culture, molecular assays have generally replaced culture as the primary mode of identification from a variety of sources including intestinal biopsies [4]. Adenovirus can be shed in stool and are

A. N. Schuetz (✉)
Department of Laboratory Medicine and Pathology, Mayo Clinic, Rochester, MN, USA
e-mail: Schuetz.audrey@mayo.edu

L. Zhang et al. (eds.), *Surgical Pathology of Non-neoplastic Gastrointestinal Diseases*,
https://doi.org/10.1007/978-3-030-15573-5_11

detectable by molecular methods for months after primary infection [5]. Detection of adenovirus in the blood is one of the mainstays of diagnosis of adenoviral infection in immunocompromised individuals. Electron microscopy is also an outmoded method of diagnosis, as it is time-consuming and requires considerable expertise to perform and interpret. Adenovirus-infected tissue shows a paracrystalline array of icosahedral capsids measuring 70–90 nm in diameter by electron microscopy. Histopathology and molecular testing of tissue or other specimens are the main means of diagnosis.

On endoscopy, mucosal erosions and ulcerations may be seen in the setting of severe intestinal disease due to adenovirus.

Pathological Features

Adenovirus infects epithelial cells and causes intranuclear inclusions. Early in infection, the inclusions are small, dense, and amphophilic. The inclusions are usually surrounded by a clear zone, and the peripheral chromatin is condensed at the edge. Late in infection, the inclusions are basophilic and smudgy (Fig. 11.1a, b). The infected nucleus is typically enlarged, with nuclear edges blurring as the inclusion matures (Fig. 11.1c). Occasionally, adenovirus is associated with Cowdry type A inclusions. In immunocompetent patients, the inflammatory background is typically lymphocytic and occasionally mixed with other inflammatory cells.

Immunohistochemistry and in situ hybridization are available to confirm the presence of adenovirus inclusions (Fig. 11.2a, b).

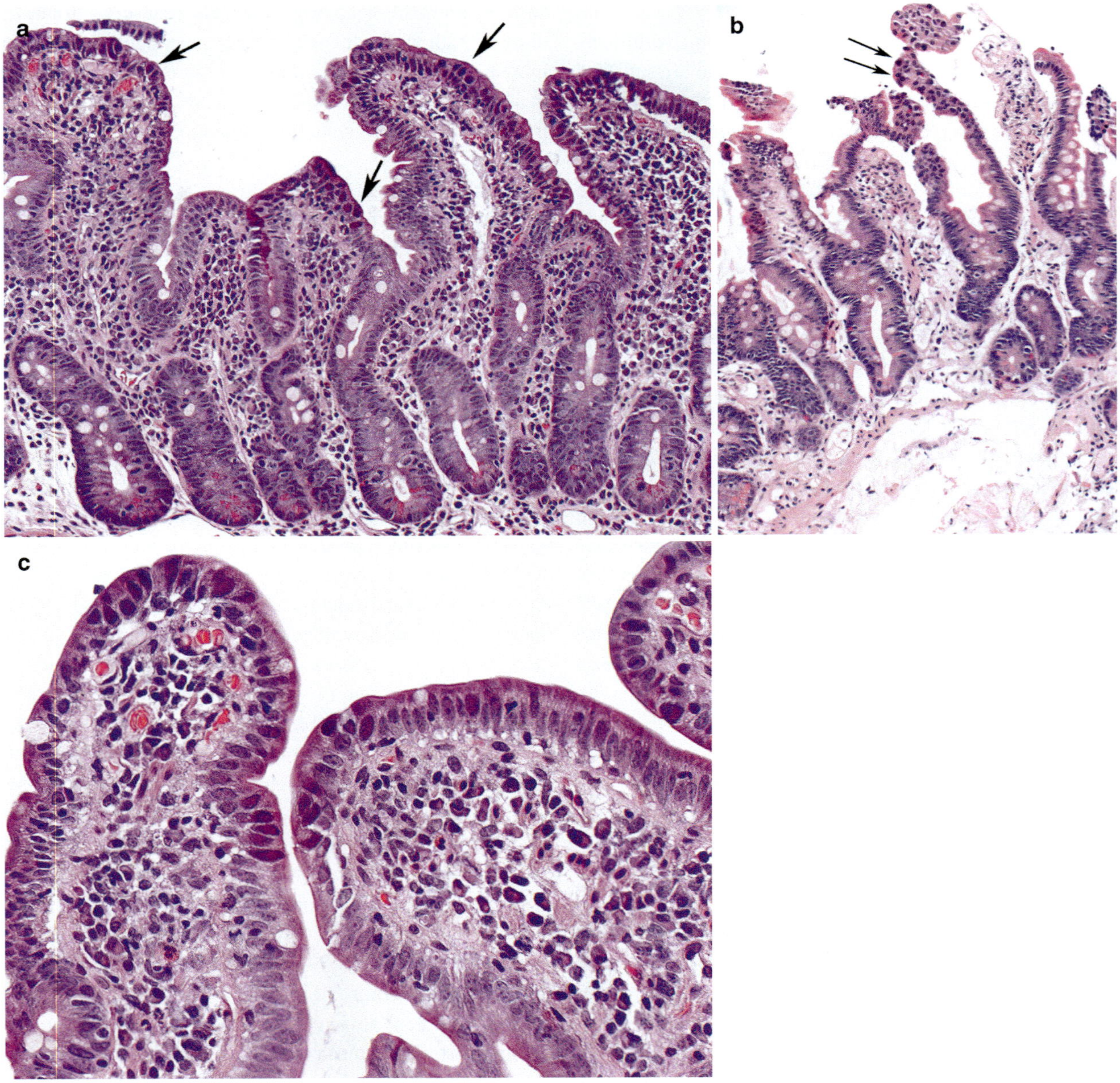

Fig. 11.1 Adenoviral duodenitis. (**a**) Scattered epithelial cells contain large adenoviral inclusions (arrows) in an inflammatory background of lymphocytes and plasma cells. (**b**) Smudgy inclusions which are typical of adenovirus are seen in some of the epithelial cells at the tips of the villi (arrows). (**c**) Several large intranuclear adenoviral inclusions are seen

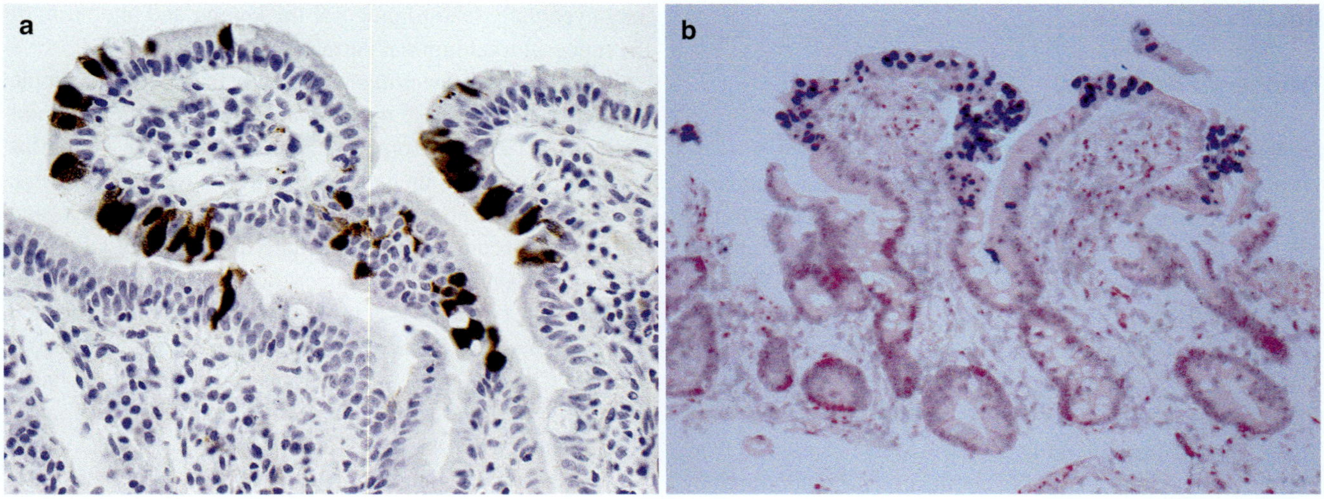

Fig. 11.2 Immunohistochemical and in situ hybridization staining for adenovirus. (**a**) Immunohistochemical stain for adenovirus highlights infected cells. (**b**) In situ hybridization for adenovirus highlights patchy distribution of infected cells

Table 11.1 Characteristics of viral infections of the small bowel

Virus	Cell type infected	Intranuclear inclusions	Cytoplasmic inclusions	Disease presentation and patient population	Comments
Adenovirus	Epithelial	Early: Small, amphophilic Late: Basophilic, smudgy	None	Enteritis Colitis Immunocompetent or immunocompromised individuals	Enlarged nucleus, nuclear contours become blurred as inclusion matures
Cytomegalovirus	Endothelial, epithelial, mesenchymal	Basophilic to amphophilic with surrounding halo	Eosinophilic to basophilic	Mucosal ulcers and erosions Enteritis and colitis Typically immunocompromised individuals	Markedly enlarged cell, characteristic Cowdry type A inclusions
Herpes simplex virus	Epithelial	Eosinophilic Cowdry type A, ground glass chromatin	None	Upper gastrointestinal tract disease Occasionally enteritis Typically immunocompromised individuals	Multinucleation common; nuclear molding and marginated chromatin; single cells not enlarged
Varicella zoster virus	Epithelial	Eosinophilic Cowdry type A, ground glass chromatin	None	Upper gastrointestinal tract disease Rarely enteritis	Multinucleation common; nuclear molding and marginated chromatin; single cells not enlarged; multinucleated cells primarily in stratified squamous epithelium

Differential Diagnosis

Various viruses cause inclusions in infected cells. Herpes simplex virus (HSV) or varicella zoster virus (VZV) may lead to intranuclear inclusions, but syncytia or multinucleated cells are often seen in infections related to these two viruses. Cytomegalovirus (CMV) causes cytoplasmic inclusions as well as intranuclear inclusions. Other viruses which lead to cytopathic effect include BK virus and JC virus, but small intestinal infection with these viruses is rare. Table 11.1 shows a comparison of the various inclusions caused by these viruses which may infect the gastrointestinal tract.

Treatment and Prognosis

Prognosis depends upon the site of infection and immune status of the host. In general, disease due to adenovirus is self-limited in immunocompetent hosts but may be associated with high mortality (>50%) in immunocompromised children and adults. In transplant recipients with disseminated adenoviral disease, treatment options are few. Cidofovir or other antiviral medications may be tried [6]. Enteric adenovirus infection in immunocompetent patients with diarrhea is self-limited and resolves without treatment.

Bacterial Diseases

Tropheryma whipplei

Definition

Tropheryma whipplei (*T. whipplei*) is the causative agent of Whipple disease, a chronic and multisystem illness characterized by macrophage infiltration of multiple organs and tissues. The small bowel is often involved in cases of Whipple disease, and small intestinal biopsies are frequently performed to establish the diagnosis.

Clinical Features

Most reported cases of Whipple disease have originated from Europe and the USA [7]. Whipple disease predominantly affects middle-aged men. Although the route of transmission of *T. whipplei* has not yet been conclusively identified, it is thought to occur via the fecal-oral route. Asymptomatic carriers are believed to be a reservoir, and *T. whipplei* DNA has been detected in stool, saliva, and biopsies from such individuals [8, 9]. There is increasing evidence of a genetic predisposition to Whipple disease [8].

The macrophages contain large numbers of bacilli in Whipple disease. Being unable to kill the bacteria, macrophages attempt to contain them within their cytoplasm. Bacteria are believed to travel through the lymphatics to the circulatory system, spreading to other organs within the body. Symptoms of intestinal disease are due to the large numbers of macrophages within the intestinal wall which may eventually lead to mucosal thickening and alteration of the mucosal tract luminal surface.

The small intestine is most frequently involved by Whipple disease, but the disease may affect any area of the gastrointestinal tract or other organs. Clinical signs and symptoms are nonspecific and include weight loss, fever, and anemia. Intestinal manifestations include diarrhea, steatorrhea, and abdominal discomfort and are usually indicative of late-stage disease. Mesenteric and retroperitoneal lymphadenopathies are common. Other areas of the body may also be affected, and multisystem disease can be a clue to the diagnosis of Whipple disease. Clinical clues include joint discomfort, lymphadenopathy, arthralgias, and hyperpigmentation. Approximately 70% of cases will have some form of joint involvement which is often the earliest manifestation of Whipple disease [8].

The small intestinal mucosa may be thickened and pale yellow or whitish in color on endoscopy; yet, it may also appear normal [10]. Erythema and other inflammatory signs of intestinal mucosa are not commonly seen. The distribution may be diffuse or patchy; therefore, several biopsies should be obtained and examined. Anemia may result from occult gastrointestinal bleeding. Molecular studies for *T. whipplei* may be performed on fresh or formalin-fixed, paraffin-embedded (FFPE) tissue, although histopathology is also definitive.

Pathological Features

The villi in small intestinal biopsies affected by Whipple disease may be swollen or flattened with dilation of the lacteals (Fig. 11.3a–c). Bacilli-containing macrophages usually

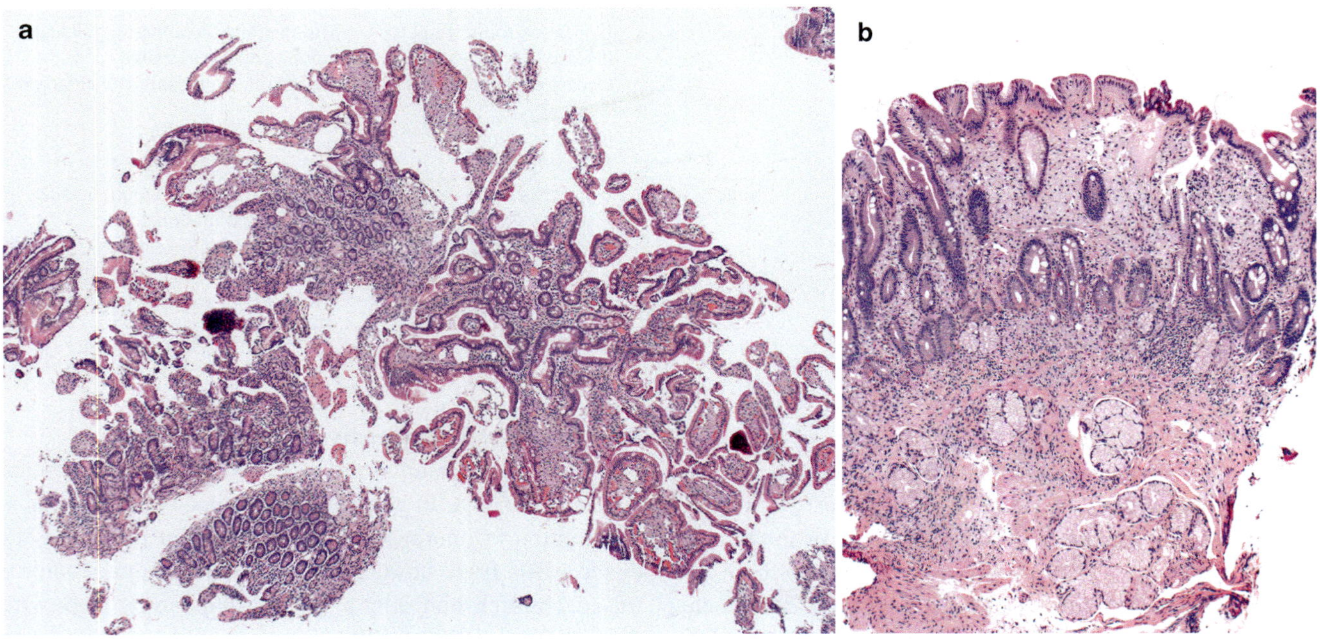

Fig. 11.3 Whipple disease involving the small intestine. (**a**) Low-power view of Whipple disease involving the small intestine. Macrophages distend some of the villi. (**b**) Blunting and infiltration of the villi with foamy macrophages are evident in this case of severe Whipple disease. (**c**) Dilated lacteals are conspicuous, and an increase in inflammatory cells is seen in this case of Whipple disease. (**d**) Foamy macrophages distend the villus. (**e**) High-power view of foamy macrophages with finely vacuolated cytoplasm

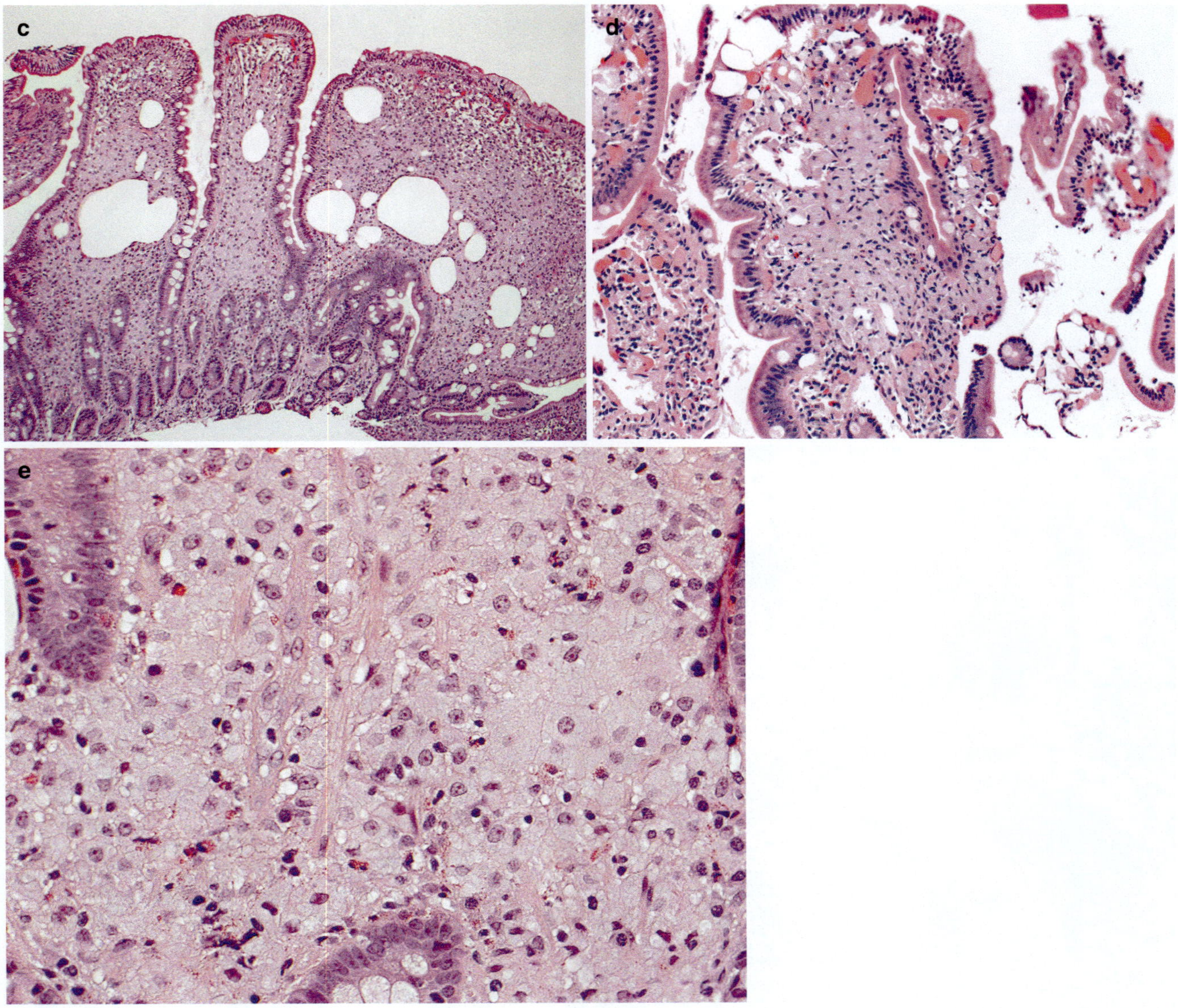

Fig. 11.3 (continued)

cluster at the apices of the villi and are primarily mucosal in location; however, they may also extend to the submucosa. Villous architecture may be maintained. Although an inflammatory component is rare, the lamina propria may contain lymphocytes, plasma cells, or eosinophils. Occasionally, non-necrotizing granulomas may be seen. More severe clinical disease may be related to the depth to which macrophages extend into the submucosa and the degree of non-macrophage inflammation and villous blunting (Fig. 11.3c).

Collections of foamy macrophages stuffed with PAS-positive bacilli are characteristic of Whipple disease. On hematoxylin and eosin stain (H&E), macrophages are polygonal in shape and contain pale-gray, finely vacuolated cytoplasm (Fig. 11.3d, e). PAS and PAS-diastase stains highlight intensely pink or magenta bacillary or rod-like forms within the cytoplasm (Fig. 11.4a, b). The intracellular forms may also appear globular, due to degradation of bacilli by the macrophages. Silver deposition stains such as Warthin-Starry may also demonstrate the small rods of *T. whipplei*. Although a Gram-negative bacillus, *T. whipplei* is not easily seen on tissue Gram stain. Electron microscopic examination can be used to confirm the presence of *T. whipplei* (Fig. 11.4c, d). On electron microscopy, *T. whipplei* bacilli are rod-shaped with an inner dense layer and an outer dense layer which is composed of a trilaminar membrane.

Following treatment, bacilli are less apparent on PAS and other stains. On the other hand, macrophages clear more slowly and may still be present after a year of antibiotic treatment [11].

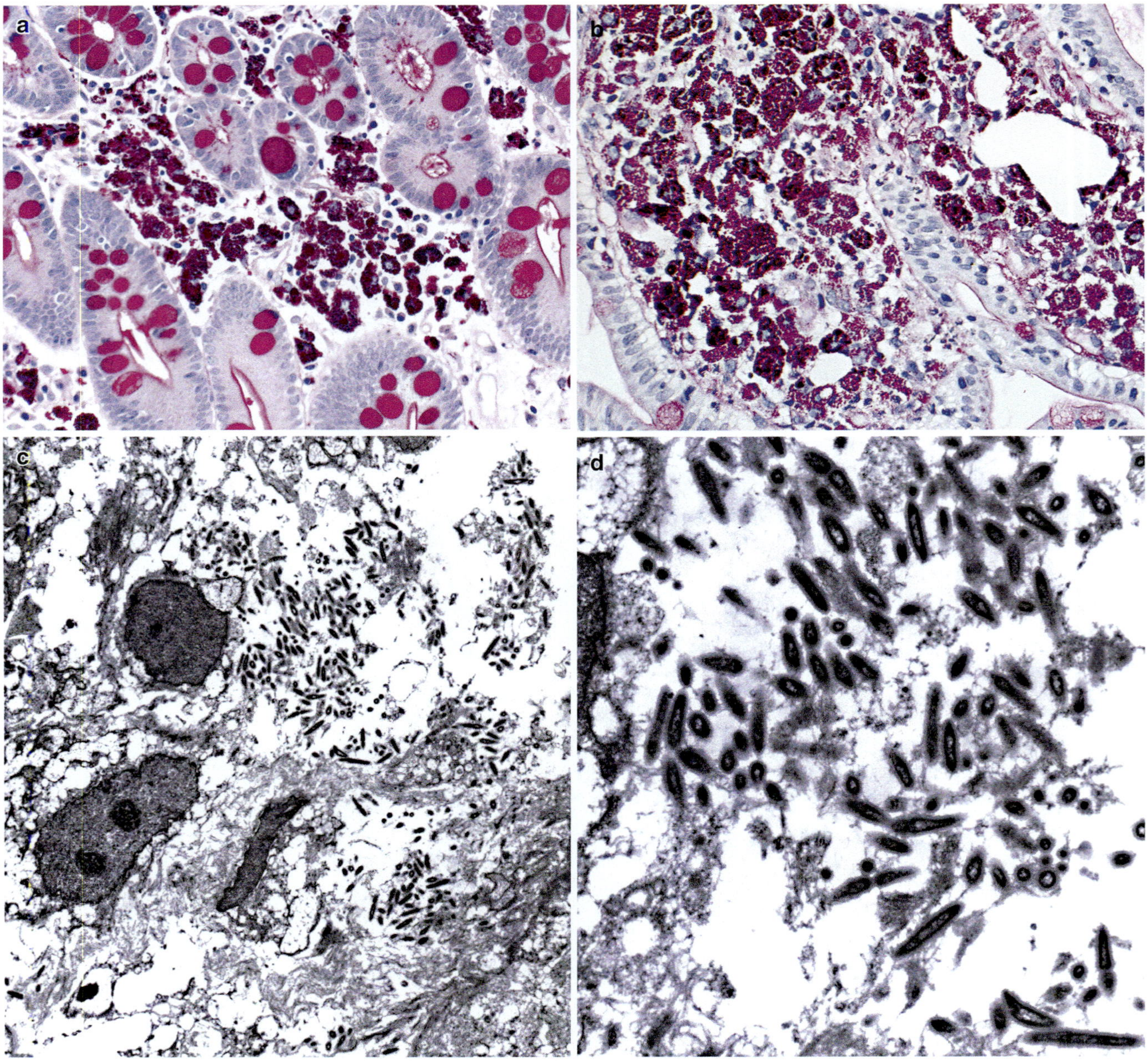

Fig. 11.4 Whipple disease of the small intestine. (**a**) Globular- and bacillary-shaped PAS-positive *T. whipplei* bacilli fill the cytoplasm of macrophages. (**b**) PAS-positive bacilli appear globular in this biopsy, due to partial degradation by the macrophages. (**c**) Electron microscopy demonstrates intracytoplasmic rod-shaped *T. whipplei* bacilli. (**d**) Higher-power view of *T. whipplei* rod-shaped bacilli

Differential Diagnosis

Due to the nonspecific nature of symptoms of intestinal Whipple disease, the clinical differential diagnosis is broad and includes malabsorption syndromes such as celiac disease and sarcoidosis.

The differential diagnosis of PAS-positive granules or bodies within foamy macrophages includes *Rhodococcus equi* or mycobacteria other than *Mycobacterium tuberculosis*. The presence of macrophages containing PAS-positive bacilli within the lamina propria may be seen in intestinal disease due to *Mycobacterium avium* complex (MAC) or other non-tuberculous mycobacteria (NTM) associated with HIV or AIDS. However, the acid-fast stain is negative in Whipple disease, while mycobacteria are acid-fast positive. *R. equi* is partially acid-fast or modified acid-fast positive (i.e., positive by the Fite stain). Macroglobulinemia is also in the differential of Whipple disease. In macroglobulinemia, PAS staining of the macrophages is faint and homogenous rather than strong and clumpy. Finally, the presence of non-necrotizing granulomas in Whipple disease is uncommon and should raise the suspicion of sarcoidosis or other granulomatous conditions.

Treatment and Prognosis

The prognosis of untreated Whipple disease is poor. Antibiotic treatment for intestinal Whipple disease consists of long-term combination antibiotics, typically 12 months of doxycycline plus hydroxychloroquine followed by lifelong suppression with doxycycline [12]. Although intestinal symptoms generally improve rapidly after therapy is begun, relapses may be frequent after discontinuation of antimicrobials. Immune reconstitution inflammatory syndrome (IRIS) may occur upon initiation of treatment [12].

Mycobacteria

Definition

Non-tuberculous mycobacteria (NTM) may cause disseminated or localized disease in immunocompromised persons. Symptoms of infection due to MAC—one of the NTM—in patients with depressed immune function are nonspecific but include diarrhea for which intestinal biopsies may be obtained.

Clinical Features

NTM are ubiquitous in the environment and have been isolated from soil, dust, fresh and salt water, and animals [13]. Disseminated disease due to MAC was common in the 1980s due to the AIDS epidemic, but dramatic declines in the incidence of MAC infection have been seen over the past 20 years due to widespread use of antiretroviral therapy [14]. A CD4 count below 100 cells/μL is a risk factor among HIV-infected patients for disseminated MAC infection. Other NTM species such as *Mycobacterium genavense* have been known to cause disseminated disease in immunocompromised patients and lead to histologic and clinical findings similar to MAC [15].

Patients who are immunocompromised due to conditions other than HIV may also develop NTM intestinal infections [16]. NTM intestinal and disseminated diseases have been documented in solid organ or bone marrow transplant recipients.

NTM intestinal infection is most common in the small intestine, particularly the duodenum. Colonic involvement may also be present, but gastric or esophageal involvement is rare. Mesenteric lymph nodes may be enlarged; there have been reports of intestinal obstruction due to massively enlarged abdominal lymphadenopathy [17]. The bone marrow is often involved in cases of disseminated infection. Disseminated MAC or other NTM can involve almost any organ. Hepatic and splenic involvement is also commonly seen in disseminated disease. Disseminated NTM infection may also present as weight loss and fever; diarrhea and abdominal pain may occur if the intestinal tract is involved. Malabsorption may occur due to structural changes in the small intestinal mucosa, such as villus flattening.

Fine white nodules of the duodenal mucosa may be seen on endoscopy in cases of intestinal NTM disease. Flattening of the villous surface may also be evident on endoscopy. Rarely, ulceration or hemorrhage may be seen [18].

Radiologic or laboratory findings associated with disseminated NTM disease are nonspecific and cause pathology in involved organs. Since the gastrointestinal tract is colonized with NTM, stool cultures should not be routinely used to diagnose intestinal NTM disease. Cultures of lymph nodes, bone marrow, or blood may aid in the diagnosis of disseminated NTM disease.

Pathological Features

In immunocompetent patients, necrotizing or non-necrotizing granulomas may be seen on intestinal biopsies in patients with disseminated NTM infection. In the immunocompetent patient with intestinal NTM disease, acid-fast smears may reveal only rare bacilli. However, in patients with AIDS or HIV infection, granulomas are usually not formed. Massive infiltrates of foamy macrophages may be seen in the small bowel and surrounding lymph nodes of HIV-positive patients with disseminated NTM infection of the small bowel (Fig. 11.5a). The macrophages are plump (Figs. 11.5b and 11.6b). Granulomas may be poorly formed or absent entirely in the immunocompromised patient population. The proximal small bowel or duodenum is often the most severely infected site of the gastrointestinal tract. In advanced cases, infected macrophages may be present throughout the entire thickness of the small intestinal wall (Fig. 11.6a). The histiocytic infiltrate may be so severe as to cause villous widening and blunting (Fig. 11.5a).

Acid-fast-positive bacilli may appear beaded but may stain homogeneously. Bacilli measure approximately 4–6 μm in length and are less than 1 μm in diameter. Macrophages are stuffed with acid-fast-positive mycobacteria in cases of disseminated NTM intestinal disease of immunocompromised patients (Figs. 11.5c and 11.6c). Mycobacteria also stain positive with PAS (Fig. 11.5d) and GMS stains.

Differential Diagnosis

Histiocytic infiltration of the lamina propria and blunting of the villi in disseminated NTM disease may resemble Whipple disease on small intestinal biopsies [19]. Both the bacilli of *T.*

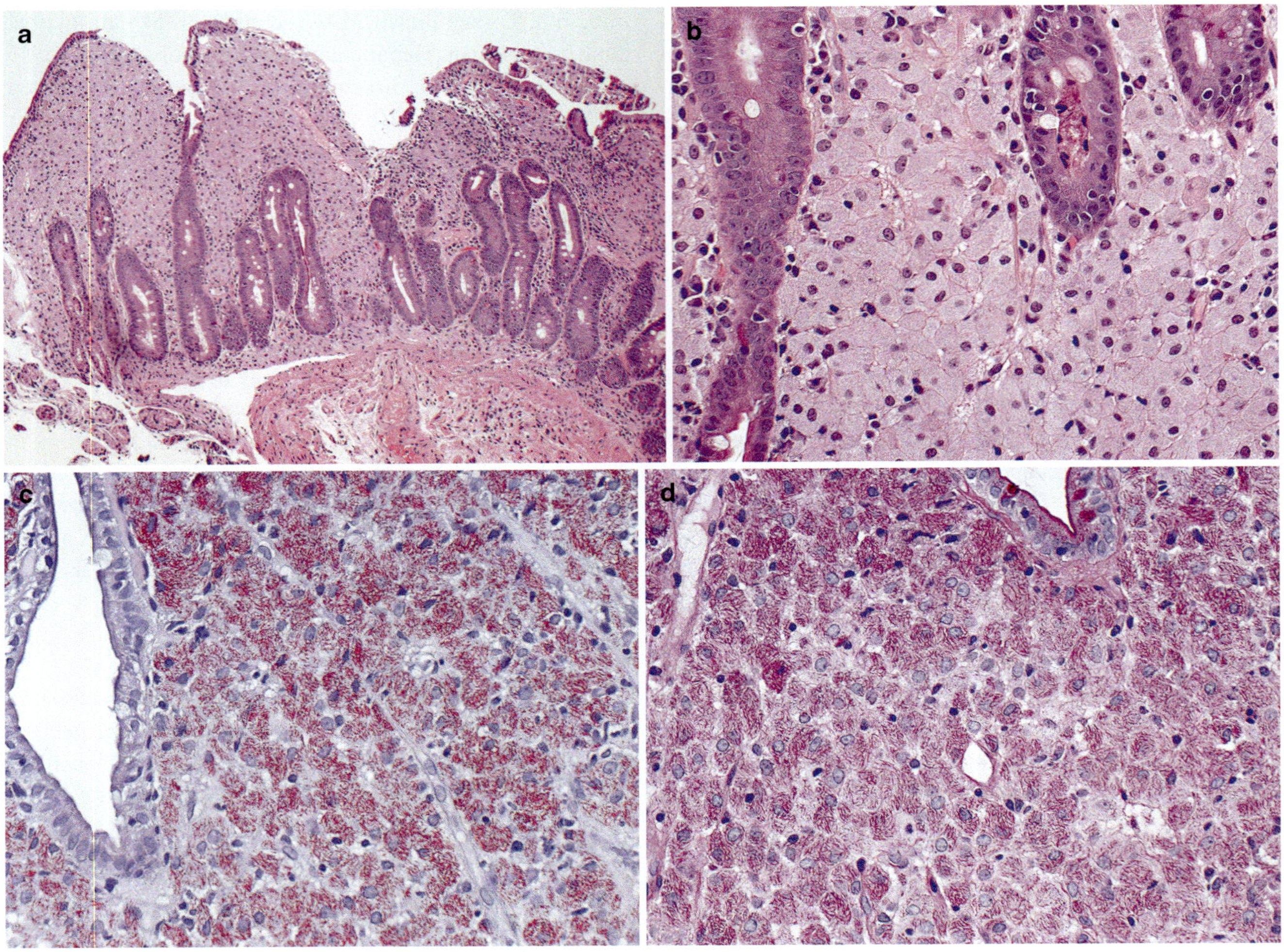

Fig. 11.5 Duodenal biopsy of an immunocompromised person with *Mycobacterium avium-intracellulare* involving the duodenum. (**a**) The villi are packed and swollen with large numbers of macrophages. (**b**) The macrophages contain foamy cytoplasm. (**c**) AFB stain demonstrates many AFB-positive mycobacteria filling the cytoplasm. (**d**) The mycobacteria also stain with PAS

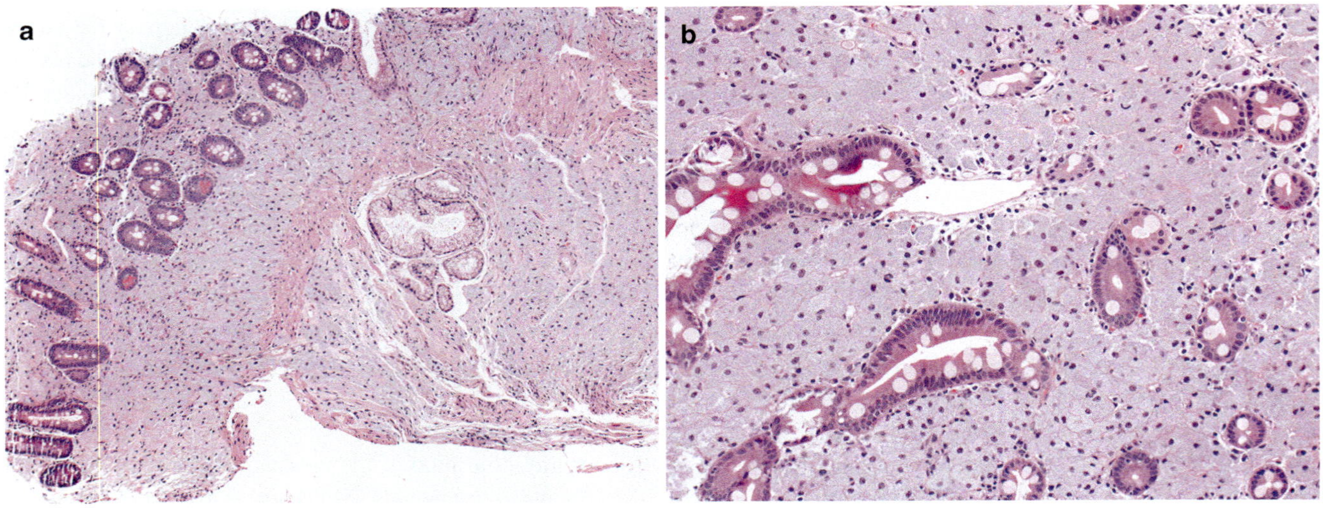

Fig. 11.6 Duodenal biopsy of an immunocompromised person with non-tuberculous mycobacterium *Mycobacterium genavense* involving the duodenum. (**a**) Large numbers of macrophages infiltrate into the submucosa. (**b**) The macrophages contain foamy cytoplasm. (**c**) AFB stain demonstrates that the macrophages are filled with AFB-positive organisms

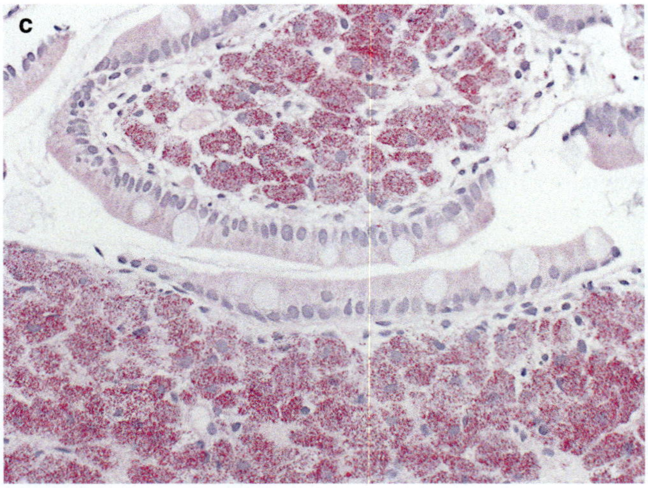

Fig. 11.6 (continued)

whipplei and mycobacteria stain positive with PAS. However, mycobacteria stain positive with acid-fast stains, while *T. whipplei* do not. Fungi also stain positive by GMS, but fungal hyphae are larger than mycobacteria (more than 1 μm in diameter) and may branch. Bacteria other than mycobacteria may also stain positive by GMS, but positive staining on acid-fast stains indicate mycobacteria rather than bacteria.

Treatment and Prognosis

Treatment regimens differ among different species of mycobacteria. Given the different treatment approaches to infections due to *M. tuberculosis*, MAC, or other NTM, it is vital to attempt to recover the organism by culture. Combination therapy is common, and treatment durations are months to years, due to the slow-growing nature of mycobacteria. The duration of therapy also depends upon recovery of immune function, immunocompromised state, and the extent of disease.

Fungal Diseases

Microsporidia

Definition

Microsporidia are obligate intracellular spore-forming fungi which infect a wide variety of cells throughout the human body. The most common clinical presentation of microsporidiosis is intestinal disease in severely immunocompromised persons due to *Enterocytozoon bieneusi* or *Encephalitozoon intestinalis*.

Clinical Features

Originally believed to be protozoan parasites, microsporidia are a complex group of unicellular fungi comprised of a variety of genera such as *Enterocytozoon*, *Encephalitozoon*, *Nosema*, and *Pleistophora*. Microsporidial species which are known to infect humans are very small in size and range from 1 to 5 μm in length. Microsporidia are also obligate parasites of a variety of animals, including insects, fish, reptiles, mammals, and birds. Microsporidial spores are ubiquitous in the environment. The spore is the infective form and survives well in the environment. Spores enter the human host through ingestion or inhalation. A coiled polar tubule present inside each spore everts once inside the host and injects its contents into the host cell, thereby infecting the cell. After maturation, the spores within the host cell burst out of the infected cell and proceed to infect neighboring cells. Pathogenesis, transmission, and life cycle of microsporidia are not fully understood.

Asymptomatic infection occurs in immunocompetent persons, while immunocompromised patients are usually symptomatic. The most common clinical presentation of microsporidiosis is intestinal disease leading to diarrhea, nausea, abdominal pain, and fever. Diarrhea can be chronic and severe in immunocompromised persons. The incidence of small intestinal microsporidiosis in HIV-infected patients has dramatically declined since the 1980s when AIDS was gaining in recognition [20]. The risk of intestinal microsporidiosis in HIV-infected patients rises when the CD4 cell count drops below 20 cells/μL [21]. Other immunocompromised states such as solid organ transplantation, chemotherapy, and immune suppression related to chronic diseases may also predispose to microsporidiosis. Microsporidia may disseminate from the intestinal tract to other areas of the body such as the brain and genitourinary and respiratory tracts

Detection of microsporidia as the cause of disease is difficult to ascertain by histopathology alone due to the very small size of the spores. Electron microscopy has historically been required for species-level identification of microsporidia; the number and arrangement of coils seen on electron micrographs differ among species. More recently, molecular techniques such as polymerase chain reaction (PCR) have been used to establish a diagnosis of microsporidiosis but are not widely used in clinical laboratories [22]. Microsporidia may also be detected in stool or other body fluid or tissue specimens with the use of special stains such as chromotrope 2R and modified trichrome.

Pathological Features

Villous atrophy is seen on small intestinal biopsies of intestinal microsporidiosis. A mild increase in macrophages, lymphocytes, and plasma cells may be seen in the lamina propria. Microsporidial spores are usually present within the apical portion of the enterocyte cytoplasm. However, some species can infect cells other than the enterocyte, such as endothelial cells and even fibroblasts. Most microsporidia that infect the intestinal tract are approximately 1 μm in size and are difficult to appreciate even on 1000× high-power magnification with oil immersion (Fig. 11.7a). Spores appear on H&E as small vacuoles in the human host cell cytoplasm, or they may appear as faintly basophilic granules within vacuoles. The spores stain strongly purple, or Gram-positive, with tissue Gram stains such as Brown-Brenn and Brown-Hopps (Fig. 11.7b, c). Spores also stain strongly with Warthin-Starry [23]. The polar tubule stains as a belt-like stripe on GMS and Ziehl-Neelsen acid-fast stains. On PAS, the spores may stain focally on one end. Under polarized light, the spores are birefringent.

Differential Diagnosis

Most microsporidial species which infect the intestinal tract are small (e.g., 1 μm) in size and are present within the apical portion of the enterocytes. Other microsporidial species which infect other areas of the body such as the respiratory tract or eye may be as large as 2–5 μm. These larger microsporidia may be mistaken for small yeasts such as *Histoplasma capsulatum*. However, in contrast to yeasts, microsporidia stain focally or weakly with GMS and do not bud. Additionally, the focal acid-fast-positive staining and birefringence of microsporidia differentiate them from small yeasts. Microsporidia must also be differentiated from enterochromaffin granules which are located basal to the nucleus in intestinal epithelial cells.

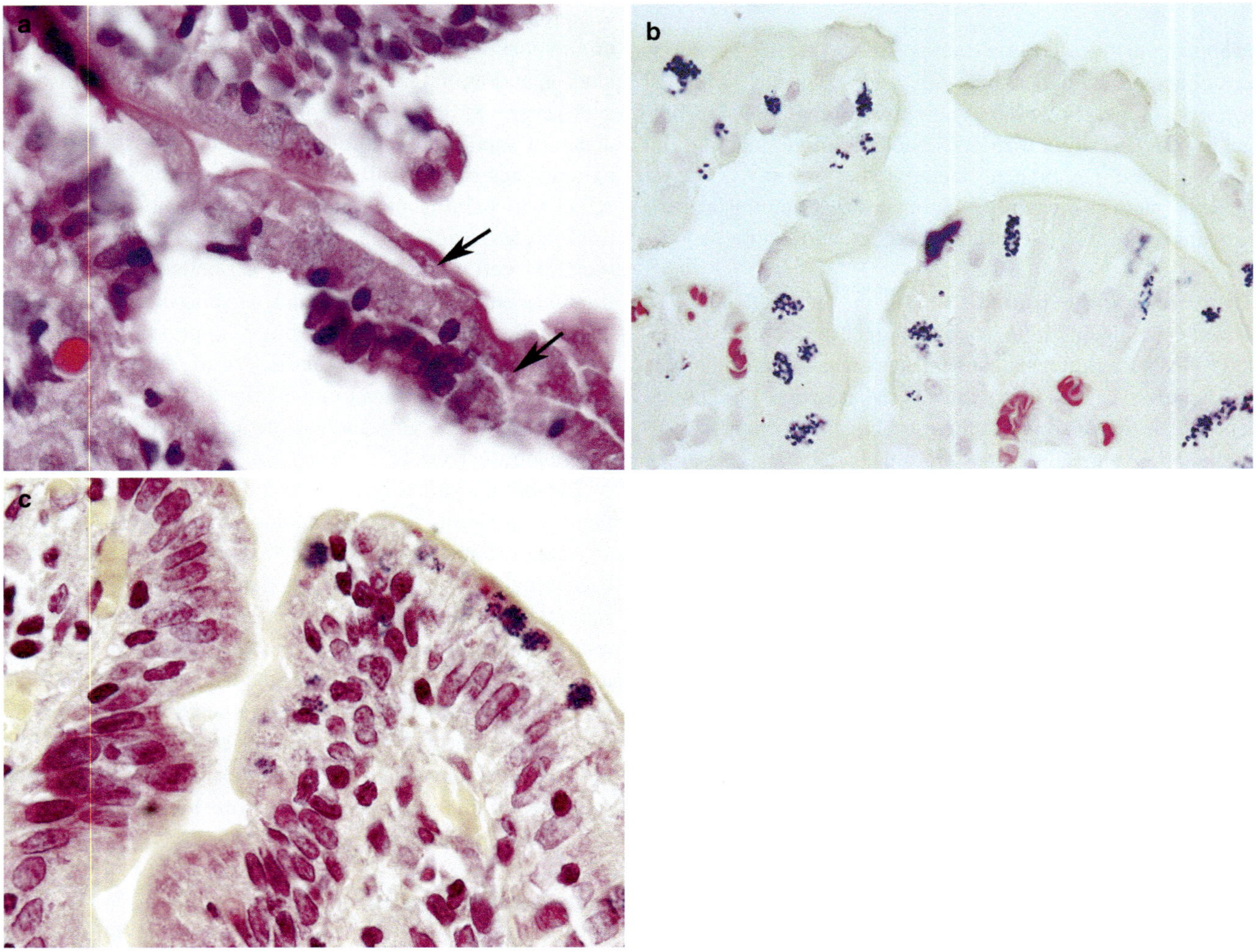

Fig. 11.7 Microsporidiosis of the small intestine. (**a**) Small intestinal mucosa with microsporidia appearing as vacuoles within apical ends of enterocytes (arrows). The microsporidia are very difficult to appreciate on H&E, even on oil immersion with 100× objective. (**b**) Brown-Brenn Gram stain demonstrates darkly staining microsporidia clustering within the apical ends of enterocytes. (**c**) Brown-Hopps Gram stain also demonstrates darkly staining microsporidia clustering within the apical ends of enterocytes

Treatment and Prognosis

Albendazole is the primary therapy for intestinal disease due to *E. intestinalis*. However, albendazole is not effective against *E. bieneusi* which also causes intestinal disease; in such cases, fumagillin is recommended [24]. Therefore, it is useful to obtain species-level identification via PCR in intestinal microsporidiosis in order to guide therapy.

Parasitic Diseases

Strongyloides

Definition

Strongyloidiasis is a multisystem disease due to the nematode *Strongyloides stercoralis*. Intestinal disease due to this parasite has become more widely recognized in recent years due to widespread use of immunosuppressive drugs in transplant or cancer patients who have developed disseminated disease [25].

Clinical Features

The roundworm *Strongyloides* is found in warm and wet soil in tropical and temperate areas. It is endemic in southern USA. The life cycle of *Strongyloides* is one of the most complicated of the nematode group. Exposure occurs when the infective filariform larvae penetrate the human skin and migrate directly either to the intestine or to the lungs through the venous circulation. The filariform larvae, which measure approximately 500–600 μm in length, may penetrate the pulmonary alveolar walls, ascend the trachea, and then reach the digestive tract after having been swallowed. The adult worm develops in the duodenum where it deposits up to 50 eggs daily [25]. The adult is a parthenogenetic female, in which reproduction occurs without fertilization of eggs. The eggs hatch within the mucosal lining of the small intestine into rhabditiform larvae which are noninfective. Rhabditiform larvae migrate into the intestinal lumen and are released into the external environment through feces. They develop within soil into filariform larvae or free-living adults within 24–36 hours; they can survive in moist soil for weeks [26]. Free-living adults produce filariform larvae. The entire period from penetration of the skin by filariform larvae to appearance of rhabditiform larvae in stool is approximately 2–4 weeks. In some cases, autoinfection may occur, during which rhabditiform larvae develop into infective filariform larvae before even leaving the body and penetrate the intestinal wall or perianal skin, leading to chronic disease that may last decades. Person-to-person transmission can also occur [27].

Although infection can occur in immunocompetent individuals, more severe and chronic disease is seen in immunocompromised individuals, such as organ transplant recipients, patients on long-term corticosteroid therapy, individuals with hematologic malignancies, and persons with human T-lymphotropic virus type 1 (HTLV-1) infection [28].

Infection due to *S. stercoralis* is usually asymptomatic in healthy individuals. Symptoms of chronic infection include abdominal discomfort, epigastric pain, diarrhea, and urticaria. Recurrent pruritic, migratory, and erythematous rashes may occur due to larval migration in the skin. Other chronic symptoms include weight loss, nausea and vomiting, weakness, and constipation. In immunocompromised hosts, wheezing and dyspnea may accompany migration of larvae through the lungs, known as Loeffler-like syndrome. In immunocompromised individuals or severely debilitated persons, complicated strongyloidiasis may occur in the form of autoinfection or hyperinfection. Hyperinfection occurs when very high numbers of filariform larvae penetrate the bowel wall and disseminate to the central nervous system or other organs.

On endoscopy, the mucosal surface of the bowel may be edematous. The bowel lumen may contain petechiae and small ulcerations. Diagnosis of strongyloidiasis is accomplished usually by microscopic analysis of stool, respiratory specimens, or occasionally duodenal aspirates for the presence of larvae. Stool or other specimens may be examined for the presence of rhabditiform or filariform larvae by microscopy or by culture on nutrient agar plates. Occasionally, repeat examinations of specimens are required for detection of organisms. Serology via enzyme immunoassay (EIA) may be performed; sensitivity ranges from 85–95% in patients with proven infection [29]. However, serology is limited by lower sensitivity in immunocompromised patients and cross-reactivity in patients with other nematode infections such as hookworm, *Ascaris* infection, and filariasis. Moderate peripheral eosinophilia of 10–25% may be seen in acute infections but is nonspecific. In cases of hyperinfection, enteric bacteria of the human intestine may accompany the filariform larvae as they penetrate the bowel wall and lead to bloodstream infection or meningitis, often with enteric Gram-negative rods or enterococci [30]. Molecular diagnostic assays are not widely used and are primarily only available at research institutions.

Pathological Features

The bowel wall may be edematous and congested in heavy infections. Chronic inflammation may be present. Granulomas may form when organisms are dead or dying. Larvae (approximately 180–380 μm in length) are the forms primarily seen in biopsies (Fig. 11.8a–d). However, eggs (30–40 μm in diameter) and adult forms (30–40 μm in diameter) may also be seen within the lamina propria (Fig. 11.9a, b). Larvae and adults may be seen in cross-section and stain

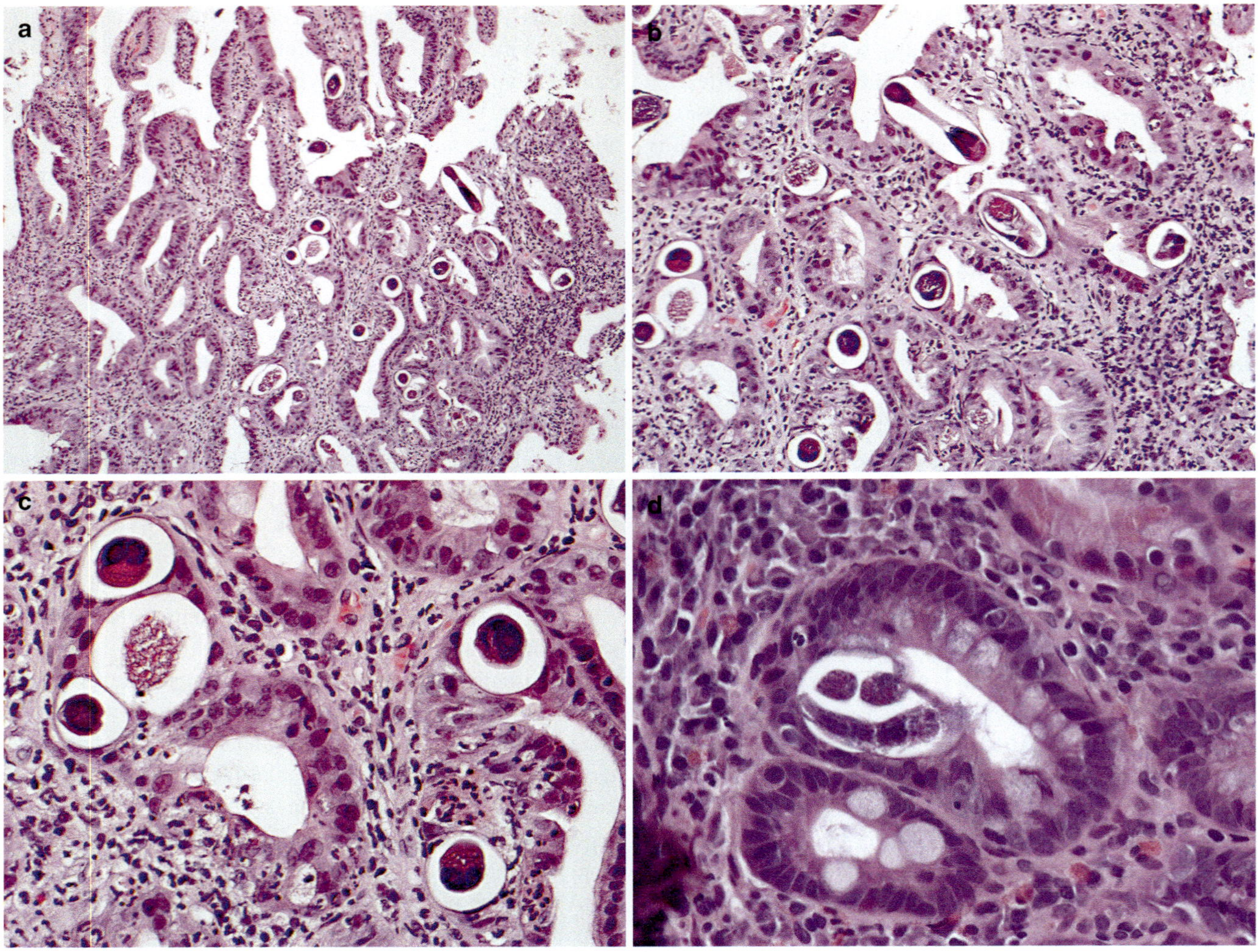

Fig. 11.8 Strongyloidiasis of the small intestine. (**a**, **b**) Multiple larvae are present throughout the duodenal mucosa. (**c**, **d**) Higher-power view of larvae

purple on H&E, with some stippling of the organism. Large numbers of larvae and eggs may be seen on biopsy in cases of hyperinfection.

Differential Diagnosis

Biopsies of most other intestinal nematode infections do not typically display larvae, eggs, and adults in the intestinal wall. The diagnosis is usually straightforward; however, strongyloidiasis should be differentiated from intestinal infection with the nematode *Capillaria philippinensis*, which is unusual in North America. Intestinal capillariasis presents with abdominal symptoms similar to strongyloidiasis. *C. philippinensis* eggs, larvae, and adult worms most commonly infect the jejunum in large numbers, and the various forms may appear morphologically similar to *Strongyloides* (Fig. 11.10a). Two features distinguish *C. philippinensis* from *S. stercoralis* on biopsy. First, the eggs of the former are peanut-shaped with flattened polar plugs and measure approximately 35–45 μm. Second, *C. philippinensis* possesses a stichosome (i.e., a longitudinal series of dark cells arranged in a row) which is lacking in *Strongyloides* [31] (Fig. 11.10b).

Treatment and Prognosis

If untreated, hyperinfection due to *Strongyloides* is fatal. Sepsis due to bacterial bloodstream infection is an independent predictor of shock and mortality in cases of disseminated infection [32]. Treatment is accomplished through ivermectin, and albendazole or mebendazole are alternative treatments. Multiple courses of therapy may be necessary in disseminated cases or in severely immunocompromised patients. In such cases, it is recommended to monitor response to therapy through the use of stool microscopy, sputum examination, or peripheral blood eosinophilia counts, as applicable [25].

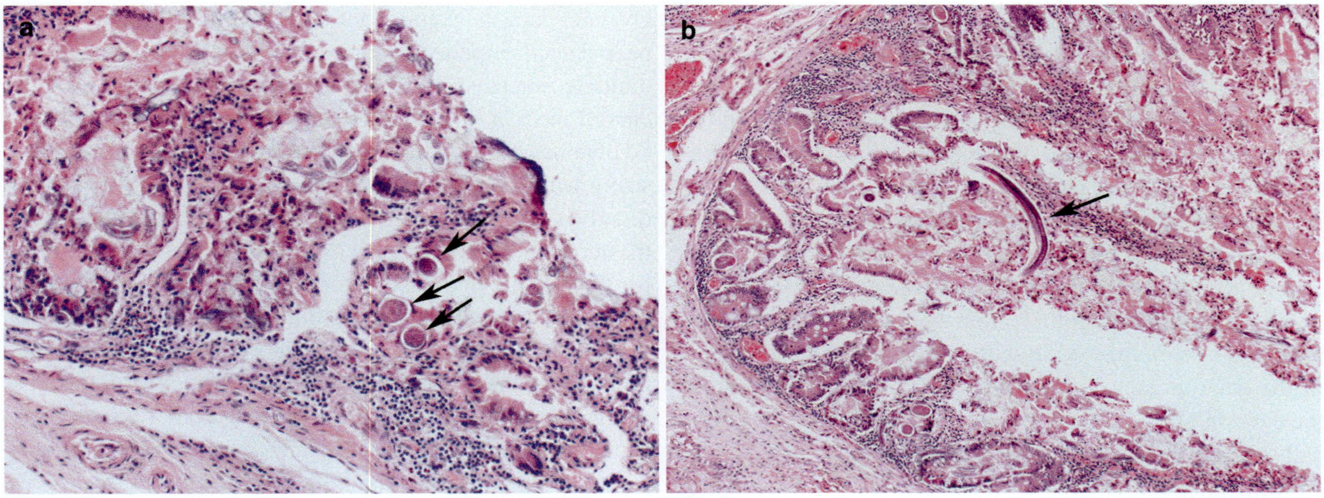

Fig. 11.9 Strongyloidiasis of the small intestine. (**a**) *Strongyloides* eggs (arrows) are noted in addition to larval forms. (**b**) An adult worm (arrow) is present in addition to larval forms

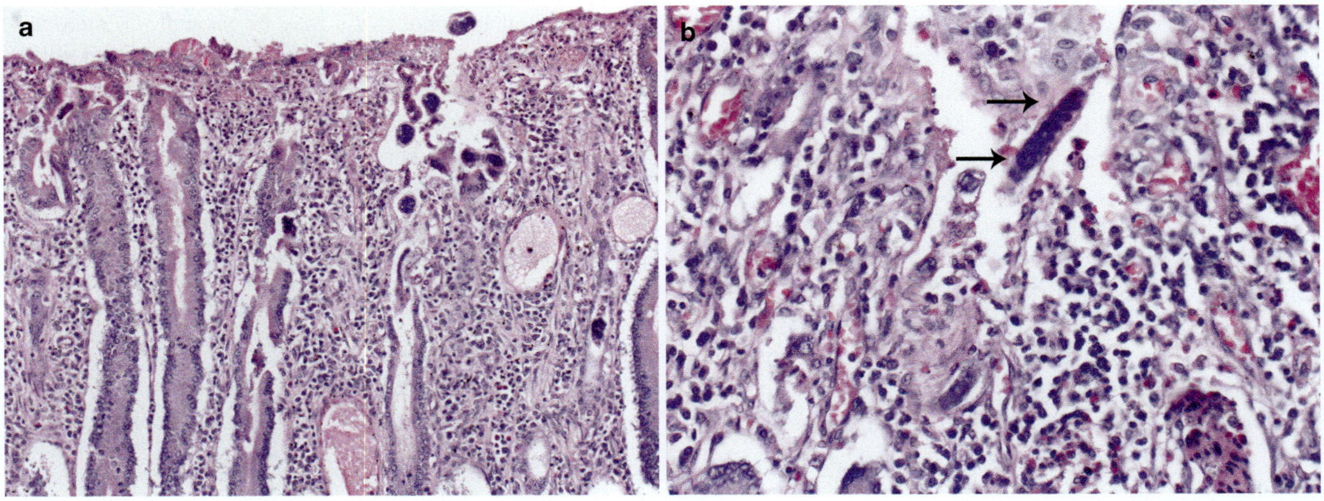

Fig. 11.10 Capillariasis of the small intestine. (**a**) *Capillaria* larvae within the small intestine resemble *Strongyloides*. (**b**) The stichosome (arrows) of *Capillaria* differentiates it from *Strongyloides* which does not contain a stichosome

Giardia

Definition

Giardiasis is a gastrointestinal infection due to the protozoan parasite *Giardia duodenalis*, also known as *Giardia intestinalis* and *Giardia lamblia*. *G. duodenalis* is the most common intestinal protozoan worldwide. The parasite is flagellated, and there are two morphologic forms of the parasite: cyst and trophozoite.

Clinical Features

The disease is cosmopolitan in nature, and the parasite is worldwide in distribution. Prevalence is higher in areas of poor sanitation and in institutional settings such as day cares in which children are not toilet-trained. Children are more often infected than adults, and disease is more common in warmer climates. The parasite is transmitted by the fecal-oral route through ingestion of cysts from the feces of an infected individual. Transmission may also occur through contaminated drinking water from unfiltered sources such as mountain streams, through swimming in bodies of contaminated water, and by consuming food which has been contaminated. Several wild and domestic animals such as beavers, cattle, dogs, and cats are possible reservoirs of *Giardia*. Outbreaks associated with recreational waters have been reported [33]. Disease has also been reported in campers who consume untreated waters from lakes or streams open to contamination from humans or animals. Anal intercourse may also be a mode of transmission for *Giardia* [34]. The chlorine- and disinfectant-resistant cysts of *Giardia* are hardy and survive for several months in cold water.

The incubation period for disease is 3–25 days, with a median period of 7–10 days. After being ingested, *Giardia* excysts in the small intestine and releases trophozoites. Each cyst releases two trophozoites. Trophozoites multiply in the lumen of the intestine and attach to the mucosa with a ventral sucking disk. The parasite causes disease by adhering to mucosa and interfering with absorption. Trophozoites may either encyst in the intestine or may be passed in the stool as free trophozoites. The cysts are infectious either when passed in stool or soon thereafter; therefore, person-to-person transmission may occur without the need for maturation in the environment. Trophozoites, which do not survive in the environment, are shed in watery diarrhea. Cysts are typically shed in stool that is not watery.

Clinical presentation of giardiasis is variable, ranging from asymptomatic carriage to severe diarrhea and malabsorption. Typical symptoms include nausea, malaise, and explosive and foul-smelling, watery diarrhea. However, chronic diarrhea may occur, with accompanying symptoms of steatorrhea, abdominal cramping, bloating, and flatulence, alternating with periods of diarrhea and constipation. Stools may be loose, pale, and greasy and may float on top of the water due to excess fats or air. Malabsorption and weight loss may occur due to loss of fat-soluble vitamins in severe cases.

On endoscopy, the small bowel may appear normal or flattened due to edema and villous blunting. Diagnosis is supported by stool studies which assess for the presence of *Giardia* cysts or trophozoites. Organisms may be shed intermittently in stool; therefore, multiple stool specimens should be collected over several days to rule out giardiasis. Up to seven stool specimens may be required for diagnosis. Ova and parasite examination of the stool shows the typical pear-shaped trophozoites or oval cysts, both of which have multiple nuclei, a longitudinal axoneme, and transverse curved median bodies. Duodenal material for analysis can be obtained by aspiration or peroral string test (i.e., a coiled string which is encapsulated; when swallowed, the capsule dissolves and the weighted string is carried by peristalsis to the duodenum). The string or aspirated contents are examined for the parasite in the laboratory. In addition to morphologic examination, stool may be submitted for antigenic studies by enzyme immunoassay or direct fluorescence. Serology has little role in the diagnosis of giardiasis. Multiplex molecular assays for stool which target *Giardia* and other microorganisms associated with diarrhea are commercially available and are promising tools for clinical laboratories [35].

Pathological Features

Villous blunting or flattening may be present. Lymphocytes and granulocytes may infiltrate the lamina propria. Mild intraepithelial lymphocytosis may be present. *G. duodenalis* trophozoites are found between normal or blunted villi in small intestinal biopsies (Fig. 11.11a, b). The organisms are small (10–20 μm) and can be mistaken for debris, especially if present in low numbers. The organisms may adhere to the mucosa and may appear crescent-like, oval, or pear-shaped (Fig. 11.11c). If the organisms are cut on ventral view, the paired nuclei of the trophozoites may occasionally be seen (Fig. 11.11d, e).

Differential Diagnosis

Histopathology via duodenal or small bowel biopsy is an uncommon method for routine diagnosis of giardiasis.

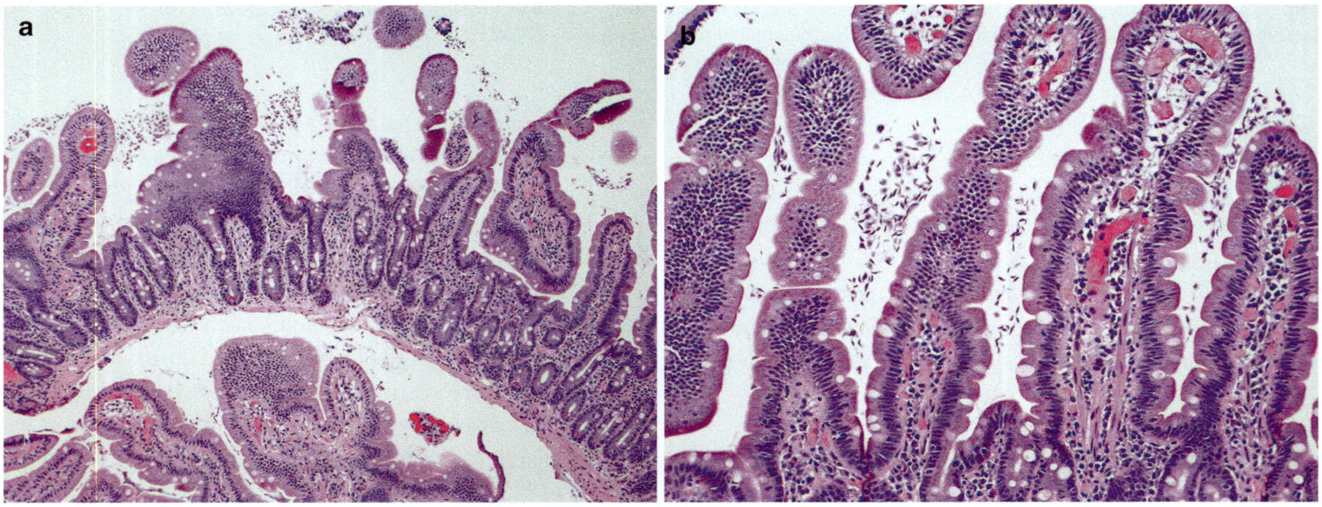

Fig. 11.11 Giardiasis of the small intestine. (**a**) Large numbers of *Giardia* organisms are seen between the villi. (**b**) Crescent-shaped *Giardia* organisms are seen between the villi. (**c**) On higher magnification, both crescent-shaped and pear-shaped forms of *Giardia* are seen. (**d**, **e**) On high magnification, the paired nuclei of the *Giardia* trophozoites are visible (arrows)

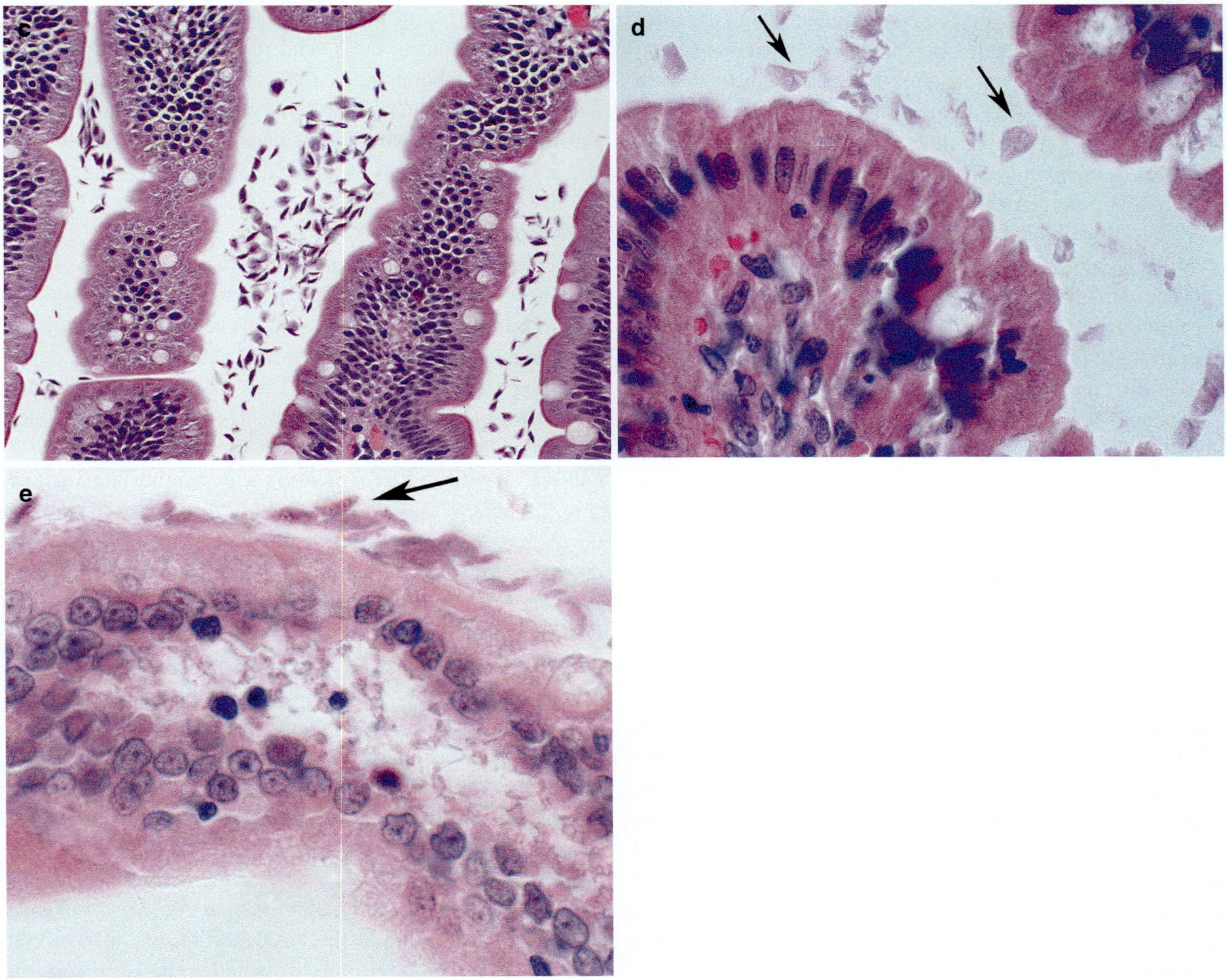

Fig. 11.11 (continued)

Biopsy is most often used in cases of chronic giardiasis, for which a broad, noninfectious clinical differential is possible such as celiac disease, irritable bowel syndrome, inflammatory bowel disease, or small bowel lymphoma. Bacterial, viral, and other parasitic causes of diarrhea should also be considered.

Giardia trophozoites are unlikely to be confused with other intestinal parasites, due to their size and location. *Cryptosporidium* are smaller (5 μm) and are present within the brush border. *Cystoisospora belli* are larger and oval in shape and are present within the cytoplasm of enterocytes. Microsporidia are much smaller in size (1–5 μm) and are intracytoplasmic within enterocytes.

Treatment and Prognosis

In chronic cases of giardiasis, symptoms may be recurrent and the disease is difficult to diagnose and treat. Acute diarrhea due to giardiasis may be self-limited at 2–4 weeks. Patient with HIV may have more severe and chronic cases of giardiasis. Drugs of choice are metronidazole or tinidazole. Nitazoxanide, paromomycin, and other antimicrobials have been used for treatment of severe, recurrent, or chronic cases [36].

Cyclospora

Definition

Cyclosporiasis is an infection of the small bowel due to the coccidian parasite *Cyclospora cayetanensis*.

Clinical Features

Cyclospora is endemic in many countries, particularly in tropical and subtropical areas of the world. Humans are the reservoirs of this parasite; there are no known animal reservoirs.

Transmission occurs by the fecal-oral route through ingestion of sporulated, infectious oocysts in contaminated drinking or swimming water, or by consumption of contaminated fruits or vegetables. Foodborne outbreaks have been associated with raspberries, basil, mesclun lettuce, and other fresh foods [37].

After an incubation period of 1 week, ingested oocysts excyst. Free sporozoites invade the epithelial cells of the small intestine and develop inside parasitophorous vacuoles within the cells into oocysts which are subsequently shed into the stool. The unsporulated oocysts of *Cyclospora* are not immediately infectious when shed in stool but require days to weeks in the environment to sporulate and become infectious. Thus, person-to-person transmission is unlikely. *Cyclospora* cysts are highly resistant to chlorination. Symptoms of cyclosporiasis consist of watery diarrhea, malaise, nausea, anorexia, abdominal cramps, and weight loss. Fever is uncommon. Symptoms may recur.

Various techniques may be used in the clinical microbiology laboratory to detect *Cyclospora* oocysts in stool. Laboratories may experience difficulty in detecting this organism by microscopy as it does not stain well with the trichrome stain typically used for the ova and parasite examination and is best seen with the modified acid-fast stain which is uncommonly used by laboratories for stool examination [38, 39]. Oocysts of *Cyclospora* may also be visualized under certain wavelengths of ultraviolet light due to their autofluorescent properties, but this technique is also infrequently used in clinical laboratories. Despite the fact that microscopy of stool is labor-intensive and requires a skilled technologist, it remains the recommended diagnostic method for *Cyclospora*. If *Cyclospora* is suspected on tissue biopsy, follow-up stool examinations should be performed. Clinicians should notify the laboratory if *Cyclospora* is on their differential, allowing the laboratory to utilize alternative methods of diagnosis mentioned above, or to send out the sample for testing at a reference laboratory, as applicable. Multiplex molecular assays for stool which target *Cyclospora* and other microorganisms associated with diarrhea are commercially available and are promising tools for clinical laboratories [40].

Pathological Features

Cyclospora primarily infects the jejunum. The microvilli may atrophy, shorten, and widen. Various inflammatory cell types infiltrate the lamina propria. Developing stages of the parasite may be seen within the host cell's cytoplasm at the apical end of the cell (Fig. 11.12a). The parasites measure approximately 8–10 μm. The parasites occupy parasitophorous vacuoles within epithelial cells near the tips of the villi and are surrounded by a clearing representing the vacuole (Fig. 11.12b). Within the vacuoles, varying stages of parasite development may be seen as spherical forms (i.e., gametocytes) or elongated forms (i.e., merozoites) (Fig. 11.12c, d).

Differential Diagnosis

Clinically, most cases of cyclosporiasis are diagnosed in travelers or from inhabitants of areas where this parasite is endemic. Due to clinical overlap of symptoms with other bacterial or parasitic causes of diarrhea, the differential diagnosis is broad.

Cystoisospora (formerly *Isospora*) *belli* are slightly larger in size (10–20 μm) than *Cyclospora*, but both parasites may appear morphologically similar in tissue sections. However, *Cyclospora* are more often found at the margin of the epithelial cell near the luminal border, while *Cystoisospora* are more often found at the basal portion of the host cell (Fig. 11.13). Cryptosporidia are smaller than *Cyclospora*, measuring approximately 4–6 μm. Cryptosporidia appear as

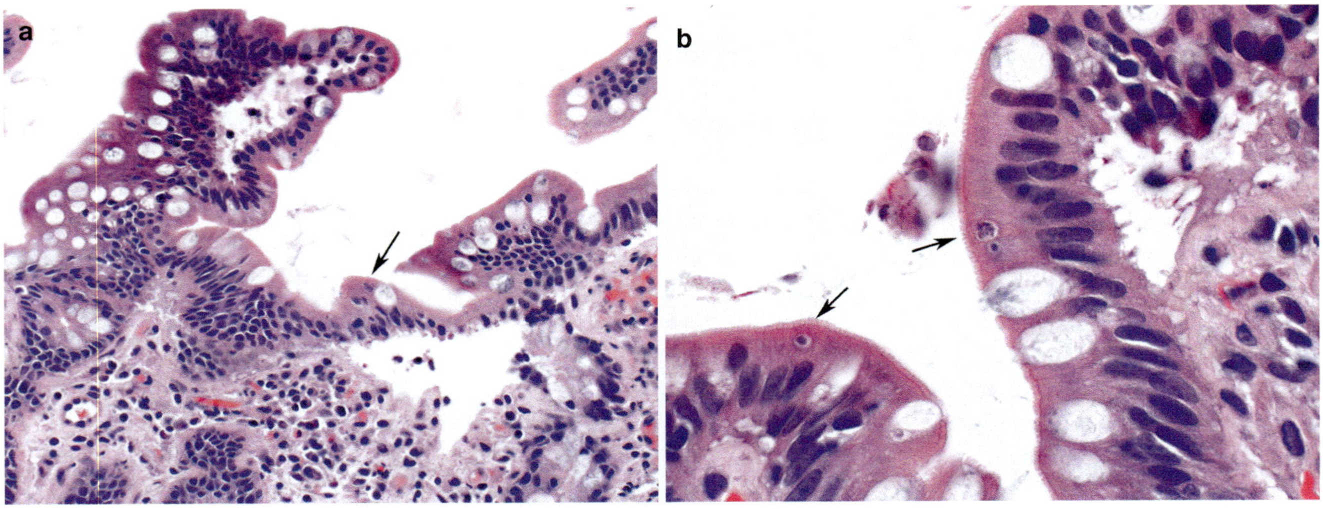

Fig. 11.12 Cyclosporiasis of the small intestine. (**a**) Several *Cyclospora* parasites seen (arrow) within vacuoles. (**b**) Several different forms of *Cyclospora* parasites (arrows) seen within the cytoplasm and surrounded by a clear vacuole at the apical ends of the enterocytes. (**c**) Elongated *Cyclospora* parasites seen within a cell (arrow). (**d**) Spherical *Cyclospora* parasites are present (arrows)

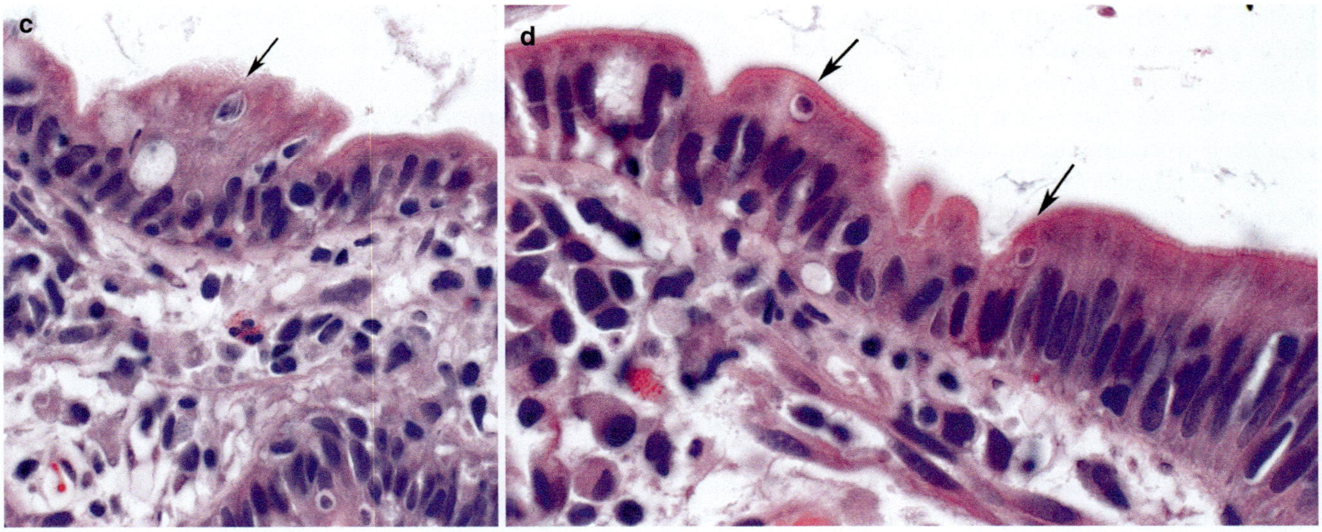

Fig. 11.12 (continued)

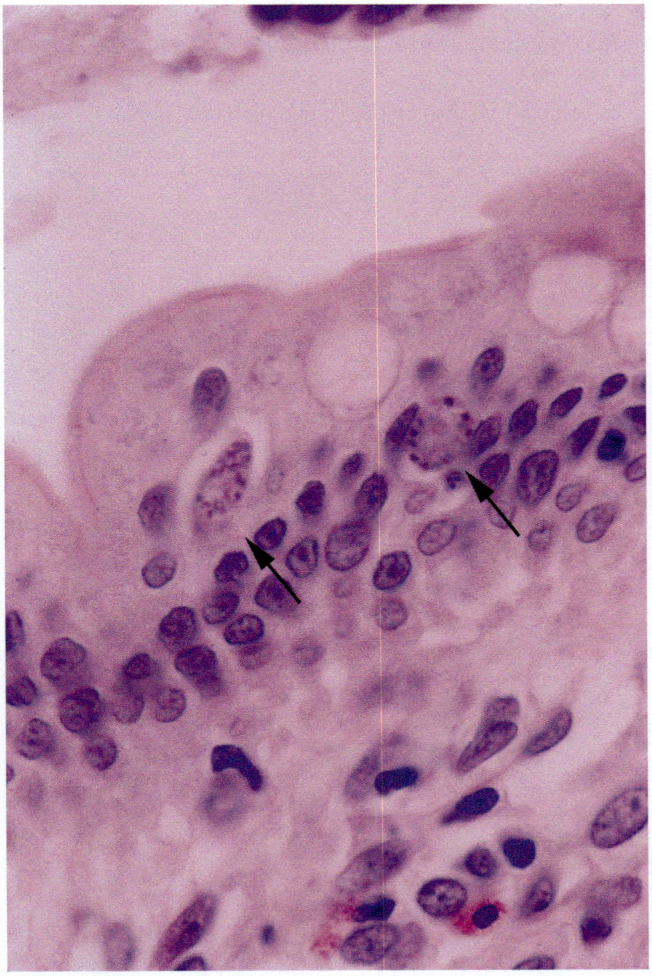

Fig. 11.13 Cystoisosporiasis of the small intestine. Several *Cystoisospora* parasites (arrows) seen at the basal portion of the host cell

small basophilic round objects which appear to line up in rows within the brush border of the epithelial cell surface. Despite this appearance, cryptosporidia are actually intracellular in location. Mucosal damage with atrophy of microvilli and inflammatory cell infiltrate within the lamina propria may be seen in infection due to any of the three organisms—*Cyclospora*, *Cystoisospora*, or *Cryptosporidium*.

Treatment and Prognosis

Treatment consists of a 7–10-day course of trimethoprim-sulfamethoxazole which is curative in the majority of cases. If sulfa drugs cannot be tolerated, patients may be offered ciprofloxacin, although such treatment is less successful. Nitazoxanide has also been explored as a treatment option [41]. Patients with HIV may require longer treatment courses. Patients may have a self-limited episode or suffer from a waxing and waning course of symptoms.

Cryptosporidium

Definition

Cryptosporidiosis is an infection of the small bowel due to the parasite *Cryptosporidium parvum* and *Cryptosporidium hominis*.

Clinical Features

Cryptosporidia infect humans and animals worldwide. In humans, *Cryptosporidium* causes sporadic outbreaks, usually waterborne in nature, or self-limited diarrhea in immunocompetent hosts. Immunocompromised patients, particularly HIV-infected individuals, may suffer from chronic illness. In developing countries, diarrhea due to cryptosporidiosis may lead to malnutrition in young children. *Cryptosporidium* may also infect mammals, reptiles, birds, and fish which may serve as reservoirs and transmission vehicles. Transmission may occur through contaminated drinking water, contaminated recreational water facilities and swimming pools, animal contact, or person-to-person contact among household members or close contacts. The largest outbreak in the USA occurred in 1993 in Milwaukee, Wisconsin, during which over 400,000 people were sickened due to contamination of a public water supply [42].

Transmission occurs through ingestion of the infective oocyst. After excystation, sporozoites are released and invade the epithelial cells of the small intestine. The parasites multiply in the intestinal tract, releasing oocysts which are then excreted in the host's stool. Structural alterations in the intestinal epithelium and inflammatory mediators released in response to the presence of the parasites lead to an osmotic diarrhea [43]. As opposed to the oocysts of *Cyclospora*, cysts of *Cryptosporidium* are immediately infectious. Therefore, person-to-person transmission can occur, as can autoinfection. Although *Cryptosporidium* is resistant to chemical disinfectants, water filters which remove particles 0.1–1.0 μm in size are effective.

After an incubation period of an average of 1 week (range 1–12 days), symptoms such as watery diarrhea, dehydration, abdominal pain, fever, nausea, and vomiting may occur. Weight loss is common in severe cases. Cryptosporidia may also invade other areas of the body such as other areas of the gastrointestinal tract, pulmonary tract, and conjunctiva.

Various techniques may be used in the clinical microbiology laboratory to detect *Cryptosporidium* oocysts. *Cryptosporidium* does not stain well with the trichrome stain typically used for the ova and parasite examination and may be confused with yeasts [43]. Other diagnostic platforms may also be used to diagnose *Cryptosporidium* in stool, such as direct fluorescent antigen tests or EIA. Multiplex molecular assays for stool which target *Cryptosporidium* and other microorganisms associated with diarrhea are commercially available and are promising tools for clinical laboratories [40].

Pathological Features

Microvilli of the small intestine may atrophy, shorten, and widen. The jejunum is typically the most heavily infected site of the small intestine. Inflammatory cells of various types infiltrate the lamina propria (Fig. 11.14a). *Cryptosporidium* oocysts appear as small basophilic round objects lining up in rows within the brush border of the epithelial cell surface (Fig. 11.14b, c). Despite the appearance of being extracellular in location, cryptosporidia are actually intracellular but

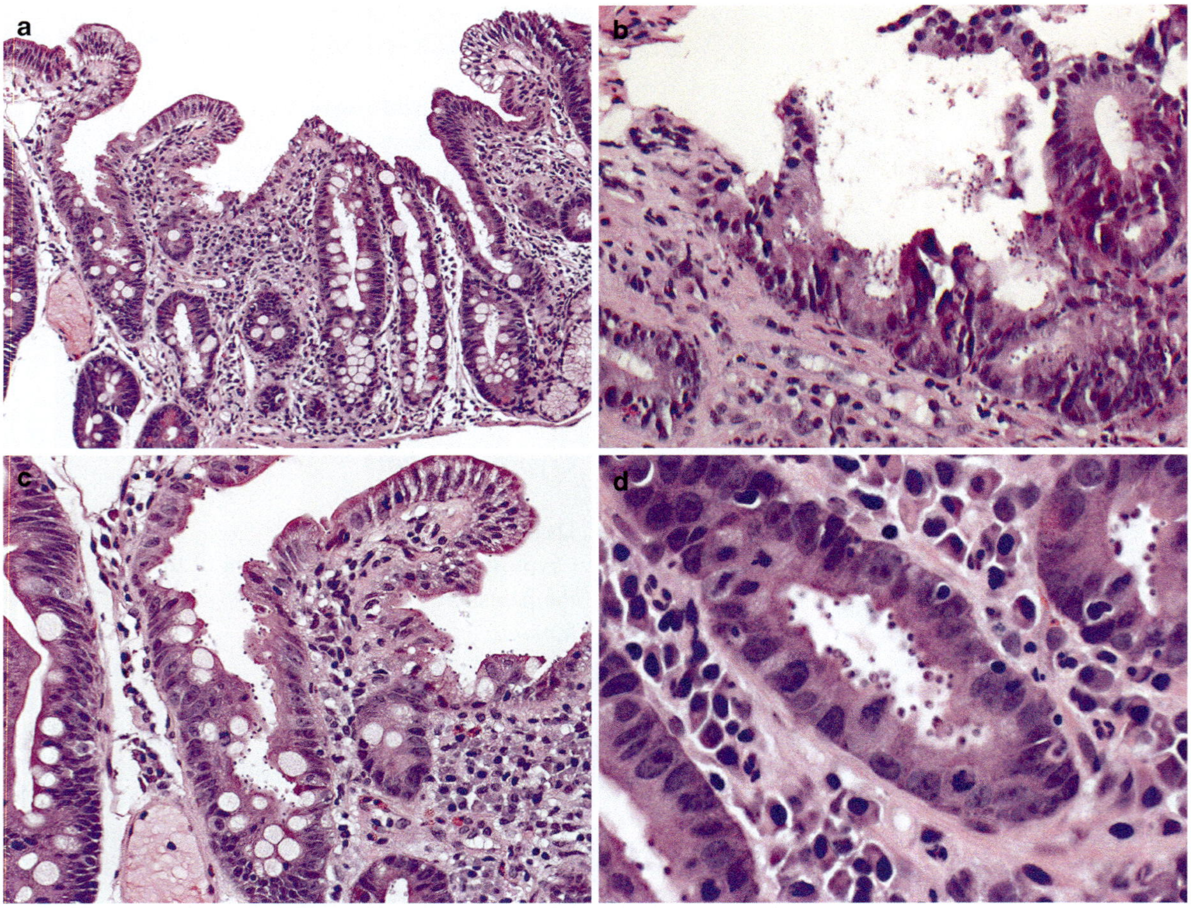

Fig. 11.14 Cryptosporidiosis of the small intestine. (**a**) Small intestinal mucosa with inflammatory cell infiltrate in lamina propria. Numerous *Cryptosporidium* parasites appear to line up on the luminal edge of epithelial cells. (**b, c**) High-power view of numerous basophilic, spherical *Cryptosporidium* parasites. (**d**) Numerous *Cryptosporidium* parasites in various stages of development are seen

extracytoplasmic. The organisms measure approximately 4–6 μm and are typically in various stages of development when examined closely (Fig. 11.14d).

Differential Diagnosis

Due to clinical overlap of symptoms with other bacterial or parasitic causes of diarrhea, differential diagnosis is broad.

Cyclospora, *Cystoisospora belli*, and *Cryptosporidium* all cause similar disease in the small intestine and may be seen on biopsy. Cryptosporidia are the smallest of the three at 4–6 μm. *Cyclospora* are the next largest in size at 8–10 μm. *Cyclospora* parasites are found within vacuoles at the apical margin of the epithelial cells but appear deeper in the cytoplasm than the intracellular but extracytoplasmic *Cryptosporidium*. Additionally, *Cyclospora* parasites can appear as elongated merozoite forms, as compared to the spherical shape of *Cryptosporidium*. *Cystoisospora* is the largest of the three at 10–20 μm and is more often found at the basal portion of the host cell (Fig. 11.13). Mucosal damage with atrophy of microvilli and inflammatory cell infiltrate within the lamina propria may be seen with any of the three organisms—*Cyclospora*, *Cystoisospora*, or *Cryptosporidium*.

Treatment and Prognosis

Cryptosporidiosis in immunocompetent hosts is usually self-limited and treated symptomatically. Nitazoxanide has been used with some success in patients without HIV. Antiretroviral therapy with control of viral load is the most effective way to control the symptoms of cryptosporidiosis in HIV patients. Diarrhea usually lasts 10–24 days if untreated in the immunocompetent host. In the immunocompromised host, symptoms may last months.

Anisakis

Definition

Anisakiasis is due to tissue invasion by larvae of the nematodes *Anisakis simplex* (and other *Anisakis* species) or *Pseudoterranova decipiens*. The parasite may attach and invade the small intestine or stomach, leading to symptoms.

Clinical Features

The disease occurs in individuals who eat undercooked or uncooked saltwater fish or squid. Most cases have been reported from Japan due to consumption of sushi and sashimi, Scandinavian countries due to consumption of gravlax, Latin America due to consumption of ceviche, the Netherlands due to consumption of herring, and Spain due to consumption of anchovies. Fish most commonly infected with anisakid larvae include mackerel, haddock, herring, cold, halibut, rockfish, and pollock. Reservoirs of *Anisakis* are saltwater fish and sea mammals. Humans are infected after eating larvae but are dead-end hosts and cannot further transmit the parasite. Hence, there is no human-to-human transmission. Marine mammals excrete eggs which hatch in the water into larvae which are then ingested by crustaceans. Fish and squid ingest infected crustaceans; larvae then migrate to the muscle tissues of the fish and squid. Finally, marine mammals ingest infected fish and squid, completing the life cycle.

Gastric symptoms of abdominal pain, nausea, and vomiting occur within several hours after ingestion of undercooked fish or squid. Larvae invade the gastric mucosa. Hematemesis may also occur. The parasite dies and resulting inflammation or tissue response may lead to a mass in the esophagus, stomach, or intestine. Some people complain of a tingling sensation when eating raw or undercooked fish or squid; this sensation is said to be the worm moving in the mouth and throat. Anisakiasis is associated with a strong allergic response with manifestations ranging from urticaria after consumption to anaphylaxis [44]. Small intestinal symptoms may occur due to inflammatory reactions around worms and usually develop within a few days or weeks after ingestion.

Diagnosis is made most commonly by endoscopy. The worm may be coiled and embedded in the gastric mucosa. Infection of the small bowel may reveal thickening, mucosal edema, and luminal narrowing on endoscopy. *A. simplex* larvae are white in color and 19 to 36 mm in length. *P. decipiens* larvae are yellow-brown in color, 20 to 25 mm in length, and slightly wider than *A. simplex*. In order to definitively identify the type of anisakid larvae, the worm should be sent to the microbiology laboratory for identification. Peripheral eosinophilia is seen more commonly with gastric anisakiasis than intestinal anisakiasis [45]. Serology may be performed, but cross-reactivity occurs with other nematodes such as *Toxocara canis* [45].

Pathological Features

Any portion of the intestine may be invaded by anisakids, but the terminal ileum is the most common. Anisakid larvae produce a strong eosinophilic reaction around the parasite (Fig. 11.15a). Abscesses may develop around dead and dying worms. Over time, granulomatous lesions may replace the abscesses, and the degenerating worm may be difficult to identify. On transverse section, *Anisakis* spp. have lateral Y-shaped cords (Fig. 11.15b) with narrow bases. The lateral chords of *Pseudoterranova* sp. have a broader base and are more compact in appearance.

Differential Diagnosis

When the worm is removed from the body by endoscopy, morphologic features combined with clinical presentation are usually adequate for diagnosis. Grossly, the worms may be confused with *Ascaris*, but *Ascaris* is usually larger in size (15–35 cm in length).

Treatment and Prognosis

Endoscopic removal of the parasite is diagnostic and therapeutic. Albendazole may be used if surgical or endoscopic therapy is not attempted.

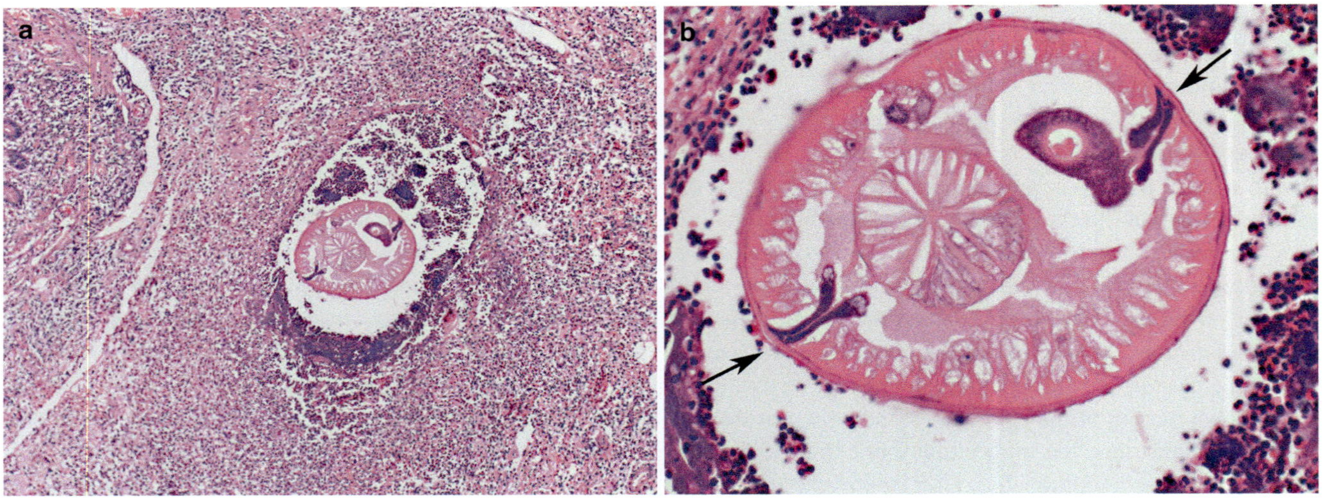

Fig. 11.15 Anisakiasis of the small intestine. (**a**) *Anisakis* larva in small intestine surrounded by dense inflammatory infiltrate composed of many eosinophils and other mixed inflammatory cells. (**b**) *Anisakis* larva demonstrating lateral Y-shaped chords (arrows)

Angiostrongylus costaricensis

Definition

Angiostrongylus costaricensis is a nematode which causes enteritis in humans, primarily in children.

Clinical Features

Angiostrongyliasis is a zoonotic disease caused by the nematode *Angiostrongylus*. Rodents such as rats are the natural hosts for *Angiostrongylus*. Snails and slugs are the intermediate hosts. Humans become infected after ingesting infected snails or slugs or after consuming raw vegetables contaminated with slugs or mollusk secretions (i.e., slime). Larvae ingested by humans develop in the intestine into adult worms which release eggs. The eggs and larvae degenerate and cause intense local inflammatory reactions. The incubation period before symptoms appear is usually 2–4 weeks.

Children between the ages of 6 and 12 are most commonly infected [46]. Most infections have been reported from Central and South America, and it is unclear whether transmission occurs outside of the Caribbean and the Americas [47].

Abdominal pain, fever, anorexia, vomiting, constipation, and diarrhea are common complaints. Abdominal tenderness and the presence of a mass in the right lower quadrant of the abdomen, right flank, or iliac fossa may be seen in children. Intestinal obstruction and perforation may occur in severe cases. Adult worms and eggs present in the mesenteric arteries may lead to inflammation and thrombosis of vessels, leading to abdominal pain and discomfort. Involvement of liver has also been reported [48].

Eggs and larvae are not shed in the stool of humans. Therefore, diagnosis is usually made on a clinical basis in concert with histopathologic appearance on biopsy or via resection specimen. Diagnosis is usually obtained through laparotomy and surgical resection of affected tissue, rather than endoscopically, due to disease presentation as a mass. Peripheral leukocytosis is common, and eosinophilia is typically above 20% [49]. Molecular diagnosis is not readily available.

Pathological Features

The intestinal wall may appear thickened and hardened, and yellow granules may be apparent on the subserosa. The appendix, distal small bowel, or colon may be involved. Histologically, the mass comprises adult worms (Fig. 11.16a) or eggs surrounded by large numbers of eosinophils. Granulomatous reaction to the worms or eggs is pronounced (Fig. 11.16b, c). Adult worms may be found in the small arteries of the ileocecal area, with surrounding eosinophils. Adult worms are large, measuring 40 to 45 mm in length. Eggs and larvae may also be found in lymph nodes, intestinal wall, and the omentum. Eggs in tissue are thin-walled and approximately 65 μm by 50 μm (Fig. 11.16d).

Differential Diagnosis

When angiostrongyliasis presents as an intestinal mass, the clinical differential diagnosis is broad and includes malignant tumors, appendicitis, inflammatory bowel disease or Meckel diverticulum. The clinical presentation of an inflammatory mass and presence of adult worms and eggs within the mesenteric arteries is distinctive for this parasite.

Treatment and Prognosis

Thiabendazole, albendazole, and diethylcarbamazine may be effective. However, intestinal angiostrongyliasis usually

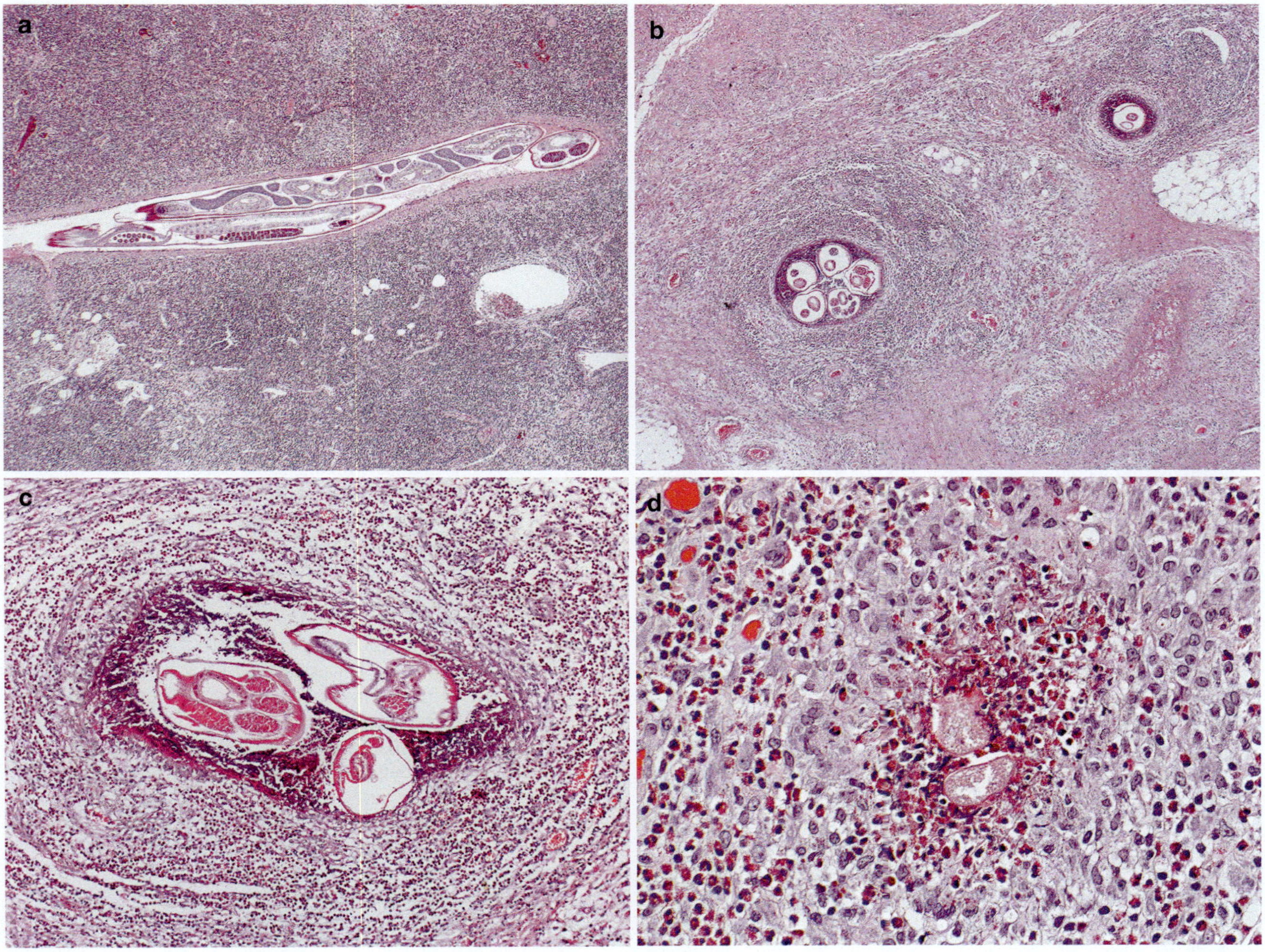

Fig. 11.16 Angiostrongyliasis of the small intestine. (**a**) Adult *Angiostrongylus costaricensis* worm in cross-section with dense surrounding inflammation. (**b**) Adult *A. costaricensis* worms with surrounding granulomatous inflammation in bowel wall. (**c**) Partially degraded adult *A. costaricensis* worms surrounded by dense eosinophilic infiltrate within bowel wall. (**d**) Thin-walled eggs of *A. costaricensis* with surrounding eosinophils and granulomatous inflammation

resolves without treatment in a few weeks to months. A surgical approach to treatment is common when lesions are large or infection is heavy.

References

1. Han G, Niu H, Zhao S, Zhu B, Wang C, Liu Y, et al. Identification and typing of respiratory adenoviruses in Guangzhou, Southern China using a rapid and simple method. Virol Sin. 2013;28(2):103–8. https://doi.org/10.1007/s12250-013-3308-7.
2. Pinchoff RJ, Kaufman SS, Magid MS, Erdman DD, Gondolesi GE, Mendelson MH, et al. Adenovirus infection in pediatric small bowel transplantation recipients. Transplantation. 2003;76(1):183–9. https://doi.org/10.1097/01.TP.0000072808.93060.0F.
3. Robin M, Marque-Juillet S, Scieux C, Peffault de Latour R, Ferry C, Rocha V, et al. Disseminated adenovirus infections after allogeneic hematopoietic stem cell transplantation: incidence, risk factors and outcome. Haematologica. 2007;92(9):1254–7.
4. McLaughlin GE, Delis S, Kashimawo L, Cantwell GP, Mittal N, Cirocco RE, et al. Adenovirus infection in pediatric liver and intestinal transplant recipients: utility of DNA detection by PCR. Am J Transplant. 2003;3(2):224–8.
5. Fox JP, Hall CE, Cooney MK. The Seattle virus watch. VII. observations of adenovirus infections. Am J Epidemiol. 1977;105(4):362–86.
6. Lion T. Adenovirus infections in immunocompetent and immunocompromised patients. Clin Microbiol Rev. 2014;27(3):441–62. https://doi.org/10.1128/cmr.00116-13.
7. Biagi F, Balduzzi D, Delvino P, Schiepatti A, Klersy C, Corazza GR. Prevalence of Whipple's disease in north-western Italy. Eur J Clin Microbiol Infect Dis. 2015;34(7):1347–8. https://doi.org/10.1007/s10096-015-2357-2.
8. Dolmans RA, Boel CH, Lacle MM, Kusters JG. Clinical manifestations, treatment, and diagnosis of Tropheryma whipplei infections. Clin Microbiol Rev. 2017;30(2):529–55. https://doi.org/10.1128/cmr.00033-16.
9. Grasman ME, Pettersson AM, Catsburg A, Koek AG, van Bodegraven AA, Savelkoul PH. Tropheryma whipplei, a potential commensal detected in individuals undergoing routine colonoscopy.

J Clin Microbiol. 2015;53(12):3919–21. https://doi.org/10.1128/jcm.02630-15.
10. Gunther U, Moos V, Offenmuller G, Oelkers G, Heise W, Moter A, et al. Gastrointestinal diagnosis of classical Whipple disease: clinical, endoscopic, and histopathologic features in 191 patients. Medicine. 2015;94(15):e714. https://doi.org/10.1097/md.0000000000000714.
11. Dobbins WO. Whipple's disease. In: Connor DH, Chandler FW, Schwartz DA, Manz HJ, Lack EE, editors. Pathology of infectious diseases. Stamford: Appleton & Lange; 1997. p. 897–903.
12. Fenollar F, Puechal X, Raoult D. Whipple's disease. N Engl J Med. 2007;356(1):55–66. https://doi.org/10.1056/NEJMra062477.
13. Reed C, von Reyn CF, Chamblee S, Ellerbrock TV, Johnson JW, Marsh BJ, et al. Environmental risk factors for infection with *Mycobacterium avium* complex. Am J Epidemiol. 2006;164(1):32–40. https://doi.org/10.1093/aje/kwj159.
14. Karakousis PC, Moore RD, Chaisson RE. *Mycobacterium avium* complex in patients with HIV infection in the era of highly active antiretroviral therapy. Lancet Infect Dis. 2004;4(9):557–65. https://doi.org/10.1016/s1473-3099(04)01130-2.
15. Santos M, Gil-Brusola A, Escandell A, Blanes M, Gobernado M. Mycobacterium genavense infections in a tertiary hospital and reviewed cases in non-HIV patients. Patholog Res Int. 2014;2014:371370. https://doi.org/10.1155/2014/371370.
16. Yamazaki R, Mori T, Nakazato T, Aisa Y, Imaeda H, Hisamatsu T, et al. Non-tuberculous mycobacterial infection localized in small intestine developing after allogeneic bone marrow transplantation. Intern Med (Tokyo, Japan). 2010;49(12):1191–3.
17. Mohar SM, Saeed S, Ramcharan A, Depaz H. Small bowel obstruction due to mesenteric abscess caused by *Mycobacterium avium* complex in an HIV patient: a case report and literature review. J Surg Case Rep. 2017;2017(7):rjx129. https://doi.org/10.1093/jscr/rjx129.
18. Cappell MS, Gupta A. Gastrointestinal hemorrhage due to gastrointestinal *Mycobacterium avium* intracellulare or esophageal candidiasis in patients with the acquired immunodeficiency syndrome. Am J Gastroenterol. 1992;87(2):224–9.
19. Roth RI, Owen RL, Keren DF, Volberding PA. Intestinal infection with *Mycobacterium avium* in acquired immune deficiency syndrome (AIDS). Histological and clinical comparison with Whipple's disease. Dig Dis Sci. 1985;30(5):497–504.
20. Field AS, Hing MC, Milliken ST, Marriott DJ. Microsporidia in the small intestine of HIV-infected patients. A new diagnostic technique and a new species. Med J Aust. 1993;158(6):390–4.
21. Dore GJ, Marriott DJ, Hing MC, Harkness JL, Field AS. Disseminated microsporidiosis due to Septata intestinalis in nine patients infected with the human immunodeficiency virus: response to therapy with albendazole. Clin Infect Dis. 1995;21(1):70–6.
22. Ghosh K, Weiss LM. Molecular diagnostic tests for microsporidia. Interdiscip Perspect Infect Dis. 2009;2009:926521. https://doi.org/10.1155/2009/926521.
23. Field AS, Milner DA Jr. Intestinal microsporidiosis. Clin Lab Med. 2015;35(2):445–59. https://doi.org/10.1016/j.cll.2015.02.011.
24. Molina JM, Tourneur M, Sarfati C, Chevret S, de Gouvello A, Gobert JG, et al. Fumagillin treatment of intestinal microsporidiosis. N Engl J Med. 2002;346(25):1963–9. https://doi.org/10.1056/NEJMoa012924.
25. Jourdan PM, Lamberton PHL, Fenwick A, Addiss DG. Soil-transmitted helminth infections. Lancet (London, England). 2017. https://doi.org/10.1016/s0140-6736(17)31930-x.
26. Baek BK, Islam MK, Matsuda K. Viability of eggs, filariform larvae and adults of Strongyloides venezuelensis (Nematoda: Strongyloidea) maintained in vitro. Korean J Parasitol. 1998;36(2):99–107.
27. Czachor JS, Jonas AP. Transmission of Strongyloides steracolis person to person. J Travel Med. 2000;7(4):211–2.
28. Izquierdo I, Briones J, Lluch R, Arqueros C, Martino R. Fatal strongyloides hyperinfection complicating a gram-negative sepsis after allogeneic stem cell transplantation: a case report and review of the literature. Case Rep Hematol. 2013;2013:860976. https://doi.org/10.1155/2013/860976.
29. Loutfy MR, Wilson M, Keystone JS, Kain KC. Serology and eosinophil count in the diagnosis and management of strongyloidiasis in a non-endemic area. Am J Trop Med Hyg. 2002;66(6):749–52.
30. Abu Omar M, Abu Ghanimeh M, Kim S, Howell G. Strongyloides hyperinfection syndrome and VRE pneumonia. BMJ Case Rep. 2017;2017. https://doi.org/10.1136/bcr-2016-216634.
31. Cross JH. Intestinal capillariasis. Clin Microbiol Rev. 1992;5(2):120–9.
32. Geri G, Rabbat A, Mayaux J, Zafrani L, Chalumeau-Lemoine L, Guidet B, et al. *Strongyloides stercoralis* hyperinfection syndrome: a case series and a review of the literature. Infection. 2015;43(6):691–8. https://doi.org/10.1007/s15010-015-0799-1.
33. McClung RP, Roth DM, Vigar M, Roberts VA, Kahler AM, Cooley LA, et al. Waterborne disease outbreaks associated with environmental and undetermined exposures to water—United States, 2013–2014. MMWR Morb Mortal Wkly Rep. 2017;66(44):1222–5. https://doi.org/10.15585/mmwr.mm6644a4.
34. Pakianathan MR, McMillan A. Intestinal protozoa in homosexual men in Edinburgh. Int J STD AIDS. 1999;10(12):780–4.
35. Parcina M, Reiter-Owona I, Mockenhaupt FP, Vojvoda V, Gahutu JB, Hoerauf A, et al. Highly sensitive and specific detection of Giardia duodenalis, Entamoeba histolytica, and Cryptosporidium spp. in human stool samples by the BD MAX Enteric Parasite Panel. Parasitol Res. 2018;117(2):447–51. https://doi.org/10.1007/s00436-017-5720-7.
36. Escobedo AA, Cimerman S. Giardiasis: a pharmacotherapy review. Expert Opin Pharmacother. 2007;8(12):1885–902. https://doi.org/10.1517/14656566.8.12.1885.
37. Ortega YR, Sanchez R. Update on Cyclospora cayetanensis, a food-borne and waterborne parasite. Clin Microbiol Rev. 2010;23(1):218–34. https://doi.org/10.1128/cmr.00026-09.
38. Visvesvara GS, Moura H, Kovacs-Nace E, Wallace S, Eberhard ML. Uniform staining of Cyclospora oocysts in fecal smears by a modified safranin technique with microwave heating. J Clin Microbiol. 1997;35(3):730–3.
39. Cann KJ, Chalmers RM, Nichols G, O'Brien SJ. Cyclospora infections in England and Wales: 1993 to 1998. Commun Dis Public Health. 2000;3(1):46–9.
40. Buss SN, Leber A, Chapin K, Fey PD, Bankowski MJ, Jones MK, et al. Multicenter evaluation of the BioFire FilmArray gastrointestinal panel for etiologic diagnosis of infectious gastroenteritis. J Clin Microbiol. 2015;53(3):915–25. https://doi.org/10.1128/jcm.02674-14.
41. Zimmer SM, Schuetz AN, Franco-Paredes C. Efficacy of nitazoxanide for cyclosporiasis in patients with sulfa allergy. Clin Infect Dis. 2007;44(3):466–7. https://doi.org/10.1086/510744.
42. MacKenzie WR, Schell WL, Blair KA, Addiss DG, Peterson DE, Hoxie NJ, et al. Massive outbreak of waterborne cryptosporidium infection in Milwaukee, Wisconsin: recurrence of illness and risk of secondary transmission. Clin Infect Dis. 1995;21(1):57–62.
43. Vanathy K, Parija SC, Mandal J, Hamide A, Krishnamurthy S. Cryptosporidiosis: a mini review. Trop Parasitol. 2017;7(2):72–80. https://doi.org/10.4103/tp.TP_25_17.
44. Audicana MT, Kennedy MW. Anisakis simplex: from obscure infectious worm to inducer of immune hypersensitivity. Clin Microbiol Rev. 2008;21(2):360–79, table of contents. https://doi.org/10.1128/cmr.00012-07.
45. Hochberg NS, Hamer DH. Anisakidosis: perils of the deep. Clin Infect Dis. 2010;51(7):806–12. https://doi.org/10.1086/656238.

46. Loria-Cortes R, Lobo-Sanahuja JF. Clinical abdominal angiostrongylosis. A study of 116 children with intestinal eosinophilic granuloma caused by Angiostrongylus costaricensis. Am J Trop Med Hyg. 1980;29(4):538–44.
47. Neafie RC, Marty AM. Unusual infections in humans. Clin Microbiol Rev. 1993;6(1):34–56.
48. Vazquez JJ, Sola JJ, Boils PL. Hepatic lesions induced by Angiostrongylus costaricensis. Histopathology. 1994;25(5):489–91.
49. Kroner PT, Argueta V. Abdominal angiostrongyliasis mimicking acute appendicitis. Encoscopy. 2015;47(Suppl 1 UCTN):E179–80. https://doi.org/10.1055/s-0034-1391501.

Drug-Induced Injury, Polyps, Congenital, and Miscellaneous Disorders

12

Vishal S. Chandan and Tsung-Teh Wu

Drug-Induced Injury

In the recent years, there has been an overwhelming increase in the number of drugs that may injure the gastrointestinal tract. However, there are certain characteristic injury patterns that should prompt consideration for drug-induced injury. The intent here is to provide a practical guide for surgical pathologists to recognize and diagnose drug-related injury to the duodenum. A subset of medications produce characteristic histopathological changes; however, most cause non-specific patterns of injury that can show considerable overlap with histological changes caused by other drugs, infections, or autoimmune diseases. The type and severity of these changes also depend on a number of factors such as the dose of the medication, drug interactions, mechanism of action, and the patients' underlying disease.

Immunomodulators and Targeted Agents

Ipilimumab is a monoclonal antibody against cytotoxic T-lymphocyte-associated antigen-4 (CTLA-4), and it can bind to CTLA-4 to block the inhibitory signal to enhance T-cell activation against cancer cells [1]. It has been approved by the food and drug administration (FDA) in 2011 and has shown significant survival benefit in patients with metastatic melanoma [2–4]. Its benefits are being currently investigated in other malignancies such as prostate cancer, renal cell carcinoma, and non-small cell lung carcinoma [5–8]. The most common gastrointestinal side effects are diarrhea and colitis, and they have been reported in up to 30% of patients [9]. The symptoms typically occur 1–2 months after initiation of the drug but may also occur earlier. However, toxicity has also been observed weeks to months after the discontinuation of the drug. Endoscopy may show small ulcers in the duodenum [10]. The enteritis may precede the colitis in some cases; hence, the examination of the small bowel may be warranted to make the diagnosis. Histological examination of the duodenum may show villous blunting with acute inflammation, crypt distortion, lymphoplasmacytic expansion of the lamina propria, hyperplasia of Brunner glands, and increased apoptotic bodies (Fig. 12.1a, b) [10, 11]. Treatment includes stopping ipilimumab, starting steroids, and followed by infliximab (anti-tumor necrosis factor alpha antibody) [12].

Programmed cell death protein 1 (PD-1) is found on T cells as a cell surface receptor and functions as an immune checkpoint to prevent cytotoxic T-cell activation by self-antigens [13]. Some tumors show high levels of PD-1 ligand (PD-L1), blunting the immune response against them. The PD-1 inhibitors circumvent this interaction facilitating cytotoxic T-cell activity against these tumors [14]. PD-1 and PD-L1 inhibitors (such as pembrolizumab, nivolumab, and atezolizumab) have proved successful in prolonging survival for patients with metastatic melanoma, lung carcinoma, renal cell carcinoma, mismatch repair-deficient colorectal carcinoma, and urothelial carcinoma. Diarrhea is one of the most common side effects of these medications and can be seen in 10–20% of patients [15, 16]. Other common side effects include nausea, vomiting, and fatigue [15, 17]. At endoscopy, the duodenum may show erythema, erosion, or small non-bleeding ulcers. Histology may show a range of findings including villous blunting, acute inflammation, increased eosinophils within the lamina propria, lymphoplasmacytic lamina propria expansion, decreased goblet cells and Paneth cells, increased intraepithelial lymphocytes, and increased crypt apoptosis [18].

Idelalisib is recently approved for treatment of relapsed chronic lymphocytic leukemia and non-Hodgkin lymphoma.

V. S. Chandan
Department of Pathology, University of California – Irvine, Irvine, CA, USA

T.-T. Wu (✉)
Department of Laboratory Medicine and Pathology, Mayo Clinic, Rochester, MN, USA
e-mail: Wu.TsungTeh@mayo.edu

L. Zhang et al. (eds.), *Surgical Pathology of Non-neoplastic Gastrointestinal Diseases*, https://doi.org/10.1007/978-3-030-15573-5_12

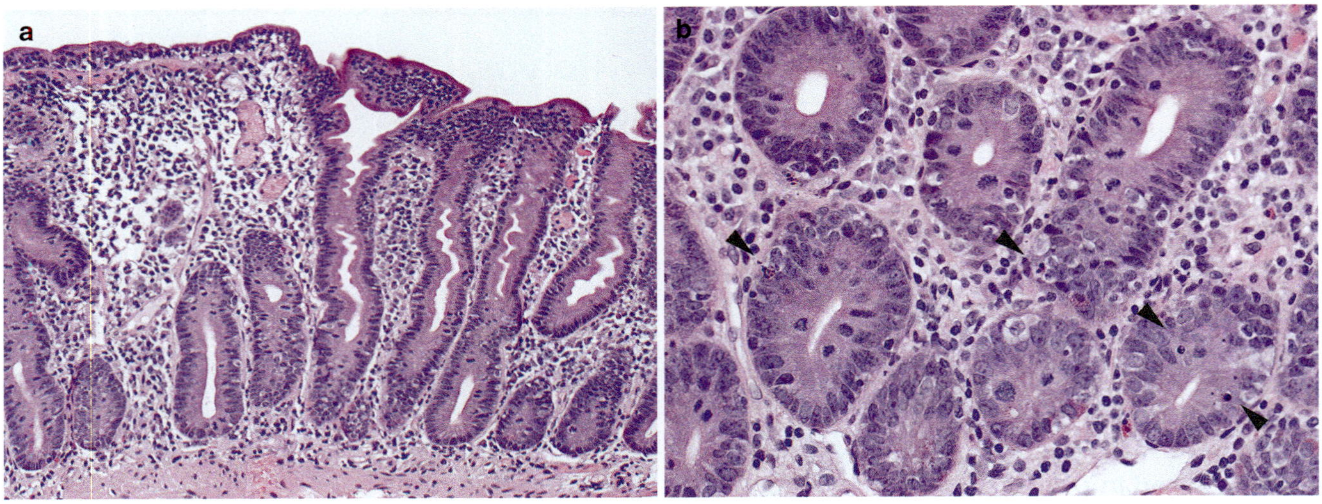

Fig. 12.1 Ipilimumab-associated injury. (**a**) Duodenal biopsy from a patient with prostate cancer presenting with watery diarrhea after three cycles of ipilimumab shows villous atrophy, increased chronic inflammation in lamina propria, increased intraepithelial lymphocytes, and reactive epithelial changes with decreased number of goblet cells and Paneth cells. (**b**) Increased apoptotic bodies (arrowheads) are also present within the crypts

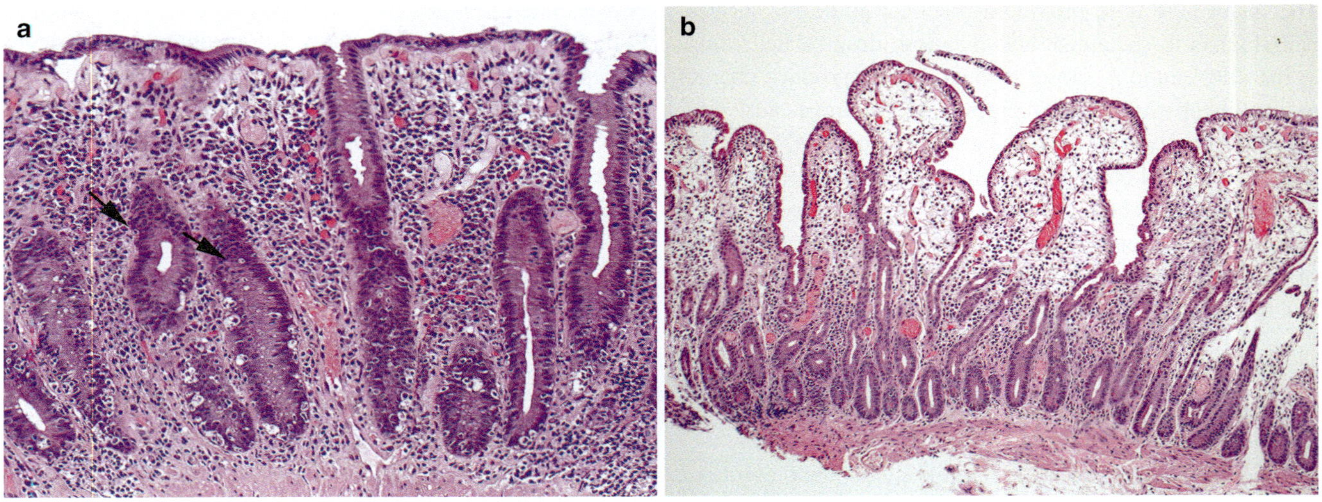

Fig. 12.2 Mycophenolate mofetil-induced injury. (**a**) Duodenal biopsy shows villous atrophy, increased lymphoplasmacytic infiltrates in lamina propria, focal cryptitis (arrows), and prominent apoptotic bodies resembling graft versus host disease. (**b**) Chronic duodenitis-like features with edema of lamina propria and marked reactive epithelial changes

It is an inhibitor of the delta isoform of phosphoinositide 3-kinase. The histologic features of idelalisib-induced injury are similar to PD-1/PD-L1 and CTLA-4 inhibitors, which include prominent intraepithelial lymphocytosis, acute inflammation, and increased apoptosis [19, 20].

Mycophenolate Mofetil (CellCept, MMF)

Mycophenolate mofetil (MMF) is an immunosuppressant used in solid organ and bone marrow as well as stem cell transplant patients to prevent allograft rejection and graft versus host disease (GVHD). The histological hallmark of MMF-induced injury is increased crypt apoptosis, characterized by an empty space surrounding the degenerated cell components comprising of condensed and fragmented blue nuclear and pink cytoplasmic material. Duodenal biopsies can show a range of histological changes including villous blunting, increased crypt apoptosis (Fig. 12.2a), chronic peptic-type injury with gastric mucinous cell metaplasia, chronic duodenitis (Fig. 12.2b), and increased intraepithelial lymphocytes [21].

Medication Associated with Mitotic Arrest (Colchicine and Taxol)

Colchicine is an alkaloid used for treatment of gout and other medical conditions including immune/rheumatologic disorders. Colchicine exhibits antimitotic activity due to its ability to bind to tubulin and to prevent the polymerization of tubulin into microtubules. Patients with renal and/or hepatic failure usually are at risk to develop colchicine toxicity. The most noticeable feature of colchicine toxicity is mitotic arrest in metaphase with absent mitotic spindles and bizarre chromatin patterns, specially ring mitosis [22, 23]. The distinct morphological features include metaphase mitoses (ring mitosis), epithelial pseudostratification, increased apoptosis, and loss of epithelial polarity (Fig. 12.3a, b). It is important for the pathologist to recognize this epithelial atypia as to be related to colchicine toxicity in order to avoid confusion with high-grade dysplasia which can also show abnormal cytologic changes. Villous atrophy and gastric mucin cell metaplasia can also be seen with colchicine-induced injury [22]. These histological changes are usually not seen in patients taking colchicine without clinical evidence of toxicity. Hence when these changes are identified by pathologists, it is important to reconcile with the patient's medication list, because if colchicine is the offending agent, then the patient is probably toxic. Of note, even therapeutic doses of colchicine may rarely cause ring mitosis, especially in colorectal polyps [24]. The histological findings of colchicine toxicity regress on cessation of the drug.

Taxol (paclitaxel) is a chemotherapy drug used to treat malignancies of lung, esophagus, and breast. Like colchicine, Taxol causes increased and arrested mitotic activity including ring mitosis [22, 25]. The mitotic figures are predominantly seen in the proliferative zone of the duodenum. Taxol effects are histologically identical to those of colchicine toxicity and morphologically indistinguishable. However, the histological features of Taxol effect can be seen in any patient undergoing chemotherapy with this drug. Unlike colchicine, mitotic arrest and ring mitosis after Taxol administration do not necessarily indicate Taxol toxicity. Rarely may patients with telomere-mediated disorders show ring mitosis and apoptosis [26].

Non-steroidal Anti-inflammatory Drugs (NSAIDs)

NSAIDs are widely used for their analgesic and anti-inflammatory effects. They prevent prostaglandin synthesis which results in mucosal ischemia and decreased mucosal integrity. Within the duodenum they can cause mucosal architectural distortion with patchy active inflammation that can resemble Crohn's disease. They can also cause increased intraepithelial lymphocytes [27]. Duodenal ulcers can occur in chronic NSAIDs' users.

Yttrium-90

Yttrium-90 microspheres injected for selective internal radiation are typically offered to patients with unresectable primary or metastatic liver cancer. They can be associated with duodenal ulceration and presence of black microspheres within the mucosal capillaries [28, 29]. This occurs when the Yttrium-labeled

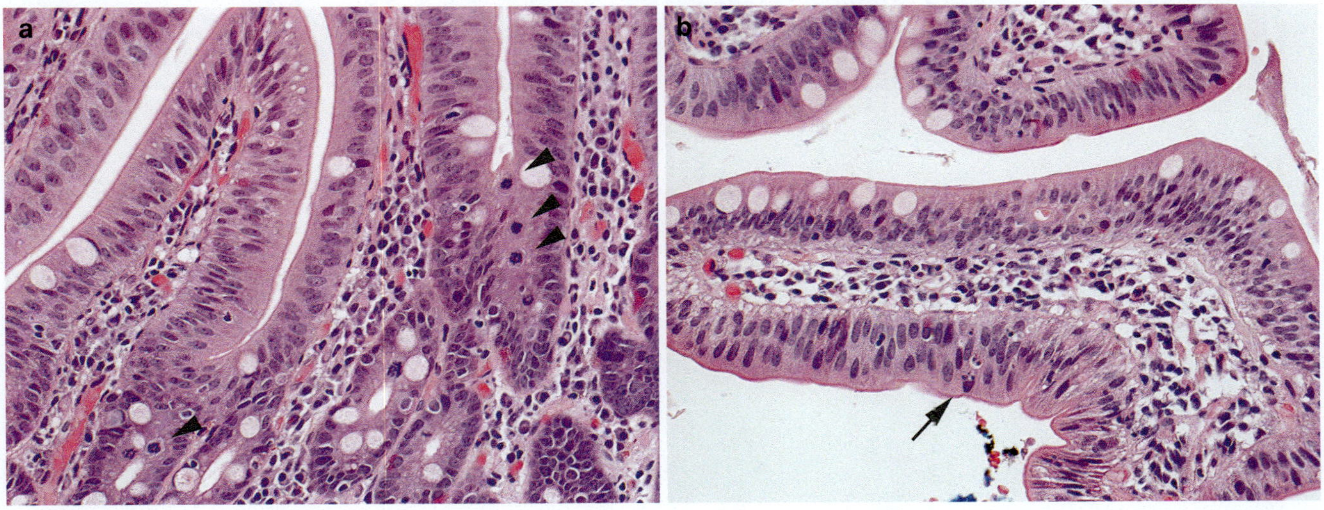

Fig. 12.3 Histological features of colchicine toxicity. (**a**) Multiple interphase (ring) mitoses (arrowheads) are present in the duodenal biopsy from a patient with chronic renal failure and taking colchicine. (**b**) Reactive epithelial changes with epithelial pseudostratification and increased apoptosis (arrow) can be present in colchicine toxicity

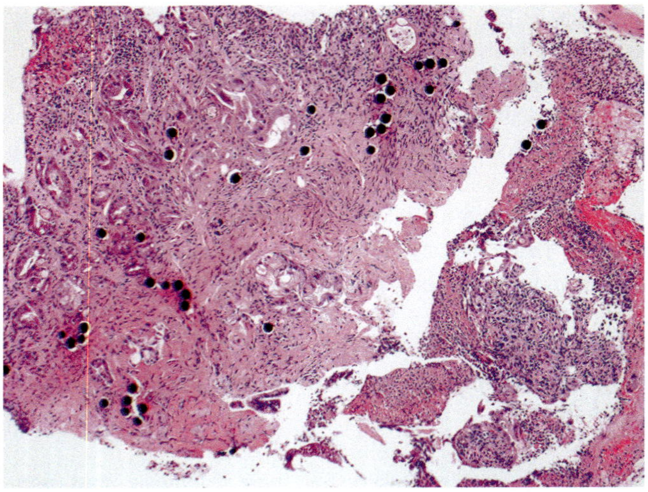

Fig. 12.4 Yttrium-90 microspheres-induced duodenal ulceration. Duodenal ulceration with marked reactive glandular epithelial atypia due to radiation-induced injury, and multiple basophilic, deep purple, uniformly round microspheres resembling psammoma bodies are present in the lamina propria and muscularis mucosae

microspheres accidentally enter the arteries supplying the duodenum, causing unintended radiation damage. The duodenum shows mucosal ulceration and granulation tissue with lamina propria hyalinization, as well as atypical stromal and endothelial cells. The microspheres, measuring about 30–40 μm in diameter, appear as basophilic, deep purple, uniformly round acellular foreign bodies resembling psammoma bodies (Fig. 12.4) [29–31]. These radiation microspheres may be found in the lamina propria, deep mucosa, or muscular layer.

Lanthanum

Lanthanum carbonate (Fosrenol) is used in patients with chronic renal failure for treatment of hyperphosphatemia. It binds with phosphate and is poorly absorbed in the gastrointestinal tract. However, a small subset of patients taking this drug can develop lanthanum deposition within mucosal histiocytes causing duodenal villous blunting and focal ulcerations (Fig. 12.5a) [32, 33]. The histiocytes show a fine to coarse granular inclusion-like

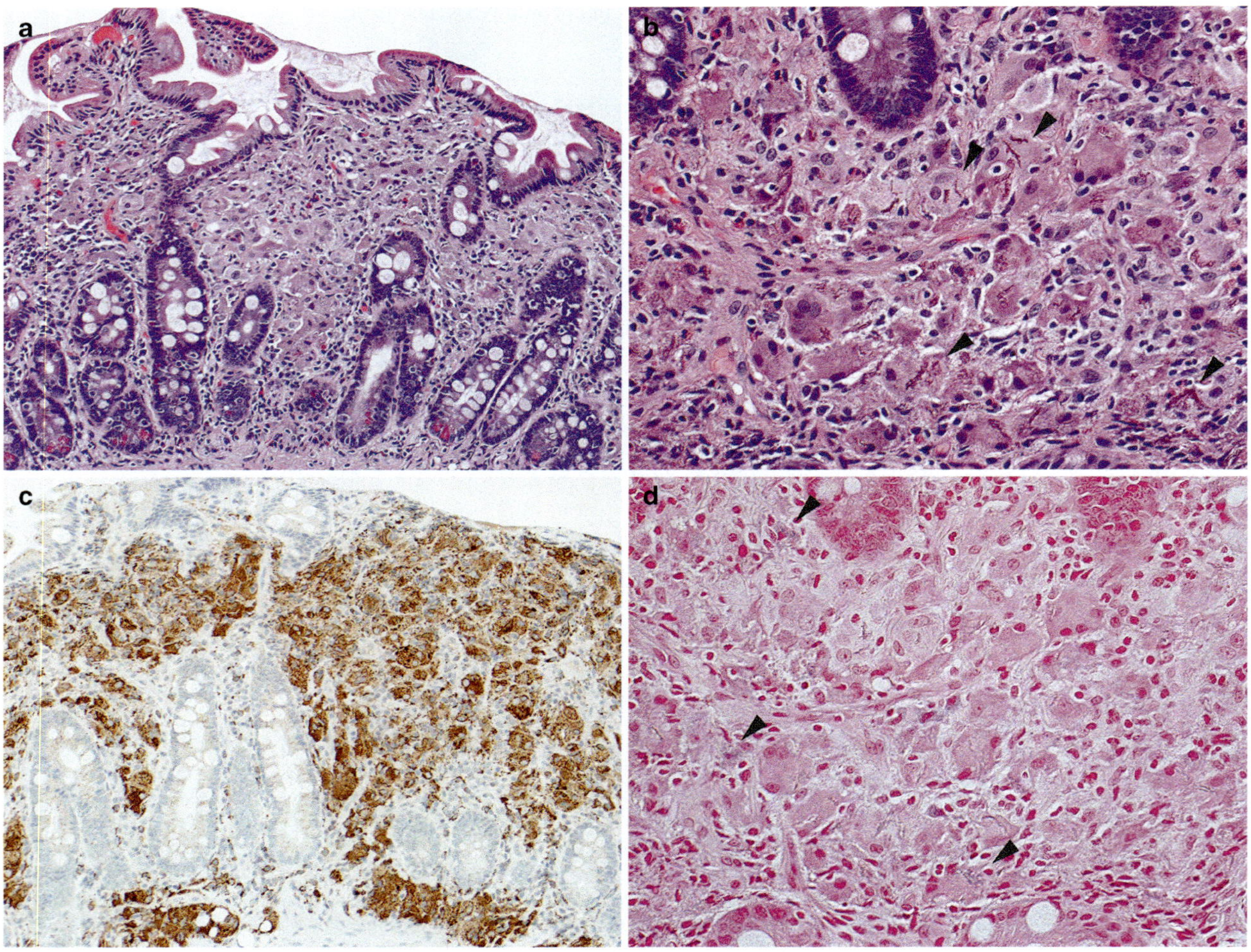

Fig. 12.5 Lanthanum deposition. (**a**) Duodenal biopsy from a chronic renal failure patient receiving lanthanum carbonate for hyperphosphatemia shows villous atrophy and marked histiocytic aggregates within lamina propria. (**b**) There are numerous cytoplasmic coarse inclusion-like brownish materials with irregular branching (arrowheads) present within the histiocytes. (**c**) The histiocytes within the lamina propria are positive for CD68 by immunohistochemical stain. (**d**) The cytoplasmic inclusion-like materials are focally weak positive (arrowheads) for Perl's Prussian blue stain

Duodenal ectopic pancreas should not be confused with paraduodenal pancreatitis (groove pancreatitis). Paraduodenal pancreatitis is a well-known complication of chronic pancreatitis with duodenal involvement and duodenal stenosis in 20–31% of cases and is typically seen in young to middle-aged men with alcohol use [67]. Paraduodenal pancreatitis has also been referred as periampullary wall cyst, cystic dystrophy of heterotopic pancreas, and pancreatic hamartoma of duodenum. Paraduodenal pancreatitis is typically centered in the duodenal wall near minor papilla with luminal stenosis, giant mucosal folds, sieve-like cystic changes, and thickening or scarring of the duodenal wall in the "groove area (the sliding plane between duodenum and pancreas)" [68, 69]. The cysts embedded in the duodenal wall can be multiple and range from 1 to 10 cm in size, and contain clear fluid, necrotic and granular materials, or stones. Histologically, the characteristic features of paraduodenal pancreatitis are the presence of pancreatic tissue with dilated ducts and cystic changes with surrounding smooth muscle and myofibroblastic proliferation in the duodenal wall, duodenal submucosal fibrosis extending into the adjacent soft tissue in the groove area and pancreas, and variable amount of duodenal Brunner gland hyperplasia (Fig. 12.12a, b) [69].

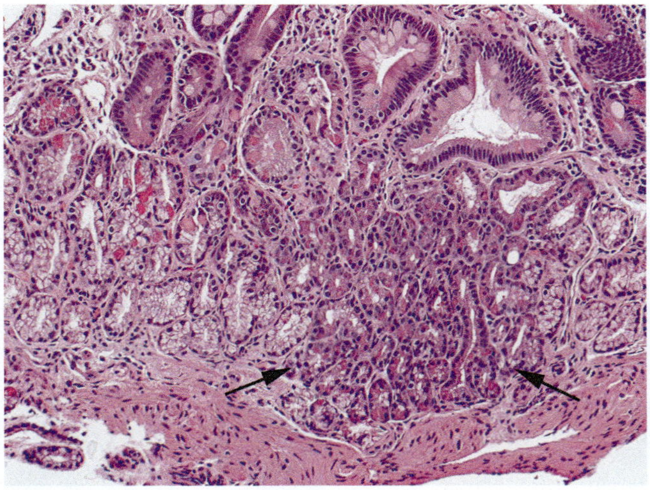

Fig. 12.11 Duodenal pancreatic acinar cell metaplasia. A small focus pancreatic acinar cell (arrows) is present in mucosa from endoscopically normal-appearing duodenal mucosa

Treatment and Prognosis

For patients with symptomatic duodenal ectopic pancreas, local resection of lesion is appropriate therapy after exclusion of malignancy [66]. Diseases occur in normal pancreas such as chronic pancreatitis, pancreatic intraepithelial neoplasia, intraductal papillary mucinous neoplasm, and mucinous neoplasm have all been reported in ectopic pancreas [70–72]. Frequency of malignant transformation in ectopic pancreas is low ranging from 0.7% to 1.8% [73, 74] and can also present in duodenal ectopic pancreas [75, 76].

Miscellaneous Disorders

Pseudomelanosis Duodeni

Definition

Pseudomelanosis duodeni (PD) is characterized by accumulation of dark pigmented granules in macrophages within the lamina propria of duodenal villi.

Clinical Features

PD is a rare entity and occurs predominately in middle-aged or over 60-year-old adults and is more common in female [77, 78]. PD can occasionally occur in pediatric

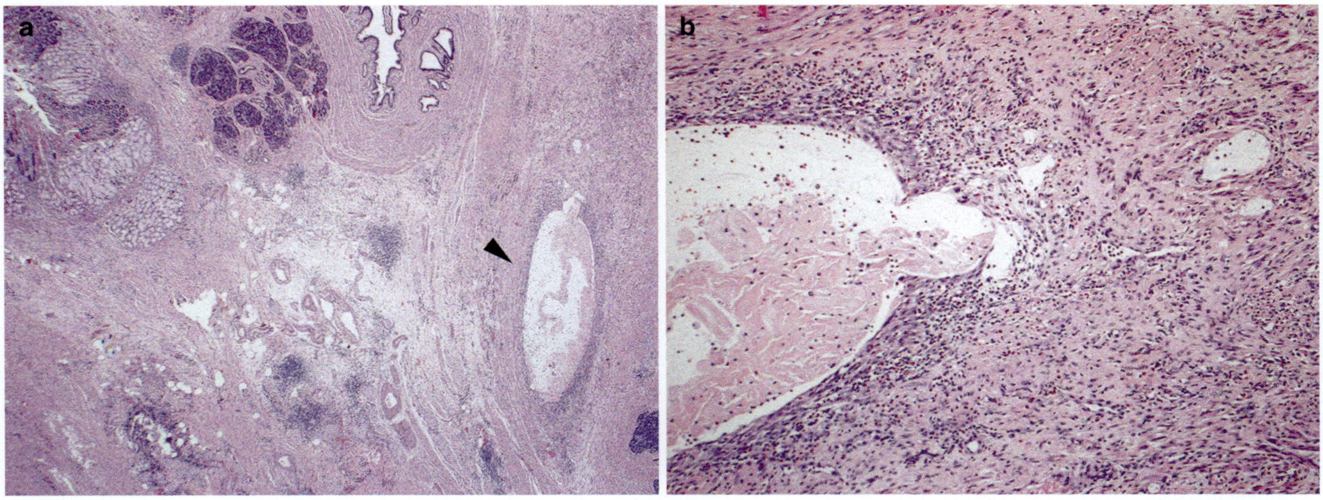

Fig. 12.12 Paraduodenal pancreatitis (groove pancreatitis). (**a**) Pancreatic tissue in the duodenal wall shows dilated ducts and cystic changes (arrow). (**b**) The dilated duct with cystic change with surrounding inflammation, smooth muscle, and myofibroblastic proliferation

patients [77, 79]. PD typically is an incidental finding without specific associated clinical symptoms. On upper gastrointestinal endoscopy, the duodenal mucosa shows multiple speckled, discrete, flat, and dark spots in duodenal bulb and second portion of the duodenum (Fig. 12.13a), and these characteristic endoscopic features are apparent in 35% of patients with histological diagnosis of PD [78]. The brownish black mucosal spots can also be present in stomach, jejunum, and ileum [80–82]. PD occurs in patients with chronic renal failure, arterial hypertension, diabetes mellitus, gastrointestinal bleeding, and use of medications such as ferrous sulfate and antihypertensive treatment including hydralazine, propranolol, hydrochlorothiazide, and furosemide [78].

Pathological Features

Duodenal biopsy demonstrates collection of brownish black granular pigments in macrophages in the lamina propria and mainly within the tip of the villi (Fig. 12.13b). These brownish black pigments are originally interpreted as melanin [83, 84], pseudomelanin, or hemosiderin; and now have been demonstrated to be mostly ferrous sulfate and small amount of calcium, potassium, aluminum, magnesium, and silica [85, 86]. Iron (Perl's Prussian blue) or melanin (Masson-Fontana) stains may be positive (Fig. 12.13c), but the stains can be variable [77, 78]. Iron stain can be negative if ferrous oxide is present instead of ferrous sulfide [86]. The exact pathogenesis for the PD is still unclear, and possible explanations include abnormal iron accumulation secondary to oral iron intake or mucosal bleeding in the upper gastrointestinal tract [86, 87]; or defect in macrophage metabolism of drugs containing cyclic compounds such as phenols, skatoles, and indoles [88]. Unlike other iron and other heavy metal depositions in other part of body, no specific fibroinflammatory reaction, fibrosis, erosion, or stricture are associated with PD.

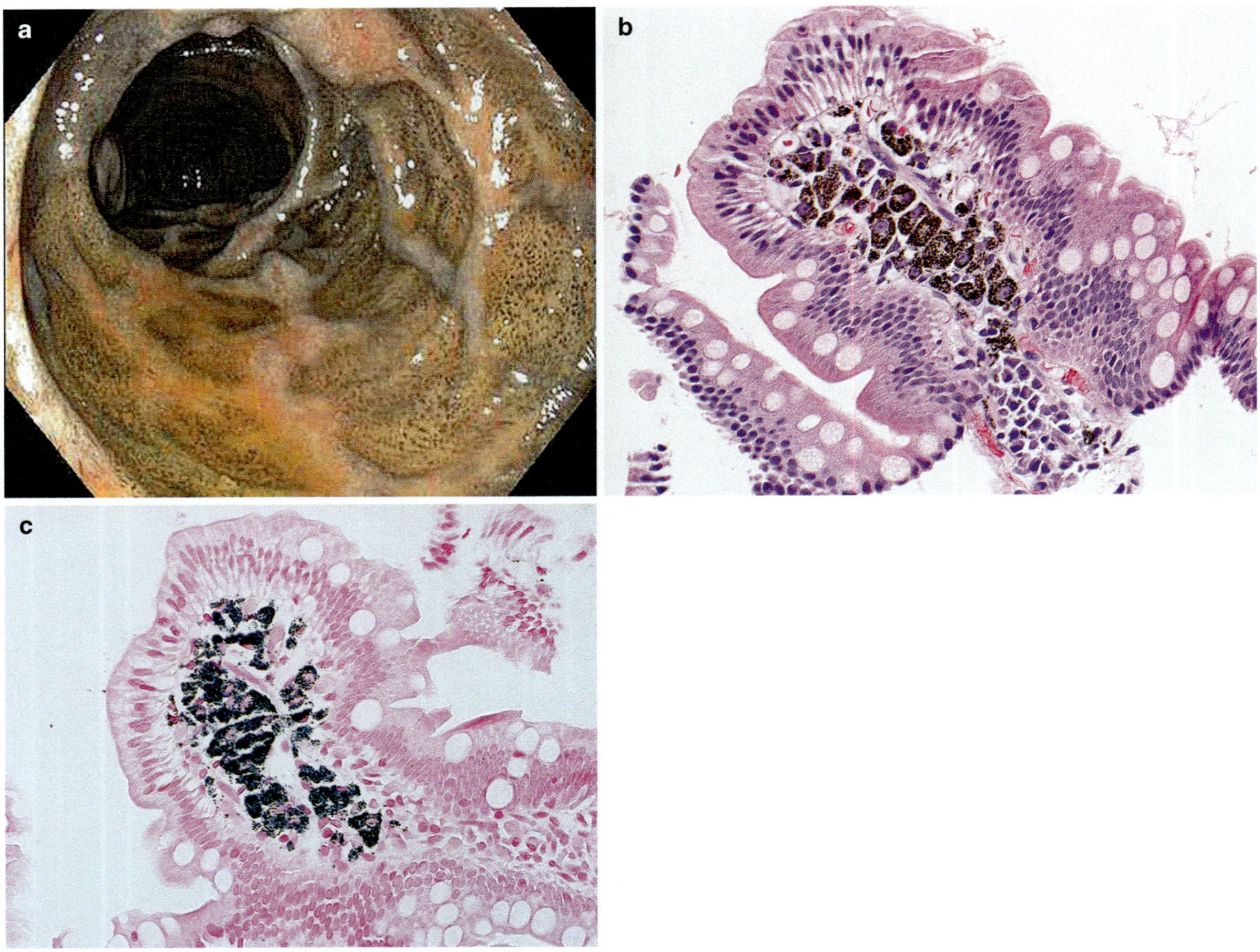

Fig. 12.13 Pseudomelanosis duodeni. (**a**) Multiple speckled, discrete, flat, and dark spots are present in the duodenum on upper gastrointestinal endoscopy. (**b**) Clusters of brownish black granular pigments in macrophages are in the lamina propria and within the tip of the villi. (**c**) In this case, these brownish black pigments are positive for Perl's Prussian blue stain

Differential Diagnosis

The presence of brownish black pigments needs to be differentiated from metastatic melanoma, hemosiderosis secondary to previous mucosal hemorrhage, and other pigmentations such as exogenous ingested barium sulfate and charcoal. The charcoal-induced pseudomelanosis in small bowel is predominately present in the terminal ileum instead of proximal duodenum [89, 90]. The pigments in hemosiderosis secondary to previous mucosal hemorrhage are brownish in color and are strongly positive on iron stain.

Treatment and Prognosis

The prognostic significance of PD is unclear and has yet to be determined. No long-term complications such as worsening of underlying medical conditions or malignant transformation are associated with patients with PD. No specific therapy or follow-up protocol is recommended [78].

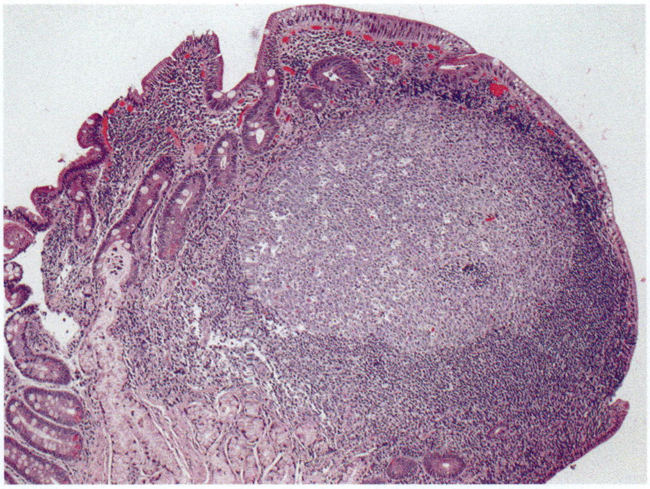

Fig. 12.14 Benign nodular lymphoid hyperplasia. A hyperplastic lymphoid follicle with a large germinal center containing tangible body macrophages and surrounded by a normal-appearing mantle zone in the lamina propria is present in the duodenum from a 9-year-old male patient with grossly unremarkable duodenum

Benign Nodular Lymphoid Hyperplasia

Definition

Benign nodular lymphoid hyperplasia (NLH) is characterized by the presence of multiple visible mucosal hyperplastic lymphoid follicles normally between 2 and 10 mm in diameter.

Clinical Features

NLH of gastrointestinal tract affects all age group but primarily in children under 10 years of age [91]. In children, NLH can occur in association with viral infections and food allergy, and tends to have a benign course and can regress spontaneously [92, 93]. NLH in gastrointestinal tract is a rare disease in adults and usually occurs in patients with congenital or acquired immunodeficiency such as IgA deficiency, common variable immunodeficiency syndrome (CVID), and acquired immunodeficiency syndrome, gastrointestinal tract infections due to Giardia or Helicobacter pylori, and celiac disease [94–100]. NLH can also occur in immunocompetent patients [101, 102]. Patients with NLH can be asymptomatic or with gastrointestinal symptoms such as abdominal pain, chronic diarrhea, bleeding, and intestinal obstruction [91]. Duodenal NLH can present as polyposis in patient with CVID [103].

Pathological Features

Benign NLH can be divided into diffuse and focal forms, and also can involve colon, terminal ileum, stomach, and small bowel [94]. The pathological features of NLH are the presence of hyperplastic lymphoid follicles with large germinal centers surrounded by a normal-appearing mantle zone in the lamina propria and superficial submucosa (Fig. 12.14) [94].

The pathogenesis of NLH is not well known. In the immunodeficiency status, the presence of NLH can be caused by accumulation of plasma cell precursors due to maturation defects in the development of B lymphocytes to compensate the functional inadequate intestinal lymphoid tissue [91]. Intestinal antigenic trigger possibly due to infections such as Giardia leading to repetitive stimulation and eventually lymphoid hyperplasia may explain the NLH occurs in the absence of immunodeficiency [91].

Differential Diagnosis

Grade 1–2 follicular lymphoma should be differentiated from NLH. Duodenal follicular lymphoma is typically an incidental finding on endoscopic examination, has an indolent clinical course [104, 105], and is distinct from follicular lymphomas involving other parts of gastrointestinal tract [105]. Follicular lymphoma has a nodular monotonous proliferation of small centrocytes positive for BCL-2, BCL-6, and CD10, and lack of tangible body macrophages and normal polarity of germinal center (Fig. 12.15a–d); in contrast to the normal germinal centers in NLH which are positive for BCL-6 and CD10 but negative for BCL-2 by immunohistochemical stains.

Treatment and Prognosis

Treatment is directed to the associated conditions, and surveillance to exclude lymphomatous transformation is necessary [91]. Malignant lymphoma has been reported to arise in NLH associated with immunodeficiency or immunocompetent conditions [106, 107].

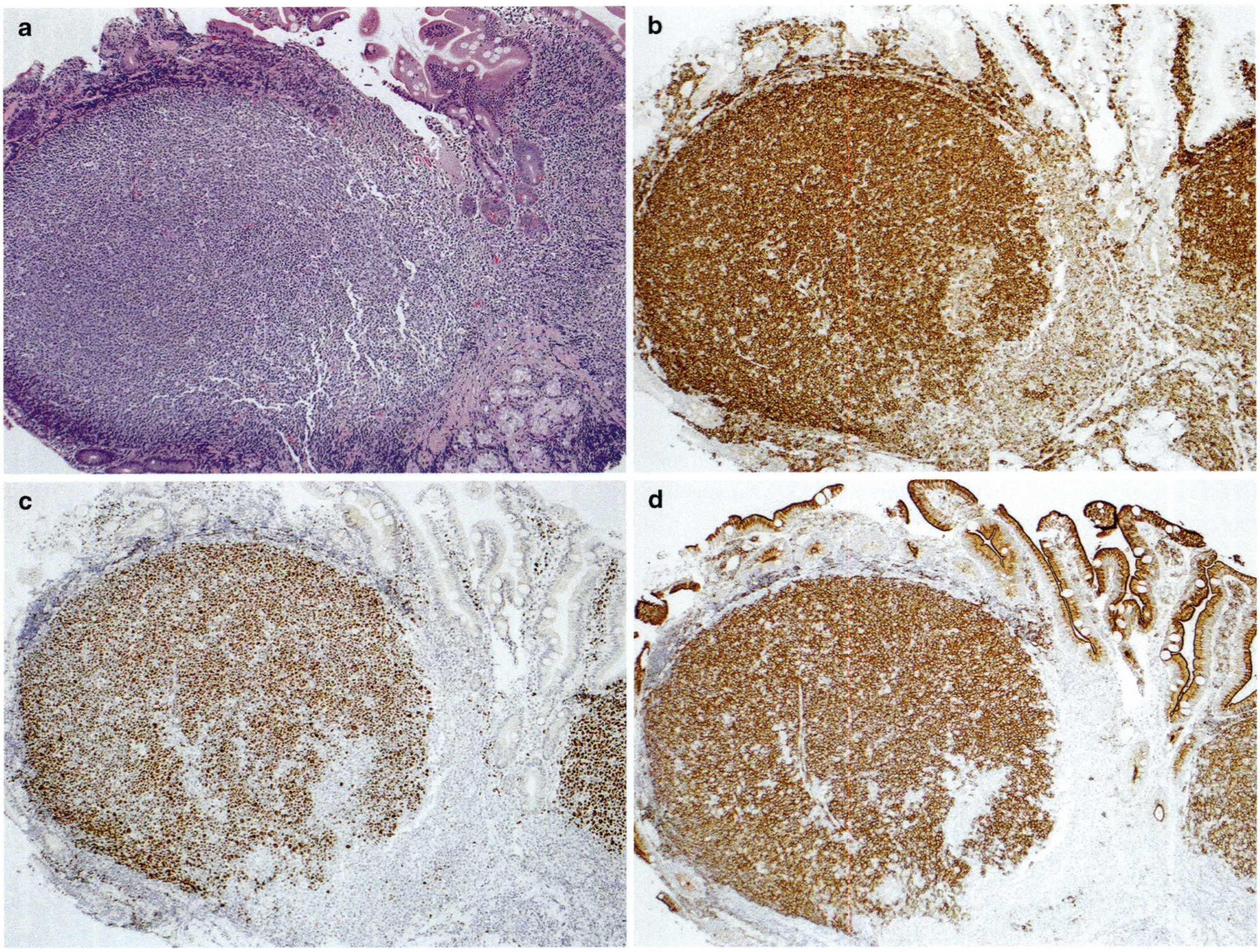

Fig. 12.15 Grade 1 follicular lymphoma. (**a**) A nodular monotonous proliferation of small centrocytes with absence of tangible body macrophages and normal polarity of germinal center in biopsy of nodular duodenal lesion. The monotonous small centrocytes are positive for BCL-2 (**b**), BCL-6 (**c**), and CD10 (**d**) by immunohistochemical stains

Brunner Gland Hyperplasia/Hamartoma

Definition

Brunner gland hyperplasia/hamartoma (BGH) is a Brunner gland proliferating lesion within the duodenal mucosa and submucosa.

Clinical Features

BGH is not an infrequent benign lesion in the proximal duodenum and can be identified in 2% of upper gastrointestinal endoscopic examinations [108]. BGH occurs mainly in adults and rarely in children [109]. Brunner gland hyperplasia has been reported more commonly in male, and Brunner gland hamartoma is more common in female [108, 110, 111]. BGH is frequently (15–55%) identified in patients with uremia [112]. Patients with BGH can be asymptomatic or have non-specific symptoms of nausea, vomiting, abdominal pain, or bloating [108]. Gastrointestinal bleeding, biliary obstructive symptom with acute pancreatitis, gastroduodenal intussusception, and gastric outlet obstruction can occur in patients with large (>2 cm) BGH [109, 110, 113, 114]. BGH is more commonly presented within the duodenal bulb but can also occur in the second or third part of duodenum [108, 110, 111].

Pathological Features

BGH can present as circumscribed nodular hyperplasia, diffuse nodular hyperplasia, and polypoid tumor-like lesion, ranging from 0.5 cm to 6 cm in size (Fig. 12.16a, b) [108, 110]. Brunner gland hyperplasia and hamartoma are often used interchangeably and share similar histological features of lobulated Brunner gland proliferation separated by fibrous septa within the mucosa and submucosa (Fig. 12.16c). Brunner gland hamartoma tends to be a solitary lesion and

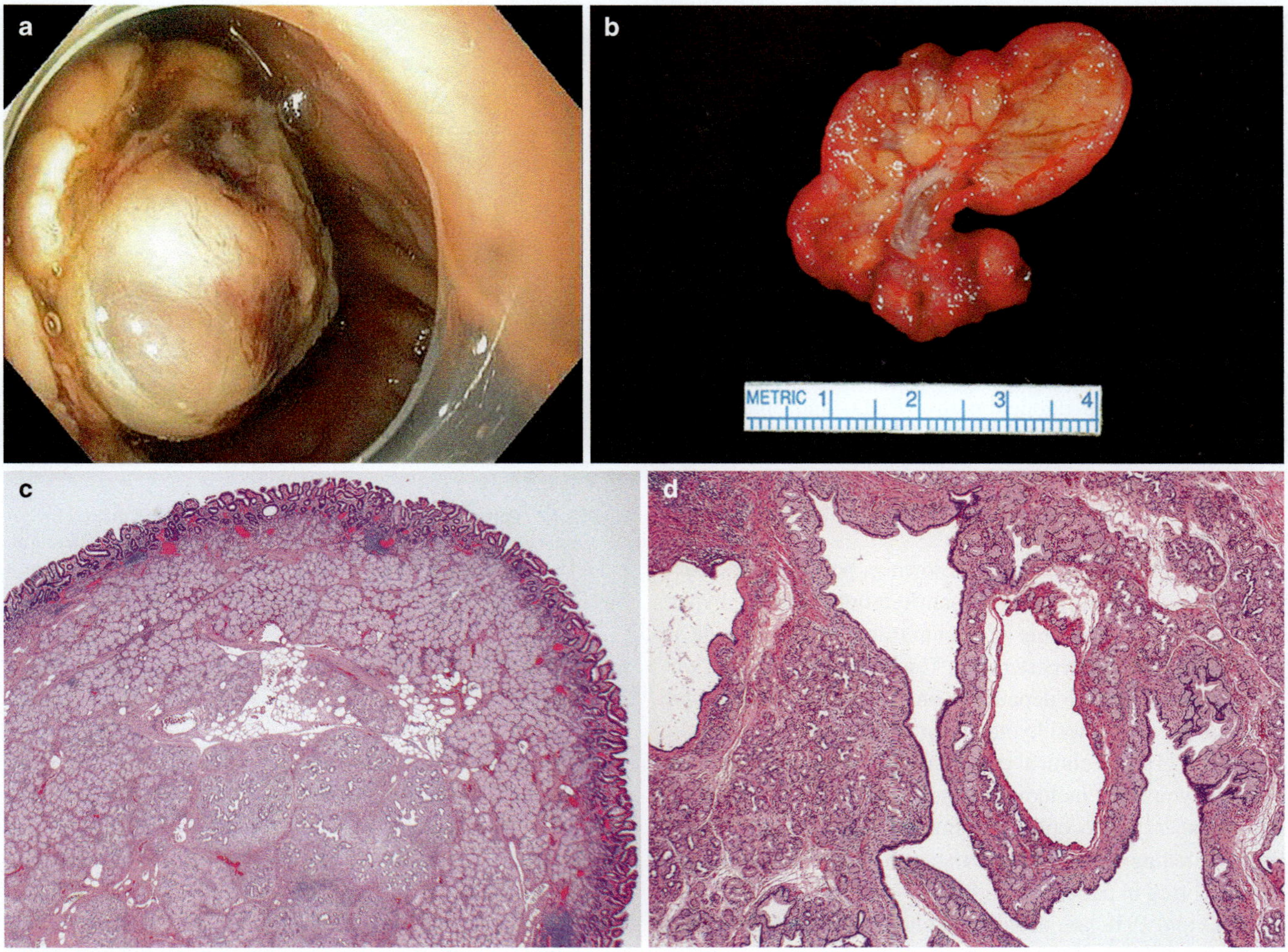

Fig. 12.16 Brunner gland hyperplasia/hamartoma. (**a**) A large polypoid lesion is present in the duodenal bulb on endoscopic examination. (**b**) Cross-section of the resected polypoid lesion shows a light yellow-colored multi-lobulated submucosal nodule. (**c**) Proliferation of lobules of Brunner glands separated by thin fibrous septa in the submucosa and mucosa at low power view. (**d**) Brunner gland cyst with multiple large cystic dilated glands is present in Brunner gland hyperplasia/hamartoma

is characterized by the presence of Brunner gland, ducts, smooth muscle, adipose tissue, and lymphoid tissue [110, 111]. The term of Brunner gland adenoma has been also used to describe Brunner gland hamartoma, and is not recommended to use to avoid confusion of rare true dysplasia arising from BGH. Brunner glands express mucin core peptide MUC6, and the Brunner ducts can occasionally express mucin core peptide MUC1 or MUC6 by immunohistochemical stain [111]. BGH can present as a cystic lesion and has been also referred as Brunner gland cyst (Fig. 12.16d), mucocele of Brunner gland, and cystic Brunner gland hamartoma [115, 116].

The pathogenesis of BGH is not fully understood. BGH was regarded as a hamartomatous lesion [117]; however, gastric acid hypersecretion and presence of Helicobacter pylori may play a significant role of developing Brunner gland hyperplasia [108].

Differential Diagnosis
Increased or proliferative intramucosal Brunner glands are often present in peptic-type duodenitis, and BGH should be reserved for Brunner gland proliferation in mucosa and submucosa when duodenal nodules are identified endoscopically. Pyloric gland adenoma arising from gastric heterotopia has proliferation of small pyloric glands, and the histological features can resemble BGH. Both pyloric glands and Brunner glands are positive for mucin core peptide MUC6, but pyloric gland adenoma is also positive for MUC5AC by immunohistochemistry and can be used to differentiate from BGH [63].

Treatment and Prognosis
BGH is not a neoplastic lesion [118]. Large or pedunculated BGH can be removed surgically or endoscopically with favorable outcome [110]. Dysplasia in Brunner gland duct

but not in Brunner glands is only rarely reported in BGH [119, 120]. Most of the reported dysplasia and adenocarcinomas in BGH are dysplasia involving the surface epithelium but not underlying BGH itself; and the adenocarcinomas may actually arise from pyloric gland adenoma but not from BGH [118, 121–123].

Portal Hypertensive Duodenopathy and Enteropathy

Definition

Portal hypertensive duodenopathy (PHD) and enteropathy (PHE) is a condition defined by mucosal pathological abnormalities occurring in patients with portal hypertension.

Clinical Features

PHD and PHE (also previously known as portal hypertensive intestinal vasculopathy) are the manifestations of portal hypertensive changes involving duodenum and small intestine in patients with portal hypertension. The prevalence of PHE varies from 15% to 82% depending on the different endoscopic methods or video capsule endoscopy (VCE) used in cirrhotic patients [124]. The clinical presentations can be asymptomatic or with symptoms including anemia, melena, hematochezia, hematemesis, and occult gastrointestinal bleeding. Fetal and life-threatening variceal hemorrhage in small bowel has also been reported in patients with PHE [125, 126].

PHD and PHE are usually diagnosed by a VCE or deep endoscopy. The endoscopic manifestations show a wide range of vascular and nonvascular mucosal changes including mucosal edema, congested and rounded blunt villi with classic "herring-roe" appearance, friability, loss of vascularization, flat red spots, angioectasia, mucosal granularity, ulcers, varices, and inflammatory polyps [124–126]. PHE can also present as polypoid lesions or polyposis in small intestine in 0.3% of patients with portal hypertension [126, 127]. There are several proposed endoscopic scoring systems for PHE; however, no standardized scoring system is currently available [128–130].

Pathological Features

The characteristic pathological features of PHD and PHE are the presence of dilated mucosal vessels with thickened walls, capillary congestion and proliferation, edema of lamina propria, fibromuscular proliferation, villous blunting, thickened muscularis mucosae, and erosion (Fig. 12.17) [131, 132].

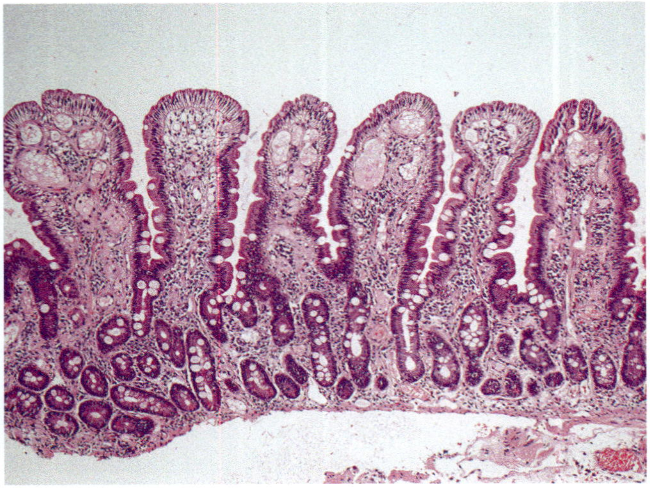

Fig. 12.17 Portal hypertensive duodenopathy. Multiple dilated mucosal vessels with thickened walls, capillary congestion and proliferation, and edema of lamina propria are present in duodenal biopsy from a patient with cirrhosis and portal hypertension

Differential Diagnosis

Small intestinal angioectasia (angiodysplasia) is the most common cause of small bowel bleeding in adults over 40 years old [133, 134]. Small bowel angioectasia is a localized vascular lesion with clusters of abnormally dilated vessels in the submucosa and mucosa and can mimic PHE in small intestinal biopsy.

Treatment and Prognosis

There are no standardized therapeutic guidelines for symptomatic PHE, and management should be individualized based on the acuity and severity of the hemorrhage, endoscopic accessibility of the lesion, and surgical risk of the patient [124]. Argon plasma coagulation is used for angioectasia, and multiple approaches including endoscopic variceal ligation, endoscopic sclerotherapy, transjugular intrahepatic portosystemic shunt, and polypectomy have been used for small bowel varices with polypoid enteropathy [124, 126, 135].

References

1. Peggs KS, Quezada SA, Korman AJ, Allison JP. Principles and use of anti-CTLA4 antibody in human cancer immunotherapy. Curr Opin Immunol. 2006;18(2):206–13. https://doi.org/10.1016/j.coi.2006.01.011.
2. Traynor K. Ipilimumab approved for metastatic melanoma. Am J Health Syst Pharm. 2011;68(9):768. https://doi.org/10.2146/news110025.
3. Hodi FS, O'Day SJ, McDermott DF, Weber RW, Sosman JA, Haanen JB, et al. Improved survival with ipilimumab in patients with metastatic melanoma. N Engl J Med. 2010;363(8):711–23. https://doi.org/10.1056/NEJMoa1003466.
4. Robert C, Thomas L, Bondarenko I, O'Day S, Weber J, Garbe C, et al. Ipilimumab plus dacarbazine for previously untreated metastatic melanoma. N Engl J Med. 2011;364(26):2517–26. https://doi.org/10.1056/NEJMoa1104621.
5. Jochems C, Tucker JA, Tsang KY, Madan RA, Dahut WL, Liewehr DJ, et al. A combination trial of vaccine plus ipilimumab in metastatic castration-resistant prostate cancer patients: immune correlates. Cancer Immunol Immunother. 2014;63(4):407–18. https://doi.org/10.1007/s00262-014-1524-0.

6. Kwon ED, Drake CG, Scher HI, Fizazi K, Bossi A, Van den Eertwegh AJM, et al. Ipilimumab versus placebo after radiotherapy in patients with metastatic castration-resistant prostate cancer that had progressed after docetaxel chemotherapy (CA184–043): a multicentre, randomised, double-blind, phase 3 trial. Lancet Oncol. 2014;15(7):700–12. https://doi.org/10.1016/S1470–2045(14)70189–5.
7. Reck M, Bondarenko I, Luft A, Serwatowski P, Barlesi F, Chacko R, et al. Ipilimumab in combination with paclitaxel and carboplatin as first-line therapy in extensivedisease-small-cell lungcancer: results from a randomized, double-blind, multicenter phase 2 trial. Ann Oncol. 2013;24(1):75–83. https://doi.org/10.1093/annonc/mds213.
8. Van den Eertwegh AJM, Versluis J, Van den Berg HP, Santegoets SJAM, Van Moorselaar RJA, Van der Sluis TM, et al. Combined immunotherapy with granulocyte-macrophage colony-stimulating factor-transduced allogeneic prostate cancer cells and ipilimumab in patients with metastatic castration-resistant prostate cancer: a phase 1 dose-escalation trial. Lancet Oncol. 2012;13(5):509–17. https://doi.org/10.1016/S1470–2045(12)70007–4.
9. Freeman HJ. Colitis associated with biological agents. World J Gastroenterol. 2012;18(16):1871–4. https://doi.org/10.3748/wjg.v18.i16.1871.
10. Messmer M, Upreti S, Tarabishy Y, Mazumder N, Chowdhury R, Yarchoan M, et al. Ipilimumab-induced enteritis without colitis: a new challenge. Case Rep Oncol. 2016;9(3):705–13. https://doi.org/10.1159/000452403.
11. Cramer P, Bresalier RS. Gastrointestinal and hepatic complications of immune checkpoint inhibitors. Curr Gastroenterol Rep. 2017;19(1):3. https://doi.org/10.1007/s11894–017–0540–6.
12. Klair JS, Girotra M, Hutchins LF, Caradine KD, Aduli F, Garcia-Saenz-de-Sicilia M. Ipilimumab-induced gastrointestinal toxicities: a management algorithm. Dig Dis Sci. 2016;61(7):2132–9. https://doi.org/10.1007/s10620–016–4042–4.
13. Keir ME, Butte MJ, Freeman GJ, Sharpe AH. PD-1 and its ligands in tolerance and immunity. Ann Rev Immunol. 2008;26:677–704.
14. McDermott DF, Atkins MB. PD-1 as a potential target in cancer therapy. Cancer Med. 2013;2(5):662–73. https://doi.org/10.1002/cam4.106.
15. Topalian SL, Hodi FS, Brahmer JR, Gettinger SN, Smith DC, McDermott DF, et al. Safety, activity, and immune correlates of anti-PD-1 antibody in cancer. N Engl J Med. 2012;366(26):2443–54. https://doi.org/10.1056/NEJMoa1200690.
16. Hamid O, Robert C, Daud A, Hodi FS, Hwu WJ, Kefford R, et al. Safety and tumor responses with lambrolizumab (anti-PD-1) in melanoma. N Engl J Med. 2013;369(2):134–44. https://doi.org/10.1056/NEJMoa1305133.
17. Ribas A, Hamid O, Daud A, Hodi FS, Wolchok JD, Kefford R, et al. Association of pembrolizumab with tumor response and survival among patients with advanced melanoma. JAMA. 2016;315(15):1600–9. https://doi.org/10.1001/jama.2016.4059.
18. Gonzalez RS, Salaria SN, Bohannon CD, Huber AR, Feely MM, Shi C. PD-1 inhibitor gastroenterocolitis: case series and appraisal of 'immunomodulatory gastroenterocolitis'. Histopathology. 2017;70(4):558–67. https://doi.org/10.1111/his.13118.
19. Weidner AS, Panarelli NC, Geyer JT, Bhavsar EB, Furman RR, Leonard JP, et al. Idelalisib-associated colitis. Am J Surg Pathol. 2015;39(12):1661–7. https://doi.org/10.1097/PAS.0000000000000522.
20. Louie CY, Dimaio MA, Matsukuma KE, Coutre SE, Berry GJ, Longacre TA. Idelalisib-associated enterocolitis. Am J Surg Pathol. 2015;39(12):1653–60. https://doi.org/10.1097/PAS.0000000000000525.
21. Nguyen T, Park JY, Scudiere JR, Montgomery E. Mycophenolic acid (cellcept and myofortic) induced injury of the upper gi tract. Am J Surg Pathol. 2009;33(9):1355–63. https://doi.org/10.1097/PAS.0b013e3181a755bd.
22. Iacobuzio-Donahue CA, Lee EL, Abraham SC, Yardley JH, Wu TT. Colchicine toxicity: distinct morphologic findings in gastrointestinal biopsies. Am J Surg Pathol. 2001;25(8):1067–73. https://doi.org/10.1097/00000478–200108000–00012.
23. Al-Daraji WI, Al-Mahmoud RM, Ilyas M. Gastric changes following colchicine therapy in patients with FMF. Dig Dis Sci. 2008;53(8):2079–82. https://doi.org/10.1007/s10620–007–0132–7.
24. Torbenson M, Montgomery EA, Iacobuzio-Donahue C, Yardley JH, Wu TT, Abraham SC. Colchicine effect in a colonic hyperplastic polyp: a lesion mimicking serrated adenoma. Arch Pathol Lab Med. 2002;126(5):615–7.
25. Daniels JA, Gibson MK, Xu L, Sun S, Canto MI, Heath E, et al. Gastrointestinal tract epithelial changes associated with taxanes: marker of drug toxicity versus effect. Am J Surg Pathol. 2008;32(3):473–7. https://doi.org/10.1097/PAS.0b013e3181582331.
26. Jonassaint NL, Guo N, Califano JA, Montgomery EA, Armanios M. The gastrointestinal manifestations of telomere-mediated disease. Aging Cell. 2013;12(2):319–23. https://doi.org/10.1111/acel.12041.
27. Kakar S, Nehra V, Murray JA, Dayharsh GA, Burgart LJ. Significance of intraepithelial lymphocytosis in small bowel biopsy samples with normal mucosal architecture. Am J Gastroenterol. 2003;98(9):2027–33. https://doi.org/10.1111/j.1572–0241.2003.07631.x.
28. Lim LC, Gibbs P, Yip D, Shapiro JD, Dowling R, Smith D, et al. A prospective evaluation of treatment with selective internal radiation therapy (SIR-spheres) in patients with unresectable liver metastases from colorectal cancer previously treated with 5-FU based chemotherapy. BMC Cancer. 2005;5 https://doi.org/10.1186/1471–2407–5–132.
29. Ogawa F, Mino-Kenudson M, Shimizu M, Ligato S, Lauwers GY. Gastroduodenitis associated with yttrium 90-microsphere selective internal radiation: an iatrogenic complication in need of recognition. Arch Pathol Lab Med. 2008;132(11):1734–8. https://doi.org/10.1043/1543–2165–132.11.1734.
30. Crowder CD, Grabowski C, Inampudi S, Sielaff T, Sherman CA, Batts KP. Selective internal radiation therapy-induced extrahepatic injury an emerging cause of iatrogenic organ damage. Am J Surg Pathol. 2009;33(7):963–75. https://doi.org/10.1097/PAS.0b013e31817ed787.
31. Konda A, Savin MA, Cappell MS, Duffy MC. Radiation microsphere-induced GI ulcers after selective internal radiation therapy for hepatic tumors: an underrecognized clinical entity. Gastrointest Endosc. 2009;70(3):561–7. https://doi.org/10.1016/j.gie.2009.03.015.
32. Rothenberg ME, Araya H, Longacre TA, Pasricha PJ. Lanthanum-induced gastrointestinal histiocytosis. ACG Case Rep J. 2015;2:187–9.
33. Haratake J, Yasunaga C, Ootani A, Shimajiri S, Matsuyama A, Hisaoka M. Peculiar histiocytic lesions with massive lanthanum deposition in dialysis patients treated with lanthanum carbonate. Am J Surg Pathol. 2015;39(6):767–71. https://doi.org/10.1097/pas.0000000000000385.
34. Hoda RS, Sanyal S, Abraham JL, Everett JM, Hundemer GL, Yee E, et al. Lanthanum deposition from oral lanthanum carbonate in the upper gastrointestinal tract. Histopathology. 2017;70(7):1072–8. https://doi.org/10.1111/his.13178.
35. Davis RL, Abraham JL. Lanthanum deposition in a dialysis patient. Nephrol Dial Transplant. 2009;24(10):3247–50. https://doi.org/10.1093/ndt/gfp364.
36. Hochter W, Weingart J, Seib HJ, Ottenjann R. Duodenal polyps. Deutsche Medizinische Wochenschrift. 1984;109(31–32):1183–6.
37. Reddy RR, Schuman BM, Priest RJ. Duodenal polyps: diagnosis and management. J Clin Gastroenterol. 1981;3(2):139–45.
38. Jepsen JM, Persson M, Jakobsen NO, Christiansen T, Skoubo-Kristensen E, Funch-Jensen P, et al. Prospective study of prevalence

and endoscopic and histopathologic characteristics of duodenal polyps in patients submitted to upper endoscopy. Scand J Gastroenterol. 1994;29(6):483–7. https://doi.org/10.3109/00365529409092458.
39. Syngal S, Brand RE, Church JM, Giardiello FM, Hampel HL, Burt RW. ACG clinical guideline: genetic testing and management of hereditary gastrointestinal cancer syndromes. Am J Gastroenterol. 2015;110(2):223–62. https://doi.org/10.1038/ajg.2014.435.
40. Brosens LAA, van Hattem WA, Jansen M, de Leng WWJ, Giardiello FM, Offerhaus GJA. Gastrointestinal polyposis syndromes. Curr Mol Med. 2007;7(1):29–46. https://doi.org/10.2174/156652407779940404.
41. Latchford AR, Phillips RKS. Gastrointestinal polyps and cancer in Peutz-Jeghers syndrome: clinical aspects. Fam Cancer. 2011;10(3):455–61. https://doi.org/10.1007/s10689-011-9442-1.
42. Westerman AM, Entius MM, De Baar E, Boor PPC, Koole R, Van Velthuysen MLF, et al. Peutz-Jeghers syndrome: 78-year follow-up of the original family. Lancet. 1999;353(9160):1211–5. https://doi.org/10.1016/S0140-6736(98)08018-0.
43. Shaco-Levy R, Jasperson KW, Martin K, Samadder NJ, Burt RW, Ying J, et al. Morphologic characterization of hamartomatous gastrointestinal polyps in Cowden syndrome, Peutz-Jeghers syndrome, and juvenile polyposis syndrome. Hum Pathol. 2016;49:39–48. https://doi.org/10.1016/j.humpath.2015.10.002.
44. Shepherd NA, Bussey HJR, Jass JR. Epithelial misplacement in Peutz-Jeghers polyps. A diagnostic pitfall. Am J Surg Pathol. 1987;11(10):743–9.
45. Van Lier MGF, Westerman AM, Wagner A, Looman CWN, Wilson JHP, De Rooij FWM, et al. High cancer risk and increased mortality in patients with Peutz—Jeghers syndrome. Gut. 2011;60(2):141–7. https://doi.org/10.1136/gut.2010.223750.
46. Giardiello FM, Brensinger JD, Tersmette AC, Goodman SN, Petersen GM, Booker SV, et al. Very high risk of cancer in familial Peutz-Jeghers syndrome. Gastroenterology. 2000;119(6):1447–53. https://doi.org/10.1053/gast.2000.20228.
47. Rosty C, Buchanan DD, Walters RJ, Carr NJ, Bothman JW, Young JP, et al. Hyperplastic polyp of the duodenum: a report of 9 cases with immunohistochemical and molecular findings. Hum Pathol. 2011;42(12):1953–9. https://doi.org/10.1016/j.humpath.2011.02.018.
48. Roche HJ, Carr NJ, Laing H, Bateman AC. Hyperplastic polyps of the duodenum: an unusual histological finding. J Clin Pathol. 2006;59(12):1305–6. https://doi.org/10.1136/jcp.2005.035022.
49. Franzin G, Novelli P, Fratton A. Hyperplastic and metaplastic polyps of the duodenum. Gastrointest Endosc. 1983;29(2):140–2. https://doi.org/10.1016/S0016-5107(83)72560-5.
50. Genta RM, Kinsey RS, Singhal A, Suterwala S. Gastric foveolar metaplasia and gastric heterotopia in the duodenum: no evidence of an etiologic role for Helicobacter pylori. Hum Pathol. 2010;41(11):1593–600. https://doi.org/10.1016/j.humpath.2010.04.010.
51. Hoedemaeker PJ. Heterotopic gastric mucosa in the duodenum. Digestion. 1970;3(3):165–73. https://doi.org/10.1159/000197027.
52. Johansen A, Hansen OH. Heterotopic gastric epithelium in the duodenum and its correlation to gastric disease and acid level. Acta Pathol Microbiol Scand A Pathol. 1973;81(5):676–80.
53. Yu L, Yang Y, Cui L, Peng L, Sun G. Heterotopic gastric mucosa of the gastrointestinal tract: prevalence, histological features, and clinical characteristics. Scand J Gastroenterol. 2014;49(2):138–44. https://doi.org/10.3109/00365521.2013.860558.
54. Vizcarrondo FJ, Wang TY, Brady PG. Heterotopic gastric mucosa: presentation as a rugose duodenal mass. Gastrointest Endosc. 1983;29(2):107–11.
55. James AH. Gastric epithelium in the duodenum. Gut. 1964;5:285–94.
56. Lessells AM, Martin DF. Heterotopic gastric mucosa in the duodenum. J Clin Pathol. 1982;35(6):591–5.
57. Terada T. Pathologic observations of the duodenum in 615 consecutive duodenal specimens: I. benign lesions. Int J Clin Exp Pathol. 2012;5(1):46–51.
58. Graham DY. Campylobacter pylori and peptic ulcer disease. Gastroenterology. 1989;96(2 Pt 2 Suppl):615–25.
59. Nakagawa M, Kitazawa R, Kondo T, Ninomiya K, Okita M, Haraguchi R, et al. Duodenal gastric heterotopia, sporadic or fundic gland polyp-associated, frequently carries beta-catenin mutation. Virchows Arch. 2014;465(3):253–6. https://doi.org/10.1007/s00428-014-1612-8.
60. Matsubara A, Ogawa R, Suzuki H, Oda I, Taniguchi H, Kanai Y, et al. Activating GNAS and KRAS mutations in gastric foveolar metaplasia, gastric heterotopia, and adenocarcinoma of the duodenum. Br J Cancer. 2015;112(8):1398–404. https://doi.org/10.1038/bjc.2015.104.
61. Conlon N, Logan E, Veerappan S, McKiernan S, O'Briain S. Duodenal gastric heterotopia: further evidence of an association with fundic gland polyps. Hum Pathol. 2013;44(4):636–42. https://doi.org/10.1016/j.humpath.2012.07.014.
62. Kushima R, Rüthlein HJ, Stolte M, Bamba M, Hattori T, Borchard F. 'Pyloric gland-type adenoma' arising in heterotopic gastric mucosa of the duodenum, with dysplastic progression of the gastric type. Virchows Archiv. 1999;435(4):452–7. https://doi.org/10.1007/s004280050425.
63. Chen ZM, Scudiere JR, Abraham SC, Montgomery E. Pyloric gland adenoma: an entity distinct from gastric foveolar type adenoma. Am J Surg Pathol. 2009;33(2):186–93. https://doi.org/10.1097/PAS.0b013e31817d7ff4.
64. Lai ECS, Tompkins RK. Heterotopic pancreas. Review of a 26 year experience. Am J Surg. 1986;151(6):697–700. https://doi.org/10.1016/0002-9610(86)90045-0.
65. Distler M, Ruckert F, Aust D, Saeger HD, Grutzmann R. Pancreatic heterotopia of the duodenum: anatomic anomaly or clinical challenge? J Gastrointest Surg. 2011;15(4):631–6. https://doi.org/10.1007/s11605-011-1420-2.
66. Betzler A, Mees ST, Pump J, Scholch S, Zimmermann C, Aust DE, et al. Clinical impact of duodenal pancreatic heterotopia—Is there a need for surgical treatment? BMC Surg. 2017;17(1):53. https://doi.org/10.1186/s12893-017-0250-x.
67. Becker V, Mischke U. Groove pancreatitis. Int J Pancreatol. 1991;10(3–4):173–82.
68. Kloppel G. Chronic pancreatitis, pseudotumors and other tumor-like lesions. Mod Pathol. 2007;20(Suppl 1):S113–31. https://doi.org/10.1038/modpathol.3800690.
69. DeSouza K, Nodit L. Groove pancreatitis: a brief review of a diagnostic challenge. Arch Pathol Lab Med. 2015;139(3):417–21. https://doi.org/10.5858/arpa.2013-0597-RS.
70. Zhang L, Sanderson SO, Lloyd RV, Smyrk TC. Pancreatic intraepithelial neoplasia in heterotopic pancreas: evidence for the progression model of pancreatic ductal adenocarcinoma. Am J Surg Pathol. 2007;31(8):1191–5. https://doi.org/10.1097/PAS.0b013e31806841e1.
71. Cates JM, Williams TL, Suriawinata AA. Intraductal papillary mucinous adenoma that arises from pancreatic heterotopia within a meckel diverticulum. Arch Pathol Lab Med. 2005;129(3):e67–9. https://doi.org/10.1043/1543-2165(2005)129<e67:IPMATA>2.0.CO;2.
72. Naqvi A, de la Roza G. Borderline mucinous cystic tumor in jejunal pancreatic heterotopia. Ann Diagn Pathol. 2004;8(3):151–5.
73. Guillou L, Nordback P, Gerbet C, Schneider RP. Ductal adenocarcinoma arising in a heterotopic pancreas situated in a hiatal hernia. Arch Pathol Lab Med. 1994;118(5):568–71.
74. Makhlouf HR, Almeida JL, Sobin LH. Carcinoma in jejunal pancreatic heterotopia. Arch Pathol Lab Med. 1999;123(8):707–11.
75. Fukino N, Oida T, Mimatsu K, Kuboi Y, Kida K. Adenocarcinoma arising from heterotopic pancreas at the third portion of the duodenum. World J Gastroenterol. 2015;21(13):4082–8. https://doi.org/10.3748/wjg.v21.i13.4082.
76. Ginori A, Vassallo L, Butorano MA, Bettarini F, Di Mare G, Marrelli D. Pancreatic adenocarcinoma in duodenal ectopic pancreas: a case report and review of the literature. Pathologica. 2013;105(2):56–8.

77. Kang JY, Wu AY, Chia JL, Wee A, Sutherland IH, Hori R. Clinical and ultrastructural studies in duodenal pseudomelanosis. Gut. 1987;28(12):1673–81.
78. Giusto D, Jakate S. Pseudomelanosis duodeni: associated with multiple clinical conditions and unpredictable iron stainability—A case series. Endoscopy. 2008;40(2):165–7. https://doi.org/10.1055/s-2007-995472.
79. Pueblitz S, Squires RH, Timmons CF. Pseudomelanosis duodeni in an adolescent male: case report and review of the literature. Pediatr Pathol Lab Med. 1997;17(1):115–23.
80. Weinstock LB, Katzman D, Wang HL. Pseudomelanosis of stomach, duodenum, and jejunum. Gastrointest Endosc. 2003;58(4):578.
81. Rustagi T, Mansoor MS, Gibson JA, Kapadia CR. Pseudomelanosis of stomach, duodenum, and jejunum. J Clin Gastroenterol. 2015;49(2):124–6. https://doi.org/10.1097/mcg.0000000000000081.
82. Sunkara T, Caughey ME, Gaduputi V. Rare finding of concomitant pseudomelanosis of stomach and duodenum; case report and literature review. Gastroenterol Hepatol from bed to bench. 2018;11(1):86–9.
83. Bisordi WM, Kleinman MS. Melanosis duodeni. Gastrointest Endosc. 1976;23(1):37–8.
84. Breslaw L. Melanosis of the duodenal mucosa. Gastrointest Endosc. 1980;26(2):45–6.
85. Ghadially FN, Walley VM. Pigments of the gastrointestinal tract: a comparison of light microscopic and electron microscopic findings. Ultrastruct Pathol. 1995;19(4):213–9.
86. Pounder DJ, Ghadially FN, Mukherjee TM, Hecker R, Rowland R, Dixon B, et al. Ultrastructure and electron-probe x-ray analysis of the pigment in melanosis duodeni. J Submicrosc Cytol. 1982;14(2):389–400.
87. Steckman M, Bozymski EM. Hemosiderosis of the duodenum. Gastrointest Endosc. 1983;29(4):326–7.
88. Leong S. Pseudomelanosis duodeni and the controversial pigment—a clinical study of 4 cases. Ann Acad Med Singap. 1992;21(3):394–8.
89. Kim J, Hwang JK, Choi WS, Lee BJ, Park JJ, Kim JS, et al. Pseudomelanosis ilei associated with ingestion of charcoal: case report and review of literature. Dig Endosc. 2010;22(1):56–8. https://doi.org/10.1111/j.1443-1661.2009.00919.x.
90. Kim SY, Koo JS, Hynun JJ, Jung SW, Choung RS, Yim HJ, et al. Charcoal-induced pseudomelanosis ilei. Endoscopy. 2011;43(Suppl 2 UCTN):E380. https://doi.org/10.1055/s-0030-1257042.
91. Albuquerque A. Nodular lymphoid hyperplasia in the gastrointestinal tract in adult patients: a review. World J Gastrointest Endosc. 2014;6(11):534–40. https://doi.org/10.4253/wjge.v6.i11.534.
92. Colon AR, DiPalma JS, Leftridge CA. Intestinal lymphonodular hyperplasia of childhood: patterns of presentation. J Clin Gastroenterol. 1991;13(2):163–6.
93. Mansueto P, Iacono G, Seidita A, D'Alcamo A, Sprini D, Carroccio A. Review article: intestinal lymphoid nodular hyperplasia in children—the relationship to food hypersensitivity. Aliment Pharmacol Ther. 2012;35(9):1000–9. https://doi.org/10.1111/j.1365-2036.2012.05062.x.
94. Ranchod M, Lewin KJ, Dorfman RF. Lymphoid hyperplasia of the gastrointestinal tract. A study of 26 cases and review of the literature. Am J Surg Pathol. 1978;2(4):383–400.
95. Ward H, Jalan KN, Maitra TK, Agarwal SK, Mahalanabis D. Small intestinal nodular lymphoid hyperplasia in patients with giardiasis and normal serum immunoglobulins. Gut. 1983;24(2):120–6.
96. Washington K, Stenzel TT, Buckley RH, Gottfried MR. Gastrointestinal pathology in patients with common variable immunodeficiency and X-linked agammaglobulinemia. Am J Surg Pathol. 1996;20(10):1240–52.
97. Daniels JA, Lederman HM, Maitra A, Montgomery EA. Gastrointestinal tract pathology in patients with common variable immunodeficiency (CVID): a clinicopathologic study and review. Am J Surg Pathol. 2007;31(12):1800–12. https://doi.org/10.1097/PAS.0b013e3180cab60c.
98. Khuroo MS, Khuroo NS, Khuroo MS. Diffuse duodenal nodular lymphoid hyperplasia: a large cohort of patients etiologically related to Helicobacter pylori infection. BMC Gastroenterol. 2011;11:36. https://doi.org/10.1186/1471-230x-11-36.
99. Elkholy S, Mogawer S, Farag A. Nodular lymphoid hyperplasia of the gastrointestinal tract: a comprehensive review. Acta Gastroenterol Belg. 2017;80(3):405–10.
100. Rubio-Tapia A, Hernandez-Calleros J, Trinidad-Hernandez S, Uscanga L. Clinical characteristics of a group of adults with nodular lymphoid hyperplasia: a single center experience. World J Gastroenterol. 2006;12(12):1945–8.
101. Rambaud JC, De Saint-Louvent P, Marti R, Galian A, Mason DY, Wassef M, et al. Diffuse follicular lymphoid hyperplasia of the small intestine without primary immunoglobulin deficiency. Am J Med. 1982;73(1):125–32.
102. Matuchansky C, Morichau-Beauchant M, Touchard G, Lenormand Y, Bloch P, Tanzer J, et al. Nodular lymphoid hyperplasia of the small bowel associated with primary jejunal malignant lymphoma. Evidence favoring a cytogenetic relationship. Gastroenterology. 1980;78(6):1587–92.
103. Sharma M, Goyal A, Ecka RS. An unusual cause of recurrent diarrhea with small intestinal "polyposis". Nodular lymphoid hyperplasia of the small intestine. Gastroenterology. 2012;142(7):e8–9. https://doi.org/10.1053/j.gastro.2011.11.053.
104. Schmatz AI, Streubel B, Kretschmer-Chott E, Püspök A, Jäger U, Mannhalter C, et al. Primary follicular lymphoma of the duodenum is a distinct mucosal/submucosal variant of follicular lymphoma: a retrospective study of 63 cases. J Clin Oncol. 2011;29(11):1445–51. https://doi.org/10.1200/JCO.2010.32.9193.
105. Swerdlow SH, Campo E, Pileri SA, Harris NL, Stein H, Siebert R, et al. The 2016 revision of the World Health Organization classification of lymphoid neoplasms. Blood. 2016;127(20):2375–90. https://doi.org/10.1182/blood-2016-01-643569.
106. Lamers CB, Wagener T, Assmann KJ, van Tongeren JH. Jejunal lymphoma in a patient with primary adult-onset hypogammaglobulinemia and nodular lymphoid hyperplasia of the small intestine. Dig Dis Sci. 1980;25(7):553–7.
107. Matuchansky C, Touchard G, Lemaire M, Babin P, Demeocq F, Fonck Y, et al. Malignant lymphoma of the small bowel associated with diffuse nodular lymphoid hyperplasia. N Engl J Med. 1985;313(3):166–71. https://doi.org/10.1056/nejm198507183130307.
108. Franzin G, Musola R, Ghidini O, Manfrini C, Fratton A. Nodular hyperplasia of Brunner's glands. Gastrointest Endosc. 1985;31(6):374–8.
109. El Faleh I, Lutz N, Osterheld MC, Reinberg O, Nydegger A. Gastric outlet obstruction by Brunner's gland hyperplasia in an 8-year-old child. J Pediatr Surg. 2009;44(4):E21–4. https://doi.org/10.1016/j.jpedsurg.2009.01.075.
110. Levine JA, Burgart LJ, Batts KP, Wang KK. Brunner's gland hamartomas: clinical presentation and pathological features of 27 cases. Am J Gastroenterol. 1995;90(2):290–4.
111. Kim K, Jang SJ, Song HJ, Yu E. Clinicopathologic characteristics and mucin expression in Brunner's gland proliferating lesions. Dig Dis Sci. 2013;58(1):194–201. https://doi.org/10.1007/s10620-012-2320-5.
112. Paimela H, Tallgren LG, Stenman S, von Numers H, Scheinin TM. Multiple duodenal polyps in uraemia: a little known clinical entity. Gut. 1984;25(3):259–63.
113. Khanna M, Ramanathan S, Ahmed A, Kumar D. Gastroduodenal intussusception secondary to a pedunculated Brunner's gland hamartoma: CT and endoscopic features. J Gastrointest Cancer. 2014;45(Suppl 1):257–60. https://doi.org/10.1007/s12029-014-9656-1.

114. Kibria R, Ali SA, Butt S, Akram S. Biliary obstruction and pancreatitis caused by diffuse nodular hyperplasia of Brunner's gland. J Gastrointest Cancer. 2009;40(3–4):128–30. https://doi.org/10.1007/s12029-009-9090-y.
115. Varnholt H, Gang DL, Desilets DJ, Pantanowitz L. Brunner gland cyst. Int J Surg Pathol. 2007;15(1):64–5. https://doi.org/10.1177/1066896906296001.
116. Park BJ, Kim MJ, Lee JH, Park SS, Sung DJ, Cho SB. Cystic Brunner's gland hamartoma in the duodenum: a case report. World J Gastroenterol. 2009;15(39):4980–3.
117. Goldman RL. Hamartomatous polyp of Brunner's glands. Gastroenterology. 1963;44:57–62.
118. Sakurai T, Sakashita H, Honjo G, Kasyu I, Manabe T. Gastric foveolar metaplasia with dysplastic changes in Brunner gland hyperplasia: possible precursor lesions for Brunner gland adenocarcinoma. Am J Surg Pathol. 2005;29(11):1442–8.
119. Fujimaki E, Nakamura S, Sugai T, Takeda Y. Brunner's gland adenoma with a focus of p53-positive atypical glands. J Gastroenterol. 2000;35(2):155–8.
120. Faller G, Kirchner T. Low-grade intraepithelial neoplasia of Brunner's gland. Histopathology. 2005;47(1):118–9. https://doi.org/10.1111/j.1365-2559.2005.02066.x.
121. Brookes MJ, Manjunatha S, Allen CA, Cox M. Malignant potential in a Brunner's gland hamartoma. Postgrad Med J. 2003;79(933):416–7.
122. Koizumi M, Sata N, Yoshizawa K, Kurihara K, Yasuda Y. Carcinoma arising from Brunner's gland in the duodenum after 17 years of observation—A case report and literature review. Case Rep Gastroenterol. 2007;1(1):103–9. https://doi.org/10.1159/000108944.
123. Ohta Y, Saitoh K, Akai T, Uesato M, Ochiai T, Matsubara H. Early primary duodenal carcinoma arising from Brunner's glands synchronously occurring with sigmoid colon carcinoma: report of a case. Surg Today. 2008;38(8):756–60. https://doi.org/10.1007/s00595-007-3707-1.
124. Mekaroonkamol P, Cohen R, Chawla S. Portal hypertensive enteropathy. World J Hepatol. 2015;7(2):127–38. https://doi.org/10.4254/wjh.v7.i2.127.
125. Jeon SR, Kim JO, Kim JB, Ye BD, Chang DK, Shim KN, et al. Portal hypertensive enteropathy diagnosed by capsule endoscopy in cirrhotic patients: a nationwide multicenter study. Dig Dis Sci. 2014;59(5):1036–41. https://doi.org/10.1007/s10620-014-3036-3.
126. Lemmers A, Evrard S, Demetter P, Verset G, Gossum AV, Adler M, et al. Gastrointestinal polypoid lesions: a poorly known endoscopic feature of portal hypertension. United European Gastroenterol J. 2014;2(3):189–96. https://doi.org/10.1177/2050640614529108.
127. Gurung A, Jaffe PE, Zhang X. Duodenal polyposis secondary to portal hypertensive duodenopathy. World J Gastrointest Endosc. 2015;7(17):1257–61. https://doi.org/10.4253/wjge.v7.i17.1257.
128. De Palma GD, Rega M, Masone S, Persico F, Siciliano S, Patrone F, et al. Mucosal abnormalities of the small bowel in patients with cirrhosis and portal hypertension: a capsule endoscopy study. Gastrointest Endosc. 2005;62(4):529–34. https://doi.org/10.1016/S0016-5107(05)01588-9.
129. Abdelaal UM, Morita E, Nouda S, Kuramoto T, Miyaji K, Fukui H, et al. Evaluation of portal hypertensive enteropathy by scoring with capsule endoscopy: is transient elastography of clinical impact? J Clin Biochem Nutr. 2010;47(1):37–44. https://doi.org/10.3164/jcbn.10-14.
130. Kodama M, Uto H, Numata M, Hori T, Murayama T, Sasaki F, et al. Endoscopic characterization of the small bowel in patients with portal hypertension evaluated by double balloon endoscopy. J Gastroenterol. 2008;43(8):589–96. https://doi.org/10.1007/s00535-008-2198-1.
131. Misra V, Misra SP, Dwivedi M, Gupta SC. Histomorphometric study of portal hypertensive enteropathy. Am J Clin Pathol. 1997;108(6):652–7.
132. Barakat M, Mostafa M, Mahran Z, Soliman AG. Portal hypertensive duodenopathy: clinical, endoscopic, and histopathologic profiles. Am J Gastroenterol. 2007;102(12):2793–802. https://doi.org/10.1111/j.1572-0241.2007.01536.x.
133. Jackson CS, Strong R. Gastrointestinal angiodysplasia: diagnosis and management. Gastrointest Endosc Clin N Am. 2017;27(1):51–62. https://doi.org/10.1016/j.giec.2016.08.012.
134. DeBenedet AT, Saini SD, Takami M, Fisher LR. Do clinical characteristics predict the presence of small bowel angioectasias on capsule endoscopy? Dig Dis Sci. 2011;56(6):1776–81. https://doi.org/10.1007/s10620-010-1506-9.
135. Dai C, Liu WX, Jiang M, Sun MJ. Endoscopic variceal ligation compared with endoscopic injection sclerotherapy for treatment of esophageal variceal hemorrhage: a meta-analysis. World J Gastroenterol. 2015;21(8):2534–41. https://doi.org/10.3748/wjg.v21.i8.2534.

Part V

Non-neoplastic Diseases of the Jejunum and Ileum

Inflammatory Bowel Disease

13

Lizhi Zhang

Introduction

Inflammatory bowel disease (IBD) consists of two different diseases, Crohn's disease (CD) and ulcerative colitis (UC). Although they are considered as a group of inflammatory disorders of gastrointestinal tract, one major difference between CD and UC is small bowel involvement. Approximately 80% of patients with CD have small bowel involvement, usually in the distal ileum, with one-third of patients having ileitis exclusively, fewer patients having involvement of the proximal small bowel, and rare with isolated jejunal CD [1]. UC only involves colon, although some histological changes in upper gastrointestinal tract such as focal gastritis or diffuse chronic duodenitis have been described in rare case reports [2]. On the other hand, in about 10–20% patients with UC, inflammation can occur in the last few centimeters of terminal ileum, known as backwash ileitis, which can cause confusion with CD. This chapter will focus on CD involving small bowel. Additional information of CD will also be introduced side-by-side with UC in the colonic IBD chapter (Chap. 15).

Crohn's Disease

Definition

CD is an idiopathic chronic, transmural, and occasionally granulomatous inflammatory disorder involving entire gastrointestinal tract from mouth to perianal area, but most commonly affecting the distal small bowel and colon.

L. Zhang (✉)
Department of Laboratory Medicine and Pathology, Mayo Clinic, Rochester, MN, USA
e-mail: Zhang.Lizhi@mayo.edu

Clinical Features

CD was named after gastroenterologist Burrill Bernard Crohn, who described a series of patients with inflammation of terminal ileum with other two colleagues in 1932 [3]. Unlike UC, the clinical presentations of CD are more variable, and patients may have symptoms years before the diagnosis. The main gastrointestinal manifestations are abdominal pain, prolonged diarrhea with or without gross bleeding, and fistulas. Crampy abdominal pain is a common feature of CD, which is caused by repeated episodes of small bowel obstruction due to fibrotic strictures. The pain is usually at right lower quadrant because in majority of patients, the disease is limited to the distal ileum or ileocecum. The diarrhea fluctuates over a long period of time. Bloody diarrhea is not common in CD, although stools are frequently positive for occult blood tests. One unique feature of CD which is different from UC is transmural inflammation leading to sinus tract formation and penetration of the serosa to form fistulas. This is a chronic and indolent process that usually does not result in acute abdomen. The common fistulas found in CD are the connection between intestine and bladder (enterovesical), skin (enterocutaneous), bowel (enteroenteric), and vagina (enterovaginal), and the clinical manifestations of the fistulas depend upon the type and area of involvement. The cumulative risk of any type of fistula in CD is 33% after 10 years and 50% after 20 years [4]. The non-penetrating sinus tracts can present as a phlegmon or an abscess. The disease in the terminal ileum can significantly affect bile acids absorption, leading to watery diarrhea and steatorrhea. In severe cases, malnutrition, clotting abnormalities, osteomalacia, and hypocalcemia may occur. If CD involves multiple sites of gastrointestinal tract simultaneously, patients also present with symptoms at the corresponding site, for example, gross bleeding in Crohn's colitis, odynophagia and dysphagia in esophageal involvement, or upper abdominal pain and nausea for gastroduodenal CD.

L. Zhang et al. (eds.), *Surgical Pathology of Non-neoplastic Gastrointestinal Diseases*,
https://doi.org/10.1007/978-3-030-15573-5_13

Patients with CD commonly have systemic symptoms such as fever, weight loss, and fatigue. Like UC, CD can also have a number of extraintestinal manifestations, including large joint arthritis, eye involvement (uveitis, iritis, and episcleritis), skin involvement (erythema nodosum and pyoderma gangrenosum), primary sclerosing cholangitis (PSC), pulmonary involvement (bronchiectasis, chronic bronchitis, interstitial lung disease, or bronchiolitis obliterans with organizing pneumonia), venous and arterial thromboembolism, and bone loss or osteoporosis.

Laboratory Findings

Serological studies in CD often reveal anemia, thrombocytosis, elevated white blood cell count, iron deficiency, and vitamin B12 deficiency. Erythrocyte sedimentation rate (ESR) and C-reactive protein (CRP) can be used to monitor disease activity and treatment response, to predict the course of the disease, and to subclassify patients. The tests of multiple antibodies against *saccharomyces cerevisiae* (ASCA), antineutrophil cytoplasmic antibodies (ANCA), CBir1, or OmpC have a limited role in diagnosing CD and differentiating CD from UC. If diarrhea is present, stool should be tested for enteric pathogens, parasites, and *Clostridium difficile* toxin. Fecal biomarkers (calprotectin and lactoferrin) can provide valuable information in diagnosing and monitoring CD [5].

Radiological Findings

Imaging studies can provide key information for diagnosing, assessing disease severity and extent, detecting complications, and guiding treatment of CD. Although plain abdominal radiographs are gradually being replaced by ultrasonography (US), computed tomography enterography (CTE), and magnetic resonance enterography (MRE), abdominal radiographs still serve as a first imaging tool for CD in the detection of bowel dilatation, obstruction, bowel perforation, and bowel wall thickening because of their portability, inexpensiveness, and low radiation exposure. US is able to detect small bowel CD with a sensitivity of 85% and a specificity of 98%, respectively [6]. The characteristic features of US in detecting small bowel CD are increased bowel wall thickness and vascularization, alterations in bowel wall stratification, and fibrofatty proliferation. Abdominal CTE is the most preferred first-line imaging study used in the assessment of small bowel CD with a sensitivity of 95%, which is commonly combined with ileocolonoscopy as the first-line diagnostic assessment of small bowel CD [7, 8]. MRE also has similar accuracy in detecting small bowel CD, with the advantage of avoiding radiation exposure [9]. The features of small bowel CD on CTE or MRE are segmental mural hyperenhancement and asymmetric wall thickening, bi- or trilaminar pattern of bowel wall, intramural edema, and presence of complications such as strictures and penetrations [10].

Endoscopic Findings

Enteroscopy plays a key role in managing CD because it can provide real-time viewing, biopsy abnormal mucosa or lesions, and therapies such as dilation or stent insertion. However, endoscopic assessment of small bowel CD remains challenging because of the limited accessibility, the length of the small bowel, and looping and tortuous nature of the small bowel anatomy. The distal 10–20 cm of the ileum can be accessible with ileocolonoscopy, but more proximal visualization is often limited by looping. Nowadays, the advances of endoscopic technology have extended our reach to the entire gastrointestinal tract, including double or single balloon enteroscope and spiral enteroscope. Wireless capsule endoscopy (WCE) provides another means to visualize the small bowel, and is being used increasingly for the evaluation of suspected and established small bowel CD prior to any invasive deep bowel enteroscopy, once small bowel strictures have been excluded. Recently, self-dissolving capsules have been developed which start to dissolve 30 hours after ingestion by digestive juice, and they can significantly reduce the risk of capsule retention and temporary intestinal occlusion [11]. The endoscopic findings in CD are highly variable and change with disease activity and duration. However, the characteristic features include aphthous ulcers (Fig. 13.1a), longitudinal or fissuring ulcers, cobble stone appearance, strictures, and fistulas (Fig. 13.1b) [12]. In early and mild disease, the small bowel mucosa may appear normal or only show scattered small punched-out aphthous ulcers. As disease severity increases, the aphthous ulcers coalesce into larger ulcers and eventually become linear and serpiginous. Deep ulcers and vertical fissures are commonly seen. Luminal narrowing with or without strictures and fistula formation are highly supportive of CD.

Pathological Features

Gross Findings

CD has some characteristic gross features that can help to establish the diagnosis. The most common finding of small bowel CD is long segmental strictures, associated with wall thickening, stiffness, wrapping fat, mucosal inflammation, and fistulas (Fig. 13.2a–f). Multiple short strictures can also occur, separated by uninvolved mucosa (skip lesions). The transition from normal-appearing bowel to the affect segment is abrupt. The thickened wall is firm and stiff, composed of transmural inflammation, hypertrophy of muscularis mucosae and propria, and submucosal fibrosis. Wrapping fat, or creeping fat (Fig. 13.2b), is a result of hyperplasia of the subserosal and mesenteric adipose tissue which extends from the mesenteric attachment and usually covers more than 50% of the small bowel circumference with loss of the bowel-mesentery angle. It is considered as a hallmark in CD and can be

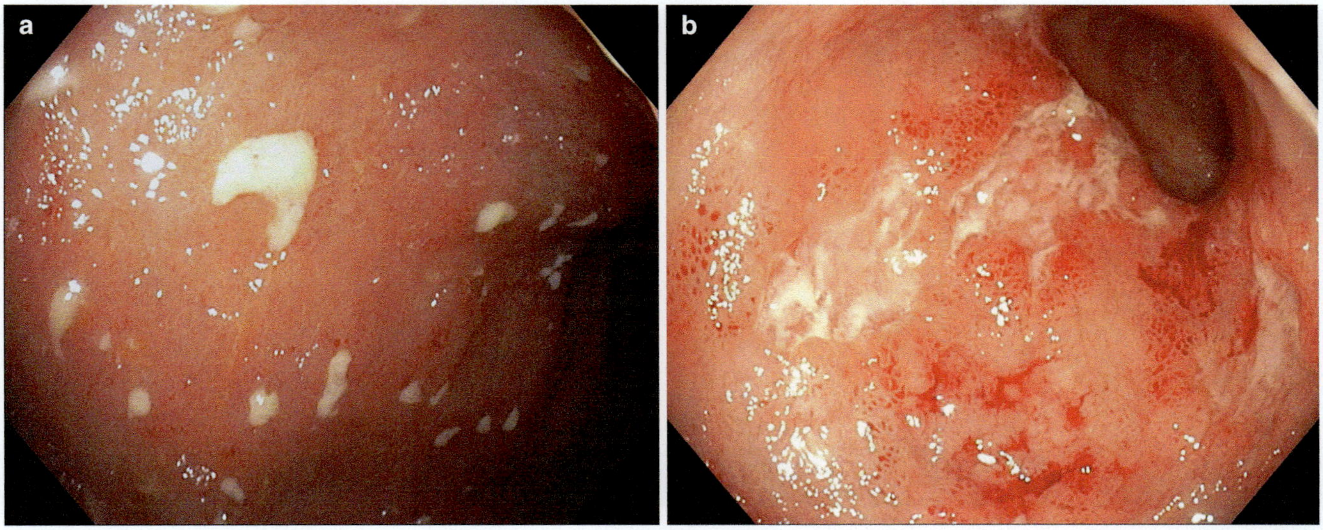

Fig. 13.1 Endoscopic features of Crohn's disease. Many small discrete aphthous ulcers in early disease (**a**); a cobble stone appearance, edema, spontaneous bleeding, and serpentine ulceration of mucosa in severe disease (**b**)

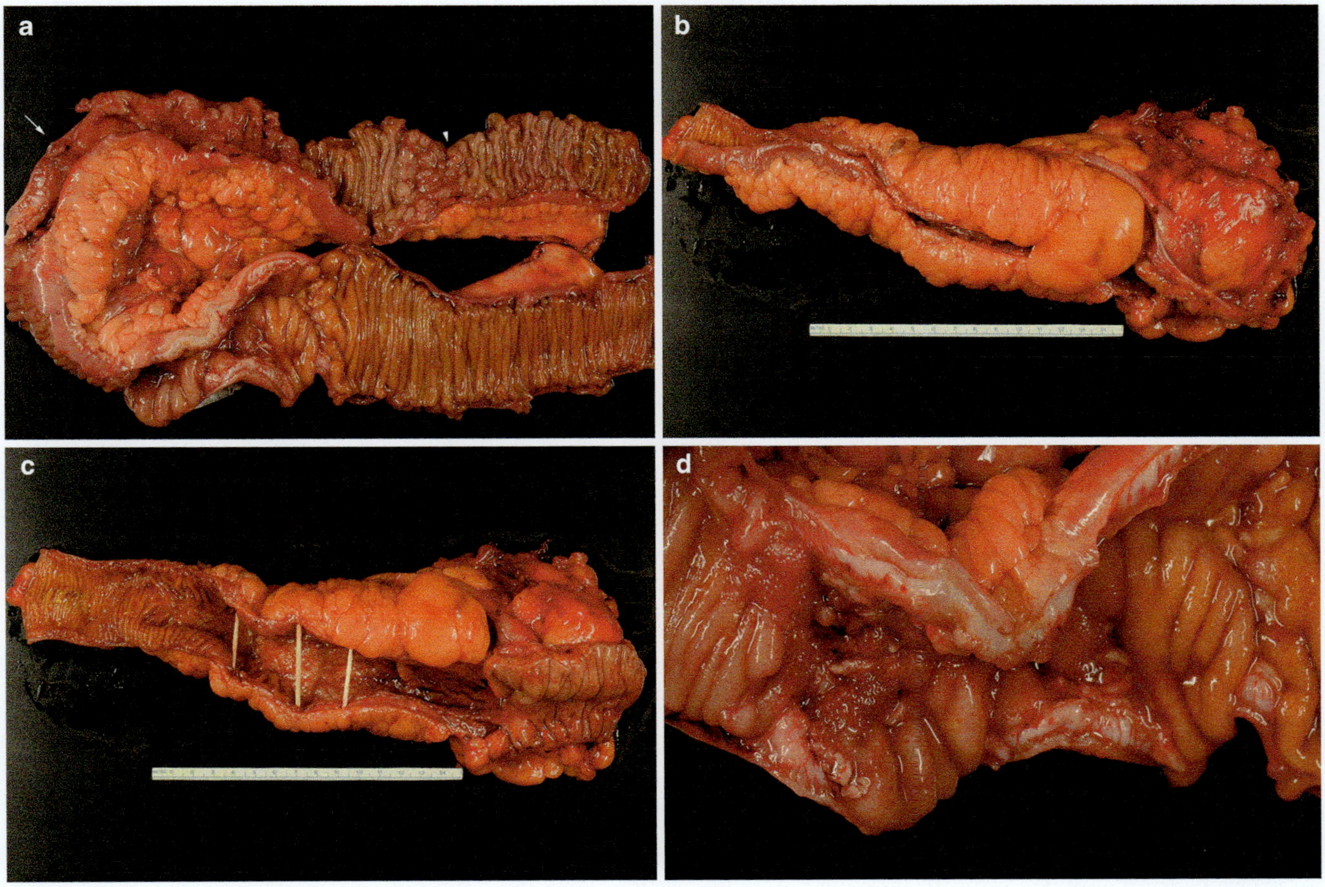

Fig. 13.2 Gross features of Crohn's disease. (**a**) a long (arrow) and a short stricture (arrowhead) separated by normal small bowel, i.e., skip areas; (**b**) stricture of terminal ileum with wrapping fat, which covers nearly the entire circumstance of the small bowel; (**c**) mucosal changes in terminal ileum, including a cobble stone appearance, bleeding, long and fissuring ulcers, and inflammatory pseudopolyp. Note the disease not involving cecum; (**d**) a close up view at stricture site. Note the wall thickening with transmural involvement, wrapping fat, deep mucosal ulceration, and adjacent unremarkable mucosa; (**e**) serpentine ulceration in mucosal changes; (**f**, **g**) ileocecal involvement with a fistula formation (arrow and probe)

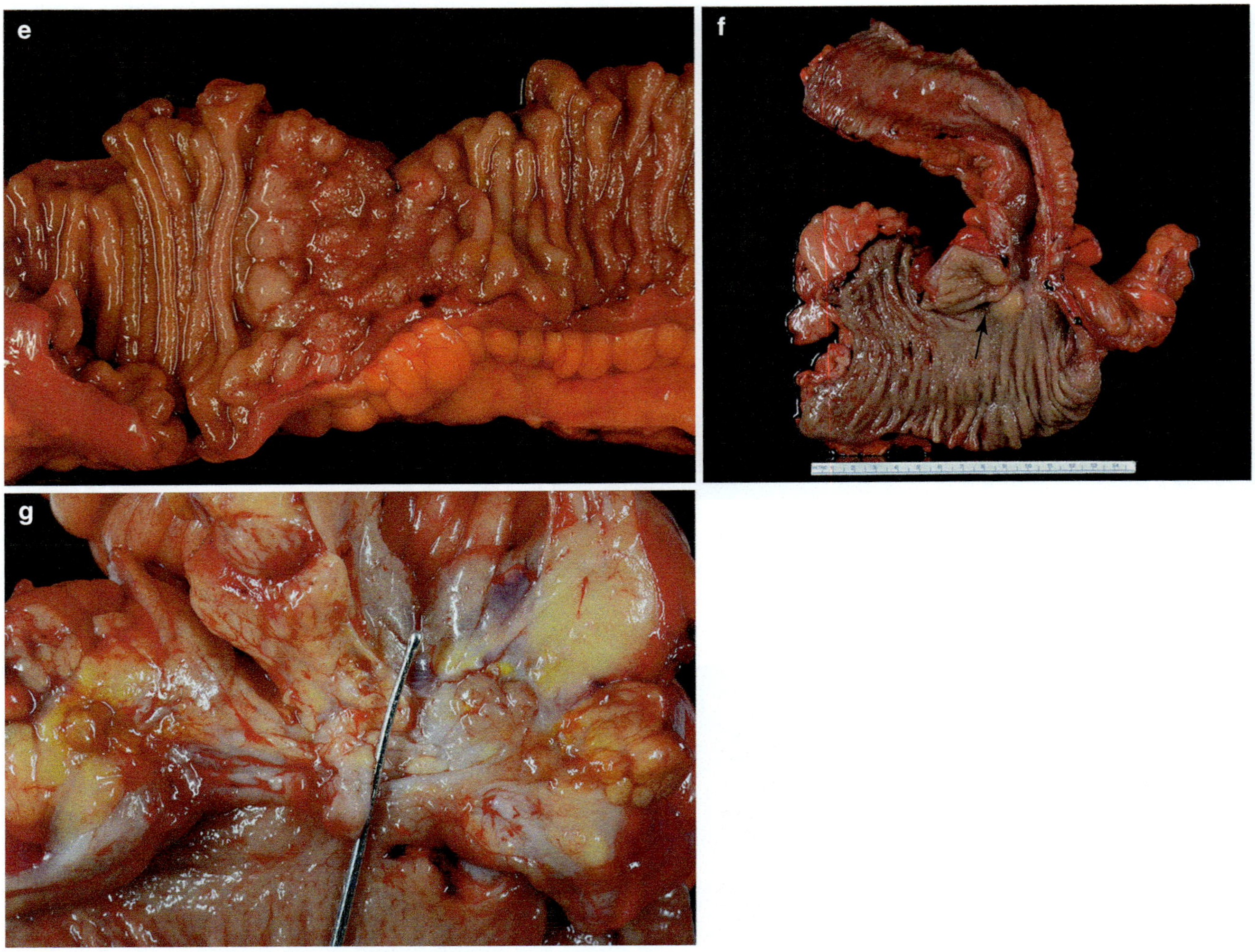

Fig. 13.2 (continued)

observed in 50–75% small bowel CD [13]. The serosa may also appear congested or fibrotic. The affected bowel loop often adheres to another segment of bowel or other organs, with or without fistula formation. Small bowel perforation is rare in CD. Abscess cavities can be found within the bowel wall or mesentery in some cases. Careful gross examination is necessary to detect these complications.

The mucosal surface shows variable changes in different disease stage and severity, but the patchy distribution pattern and sharply delineated injured areas surrounded by normal mucosa are unique in CD. The earliest mucosal change in CD is small punched-out shallow aphthous ulcers. They can also occur at a distance from the region with more obvious disease. They can range from tiny ulcers that are difficult to be found to small well-demarcated ulcer with white base. With disease progressing, the aphthous ulcers become bigger and coalesce to develop longitudinal, linear, and serpiginous ulcers (Fig. 13.2e). The patchy intervening intact mucosa with edema and submucosal damage between these ulcers gives a classic "cobblestoned" gross appearance (Fig. 13.2c). Inflammatory pseudopolyps are often present. The ulcers also deepen and become fissuring, extending to submucosa and then penetrating into or through muscularis propria. The mucosa depressions without apparent inflammatory changes represent scars of healed ulcers. Sections are usually taken every 5 cm for shorter bowel segments and every 10 cm for longer segments including the margins, in addition to other lesional areas such as strictures, fistula tracts, and polypoid or mass lesions. Sections from ileocecal valve and colon are also necessary to document colon involvement if available.

Microscopic Findings

The microscopic diagnostic features of CD in small bowel are focal transmural inflammation and lymphoid aggregates (in resection specimens), mucosal active chronic inflammation, deep or fissuring ulceration, villous architectural distortion, epithelioid granulomas, pseudopyloric metaplasia, muscular hypertrophy, and some stromal changes such as fibrosis, neural hyperplasia, or vasculitis. The distribution of these changes is patchy or segmental, which is also another feature of CD. Although it has been suggested that presence of granulomas with one other feature or presence of three features in the absence of granulomas is reliable for diagnosing CD in both biopsy and resection specimens [14], pathologists should be cautious to try to give a definitive diagnosis, especially for biopsy specimens, without correlation with clinical, endoscopic, and radiological information, because none of above features are entirely specific for CD.

Mucosal Changes In CD, the small bowel mucosa shows patchy active and chronic changes (Fig. 13.3). The active disease refers to neutrophil infiltrate, epithelial injury, erosion, and ulcerations, which can be graded as mild, moderate, and severe (Fig.13.4a–c). Neutrophils first appear in lamina propria, but the activity is more readily determined when they infiltrate in the surface and tips of the villi in mild disease. The earliest epithelial injury in CD is known as aphthous ulcer or aphthous lesion (Fig. 13.5). It is characterized by focal surface neutrophilic infiltrate and erosion, usually 1–2 mm, which is often associated with an underlying lymphoid aggregate/follicle. The mucosa adjacent to the ulcer

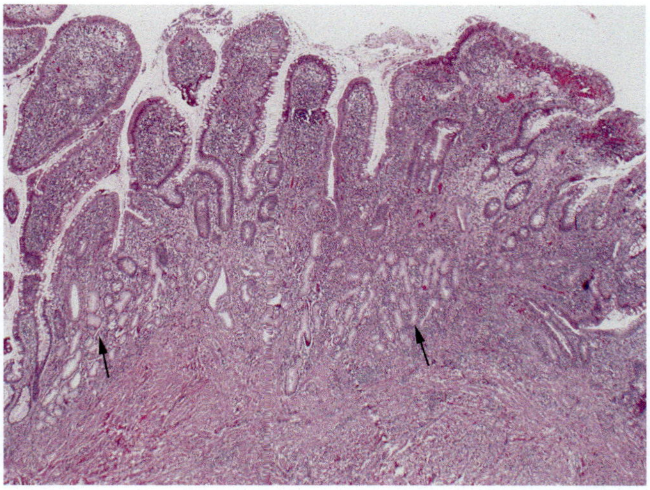

Fig. 13.3 Active chronic ileitis in Crohn's disease. The mucosal changes include increased lamina propria inflammatory infiltrate, neutrophil infiltrate, villous architectural distortion, focal erosion, and pseudopyloric metaplasia (arrows)

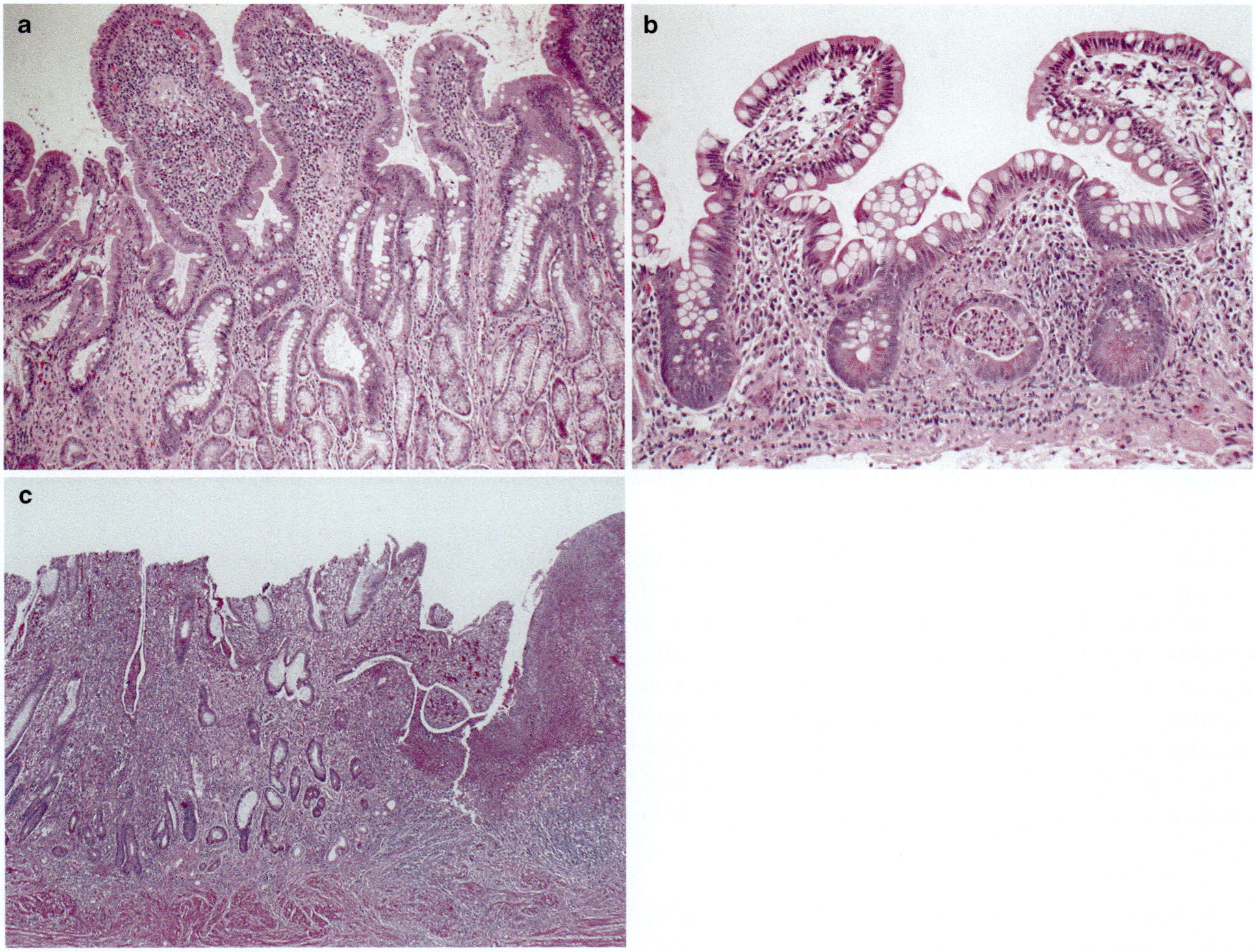

Fig. 13.4 Disease activity. (**a**) mild activity, with lamina propria expansion by mononuclear cells and eosinophils, and only focal neutrophil infiltrate in the epithelium; (**b**) moderate activity, showing more neutrophil infiltrate with cryptitis and crypt abscess; (**c**) severe activity, with marked epithelial injury, deepening and broadening ulcers

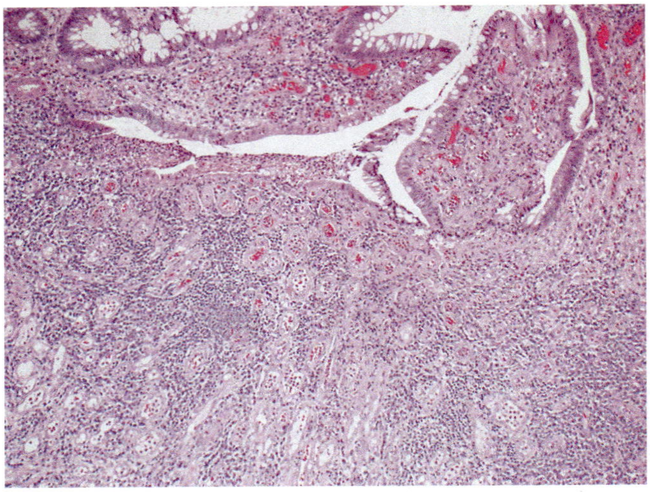

Fig. 13.5 Aphthous ulcer. Surface neutrophil infiltrate and erosion, associated with an underlying lymphoid aggregate

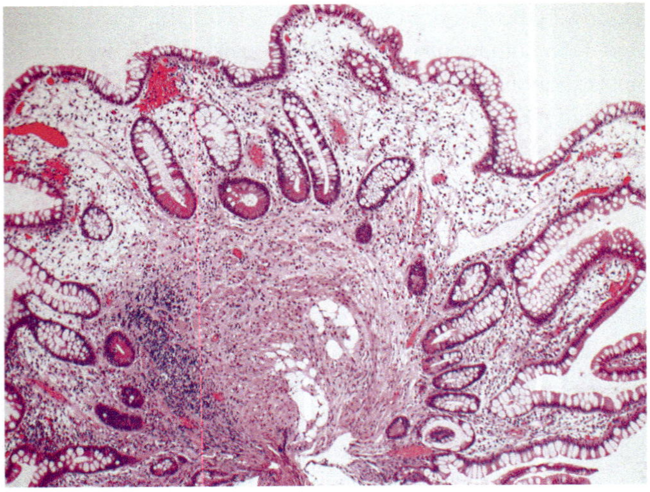

Fig. 13.6 Small bowel villous architectural distortion, characterized by shortening, broadening, and variable size and shape

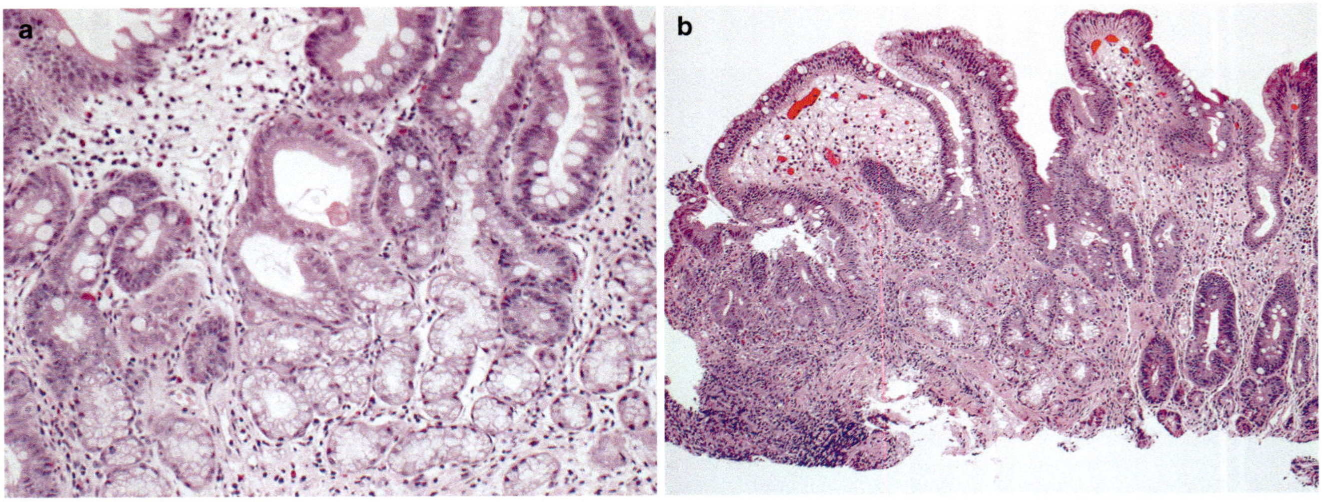

Fig. 13.7 Pseudopyloric metaplasia. (**a**) characterized by small round glands in the deep mucosa composed of cuboidal or columnar cells with abundant pale cytoplasm and small basal nuclei; (**b**) pseudopyloric metaplasia and gastric foveolar metaplasia in terminal ileum

typically shows no significant abnormalities or mild reactive changes such as mucin depletion. Of note, scattered neutrophils in intact epithelium overlying lymphoid aggregates can be observed in patients with no ileitis. In moderately active disease, neutrophil infiltrate becomes more prominent with cryptitis, occasional crypt abscesses, and focal epithelial erosion/ulceration. Most mucosal surface is involved, but ulceration is focal. Diffuse inflammatory infiltrate, epithelial loss, deep circumferential ulcers, and deep fissures are seen in severe Crohn's ileitis.

The chronicity is manifested by chronic inflammatory infiltrate, villous architectural changes, and pseudopyloric metaplasia (Fig. 13.3). The lamina propria is expanded by edema and increased inflammatory cells, mainly lymphocytes and plasma cells. Increased eosinophils and intraepithelial lymphocytes can be seen in some cases. Reactive lymphoid aggregates and follicles are common, and some can become prominent. The inflammation is not only transmucosal, but also extends into muscularis mucosae and submucosa with similar density to the inflammatory infiltrate at the upper and lower parts of the mucosa. This finding can even be appreciated in mucosal biopsy specimens, reflecting the transmural nature of the disease. The villous architecture is distorted by shortening, broadening, and variable shapes (Fig. 13.6). The mucosa can be totally flat. The crypts are hyperplastic with irregular distribution, shapes, and sizes. The muscularis mucosae are hypertrophic focally. Pseudopyloric metaplasia is a reliable marker indicating chronic mucosal injury (Fig. 13.7a). Although it is not specific for CD and can occur in other chronic conditions such as chronic infection, chronic ischemic injury, or NSAIDs-induced injury, the finding of pseudopyloric metaplasia would be highly suggestive of CD in a proper clinical setting, especially when distinguishing Crohn's ileitis from backwash ileitis in UC [15, 16]. Detecting pseudopyloric metaplasia can be challenging in biopsy specimens, and multiple deep levels should be examined in cases with suspicion of CD. It is located deep in the mucosa and can be very focal, and sometimes present as a single gland. The atrophic crypts may mimic pseudopyloric metaplasia, but they usually have less abundant and eosinophilic cytoplasm, rather than pale-stained mucinous cytoplasm in pseudopyloric metaplasia. Gastric foveolar metaplasia is rarely seen and is also indicative of chronicity (Fig. 13.7b).

Mural Changes Unlike UC, CD involves all layers of intestinal wall. The mural changes are also helpful in the diagnosis, but they can only be assessed on resection specimens. Although the active chronic inflammation predominantly locates in mucosa, the mononuclear cells and eosinophils can be seen throughout the intestinal wall, known as transmural inflammation. However, the density of inflammatory infiltrate in deep levels is much less than in mucosa (Fig. 13.8). The transmural inflammation is also manifested as transmural lymphoid aggregates, i.e., lymphoid aggregates with or without germinal centers present in all layers. In particular, the lymphoid aggregates in subserosal space along the muscularis propria, sometimes in submucosa, tend to regularly arrange one by one, a pattern described as "a string of beads," which is considered as a hallmark of CD (Fig. 13.9a, b). Often time, the string of beads is only composed by a few lymphoid aggregates, and the lymphoid aggregates are also loosely formed. These findings may be overlooked by pathologists so that one of the most important diagnostic features of CD may be missed.

In moderate and severe active disease, the ulcers begin deepening from the base of the aphthous ulcers and extending beyond mucosa into submucosa and muscularis propria to form deep ulcers and fissures. The ulcers may show broad base, but more often present as knifelike deep ulcers/fissures, associated with active and chronic inflammation, granulation tissue, and fibrosis (Fig. 13.10a, b).

The intestinal wall is thickened, especially at the stricture sites, which is resulted from fibrosis and hypertrophy of muscular layers (Fig. 13.11a). The fibrostenotic change is a major pathological event in CD and a main contributor of CD-related complications and mortality. The fibrosis is also

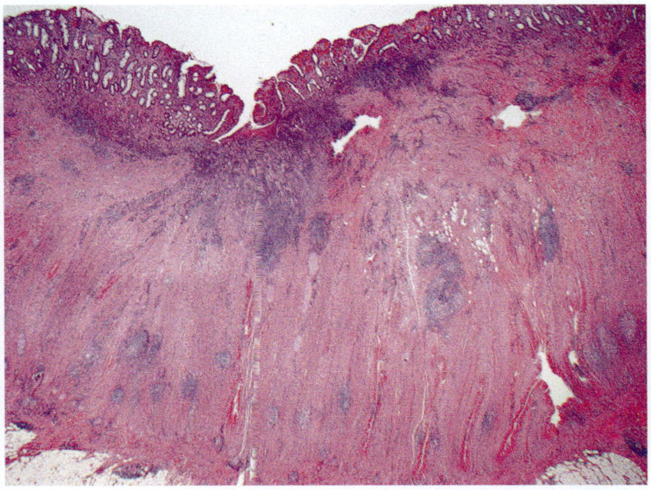

Fig. 13.8 Transmural inflammation and lymphoid aggregates

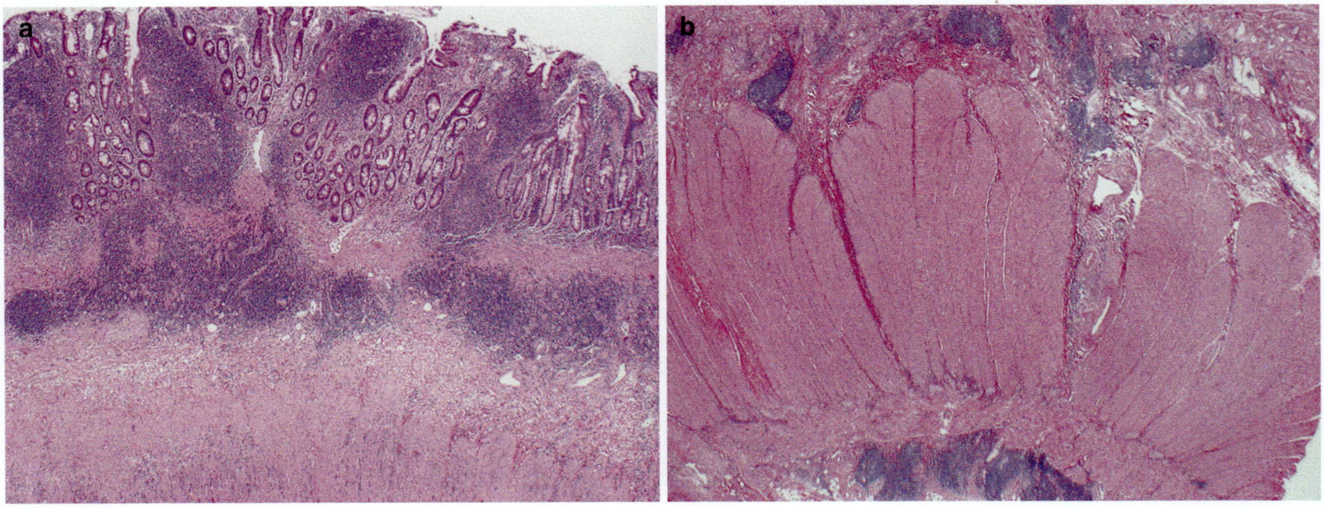

Fig. 13.9 Transmural lymphoid aggregates. Mucosal and submucosal lymphoid aggregates and follicles (**a**); "a string of beads" of lymphoid aggregates in subserosa and submucosa along the muscularis propria (**b**)

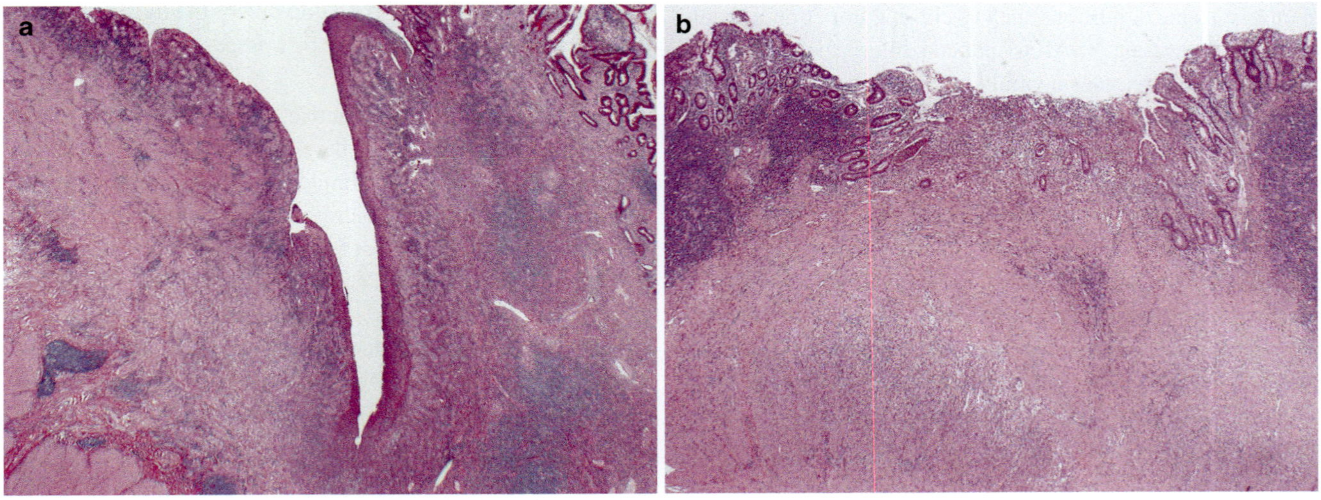

Fig. 13.10 A deep knife-like fissuring ulcer (**a**) and a broad-based ulcer (**b**) associated with active and chronic inflammation, granulation tissue, and fibrosis

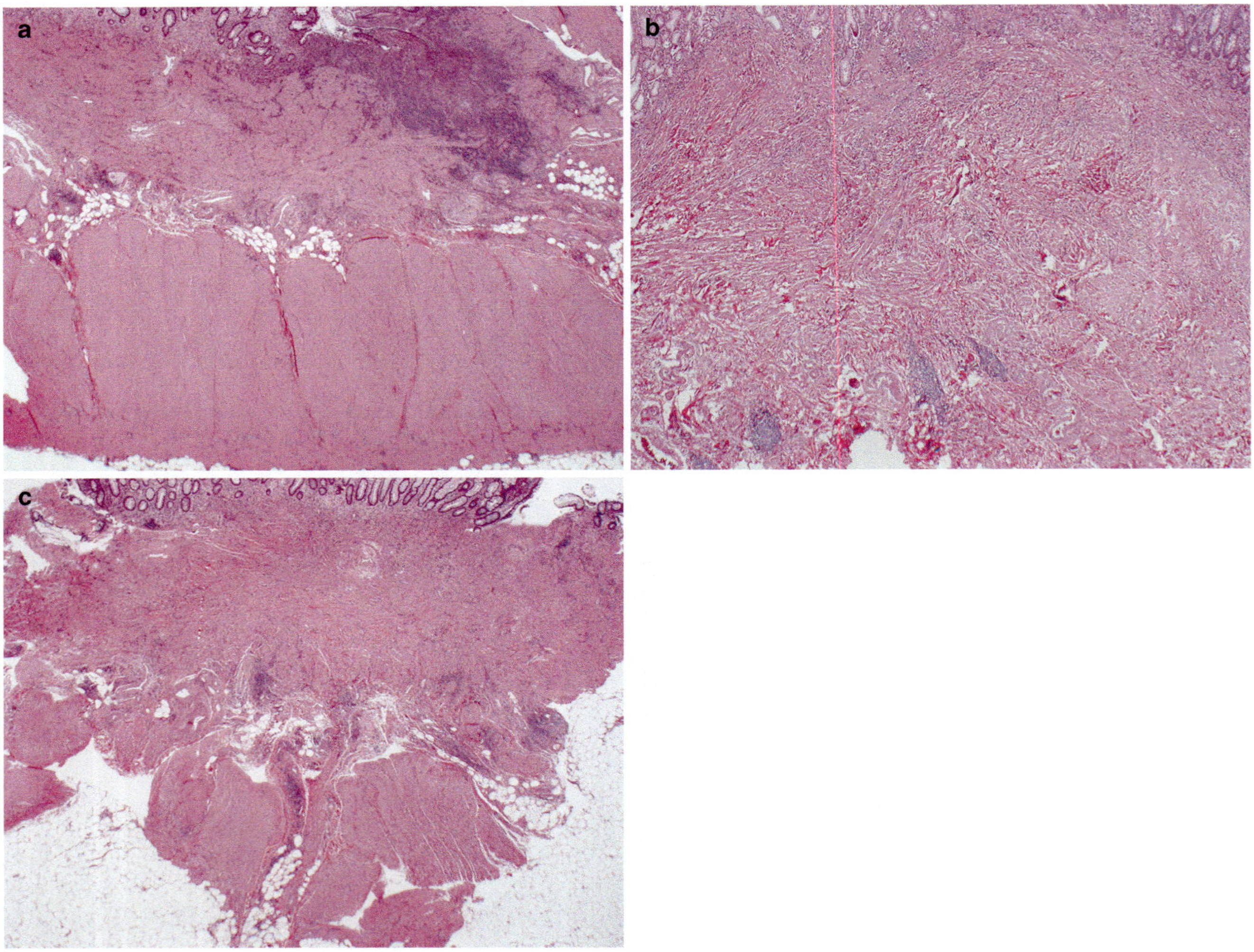

Fig. 13.11 The intestinal wall thickening with fibrosis, hypertrophy of muscular layers, and obliterative muscularization of submucosa (**a**); prominent submucosal fibrosis (**b**); hypertrophic muscularis propria, obliterative muscularization of submucosa, and overgrowth of mesenteric fat wrapping intestinal wall (**c**)

transmural, but it is not prominent in mucosa. The submucosa is the main fibrotic site with dense collagen deposition (Fig. 13.11b). The fibrosis is also associated with muscular hypertrophy. In submucosa, the focal smooth muscle proliferation surrounded by dense collagen may become so extensive that it obliterates the submucosa, known as obliterative muscularization of submucosa (Fig. 13.11a) [17]. The muscularis propria is also thickened, especially the inner layer, showing significant hypertrophy with deposition of collagen. The overgrowth of subserosal fat and hypertrophy of the mesenteric fat, corresponding to fat wrapping grossly, may also contribute to the strictures, and the extent of fat wrapping is correlated significantly with the degree of active chronic inflammation and extent of transmural lymphoid aggregates (Fig. 13.11c). Other histological abnormalities have been observed in mesentery in CD include fibrosis, perivascular and perineuronal chronic inflammation, thickened lymphatic vessels, and small-sized adipocytes [18].

Granulomas Epithelioid non-necrotizing granuloma is another hallmark of CD, although it is not entirely specific. Granulomas can be detected in approximately 50% of resection specimens and 30% of biopsy samples. The frequency of detection of granulomas increases with increasing numbers of submitted sections or biopsy samples and by examining multiple serial sections. They are usually small and with less well-defined outlines (Fig. 13.12a). The granulomas can be recognized by their eosinophilic color in a blue background containing many lymphocytes and plasma cells, because of abundant pale eosinophilic cytoplasm of the epithelioid histiocytes. Multinucleated giant cells can be present (Fig. 13.12a). The granulomas can be found throughout the intestinal wall, but they are more often situated in mucosa, submucosa, subserosa, and ulcer areas. The granulomas can also be found in mesenteric lymph nodes in CD. But if the granulomas are only present in lymph nodes, other possibilities have to be considered besides CD. Small clusters of

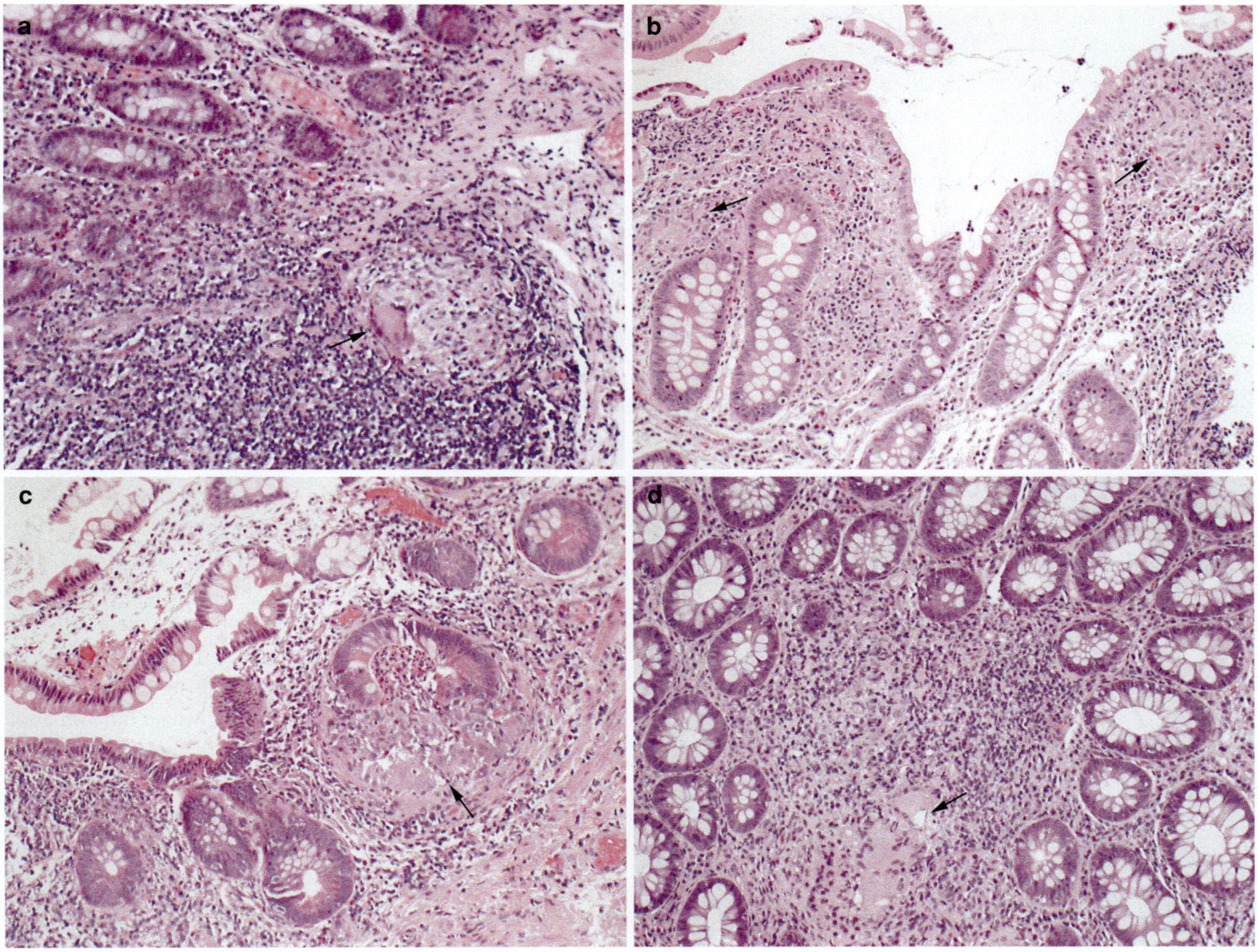

Fig. 13.12 Epithelioid non-necrotizing granuloma is a hallmark of CD (**a**) multinucleated giant cells can be present (arrow); micrgranulomas (arrows) are also frequently identified (**b**); crypt rupture granulomas (**c**) or foreign body granulomas (arrow) (**d**) are less reliable for diagnosing Crohn's disease

loosely arranged histiocytes (typically less than 20 cells), also known as microgranulomas or poorly formed granulomas, are also frequently seen in mucosa, which can provide diagnostic value for CD as well (Fig. 13.12b) [19]. Granulomas associated with crypt rupture or foreign bodies are a less reliable diagnostic marker for CD (Fig. 13.12c, d). Being aware of some mimickers can avoid misdiagnosis, such as small germinal centers, crushed small vessels with plumped endothelial cells, or tangential cuts at the peripheral of glands, and they can usually be differentiated from true granulomas after examining multiple levels.

Neural Changes Changes of enteric nervous system are common in CD. The main abnormalities include patchy hypertrophy and hyperplasia of nerve fibers in submucosa and muscularis propria, and increased number of neurons, ganglion cells, and interstitial cells of Cajal (Fig. 13.13). These abnormalities are absent in uninvolved regions and can be used as a diagnostic feature for CD [20, 21].

Vascular Changes In CD, granulomas associated with both arteries and veins are occasionally seen. A majority of granulomas are located at perivascular area without direct involvement of vessel wall and lumen. This is believed to represent a secondary phenomenon due to granulomas involving lymphatic vessels adjacent to blood vessels. However, granulomatous vasculitis can occur in approximately 6–10% of patients with CD (Fig. 13.14), which is also considered as a secondary change [22, 23]. Other abnormalities include perivascular and intramural inflammatory infiltrate, intimal proliferation, fibrosis of the vessel wall, or obliterative lesions.

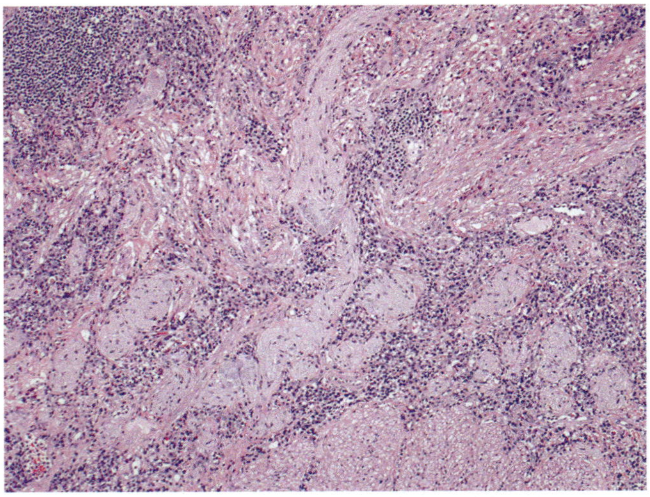

Fig. 13.13 Marked neural hyperplasia in submucosa

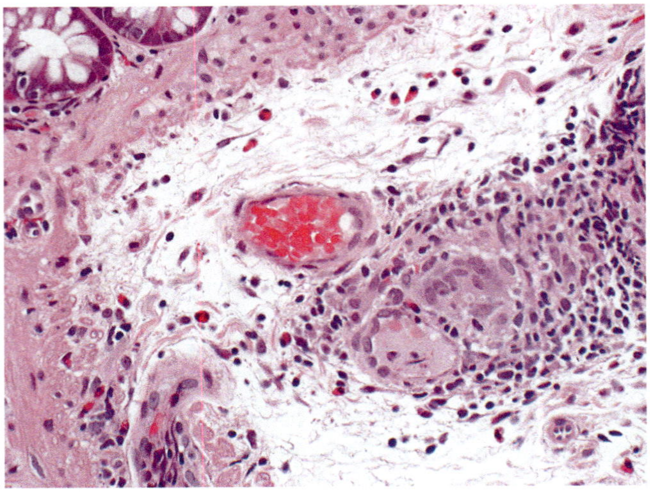

Fig. 13.14 Vasculitis and granulomatous inflammation with multinucleated giant cells in submucosa

Differential Diagnosis

The diagnosis of CD requires combination of clinical, endoscopic, radiological, and pathological assessment. The common differential diagnoses of small bowel CD are listed in Table 13.1, and infections are the main concern. The pathological diagnosis of small bowel CD is usually straightforward on resection specimens, based on characteristic gross findings (wrapping fat, strictures, skip lesions, deep ulceration, and fistulas) and microscopic features (transmural inflammation and lymphoid aggregates, granulomas, mucosal active chronic inflammation and architectural changes, and muscular and neural hyperplasia). However, on biopsy samples, most of these diagnostic features are absent or are not easily identified because of superficial nature, small sample size, and artifacts of the mucosal biopsy. A specific diagnosis of CD is occasionally given on biopsy in cases with an established diagnosis of CD or unequivocal evidence such as non-necrotizing granuloma with a proper clinical setting. More often, a descriptive diagnosis is used to reflect the pathological findings in ileal biopsy, such as active chronic ileitis with or without granulomas or ulcerations, if the chronicity is identified; or, if the chronic changes are not convincing, it may be described as non-specific active chronic inflammation or focal acute ileitis (Fig. 13.15), and a list of differential diagnosis may be followed. The main histological patterns of CD on biopsy that can be confused with other disorders are non-specific active chronic inflammation or active chronic ileitis, granulomatous inflammation, and ileal ulceration.

Active Chronic Ileitis This is a preferred term to describe the pattern of histological changes in ileal CD on biopsy

Table 13.1 Differential diagnosis of Crohn's disease involving small intestine

Classifications	Conditions
Granulomatous inflammation	Infection (*Mycobacterium tuberculosis*, Yersinia, fungal, chlamydial, and parasitic); sarcoidosis; foreign bodies; chronic granulomatous disease; granulomatosis with polyangiitis
Inflammatory disease	Backwash ileitis (terminal ileitis in ulcerative colitis); isolated terminal ileal ulceration; eosinophilic enteritis; cryptogenic multifocal ulcerous stenosing enteritis; ulcerative jejunoileitis
Infection	Mycobacterium tuberculosis; cytomegalovirus; Actinomycosis; Anisakiasis; *Clostridium difficile*; *Cryptococcus neoformans*; neutropenic enterocolitis; Salmonella spp.; Yersinia enterocolitica; Yersinia pseudotuberculosis
Vascular disorders	Ischemia; Behcet's disease; giant cell arteritis; Henoch-Schonlein purpura; polyarteritis nodosa; systemic lupus erythematosus; granulomatosis with polyangiitis
Drug injury	NSAIDs; antihypertensives; digoxin; diuretics; ergotamine; oral contraceptives
Neoplasm	Neuroendocrine tumor; adenocarcinoma; lymphoma; systemic mastocytosis; metastatic cancer
Other	Lymphoid nodular hyperplasia; focal mechanical injury; radiation enteritis; amyloidosis; Meckel's diverticulum

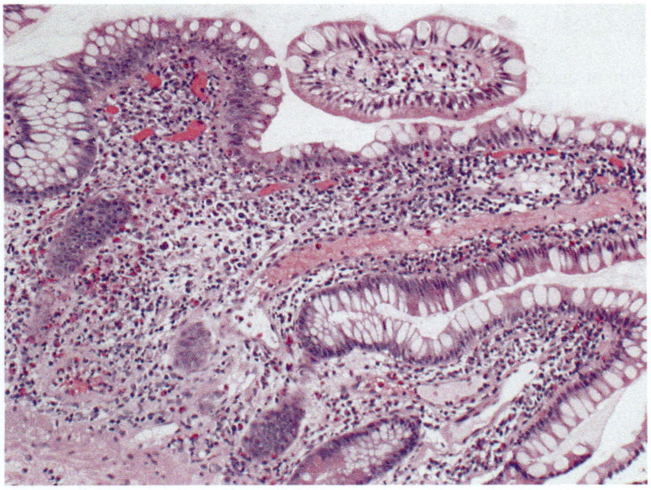

Fig. 13.15 Focal mild active ileitis. A non-specific histological finding can be due to a variety of causes

samples, but it is not specific for CD, especially when granulomas are absent. If the chronicity is not obvious, non-specific active chronic inflammation or focal acute ileitis can be used as well. Besides CD, other common considerations include infections, ischemia, NSAIDs-induced injury, and backwash ileitis. Infections must be ruled out at first. A number of pathogens are list in Table 13.1. Infectious ileitis typically shows active or acute ileitis. The chronic changes such as mucosal architectural changes or pseudopyloric metaplasia are usually absent, unless the infection is in a chronic and persistent form, for example, intestinal histoplasmosis (Fig. 13.16a, b), tuberculosis, or CMV infection in immunocompromised patients. Ischemic enteritis, especially chronic ischemia, can mimic CD, because of mucosal chronic injury, strictures, and fibrosis. The presence of hemosiderin-laden macrophages, prominent fibrosis, and vascular changes favors an ischemic etiology (Fig. 13.17), while the granulomas and involvement of other part of gastrointestinal tract would support CD. NSAIDs-induced small bowel injury is common nowadays because enteric-coated aspirin can cause damages in more distal part of small intestine. The morphological changes in NSAIDs-induced enteropathy are non-specific, including villous blunting, increased inflammatory infiltrate in lamina propria, including neutrophils and eosinophils, occasional cryptitis or crypt abscesses, and erosion/ulceration. Pseudopyloric metaplasia can occur. But NSAIDs-induced mucosal injury does not show prominent mucosal architectural distortion, and the ulcers tend to have more fibrosis and less inflammation rather than the deep or fissuring ulcers seen in CD (Fig. 13.18). Granulomas are typically absent in NSAIDs-induced enteropathy. Active chronic ileitis can be seen in up to 75% of patients with autoimmune enteropathy, including villous atrophy, lamina propria lymphoplasmacytic infiltrate, cryptitis, crypt abscesses, and rarely pseudopyloric metaplasia, but increased intraepithelial lymphocytes, apoptosis, absence or diminishing goblet cells and/or Paneth cells would argue against CD (Fig. 13.19) [24]. Distinguishing CD and backwash ileitis is of clinical significance, which can be difficult based on terminal ileum biopsy alone. If active chronic ileitis is seen beyond 5 cm from ileocecal valve, backwash ileitis would be very unlikely. Determination of chronicity is important since profound mucosal architectural distortion and pseudopyloric metaplasia are not typically seen in backwash ileitis.

Behçet disease has many overlap features with CD, and the differential diagnosis is mainly based on clinical findings [25]. Ileocecal area is the most common location of intestinal Behçet disease. There are discrete single or multiple ulcers with crater formation. The mucosal changes are mild and non-specific. The ulcers usually involve underlying Peyer's patches or lymphoid follicles. Granulomas are absent. The finding of necrotizing lymphocytic vasculitis in small veins and venules, with perivenulitis, intimal thickening, and thrombosis can help in

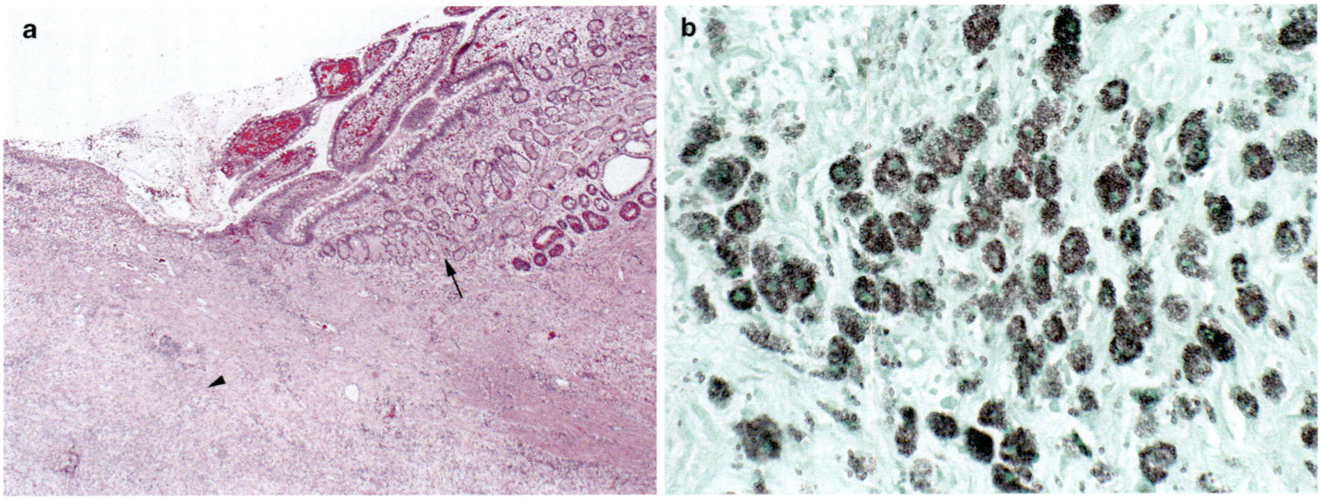

Fig. 13.16 Chronic intestinal histoplasmosis mimicking Crohn's disease. There are ulceration and mucosal active chronic inflammation and pseudopyloric gland metaplasia (arrow) (**a**); note the histiocytic infiltrate at ulcer base (arrowhead) and intracytoplasmic *Histoplasma capsulatum* identified by GMS stain (**b**)

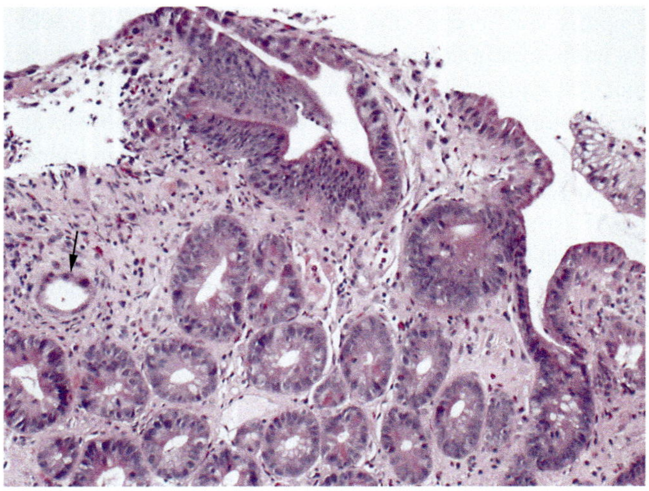

Fig. 13.17 Chronic ischemia. The mucosal chronic injury manifested with surface epithelial damage, mild villous architectural change, vascular ectasia, a withered crypt (arrow), and fibrosis

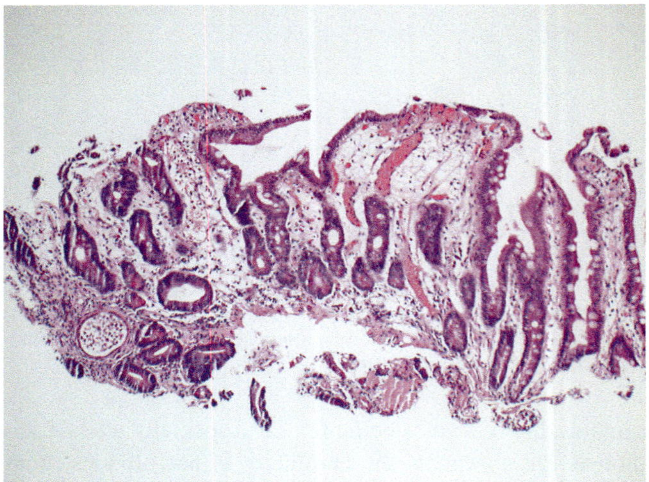

Fig. 13.18 NSAIDs-induced non-specific small bowel mucosal injury, including mild inflammation, edema, epithelial injury, and mild architectural change

the diagnosis, although they are not pathognomonic for Behçet disease (see Chap. 15, Fig. 15.43).

Granulomatous Inflammation Although identifying granulomas is particular helpful in diagnosing CD, they are not entirely specific. Some infections can have granulomatous inflammation, especially intestinal tuberculosis. Distinguishing CD from tuberculosis is a clinical and pathological dilemma, especially in developing countries. However, the incidence of tuberculosis is also increasing in North America due to AIDS epidemic, drug-resistant tuberculosis, more immunocompromised patients, and immigrants. Microscopically, the typical features in tuberculosis are the large, multiple, and confluent granulomas with central caseating necrosis and peripheral palisading histiocytes and lymphocytes, associated with marked active chronic inflammation, mucosal damage, multinucleated giant cells, and ulceration (Fig. 13.20a). In older cases, the granulomas become hyalinized and calcified. But small non-caseating epithelioid granulomas can be seen in tuberculosis which are indistinguishable from the granulomas in CD. The diagnosis of tuberculosis is based on identifying acid-fast bacilli on special stains such as Ziehl–Neelsen stain (Fig. 13.20b). The organisms are usually located in necrotic areas or within macrophages. However, acid-fast bacilli may only be identified in less than 30% of biopsies. Real-time PCR test is also used in conjunction with histological examination, with a moderate sensitivity of 40–75%. Bacterial culture of biopsy tissue is the gold standard, but it takes 3–8 weeks to provide conclusive results [26, 27].

Chronic granulomatous disease (CGD) is a rare primary immunodeficiency disease caused by a defect in a subunit of nicotinamide dinucleotide phosphate (NADPH) oxidase, and some patients may have granulomas in gastrointestinal tract mimicking CD. Non-necrotizing granulomas, usually micro-granulomas, can be observed in small bowel biopsies in about 25% of patients with CGD. Other mucosal changes include chronic inflammation with eosinophilia, villous blunting, focal acute inflammation, and ulceration. The presence of pigmented macrophages in all levels of intestinal wall is considered as a hallmark of CGD (see Chap. 15, Fig. 15.41). The macrophages contain brown granular pigmented cytoplasm which represents a by-product of ineffective digestion of microorganisms, membranes, and lipids [28].

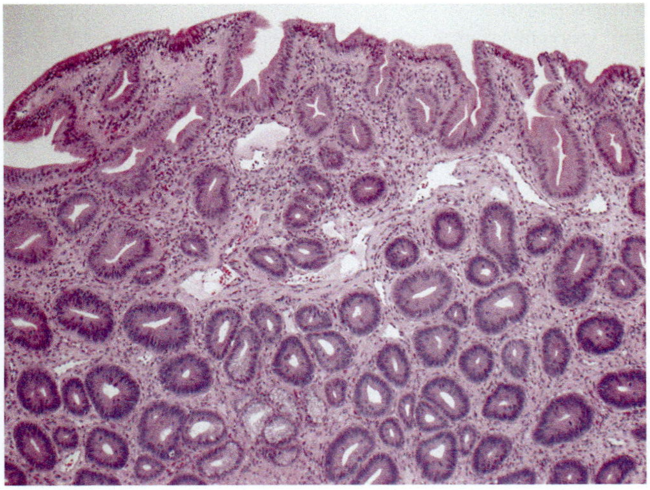

Fig. 13.19 Autoimmune enteropathy involving terminal ileum. Active chronic ileitis with villous atrophy, lamina propria inflammation, pseudopyloric gland metaplasia, increased apoptosis, and absence of goblet cells and Paneth cells

Terminal Ileal Ulcers Isolated terminal ileal ulcer (ITIU) is not an uncommon endoscopic finding. Although most patients with ITIU are asymptomatic or non-specific, CD is the commonest cause in symptomatic patients, followed by NSAIDs-induced ulcers, intestinal tuberculosis, and eosinophilic enteritis [29, 30]. There are many other conditions that can cause small ulcerations as well. The ulcer itself is not etiologic specific. Pathologists need to give differential diagnoses rather than a specific diagnosis when evaluating such cases. Some helpful features in the differential diagnosis of small bowel ulcerations are listed in Table 13.2.

Treatment and Prognosis

The recently developed therapies, targeting either a specific location or a specific immunological pathway, have significantly improved the treatment of CD. The medical treatment of CD mainly includes aminosalicylates, antibiotics, corticosteroids, immunomodulators, and biologics. Aminosalicylates contain 5-aminosalicylate acid (5-ASA), including sulfasalazine, mesalamine, olsalazine, and balsalazide. However, 5-ASA is only effective in a small subset of patients with CD. Sulfasalazine is mainly used in colonic disease but not alleviate small bowel CD because 5-ASA is released in colon by bacterial degradation. Mesalamine can release 5-ASA in the distal small bowel and is more effective in patients with small bowel CD. Antibiotics such as metronidazole,

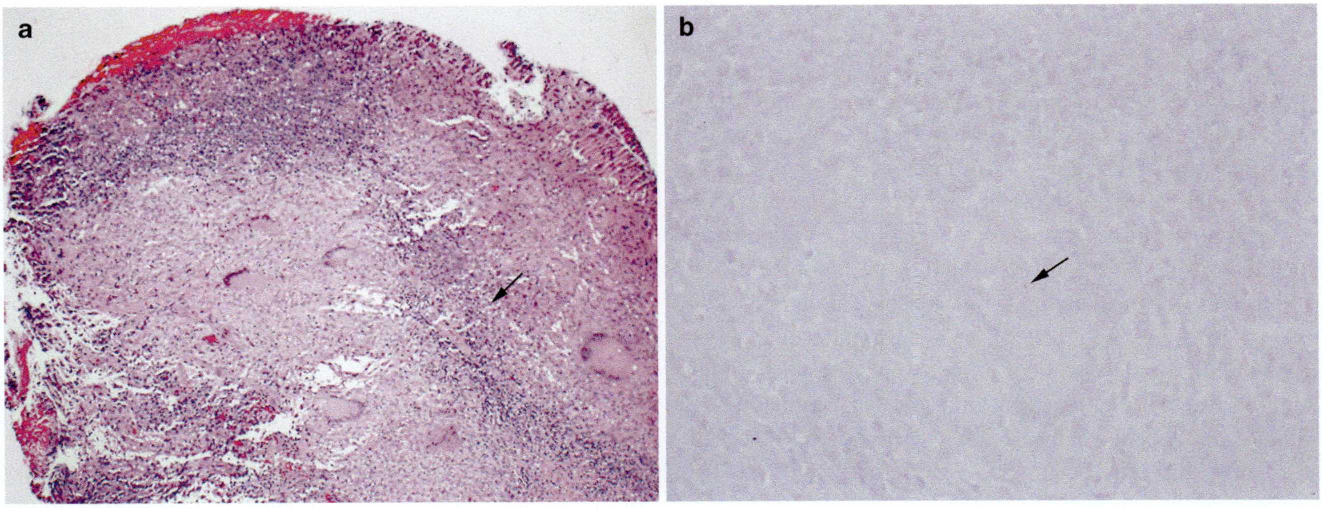

Fig. 13.20 Intestinal tuberculosis. Marked active chronic inflammation, ulceration, confluent large granulomas with giant cells, and focal necrosis (arrow) (**a**); a single acid-fast bacteria (arrow) identified on Ziehl–Neelsen (AFB) stain (**b**)

Table 13.2 Differential diagnosis of small bowel ulcerations

Disorders	Main features of ulcers
Crohn's disease	Aphthous ulcer: small, superficial, often overlying lymphoid follicles Fissuring ulcer: orientated at right angle to the long axis of the bowel, narrow, deep and may extending through bowel wall to form fissures Adjacent unaffected mucosa normal Non-necrotizing granulomas
NSAIDs-induced enteropathy	Wild variations in number, size, shape, and depth. Deep, but not fissuring, ulcers may be associated with perforation Diffuse erosion with pseudomembrane Healing ulcers with dense vertical fibrosis and less inflammatory infiltrate at the base Adjacent mucosa with inflammation and villous atrophy
Ischemia/vasculitis	Mucosal sloughing, hemorrhage, necrosis Adjacent mucosa with ischemic changes May have transmural necrosis or pseudomembrane Vasculitis, fibrin thrombi Hemosiderin-laden macrophages
Behçet disease	Oval or round deep ulcers with discrete margins and carters Normal circumferential mucosa surrounding ulceration Necrotizing lymphocytic vasculitis in small veins and venules Non-specific mucosal inflammation No granulomas
Cryptogenic multifocal ulcerous stenosing enteritis (CMUSE)	Multiple (>20) Circular or irregular with clear border; fused multiple ulcers with a geographic configuration Superficial, restricted to the mucosa or submucosa, with mild mixed inflammatory infiltrate and fibrosis Associated with multiple stenosis Intervening mucosa unremarkable
Ulcerative jejunoileitis (UJI)	Associated with celiac disease or enteropathy-associated T-cell lymphoma Restricted to small intestine Transversely oriented with variable depth Acute and chronic inflammation, granulation tissue, and overlying fibrinopurulent exudates Perforation may present Scar and strictures in chronic phase Adjacent mucosa with villous atrophy
Infections	Marked acute, chronic, or granulomatous inflammation Ulcers due to bacterial infections (Campylobacter, Shigella, Yersinia, or Salmonella) are superficial, self-limited, and with no stricture formation Ulcers in tuberculosis and cytomegalovirus can be persistent with chronic changes Special stains, tissue culture, or molecular tests may be needed for diagnosis
Neoplasm	Irregular shape and border Mass-forming or polypoid Dirty necrosis and bleeding Neoplastic cells (lymphoma and carcinoma are most common)

rifaximin, or ciprofloxacin may help control symptoms by reducing intestinal bacteria and by directly suppressing the intestine's immune system. Corticosteroid is indicated in patients with severe systemic symptoms or in those who do not respond to anti-inflammatory agents. Immunomodulators such as azathioprine and methotrexate are helpful in maintaining but not in inducing remission in CD. The biologic agents, especially anti-TNF alpha agents (infliximab, adalimumab, golimumab, and certolizumab pegol), have significantly advanced the treatment, improved the induction and maintenance of clinical remission in patients with moderate-to-severe disease, and are particularly helpful in corticosteroid-dependent patients.

A "step-up" approach is used for treating mild CD, in which less aggressive and less toxic treatments are initiated first, followed by more potent medications or surgeries if the initial therapy fails. For the treatment of moderate-to-severe CD, current recommendations include a "top-down" approach, which differs from the conventional "step-up" approach, in which the more potent agents are administered initially, including biologic agents and steroids as needed or combination therapy with both biologics and immunomodulators. For extensive small bowel CD, which refers to patients with >100 cm small bowel involvement, aggressive treatment should be initiated with systemic corticosteroids along with concomitant immunomodulators and nutritional support, because of the severity of the disease, the higher incidence of nutritional deficiencies, and the high chance to develop short bowel syndrome.

Surgery plays a critical role in controlling the symptoms and treating the complications of CD, but operative resection is not curative. Most patients with CD require surgical intervention during their lifetime, and many of them need multiple surgical procedures. Repeated intestinal resection is a major cause of short bowel syndrome in CD. Therefore, it is important to preserve the intestinal length and function to avoid short bowel syndrome. The indications for surgery are failed medical therapy, perforation, obstruction, hemorrhage, abscesses, fistulas, and neoplasia. Surgical procedures include bowel resection, stricturoplasty, and drainage of abscesses. Endoscopic therapy has also been applied for managing some complications to avoid surgeries, such as endoscopic balloon dilation or self-expanding stent implantation, endoscopic fistulotomy, and endoscopic incision and drainage of abscesses [31].

CD is a chronic condition with no known cure, and the general goals of treatment are to achieve and maintain remission to allow patients to function as normally as possible. Most patients experience periods of improvement followed by episodes of flares. The mortality rate of patients with small bowel CD is similar to the background populations, but it is associated with increased risk of adenocarcinoma [32]. One critical issue is recurrence after segmental small bowel resection, and approximately 85–90% of patients develop disease recurrence within the first postoperative year. The postoperative recurrence of CD is defined in different forms. Endoscopic recurrence can be observed in up to 90% of patients at the neoterminal ileum within the first year of surgery. It is graded using Rutgeerts' score system, including the presence of >5 aphthous lesions, inflamed mucosa, larger ulcers, nodules, and/or narrowing [33]. Surgical recurrence refers to patients with CD who require another intestinal resection after initial surgery, and occurs in approximately 25% of patients by 5 years and 35% of patients by 10 years. Clinical recurrence is defined using the Crohn's Disease Activity Index, which develops in 20–40% of patients within the first year of surgery and in 35–50% of patients by 5 years. Several risk factors may be associated with postoperative recurrence, including penetrating disease, a history of two previous CD-related surgeries, young age at disease diagnosis (<30 years), extensive small bowel resection, and cigarette smoking. Patients with endoscopic recurrence are at high risk to develop clinical and surgical recurrence, and endoscopic remission is considered to be an appropriate surrogate marker for preventing future surgical recurrence. Early postoperative pharmacological prophylaxis, routine endoscopic monitoring 6–12 months after surgical resection, and anti-TNF alpha or thiopurine monotherapy can probably reduce the risk of recurrence [34].

Stem cell therapy has been developed and showed promising results for refractory CD and fistulizing CD [35]. Hematopoietic stem cells transplantation (HSCT) is used to immediately shut down the immune response and allow the transplanted stem cells to develop into self-tolerant lymphocytes. Mesenchymal stromal cell (MSC) therapy is to deposit MSC into the fistulizing tracts to control the local inflammation and promote wound healing.

Crohn's Disease-Associated Small Bowel Dysplasia and Adenocarcinoma

Although few studies on small bowel dysplasia and small bowel adenocarcinoma (SBA) associated with CD are available, an inflammation–dysplasia–adenocarcinoma sequence similar to that described in IBD-related colorectal carcinoma has been suggested [36, 37]. Most SBA develops on a chronically inflamed area and is associated with dysplasia [36]. The risk of SBA is 20–30 times higher in patients with small bowel CD than in the general population. The incidence of SBA in patients with long-standing small bowel CD is approximately 0.2–4%, and CD-associated SBA carries a poor prognosis [37–40]. Small bowel resection and prolonged salicylates use may protect against SBA in CD patients [41]. Unlike endoscopic screening for dysplasia in colon, there is no guideline for endoscopic surveillance of small bowel dysplasia and adenocarcinoma in CD because of low sensitivity [39]. Surgical resection should first be considered in patients with long-term small bowel disease who develop recent obstructive symptoms or treatment-refractory strictures.

Dysplasia in small bowel can be flat or raised, adjacent to or at distance from SBA. Dysplasia is rarely encountered in random ileal mucosal biopsies. However, once present, it is very likely that SBA would be detected at the same time or on a subsequent resection. One prospective study found only two cases showing indefinite dysplasia on ileal biopsy among 101 patients, but one of the two cases had SBA on small bowel resection [39]. Dysplasia can be identified in approximately 50% SBA cases, and most are high grade and adjacent to the tumor, either flat or raised. In cases without SBA, the dysplastic lesions tend to be low grade and flat [36]. The microscopic features of dysplasia are similar to those in colon, and it is also graded as low, high, or indefinite. The common features of low-grade dysplasia include increased N/C ratio, nuclear pleomorphism, stratification, and atypia, mucin loss, and lack of surface maturation (Fig. 13.21). High-grade dysplasia is characterized by complex glandular architecture. If the atypical features are not convincing, especially in a background with active chronic inflammation or ulceration, indefinite for dysplasia can be considered. Unusual forms of dysplasia such as villiform or hypermucinous dysplasia can occur in small bowel as well. The CD-related SBA is typical intestinal type and at advanced stage at the time of

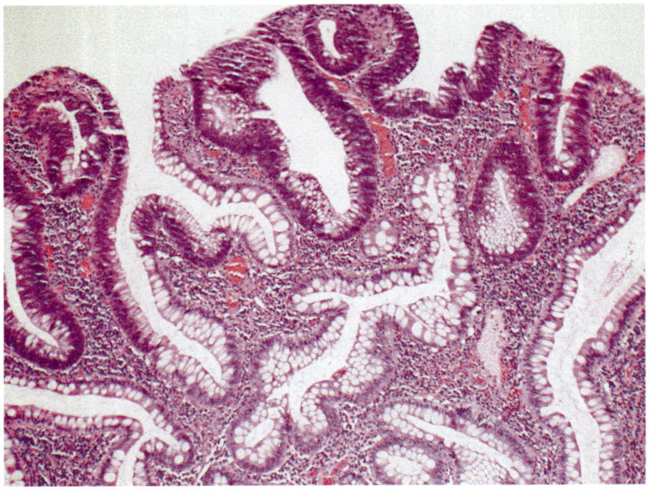

Fig. 13.21 Low-grade dysplasia associated small bowel Crohn's disease

diagnosis. Other morphologic types include mucinous adenocarcinoma and signet ring cell carcinoma. One study showed that 35% of CD-associated SBA had signet ring cell feature while it was absent in patients with SBA *de novo* [40]. Immunohistochemical and molecular studies of small bowel dysplasia and SBA in CD showed p53 overexpression in about 60% cases, which can be used to facilitate diagnosis of high-grade dysplasia and invasive carcinoma in daily practice. A subset of cases carries *KRAS* mutations, but *BRAF* and *PIK3CA* mutations as well as microsatellite instability are rare [36, 37].

Backwash Ileitis (Terminal Ileitis in Ulcerative Colitis)

Definition

Backwash ileitis refers to mild inflammation involving the very distal portion of terminal ileum in patients with UC.

Clinical Features

Although UC is considered as a disease restricted in colon, the reported incidence of terminal ileitis in UC ranges from 2% to 100% in the literature; however, most of cases in the earlier studies were CD rather than UC [42]. More recent studies showed that 10–20% of patients with confirmed diagnosis of UC may have inflammation in the terminal ileum [16, 43–45]. Terminal ileitis is more commonly seen in patients with severe pancolitis or severe right-sided colitis, younger age, and concurrent PSC [46, 47].

The term "backwash" implies a presumed etiology, in which the colonic contents retrograde flow into the distal ileum through incompetent ileocecal valve in severe UC involving ileocecal region [48, 49]. This theory has been contested because: (1) the fact that backwashed colonic contents can lead to inflammation in ileum has never been proved. The cecoileal reflux could occur in 25% normal individuals, but no abnormalities were observed in the terminal ileum in both normal and IBD patients [50]; (2) terminal ileitis was frequently seen in UC patients whose ileocecal involvement was either absent or only with mild activity [16, 43–45]; and (3) other factors such as infections, NSAIDs, or alcohol may also contribute to the ileitis in both IBD and non-IBD patients. Therefore, some authors considered that backwash ileitis may represent primary involvement or direct extension of UC in terminal ileum and a term of UC-associated ileitis has been proposed [42]. Further studies are needed to demonstrate the nature of this type of inflammation in the terminal ileum in some patients with UC.

There are no specific clinical symptoms or signs associated with backwash ileitis. The diagnosis is made based on endoscopic and/or histological findings. Endoscopically, the backwash ileitis is limited within only a few centimeters beyond ileocecal valve. The ileocecal valve is usually widely open. The mucosa inflammatory changes are similar to those in colon, including edema, erythema, granularity, and loss of vascular pattern. Erosion and ulceration are occasionally seen. If the inflammation extends more than 5 cm in the terminal ileum, or with strictures or distinct ulcers, CD is possible.

Pathological Features

The length of distal terminal ileum attached to the colectomy specimens in UC patients is variable. In modern era, the mean length of ileum is approximately 3 cm (range, 1.2–5 cm) [16]. Mild and moderate backwash ileitis is manifested with mucosal edema and erythema, with or without focal erosions, involving <2 cm of distal ileum. In severe cases, the injury can extend to a few centimeters but rarely go beyond 5 cm, with extensive mucosal ulceration and a surface layer of fibrinopurulent exudates. The injury also shows a zonal distribution, which is more prominent in the distal end and gradually becomes less active in the more proximal mucosa. Strictures or discrete ulcers are absent.

Microscopically, backwash ileitis is characterized by lamina propria expansion by edema and increased inflammatory infiltrate, neutrophil infiltrate in lamina propria and epithelium, variable degree of villous and crypt architectural disarray, and mucosal erosions/ulcerations in more severe cases (Fig. 13.22). The distribution of inflammation can be in a

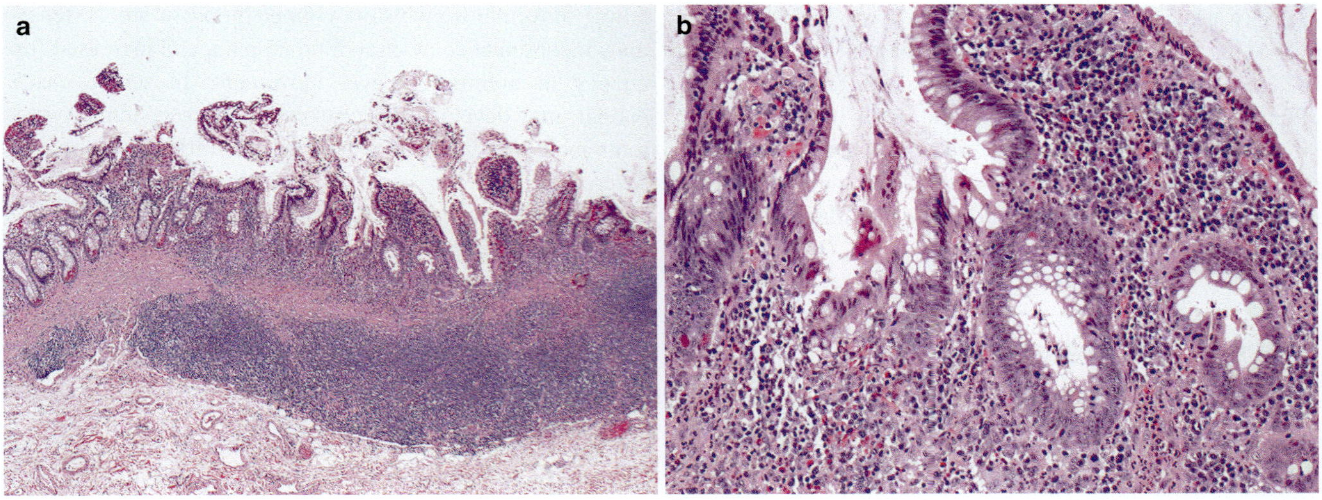

Fig. 13.22 Backwash ileitis. (**a**) The ileal mucosa shows lamina propria expansion by mixed inflammatory infiltrate, focal epithelial injury, mild villous and crypt architectural disarray, and no granulomas or pseudopyloric metaplasia. (**b**) Another example shows lamina propria inflammation with neutrophil infiltrate

continuous pattern from ileocecal valve or patchy. The inflammation is confined in the mucosa, but it can extend down through the muscularis mucosae into submucosa, which is typical at the ulceration site. The inflammatory activity is graded based on the neutrophil infiltrate and mucosal injury, ranging from no, mild, moderate, to severe active inflammation. In cases with no activity, the ileal mucosa shows increased lamina propria mononuclear cell infiltrate but no neutrophils, mild villous atrophy, and epithelial regenerative changes. Majority cases show mild-to-moderate active ileitis (Fig. 13.22). There are scattered neutrophils within lamina propria and the tips of villi in mild cases, while the moderate activity shows increased neutrophil infiltrate with cryptitis, crypt abscesses, and focal erosion. Severe backwash ileitis is not common, in which the mucosa is extensively inflamed with ulceration and surface fibrinopurulent exudates. Granulomas, deep ulcerations, and transmural inflammation and lymphoid aggregates are absent in backwash ileitis, which are important features in distinguishing CD.

The determination of chronicity in backwash ileitis is an important issue when considering a differential diagnosis of CD. Besides lamina propria inflammatory infiltrate, the other two features in chronicity are villous and crypt architectural distortion and pseudopyloric metaplasia. Backwash ileitis can show mucosal architectural disarray, but it is usually in a milder form compared to that in CD. The villi can become shortened, broadened, or fused due to lamina propria inflammation and edema. The crypts appear atrophic or hyperplastic, with variation in size, shape, and distribution. The presence of pseudopyloric metaplasia in backwash ileitis is controversial. For example, Goldstein et al. did not identify a single case with pseudopyloric metaplasia in their cohort of 143 backwash ileitis cases, but it was present in 27% cases with CD [16]. Other studies also did not reveal pseudopyloric metaplasia in backwash ileitis, although case numbers were small [44, 45, 51, 52]. But Haskell et al. found pseudopyloric metaplasia in nearly 10% (4/34) cases with backwash ileitis [43]. Nevertheless, pseudopyloric metaplasia, the most unequivocal histologic evidence of chronicity in ileitis, is a rare finding in backwash ileitis. Whenever it is present in patients with IBD, especially in biopsy specimens, CD should always be considered, unless there is compelling clinical evidence to support UC.

Differential Diagnosis

The main differential diagnosis is CD. On resection specimens, the gross findings of disease extent, strictures, fistulas, or fissuring ulcers, in conjunction with microscopic features such as transmural inflammation and lymphoid aggregates and granulomas, can help to distinguish CD from backwash ileitis without much difficulty. However, the differentiation between these two disorders is difficult based on terminal ileum biopsy alone. The main histological features such as active chronic mucosal inflammation, mucosal architectural distortion, or erosions/ulcerations can be seen in both CD and backwash ileitis. Determination of chronicity is an important approach in this setting. Although the common features of chronicity, including mucosal architectural distortion, and lymphoplasmacytic inflammation in lamina propria can also be seen in backwash ileitis, the degree and extent of architectural distortion and lamina propria lymphoplasmacytic inflammation tend to be less than those in CD. As mentioned above, pseudopyloric metaplasia is rare in backwash ileitis. The positive predictive value of pseudopyloric metaplasia is nearly 98% in distinguishing CD versus UC [15]. The presence of this feature would favor CD, so do granulomas. Other causes of terminal ileitis in patients with UC, other than backwash ileitis, are needed to rule out sometimes, which include infection or NSAIDs, and correlation with clinical information and other ancillary tests are necessary.

Treatment and Prognosis

No particular therapy is required for backwash ileitis. The presence of backwash ileitis does not affect pouch outcome in UC patients with an ileal pouch-anal anastomosis (IPAA) after a total proctocolectomy [43, 53]. It is not contraindicated to use the inflamed terminal ileum for construction of the ileal pouch and anastomosis. One study showed that patients with backwash ileitis had a significantly higher risk to develop dysplasia and colorectal cancer than those without backwash ileitis in UC [54].

Pouchitis

Definition

Pouchitis refers to idiopathic inflammation of ileal pouch which is created in IPAA procedure mainly performed in patients with UC and familial adenomatous polyposis (FAP).

Clinical Features

Pouchitis is the most common complication of IPAA. Approximately 50% of patients who have had an IPAA experience at least one episode of pouchitis. The etiology of pouchitis remains poorly understood, and the dysfunction of mucosal immune response to the altered mucosal and luminal microbiota is believed to play an important role in the pathogenesis of pouchitis [55]. There are several factors related to high risk of developing acute or chronic pouchitis, such as extensive colonic disease, smoking, concomitant autoimmune disorder or PSC, use of NSAIDs, and *NOD2insC* variant [56, 57]. Although the previous reports believed that pouchitis almost exclusively occurred in patients with UC or other forms of chronic colitis, but not in FAP patients, the recent studies have showed that pouchitis is very common in FAP, even though it usually occurs later and has a milder course than those with UC [58]. Patients with pouchitis present with increased frequency of bowel movements (with or without blood in stool), tenesmus, incontinence, lower abdominal pain, and increased frequency in nighttime bowel movement. In severe cases, patients may develop extragastrointestinal or systemic symptoms including fever, dehydration, malnutrition, anemia, or severe joint pain. Occasionally, patients can develop CD-like complications such as proximal ileal or pouch strictures or fistulas and perianal fissures or fistulas, which may raise concern to change the initial diagnosis of UC to CD [59].

The clinical presentations of pouchitis are not specific and range widely. The diagnosis of pouchitis requires a combined assessment of clinical symptoms, endoscopic findings (Fig. 13.23), and histologic features. Pouch endoscopy can evaluate mucosal inflammation in pouch and proximal ileum, structural abnormalities such as strictures or fistulas, and cuffitis. The pouchitis disease activity index and score systems have been developed, but they are mainly used for clinical trials [60]. There are several clinical classifications for pouchitis based on different factors which are useful for the management. For example, pouchitis can be acute (<4 weeks) or chronic (≥4 weeks) based on the duration of symptoms; antibiotic-responsive or antibiotic-dependent pouchitis based on response to antibiotics; frequent pouchitis (<3 episodes/year) or relapsing pouchitis (≥3 episodes/year) based on the frequency of flares; idiopathic or secondary (infection, concurrent inflammatory or structural pouch disorder, autoimmune-related, or luminal or vascular factor-associated) based on the etiology [61].

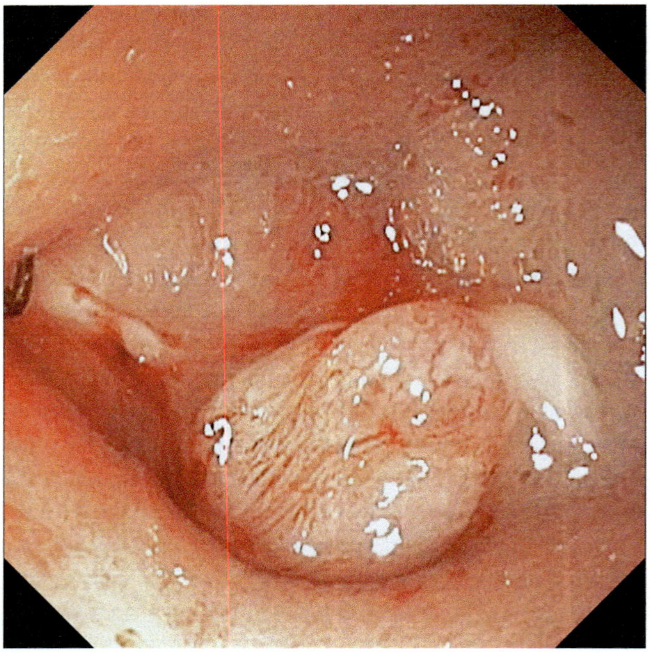

Fig. 13.23 Endoscopic features of pouchitis. Fragile mucosa with edema, erythema, and many small ulcers

Pathological Features

Gross Findings

Failure of pouch resulting in pouch excision occurs in a small portion of patients. There are several forms of ileal pouch. J and S pouches are commonly used nowadays; Kock pouch or K pouch is used in patients with poor anal sphincter; W pouch is essentially abandoned because of complications. Understanding the anatomy of pouch construction and reasons for pouch excision is necessary for gross examination. The mucosa of pouchitis typically shows edema, erythema, loss of vascular pattern, friability, hemorrhage, erosion, and ulceration. Pseudomembranous material and ischemic necrosis may be present. Findings such as strictures, fissuring ulcers, fistulas, or sinus tract are suggestive of CD. Polypoid lesions and malignancy rarely develop in pouch.

Microscopic Findings

The normal morphology of ileal mucosa is slightly altered in pouch mucosa in all cases due to the adaptive changes to the new luminal environment, which includes mild lamina propria inflammation, shortening of villi, crypt hyperplasia, increased Paneth cells, but no neutrophil infiltrate (Fig. 13.24) [62]. The histologic changes in pouchitis are similar to active chronic ileitis in CD, except that granulomas and pseudopyloric metaplasia are rare. The term chronic pouchitis or active chronic pouchitis is used for pathological diagnosis. The chronicity is manifested by lamina propria expansion by mixed inflammatory infiltrate, predominantly by mononuclear cells, with many eosinophils and few neutrophils. The villous architecture is distorted by shortening, broadening, and variable shapes. The crypts appear hyperplastic with uneven distribution and variable sizes. Granulomas, mostly non-caseating, can be rarely seen in pouchitis, but they are not specific for CD. Granulomas can also be associated with foreign body, infections, or ruptured crypts. The presence of neutrophils represents active disease, which can be graded as mild, moderate, and severe, based on the degree of inflammation and mucosal injury. In mild active pouchitis, the neutrophils may be in the lamina propria, but they are readily recognized when infiltrating in the epithelium, which is typically more prominent in the surface epithelium. Cryptitis and crypt abscesses can be seen in moderate and severe active pouchitis, along with erosion and ulceration (Fig. 13.25a–c). The histology has a limited role in assessing disease activity because it does not correlate with the clinical and endoscopic activity scores [63]. The pouch biopsy is probably more important in identifying CD-like features (granulomas and pseudopyloric gland metaplasia), ruling out other conditions (infections, ischemia), and detecting dysplasia or cancer.

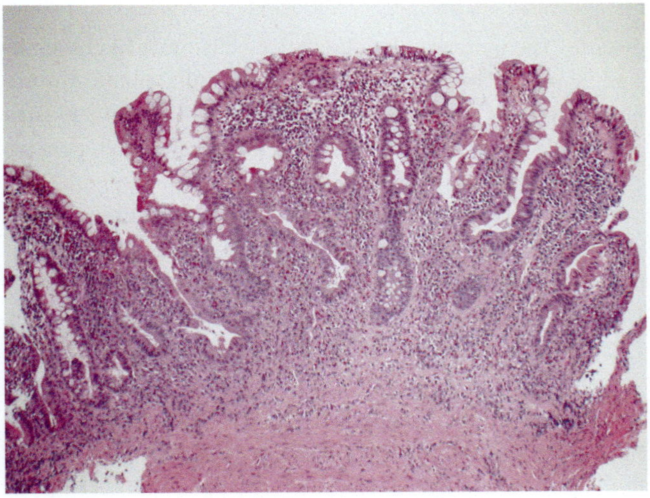

Fig. 13.24 Adaptive changes of ileal mucosa in pouch, including mild lamina propria inflammation with no neutrophils, mild villous atrophy, and crypt hyperplasia

The biopsy from the afferent limb proximal to the pouch and rectal cuff is also obtained during pouch endoscopy. The proximal ileum usually also has mild non-specific changes. But the presence of ulcers, granulomas, or pseudopyloric metaplasia is suggestive of CD (Fig. 13.26). The rectal cuff typically shows changes of UC which is referred to cuffitis and will be discussed in the corresponding chapter in this book.

Differential Diagnosis

Non-specific mild chronic inflammation, mild villous shortening, and mucosal architectural changes are commonly seen in pouch biopsies, and they should not be reported as active chronic pouchitis. These findings represent adaptive changes of the ileal mucosa to the new luminal environment [62]. The biopsy from anastomosis also shows marked mucosal inflammation and distortion, often with ulceration, and they are procedure-related mucosal damage rather than pouchitis. Infectious pouchitis is needed to be ruled out in the initial workup in all cases. Stool culture and *Clostridium difficile* toxin assay are required. CMV infection can be *de novo* or superimposed, and CMV immunostain is necessary in some cases. Ischemic pouchitis shows similar mucosal changes of ischemic injury to ischemic enterocolitis in other site. IgG4-associated pouchitis has been proposed for patients with refractory or recurrent pouchitis who had >10 IgG4 positive plasma cells/HPF in pouch mucosal biopsy [64, 65]. However, there is no correlation between serum IgG4 level and tissue IgG4 positive cells. The significance of this finding remains unclear. It is unlikely that IgG4-associated pouchitis belongs to the family of IgG4-related

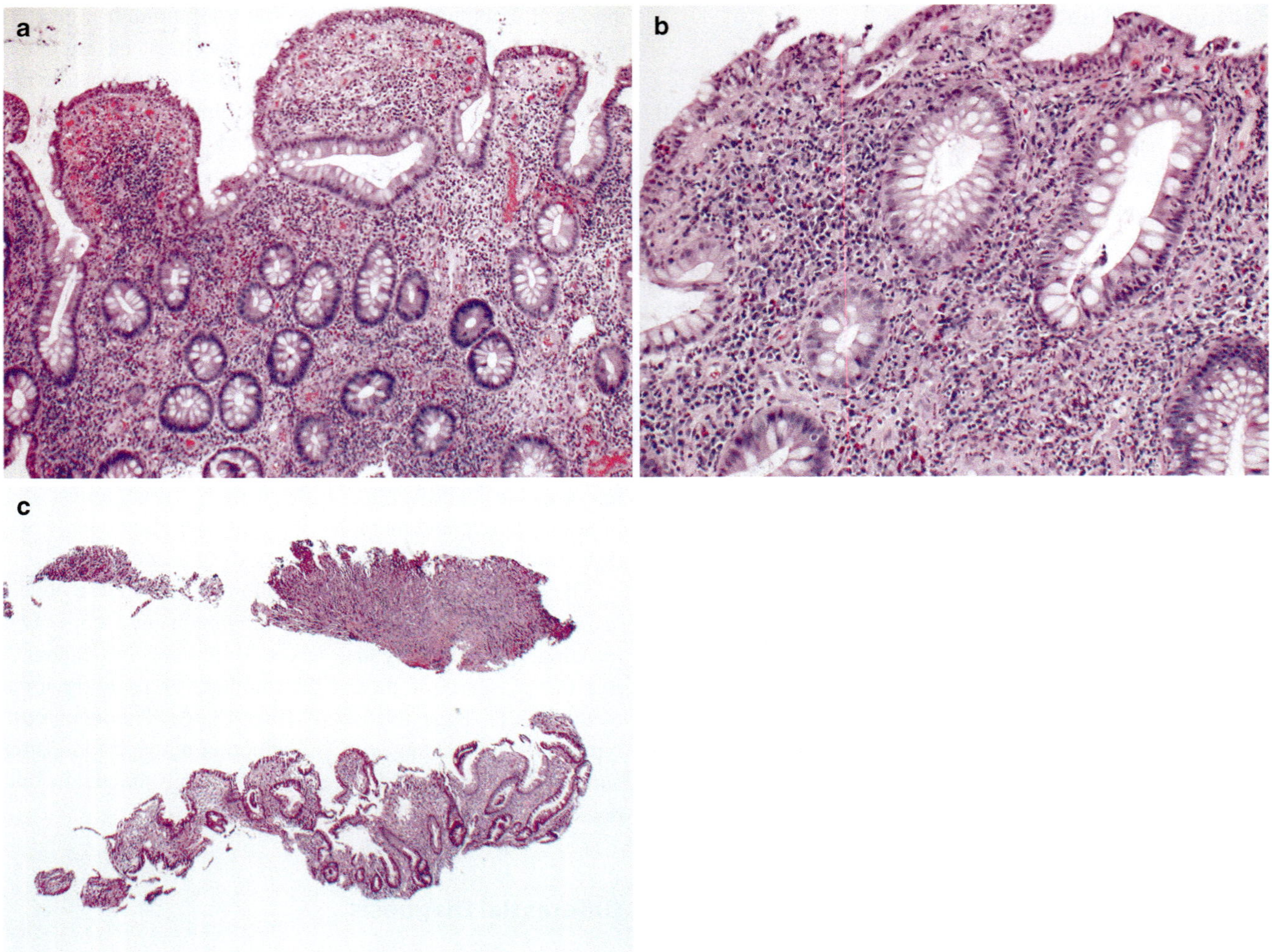

Fig. 13.25 Pouchitis. Mild active chronic pouchitis is characterized by lamina propria inflammation, focal neutrophilic infiltrate, and mild architectural changes (**a**); marked neutrophilic infiltrate and ulceration in more severe disease (**b**, **c**)

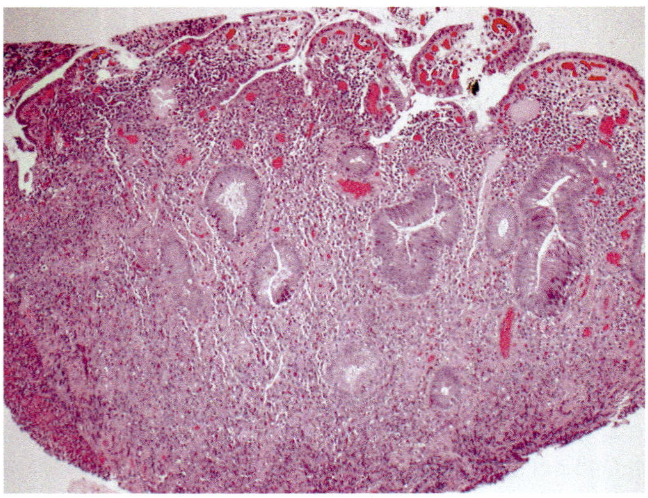

Fig. 13.26 Recurrent Crohn's disease in afferent limb. The ileum proximal to the pouch shows active chronic ileitis with ulceration and pseudopyloric gland metaplasia

disease. The increased IgG4 positive cells more likely represent a secondary change in mucosal inflammation since nearly 40% UC patients also had >10 IgG4 positive plasma cells/HPF in colonic biopsy, and the mean IgG4 positive cells in UC was 12.8/HPF [66].

The distinction of pouchitis from CD is of clinically significance. Nearly one-third of patients may be reclassified as CD after IPAA because of preoperative misclassification of UC, indeterminate colitis, and fulminant colitis [67]. Histologic evaluation of biopsy specimens may provide valuable information for confirming the diagnosis in patients developing CD-like complications. Chronic active inflammation with or without ulceration in afferent limb proximal to the pouch is more common in CD (Fig. 13.26). The presence of pseudopyloric gland metaplasia in the pouch was identified in 77% of cases who subsequently diagnosed with CD, while only 22% of chronic pouchitis had pseudopyloric gland metaplasia [68]. The granulomas in pouch biopsies, especially those not related to foreign bodies and crypt

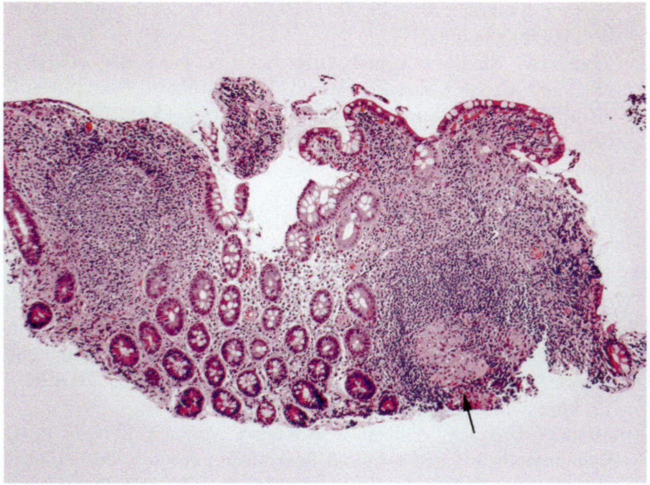

Fig. 13.27 Recurrent Crohn's disease in pouch. Active chronic ileitis with non-necrotizing granuloma (arrow)

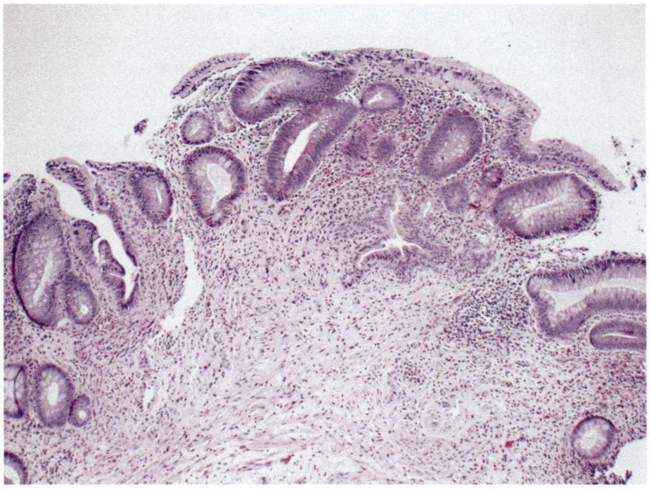

Fig. 13.28 Low grade dysplasia in pouch

injury, are also suggestive of CD, although they are not entirely specific (Fig. 13.27). Transmural inflammation can be seen in resected pouch which is not necessarily indicative of CD.

Treatment and Prognosis

Antibiotics is the first-line treatment, specifically with ciprofloxacin and metronidazole. Acute pouchitis typically responds well to antibiotic therapy. If patients develop symptoms of pouchitis shortly after pouch construction but do not respond to antibiotics, surgery-related complications such as leaking should be suspected. Probiotic VSL#3, which contains viable lyophilized bacteria with 4 strains of *Lactobacillus*, 3 strains of *Bifidobacterium* species, and *Streptococcus salivarius* subsp. *thermophilus*, has shown promising effect in prophylaxis and treating relapsing and chronic antibiotic-refractory pouchitis [69]. For immune-mediated pouchitis, oral or topical mesalamine agents and topical corticosteroid (budesonide) are preferred. Patients with underlying CD may benefit from immunomodulators and biologics. Although pouch-related adenocarcinomas are rare, endoscopic surveillance of the pouch is required for patients with underlying IBD because detection of dysplasia (Fig. 13.28) in the pouch presumably can offer a time window for cancer prevention. The guideline is similar to that of IBD. The pouchoscopy with biopsy begins 10 years after the initial diagnosis of UC and then in every 3 years. For patients with high-risk factors, such as chronic pouchitis or cuffitis, family history of colon cancer, or PSC, the pouchoscopy is needed every 1–3 years. For those with a preoperative diagnosis of colon cancer, pouchoscopy and biopsy are performed annually.

The prognosis of pouchitis is determined by the frequency of the need for antibiotics and the development of refractory pouchitis. Approximately 5–19% of patients with acute pouchitis develop refractory or relapsing disease. Failure of the pouch is defined as permanent diversion or pouch excision, which can occur in 1–12% of patients. The main causes of pouch excision are sepsis (due to anastomotic leak or fistula); mechanical or functional problems (stricture or obstruction); disease-related failure (CD being the most common); and cancer development [70].

References

1. Farmer RG, Hawk WA, Turnbull RB Jr. Clinical patterns in Crohn's disease: a statistical study of 615 cases. Gastroenterology. 1975;68(4 Pt 1):627–35.
2. Lin J, McKenna BJ, Appelman HD. Morphologic findings in upper gastrointestinal biopsies of patients with ulcerative colitis: a controlled study. Am J Surg Pathol. 2010;34(11):1672–7. https://doi.org/10.1097/PAS.0b013e3181f3de93.
3. Crohn BB, Ginzburg L, Oppenheimer GD. Regional ileitis: a pathologic and clinical entity. 1932. Mt Sinai J Med. 2000;67(3):263–8.
4. Schwartz DA, Loftus EV Jr, Tremaine WJ, Panaccione R, Harmsen WS, Zinsmeister AR, et al. The natural history of fistulizing Crohn's disease in Olmsted County, Minnesota. Gastroenterology. 2002;122(4):875–80.
5. Wright EK, De Cruz P, Gearry R, Day AS, Kamm MA. Fecal biomarkers in the diagnosis and monitoring of Crohn's disease. Inflamm Bowel Dis. 2014;20(9):1668–77. https://doi.org/10.1097/MIB.0000000000000087.
6. Calabrese E, La Seta F, Buccellato A, Virdone R, Pallotta N, Corazziari E, et al. Crohn's disease: a comparative prospective study of transabdominal ultrasonography, small intestine contrast ultrasonography, and small bowel enema. Inflamm Bowel Dis. 2005;11(2):139–45.
7. Siddiki HA, Fidler JL, Fletcher JG, Burton SS, Huprich JE, Hough DM, et al. Prospective comparison of state-of-the-art MR enterography and CT enterography in small-bowel Crohn's disease. AJR Am J Roentgenol. 2009;193(1):113–21. https://doi.org/10.2214/AJR.08.2027.

8. Solem CA, Loftus EV Jr, Fletcher JG, Baron TH, Gostout CJ, Petersen BT, et al. Small-bowel imaging in Crohn's disease: a prospective, blinded, 4-way comparison trial. Gastrointest Endosc. 2008;68(2):255–66. https://doi.org/10.1016/j.gie.2008.02.017.
9. Fiorino G, Bonifacio C, Peyrin-Biroulet L, Minuti F, Repici A, Spinelli A, et al. Prospective comparison of computed tomography enterography and magnetic resonance enterography for assessment of disease activity and complications in ileocolonic Crohn's disease. Inflamm Bowel Dis. 2011;17(5):1073–80. https://doi.org/10.1002/ibd.21533.
10. Bruining DH, Zimmermann EM, Loftus EV Jr, Sandborn WJ, Sauer CG, Strong SA, et al. Consensus recommendations for evaluation, interpretation, and utilization of computed tomography and magnetic resonance enterography in patients with small bowel Crohn's disease. Radiology. 2018;286(3):776–99. https://doi.org/10.1148/radiol.2018171737.
11. Rommele C, Brueckner J, Messmann H, Golder SK. Clinical experience with the PillCam patency capsule prior to video capsule endoscopy: a real-world experience. Gastroenterol Res Pract. 2016;2016:9657053. https://doi.org/10.1155/2016/9657053.
12. Lee SD, Cohen RD. Endoscopy of the small bowel in inflammatory bowel disease. Gastrointest Endosc Clin N Am. 2002;12(3):485–93.
13. Sheehan AL, Warren BF, Gear MW, Shepherd NA. Fat-wrapping in Crohn's disease: pathological basis and relevance to surgical practice. Br J Surg. 1992;79(9):955–8.
14. Magro F, Langner C, Driessen A, Ensari A, Geboes K, Mantzaris GJ, et al. European consensus on the histopathology of inflammatory bowel disease. J Crohns Colitis. 2013;7(10):827–51. https://doi.org/10.1016/j.crohns.2013.06.001.
15. Doumit J, Shen B, Goldblum J, et al. Pyloric gland metaplasia- a specific histopathologic marker for Crohn's disease. Am J Gastroenterol. 2003;98(9):S260.
16. Goldstein N, Dulai M. Contemporary morphologic definition of backwash ileitis in ulcerative colitis and features that distinguish it from Crohn disease. Am J Clin Pathol. 2006;126(3):365–76. https://doi.org/10.1309/UAXMW3428PGN9HJ3.
17. Koukoulis G, Ke Y, Henley JD, Cummings OW. Obliterative muscularization of the small bowel submucosa in Crohn disease: a possible mechanism of small bowel obstruction. Arch Pathol Lab Med. 2001;125(10):1331–4. https://doi.org/10.1043/0003–9985(2001)125<1331:OMOTSB>2.0.CO;2.
18. Borley NR, Mortensen NJ, Jewell DP, Warren BF. The relationship between inflammatory and serosal connective tissue changes in ileal Crohn's disease: evidence for a possible causative link. J Pathol. 2000;190(2):196–202. https://doi.org/10.1002/(SICI)1096–9896(200002)190:2<196::AID-PATH513>3.0.CO;2–5.
19. Pulimood AB, Ramakrishna BS, Kurian G, Peter S, Patra S, Mathan VI, et al. Endoscopic mucosal biopsies are useful in distinguishing granulomatous colitis due to Crohn's disease from tuberculosis. Gut. 1999;45(4):537–41.
20. Geboes K, Collins S. Structural abnormalities of the nervous system in Crohn's disease and ulcerative colitis. Neurogastroenterol Motil. 1998;10(3):189–202.
21. Villanacci V, Bassotti G, Nascimbeni R, Antonelli E, Cadei M, Fisogni S, et al. Enteric nervous system abnormalities in inflammatory bowel diseases. Neurogastroenterol Motil. 2008;20(9):1009–16. https://doi.org/10.1111/j.1365–2982.2008.01146.x.
22. Mooney EE, Walker J, Hourihane DO. Relation of granulomas to lymphatic vessels in Crohn's disease. J Clin Pathol. 1995;48(4):335–8.
23. Matson AP, Van Kruiningen HJ, West AB, Cartun RW, Colombel JF, Cortot A. The relationship of granulomas to blood vessels in intestinal Crohn's disease. Mod Pathol. 1995;8(6):680–5.
24. Masia R, Peyton S, Lauwers GY, Brown I. Gastrointestinal biopsy findings of autoimmune enteropathy: a review of 25 cases. Am J Surg Pathol. 2014;38(10):1319–29. https://doi.org/10.1097/PAS.0000000000000317.
25. Yazisiz V. Similarities and differences between Behcet's disease and Crohn's disease. World J Gastrointest Pathophysiol. 2014;5(3):228–38. https://doi.org/10.4291/wjgp.v5.i3.228.
26. Gan HT, Chen YQ, Ouyang Q, Bu H, Yang XY. Differentiation between intestinal tuberculosis and Crohn's disease in endoscopic biopsy specimens by polymerase chain reaction. Am J Gastroenterol. 2002;97(6):1446–51. https://doi.org/10.1111/j.1572–0241.2002.05686.x.
27. Tandon HD, Prakash A. Pathology of intestinal tuberculosis and its distinction from Crohn's disease. Gut. 1972;13(4):260–9.
28. Alimchandani M, Lai JP, Aung PP, Khangura S, Kamal N, Gallin JI, et al. Gastrointestinal histopathology in chronic granulomatous disease: a study of 87 patients. Am J Surg Pathol. 2013;37(9):1365–72. https://doi.org/10.1097/PAS.0b013e318297427d.
29. Mehta V, Gupta A, Mahajan R, Narang V, Midha V, Sood N, et al. Symptomatic isolated terminal ileal ulcers: etiology and clinical significance. Endosc Int Open. 2017;5(7):E539–E46. https://doi.org/10.1055/s-0043–100688.
30. Courville EL, Siegel CA, Vay T, Wilcox AR, Suriawinata AA, Srivastava A. Isolated asymptomatic ileitis does not progress to overt Crohn disease on long-term follow-up despite features of chronicity in ileal biopsies. Am J Surg Pathol. 2009;33(9):1341–7. https://doi.org/10.1097/PAS.0b013e3181ad25b6.
31. Shen B. Exploring endoscopic therapy for the treatment of Crohn's disease-related fistula and abscess. Gastrointest Endosc. 2017;85(6):1133–43. https://doi.org/10.1016/j.gie.2017.01.025.
32. Munkholm P, Langholz E, Davidsen M, Binder V. Intestinal cancer risk and mortality in patients with Crohn's disease. Gastroenterology. 1993;105(6):1716–23.
33. Rutgeerts P, Geboes K, Vantrappen G, Beyls J, Kerremans R, Hiele M. Predictability of the postoperative course of Crohn's disease. Gastroenterology. 1990;99(4):956–63.
34. Regueiro M, Velayos F, Greer JB, Bougatsos C, Chou R, Sultan S, et al. American gastroenterological association institute technical review on the management of Crohn's disease after surgical resection. Gastroenterology. 2017;152(1):277–95 e3. https://doi.org/10.1053/j.gastro.2016.10.039.
35. Hawkey CJ, Hommes DW. Is stem cell therapy ready for prime time in treatment of inflammatory bowel diseases? Gastroenterology. 2017;152(2):389–97 e2. https://doi.org/10.1053/j.gastro.2016.11.003.
36. Svrcek M, Piton G, Cosnes J, Beaugerie L, Vermeire S, Geboes K, et al. Small bowel adenocarcinomas complicating Crohn's disease are associated with dysplasia: a pathological and molecular study. Inflamm Bowel Dis. 2014;20(9):1584–92. https://doi.org/10.1097/MIB.0000000000000112.
37. Grolleau C, Pote NM, Guedj NS, Zappa M, Theou-Anton N, Bouhnik Y, et al. Small bowel adenocarcinoma complicating Crohn's disease: a single-centre experience emphasizing the importance of screening for dysplasia. Virchows Arch. 2017;471(5):611–7. https://doi.org/10.1007/s00428–017–2125-z.
38. Elriz K, Carrat F, Carbonnel F, Marthey L, Bouvier AM, Beaugerie L, et al. Incidence, presentation, and prognosis of small bowel adenocarcinoma in patients with small bowel Crohn's disease: a prospective observational study. Inflamm Bowel Dis. 2013;19(9):1823–6. https://doi.org/10.1097/MIB.0b013e31828c84f2.
39. Simon M, Cosnes J, Gornet JM, Seksik P, Stefanescu C, Blain A, et al. Endoscopic detection of small bowel dysplasia and adenocarcinoma in Crohn's disease: a prospective cohort-study in high-risk patients. J Crohns Colitis. 2017;11(1):47–52. https://doi.org/10.1093/ecco-jcc/jjw123.
40. Palascak-Juif V, Bouvier AM, Cosnes J, Flourie B, Bouche O, Cadiot G, et al. Small bowel adenocarcinoma in patients with

Crohn's disease compared with small bowel adenocarcinoma de novo. Inflamm Bowel Dis. 2005;11(9):828–32.
41. Piton G, Cosnes J, Monnet E, Beaugerie L, Seksik P, Savoye G, et al. Risk factors associated with small bowel adenocarcinoma in Crohn's disease: a case-control study. Am J Gastroenterol. 2008;103(7):1730–6. https://doi.org/10.1111/j.1572–0241.2008.01847.x.
42. Patil DT, Odze RD. Backwash is hogwash: the clinical significance of ileitis in ulcerative colitis. Am J Gastroenterol. 2017;112(8):1211–4. https://doi.org/10.1038/ajg.2017.182.
43. Haskell H, Andrews CW Jr, Reddy SI, Dendrinos K, Farraye FA, Stucchi AF, et al. Pathologic features and clinical significance of "backwash" ileitis in ulcerative colitis. Am J Surg Pathol. 2005;29(11):1472–81.
44. Hamilton MJ, Makrauer FM, Golden K, Wang H, Friedman S, Burakoff RB, et al. Prospective evaluation of terminal ileitis in a surveillance population of patients with ulcerative colitis. Inflamm Bowel Dis. 2016;22(10):2448–55. https://doi.org/10.1097/MIB.0000000000000911.
45. Yamamoto T, Maruyama Y, Umegae S, Matsumoto K, Saniabadi AR. Mucosal inflammation in the terminal ileum of ulcerative colitis patients: endoscopic findings and cytokine profiles. Dig Liver Dis. 2008;40(4):253–9. https://doi.org/10.1016/j.dld.2007.11.020.
46. Yamaguchi N, Isomoto H, Shikuwa S, Ohnita K, Mizuta Y, Ito M, et al. Proximal extension of backwash ileitis in ulcerative-colitis—associated colon cancer. Med Sci Monit. 2010;16(7):CS87–91.
47. Navaneethan U, Jegadeesan R, Gutierrez NG, Venkatesh PG, Arrossi AV, Bennett AE, et al. Backwash ileitis and the risk of colon neoplasia in ulcerative colitis patients undergoing restorative proctocolectomy. Dig Dis Sci. 2013;58(7):2019–27. https://doi.org/10.1007/s10620–013–2571–7.
48. Mc CF, Bargen JA, et al. Involvement of the ileum in chronic ulcerative colitis. N Engl J Med. 1949;240(4):119–27. https://doi.org/10.1056/NEJM194901272400401.
49. Saltzstein SL, Rosenberg BF. Ulcerative colitis of the ileum, and regional enteritis of the colon. A comparative histopathologic study. Am J Clin Pathol. 1963;40:610–23.
50. Machado WM, Miranda JR, Morceli J, Padovani CR. The small bowel flora in individuals with cecoileal reflux. Arq Gastroenterol. 2008;45(3):212–8.
51. Geboes K, Ectors N, D'Haens G, Rutgeerts P. Is ileoscopy with biopsy worthwhile in patients presenting with symptoms of inflammatory bowel disease? Am J Gastroenterol. 1998;93(2):201–6. https://doi.org/10.1111/j.1572–0241.1998.00201.x.
52. Koukoulis GK, Ke Y, Henley JD, Cummings OW. Detection of pyloric metaplasia may improve the biopsy diagnosis of Crohn's ileitis. J Clin Gastroenterol. 2002;34(2):141–3.
53. Arrossi AV, Kariv Y, Bronner MP, Hammel J, Remzi FH, Fazio VW, et al. Backwash ileitis does not affect pouch outcome in patients with ulcerative colitis with restorative proctocolectomy. Clin Gastroenterol Hepatol. 2011;9(11):981–8. https://doi.org/10.1016/j.cgh.2011.07.018.
54. Heuschen UA, Hinz U, Allemeyer EH, Stern J, Lucas M, Autschbach F, et al. Backwash ileitis is strongly associated with colorectal carcinoma in ulcerative colitis. Gastroenterology. 2001;120(4):841–7.
55. Landy J, Al-Hassi HO, McLaughlin SD, Knight SC, Ciclitira PJ, Nicholls RJ, et al. Etiology of pouchitis. Inflamm Bowel Dis. 2012;18(6):1146–55. https://doi.org/10.1002/ibd.21911.
56. Achkar JP, Al-Haddad M, Lashner B, Remzi FH, Brzezinski A, Shen B, et al. Differentiating risk factors for acute and chronic pouchitis. Clin Gastroenterol Hepatol. 2005;3(1):60–6.
57. Tyler AD, Milgrom R, Stempak JM, Xu W, Brumell JH, Muise AM, et al. The NOD2insC polymorphism is associated with worse outcome following ileal pouch-anal anastomosis for ulcerative colitis. Gut. 2013;62(10):1433–9. https://doi.org/10.1136/gutjnl-2011–301957.
58. Quinn KP, Lightner AL, Pendegraft RS, Enders FT, Boardman LA, Raffals LE. Pouchitis is a common complication in patients with familial adenomatous polyposis following ileal pouch-anal anastomosis. Clin Gastroenterol Hepatol. 2016;14(9):1296–301. https://doi.org/10.1016/j.cgh.2016.04.010.
59. Goldstein NS, Sanford WW, Bodzin JH. Crohn's-like complications in patients with ulcerative colitis after total proctocolectomy and ileal pouch-anal anastomosis. Am J Surg Pathol. 1997;21(11):1343–53.
60. Heuschen UA, Allemeyer EH, Hinz U, Autschbach F, Uehlein T, Herfarth C, et al. Diagnosing pouchitis: comparative validation of two scoring systems in routine follow-up. Dis Colon Rectum. 2002;45(6):776–86; discussion 86–8.
61. Pardi DS, D'Haens G, Shen B, Campbell S, Gionchetti P. Clinical guidelines for the management of pouchitis. Inflamm Bowel Dis. 2009;15(9):1424–31. https://doi.org/10.1002/ibd.21039.
62. Shen B, Fazio VW, Remzi FH, Delaney CP, Bennett AE, Achkar JP, et al. Comprehensive evaluation of inflammatory and noninflammatory sequelae of ileal pouch-anal anastomoses. Am J Gastroenterol. 2005;100(1):93–101. https://doi.org/10.1111/j.1572–0241.2005.40778.x.
63. Shen B. Pouchitis: what every gastroenterologist needs to know. Clin Gastroenterol Hepatol. 2013;11(12):1538–49. https://doi.org/10.1016/j.cgh.2013.03.033.
64. Shen B, Bennett AE, Navaneethan U. IgG4-associated pouchitis. Inflamm Bowel Dis. 2011;17(5):1247–8. https://doi.org/10.1002/ibd.21441.
65. Navaneethan U, Bennett AE, Venkatesh PG, Lian L, Hammel J, Patel V, et al. Tissue infiltration of IgG4+ plasma cells in symptomatic patients with ileal pouch-anal anastomosis. J Crohns Colitis. 2011;5(6):570–6. https://doi.org/10.1016/j.crohns.2011.05.011.
66. Virk R, Shinagare S, Lauwers GY, Yajnik V, Stone JH, Deshpande V. Tissue IgG4-positive plasma cells in inflammatory bowel disease: a study of 88 treatment-naive biopsies of inflammatory bowel disease. Mod Pathol. 2014;27(3):454–9. https://doi.org/10.1038/modpathol.2013.121.
67. Wolf JM, Achkar JP, Lashner BA, Delaney CP, Petras RE, Goldblum JR, et al. Afferent limb ulcers predict Crohn's disease in patients with ileal pouch-anal anastomosis. Gastroenterology. 2004;126(7):1686–91.
68. Agarwal S, Stucchi AF, Dendrinos K, Cerda S, O'Brien MJ, Becker JM, et al. Is pyloric gland metaplasia in ileal pouch biopsies a marker for Crohn's disease? Dig Dis Sci. 2013;58(10):2918–25. https://doi.org/10.1007/s10620–013–2655–4.
69. Shen B, Brzezinski A, Fazio VW, Remzi FH, Achkar JP, Bennett AE, et al. Maintenance therapy with a probiotic in antibiotic-dependent pouchitis: experience in clinical practice. Aliment Pharmacol Ther. 2005;22(8):721–8. https://doi.org/10.1111/j.1365–2036.2005.02642.x.
70. Conway R, Byrne DG, O'Riordan D, Silke B. Improved outcomes of high-risk emergency medical admissions cared for by experienced physicians. QJM. 2015;108(2):119–25. https://doi.org/10.1093/qjmed/hcu171.

14 Drug-Induced Injury, Vascular, Congenital, and Miscellaneous Disorders

Lizhi Zhang

Drug-Induced Injury

Nonsteroidal Anti-inflammatory Drugs (NSAIDs)-Induced Enteropathy

Definition

NSAIDs-induced enteropathy is a small intestinal injury caused by NSAIDs use which has some different clinicopathological features compared to NSAIDs-induced injuries in other sites of gastrointestinal tract.

Clinical Features

The incidence of NSAIDs-induced enteropathy has continuously increased over the last decades because of increased prescriptions and advances in endoscopic techniques which enable direct visualization of the small bowel such as capsule endoscopy and double balloon endoscopy. The earlier reports showed that small intestinal ulcerations occurred in less than 10% of the NSAIDs users [1]; however, recent studies using advanced endoscopy have reported the prevalence of small bowel injuries induced by NSAIDs ranging from 50% to 80% [2–4]. Another reason that the importance of NSAIDs-induced enteropathy is underestimated is because most of the cases have subclinical and nonspecific signs and symptoms compared with NSAIDs-induced injuries in stomach, duodenum, and colon [5]. When present, patients may have various manifestations, including abdominal pain, diarrhea, indigestion, and more severe complications such as iron-deficiency anemia due to occult or overt bleeding, hypoalbuminemia or malabsorption from enteropathy, small bowel stricture and obstruction due to ulceration or intestinal diaphragm, acute abdomen from perforation, or even death [4, 6–9].

While the mechanisms of NSAIDs-induced gastric and duodenal injuries have been clearly illustrated, the pathogenesis of NSAIDs-induced enteropathy has not been well understood because it is believed that there are multiple factors contributing to the mucosal damages in more distal end of the small bowel. The common pathway of NSAIDs-induced mucosal injury is through inhibiting cyclooxygenase (COX) to decrease prostaglandin synthesis leading to the reduction of mucosal blood flow, direct damage of the small bowel epithelium, and increase in intestinal permeability of bile acid, bacteria, proteolytic enzymes, and toxins, and then inflammation is induced and causes the tissue damages such as erosion, ulceration, and bleeding. There are two isoforms of COX, COX-1 and COX-2. Even though it was thought that only the COX-1 inhibition was associated with mucosal injuries, recent studies have shown that both types of COX are probably equally important in maintaining the mucosal integrity, repairing tissue injury, and resolving inflammation. Therefore, nonselective NSAIDs and selective COX-2 inhibitors are not significantly different in inducing small bowel injuries [10, 11].

Besides the mucosal injury induced by decreasing prostaglandin synthesis by NSAIDs, other two factors which also play important role in NSAIDs-induced enteropathy are intestinal bacteria and enterohepatic circulation. Animal studies have shown that no NSAIDs-induced injury occurred in germ-free rats or mice, but the small intestine was susceptible to injuries after recolonization of gram-negative bacteria [12, 13]. In addition, some antibiotics were able to reduce NSAIDs-induced enteropathy, and probiotics could also decrease the severity of NSAIDs-induced enteropathy [14, 15]. On the other hand, bacterial overgrowth induced by chronic acid suppression by proton pump inhibitors (PPI) can exacerbate the NSAIDs-induced enteropathy through dysbiosis [16–18], although it is also well established that PPI can reduce the risk for gastroduodenal ulceration and bleeding from NSAIDs [19].

L. Zhang (✉)
Department of Laboratory Medicine and Pathology, Mayo Clinic, Rochester, MN, USA
e-mail: Zhang.Lizhi@mayo.edu

L. Zhang et al. (eds.), *Surgical Pathology of Non-neoplastic Gastrointestinal Diseases*,
https://doi.org/10.1007/978-3-030-15573-5_14

Enterohepatic circulation can prolong exposure of some NSAIDs which is also important in the pathogenesis of NSAIDs-induced enteropathy. Studies have shown that NSAIDs-induced small bowel mucosal injuries could not occur if NSAIDs did not undergo enterohepatic circulation [20–22]. This is particularly important after introducing enteric-coated aspirin because regular aspirin is rapidly absorbed in the stomach and duodenum with no enterohepatic recirculation; however, enteric-coated aspirin dissolves mainly in small bowel and enters the enterohepatic circulation which causes damage in more distal part of the small intestine [23, 24]. The clinicians and pathologists may be confused by mucosal injuries and ulceration in terminal ilium caused by NSAIDs because they can mimic Crohn's disease.

The clinical diagnosis of NSAIDs-induced enteropathy is mainly relied on the history of NSAIDs use, endoscopic findings, and ruling out other conditions such as infection or inflammatory bowel disease [25]. Endoscopically, NSAIDs-induced enteropathy can present with petechiae, erosions, ulcerations, bleeding, or strictures. Diaphragm-like stricture is a rare but pathognomonic feature of NSAIDs-induced enteropathy, although it has also been reported in cases with no use of NSAIDs [26]. It is characterized by concentric luminal projections of mucosal and submucosal tissue causing strictures with or without obstructive symptoms [27, 28].

Pathological Features

Segmental small bowel resections of NSAIDs-induced enteropathy are occasionally encountered in surgical pathology, which are usually due to small bowel obstruction with unclear causes, perforation, or diaphragm disease. Grossly, the disease can involve the entire small bowel or can be patchy. The mucosal abnormalities include villous atrophy, erosions, bleeding, and ulcerations. The ulcerations occur more frequently in ileum which can be single or multiple, with variable sizes, ranging from aphthoid lesions and small punched-out ulcers to extensive deep ulcerations (Fig. 14.1). The ulcerations may undergo perforation. Fibrosis is usually associated with ulcerations which may cause stenosis and strictures. The serosa is typically unremarkable, except for diaphragm disease in which ring-like serosal constrictions have been observed (Fig. 14.2a) [26, 29]. Fat wrapping or bowel adhesion is not present. Diaphragm disease is unique in NSAIDs-induced enteropathy. The diaphragms are usually multiple with variable shapes and heights which represent different stages of diaphragm formation (Fig. 14.2b). The fully formed diaphragms are thin circumferential mucosal projections with narrowed-lumen that divide the small bowel into multiple compartments; or they can look like tall plicae circularis, broad based humps, or flat strictures [29, 30]. Linear ulcerations are always present at the tip of the diaphragms. Indeed, the linear circumferential ulcerations were considered as the precursors of the diaphragms [31].

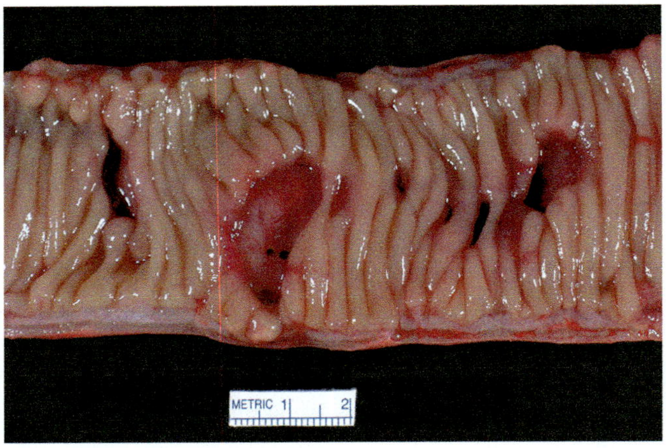

Fig. 14.1 NSAIDs-induced enteropathy. Multiple discrete ulcerations and intertwining mucosa with normal appearance

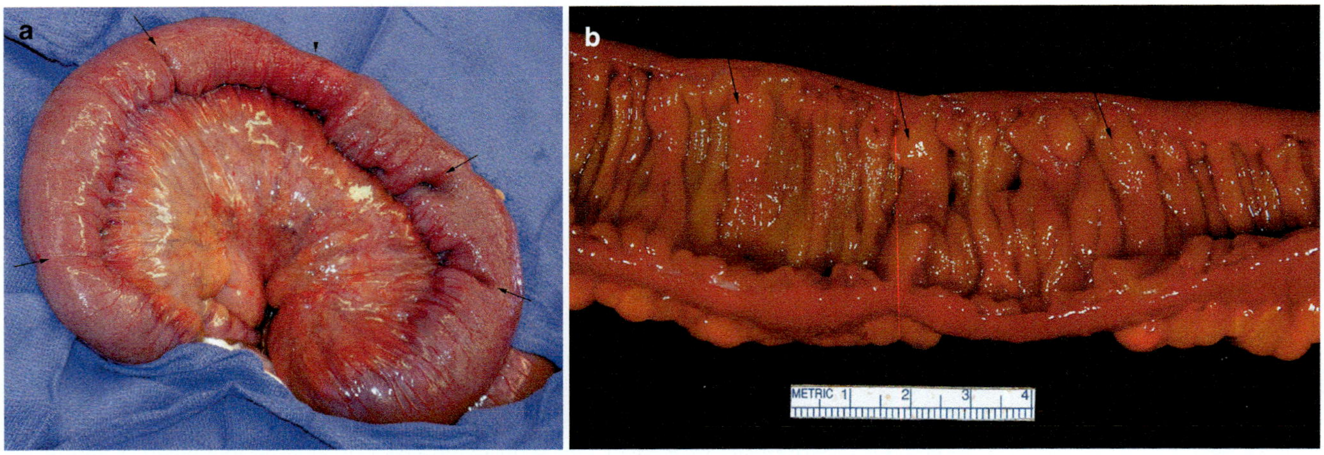

Fig. 14.2 Diaphragm disease. (**a**) Multiple ring-like serosal constrictions (arrows) and a short segment of stricture (arrowhead). (**b**) The open specimen shows multiple diaphragms (arrows) formed by circumferential mucosal projections with superficial ulcerations and narrow lumen

Microscopically, there are various nonspecific morphological changes in NSAIDs-induced enteropathy. The early epithelial damage may be manifested as cytoplasmic vacuolization or mucin depletion at the tips of villi, mild villous blunting, and increased inflammatory infiltrate in lamina propria, including neutrophils and eosinophils (Fig. 14.3a). Cryptitis or crypt abscess is rarely seen. In severe cases, total villous atrophy can develop, but there is no intraepithelial lymphocytosis. Erosions and ulcerations are very common. Widespread erosion with pseudomembrane formation can occur. The ulcerations are usually superficial with dense vertical fibrosis and less inflammatory infiltrate at the base (Fig. 14.3b). Deeper ulceration, but not fissuring-type ulceration seen in Crohn's disease, may occur and can be associated with perforation (Fig. 14.3c).

Features of chronicity are often present, which are typically seen in the mucosa adjacent to the ulcers or diaphragms. Mild crypt architectural distortion, pylori gland metaplasia, or crypt dropout is frequently seen. Mucosal and submucosal fibrosis is common and typically associated with ulceration (Fig. 14.3d). Neuromuscular changes due to chronic injuries are also present, such as duplication of muscularis mucosae or increased nerve fibers and ganglion cells, especially in diaphragm disease.

Unlike the characteristic endoscopic and gross appearances of diaphragms in NSAIDs-induced enteropathy, the microscopic features of diaphragms are less impressive which may look like taller and thickened plicae circularis. Erosions and ulcerations are always present at the overlying epithelium. The mucosa and submucosa contain fibrosis, proliferative small vessels, and abundant connective tissue, which are usually perpendicular to the luminal surface. These features were initially described as neuromuscular and vascular hamartoma-like changes [32] and then were proved

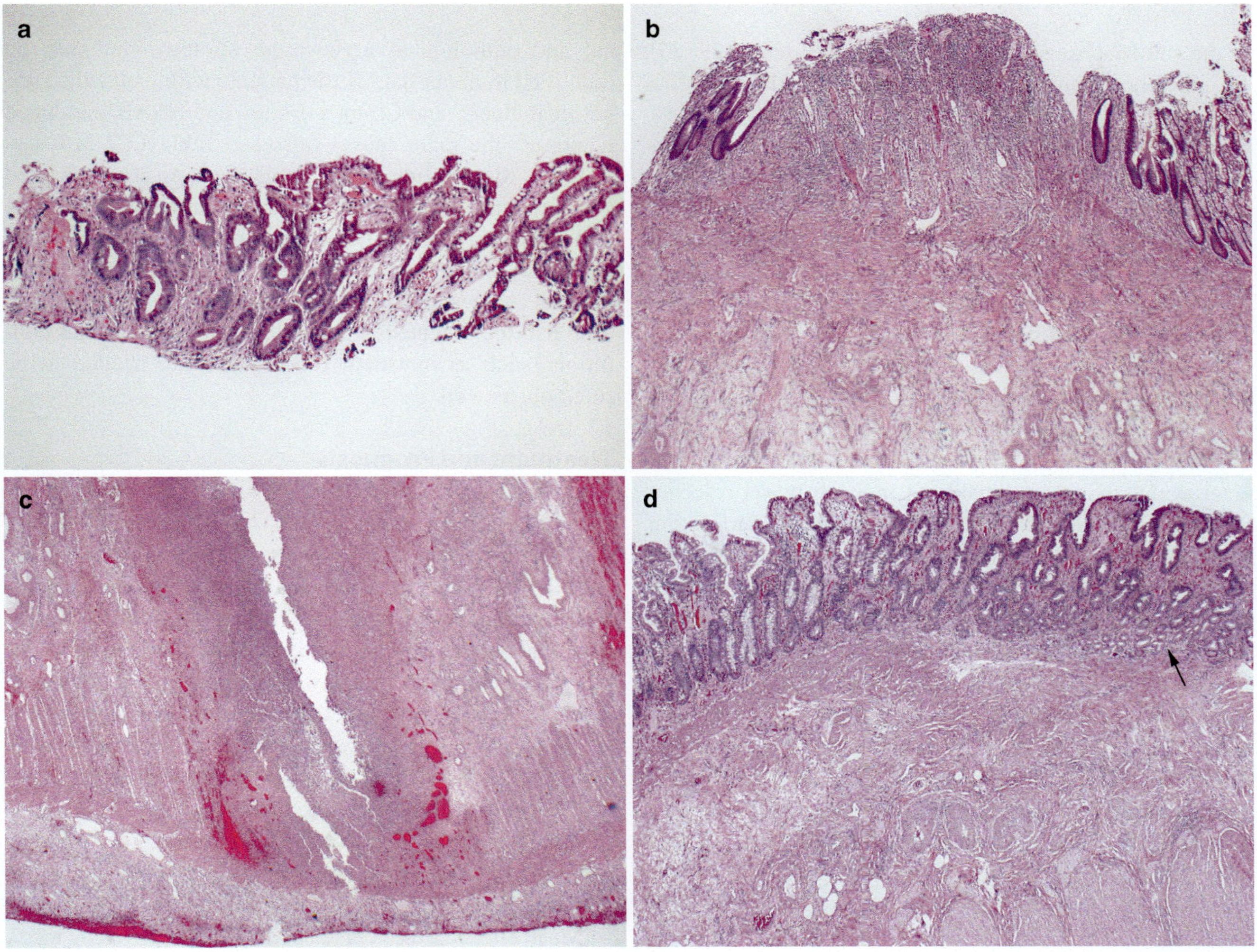

Fig. 14.3 NSAIDs-induced enteropathy. (**a**) Epithelial damages include mucin depletion at the tips of villi, villous blunting, increased inflammatory infiltrate in lamina propria, and focal erosion. (**b**) Ulceration with dense vertical fibrosis and less inflammatory infiltrate at the base. (**c**) Deep penetration ulceration. (**d**) Chronic mucosa injury with architectural distortion, villous atrophy, pseudopyloric metaplasia (arrow), and fibrosis in mucosa and submucosa

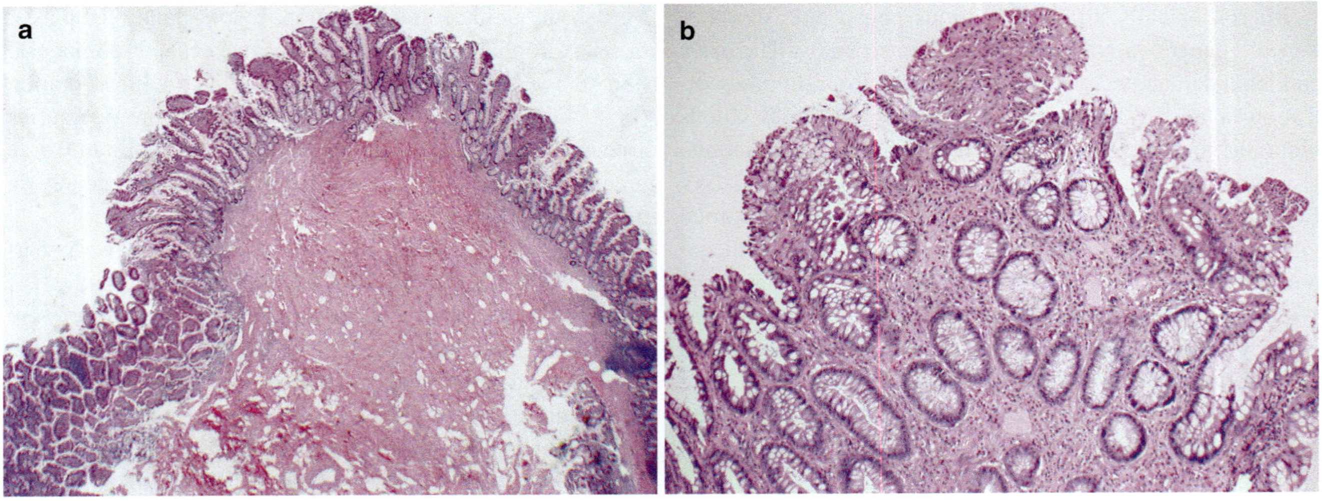

Fig. 14.4 Diaphragm in NSAIDs-induced enteropathy. (**a**) A broad-based mucosal projection, perpendicular to the luminal surface, consists of mucosa and submucosa fibrosis, proliferative small vessels, and abundant connective tissue. (**b**) Surface epithelial injury at the tip of a diaphragm, with increased inflammation, architectural distortion, focal erosion, and reactive/regenerative change

as the similar changes seen in diaphragm disease [29, 33]. The diaphragms may be also broad-based without obvious projections (Fig. 14.4). The overlying epithelium can be erosive or shows marked reactive/regenerative atypia, in association with significant architectural distortion, inflammation, and dense fibrosis. Features in Crohn's disease such as granulomas or transmural inflammation are not identified in diaphragm disease [29].

Differential Diagnosis

Establishing a histological diagnosis of NSAIDs-induced enteropathy requires clinical and endoscopic correlation, since there are no specific histopathological features besides diaphragm disease. The possibility of NSAIDs-induced enteropathy should be considered in small bowel resection for unknown cause of obstruction, bleeding, or perforation. Biopsy specimens for endoscopically accessible strictures or ulcerations, typically from distal and terminal ilium, are often obtained for pathological evaluation as well. The differential diagnoses of above-mentioned changes in small bowel can be broad, including Crohn's disease, ischemic enteropathy, mechanical injury, other drugs such as Kayexalate or slow-release potassium, infections, Behçet's disease, or even tumor. Often time, pathologists can only give a descriptive report and then list some main considerations to help clinicians to identify the underlying cause with proper clinical context.

Nowadays, ileoscopy at colonoscopy is performed routinely for the completeness of the procedure and improves the diagnostic yield. It is not uncommon to find isolated terminal ileal ulcers during the procedures that are biopsied for pathological evaluation. Even with thorough clinical and pathological review, the etiology can only be identified in about half of the patients with isolated terminal ileal ulcers, and Crohn's disease and NSAIDs-induced ulcers are the main causes (also see Table 13.2 in Chap. 13) [34]. Microscopically, if the ileal ulcers are associated with more profound inflammation and architectural distortion, especially when granulomas present, Crohn's disease is favored. NSAIDs-induced ulcers tend to have more fibrosis and less inflammation. However, it is difficult to establish the diagnosis by histology alone, and other conditions such as intestinal tuberculosis are needed to be ruled out as well.

Treatment and Prognosis

Even though majority of NSAIDs-induced enteropathy is subclinical, severe complications such as bleeding, obstruction, or perforation may be as frequent and severe as NSAIDs-induced gastroduodenal injuries. The most important and effective method to prevent or cure NSAIDs-induced enteropathy is to discontinue the NSAIDs. The nonobstructive symptoms can be quickly improved after withdrawal of NSAIDs. However, obstructive symptoms due to strictures are unlikely to resolve, which usually require endoscopic interventions such as through-the-scope balloon dilation or needle-knife electroincision. Resections are also indicated if there are endoscopically inaccessible strictures, multiple diaphragm-like strictures, significant bleeding, or perforation.

Much effort has been made to develop prophylactic medications for chronic NSAIDs users, but only with limited success. Medications used for managing gastroduodenal injuries caused by NSAIDs, such as PPIs, H2 antagonists, or sucralfate, are not effective in preventing the small intestine injuries [5]; COX-2 inhibitors are supposedly to cause less gastroduodenal ulceration and bleeding, compared with nonselective NSAIDs, but there is no significant difference in the incidence of small bowel between these two in the long-term users [10, 11]; medications either promoting prostaglandin synthesis or simulating prostaglandin, such as rebamipide and misoprostol, may reduce NSAIDs-induced injury, but additional studies are required to verify the effectiveness, and some severe adverse effects also limit their usage [35, 36]; antibiotics such as metronidazole or probiotic formulation may be effective against NSAIDs-induced injury, and more clinical studies are necessary [37, 38].

Other Drugs-Induced Injury

Other drugs-induced injuries in the jejunum and ileum are less recognized and documented than those in the stomach, duodenum, and colon, probably because of limited accessibility. Some medications such as chemotherapeutic agents, immunosuppressants, and antibiotics, which commonly cause damages in other sites of gastrointestinal tract, can also affect the small intestine.

Chemotherapy

Chemotherapy-related gastrointestinal complications are common. The mucosa of the small intestine is most sensitive to chemotherapeutic agents-induced injury because of rapidly divided cells. The severity of mucosal injury is related to the dosage, route, combination of drugs, and concomitant use of radiation. Endoscopically, the small intestinal mucosal injury can be manifested as widespread ulceration, erosion, or active bleeding [39]. Microscopically, the early changes of surface epithelial cells include mucin depletion, loss of brush border, vacuolation of cytoplasm, and enlarged nuclei. The cells may transform to a more cuboidal shape. The cells at the crypt bases show significantly increased apoptosis [40–42]. Inflammatory infiltration including eosinophils may increase. The mucosa shows edema and congestion. Villous atrophy and crypt hypoplasia develop after a few days of chemotherapy. The villous blunting can range from mild to complete atrophy. In severe cases, the small bowel mucosa can be completely destroyed with ulcerations and only scattered crypts in the lamina propria. The remaining crypts are smaller in size with a withered appearance. Chemotherapy can induce mild atypia of the epithelial cells and stromal cells. It can also reduce lymphoid tissue and cellularity in lamina propria, and Peyer patches in distal ileum may be depleted. Regeneration typically occurs within 2 weeks after chemotherapy. The villi and crypts can grow back to normal length at day 16 [42]. Mitoses are numerous and the regenerative cells can show significant cytological atypia. The crypts may be dilated with hyperplastic changes. The differential diagnosis mainly includes infection and ischemia. The presence of apoptotic cells, crypt dropout, and cytological atypia suggests chemotherapy-induced injury. Concomitant infections such as CMV or *Candida* are not uncommon given the immunocompromised status. Special stains are usually ordered to exclude these possibilities.

Immunosuppressants

Immunosuppressants are widely used in organ transplantation, inflammatory bowel disease, and autoimmune disorders. The commonly used agents include corticosteroids, TNF antagonists, cyclosporine, tacrolimus, mycophenolate, azathioprine, and methotrexate. All these agents can be associated with gastrointestinal complications. However, their effect on jejunum and ileum is largely unknown. Corticosteroids may deplete lymphoid tissue and inflammatory cells in lamina propria in the ileum (Fig. 14.5); mycophenolate-induced upper and lower gastrointestinal mucosa injury has been well described [43–45], which is typically characterized with graft versus host disease (GVHD)-like changes including increased apoptosis, crypt architectural disarray, lamina propria edema and increased inflammation, cryptitis, and crypt dropout. Terminal ileum changes were described in one of the studies [44]. Four of the 5 terminal ileum biopsies showed abnormalities. Two cases had GVHD-like features, but there was one case also showing Crohn-like features including granulomatous inflammation. Focal active ileitis was found in the other abnormal cases.

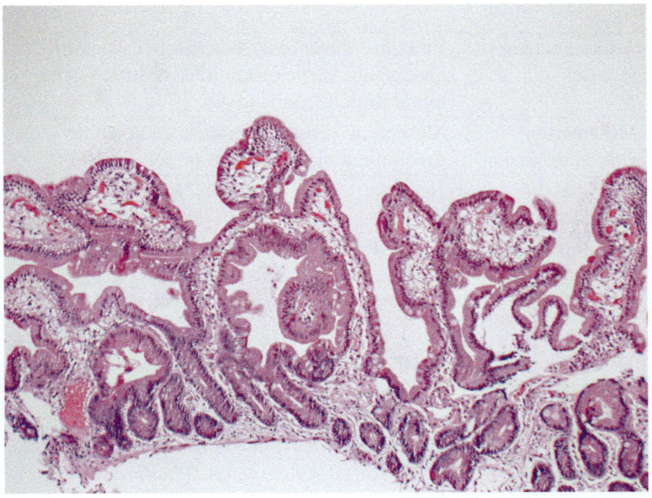

Fig. 14.5 Corticosteroid-related changes in ileum. Note the empty lamina propria with no lymphoid tissue and rare inflammatory cells

Ischemic, Vascular, and Structural Disorders

Ischemic Enteritis

Definition

Ischemic enteritis is inflammation, injury, or necrosis of small intestine caused by sudden loss or chronic insufficient intestinal blood supply.

Clinical Features

Ischemic enteritis is rare and predominantly occurs in elderly person with underlying cardiovascular disease. However, it may affect individuals of any age, including infants. The etiology of small intestine ischemia is heterogeneous, and it can be acute or chronic, occlusive or nonocclusive, and intrinsic or extrinsic to the bowel. The arterial ischemia is more common than venous ischemia, and the common causes are listed in the Table 14.1.

The clinical presentations of ischemic enteritis are nonspecific, and they vary with different etiologies. The severity and clinical course of ischemic enteritis range widely from asymptomatic transient minimal ischemic episodes to massive and sometimes fatal hemorrhagic infarctions. Generally, patients with acute occlusive ischemia of small intestine present with an acute abdomen and become abruptly ill with colicky abdominal pain and bloody diarrhea. As the ischemia persists and infarction develops, the patients often develop fever, paralytic ileus, peritonitis, hypotension, and an elevated white blood count. In the chronic setting, the patients may or may not have abdominal pain, but rather weight loss and food-fear because of increased demand of blood flow at postprandial period. The patients may also develop nausea, vomiting, bloody stool, or ascites.

Table 14.1 Common causes of small intestinal ischemia

Causes	Diseases
Systemic low flow status	Low cardiac output, hypotension, and shock
Arterial occlusive disease	Embolus, thrombosis, atherosclerosis, aortic aneurysms, aortic dissections, obstruction by mural thrombi, and tumors
Mesenteric venous occlusion	Mesenteric venous thrombosis, idiopathic myointimal hyperplasia of mesenteric veins
Necrotizing enterocolitis	Neonatal, tropical (enteritis Necroticans)
Vasculitis	Polyarteritis nodosa, Henoch-Schonlein Purpura, microscopic polyangiitis, Churg-Strauss syndrome, and Kawasaki disease
Mechanical vascular compression	Torsion, volvulus, intussusception, hernias, and celiac compression
Drugs	Oral contraceptives, cocaine, digitalis, vasopressors, and potassium chloride
Infections	CMV, fungal, *Clostridium difficile*, and Enterotoxigenic *E. coli*
Others	Amyloidosis, collagen vascular diseases, radiation damage, coagulation disorders, and dialysis

Endoscopic findings of ischemic enteritis include mucosal congestion, edema, or ulceration, but these features are not specific for ischemic injury. Laboratory tests for bowel ischemia are generally nonspecific. Imaging studies are particularly important in establishing the diagnosis and identifying the etiology. The blood flow in major vessels can be evaluated by duplex ultrasonography. Contrast-enhanced CT scan may find evidence of ischemia such as vessel filling defect, arterial narrowing, thickened and edematous bowel wall, variable bowel enhancement, mesenteric fat stranding, and free fluid in ischemic enteritis [46]. CT angiography remains the standard test to assess both acute and chronic mesenteric ischemia. It is a fast and noninvasive test with high sensitivity and specificity [47]. Magnetic resonance arteriography is occasionally used to evaluate the patency of the superior mesenteric artery and inferior mesenteric artery, but its role is limited in evaluating distal arterial stenosis and nonocclusive mesenteric ischemia.

Pathological Features

The pathological changes of ischemic enteritis range widely on both gross and microscopic examination, which would depend on the underlying causes, the onset and duration of ischemia, the size and severity of vascular occlusion, and reperfusion. Therefore, ischemic enteritis may vary from minimal changes to extensive transmural infarction and perforation. Resection specimens are more commonly encountered than mucosal biopsies in small bowel ischemic enteritis. The gross examination not only documents the presence of ischemic injury but also is important in determining the extent of ischemia, the margin status, the associated disorders, and possible etiology (Fig. 14.6a, b). The earlier changes of ischemic bowel include edema, congestion, focal hemorrhage, and mucosal sloughing. With prolonged and persistent ischemia, the mucosa shows diffuse ulceration, hemorrhage, and necrosis. The serosa becomes dusky with dark red or blue-brown discoloration. Transmural necrosis with blue-black color, pneumatosis intestinalis, and perforation develop at advanced stage. The bowel wall becomes very thin and friable and the lumen usually contains a large amount of blood. The ischemic injury is usually geographic which depends on the distribution of blood flow in the affected bowel. The ischemic bowel can be sharply demarked from the unaffected bowel. Identifying associated disorders such as volvulus, herniation, or intussusception can help in determining the causes. The attached mesentery should also be carefully examined and sections containing vessels should be submitted to identify emboli, thrombosis, atherosclerosis, amyloidosis, or vasculitis (Fig. 14.7). For chronic ischemic enteritis, fibrosis and multiple stricture formation are the main features.

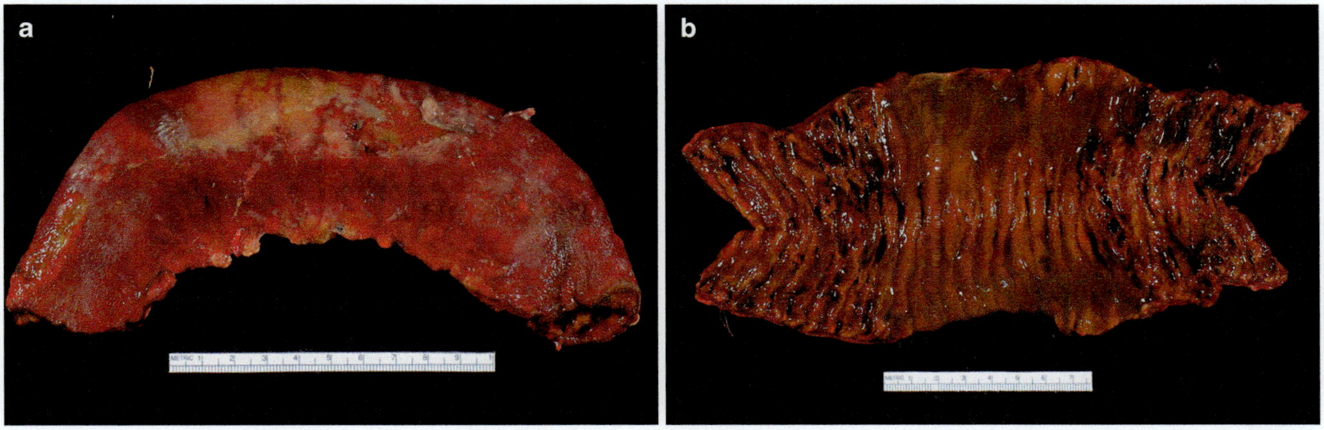

Fig. 14.6 Ischemic enteritis. (**a**) The segment of small bowel shows edema, congestion, focal hemorrhage, and dusky serosa. (**b**) The open specimen shows diffuse mucosal ulceration, hemorrhage, and necrosis

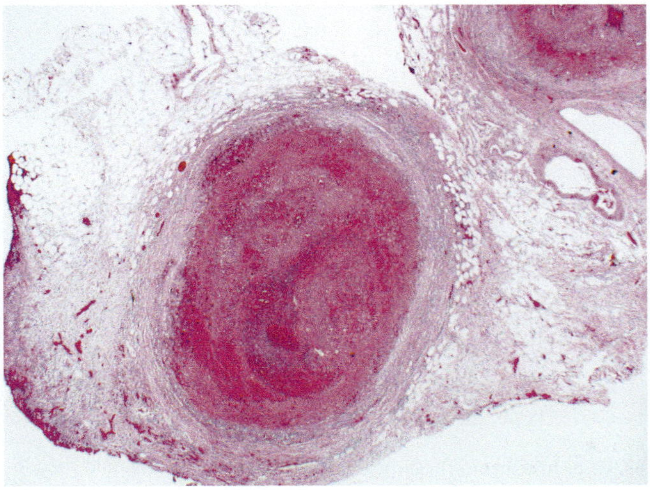

Fig. 14.7 Thrombi in mesenteric vessels causing ischemic enteritis

The microscopic changes in ischemic enteritis are similar to the ischemic injury at the other site of gastrointestinal tract (Fig. 14.8). The mucosa is the most vulnerable to ischemia and is damaged first. Within the first few hours of total vascular occlusion, the epithelial cells lining the villi start lifting off the basement membrane, and the mucosa becomes denuded with ulceration. This process advances from the villous tips to the crypt bases. The crypt may be intact initially but become dilated and atrophic later. The lamina propria contains edema and congested capillaries with fibrin and red cell extravasation (Fig. 14.8a). A few hours after acute total occlusion, the epithelium is completely lost and entire intestinal wall appears necrotic and perforation may occur (Fig. 14.8b, c). The inflammation accompanying the coagulation necrosis is typically not prominent which mimics autolysis. Fibrin thrombi in mucosal capillaries are often identified. If partial blood flow is maintained, the ischemic changes are often superimposed with the effects of the reperfusion. The lamina propria is edematous and hemorrhagic, with telangiectasia, emigration of neutrophils, and cryptitis. The crypts fill with necrotic and inflammatory debris, and eventually pseudomembrane composed of necrotic epithelium, fibrinous exudates, and inflammatory cells develops. If the affected segment is small and with collateral circulation, a healing process may develop simultaneously with superimposed regenerative changes.

After the initial ischemic injury, the ulcerated region is replaced by granulation tissue with chronic inflammation, and then becomes fibrotic (Fig. 14.8d). The degree of fibrosis in chronic ischemia depends on the extent of the ischemic damage that may lead to stricture formation. Macrophages containing hemosiderin after removing red blood cells in the hemorrhagic area is an important diagnostic clue for ischemic injury. The regenerative epithelium shows architectural distortion, increased mitotic activity, and endocrine cell hyperplasia. The lamina propria has variable degrees of fibrosis, mixed inflammation, and dilated prominent capillaries.

Differential Diagnosis

Most diagnoses of ischemic enteritis are made upon examining resected small intestinal specimens without any difficulties. Mucosal biopsies for small intestinal ischemia are not frequently encountered by pathologists. The diagnostic challenges are determined by the underlying causes of ischemia, early or chronic ischemic changes, and associated complications. Correlation with clinical history, imaging, gross and microscopic examination of mesentery and small bowel wall is necessary to determine or confirm the cause. For example, identifying vasculitis with fibrinoid necrosis in submucosa in patient with systemic lupus erythematosus (SLE) who presents with ischemic enteritis is diagnostic for SLE-related gastroenteropathy (Fig. 14.9a, b). The early changes, especially with partial vascular occlusion, may be mild and nonspecific. The small bowel

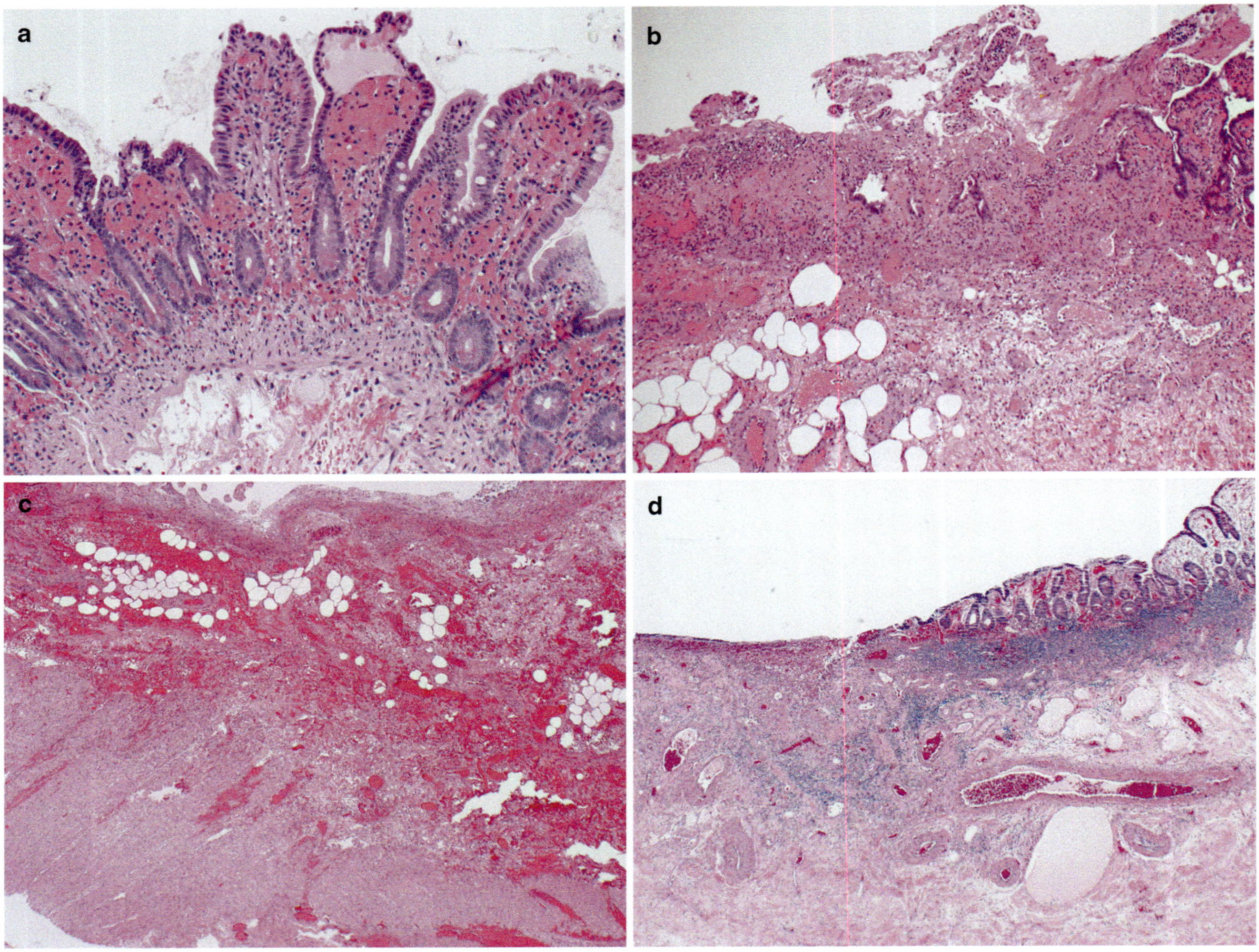

Fig. 14.8 Ischemic enteritis. (**a**) Early changes in acute ischemic injury, characterized by lifting of the epithelial cells lining the villi and crypt atrophy, with lamina propria edema, congestion, and red cell extravasation. (**b**) Severe acute ischemic enteritis with epithelial necrosis, crypt loss, hemorrhage, less prominent inflammation, and pseudomembranous material. (**c**) Full-thickness necrosis. (**d**) Chronic ischemic enteritis with ulceration. Note the chronic ischemic injury in the epithelium next to the ulcer

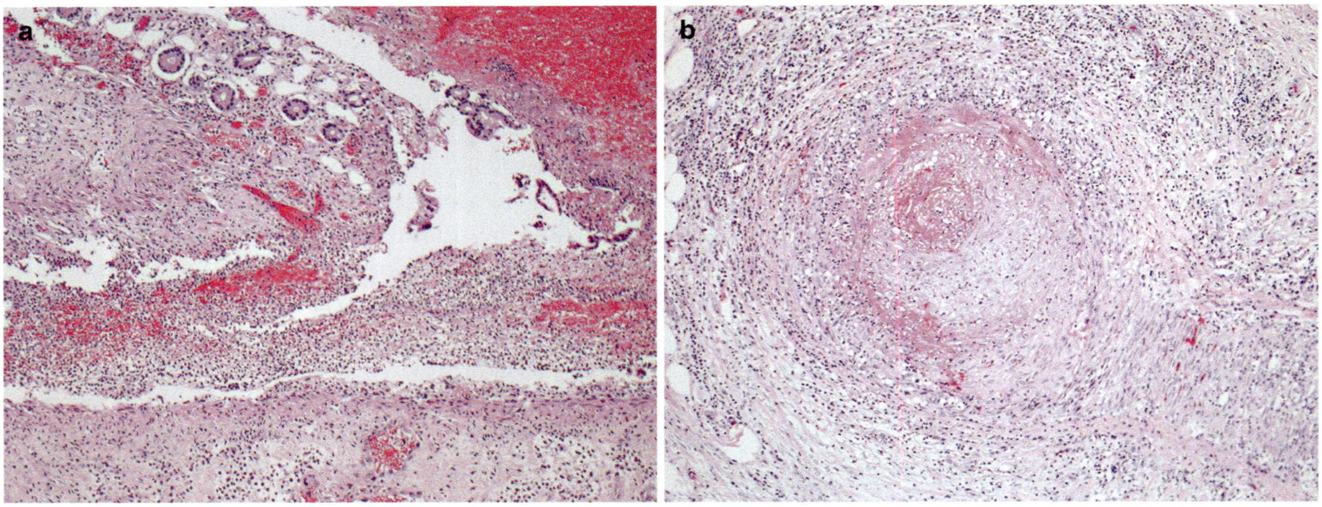

Fig. 14.9 Systemic lupus erythematosus-related ischemic enteritis. (**a**) The small bowel shows acute ischemic injury. (**b**) Lupus vasculitis with fibrinoid necrosis and luminal deposits of eosinophilic and homogeneous proteinaceous material in mesenteric vessels

may only show edema, congestion, and patchy superficial loss of epithelium at the villous tips, and other possible causes such as infection, drug injury, or even artifacts are needed to rule out. The chronic ischemia may mimic Crohn's disease because of the presence of mucosal ulceration, strictures, and fibrosis. The findings of hemosiderin-laden macrophages, prominent fibrosis, and vascular changes support an ischemic etiology, while Crohn's disease shows transmural inflammation, granulomas, and involvement of other part of gastrointestinal tract.

Treatment and Prognosis

The treatment of ischemic enteritis relies on the specific etiology. Besides general management such as pain control and antibiotics, mesenteric arterial occlusion can be treated with surgical laparotomy with embolectomy, revascularization, or thrombolysis with endovascular angioplasty and stenting; and for nonocclusive mesenteric ischemia, the management focuses on treating underlying causes with hemodynamic support. The prognosis is also related to the etiology. In general, patients with an arterial etiology have worse outcome than those with a venous etiology. The reported mortality rates are nearly 50% for patients with acute mesenteric ischemia [48].

Small Intestine in Systemic Vasculitis

Systemic vasculitis can involve vessels in both mesentery and small bowel wall and lead to intestinal ischemia. Most of cases have chronic clinical presentations, but acute mesenteric ischemia may occur. The clinical features and pathological findings vary with different types of vasculitis. Large vessel vasculitis (Takayasu arteritis and giant cell arteritis) rarely affects gastrointestinal tract. Medium and small vessel vasculitis frequently involves small bowel. It is most prevalent in patients with Henoch-Schönlein purpura, polyarteritis nodosa, antineutrophil cytoplasmic autoantibody (ANCA)-associated vasculitis (Eosinophilic granulomatosis with polyangiitis, granulomatosis with polyangiitis, and microscopic polyangiitis). Some extremely rare idiopathic systemic vasculopathy such as Degos disease can also involve small bowel and lead to infarct (Fig. 14.10a, b) [49, 50]. However, the diagnosis of gastrointestinal tract involvement is primarily relied on the established diagnosis of systemic vasculitis and extraintestinal manifestations, and pathological confirmation is typically made on resection tissue but not biopsies.

Polyarteritis Nodosa

Polyarteritis nodosa (PAN) is a systemic necrotizing vasculitis affecting medium-sized muscular arteries, with occasional involvement of small muscular arteries. PAN is not associated with ANCA. Patients with PAN typically present with systemic symptoms such as fever, fatigue, and weight loss, and signs of multisystem involvement [51]. Gastrointestinal involvement occurs in 14–65% of patients with PAN, and abdominal pain, especially postprandial abdominal pain, is the most common symptom [52]. Patients may also develop nausea, vomiting, bloody or nonbloody diarrhea, or even more severe complications including bowel infarction, perforation, or life-threatening gastrointestinal bleeding. Mesenteric vasculitis affects the small intestine more commonly than other parts of the gastrointestinal tract. Immunosuppression such as using corticosteroid or cyclophosphamide is the mainstay of treatment which has decreased mortality dramatically.

Although PAN commonly involves small intestine and ischemic lesions such as ulcerations are often found endoscopically, diagnosis of PAN is rarely made based on gastro-

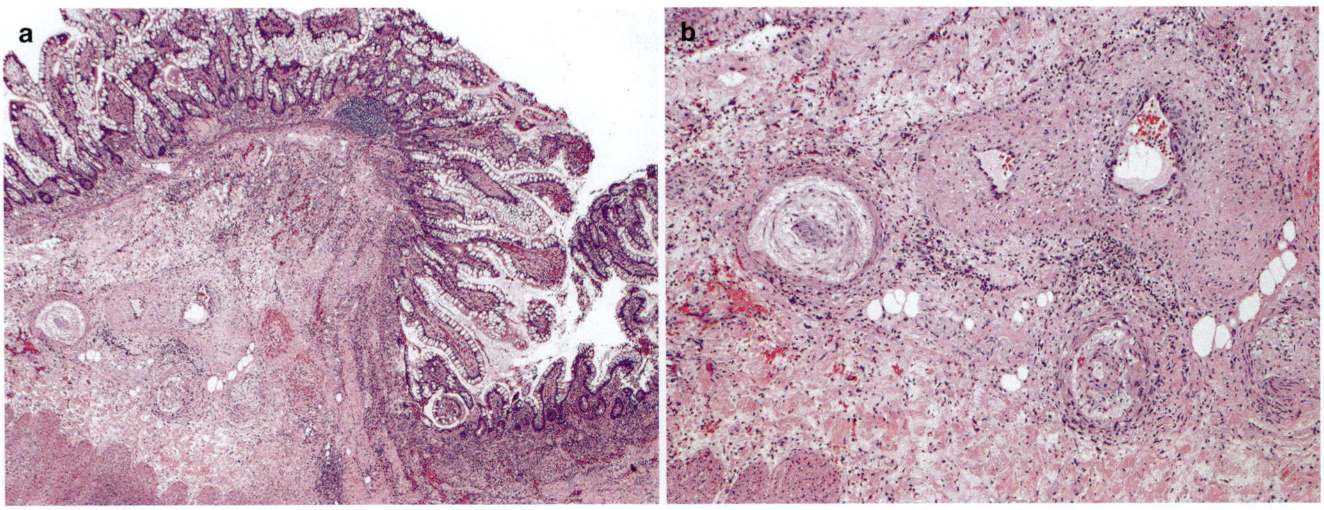

Fig. 14.10 Degos disease involving small intestine. (**a**) Obliterative vasculopathy in submucosal vessels with focal ischemic injury of small bowel mucosa. (**b**) The obliterative vasculopathy is characterized by occlusion by acellular mucinous fibrous plugs and luminal thrombus, with expansion of the intima, endothelial cell injury, and perivascular inflammation

intestinal biopsies. Features of vasculitis are usually absent due to the superficial nature of the biopsy [53]. Resection specimens show changes of ischemic injury. Microscopically, the vasculitis is limited to small and medium arteries. The veins are not involved. The characteristic features of PAN are transmural inflammatory infiltration and fibrinoid necrosis of the arterial wall (Fig. 14.11). The inflammation is predominantly composed of neutrophils and eosinophils. Thrombi are often present. The inflammation also extends to the surrounding soft tissue. The bowel wall shows variable ischemic changes, ranging from mucosal congestion, edema, ulceration, to necrosis and infarction. After acute phase, the inflammation and destruction of arterial wall are replaced by mononuclear cell infiltrate, granulation tissue, and fibrosis.

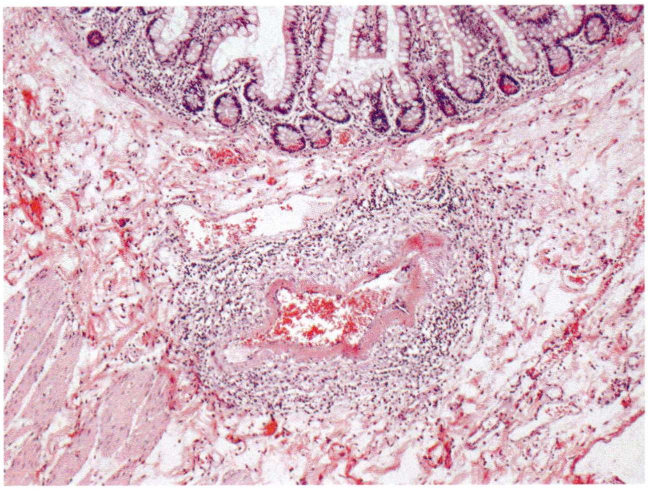

Fig. 14.11 Polyarteritis nodosa. The submucosal artery shows transmural neutrophilic and eosinophilic infiltration with fibrinoid necrosis of the arterial wall and inflammation in the surrounding area

Henoch-Schönlein Purpura

Henoch-Schönlein purpura (HSP), also known as IgA vasculitis, anaphylactoid purpura, or purpura rheumatica, is a systemic small vessel vasculitis characterized by deposition of immune complexes containing IgA and C3. HSP most commonly affects children and is the most common vasculitis in children, although it can occur in any age. The characteristic clinical presentations are purpura, arthritis, and abdominal pain which are known as the "classic triad" of HSP [54]. Purpura occurs in all patients, while joint pains, arthritis, and abdominal pain in 60–80% of cases. Some patients with HSP may also develop gastrointestinal bleeding, nephritis, or hematuria. Most patients do not need therapy because of the high spontaneous recovery rate, and the overall prognosis of HSP is good, but recurrence can occur which is more common in older children and adults [55].

Gastrointestinal involvement can occur in 50–75% of patients with HSP, and the small intestine is more commonly affected than other sites of the gastrointestinal tract. The endoscopic findings include diffuse mucosal redness, small ring-like petechiae, erosions, irregular ulcers, or hematoma-like protrusions. The resected small bowel may reveal intramural hemorrhages with edema, congestion, ulceration, and mottling. Submucosal hemorrhage is often present which can become the leading point of small bowel intussusception. Massive gastrointestinal hemorrhage, perforation, or stricture is rarely seen [56]. Microscopically, variable degrees of ischemic injury (Fig. 14.12a) are present. The villus architecture is usually preserved, and neutrophilic and eosinophilic infiltrates can be seen in lamina propria. The vasculitis in small vessels is so-called leukocytoclastic vasculitis which is manifested with neutrophilic and mononuclear cell infiltrates, fibrinoid necrosis, and

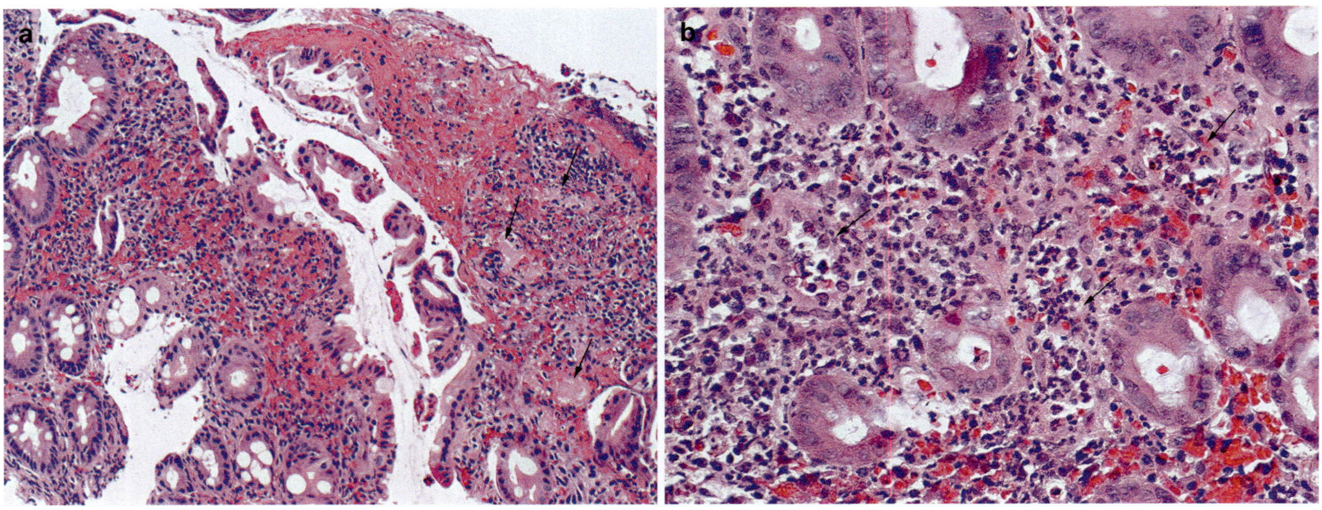

Fig. 14.12 Henoch-Schönlein purpura (HSP). (**a**) Ischemic injury of small bowel mucosa with inflammation, erosion, hemorrhage, and fibrin thrombi (arrows). (**b**) Leukocytoclastic vasculitis involving small capillaries within the lamina propria (arrows) may be observed in about one third of cases

fibrin thrombi (Fig. 14.12b). The vasculitis is also present in nonnecrotic area which is an important feature to exclude secondary changes. In fact, the vasculitis is not commonly seen in mucosal biopsies. Instead, there are a spectrum of changes in mucosa including erosion, lamina propria hemorrhage, fibrin deposition with red cell sludging, and focal active inflammation. Leukocytoclastic vasculitis involving small capillaries within the lamina propria may be observed in about one third of cases [57].

Eosinophilic Granulomatosis with Polyangiitis (Churg-Strauss Syndrome)

Eosinophilic granulomatosis with polyangiitis (EGPA), previously known as Churg-Strauss syndrome (CSS), is a systemic disorder characterized by eosinophil-rich and necrotizing granulomatous inflammation and necrotizing vasculitis predominantly affecting small to medium vessels, associated with chronic rhinosinusitis, asthma, and prominent peripheral blood eosinophilia [58]. ANCA is more frequent when glomerulonephritis is present. If appropriately treated, the outcome of EGPA is good. Treatment for EGPA mainly includes corticosteroid and other immunosuppressive drugs. Recently, an anti-interleukin-5 monoclonal antibody mepolizumab has been shown to significantly improve EGPA patients' symptoms [59].

Gastrointestinal involvement is frequent in patients with EGPA who may present with abdominal pain, diarrhea, or bleeding. Microscopically, the major histological features of EGPA involving small bowel are transmural eosinophilic infiltration, vasculitis in small arteries and veins, necrotizing granulomas in interstitial and perivascular area, and ischemic changes (Fig. 14.13). However, the diagnosis of EGPA in the gastrointestinal tract requires high clinical suspicion as histologic evidence of vasculitis may not be present because of sampling issues related to endoscopic biopsy or absent of vasculitis in prevasculitic phase of the disease, and eosinophilia may be the only finding [60]. The vasculitis is characterized by transmural eosinophilic infiltration and fibrinoid necrosis. Granulomatous inflammation occasionally involves vascular wall but more often at perivascular area which is composed of central necrotic eosinophilic material surrounded by palisading lymphocytes, histiocytes, and multinucleated giant cells. In the later phase, the healed necrotizing vasculitis resembles organized thrombi, and tissue eosinophilic infiltration may be absent.

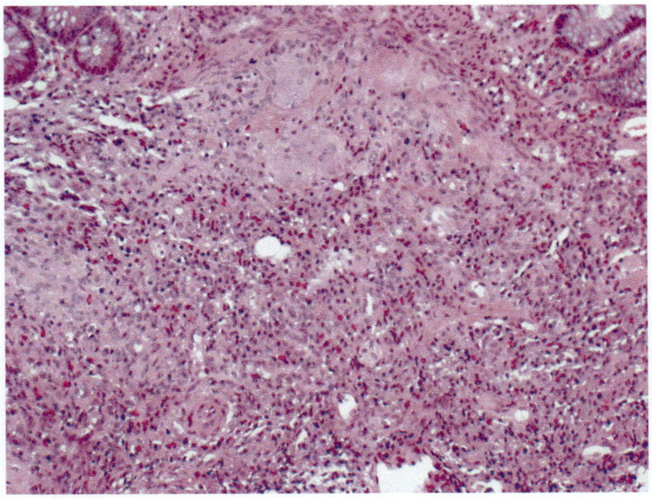

Fig. 14.13 Eosinophilic granulomatosis with polyangiitis (Churg-Strauss syndrome). Marked eosinophilia and submucosal vasculitis characterized by transmural eosinophilic infiltrate and granulomatous inflammation

Granulomatosis with Polyangiitis

Granulomatosis with polyangiitis (GPA), formerly known as Wegener's granulomatosis, is a c-ANCA associated systemic disorder characterized by granulomatosis and necrotizing vasculitis of small- and medium-size vessels in many organs. The initial clinical presentations of GPA are variable and nonspecific and diagnosis can be severely delayed. The respiratory system is most commonly affected and is related to the earliest symptoms such as rhinitis, sinus pain, nasal ulceration, serous otitis media, cough, hemoptysis, or dyspnea. The other organ site involvement includes kidneys, skin, eyes, nerve system, and gastrointestinal tract. The multidisciplinary management and collaboration between different medical specialties is crucial for the treatment of GPA. Although the prognosis of GPA has dramatically improved with immunotherapy, there is still significant morbidity from the disease itself or side effects from the therapy [61].

Gastrointestinal tract involvement is less common in GPA, and rarely can the gastrointestinal manifestation be the first symptom of GPA. The common symptoms are nonspecific including abdominal pain, nausea or vomiting, diarrhea, hematochezia, or melena. Intestinal wall necrosis and perforations (Fig. 14.14a) can occur. The endoscopic biopsy rarely reveals diagnostic features besides nonspecific inflammatory changes and ulcerations because of the superficial nature of the tissue. The small and medium diameter vessels are located deeper in the submucosa. The necrotizing vasculitis involves both arteries and veins with neutrophilic infiltration and fibrinoid necrosis of the vessel wall (Fig. 14.14b, c). The granulomas are necrotizing with palisading epithelioid histiocytes surrounding the necrotic core, and multinucleated giant cells are present in both vasculitis and granulomas (Fig. 14.14b). The differential diagnoses include infections or Crohn's disease, and the diagnosis of GPA in small intestine depends largely on clinical workup.

Microscopic Polyangiitis

Microscopic polyangiitis (MPA) is also an ANCA-associated systemic necrotizing vasculitis of small vessels

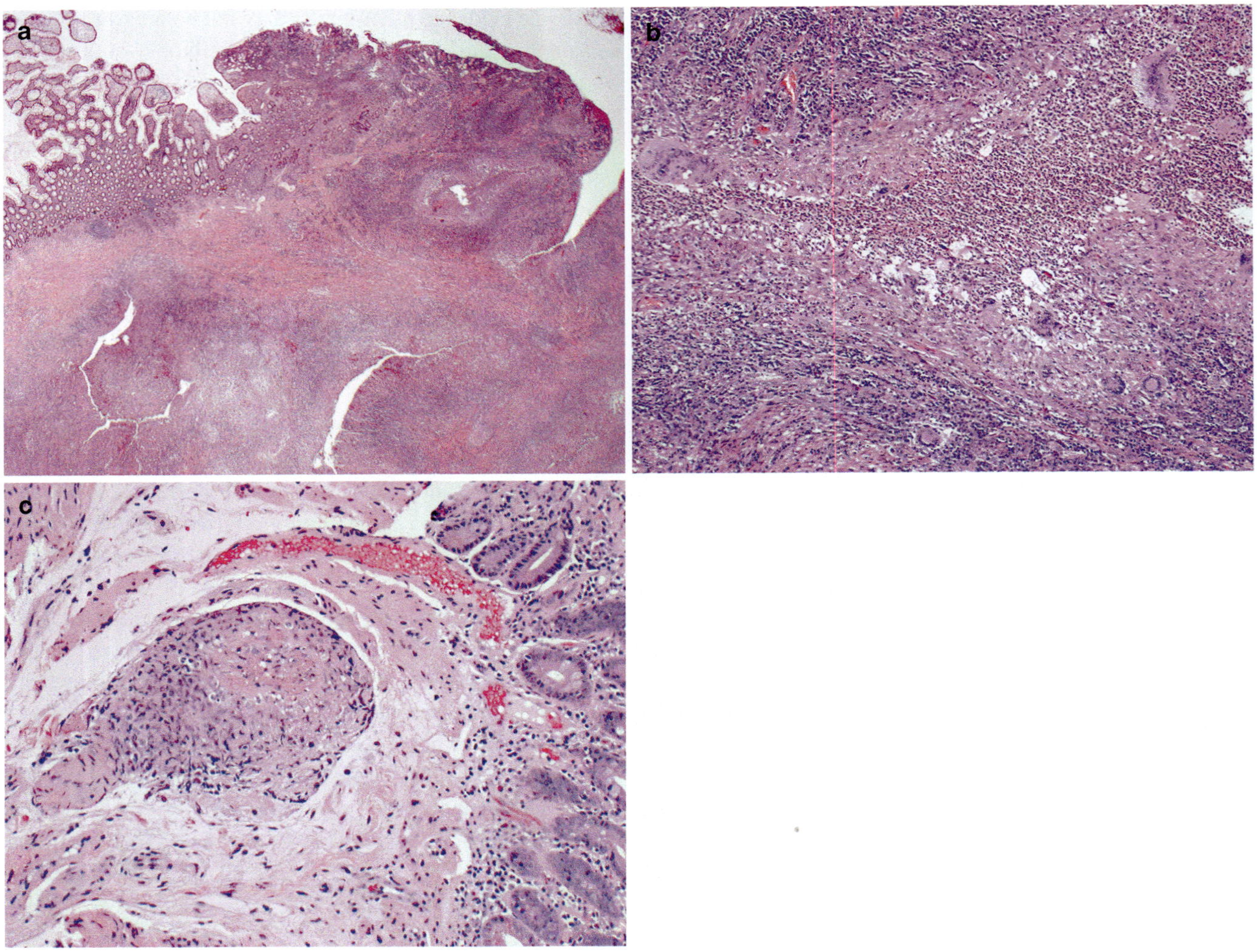

Fig. 14.14 Granulomatosis with polyangiitis. (**a**) Necrotizing granulomatous inflammation with focal deep ulceration. (**b**) Necrotizing vasculitis involves medium-sized vessels with neutrophilic infiltration, fibrinoid necrosis, granulomas, and multinucleated giant cells. (**c**) Necrotizing vasculitis involves a submucosal small artery with occlusion, neutrophilic infiltration, and fibrinoid necrosis of the vessel wall

with no necrotizing granulomatous inflammation. Because of many organ system involvements, the symptoms of MPA vary widely, but most patients have constitutional symptoms like fever, weight loss, fatigue, and kidney failure. Abdominal pain can present in up to 50% of MPA patients [52]. Other gastrointestinal symptoms include intestinal ischemia, bleeding, or bowel perforation. Microscopic features of vasculitis in small submucosal vessels are those of leukocytoclastic vasculitis, with neutrophilic infiltrates and fibrinoid necrosis of vessel wall. Medium-sized vessels are not involved. The small bowel mucosa shows secondary ischemic injury.

Intestinal Transplant-Associated Thrombotic Microangiopathy

Transplantation-associated thrombotic microangiopathy occurs after hematopoietic stem cell transplantation that can involve multiple organ systems and is associated with a poor outcome. Intestinal transplant-associated thrombotic microangiopathy (iTMA) develops when mesenteric and intestinal vasculature is involved. Since the gastrointestinal symptoms of iTMA, including diarrhea, bleeding, and pain, are more often due to GVHD, infection, or drug-induced injury after stem cell transplantation, iTMA has been thought to be underdiagnosed [62]. The possibility of iTMA should be considered in those patients with GVHD but not respond to immunosuppression.

The etiology of iTMA remains largely unknown, but endothelial cell damage induced by T-cell activation and complement activation plays an important role. Various degrees of endothelial cell injury are observed in iTMA. In resection specimens, the endothelial cells of small- to medium-sized arteries in the mesentery can show endothelial irregularities, intimal hyperplasia, myxoid degeneration of the vessel wall, fibrin thrombi, and expansion of the subendothelial spaces [63]. Although endoscopic biopsy tissue usually does not contain submucosal larger vessels, the histopathological features have been described in intestinal mucosa [62, 64, 65]. The evidence of endothelial injury in the intestinal mucosa includes endothelial cell swelling and detachment from the basement membrane, intraluminal schitosytes, intraluminal fibrin, red blood cell extravasation of mucosal capillaries, and microthrombi. The mucosal injury is secondary to ischemia including crypt dropout and mucosal denudation. The inflammation is usually not significant.

The mucosal injury in iTMA may have overlap features to GVHD, but GVHD will show more prominent apoptosis, cryptitis and crypt abscesses, crypt destruction and loss, and ulceration, while endothelial cell injury, especially fibrin microthrombi, is not typically seen in GVHD. Cytomegalovirus (CMV) infection is also frequently seen after stem cell transplantation. The infected endothelial cells may mimic endothelial injury, but they contain characteristic cytoplasmic and nuclear viral inclusions, and routine CMV immunostain can confirm the diagnosis.

Intussusception

Definition

Intussusception is a disorder in which one portion of the intestine slides into the section next to it, causing bowel obstruction.

Clinical Features

Intussusception is the most common cause of intestinal obstruction in younger children. It typically occurs between 6 and 36 months of age. Approximately 60% of children with intussusception are younger than 1 year old, and 80–90% are younger than 2 years [66]. Most cases of intussusception are idiopathic although viral infections may play a role in some children. The pathological leading point where the bowel invagination occurs, including Meckel diverticulum, polyp, duplication cyst, tumor, or hematoma, can only be identified in approximately 25% of patients. The intussusception is classified by the location: (1) ileocolic intussusception is the prolapse of the terminal ileum within the ascending colon and accounts for 90% of all cases; (2) entero-enteric, confined to the small bowel, such as jejuno-jejunal or jejunoileal intussusception; (3) colo-colic, involving the large bowel only. The classic presentation of intussusception in infants and younger children is described as a triad of cramping abdominal pain, bloody diarrhea, and a palpable sausage-shaped tender abdominal mass. However, only 15% of cases have such classical symptoms at the time of presentation. Many older children have pain alone without other signs or symptoms, and about 20% of cases even do not have obvious abdominal pain. Occasionally, the initial presenting sign is lethargy or altered consciousness alone that may be confused with sepsis clinically.

Intussusception in adults is different from pediatric intussusception in many aspects [67]. Adult intussusception only accounts for less than 5% of all cases of intussusception. Almost 90% of intussusception in adults are secondary to a pathologic condition that serves as a lead point, such as tumor, polyp, Meckel's diverticulum, colonic diverticulum, or strictures. The clinical presentation of adult intussusception varies considerably, and the classic triad in pediatric intussusception is rare in adults. The majority of cases in adults have either nonspecific symptoms or partial chronic obstruction.

Both radiology and endoscopy are very useful in diagnosing intussusception. Plain abdominal films show signs of bowel obstruction; ultrasonography may identify classical imaging features such as "target" or "doughnut" signs on the transverse view and the "pseudo-kidney" sign in the longitudinal view, but the presence of massive air in the distended bowel loops limit its accuracy; CT is the most sensitive radiologic method to confirm intussusception, and the characteristic features of CT scan include a "target" or "sausage"-shaped soft tissue mass with a layering effect and mesenteric vessels within the bowel lumen. Endoscopy can confirm the intussusception, localize the disease, and demonstrate the underlying organic lesion serving as a lead point.

Pathological Features

Gross examination revealing the invaginated small bowel confirms the diagnosis (Fig. 14.15). The ileocolic intussusception is most commonly seen in which the terminal ileum invaginates into the colon. The ischemic injury is the main feature, ranging from petechiae to necrosis. The serosa of the intus-

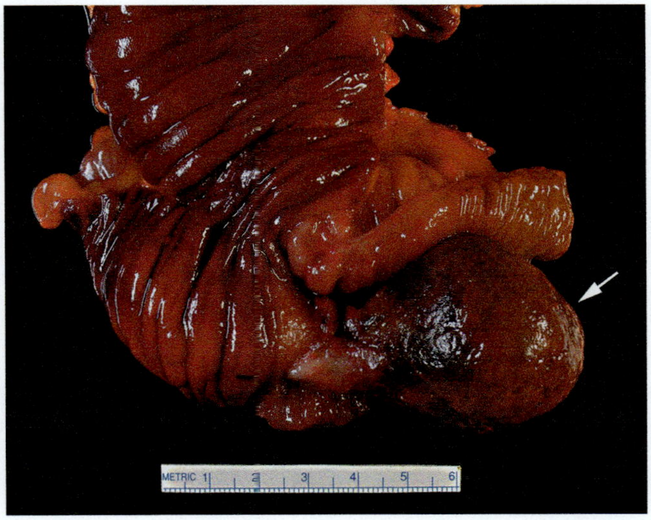

Fig. 14.15 Intussusception. The terminal ileum invaginates into the cecum, associated a big inflammatory fibroid polyp (arrow) as the leading point

susceptedbowel has a granular and dusky appearance. Upon opening the bowel, the invaginated section of the small bowel is present in the lumen with ischemic damage. The leading point often shows edema and hemorrhage, and it is very important to thoroughly examine the leading point to identify possible underlying lesions, especially in adult patients because over 50% of these patients may have an associated malignancy [68]. Carefully grossing those specimens with an underlying malignancy is important to ensure complete resection and proper tumor staging. Small bowel invagination may be absent in recurrent or old intussusception in which the intussusception can be spontaneously reduced. Evidence of chronic injury such as bowel adhesion, bowel kinking, or patchy thickening of bowel wall may be seen and identifying pathological leading point is also helpful.

The microscopic features of intussusception are variable, which include bowel injury due to intussusception, secondary ischemic changes, and predisposing disorders (Fig. 14.16a, b). In the acute setting, the bowel shows variable degree of ischemic injury, depending on the length of ischemia and degree of vascular compromise. The histological changes are similar to gastrointestinal ischemia due to other causes, ranging from mucosal congestion, edema, and ulceration to full-thickness bowel necrosis. In pediatric intussusception, the terminal ileum may show significant lymphoid hyperplasia which can service as the leading point. The lymphoid hyperplasia can be associated with viral infections such as adenovirus. Characteristic viral inclusions may be found and confirmed using immunohistochemistry. Other predisposing disorders may also be identified such as polyps, diverticulum, benign or malignant neoplasms.

For chronic or recurrent intussusception, besides the ischemic injury, the changes due to intussusception become obvious and a diagnosis of intussusception can be made sometimes based on microscopic examination when spontaneous reduction occurs. The pulling force can cause significant changes in all layers of bowel wall, especially at the leading point. The mucosa, muscular layers, and vessels may show "pulling artifact" in which they appear to be dragged toward one direction. The muscularis propria is thickened and disorganized and can be fused with muscularis mucosae, which can be an important clue of chronic or recurrent intussusception. The mucosa can show changes of chronic injury such as fibrosis, villous architectural distortion, atrophy, or hyperplasia. The serosa also shows chronic changes with fibrosis and adhesions. Vessels are usually significantly dilated throughout all layers of intestinal wall.

Differential Diagnosis

The clinical differential diagnosis of small intestinal intussusception is among other conditions that can cause bowel obstruction such as volvulus, Meckel diverticulum, tumor, or small intestinal atresia and stenosis, etc. The pathological diagnosis can be established if the small bowel invagination can be identified grossly. For the spontaneously reduced intussusception, some microscopic features can be helpful to distinguish the small bowel injury caused by intussusception versus other causes such as chronic ischemia, NSAIDs, or Crohn's disease. If a pathological lesion-associated bowel injury can be identified, it is very likely that this is the leading point of the intussusception. The portion of invaginated bowel usually shows some degree of "pulling artifact." The disorganization of muscularis propria and fusion of muscularis propria with muscularis mucosae are suggestive of intussusception. Intact circular and longitudinal layers of the muscularis propria may be occasionally seen in the submucosa in a polypoid lesion that can also confirm the intussusception.

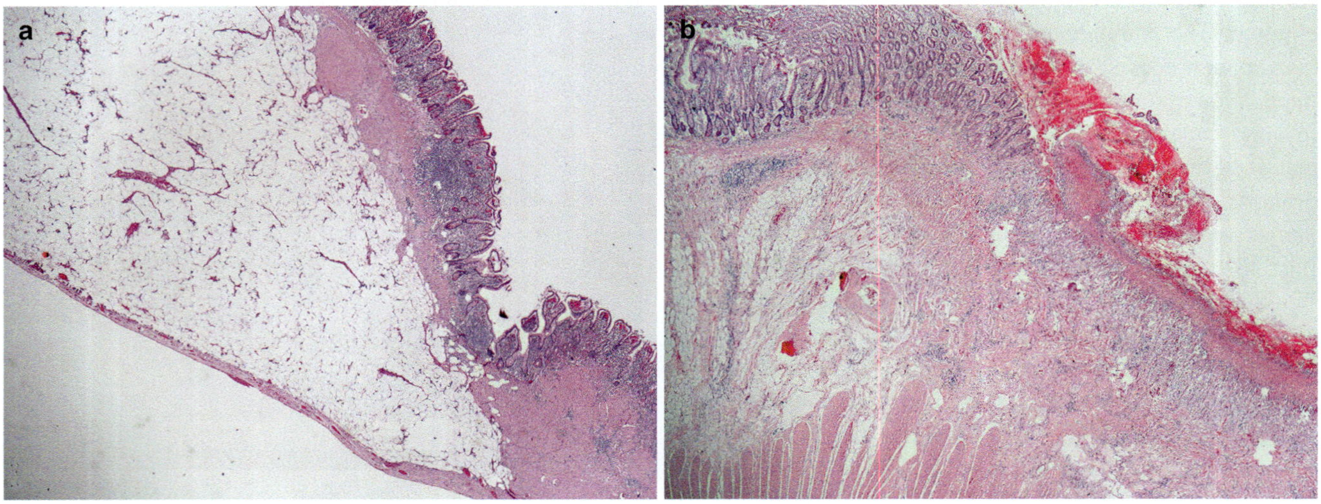

Fig. 14.16 Intussusception. The intussusception is associated with a large submucosal benign lipoma (**a**) with mucosal ischemic injury at the leading point (**b**)

Treatment and Prognosis

Some intussusception can spontaneously reduce with supportive care and intestinal decompress. Nonsurgical reduction using barium or air enema is very effective in children but rarely used in adults. Recurrence can occur in 10% of patients and repeated reduction may be necessary. Surgical correction includes manual reduction and resection. Surgical resection is mainly indicated for adults, especially for those significantly ill patients or those with perforation, infarction, or an underlying malignancy.

Volvulus

Definition

Volvulus occurs when the small intestine twists around itself and its supporting mesentery causing bowel obstruction.

Clinical Features

Volvulus of the small bowel is different in age distribution and causes. It is more common in children and is most often due to intestinal malrotation. Most small intestine volvulus of malrotated bowel occurs within the first 3 weeks of birth and 90% within 1 year [69]. The volvulus is caused by axial rotation of the small intestine with nonrotation, incomplete rotation, or lack of fixation. Other uncommon causes in pediatric volvulus are Meckel's diverticulum, meconium ileus, mesenteric and duplication cysts, or jejunal atresia. Newborns with small bowel volvulus present as acute onset of bilious vomiting, whereas older infants and children may have more variable symptoms, including abdominal pain and constipation. Small bowel volvulus is uncommon in adults and is more likely caused by postoperative adhesive bands, and the patients usually present with an acute small bowel obstruction clinically. With disease progression, ischemia of the affected portion of intestine occurs and leads to necrosis, acidosis, and death.

Imaging studies play an important role in diagnosing volvulus. Plain radiography may show signs of bowel obstruction but usually yields nonspecific findings. Fluoroscopic upper gastrointestinal and small-bowel examinations are preferred imaging tests when volvulus is suspected, which may reveal the abnormal position of the small bowel, abnormal location of the ligament of Treitz, corkscrew sign, or tapering of beaking of the bowel in complete obstruction. CT scan may find some abnormalities suggesting volvulus, such as whirlpool sign (swirling appearance of the mesentery and superior mesenteric vein around the superior mesenteric artery), inverted relationship between the superior mesenteric artery and vein, and malrotated bowel configuration.

Pathological Features

The twisted segment of small bowel in volvulus shows dilation and ischemic changes with a dusky appearance

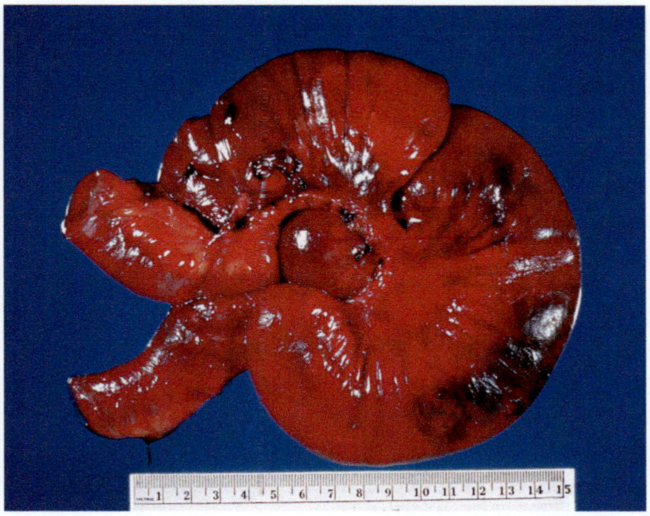

Fig. 14.17 Volvulus. The segment of small bowel twisted at the bowel adhesion site with dilation and ischemic changes

(Fig. 14.17). Intestinal strangulation, gangrene, perforation, and adhesion can also present. Microscopically, the affected bowel shows variable degrees of ischemia and necrosis. Volvulus associated with other pathological abnormalities such as Meckel's diverticulum, mesenteric and duplication cysts, intestinal atresia, or tumor may be seen occasionally.

Differential Diagnosis

The differential diagnosis of small intestinal volvulus includes other causes of bowel obstruction such as due to intussusception, small intestinal atresia and stenosis, tumor, etc. This is primarily relied on clinical, radiological, and surgical findings because of relatively nonspecific ischemic changes under microscopic examination.

Treatment and Prognosis

Emergent surgery is required to prevent ischemia, resect infarcted bowel loops, and correct the underlying cause as appropriate, if volvulus cannot be resolved by conservative management. Prognosis is dependent on the state of the small bowel and presence of systemic shock. If no ischemia of the bowel is present, the prognosis is very good.

Congenital and Neonatal Disorders

Meckel's Diverticulum

Definition

Meckel's diverticulum is a congenital disorder caused by incomplete obliteration of omphalomesenteric duct (also called vitelline duct) which results in a true diverticulum typically located in the ileum within 100 cm from the ileocecal valve.

Clinical Features

Meckel's diverticulum was first described in the fifteenth century and named by Johann Friedrich Meckel in 1809 [70] and is the most common congenital malformation of the gastrointestinal tract that affects 2–4% of the population. Meckel's diverticulum is a remnant of the omphalomesenteric duct, which connects the yolk sac with the developing midgut in fetal life. It normally regresses by the seventh to eighth week of gestation. The incomplete obliteration of the omphalomesenteric duct results in Meckel's diverticulum. Other rare variants of omphalomesenteric remnants include Meckel's diverticulum attached to umbilicus by a fibrous band, omphalomesenteric duct cyst, patent omphalomesenteric fistula, umbilical sinus, and umbilical polyp. The majority of patients with a Meckel's diverticulum are asymptomatic. Complications of Meckel's diverticulum only occur in about 4% of cases, which are often due to ectopic tissue and umbilical or mesodiverticular bands. The most frequent complications are bleeding from ectopic gastric mucosa and bowel obstruction due to the intussusception, volvulus, or adhesive band. Other uncommon complications include ulceration, diverticulitis, and perforation. It can also be present in an external hernia, typically on the right side, known as a "Hernia of Littre."

The asymptomatic Meckel's diverticulum is often incidentally diagnosed during laparoscopy or laparotomy. However, the preoperative diagnosis of Meckel's diverticulum is still challenging, as Dr. Charles Mayo stated: "Meckel's diverticulum is frequently suspected, often looked for and seldom found." Technetium-99 m pertechnetate scan, also called Meckel scan, detecting gastric mucosa, has become the most common and accurate noninvasive test to diagnose Meckel's diverticulum in children, with a 95% specificity and 85% sensitivity; however, this test is only 9% specific and 62% sensitive in adults [71]. Other tests such as colonoscopy or CT scan have limited role in diagnosing Meckel's diverticulum, but they may be helpful to rule out other disorders.

Pathological Features

Variations in location, size, and shape are very common in Meckel's diverticulum. The diverticulum usually occurs within 100 cm from the ileocecal valve at the antimesenteric border of the ileum. In children under 2 years of age, the average distance is 34 cm from the ileocecal valve and for adults is 67 cm [72]. The average length of the diverticulum is about 3 cm, but it can be longer than 10 cm and the longest record of Meckel's diverticulum is 100 cm. Giant Meckel's diverticulum is referred to those longer than 5 cm (Fig. 14.18). The diameter of the diverticulum is usually smaller than that of the ilium, but some may have a greater lumen diameter. Other lesions may be also identified by gross examinations such as umbilical bands or omphalomesenteric duct cyst.

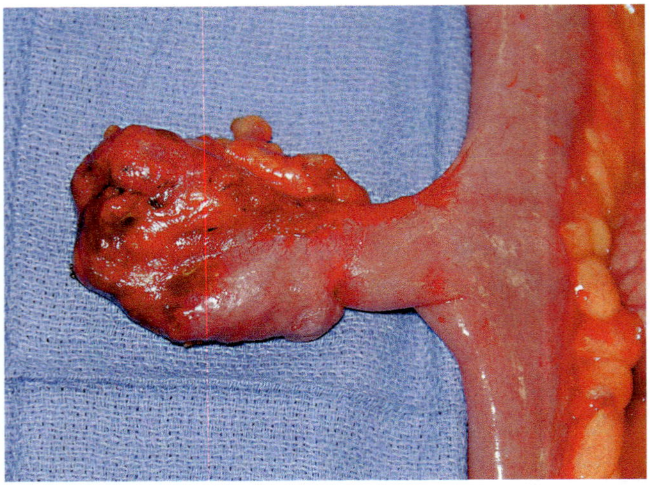

Fig. 14.18 A giant Meckel's diverticulum

The symptomatic Meckel's diverticulum may show diverticulitis, bleeding, perforation, bowel adhesion, ischemic injury, or tumors.

Microscopically, the diverticulum consists of all layers of intestinal wall. The common abnormalities in symptomatic Meckel's diverticulum are ectopic tissue, diverticulitis, enterolith, and tumors. The most common ectopic tissue seen in Meckel's diverticulum is gastric mucosa (Fig. 14.19a) which is found in 30–60% patients with symptomatic Meckel's diverticulum [72, 73]. The ectopic gastric mucosa can result in peptic ulceration, bleeding, or perforation. Helicobacter pylori has also been found in the ectopic gastric mucosa [74]. The second most common ectopic tissue seen in Meckel's diverticulum is pancreatic tissue (Fig. 14.19b). Other rare ectopic tissue includes jejunal, duodenal mucosa or Brunner's tissue, colonic mucosa, endometriosis, or hepatobiliary tissue. A variety of benign or malignant tumors can rarely occur in the ectopic tissue in Meckel's diverticulum with neuroendocrine tumor and lipoma being the most common types. Other rare tumors in the literatures include adenocarcinoma, gastrointestinal stromal tumor, intraductal papillary mucinous neoplasm or pancreatic intraepithelial neoplasm, leiomyosarcoma, peripheral nerve sheath tumor, and desmoplastic small round cell tumor [73, 75–79].

Differential Diagnosis

The differential diagnosis is a clinical dilemma because symptomatic Meckel's diverticulum can mimic many conditions causing bleeding and acute abdomen such as acute appendicitis or intussusception. When examining small bowel resection for obstruction, bleeding, or perforation, identifying an outpouching of the small bowel and ectopic tissue can indicate Meckel's diverticulum as the underlying cause of these complications. Intestinal duplication or duplication cyst is also consisted with full layers of small bowel

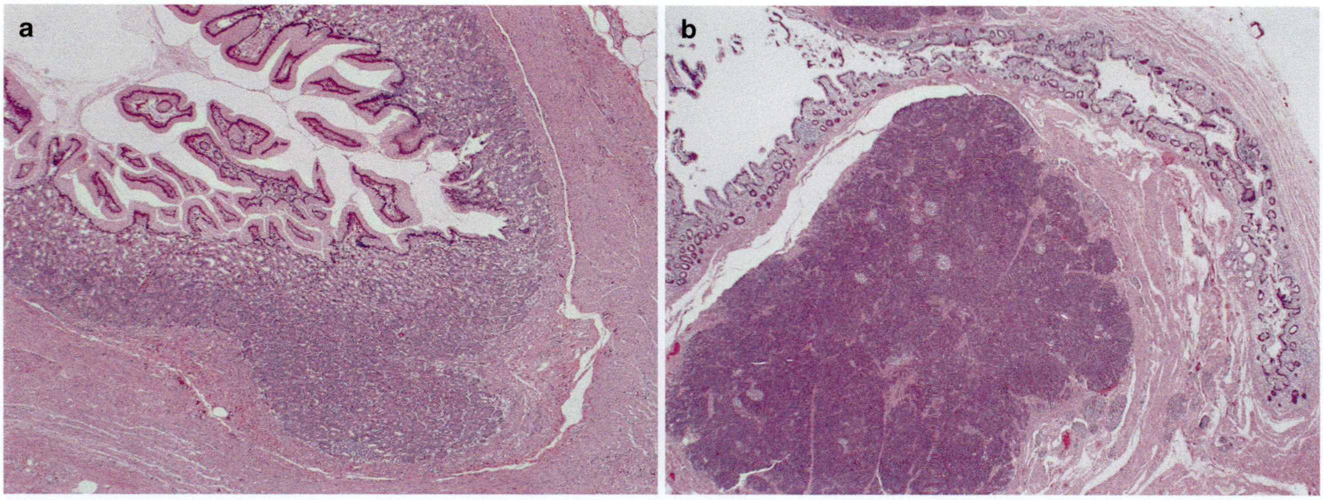

Fig. 14.19 Meckel's diverticulum. (**a**) The diverticulum consists of all layers of intestinal wall and ectopic gastric tissue. (**b**) Ectopic pancreatic tissue present in the diverticulum

wall and ectopic tissue, but they are typically presented as a tubular or cystic structure located at the mesenteric side.

Treatment and Prognosis

The treatment for the symptomatic Meckel's diverticulum is the surgical resection. Prophylactic diverticulectomy is recommended for incidental asymptomatic Meckel's diverticulum to reduce the risk of postoperative morbidity and the lifetime complications, when compared to resection of a complicated Meckel's diverticulum [73].

Omphalomesenteric Duct Cyst

The omphalomesenteric duct cyst is a rare variant of remnant of the omphalomesenteric duct, in which the middle portion omphalomesenteric duct remains patent. It resembles Meckel's diverticulum except for no communication between the cyst and the ileum. It is located between the ileum and anterior abdominal wall and may be connected at each end by fibrous bands. The cysts range from 0.4 to 6.0 cm in diameter. The cystic wall is composed of fibromuscular tissue and is lined by a columnar mucin-secreting intestinal or gastric type epithelium. Islands of pancreatic tissue may be associated with the cyst lining [80, 81].

Intestinal Duplication and Duplication Cyst

Definition

Intestinal duplication is a rare congenial malformation of partial or complete doubling of a portion of gastrointestinal tract located in, or immediately adjacent to, the small bowel. The most common site of gastrointestinal duplication is the ileum, followed by the esophagus, colon, jejunum, stomach, duodenum, and rectum [82]. The cystic form is referred as duplication cyst. The duplication cyst with no communication with the main intestinal lumen is also known as enterogenous cyst.

Clinical Features

Intestinal duplications are rare, occurring in about 1 in 100,000 live births, with a male predominance. About one third of affected children have associated congenital anomalies. The etiology of intestinal duplications is unknown. Several theories have been proposed, such as split notochord syndrome, aberrant luminal recanalization, an intrauterine vascular accident, persistent embryonic diverticula, and partial twinning, but there is no single theory can explain all duplications in all locations. Most intestinal duplications are asymptomatic and incidentally diagnosed. The clinical presentations of symptomatic intestinal duplications are variable, and most of them present with a combination of pain and obstructive symptoms.

Pathological Features

Most small intestine duplications are located in the ileum [83]. Grossly, duplications may be cystic or tubular and are located at the mesenteric side, sometimes intramural (Fig. 14.20a, b). The duplications often share a common muscular wall and blood supply with the native intestine. They can be completely separated from the native intestine, but often time communicate with the intestinal lumen at proximal or distal end of the duplications or at both ends. Multiple small intestine duplications may be present. Microscopically, the wall of duplications is lined with intestinal mucosa and contains its own smooth muscle layers (Fig. 14.20c) or shares with the native intestine. However, the gastric or ciliated mucosa lining can occur. Of note, the

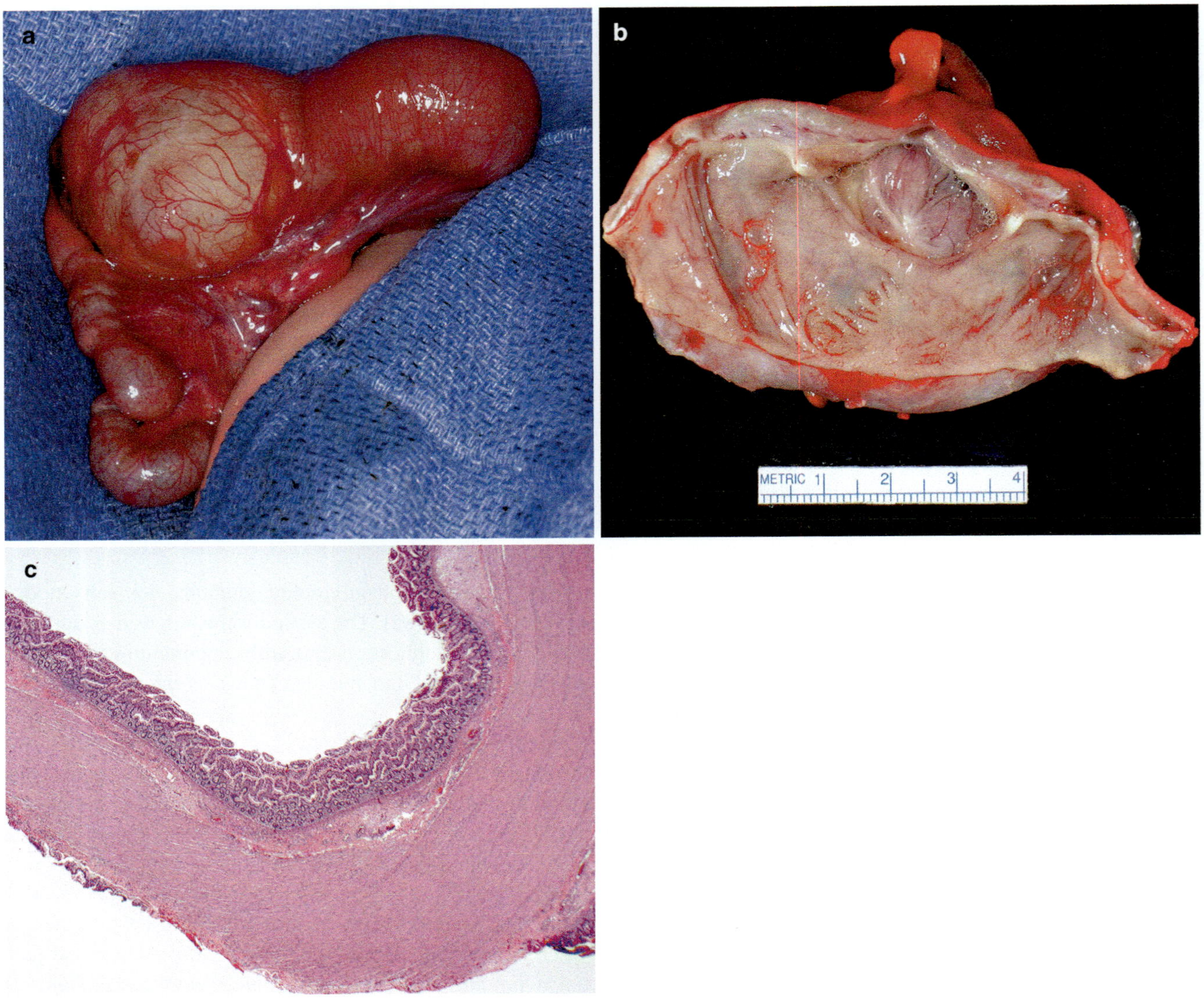

Fig. 14.20 Intestinal duplication cyst. (**a**) A cystic mass sitting between two segments of small bowel. (**b**) The cyst consists of enteric mucosa and intestinal wall. (**c**) Microscopically, the duplications cyst is lined with intestinal mucosa and shares the muscular layers with the native intestine

current nomenclature of duplications relies on the anatomic location of the duplication in relation to the normal intestinal tract but not on the histologic types of the mucosal lining. Ectopic gastric mucosa and pancreatic tissue are common. Other types of ectopic tissue include squamous or transitional epithelium, ciliated bronchial epithelium, lung tissue, cartilage, thyroid stroma, or lymphoid aggregates resembling Peyer patches [84, 85].

Differential Diagnosis

Intestinal duplications more often present as noncommunicating spherical cysts of varying size in the mesentery, i.e., duplication cysts or enterogenous cysts. Therefore, the differential diagnosis includes other cystic lesions in the mesentery, including mesenteric cysts and cystic lymphangiomas. A mesenteric cyst is referred to any cyst that is located in the mesentery and may or may not extend into the retroperitoneum, which is lined with endothelial or mesothelial cells with no smooth muscle in the wall; cystic lymphangioma is also lined with endothelial cells but with thin walls contain foamy cells, lymphatic spaces, lymphoid tissue, and smooth muscle.

Treatment and Prognosis

Complete resection of the duplicated portion is the standard management if feasible. The outcome is good in patients in whom it is an isolated congenital abnormality.

Intestinal Malrotation

Intestinal malrotation is a congenital disorder occurring at any stage of rotation and fixation of the gastrointestinal tract during embryologic development. The development of gastrointestinal tract involves three stages of rotation and fixation. Normally, stage 1 occurs between 5 and 10 weeks' gestation in which a 270° counterclockwise rotation takes place around the superior mesenteric artery as the axis for the bowel to return to the abdominal cavity; stage 2 occurs at 10 weeks' gestation, as the bowel returns to the abdominal cavity, it undergoes additional rotations with fixation of the duodenojejunal loop to the left of the midline; and stage 3 lasts from 11 weeks' gestation until term with the descent of the cecum to the right lower quadrant and fixation of the mesenteries. There are many forms of intestinal malrotation, and four main types are: nonrotation, incomplete rotation, reversed rotation, and incomplete fixation [86]. Briefly, nonrotation refers to complete failure of rotation at stage 1 resulting in a right-sided small intestine and left-sided colon in the abdomen (Fig. 14.21); incomplete rotation, also known as mixed rotation, is the most common type due to stage 2 arrest, with misplaced cecum and small intestine mainly at right side. Duodenal obstruction and internal herniation are common in incomplete rotation; reversed rotation is rare, in which the midgut loop rotates an additional 180° resulting in the duodenum and superior mesenteric artery located anterior to the transverse colon; incomplete rotation occurs when the mesentery of the right and left colon and the duodenum do not become fixed to the retroperitoneum, which may cause mesocolic hernia and volvulus.

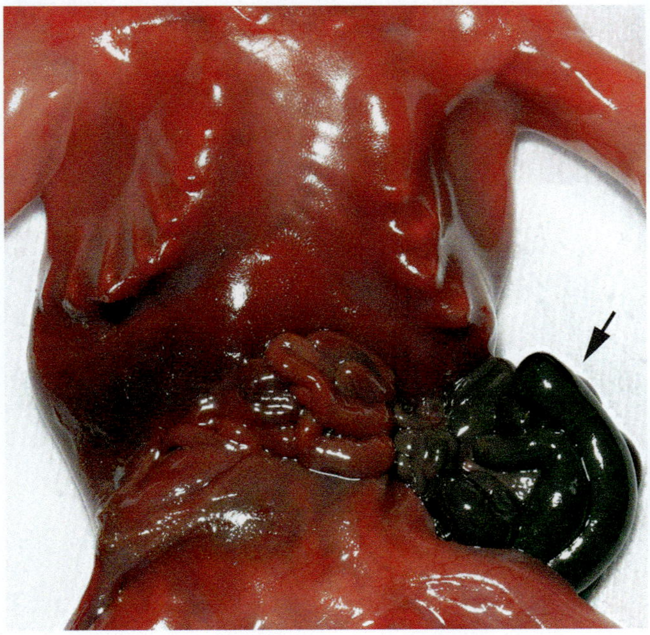

Fig. 14.21 Intestinal malrotation and gastroschisis. This premature infant shows gastroschisis with the entire gastrointestinal tract being outside the abdomen due to abdominal wall defect. The gut also shows nonrotation with a right-sided small intestine and left-sided colon (arrow)

Intestinal malrotation occurs approximately 1 in 200–500 live births. However, most patients are asymptomatic and the frequency of symptomatic malrotation is about 1 in 6000 live births [87]. The symptoms depend on the types of malrotations and acute or chronic process, which may include acute or chronic volvulus, duodenal obstruction, or internal herniation. Symptoms and diagnosis may occur at any age, and about 40–50% patients diagnosed with malrotations are adults [88, 89]. The gross examination identifying the misplaced intestine within the abdomen establishes the diagnosis. The affected bowel shows normal histology unless there are associated abnormalities such as volvulus with ischemia. The Ladd's procedure is the surgical approach for intestinal malrotation in both children and adults, consisting of division of mesenteric bands (Ladd's bands), reduction of volvulus, appendectomy, and functional positioning of the intestine with or without fixation.

Atresia and Stenosis

Definition

Intestinal atresia and stenosis are congenital obstruction with complete or partial occlusion of the intestinal lumen.

Clinical Features

The jejunoileal atresia and stenosis affect jejunum and ileum equally, and multiple atresias can occur in 6–20% of cases [90]. Although the incidence of jejunoileal atresia and stenosis is similar to that of duodenal involvement [91], the pathophysiology of stenosis and atresia is different in two sites. The duodenal atresia is due to a failure of recanalization of intestinal tube and occurs at 8–10 weeks' gestation, and incomplete recanalization can lead to duodenal stenosis or duodenal web. On the other hand, jejunoileal atresia and stenosis are secondary to an intrauterine vascular event and occur after intestinal development because of the presence of bile droplets, meconium, or lanugo distal to the site of obstruction. Jejunoileal atresia is often associated with other conditions such as malrotation, volvulus, perforation, internal hernias, gastroschisis, and omphalocele.

Jejunoileal atresia or stenosis is one of the most common causes of neonatal intestinal obstruction. The patients with jejunoileal atresia and stenosis are often associated with polyhydramnios, prematurity, and low birth weight. Most patients present with bilious emesis, abdominal distention, jaundice, and failure to pass meconium in the first 24 hours. Jejunoileal atresia and stenosis may be detected on antenatal ultrasonography. Plain radiograph of the abdomen in newborns shows the classic double-bubble sign.

Pathological Features

In atresia, there is an entirely missing segment of bowel, and there are gaps or fibrous cords between the two blind ends (Fig. 14.22a). The commonly used classification scheme describes four types in jejunoileal atresia listed in Table 14.2 [92]. The atresia causes complete occlusion of the small bowel. The proximal segment from the point of obstruction is markedly dilated and ischemic necrosis or perforation may occur. The distal portion is collapsed or mildly distended containing meconium. Stenosis occurs much less frequently than atresia. The small bowel is in continuity with dilated proximal part at the stenotic site where a narrowed segment with a minute lumen is present (Fig. 14.22b, c). The mesentery is intact.

Microscopically, a spectrum of histological features indicating bowel injury have been observed, including mucosal and submucosal edema, mucosal denudation, congestion, ulceration, submucosal fibrosis, prominent vascular proliferation and perivascular fibrosis, granulation tissue, hemosiderin-laden macrophages, and foreign body giant cell reaction [93]. The proximal dilated bowel may be gangrenous. The villi are atrophic with abnormal configuration or totally flattening. The muscularis mucosae is thickened. The muscularis propria can be thickening or thinning with fibrosis and vascular proliferation. Segmental absence of muscularis propria has been reported. The serosa may show congestion, serositis with exudates, or fibrosis. In stenosis, the stenotic portion of the bowel usually shows irregular muscle layers and thickened submucosa (Fig. 14.23a, b).

Differential Diagnosis

The differential diagnosis is among other causes of neonatal intestinal obstruction. Radiologic findings are critical. Rectal biopsy may be required to rule out Hirschsprung disease, when a neonate does not pass meconium in the first 24 hours of life.

Treatment and Prognosis

Surgical treatment of intestinal atresia and stenosis is individualized according to the site of the lesion, the specific

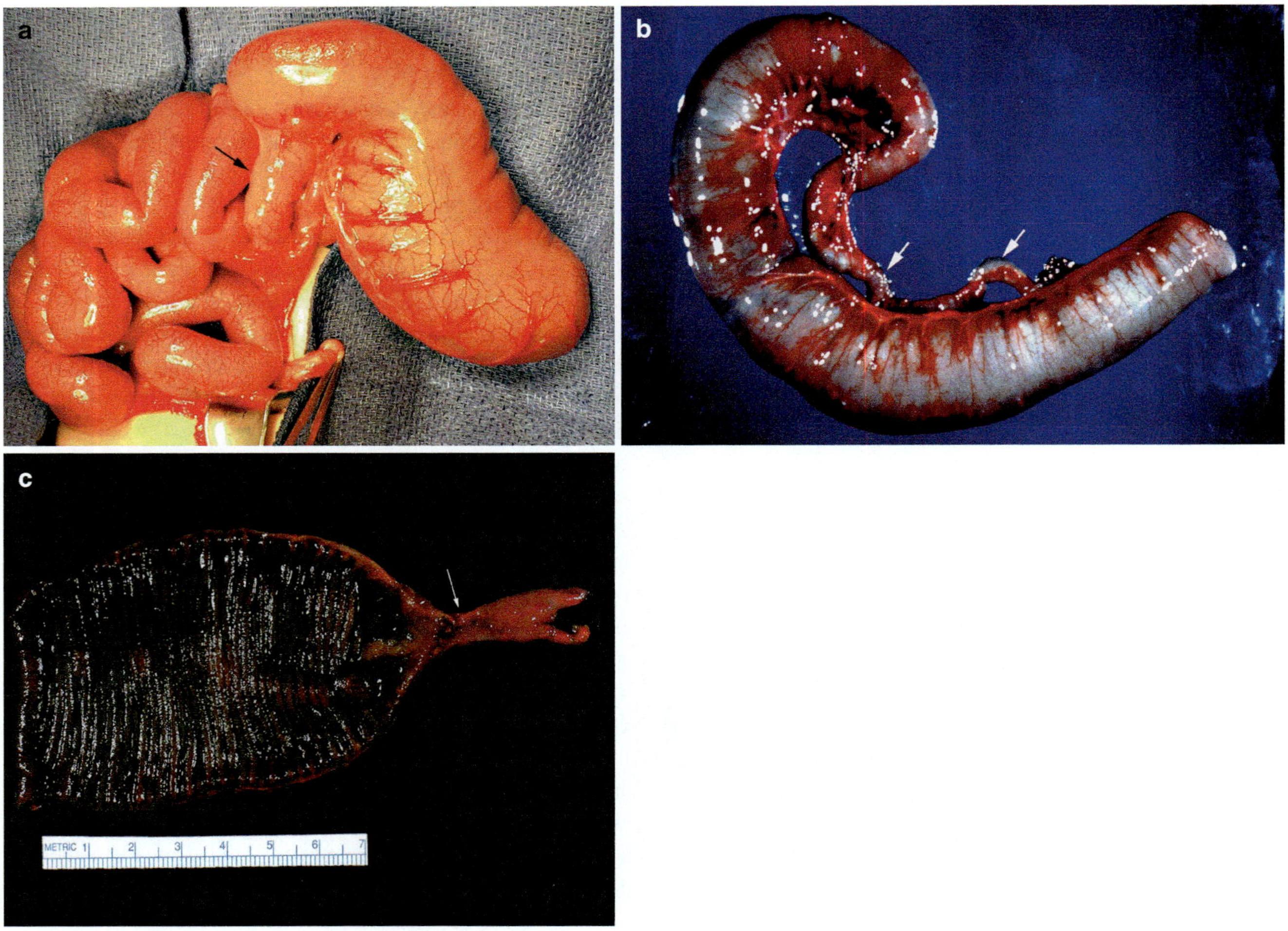

Fig. 14.22 Intestinal atresia and stenosis. (**a**) Type II atresia, the small bowel is separated by a fibrous band (arrow) with dilated proximal end. (**b**) Small intestinal stenosis. A long segment of stenotic bowel (arrows) and dilated proximal part. (**c**) Small intestinal stenosis with luminal continuity, but with a narrowed segment and minute lumen (arrow)

anatomical findings, and associated conditions. Long-term prognosis is generally good. Patients with short or ultrashort bowel syndrome need long-term total parenteral nutrition or small bowel transplantation.

Omphalocoele, Gastroschisis, and Umbilical Hernia

Omphalocele, gastroschisis, and umbilical hernia are most common fetal abdominal wall defects [94]. An omphalocele is a midline abdominal wall defect at the base of the umbilical cord with extraembryonic gut failing to return to the abdominal cavity. The abdominal viscera are within a sac composed of a membrane of amnion and peritoneum with Wharton's jelly between the two layers. The size varies from a few centimeters to lesions involving almost entire abdominal wall. Gastroschisis is truly an abdominal wall defect characterized by free-floating loops of bowel (Fig. 14.21). However, in case of omphaloceles with ruptured membrane, distinguishing omphalocele from gastroschisis relies on the location of the liver and cord insertion site. Omphalocele is often associated with an extracorporeal liver and cord insertion site is umbilical, while the liver is often intracorporeal and cord insertion is paraumbilical in gastroschisis. Both omphalocele and gastroschisis are often associated with other abnormalities [95]. Umbilical hernia is abdominal wall defects less than 2 cm which present as a protrusion of the umbilicus covered by peritoneum and skin. They are not associated with other anomalies or genetic syndromes. The histology of displaced organs is normal unless there are associated abnormalities.

Table 14.2 Different types of jejunoileal atresia and stenosis

	Types	Features
Atresia	Type I	Blockage caused by a membrane (mucosal septa or web) within the lumen of the intestine with intact wall; normal bowel length
	Type II	Proximal dilated end separated from distal narrow bowel by a fibrous cord; normal bowel length
	Type IIIa	Completely separated two segments with V-shaped mesentery gap; reduced bowel length
	Type IIIb	Completely separated near the ligament of Treitz with large mesentery gap and distal segment helically encircles a small vessel (apple peel deformity); reduced bowel length
	Type IV	Multiple atresia, combination of types I, II, and III; reduced bowel length, may be very short
Stenosis		Localized narrowing of the bowel with luminal continuity and intact mesentery

Neonatal Necrotizing Enterocolitis

Definition

Neonatal necrotizing enterocolitis (NNEC) is a severe acute inflammatory bowel necrosis that primarily affects premature infants after the initiation of enteral feeding.

Clinical Features

NNEC is one of the most common gastrointestinal emergencies in the newborn infants, which occurs in 1–3 per 1000 live births, about 10% of premature infants <1500 grams, or 1–5% of all neonatal intensive care unit admissions [96, 97]. The four main risk factors resulting in the

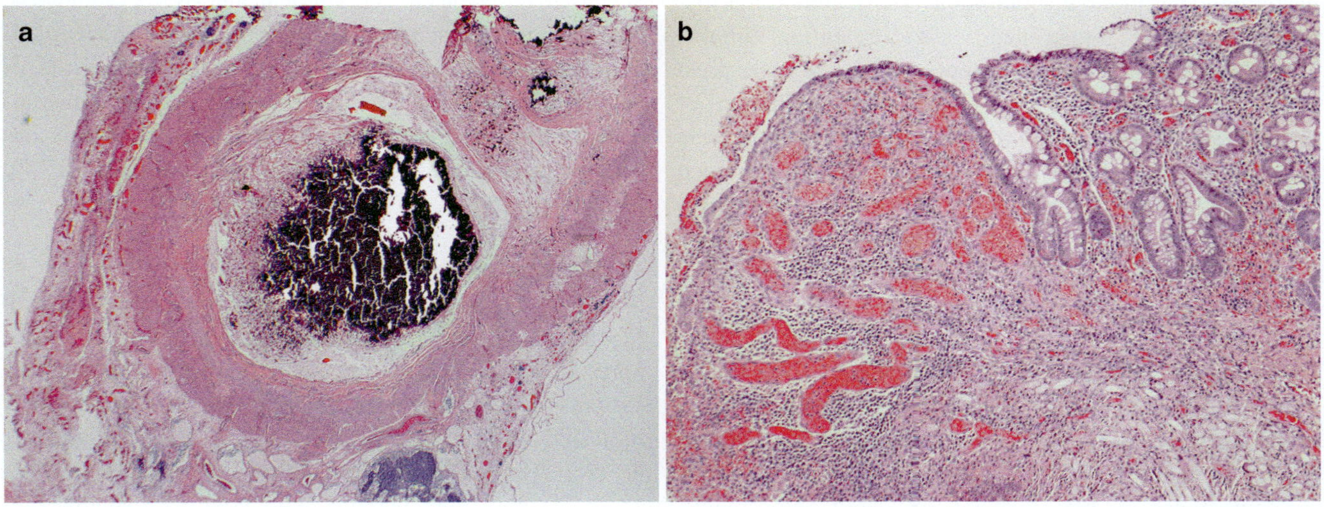

Fig. 14.23 Intestinal stenosis. (**a**) Microscopically, the stenotic site shows small bowel with a minute lumen filled with meconium, mucosal denudation, and fibrotic submucosa. (**b**) The proximal part shows ischemic injury with villous atrophy and architectural changes

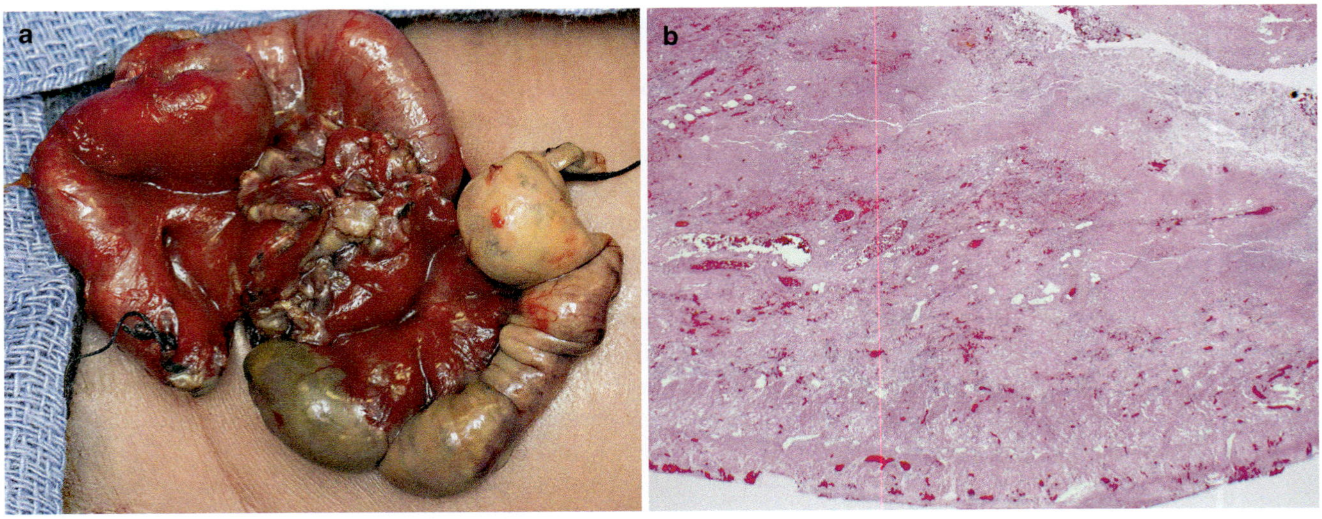

Fig. 14.24 Neonatal necrotizing enterocolitis. (**a**) Grossly, a segment of discolored small bowel is completely necrotic. (**b**) Full-thickness necrosis microscopically

mucosal injuries in NNEC are prematurity, bacterial colonization, hypoxia and compromised intestinal blood flow, and enteral feeding [98]. Although NNEC predominantly affects premature infants, approximately 13% of cases occur in term infants [99], who are typically associated with preexisting diseases such as congenital heart disease, hypoxic event, infection, seizures, hypoglycemia, or genetic disorders [100, 101].

The clinical presentations of NNEC are variable and nonspecific. The timing of the onset of symptoms appears to be inversely related to gestational age [97]. Term infants develop NNEC much earlier, usually within the first week or even the first 1–2 days of life. The estimated average age of onset for babies born at less than 30 weeks' gestational age is about 20 days, 14 days for babies born at 31–33 weeks, and 5.4 days for babies born after 34 weeks' gestation. The affected infants may show abdominal distension, feeding intolerance, gastric retention, bilious vomiting and hematochezia. About one-third of cases present with nonspecific signs with clinical suspicion of NNEC, and symptoms may resolve gradually. However, in about 40% of cases, the disease progression is fulminant with signs of peritonitis, sepsis, shock, DIC, and rapid death in severe cases. Abdominal radiograph may reveal pneumatosis intestinalis which is considered as a pathognomonic feature for NNEC.

Pathological Features

The terminal ileum and the proximal ascending colon are most commonly involved in NNEC. However, any segment of the intestine or even the entire bowel can be affected. In the acute phase, the bowel appears distended, hemorrhagic, and gangrenous necrosis (Fig. 14.24a). Gas-filled cysts can be present at submucosa and subserosa along the mesenteric border. Bowel perforation may be present. After healing, the intestinal wall is thickened with fibrinous adhesions and focal stenosis. Microscopically, the bowel shows variable degrees of ischemic injury. The early changes occur in mucosa with edema, hemorrhage, and necrosis, and then full-thickness bowel gangrenous necrosis develops (Fig. 14.24b). Pneumatosis cystoides intestinalis characterized by cyst-like spaces in the bowel wall and mesentery is a common finding. After recovery, the bowel shows reparative changes such as epithelial regeneration, Paneth cell hyperplasia and metaplasia, granulation tissue formation, and fibrosis [102, 103].

Differential Diagnosis

Intestinal ischemic necrosis due to other causes such as bowel obstruction, volvulus, or strangulated hernia can be diagnosed based on clinical, surgical, and gross examination. NNEC may be related to an infectious etiology, and recognition of the underlying pathogens such as *Candida*, virus, or pathogenic enteric bacteria is particularly important in clinical management [104, 105]. *Clostridium perfringens* has been detected in about 25% of newborns with NNEC by molecular tests of stool samples [106, 107].

Treatment and Prognosis

Nonoperative management including stopping enteral feeding, antibiotics, respiratory and cardiovascular support, and fluid resuscitation is the mainstay treatment for patients with early stage of NNEC. Surgical treatment is indicated when signs of perforated or necrotic intestine develop. The overall survival rate of infants with NNEC is about 70–80%, and patients with nonoperative management have a better survival compared to surgical management [108].

Meconium Ileus and Meconium Plug Syndrome

Meconium ileus and meconium plug syndrome are common causes of intestinal obstruction in newborn due to meconium obstruction [109]. Meconium ileus is obstruction at the terminal ileum caused by viscid, thick, and protein-rich inspissated meconium, and the majority of patients are associated with cystic fibrosis. Meconium plug syndrome is more commonly seen in premature infants, is characterized by colonic obstruction, and some cases are associated with small left colon syndrome and Hirschsprung disease, and it is only rarely associated with cystic fibrosis. The clinical presentations of meconium ileus and meconium plug syndrome are similar, including failure to pass meconium, bilious vomiting, and abdominal distention. Plain abdominal radiographs show with an obstructive pattern. Surgical intervention may be required for those patients with complications such as volvulus, atresia, gangrene, perforation, and meconium peritonitis. The resected bowel is dilated and obstructed by inspissated firm green or tarry meconium in the lumen. Since 13% of patients with meconium plug syndrome can be associated with Hirschsprung disease, a rectal biopsy has been recommended to rule out Hirschsprung disease [110].

Polypoid Lesions

Nonneoplastic polypoid lesions are occasionally encountered in jejunum and ileum, and most of them are inflammatory/hyperplastic or hamartomatous in nature. The lesions may be single, multiple, or widespread (for example, as part of a polyposis syndrome). The clinical presentations are nonspecific, and the possible signs and symptoms include abdominal pain, bowel obstruction, volvulus, intussusception, or gastrointestinal bleeding. They can be either sporadic or syndromic. However, histologic evaluation alone typically cannot distinguish those two types, and correlation with clinical findings, family history, lesions in other part of gastrointestinal tract and organ, or genetic testing is necessary. The clinicopathological features of some of these nonneoplastic polypoid lesions in jejunum and ileum, especially hamartomatous polyps, overlap with their counterparts in stomach, duodenum, and colon, which are introduced in detail elsewhere in this book.

Inflammatory Polyp

Inflammatory polyps are most commonly associated with Crohn's disease seen at terminal ileum [111], and they can be occasionally seen at terminal ileum in the setting of backwash ileitis in patients with ulcerative colitis [112]. They may also be secondary to other causes of small bowel mucosal injury such as infection, anastomotic sites, or ulcers. Endoscopic examination reveals polypoid inflammatory mucosa with surface erosion and ulceration which can be single or multiple. Microscopically, the small bowel mucosa shows variable degrees of acute and chronic inflammation, edema and congestion in lamina propria, villous architectural distortion, pyloric gland metaplasia, and surface erosion and ulceration (Fig. 14.25). The epithelium shows reactive/regenerative changes, and it may be difficult to rule out dysplasia in some cases with severe reactive atypia. In addition, some inflammatory polyps may contain large bizarre stromal cells mimicking malignant tumors in carcinomas or sarcomas. The bizarre stromal cells may be spindled, stellate, or epithelioid with marked nuclear pleomorphism. They are positive for vimentin and occasionally positive for smooth muscle actin. They are considered to be reactive fibroblasts or myofibroblasts which are related to the degenerative effects of inflammatory or hypoxic-induced changes [113]. Some inflammatory polyps may be predominantly composed of granulation tissue containing exuberant capillary proliferation, and terms such as pyogenic granuloma or lobular capillary hemangioma have been used to describe this type of inflammatory polyps in gastrointestinal tract because they share similar features with the lesions which more commonly occur in oral cavity or skin [114].

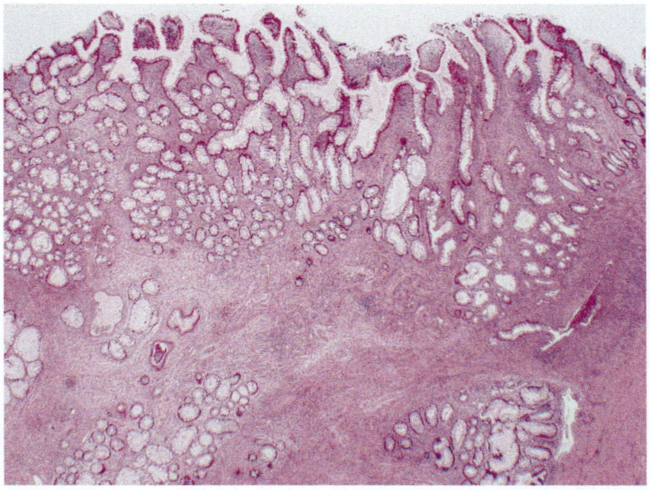

Fig. 14.25 Inflammatory polyp. An inflammatory polyp in terminal ileum associated with Crohn's disease

Hyperplastic Polyp

Hyperplastic polyps of small intestine occur much less frequently than colorectal hyperplastic polyp. They more commonly arise in the duodenum and proximal jejunum which can be single or multiple. Microscopically, they show some features of colorectal hyperplastic polyp including prominent epithelial serration and elongation and cystic dilation of glands (see Fig. 12.8 in Chap. 12). However, the hyperplastic epithelium is usually not rich in mucin or goblet cells, which has been described as resembling colonic microvesicular hyperplastic polyps with abundant eosinophilic cytoplasm and small mucin droplets [115]. The hyperplastic polyps are predominantly composed of intestinal epithelium, but some may have gastric type epithelium with variable expression patterns of different mucin (MUC2, MUC5AC, or MUC6) [115]. Some hyperplastic polyp may also have stromal overgrowth, stromal edema, surface erosion, and acute and chronic inflammation, and they can be confused with inflammatory polyp. However, the prominent epithelial hyperplasia and serration argue against inflammatory polyp [116]. *BRAF* (V600E) and *KRAS* mutations have been reported in a subset of duodenal hyperplastic polyps [115].

Peutz-Jeghers Polyp

Peutz-Jeghers polyps can develop throughout the gastrointestinal tract, but are mainly located in the small intestine, usually in the jejunum. Depending on the size and number of the polyps present within the bowel, patients with Peutz-Jeghers polyps can complicate with abdominal pain, gastrointestinal bleeding, and obstruction, and larger polyps can increase the risk of intussusception [117]. Patients with Peutz-Jeghers syndrome carry a significant overall increased lifetime risk of small bowel adenocarcinoma, with patients aged through 30 years harboring a 5% cumulative risk of cancer that rises to 85% by age 70 years, and small bowel adenocarcinoma has been reported in a child as young as 13 years [118]. Therefore, small bowel surveillance is recommended every 2–3 years for patients with Peutz-Jeghers syndrome from the age of 8–10 years. MRI enteroclysis could be the first step for small bowel surveillance, followed by balloon-assisted enteroscopy for patients with large polyps (>10 mm) or have a high polyp load [119]. Removal of large small bowel Peutz-Jeghers polyps can reduce the risk of complications.

Peutz-Jeghers polyps are often pedunculated and have characteristic morphological features, which are often described as branched, arborizing, tree-like smooth muscle cores covered with normal intestinal epithelium (Fig. 14.26a). The smooth muscle bundles arise from the muscularis mucosae and penetrate the polyps extending toward the surface to support each finger-like frond. On horizontal cuts, the smooth muscle fibers separate the epithelium into islands with less prominent arborizing feature. The villi are elongated and the crypts appear hyperplastic or mildly dilated. All types of intestinal epithelial cells are present including goblet cells, Paneth cells, absorptive cells, and endocrine cells. The lamina propria can be expanded by mild edema and inflammation, but they are in less degrees compared to inflammatory or hyperplastic polyps. Epithelium misplaced into submucosa or even muscularis propria is not an uncommon finding which can mimic invasive carcinoma (Fig. 14.26b). This is probably due to mucosal prolapse and tangential cuts, in particular for polyps with larger sizes.

Epithelial dysplasia is rare in Peutz-Jeghers polyps. When present, the dysplasia is classified as low or high grade according to the degree of cytoarchitectural atypia. However,

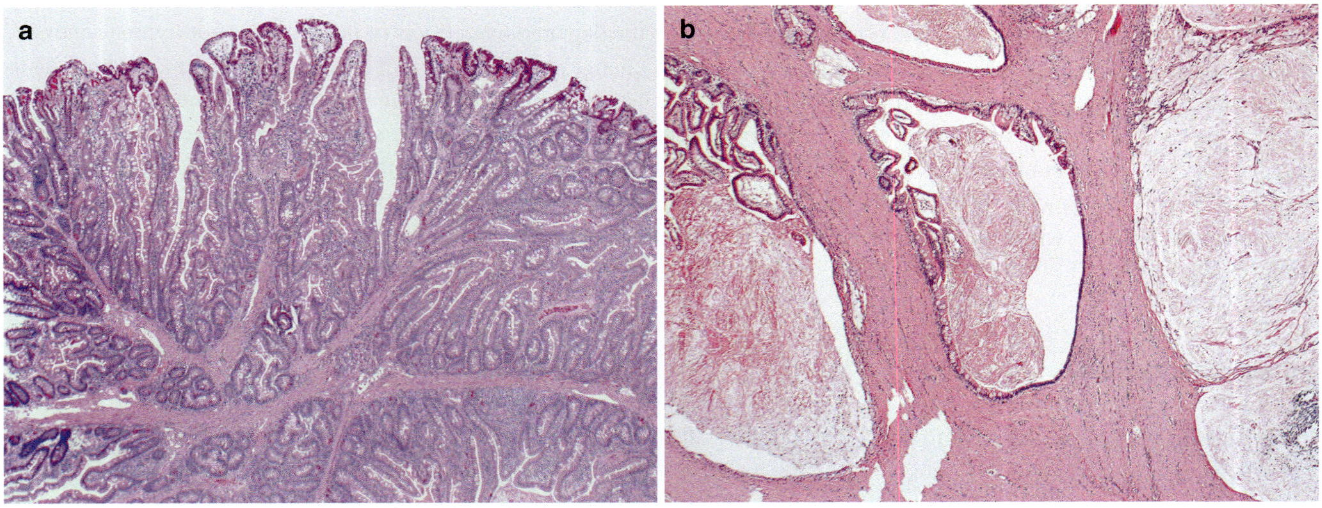

Fig. 14.26 Peutz-Jeghers polyp (PJP). (**a**) A PJP in jejunum is characterized by branched or tree-like smooth muscle cores covered with normal intestinal epithelium. (**b**) Pseudoinvasion in a PJP with epithelium misplaced into submucosa and muscularis propria

it is still controversial whether the malignancy follows the hamartoma-adenoma-carcinoma sequence or originates from coexisting adenomas or adjacent normal mucosa in Peutz-Jeghers polyps [120]. Therefore, hamartomatous polyps in Peutz-Jeghers syndrome are currently not considered precancerous lesions.

Juvenile Polyp

Juvenile polyps are a type of hamartomatous polyps that occur most commonly in juvenile polyposis syndrome and predominantly in colorectum, but they can be sporadic or are associated with other syndromes such as Cowden syndrome [121]. The upper gastrointestinal tract involvement in juvenile polyposis has been referred as generalized juvenile gastrointestinal polyposis, and the incidence of juvenile polyps in small bowel has been reported ranging 14–20% in several reports [122, 123]. Recurrent juvenile polyps have been observed in the ileal pouch of juvenile polyposis patients who have undergone proctocolectomy [124]. In addition, the risk of small bowel carcinoma associated with juvenile polyposis has also been well documented, and several such cases have been described in the literature [122, 125]. One study suggested that the incidence of gastric and small bowel carcinoma, together, was about one-fifth of the frequency of colorectal cancers in patients with juvenile polyposis syndrome [126].

Endoscopically, juvenile polyps are typically lobulated and pedunculated with surface erosion and size ranging from 5 mm to 50 mm. Histologically, juvenile polyps in small bowel are characterized by an abundance of edematous lamina propria containing inflammatory cells and cystically dilated glands (see Fig. 12.7 in Chap. 12). The dilated glands are variable in size and often filled with mucin. Surface erosion and crypt abscesses are frequently seen. The dilated glands in small bowel juvenile polyps are less rounded and organized and more compacted than those in colorectal juvenile polyps. The glands are lined by cuboidal to columnar intestinal epithelium with reactive changes, and dysplasia can be frequently identified. The smooth muscle bundles seen in Peutz-Jeghers polyps are absent. It is difficult to distinguish between an inflammatory polyp and a juvenile polyp. Indeed, if a diagnosis of juvenile polyposis syndrome has not been established clinically, the reasonable approach for pathologists for such polyps is to classify them as inflammatory polyps that could represent either inflammatory polyps or hamartomatous polyp of juvenile inflammatory type. In addition, the syndromic juvenile polyps are also similar to sporadic solitary juvenile polyps. Although a few features have been described that may favor syndromic polyps, such as multiple polyps, a frond-like growth pattern with fewer stroma, fewer dilated glands, more proliferative smaller glands, pure intestinal epithelial lining, presence of dysplasia, and prominent vessels, a consideration of juvenile polyposis syndrome must be relied on a proper clinical context [116].

Miscellaneous Disorders

Radiation Enteritis

The radiation therapy is widely used nowadays to treat gastrointestinal and pelvic malignancies and can cause direct injury on the gastrointestinal mucosa leading to radiation enteritis [127, 128]. The gastrointestinal mucosa is sensitive to radiation effect because of a high mitotic rate. The severity of the intestinal injury is related to concomitant chemotherapy, the total radiation dose, the fractionation, and the exposure in tissues peripheral to the target region. Acute radiation enteritis occurs in virtually all patients who receive abdominal or pelvic radiation, and approximately 5–15% of these patients can develop chronic radiation enteritis.

Acute radiation enteritis typically develops during the second week of treatment and peak by the fourth to fifth week. The patients usually present with cramping abdominal pain, tenesmus, nausea and vomiting, diarrhea, and hematochezia. Most of the patients are self-limiting or only require supportive management, but 15–20% of patients may be too severe to continue with the therapy. The modern technology and other preventive management to minimize radiation exposure have significantly reduced radiation injury. Histologically, the degree of small intestinal mucosa injury in acute radiation enteritis varies from nearly unrecognizable changes to severe mucosal inflammation, ulceration, hemorrhage, necrosis, or even perforation. The surface epithelial cells show mucin depletion and sloughing. The lamina propria contains edema, fibrin deposition, and increased inflammatory infiltration including neutrophils and eosinophils (Fig. 14.27a). There are cryptitis or crypt abscesses. Apoptosis is frequent. Radiation-induced cytological atypia can be seen in epithelial cells, stromal cells, and endothelial cells, which is characterized by nuclear pyknosis or nuclear enlargement with prominent nucleoli and bizarre shape (Fig. 14.27b); however, these atypical cells still keep low N/C ratio, with smooth nuclear membrane and chromatin pattern and no mitosis, which are different features from malignant tumor cells [129]. Even with severe necroinflammatory changes, the overall mucosal architectural is preserved, but with loss of epithelial cells from the tip of the villi, severe villous atrophy with crypt hyperplasia or crypt dropout is present. In patients who undergo total lymphoid radiation for preparing bone marrow transplantation, there is depletion of lymphoid follicles in Peyer patches in the ileum. Recovery of the damaged mucosa occurs within

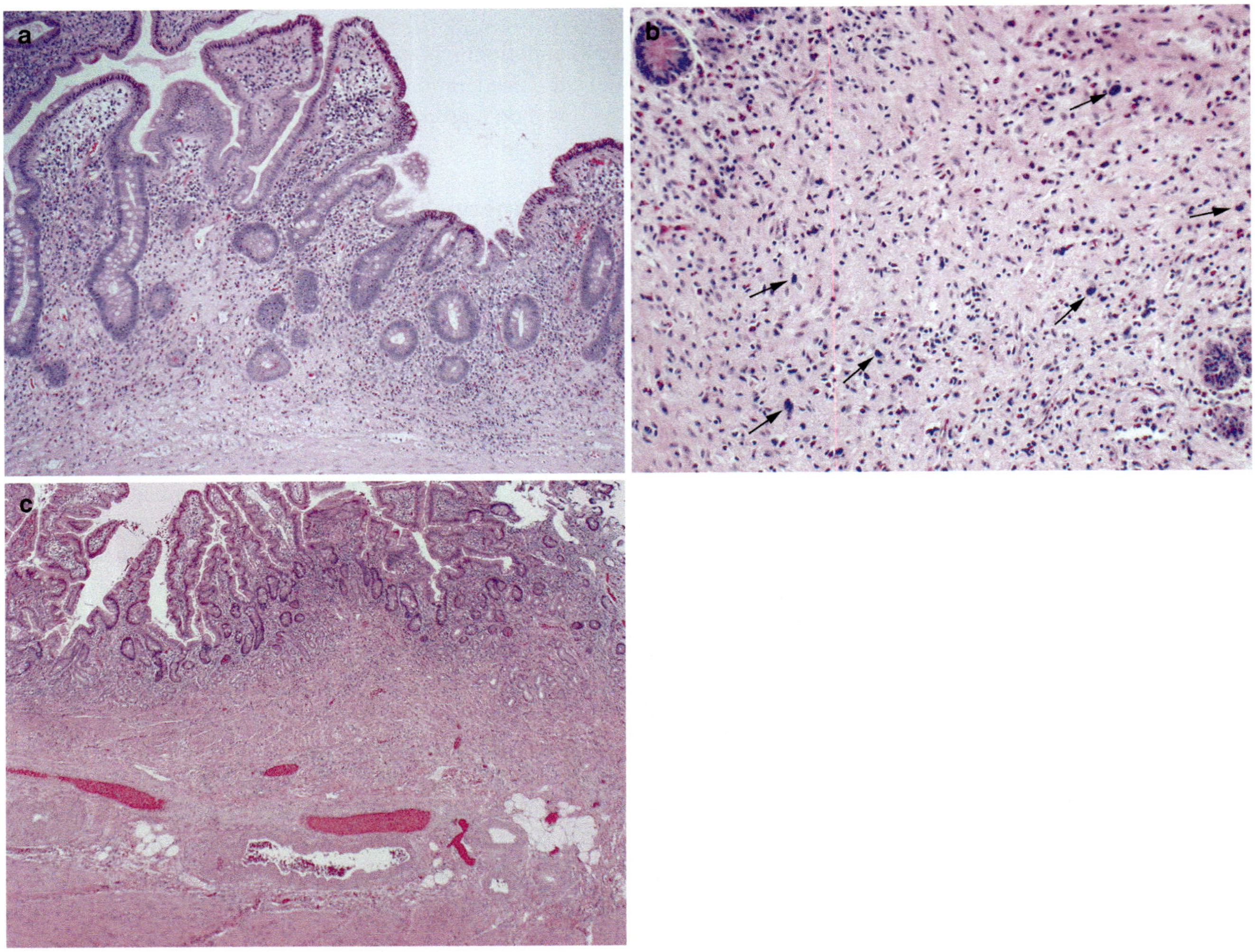

Fig. 14.27 Radiation enteritis. (a) Acute radiation-induced injury includes mucosal inflammation, edema, fibrin deposition, surface epithelial damage, and mild villous architectural change. (b) Radiation-induced cytological atypia. The atypical cells (arrows) show hyperchromatic, pleomorphic, and enlarged nuclei. (c) Chronic radiation enteritis, characterized by submucosal fibrosis, mucosal architectural changes, pseudopyloric metaplasia, and thickened wall vessels

2–3 weeks after the cessation of radiation therapy, but evidence of injury is present, such as distorted villous and crypt architecture, villous atrophy, persistent ulceration, and fibrosis [130].

Chronic radiation enteritis can develop months, years, or even decades after radiotherapy, and patients can present with a variety of gastrointestinal symptoms such as with postprandial pain, small bowel obstruction, bloating, diarrhea, steatorrhea, or malabsorption. The main histological features of chronic radiation enteritis are progressive fibrosis and vascular changes (Fig. 14.27c). The fibrosis is typically prominent in submucosa and can be hyalinized. The fibrosis can extend and involve lamina propria, muscularis mucosae and propria, which is associated with mucosal and muscular atrophy. The vascular changes include telangiectasia, endothelial cell injury, vasculitis, and eventually developing obliterative arteritis, which is characterized by intimal fibrosis, accumulation of foamy macrophages, and thickening of the vessel walls with hyalinization. Of note, the vascular changes tend to be focal and patchy, and examination of multiple sections is required to identify the characteristic vascular lesions. The progressive vascular changes lead to intestinal ischemia. The radiation-induced nuclear atypia is also present in chronic radiation enteritis which affects all cell types including ganglion cells. The presence of atypical radiation fibroblasts is a clue to chronic radiation enteritis.

Neutropenic Enterocolitis

Neutropenic enterocolitis (NEC) is a severe necrotizing enterocolitis primarily affecting immunocompromised patients with severe neutropenia. NEC more frequently occurs in patients with hematologic malignancies undergoing chemotherapy, but NEC cases after immunosuppressive therapy for solid malignancies and transplants have also been described [131]. Of note, although NEC has been described as "necrotizing enterocolitis", it is a different intestinal necroinflammatory disease from the "neonatal necrotizing enterocolitis" seen in newborns. The pathogenesis of NEC is not completely understood and is probably multifactorial. The intestinal mucosal injury resulting from cytotoxic drugs, superimposed infections, and leukemic infiltration, in conjunction with neutropenia and the immunocompromised state, makes the patients more vulnerable to bacterial intramural invasion leading to necrotizing enterocolitis. Patients with absolute neutrophil counts <500/μL are at increased risk for developing NEC, and the symptoms usually develop coinciding with the low leukocyte count following chemotherapy. The most common symptoms are abdominal pain, diarrhea, and fever. The management of NEC has not been standardized, and surgical intervention is preserved for patients with bowel perforation, uncontrolled bleeding, and other surgical implications. NEC is still a life-threatening condition, and the mortality rate can be as high as 50% [132]. Patients with normalized leukocyte count tend to have better prognosis [131, 133].

The cecum is most commonly involved in NEC, and the disease can extend into the ascending colon and terminal ileum. On resection or autopsy specimens, the bowel shows diffuse wall thickening with hemorrhage, necrosis, and possible perforation. The mucosa is markedly edematous with ulceration and necrosis. The mucosa may be completely lost and covered with fibrinous exudates (Fig. 14.28a). The wall of affected bowel has intramural edema, hemorrhage, necrosis, and often with various bacterial and/or fungal organism infiltrations. One striking feature is essentially absence of neutrophils and lymphoid inflammatory cells (Fig. 14.28b) [134].

Collagenous Ileitis

A handful of cases of collagenous ileitis have been reported in the literature, and most of them are associated collagenous or lymphocytic diseases elsewhere in the gastrointestinal tract, such as collagenous sprue and collagenous or lymphocytic gastritis and/or colitis [135–138]. Rare isolated collagenous ileitis has been reported, but the clinical significance remains unclear [137]. Diarrhea is the main clinical symptom. Similar to the collagenous disease in other sites of the gastrointestinal tract, collagenous ileitis is also characterized by thickening of subepithelial collagen bands, associated with other histological changes including mild intraepithelial lymphocytosis, lamina propria expansion by mild chronic inflammation, surface epithelium sloughing, focal neutrophil infiltration, and villous atrophy (Fig. 14.29a). In one report, the average thickness of subepithelial collagen bands in 13 cases is 32 μm, ranging from 15 to 100 μm [137]. The thickened collagenous bands tend to be patchy or even have a nodular pattern. The involved subepithelial area in that report ranges from 5% to 80%. Trichrome stain can be performed to confirm the diagnosis (Fig. 14.29b).

Cryptogenic Multifocal Ulcerating Stenosing Enteritis

Cryptogenic multifocal ulcerous stenosing enteritis (CMUSE) is an extremely rare and underdiagnosed disease characterized by chronic nonspecific ulcers and strictures of the small intestine leading to chronic intermittent gastrointestinal bleeding and small bowel obstruction [139–141]. The patients are frequently misdiagnosed with other diseases

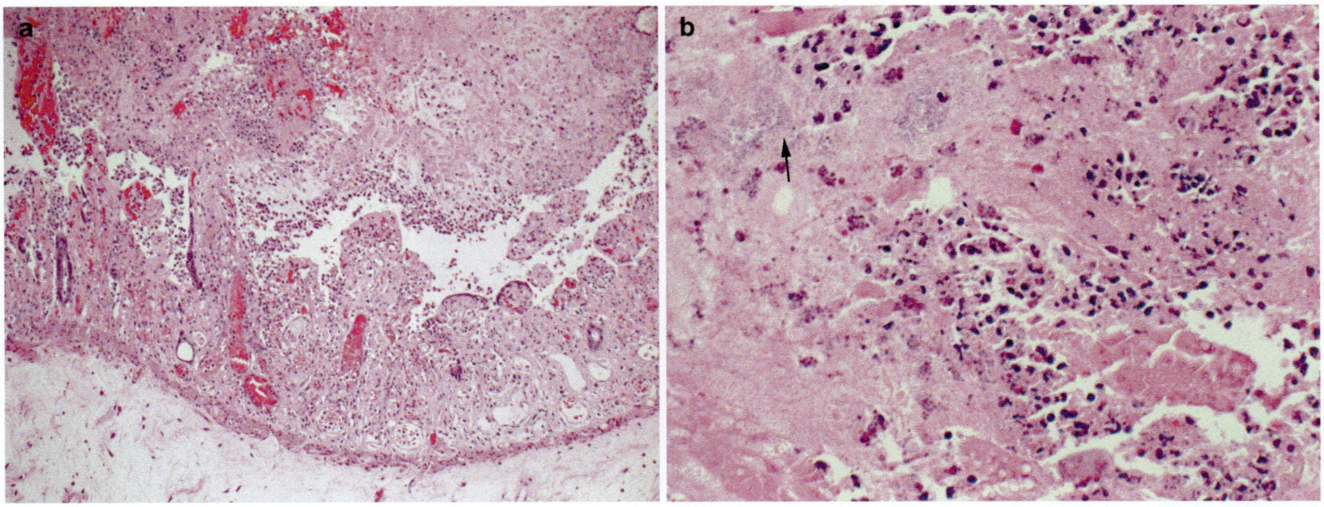

Fig. 14.28 Neutropenic enterocolitis. (**a**) Necrotic mucosa covered with fibrinous exudates. (**b**) Necrotic epithelial cells intermixed with exudates and bacterial colonies (arrow). Note the absence of neutrophils

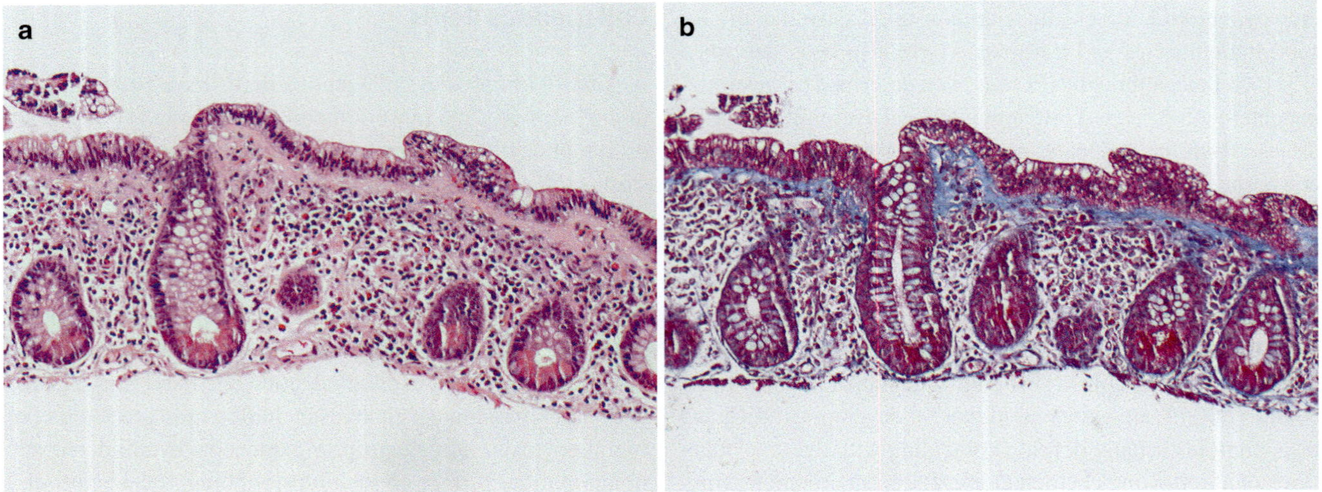

Fig. 14.29 Collagenous ileitis. (**a**) The terminal ileum biopsy shows thickening of subepithelial collagen band, with mild intraepithelial lymphocytosis, lamina propria inflammation, and villous atrophy. (**b**) Trichrome stain confirms the thickened subepithelial collagen band

in the small intestine especially Crohn's disease. The pathogenesis of CMUSE is still poorly understood. There is no specific treatment for CMUSE. Symptomatic management includes enteral and parenteral nutrition along with iron supplementation. Patients do not respond to 5-aminosalicylic acid and azathioprine. Some may respond to systemic glucocorticosteroids.

Diagnosis of CMUSE is to exclude other small bowel diseases which rely on clinical, radiological, endoscopic, and histological findings. The small intestinal ulcers in CMUSE occur predominantly in the ileum with only rare involvement in the terminal ileum. The ulcers are multiple (>20) and superficial. The multiple ulcers may fuse which gives a geographic configuration. There is no cobblestone appearance, fissuring, or fistula formation. Strictures are present in advanced cases, which are usually multiple, short, and separated by 2–10 cm of normal mucosa [142]. Microscopically, the ulcers are restricted to the mucosa or submucosa, usually associated with mild mixed inflammatory infiltrates and fibrosis (Fig. 14.30). The mucosa adjacent to the ulcers is usually unremarkable. There is no transmural inflammation or granulomas [141].

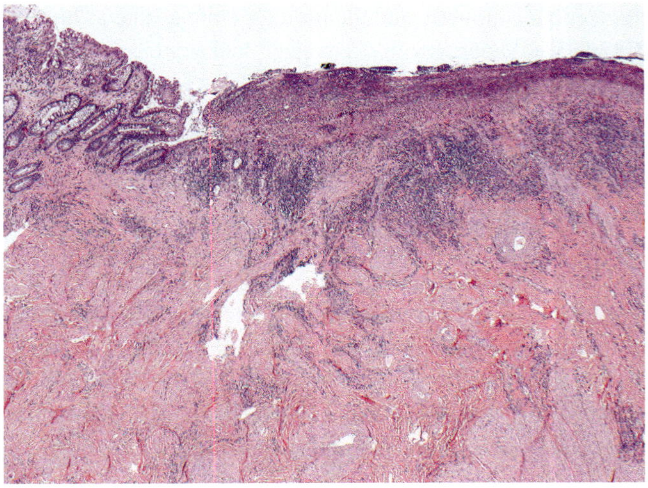

Fig. 14.30 Cryptogenic multifocal ulcerous stenosing enteritis. There is a discrete ulcer which is restricted to the mucosa and submucosa, associated with mild mixed inflammatory infiltrate and fibrosis

The main differential diagnosis of CMUSE is to exclude Crohn's disease. It is unusual for Crohn's disease to occur in the jejunum without active disease elsewhere. The histological features of Crohn's disease, such as transmural inflammation, fissuring, fistula, and granulomas, are absent in CMUSE. NSAIDs-induced enteropathy shares some clinicopathological features of CMUSE, such as anemia with fecal occult blood, ulcers, stricture formation, but NSAIDs-induced enteropathy responds dramatically after discontinuance of the causative drugs. Intestinal infection, especially tuberculosis, is also needed to rule out. Intestinal tuberculosis typically involves the ileocecal region. The ulcers in tuberculosis are irregular and at various stages. Caseating granulomatous inflammation is characteristic. Nonspecific small intestinal ulcers with no multiple strictures should not be considered as CMUSE. Other rare diseases in the differential diagnosis include Behçet's disease, or other drugs such as thiazides or potassium chloride induced small intestinal injury. Some main diagnostic features of small bowel ulcers in different disorders are summarized in Table 13.2 in Chap. 13.

Ulcerative Jejunoileitis

Ulcerative jejunoileitis, also known as chronic nongranulomatous ulcerative jejunitis, is a rare disorder characterized

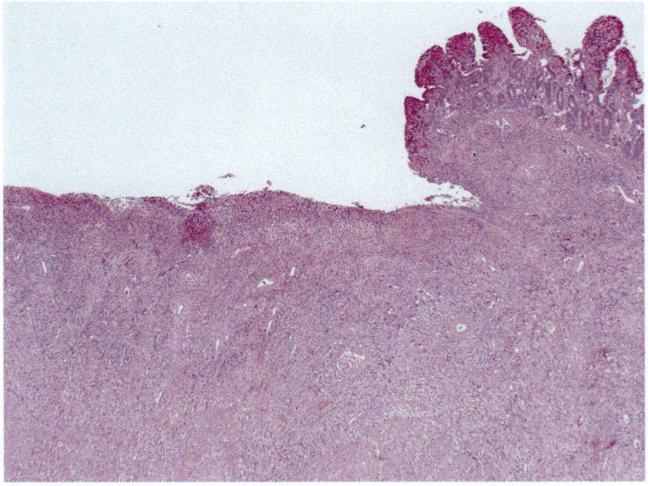

Fig. 14.31 Ulcerative jejunoileitis. A big ulceration with broad ulcer bed containing acute and chronic inflammation, granulation tissue, and fibrosis

by chronic multiple ulcerations with scarring and strictures in the small bowel, especially the jejunum [143]. The patients usually present with abdominal pain, weight loss, and diarrhea. Most of cases are associated with celiac disease and has been considered as a complication of celiac disease; some are affected by enteropathy-associated T-cell lymphoma [144]. Although the pathogenesis is still poorly understood, the mucosal infiltration by activated T-cells may play an important role. Indeed, monoclonal T-cell populations were detected in ulcers and normal mucosa [145], and patients with ulcerative jejunoileitis response to anti-TNF-α monoclonal antibody have been reported [146].

Histologically, the small bowel shows multiple ulcers which are usually transversely oriented with variable depth. The ulcer bed contains acute and chronic inflammation, granulation tissue, and overlying fibrinopurulent exudates (Fig. 14.31). Perforation may present. The adjacent mucosa shows villous atrophy. In chronic phase, there may be scar formation leading to strictures. Transmural inflammation and granulomas are absent. The differential diagnosis includes other conditions that can cause small bowel ulcerations, especially Crohn's disease. The other considerations may include CMUSE, NSAIDs-induced enteropathy, ischemia, vasculitis, or infection (see Table 13.2 in Chap. 13).

Pneumatosis Cystoides Intestinalis

Pneumatosis cystoides intestinalis (PCI) is a rare disorder characterized by the presence of gas in cyst-like spaces within the submucosa or subserosa of the intestine [147]. It occurs more commonly in males. More than half of the cases involve the colon, about one-third in the small intestine, and a small percentage of patients in both colon and small intestine [148]. The common symptoms of PCI are abdominal pain, diarrhea, abdominal distention, nausea and vomiting, and constipation. The pathogenesis of PCI is still poorly understood, and several theories have been proposed since majority of cases have underlying diseases, including intestinal wall injury or increased intraluminal pressure due to obstruction, inflammation, or ischemia; pulmonary diseases; gas-forming bacteria; production of large volume of gas in malnutrition; and other disorders such as connective tissue disease [149].

PCI shows characteristic radiographic features that have been described as linear, curvilinear, small bubbles, or collections of larger cysts of radiolucency along the wall of the intestine. Histologically, it is characterized by variable sizes of open spaces and cyst-like structures predominantly in submucosa (Fig. 14.32a), and they can be identified in subserosa at the same time. The cyst-like spaces do not have true cellular lining, but there are surrounded by a variety of cells including multinucleated giant cells, macrophages, eosinophils, and lymphocytes (Fig. 14.32b) [150]. The overlying mucosa may show some histological changes such as mild villous atrophy, mild crypt architectural distortion, or mild active chronic inflammation [151]. The much smaller empty spaces in mucosa and superficial submucosa on biopsy samples are frequently overlooked because they resemble fat cells. Recognizing the absence of eccentrically located nuclei as seen in the fat cells, significant size variation of the open spaces, and the multinucleated giant cells can help to distinguish them.

Brown Bowel Syndrome

Brown bowel syndrome, also known as intestinal lipofuscinosis or intestinal ceroidosis, is a rare disorder characterized by brown discoloration of the intestinal wall resulting from the deposition of lipofuscin in the intestinal smooth muscle cells. The lipofuscin is released from the degenerated mitochondria. Brown bowel syndrome is typically association with various malabsorption syndromes and malnutrition causing vitamin E deficiency, such as celiac disease, chronic pancreatitis, tropical sprue, intestinal lymphangiectasia, and Whipple's disease. Most patients with Brown bowel syndrome are asymptomatic, but severe clinical implications such as massive intestinal dilation and pseudo-obstruction may occur, especially in children and young adults [152, 153].

Microscopically, diffuse light-brown, granular pigmentation is identified in otherwise unremarkable smooth muscle cells of both muscularis propria and muscularis mucosae (Fig. 14.33). The same pigment is also present in the macrophages within the mesenteric lymph nodes. The architecture of intestinal villi is preserved with no increased inflammation, unless the disease is associated with other conditions such as

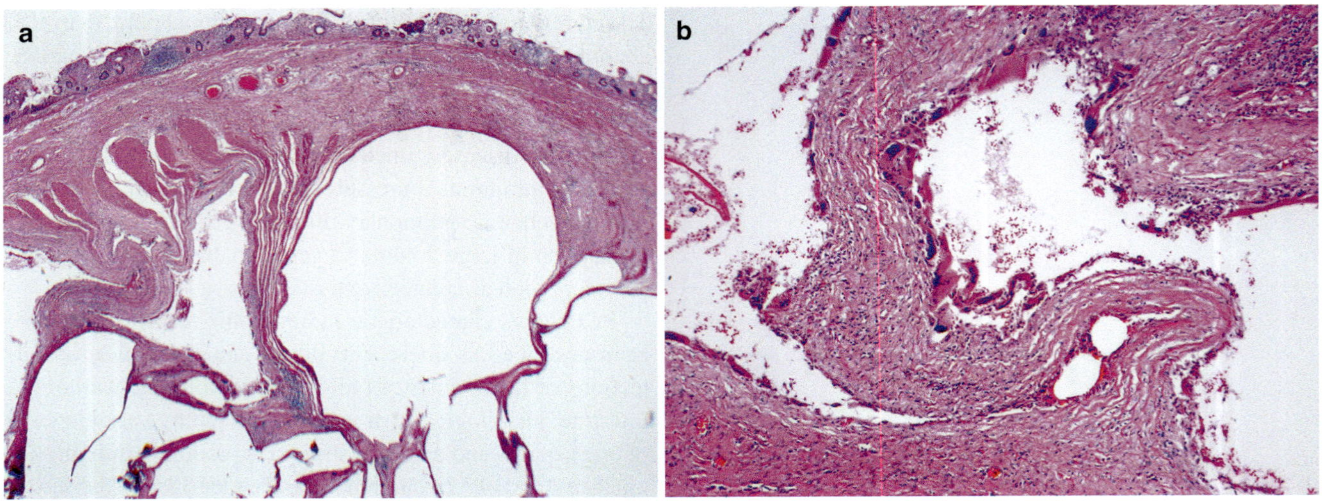

Fig. 14.32 Pneumatosis cystoids intestinalis (PCI). (**a**) There are many variable sizes of open spaces and cyst-like structures in submucosa. (**b**) The open spaces are surrounded by macrophages, eosinophils, lymphocytes, and multinucleated giant cells

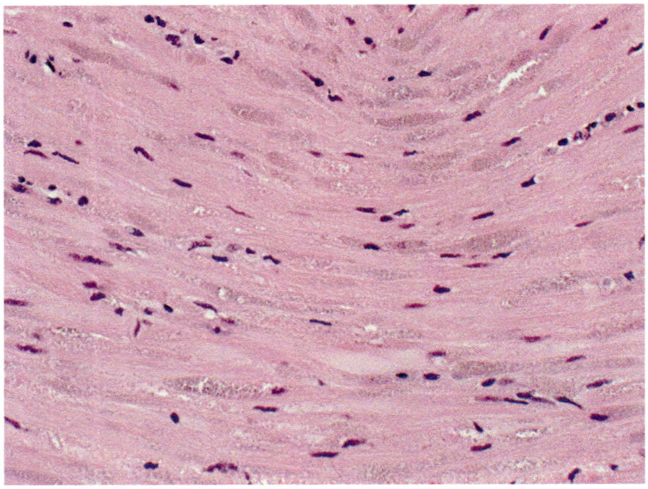

Fig. 14.33 Brown bowel syndrome. Diffuse light-brown, granular pigmentation in smooth muscle cells of muscularis propria

celiac disease. The brown pigment is positive on a PAS stain and is resistant to diastase digestion. It also stains with Masson-Fontana, methylene blue, and methenamine silver. The pigment is negative on iron and melanin stains. The other brown pigments that are occasionally seen in small intestine disorders include hemosiderin pigment, iron pill-induced injury, Whipple's disease, and melanosis intestini. However, these pigments are only present within macrophages in the lamina propria.

Lymphoid Hyperplasia in the Terminal Ileum

Normal terminal ileum is rich in lymphoid tissue such as Peyer's patches and small lymphoid aggregates in both lamina propria and submucosa, which are more prominent in children and young adults. The prominent lymphoid hyperplasia in the terminal ileum can have a nodular appearance, referred as nodular lymphoid hyperplasia or lymphoid polyp. Some patients may have symptoms such as diarrhea, lower abdominal pain, and weight loss, mimicking Crohn's disease, and intussusception may occur in children.

Microscopically, the lamina propria and submucosa are filled with lymphoid follicles with reactive germinal centers and lymphoid aggregates (Fig. 14.34). The overlying small intestinal epithelium is usually flattened or with short villi, and may contain increased lymphocytes or even scattered neutrophils. The sizes of lymphoid follicles and aggregates are variable, but they are in regular shapes, distributed evenly, and composed of small lymphocytes without cytological atypia. On immunochemical stains, CD-20 positive B-cells in the germinal centers are surrounded by CD-3 positive T-cells, and B-cell population may be expended. Concerns for lymphoma are often raised. Younger patients with history of inflammatory bowel disease or other infections, normal distribution and proportion of B- and T-cells, presence of tangible body macrophages in the germinal center favor reactive lymphoid hyperplasia. On the other hand, the presence of sheet-like monomorphic lymphocytes and lymphoepithelial lesions in older patients would be concerning for lymphoma. Immunostain workup identifying aberrant markers such as B-cells co-expressing CD5 or CD43 and detection of a monoclonal B-cell population by immunoglobin gene rearrangement test support lymphoma. Of note, abnormal immunostain patterns and clonal B-cell populations can occasionally be observed in reactive lymphoid hyperplasia, but the clones are usually different in the repeat biopsy

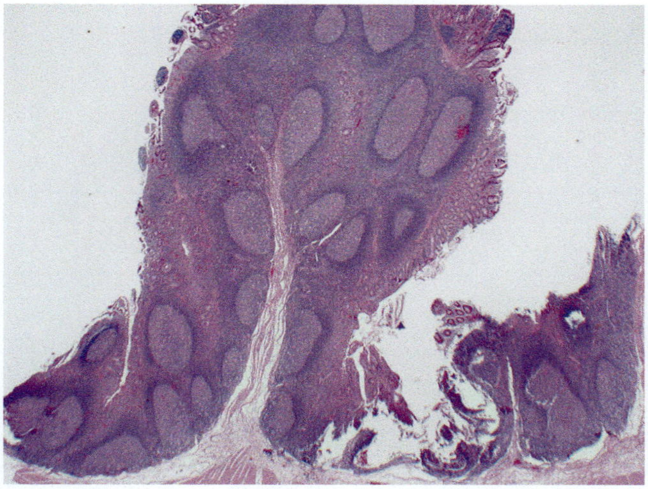

Fig. 14.34 Lymphoid hyperplasia in the terminal ileum. There are numerous lymphoid follicles with reactive germinal centers and lymphoid aggregates in lamina propria and submucosa, with flat overlying small intestinal epithelium. The shape, distribution, and orientation of these lymphoid follicles are regular

specimens. To avoid misdiagnosis of lymphomas, clonal tests should be preserved for those patients with strong clinical suspicion and compelling morphological and immunephenotypical features for lymphoma [154]. Other conditions that are needed to be ruled out in the setting of prominent lymphoid hyperplasia are infections and Crohn's disease, but they are typically associated with other histological changes such as marked inflammation and caseating granulomas in tuberculosis, viral inclusions, or mucosal changes in Crohn's disease.

Intestinal Transplantation

Intestinal transplantation is considered as the only therapeutic option for patients with irreversible intestinal failure and complications associated with the long-term use of parenteral nutrition. Short gut syndrome and functional bowel problems due to a variety of conditions are the two main causes [155]. Although intestinal transplantation is the rarest type of solid organ transplantation which is mainly due to the limitation of transplantable intestines, the number of intestinal transplants has increased significantly in the USA, from a few cases in the early 1990s to 100 to nearly 200 cases performed each year in the last decade because of the improvement in organ preservation, surgical technique, immunosuppression, postoperative management, and outcome. The pathologists may encounter four issues when participating in the management of intestinal transplantation patients: rejection, GVHD, infection, and posttransplant lymphoproliferative disorder (PTLD) [156].

Rejection Intestinal allograft rejection is a major challenge in small intestine transplantation which is associated with high morbidity and mortality because of rich lymphoid tissue in the intestine. It is mainly in a form of acute cellular rejection although antibody-mediated rejection may occur which still remains poorly defined [157, 158]. The rejection can occur at any time after transplantation but is most common in the first 6–12 months. The pathologic evaluation by biopsy is considered as the gold standard in diagnosing rejection. The protocol allograft biopsies are performed 2 or 3 times per week for the first month and 1–2 times per week for the following 2 months. Multiple biopsies from both abnormal and normal-appearing mucosa should be taken for pathological evaluation because the rejection changes can be patchy. Of note, biopsies near the stoma should be avoided where the mucosa often shows nonspecific changes.

Microscopically, the histologic features of acute cellular rejection in small intestine include increased inflammatory infiltration in lamina propria, apoptosis, endotheliitis, and mucosal damage such as cryptitis, crypt dropout, loss of villous architecture, and mucosal necrosis (Fig. 14.35a, b). An international grading scheme has been developed to evaluate the degree of acute cellular rejection in intestinal transplants [159]. There are five categories in this grading system: no evidence of acute rejection (grade 0); indeterminate for acute rejection (grade IND); mild acute cellular rejection (grade 1); moderate acute cellular rejection (grade 2); and severe acute cellular rejection (grade 3). The grading is based on main three features: (1) the crypt apoptotic body count; (2) the degree of inflammatory infiltration; and (3) the extent of mucosal injury. The apoptotic count is determined by counting the total number of apoptotic bodies in ten consecutive crypts. The inflammatory infiltration is predominantly composed of mononuclear cells intermixed with eosinophils and occasional neutrophils and is scored as mild, moderate, and severe based on the intensity. The eosinophilic infiltrate is not a reliable feature in grading the rejection. The mucosal injury is manifested from congestion, edema, epithelial cell injury, to extensive erosion, crypt dropout, ulceration, and sloughing. The diagnostic criteria of different categories of intestinal allograft rejection are summarized in Table 14.3.

Chronic rejection can also occur in small intestine transplantation which is the main cause of late intestinal graft failure. Chronic rejection is often preceded by repeated episodes of acute rejection. The patients present with persistent diarrhea with nonhealing mucosal ulceration. Pathological evaluation of mucosal biopsy in patients with chronic rejection often reveals nonspecific findings such as mild lamina propria fibrosis or ischemic changes which are not specific for diagnosing chronic rejection because they can be secondary to a variety of other causes. Obliterative vasculopathy in medium to large vessels is pathognomonic for chronic rejection, but it is rarely seen in mucosal biopsies. Therefore,

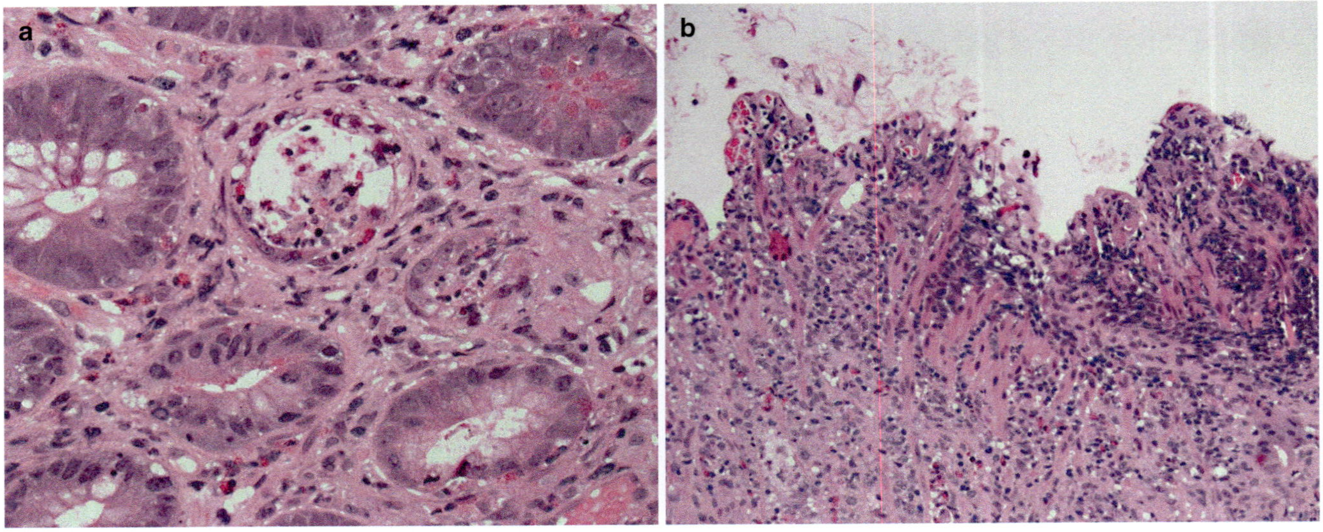

Fig. 14.35 Acute cellular rejection in small intestine transplant. (a) Moderate rejection, with prominent apoptosis, crypt loss, and inflammation. (b) Severe rejection, with complete loss of epithelium. (Courtesy from Dr. Xiuli Liu at University of Florida)

Table 14.3 Histologic grading of acute cellular rejection in intestinal allograft

Degree of acute cellular rejection	Apoptotic count (ten consecutive crypts)	Inflammatory infiltration	Mucosal damage
No rejection (grade 0)	None or<2	No increase	None or mild congestion
Indeterminate rejection (grade IND)	<6	Focal and minimal	Mild edema, congestion, villous blunting
Mild rejection (grade 1)	≥6	Mild to focal moderate	Epithelial injury with mild villus blunting and architectural distortion.
Moderate rejection (grade 2)	Frequent to confluent apoptosis	Moderate to severe	Obvious crypt destruction with villus blunting, architectural distortion, focal erosion
Severe rejection (grade 3)	Confluent apoptosis in the surviving crypts	Moderate to severe	Extensive erosion and ulceration, extensive crypt dropout and architectural distortion

chronic rejection is usually confirmed only in full-thickness biopsies or in failed grafts, where obliterative vasculopathy can be identified [160].

Graft versus host disease GVHD occurs in 7–9% of intestinal transplants because of the large volume of lymphatic tissue accompanying the intestinal allograft [161]. The patients who develop GVHD may be subclinical or can present with fever, leukopenia, diarrhea, abdominal pain, and rash. The diagnosis requires histological confirmation in skin or bowel biopsy. A sigmoidoscopy is recommended to evaluating GVHD because a study has shown that any signs of GVHD present above the sigmoid were also present at the level of the sigmoid [162].

Infections Infection is the leading cause of death in intestinal transplantation patients which accounts for nearly 50% of all deaths within 5 years of transplant [163]. The bacterial infection is the most common, followed by viral and fungal infections. The most common sites of infection are the abdominal cavity, lungs, wounds, and urinary tract. CMV infection is particularly important because it often involves the allografts leading to allograft loss and even death. The incidence of CMV infection is about 15–30% and is highest in CMV-negative recipients who receive CMV-positive grafts. The diagnosis needs histological identification of CMV-infected cells characterized by larger cells containing basophilic intranuclear inclusions (Cowdry bodies) surrounded by a clear halo and basophilic/amphophilic cytoplasmic inclusions, and this can be confirmed with immunohistochemical stain. Other pathogens that may be occasionally seen in the allograft include adenovirus and *Candida*.

Posttransplant lymphoproliferative disorder PTLDs are lymphocytic and/or plasmacytic proliferations in the setting of transplant in which the majority cases are related to

Epstein-Barr virus (EBV), but EBV-negative disease does occur. The incidence of PTLD is higher in intestinal transplant recipients than other solid organ transplantations, and the incidence is also higher in children and recipients with multivisceral transplantation [164]. The diagnosis of PTLD usually requires a biopsy, which is often taken from superficial lymph nodes or tissue with clinical or radiological suspicion of involvement. The commonly affected sites are allograft bowel, lymph nodes, and liver. If the biopsy comes from the intestine graft itself, it can be difficult to differentiate PTLD from rejection or infection. The possibility of PTLD should always be considered whenever there is a lymphoid infiltrate in patients with intestinal transplantation. The detailed histopathologic features of PTLD are beyond the scope of this book. Proper workup, including immunohistochemistry, EBV tests, B-cell or T-cell gene rearrangement studies, and consultation from an experienced hematopathologist, can help with the diagnosis.

References

1. Allison MC, Howatson AG, Torrance CJ, Lee FD, Russell RI. Gastrointestinal damage associated with the use of nonsteroidal antiinflammatory drugs. N Engl J Med. 1992;327(11):749–54. https://doi.org/10.1056/NEJM199209103271101.
2. Leung WK, Bjarnason I, Wong VW, Sung JJ, Chan FK. Small bowel enteropathy associated with chronic low-dose aspirin therapy. Lancet. 2007;369(9561):614. https://doi.org/10.1016/S0140-6736(07)60282-7.
3. Matsumoto T, Kudo T, Esaki M, Yano T, Yamamoto H, Sakamoto C, et al. Prevalence of non-steroidal anti-inflammatory drug-induced enteropathy determined by double-balloon endoscopy: a Japanese multicenter study. Scand J Gastroenterol. 2008;43(4):490–6. https://doi.org/10.1080/00365520701794121.
4. Maiden L, Thjodleifsson B, Theodors A, Gonzalez J, Bjarnason I. A quantitative analysis of NSAID-induced small bowel pathology by capsule enteroscopy. Gastroenterology. 2005;128(5):1172–8.
5. Lim YJ, Yang CH. Non-steroidal anti-inflammatory drug-induced enteropathy. Clin Endosc. 2012;45(2):138–44. https://doi.org/10.5946/ce.2012.45.2.138.
6. Park SC, Chun HJ, Kang CD, Sul D. Prevention and management of non-steroidal anti-inflammatory drugs-induced small intestinal injury. World J Gastroenterol. 2011;17(42):4647–53. https://doi.org/10.3748/wjg.v17.i42.4647.
7. Lanas A, Garcia-Rodriguez LA, Polo-Tomas M, Ponce M, Alonso-Abreu I, Perez-Aisa MA, et al. Time trends and impact of upper and lower gastrointestinal bleeding and perforation in clinical practice. Am J Gastroenterol. 2009;104(7):1633–41. https://doi.org/10.1038/ajg.2009.164.
8. Kameda N, Higuchi K, Shiba M, Machida H, Okazaki H, Yamagami H, et al. A prospective, single-blind trial comparing wireless capsule endoscopy and double-balloon enteroscopy in patients with obscure gastrointestinal bleeding. J Gastroenterol. 2008;43(6):434–40. https://doi.org/10.1007/s00535-008-2182-9.
9. Lanas A, Sopena F. Nonsteroidal anti-inflammatory drugs and lower gastrointestinal complications. Gastroenterol Clin North Am. 2009;38(2):333–52. https://doi.org/10.1016/j.gtc.2009.03.007.
10. Maiden L, Thjodleifsson B, Seigal A, Bjarnason II, Scott D, Birgisson S, et al. Long-term effects of nonsteroidal anti-inflammatory drugs and cyclooxygenase-2 selective agents on the small bowel: a cross-sectional capsule enteroscopy study. Clin Gastroenterol Hepatol. 2007;5(9):1040–5. https://doi.org/10.1016/j.cgh.2007 04.031.
11. Sigthorsson G, Simpson RJ, Walley M, Anthony A, Foster R, Hotz-Behoftsitz C, et al. COX-1 and 2, intestinal integrity, and pathogenesis of nonsteroidal anti-inflammatory drug enteropathy in mice. Gastroenterology. 2002;122(7):1913–23.
12. Robert A, Asano T. Resistance of germfree rats to indomethacin-induced intestinal lesions. Prostaglandins. 1977;14(2):333–41.
13. Uejima M, Kinouchi T, Kataoka K, Hiraoka I, Ohnishi Y. Role of intestinal bacteria in ileal ulcer formation in rats treated with a nonsteroidal antiinflammatory drug. Microbiol Immunol. 1996;40(8):553–60.
14. Watanabe T, Higuchi K, Kobata A, Nishio H, Tanigawa T, Shiba M, et al. Non-steroidal anti-inflammatory drug-induced small intestinal damage is Toll-like receptor 4 dependent. Gut. 2008;57(2):181–7. https://doi.org/10.1136/gut.2007.125963.
15. Endo H, Higurashi T, Hosono K, Sakai E, Sekino Y, Iida H, et al. Efficacy of Lactobacillus casei treatment on small bowel injury in chronic low-dose aspirin users: a pilot randomized controlled study. J Gastroenterol. 2011;46(7):894–905. https://doi.org/10.1007/s00535-011-0410-1.
16. Lombardo L, Foti M, Ruggia O, Chiecchio A. Increased incidence of small intestinal bacterial overgrowth during proton pump inhibitor therapy. Clin Gastroenterol Hepatol. 2010;8(6):504–8. https://doi.org/10.1016/j.cgh.2009.12.022.
17. Wallace JL, Syer S, Denou E, de Palma G, Vong L, McKnight W, et al. Proton pump inhibitors exacerbate NSAID-induced small intestinal injury by inducing dysbiosis. Gastroenterology. 2011;141(4):1314–22. 22 e1–5. https://doi.org/10.1053/j.gastro.2011.06.075.
18. Washio E, Esaki M, Maehata Y, Miyazaki M, Kobayashi H, Ishikawa H, et al. Proton pump inhibitors increase incidence of nonsteroidal anti-inflammatory drug-induced small bowel injury: arandomized, placebo-controlled trial. Clin Gastroenterol Hepatol. 2016;14(6):809–15e1 https://doi.org/10.1016/j.cgh.2015.10.022.
19. Hawkey CJ, Karrasch JA, Szczepanski L, Walker DG, Barkun A, Swannell AJ, et al. Omeprazole compared with misoprostol for ulcers associated with nonsteroidal antiinflammatory drugs. Omeprazole versus Misoprostol for NSAID-induced Ulcer Management (OMNIUM) Study Group. N Engl J Med. 1998;338(11):727–34. https://doi.org/10.1056/NEJM199803123381105.
20. Jacob M, Foster R, Sigthorsson G, Simpson R, Bjarnason I. Role of bile in pathogenesis of indomethacin-induced enteropathy. Arch Toxicol. 2007;81(4):291–8. https://doi.org/10.1007/s00204-006-0149-2
21. Lichtenberger LM, Phan T, Okabe S. Aspirin's ability to induce intestinal injury in rats is dependent on bile and can be reversed if pre-associated with phosphatidylcholine. J Physiol Pharmacol. 2011;62(4):491–6.
22. Reuter BK, Davies NM, Wallace JL. Nonsteroidal anti-inflammatory drug enteropathy in rats: role of permeability, bacteria, and enterohepatic circulation. Gastroenterology. 1997;112(1):109–17
23. Endo H, Hosono K, Inamori M, Nozaki Y, Yoneda K, Fujita K, et al. Characteristics of small bowel injury in symptomatic chronic low-dose aspirin users: the experience of two medical centers in capsule endoscopy. J Gastroenterol. 2009;44(6):544–9. https://doi.org/10.1007/s00535-009-0040-z.
24. Endo H, Sakai E, Kato T, Umezawa S, Higurashi T, Ohkubo H, et al. Small bowel injury in low-dose aspirin users. J Gastroenterol. 2015;50(4):378–86. https://doi.org/10.1007/s00535-014-1028-x.

25. Hayashi Y, Yamamoto H, Kita H, Sunada K, Sato H, Yano T, et al. Non-steroidal anti-inflammatory drug-induced small bowel injuries identified by double-balloon endoscopy. World J Gastroenterol. 2005;11(31):4861–4.
26. Onwudike M, Sundaresan M, Melville D, Wood JJ. Diaphragm disease of the small bowel—a case report and literature review. Dig Surg. 2002;19(5):410–3. https://doi.org/10.1159/000065824.
27. Lee FD. Drug-related pathological lesions of the intestinal tract. Histopathology. 1994;25(4):303–8.
28. Speed CA, Bramble MG, Corbett WA, Haslock I. Non-steroidal anti-inflammatory induced diaphragm disease of the small intestine: complexities of diagnosis and management. Br J Rheumatol. 1994;33(8):778–80.
29. De Petris G, Lopez JI. Histopathology of diaphragm disease of the small intestine: a study of 10 cases from a single institution. Am J Clin Pathol. 2008;130(4):518–25. https://doi.org/10.1309/7DDT5TDVB5C6BNHV.
30. Lang J, Price AB, Levi AJ, Burke M, Gumpel JM, Bjarnason I. Diaphragm disease: pathology of disease of the small intestine induced by non-steroidal anti-inflammatory drugs. J Clin Pathol. 1988;41(5):516–26.
31. Going JJ, Canvin J, Sturrock R. Possible precursor of diaphragm disease in the small intestine. Lancet. 1993;341(8845):638–9.
32. Fernando SS, McGovern VJ. Neuromuscular and vascular hamartoma of small bowel. Gut. 1982;23(11):1008–12.
33. Cortina G, Wren S, Armstrong B, Lewin K, Fajardo L. Clinical and pathologic overlap in nonsteroidal anti-inflammatory drug-related small bowel diaphragm disease and the neuromuscular and vascular hamartoma of the small bowel. Am J Surg Pathol. 1999;23(11):1414–7.
34. Mehta V, Gupta A, Mahajan R, Narang V, Midha V, Sood N, et al. Symptomatic isolated terminal ileal ulcers: etiology and clinical significance. Endosc Int Open. 2017;5(7):E539–E46. https://doi.org/10.1055/s-0043-100688.
35. Fujimori S, Takahashi Y, Gudis K, Seo T, Ehara A, Kobayashi T, et al. Rebamipide has the potential to reduce the intensity of NSAID-induced small intestinal injury: a double-blind, randomized, controlled trial evaluated by capsule endoscopy. J Gastroenterol. 2011;46(1):57–64. https://doi.org/10.1007/s00535-010-0332-3.
36. Fortun PJ, Hawkey CJ. Nonsteroidal antiinflammatory drugs and the small intestine. Curr Opin Gastroenterol. 2007;23(2):134–41. https://doi.org/10.1097/MOG.0b013e328020045a.
37. Bjarnason I, Hayllar J, Smethurst P, Price A, Gumpel MJ. Metronidazole reduces intestinal inflammation and blood loss in non-steroidal anti-inflammatory drug induced enteropathy. Gut. 1992;33(9):1204–8.
38. Montalto M, Gallo A, Curigliano V, D'Onofrio F, Santoro L, Covino M, et al. Clinical trial: the effects of a probiotic mixture on non-steroidal anti-inflammatory drug enteropathy—a randomized, double-blind, cross-over, placebo-controlled study. Aliment Pharmacol Ther. 2010;32(2):209–14. https://doi.org/10.1111/j.1365-2036.2010.04324.x.
39. Dore MP, Pes GM, Murino A, Quarta Colosso B, Pennazio M. Short article: small intestinal mucosal injury in patients taking chemotherapeutic agents for solid cancers. Eur J Gastroenterol Hepatol. 2017;29(5):568–71. https://doi.org/10.1097/MEG.0000000000000828.
40. Trier JS. Morphologic alterations induced by methotrexate in the mucosa of human proximal intestine. I. Serial observations by light microscopy. Gastroenterology. 1962;42:295–305.
41. Cunningham D, Morgan RJ, Mills PR, Nelson LM, Toner PG, Soukop M, et al. Functional and structural changes of the human proximal small intestine after cytotoxic therapy. J Clin Pathol. 1985;38(3):265–70.
42. Keefe DM, Brealey J, Goland GJ, Cummins AG. Chemotherapy for cancer causes apoptosis that precedes hypoplasia in crypts of the small intestine in humans. Gut. 2000;47(5):632–7.
43. Nguyen T, Park JY, Scudiere JR, Montgomery E. Mycophenolic acid (cellcept and myofortic) induced injury of the upper GI tract. Am J Surg Pathol. 2009;33(9):1355–63. https://doi.org/10.1097/PAS.0b013e3181a755bd.
44. Parfitt JR, Jayakumar S, Driman DK. Mycophenolate mofetil-related gastrointestinal mucosal injury: variable injury patterns, including graft-versus-host disease-like changes. Am J Surg Pathol. 2008;32(9):1367–72.
45. Selbst MK, Ahrens WA, Robert ME, Friedman A, Proctor DD, Jain D. Spectrum of histologic changes in colonic biopsies in patients treated with mycophenolate mofetil. Mod Pathol. 2009;22(6):737–43. https://doi.org/10.1038/modpathol.2009.44.
46. Dhatt HS, Behr SC, Miracle A, Wang ZJ, Yeh BM. Radiological evaluation of bowel ischemia. Radiol Clin North Am. 2015;53(6):1241–54. https://doi.org/10.1016/j.rcl.2015.06.009.
47. Horton KM, Fishman EK. Multidetector CT angiography in the diagnosis of mesenteric ischemia. Radiol Clin North Am. 2007;45(2):275–88. https://doi.org/10.1016/j.rcl.2007.03.010.
48. Cudnik MT, Darbha S, Jones J, Macedo J, Stockton SW, Hiestand BC. The diagnosis of acute mesenteric ischemia: a systematic review and meta-analysis. Acad Emerg Med. 2013;20(11):1087–100. https://doi.org/10.1111/acem.12254.
49. Amaravadi RR, Tran TM, Altman R, Scheirey CD. Small bowel infarcts in Degos disease. Abdom Imaging. 2008;33(2):196–9. https://doi.org/10.1007/s00261-007-9225-1.
50. Magro CM, Poe JC, Kim C, Shapiro L, Nuovo G, Crow MK, et al. Degos disease: a C5b-9/interferon-alpha-mediated endotheliopathy syndrome. Am J Clin Pathol. 2011;135(4):599–610. https://doi.org/10.1309/AJCP66QIMFARLZKI.
51. Pagnoux C, Seror R, Henegar C, Mahr A, Cohen P, Le Guern V, et al. Clinical features and outcomes in 348 patients with polyarteritis nodosa: a systematic retrospective study of patients diagnosed between 1963 and 2005 and entered into the French Vasculitis Study Group Database. Arthritis Rheum. 2010;62(2):616–26. https://doi.org/10.1002/art.27240.
52. Ebert EC, Hagspiel KD, Nagar M, Schlesinger N. Gastrointestinal involvement in polyarteritis nodosa. Clin Gastroenterol Hepatol. 2008;6(9):960–6. https://doi.org/10.1016/j.cgh.2008.04.004.
53. Pagnoux C, Mahr A, Cohen P, Guillevin L. Presentation and outcome of gastrointestinal involvement in systemic necrotizing vasculitides: analysis of 62 patients with polyarteritis nodosa, microscopic polyangiitis, Wegener granulomatosis, Churg-Strauss syndrome, or rheumatoid arthritis-associated vasculitis. Medicine (Baltimore). 2005;84(2):115–28.
54. Kraft DM, McKee D, Scott C. Henoch-Schonlein purpura: a review. Am Fam Physician. 1998;58(2):405–8. 11
55. Saulsbury FT. Henoch-Schonlein purpura. Curr Opin Rheumatol. 2001;13(1):35–40.
56. Chen SY, Kong MS. Gastrointestinal manifestations and complications of Henoch-Schonlein purpura. Chang Gung Med J. 2004;27(3):175–81.
57. Louie CY, Gomez AJ, Sibley RK, Bass D, Longacre TA. Histologic features of gastrointestinal tract biopsies in IgA vasculitis (Henoch-Schonlein Purpura). Am J Surg Pathol. 2018;42(4):529–33. https://doi.org/10.1097/PAS.0000000000001036.
58. Jennette JC, Falk RJ, Bacon PA, Basu N, Cid MC, Ferrario F, et al. 2012 revised international chapel hill consensus conference nomenclature of vasculitides. Arthritis Rheum. 2013;65(1):1–11. https://doi.org/10.1002/art.37715.
59. Wechsler ME, Akuthota P, Jayne D, Khoury P, Klion A, Langford CA, et al. Mepolizumab or placebo for eosinophilic granulomatosis with polyangiitis. N Engl J Med. 2017;376(20):1921–32. https://doi.org/10.1056/NEJMoa1702079.

60. Franco DL, Ruff K, Mertz L, Lam-Himlin DM, Heigh R. Eosinophilic granulomatosis with polyangiitis and diffuse gastrointestinal involvement. Case Rep Gastroenterol. 2014;8(3):329–36. https://doi.org/10.1159/000369129.
61. Berden A, Goceroglu A, Jayne D, Luqmani R, Rasmussen N, Bruijn JA, et al. Diagnosis and management of ANCA associated vasculitis. BMJ. 2012;344:e26. https://doi.org/10.1136/bmj.e26.
62. Inamoto Y, Ito M, Suzuki R, Nishida T, Iida H, Kohno A, et al. Clinicopathological manifestations and treatment of intestinal transplant-associated microangiopathy. Bone Marrow Transplant. 2009;44(1):43–9. https://doi.org/10.1038/bmt.2008.419.
63. Selby DM, Rudzki JR, Bayever ES, Chandra RS. Vasculopathy of small muscular arteries in pediatric patients after bone marrow transplantation. Hum Pathol. 1999;30(7):734–40.
64. Nishida T, Hamaguchi M, Hirabayashi N, Haneda M, Terakura S, Atsuta Y, et al. Intestinal thrombotic microangiopathy after allogeneic bone marrow transplantation: a clinical imitator of acute enteric graft-versus-host disease. Bone Marrow Transplant. 2004;33(11):1143–50. https://doi.org/10.1038/sj.bmt.1704512.
65. Warren M, Jodele S, Dandoy C, Myers KC, Wallace G, Nelson A, et al. A complete histologic approach to gastrointestinal biopsy from hematopoietic stem cell transplant patients with evidence of transplant-associated gastrointestinal thrombotic microangiopathy. Arch Pathol Lab Med. 2017;141(11):1558–66. https://doi.org/10.5858/arpa.2016–0599-RA.
66. Mandeville K, Chien M, Willyerd FA, Mandell G, Hostetler MA, Bulloch B. Intussusception: clinical presentations and imaging characteristics. Pediatr Emerg Care. 2012;28(9):842–4. https://doi.org/10.1097/PEC.0b013e318267a75e.
67. Marinis A, Yiallourou A, Samanides L, Dafnios N, Anastasopoulos G, Vassiliou I, et al. Intussusception of the bowel in adults: a review. World J Gastroenterol. 2009;15(4):407–11.
68. Haas EM, Etter EL, Ellis S, Taylor TV. Adult intussusception. Am J Surg. 2003;186(1):75–6.
69. Fischer JE, Bland KI. Mastery of surgery. Philadelphia: Lippincott Williams & Wilkins; 2007.
70. Meckel J. Uber die divertikel am darmkanal. Arch Physiol. 1809;9:421–53.
71. Uppal K, Tubbs RS, Matusz P, Shaffer K, Loukas M. Meckel's diverticulum: a review. Clin Anat. 2011;24(4):416–22. https://doi.org/10.1002/ca.21094.
72. Takeda K, Kinumaki A, Furumai T, Yamaguchi T, Ohshima S, Ito Y. Mutational biosynthesis of butirosin analogs. J Antibiot (Tokyo). 1978;31(3):247–9.
73. Park JJ, Wolff BG, Tollefson MK, Walsh EE, Larson DR. Meckel diverticulum: the Mayo Clinic experience with 1476 patients (1950–2002). Ann Surg. 2005;241(3):529–33.
74. Hill P, Rode J. Helicobacter pylori in ectopic gastric mucosa in Meckel's diverticulum. Pathology. 1998;30(1):7–9.
75. Cates JM, Williams TL, Suriawinata AA. Intraductal papillary mucinous adenoma that arises from pancreatic heterotopia within a meckel diverticulum. Arch Pathol Lab Med. 2005;129(3):e67–9. https://doi.org/10.1043/1543–2165(2005)129<e67:IPMATA>2.0.CO;2.
76. Carpenter SS, Grillis ME. Meckel's diverticulitis secondary to carcinoid tumor: an unusual presentation of the acute abdomen in an adult. Curr Surg. 2003;60(3):301–3. https://doi.org/10.1016/S0149–7944(02)00745–6.
77. Leijonmarck CE, Bonman-Sandelin K, Frisell J, Raf L. Meckel's diverticulum in the adult. Br J Surg. 1986;73(2):146–9.
78. Qureshi SS, Ramadwar MR, Viswanathan S, Bakshi AV, Arora B, Gupta T, et al. Desmoplastic small round cell tumor of Meckels diverticulum. J Clin Oncol. 2007;25(22):3372–4. https://doi.org/10.1200/JCO.2007.11.9487.
79. Zhang L, Sanderson SO, Lloyd RV, Smyrk TC. Pancreatic intraepithelial neoplasia in heterotopic pancreas: evidence for the progression model of pancreatic ductal adenocarcinoma. Am J Surg Pathol. 2007;31(8):1191–5. https://doi.org/10.1097/PAS.0b013e31806841e1.
80. Heifetz SA, Rueda-Pedraza ME. Omphalomesenteric duct cysts of the umbilical cord. Pediatr Pathol. 1983;1(3):325–35.
81. Sawada F, Yoshimura R, Ito K, Nakamura K, Nawata H, Mizumoto K, et al. Adult case of an omphalomesenteric cyst resected by laparoscopic-assisted surgery. World J Gastroenterol. 2006;12(5):825–7.
82. Macpherson RI. Gastrointestinal tract duplications: clinical, pathologic, etiologic, and radiologic considerations. Radiographics. 1993;13(5):1063–80. https://doi.org/10.1148/radiographics.13.5.8210590.
83. Arias MP, Lorenzo FG, Sanchez MM, Vellibre RM. Enteric duplication cyst resembling umbilical cord cyst. J Perinatol. 2006;26(6):368–70. https://doi.org/10.1038/sj.jp.7211520.
84. Johnson JA 3rd, Poole GV. Ileal duplications in adults.Presentation and treatment. Arch Surg. 1994;129(6):659–61.
85. Baumann JL, Patel C. Enteric duplication cyst containing squamous and respiratory epithelium: an interesting case of a typically pediatric entity presenting in an adult patient. Case Rep Gastrointest Med. 2014;2014:790326. https://doi.org/10.1155/2014/790326.
86. Estrada R. Anomalies of intestinal rotation and fixation. 1st ed. Springfield: Thomas; 1958.
87. Stockmann P. Malrotation. In: Oldham KT, Colombani PM, Foglia RP, Skinner MA, editors. Principles and practice of pediatric surgery. 2nd ed. Philadelphia: Lippincott Williams & Wilkings; 2005. p. 1283.
88. Nehra D, Goldstein AM. Intestinal malrotation: varied clinical presentation from infancy through adulthood. Surgery. 2011;149(3):386–93. https://doi.org/10.1016/j.surg.2010.07.004.
89. Durkin ET, Lund DP, Shaaban AF, Schurr MJ, Weber SM. Age-related differences in diagnosis and morbidity of intestinal malrotation. J Am Coll Surg. 2008;206(4):658–63. https://doi.org/10.1016/j.jamcollsurg.2007.11.020.
90. Puri P, Fujimoto T. New observations on the pathogenesis of multiple intestinal atresias. J Pediatr Surg. 1988;23(3):221–5.
91. Dalla Vecchia LK, Grosfeld JL, West KW, Rescorla FJ, Scherer LR, Engum SA. Intestinal atresia and stenosis: a 25-year experience with 277 cases. Arch Surg. 1998;133(5):490–6; discussion 6–7.
92. Grosfeld JL, Ballantine TV, Shoemaker R. Operative mangement of intestinal atresia and stenosis based on pathologic findings. J Pediatr Surg. 1979;14(3):368–75.
93. Subbarayan D, Singh M, Khurana N, Sathish A. Histomorphological features of intestinal atresia and its clinical correlation. J Clin Diagn Res. 2015;9(11):EC26–9. https://doi.org/10.7860/JCDR/2015/13320.6838.
94. Kelly KB, Ponsky TA. Pediatric abdominal wall defects. Surg Clin North Am. 2013;93(5):1255–67. https://doi.org/10.1016/j.suc.2013.06.016.
95. Hwang PJ, Kousseff BG. Omphalocele and gastroschisis: an 18-year review study Genet Med. 2004;6(4):232–6. http://dx.doi.org/10.109701.GIM.0000133919.68912.A3.
96. Kosloske AM. Epidemiology of necrotizing enterocolitis. Acta Paediatr Suppl. 1994;396:2–7.
97. Yee WH, Soraisham AS, Shah VS, Aziz K, Yoon W, Lee SK, et al. Incidence and timing of presentation of necrotizing enterocolitis in preterm infants. Pediatrics. 2012;129(2):e298–304. https://doi.org/10.1542/peds.2011–2022.
98. Claud EC, Walker WA. Hypothesis: inappropriate colonization of the premature intestine can cause neonatal necrotizing enterocolitis. FASEB J. 2001;15(8):1398–403.
99. Wiswell TE, Robertson CF, Jones TA, Tuttle DJ. Necrotizing enterocolitis in full-term infants.A case-control study. Am J Dis Child. 1988;142(5):532–5.

100. Short SS, Papillon S, Berel D, Ford HR, Frykman PK, Kawaguchi A. Late onset of necrotizing enterocolitis in the full-term infant is associated with increased mortality: results from a two-center analysis. J Pediatr Surg. 2014;49(6):950–3. https://doi.org/10.1016/j.jpedsurg.2014.01.028.
101. Lambert DK, Christensen RD, Henry E, Besner GE, Baer VL, Wiedmeier SE, et al. Necrotizing enterocolitis in term neonates: data from a multihospital health-care system. J Perinatol. 2007;27(7):437–43. https://doi.org/10.1038/sj.jp.7211738.
102. Ballance WA, Dahms BB, Shenker N, Kliegman RM. Pathology of neonatal necrotizing enterocolitis: a ten-year experience. J Pediatr. 1990;117(1 Pt 2):S6–13.
103. Puiman PJ, Burger-Van Paassen N, Schaart MW, De Bruijn AC, De Krijger RR, Tibboel D, et al. Paneth cell hyperplasia and metaplasia in necrotizing enterocolitis. Pediatr Res. 2011;69(3):217–23. https://doi.org/10.1203/PDR.0b013e3182092a9a.
104. Parra-Herran CE, Pelaez L, Sola JE, Urbiztondo AK, Rodriguez MM. Intestinal candidiasis: an uncommon cause of necrotizing enterocolitis (NEC) in neonates. Fetal Pediatr Pathol. 2010;29(3):172–80. https://doi.org/10.3109/15513811003777342.
105. Turcios-Ruiz RM, Axelrod P, St John K, Bullitt E, Donahue J, Robinson N, et al. Outbreak of necrotizing enterocolitis caused by norovirus in a neonatal intensive care unit. J Pediatr. 2008;153(3):339–44. https://doi.org/10.1016/j.jpeds.2008.04.015.
106. de la Cochetiere MF, Piloquet H, des Robert C, Darmaun D, Galmiche JP, Roze JC. Early intestinal bacterial colonization and necrotizing enterocolitis in premature infants: the putative role of Clostridium. Pediatr Res. 2004;56(3):366–70. https://doi.org/10.1203/01.PDR.0000134251.45878.D5.
107. Dittmar E, Beyer P, Fischer D, Schafer V, Schoepe H, Bauer K, et al. Necrotizing enterocolitis of the neonate with *Clostridium perfringens*: diagnosis, clinical course, and role of alpha toxin. Eur J Pediatr. 2008;167(8):891–5. https://doi.org/10.1007/s00431-007-0614-9.
108. Snyder CL, Gittes GK, Murphy JP, Sharp RJ, Ashcraft KW, Amoury RA. Survival after necrotizing enterocolitis in infants weighing less than 1,000 g: 25 years' experience at a single institution. J Pediatr Surg. 1997;32(3):434–7.
109. Olsen MM, Luck SR, Lloyd-Still J, Raffensperger JG. The spectrum of meconium disease in infancy. J Pediatr Surg. 1982;17(5):479–81.
110. Keckler SJ, St Peter SD, Spilde TL, Tsao K, Ostlie DJ, Holcomb GW 3rd, et al. Current significance of meconium plug syndrome. J Pediatr Surg. 2008;43(5):896–8. https://doi.org/10.1016/j.jpedsurg.2007.12.035.
111. Kahn E, Daum F. Pseudopolyps of the small intestine in Crohn's disease. Hum Pathol. 1984;15(1):84–6.
112. Gardiner GA. "Backwash ileitis" with pseudopolyposis. AJR Am J Roentgenol. 1977;129(3):506–7. https://doi.org/10.2214/ajr.129.3.506.
113. Dhungel BM, De Petris G. Bizarre stromal cells in the esophagus: report of 2 cases and literature review. Int J Surg Pathol. 2013;21(4):368–72. https://doi.org/10.1177/1066896913489347.
114. Meeks MW, Kamal UM, Hammami MB, Taylor JR, Omran ML, Chen Y, et al. Gastrointestinal pyogenic granuloma (Lobular Capillary Hemangioma): an underrecognized entity causing iron deficiency Anemia. Case Rep Gastrointest Med. 2016;2016:4398401. https://doi.org/10.1155/2016/4398401.
115. Rosty C, Buchanan DD, Walters RJ, Carr NJ, Bothman JW, Young JP, et al. Hyperplastic polyp of the duodenum: a report of 9 cases with immunohistochemical and molecular findings. Hum Pathol. 2011;42(12):1953–9. https://doi.org/10.1016/j.humpath.2011.02.018.
116. Liu X, Chen D, Dugum M, Horvath B, Yuan L, Xiao SY. Syndromic and sporadic inflammatory/hyperplastic small-bowel polyps: a comparative study. Gastroenterol Rep (Oxf). 2015;3(3):222–7. https://doi.org/10.1093/gastro/gov020.
117. van Lier MG, Mathus-Vliegen EM, Wagner A, van Leerdam ME, Kuipers EJ. High cumulative risk of intussusception in patients with Peutz-Jeghers syndrome: time to update surveillance guidelines? Am J Gastroenterol. 2011;106(5):940–5. https://doi.org/10.1038/ajg.2010.473.
118. Wangler MF, Chavan R, Hicks MJ, Nuchtern JG, Hegde M, Plon SE, et al. Unusually early presentation of small-bowel adenocarcinoma in a patient with Peutz-Jeghers syndrome. J Pediatr Hematol Oncol. 2013;35(4):323–8. https://doi.org/10.1097/MPH.0b013e318282db11.
119. Korsse SE, Dewint P, Kuipers EJ, van Leerdam ME. Small bowel endoscopy and Peutz-Jeghers syndrome. Best Pract Res Clin Gastroenterol. 2012;26(3):263–78. https://doi.org/10.1016/j.bpg.2012.03.009.
120. Gruber SB, Entius MM, Petersen GM, Laken SJ, Longo PA, Boyer R, et al. Pathogenesis of adenocarcinoma in Peutz-Jeghers syndrome. Cancer Res. 1998;58(23):5267–70.
121. Merg A, Howe JR. Genetic conditions associated with intestinal juvenile polyps. Am J Med Genet C Semin Med Genet. 2004;129C(1):44–55. https://doi.org/10.1002/ajmg.c.30020.
122. Woodford-Richens K, Bevan S, Churchman M, Dowling B, Jones D, Norbury CG, et al. Analysis of genetic and phenotypic heterogeneity in juvenile polyposis. Gut. 2000;46(5):656–60.
123. Postgate AJ, Will OC, Fraser CH, Fitzpatrick A, Phillips RK, Clark SK. Capsule endoscopy for the small bowel in juvenile polyposis syndrome: a case series. Endoscopy. 2009;41(11):1001–4. https://doi.org/10.1055/s-0029-1215175.
124. Oncel M, Church JM, Remzi FH, Fazio VW. Colonic surgery in patients with juvenile polyposis syndrome: a case series. Dis Colon Rectum. 2005;48(1):49–55; discussion -6.
125. Howe JR, Mitros FA, Summers RW. The risk of gastrointestinal carcinoma in familial juvenile polyposis. Ann Surg Oncol. 1998;5(8):751–6.
126. Brosens LA, van Hattem A, Hylind LM, Iacobuzio-Donahue C, Romans KE, Axilbund J, et al. Risk of colorectal cancer in juvenile polyposis. Gut. 2007;56(7):965–7. https://doi.org/10.1136/gut.2006.116913.
127. Stacey R, Green JT. Radiation-induced small bowel disease: latest developments and clinical guidance. Ther Adv Chronic Dis. 2014;5(1):15–29. https://doi.org/10.1177/2040622313510730.
128. Hauer-Jensen M, Denham JW, Andreyev HJ. Radiation enteropathy—pathogenesis, treatment and prevention. Nat Rev Gastroenterol Hepatol. 2014;11(8):470–9. https://doi.org/10.1038/nrgastro.2014.46.
129. Leupin N, Curschmann J, Kranzbuhler H, Maurer CA, Laissue JA, Mazzucchelli L. Acute radiation colitis in patients treated with short-term preoperative radiotherapy for rectal cancer. Am J Surg Pathol. 2002;26(4):498–504.
130. Carr KE. Effects of radiation damage on intestinal morphology. Int Rev Cytol. 2001;208:1–119.
131. Nesher L, Rolston KV. Neutropenic enterocolitis, a growing concern in the era of widespread use of aggressive chemotherapy. Clin Infect Dis. 2013;56(5):711–7. https://doi.org/10.1093/cid/cis998.
132. Ullery BW, Pieracci FM, Rodney JR, Barie PS. Neutropenic enterocolitis. Surg Infect (Larchmt). 2009;10(3):307–14. https://doi.org/10.1089/sur.2008.061.
133. Kouroussis C, Samonis G, Androulakis N, Souglakos J, Voloudaki A, Dimopoulos MA, et al. Successful conservative treatment of neutropenic enterocolitis complicating taxane-based chemotherapy: a report of five cases. Am J Clin Oncol. 2000;23(3):309–13.
134. Katz JA, Wagner ML, Gresik MV, Mahoney DH Jr, Fernbach DJ. Typhlitis.An 18-year experience and postmortem review. Cancer. 1990;65(4):1041–7.

135. Lewis FW, Warren GH, Goff JS. Collagenous colitis with involvement of terminal ileum. Dig Dis Sci. 1991;36(8):1161–3.
136. Padmanabhan V, Callas PW, Li SC, Trainer TD. Histopathological features of the terminal ileum in lymphocytic and collagenous colitis: a study of 32 cases and review of literature. Mod Pathol. 2003;16(2):115–9. https://doi.org/10.1097/01.MP.0000051990.80904.AF.
137. O'Brien BH, McClymont K, Brown I. Collagenous ileitis: a study of 13 cases. Am J Surg Pathol. 2011;35(8):1151–7. https://doi.org/10.1097/PAS.0b013e3182206ef5.
138. Kung VL, Liu TC, Ma C. Collagenous enteritis is unlikely aform of aggressive celiac disease despite sharing HLA-DQ2/DQ8 genotypes. Am J Surg Pathol. 2018;42(4):545–52. https://doi.org/10.1097/PAS.0000000000001022.
139. Debray C, Besancon F, Hardouin JP, Martin E, Marche C, Khoury K. Cryptogenetic plurifocal ulcerative stenosing enteritis. Arch Mal Appar Dig Mal Nutr. 1964;53:193–206.
140. Kohoutova D, Bartova J, Tacheci I, Rejchrt S, Repak R, Kopacova M, et al. Cryptogenic multifocal ulcerous stenosing enteritis: a review of the literature. Gastroenterol Res Pract. 2013;2013:918031. https://doi.org/10.1155/2013/918031.
141. Matsumoto T, Iida M, Matsui T, Yao T. Chronic nonspecific multiple ulcers of the small intestine: a proposal of the entity from Japanese gastroenterologists to Western enteroscopists. Gastrointest Endosc. 2007;66(3 Suppl):S99–107. https://doi.org/10.1016/j.gie.2007.01.004.
142. Perlemuter G, Guillevin L, Legman P, Weiss L, Couturier D, Chaussade S. Cryptogenetic multifocal ulcerous stenosing enteritis: an atypical type of vasculitis or a disease mimicking vasculitis. Gut. 2001;48(3):333–8.
143. Biagi F, Lorenzini P, Corazza GR. Literature review on the clinical relationship between ulcerative jejunoileitis, coeliac disease, and enteropathy-associated T-cell. Scand J Gastroenterol. 2000;35(8):785–90.
144. Biagi F, Corazza GR. (2001). La jéjuno-iléite ulcéreuse: Revue de la littérature. Acta Endoscopica, 31(3):265–69.
145. Ashton-Key M, Diss TC, Pan L, Du MQ, Isaacson PG. Molecular analysis of T-cell clonality in ulcerative jejunitis and enteropathy-associated T-cell lymphoma. Am J Pathol. 1997;151(2):493–8.
146. Seven G, Assaad A, Biehl T, Kozarek RA. Use of anti tumor necrosis factor-alpha monoclonal antibody for ulcerative jejunoileitis. World J Gastroenterol. 2012;18(36):5135–7. https://doi.org/10.3748/wjg.v18.i36.5135.
147. Rodriguez-Sanchez D, Saez-Martinez ME, Sanchez-Jimenez RM, de-Dios-Berna-Mestre J, Guzman-Aroca F. Pneumatosis cystoides, CT colonoscopy and endoscopic correlation. Rev Esp Enferm Dig. 2013;105(8):486–7.
148. Wu LL, Yang YS, Dou Y, Liu QS. A systematic analysis of pneumatosis cystoids intestinalis. World J Gastroenterol. 2013;19(30):4973–8. https://doi.org/10.3748/wjg.v19.i30.4973.
149. St Peter SD, Abbas MA, Kelly KA. The spectrum of pneumatosis intestinalis. Arch Surg. 2003;138(1):68–75.
150. Hoer J, Truong S, Virnich N, Fuzesi L, Schumpelick V. Pneumatosis cystoides intestinalis: confirmation of diagnosis by endoscopic puncture a review of pathogenesis, associated disease and therapy and a new theory of cyst formation. Endoscopy. 1998;30(9):793–9. https://doi.org/10.1055/s-2007-1001424.
151. Gagliardi G, Thompson IW, Hershman MJ, Forbes A, Hawley PR, Talbot IC. Pneumatosis coli: a proposed pathogenesis based on study of 25 cases and review of the literature. Int J Colorectal Dis. 1996;11(3):111–8.
152. Bialas M, Demczuk S, Dyduch G, Drabik G, Chrupek M, Okon K. Brown bowel syndrome (intestinal lipofuscinosis)—a case report and review of the literature. Pol J Pathol. 2013;64(3):228–31.
153. Horn T, Svendsen LB, Nielsen R. Brown-bowel syndrome. Review of the literature and presentation of cases. Scand J Gastroenterol. 1990;25(1):66–72.
154. Mojtahed A, Pai RK Anderson MW, Arber DA, Longacre TA. Reactive lymphoid hyperplasia of the terminal ileum: a benign (lymphoma-like) condition that may harbor aberrant immunohistochemical patterns or clonal immunoglobulin heavy chain gene rearrangements. Appl Immunohistochem Mol Morphol. 2014;22(8):585–92. https://doi.org/10.1097/01.pai.0000446497.93867.98.
155. Varkey J, Simren M, Jalanko H, Oltean M, Saalman R, Gudjonsdottir A, et al. Fifteen years' experience of intestinal and multivisceral transplantation in the Nordic countries. Scand J Gastroenterol. 2015;50(3):278–90. https://doi.org/10.3109/00365521.2014.999255.
156. Remotti H, Subramanian S, Martinez M, Kato T, Magid MS. Small-bowel allograft biopsies in the management of small-intestinal and multivisceral transplant recipients: histopathologic review and clinical correlations. Arch Pathol Lab Med. 2012;136(7):761–71. https://doi.org/10.5858/arpa.2011-0596-RA.
157. Ruiz P, Garcia M, Pappas P, Esquenazi V, Kato T, Mittal N, et al. Mucosal vascular alterations in the early posttransplant period of small bowel allograft recipients may reflect humoral-based allograft rejection. Transplant Proc. 2002;34(3):869–71.
158. Tsai HL, Island ER, Chang JW, Gonzalez-Pinto I, Tryphonopoulos P, Nishida S, et al. Association between donor-specific antibodies and acute rejection and resolution in small bowel and multivisceral transplantation. Transplantation. 2011;92(6):709–15. https://doi.org/10.1097/TP.0b013e318229f752.
159. Ruiz P, Bagni A, Brown R, Cortina G, Harpaz N, Magid MS, et al. Histological criteria for the identification of acute cellular rejection in human small bowel allografts: results of the pathology workshop at the VIII International Small Bowel Transplant Symposium. Transplant Proc. 2004;36(2):335–7. https://doi.org/10.1016/j.transproceed.2004.01.079.
160. Parizhskaya M, Redondo C, Demetris A, Jaffe R, Reyes J, Ruppert K, et al. Chronic rejection of small bowel grafts: pediatric and adult study of risk factors and morphologic progression. Pediatr Dev Pathol. 2003;6(3):240–50. https://doi.org/10.1007/s10024-002-0039-4.
161. Mazariegos GV, Abu-Elmagd K, Jaffe R, Bond G, Sindhi R, Martin L, et al. Graft versus host disease in intestinal transplantation. Am J Transplant. 2004;4(9):1459–65. https://doi.org/10.1111/j.1600-6143.2004.00524.x.
162. Crowell KR, Patel RA, Fluchel M, Lowichik A, Bryson S, Pohl JF. Endoscopy in the diagnosis of intestinal graft-versus-host disease: is lower endoscopy with biopsy as effective in diagnosis as upper endoscopy combined with lower endoscopy? Pediatr Blood Cancer. 2013;60(11):1798–800. https://doi.org/10.1002/pbc.24634.
163. Abu-Elmagd KM, Kosmach-Park B, Costa G, Zenati M, Martin L, Koritsky DA, et al. Long-term survival, nutritional autonomy, and quality of life after intestinal and multivisceral transplantation. Ann Surg. 2012;256(3):494–508. https://doi.org/10.1097/SLA.0b013e318265f310.
164. Mynarek M, Schober T, Behrends U, Maecker-Kolhoff B. Posttransplant lymphoproliferative disease after pediatric solid organ transplantation. Clin Dev Immunol. 2013;2013:814973. https://doi.org/10.1155/2013/814973.

Part VI

Non-neoplastic Diseases of the Colon

Inflammatory Bowel Disease

15

Lizhi Zhang and Tsung-Teh Wu

Introduction

Among dozens of different types of inflammatory disorders in the colon, inflammatory bowel disease (IBD) is a term specifically referring to two idiopathic chronic inflammatory diseases involving the colon: ulcerative colitis (UC) and Crohn's disease (CD). Although UC and CD are two distinct entities, they share some clinical and pathological features, and distinction between these two diseases can be difficult in some cases, especially in fulminant phase, and it can be classified as indeterminate colitis under this circumstance.

Since the first IBD case was reported by Wilks and Moxon in 1859 [1], IBD has been evolving in many aspects over the centuries. Especially since the last decade, the landscape of IBD has been changed dramatically, which is stemmed from Westernizaton in diet and lifestyles in developing countries, personalized management, treat-to-target strategy, new therapeutic agents, new surveillance guidelines, advances in endoscopic techniques, and progression of basic research understanding the genetic abnormalities, dysfunction of immunity, and intestinal microbiome [2]. Therefore, pathologists are also facing new challenges in diagnosing and managing IBD in the current era.

IBD is a lifelong disease which requires multidisciplinary management including patients themselves, gastroenterologists, surgeons, radiologists, and pathologists. Pathologists can provide valuable information for the patients' management by performing histopathological examination on either resection or biopsy specimens to (1) help confirming the diagnosis of IBD and distinguishing UC versus CD, (2) determine the extent and severity of IBD, (3) rule out the possibility of other types of colitis, (4) evaluate superimposed conditions, and (5) detect dysplasia or malignancy. On the other hand, it is important to realize the limitations of the histopathological evaluation. Oftentimes, the pathologists would be asked to distinguish UC versus CD. However, because of the overlapping features of UC and CD, fulminant phase of the disease, limited specimens from endoscopic biopsy, or treatment-related changes of disease distribution and pattern, a definitive diagnosis cannot be rendered unless unequivocal diagnostic features are identified, such as transmural lymphoid aggregates and granulomas in active chronic ileitis/colitis for CD. The final diagnosis usually requires combination of clinical, radiological, and pathological findings. It is also important to keep in mind that the features of chronicity in the colon, such as crypt architectural distortion, basal plasmacytosis, and Paneth cell metaplasia in left colon, which are commonly used by pathologists in daily practice, are not specific for IBD. There are many types of non-IBD colitis that can show similar chronic changes such as chronic ischemic/mechanical injury, infection, radiation colitis, diverticular disease-associated colitis, or drug-induced injury.

Evaluation of disease activity and dysplasia on endoscopic mucosal biopsy specimens from patients with established diagnosis of IBD accounts for a significant part of pathologists' daily practice. However, one major limitation of pathology is the lack of standardized criteria for evaluating disease activity and dysplasia in IBD. The pathological examination is subjective with significant variability among different pathologists. The severity of active colitis is usually graded as mild, moderate, and severe based on the findings of cryptitis, crypt abscesses, and mucosal erosion/ulceration. Although there are several scoring systems for assessing histologic disease activity in IBD, none of them have been validated, and no correlation between histologic activity and clinical disease severity has been shown. Each pathologist seems to have their "own" standard which would depend on their experience and training background. Some may think this limitation is less important because clinical impression of disease activity, which is classified primarily based on

L. Zhang (✉) · T.-T. Wu
Department of Laboratory Medicine and Pathology, Mayo Clinic, Rochester, MN, USA
e-mail: Zhang.Lizhi@mayo.edu

L. Zhang et al. (eds.), *Surgical Pathology of Non-neoplastic Gastrointestinal Diseases*,
https://doi.org/10.1007/978-3-030-15573-5_15

symptoms and/or endoscopic findings, correlates poorly with histologic activity [3]. However, recent studies have suggested that determination of microscopic mucosal activity may influence the management and surveillance of IBD. Although successful management of IBD is usually judged by endoscopic mucosal healing, a growing evidence has shown that the severity of microscopic inflammation in IBD is associated with risk of developing high-grade dysplasia and cancer, even for those with normal endoscopic findings [4–6]. Therefore, microscopic disease activity determined by pathologists on surveillance endoscopic biopsies may become more and more clinically relevant in IBD management.

The main goal of endoscopic surveillance in IBD patients is to detect dysplasia and colon cancer and to treat high-risk patients. The histological diagnosis of dysplasia in the setting of chronic colitis is very difficult, and sometimes it is almost impossible to distinguish marked reactive/regenerative atypia from true dysplasia, even for experienced pathologists who are specialized in gastrointestinal pathology. Nowadays, it is even more challenging for pathologists because of the evolving definition, subtypes, and management of IBD-associated dysplasia. The traditional terms such as dysplasia-associated lesion or mass (DALM) and adenoma-like and non-adenoma-like dysplasia are not recommended to use according to a recent SCENIC international consensus statement on surveillance and management of dysplasia in IBD [7]. This chapter will focus on the pathological features and associated complications of IBD in the colon.

Ulcerative Colitis

Definition

Ulcerative colitis (UC) is an idiopathic long-lasting inflammatory condition primarily involving the colon and rectum characterized by relapsing and remitting mucosal inflammation and ulceration.

Epidemiology

The incidence of UC has increased since the World Word II with the highest prevalence in Western countries [8]. However, recent population-based studies have shown stabilization or even a decreasing incidence since 2000 [9, 10]. On the other hand, as the onset of globalization and more industrialized countries in Asia, the Middle East, and South America, the incidence of IBD is increasing rapidly in those regions since the beginning of the twenty-first century [11]. The estimated annual incidence of UC in North America and Europe ranges from 4 to 20 per 100,000 individuals, while it is less than 2 per 100,000 individuals in Asia [12]. Meanwhile, the incidence of IBD in Central and South America has increased from 4.5 per 100,000 (1991–1995) to near 10 per 100,000 (2001–2005) [13, 14]. The highest prevalence rate of UC is in Europe (505 per 100,000), followed by North America (214–248 per 100,000) and 5–168 per 100,000 in Asia and the Middle East [11]. The risk of developing UC in children of migrants from low-incidence to high-incidence countries is similar to nonimmigrants [15].

UC has no sex predominance and can occur in all ages, but it is rare in younger than 5 or older than 75 years old [16]. The major incidence is in the adolescence and younger adults with the highest incidence among 20–29 years old. There seems a second modest rise in the incidence during the fifth and seventh decades which is considered as a second peak in the incidence [16, 17]. However, this bimodal pattern has been less apparent in recent studies [18]. The epidemiology of UC is more or less similar to that of CD, but there are also some differences between these two diseases which will be discussed later.

Etiology and Pathogenesis

The exact etiology and pathogenesis of IBD remain unknown. It is believed that IBD develops from the complex interaction among genetic predispositions, environmental risk factors, intestinal microbiota, and dysfunctional immune system. Although the literature usually discusses the etiology and pathogenesis of UC and CD side by side, significant differences do exist between them.

Genetic Factors

Population-based studies support the role of genetic factors in UC. About 8–14% of UC patients have a family history of IBD; first-degree relatives have 2–4 times higher risk of developing the disease; twin studies have shown a higher disease concordance in monozygotic, but not in dizygotic, twins; and Jewish populations have higher incidence of UC [19–22]. Genome-wide association studies and meta-analyses have identified more than 200 risk loci for IBD, and most loci contribute to both UC and CD phenotypes [23, 24]. For example, the *IBD2* locus on chromosome 12 plays a major role in UC susceptibility, but only has a relatively minor effect on CD [25]. Genes implicated in mucosal barrier function *(ECM1, CDH1, HNF4α,* and *laminin B1)* are associated with increased UC susceptibility [26]. Significantly increased frequencies of the 3435T single nucleotide polymorphism and the 3435TT genotype of multidrug resistance 1 (*MDR1*) gene have been observed in patients with UC [27]. Associations of UC with human leukocyte antigen (HLA) complex on chromosome 6p21 have also been demonstrated, in which the *DRB1*0103* and *DRB1*1502* alleles show positive associations and *DRB1*0401* with a negative association [28, 29]. However, a large effort is still required to validate and translate these new gene discoveries into useful knowledge for us to understand the pathogenesis of IBD and to develop novel therapies.

Immunologic Factors and Intestinal Microbiota

Recent research has suggested that the interaction between dysbiotic intestinal microbiota and a dysregulated immune response may play a fundamental role in the pathogenesis of IBD [30]. The immunopathogenesis of IBD is a complex and quickly evolving area, and the details are referred to the reviews in the literature elsewhere [31]. Both innate and adaptive immune systems contribute to the pathogenesis of IBD, and the IBD inflammation results from a complex cross talk between innate and adaptive cytokine networks.

The adaptive immune system is highly specific, and the key components of the adaptive immune response are T cells. In IBD, a dysregulated T-cell response with abnormal development of activated T-cell subsets leads to the onset of inflammation by an excessive release of cytokines and chemokines. T-helper cells (Th_0) can be activated and differentiated into Th_1, Th_2, or Th_{17} cells. Th_1 cells are essential in the elimination of intracellular pathogens, and Th_2 cells are protective against parasites and mediate allergic reactions. Th_{17} may contribute to the clearance of extracellular bacteria and fungi. Studies have shown that CD and UC are associated with different subtypes of proinflammatory immune responses, and UC has been considered as a Th_2-mediated disease, with excessive production of IL-5 and IL-13, and CD has been considered to be driven by a Th_1 response [32, 33]. The role of Th_{17} cells in IBD has emerged recently [34]. Th_{17} cells are induced by a combination of IL-6 and transforming growth factor (TGF)-β and are expanded by IL-23. Th_{17} cells are an important source of IL-21 and IL-17 that both are upregulated in inflamed IBD mucosa [35]. Regulatory T cells (Treg) suppress Th_0 cell proliferation and are important in the maintenance of mucosal homeostasis by producing the anti-inflammatory cytokines IL-10 and TGF-β and by suppressing or downregulating the induction and proliferation of effector T cells. The decrease in anti-inflammatory activity of Treg is equally as important as the enhancement of effector mechanisms in contributing to IBD pathogenesis [36, 37].

While most studies in the past have focused on the role of abnormal adaptive immune responses in the pathogenesis of IBD, recent advances in genome-wide association studies and immunological studies have revealed the important role of mucosal innate immune responses in IBD, such as mucosal epithelial barrier, innate microbial sensing (by natural immune cells, epithelial and stroma cells, and innate immune molecules), autophagy, and unfolded protein response. The mucosal innate immune system also regulates immune functions by regulating maturity, differentiation, and homing of immune cells in adaptive immunity. Mucous layer and epithelial barrier represent the first line of defense against bacterial invasion. In IBD, the impaired intestinal mucosal barrier function and increasing intestinal epithelial permeability allow pathogens entering the lamina propria to activate immune cells and produce a large number of inflammatory cytokines [38]. Although this phenomenon has been observed for a long time in IBD, it is not clear that these alterations represent the cause or consequence of chronic inflammation, until recent genome-wide association studies suggested that epithelial barrier defects may be a primary pathogenetic mechanism in IBD [26, 39]. Besides being a physical barrier against bacteria invasion, epithelial cells also secrete antimicrobial peptides such as defensins (α-defensins produced by Paneth cells and β-defensins produced by most epithelial cells) to limit bacterial growth and invasion. Some of them are secreted constitutively, while others are induced by the recognition of bacterial components by pattern recognition receptors (PRRs) in epithelial cells. Defection of antimicrobial peptide production is associated with the risk of IBD [40]. Innate immune cells, such as macrophages and dendritic cells, can also sense invading bacteria through extracellular and intracellular PRRs and initiate rapid inflammatory responses mediated by the secretion of cytokines and chemokines and recruitment of inflammatory cells. IL-23 has been identified as a key cytokine in the cross talk between innate and adaptive immunity, and genome-wide association studies have demonstrated the important role of IL-23/IL-17 pathway in IBD [41]. Besides its activity on Th_{17} cells, IL-23 can act on innate lymphoid cells in the human lamina propria where they contribute to mucosal inflammation by secreting cytokines, such as IL-17 and IFN-γ, and recruiting of other inflammatory cells [42].

The gastrointestinal tract harbors the largest microbial community of the human body, including bacteria, viruses, fungi, and protozoa. The gut microbiota is important in host defense, nutrition, and the development of the immune system. Dysbiosis is referred as alterations of the composition and function of the gut microbiota leading to changes in host–microbiota interaction and the host immune system, and a growing evidence has suggested that dysbiosis of the gut microbiota is associated with many human diseases including IBD [30, 43, 44], even though a direct causal relationship between dysbiosis and IBD has not been established in humans yet. Dysbiosis in IBD includes reduced diversity of the microbiota (decrease of *Firmicutes*, *Candida* spp., etc.), decrease of short-chain fatty acid-producing bacteria (*Clostridium* cluster IV, XIVa, and XVII), increase of mucolytic bacteria (*Ruminococcus gnavus* and *Ruminococcus torques*), increase of sulfate-reducing bacteria (*Desulfovibrio*), and increase of pathogenic bacteria (adhesion/invasive *E. coli*). These alterations affect the activity of the immune response and mucosal homeostasis, including increase of mucosal permeability, epithelial cell damage, degradation of mucus, and bacterial invasion, and finally activate T-helper cells, leading to mucosal inflammation and tissue injury [45].

Environmental Factors

Epidemiologic studies have suggested a strong role for the environmental factors in IBD [16, 46]. The risk of IBD in the immigrant population resembles that of country of residence rather than the country of origin [15, 47]. The developing countries with Westernizaton in diet and lifestyles and rapidly changing environment have shown an increase in the incidence of IBD over the past few decades [8]. The environmental risk factors that may contribute to the development of IBD include smoking, diet, breastfeeding, medications (such as NSAIDs), stress, appendectomy, air pollution, family sanitary conditions, etc. [48–50]. However, the understanding of the effect of the environmental factors in IBD has many limitations, because of a lack of high-quality and large cohorts of prospective studies and heterogeneity in the effect of many environmental influences. The integration of genetics may provide valuable information to understand that some individuals are more susceptible to the effect of a specific environmental factor.

Smoking is the most widely studied and the only confirmed environmental risk factor. Interestingly, smoking seems playing different roles in UC and CD. Many studies have confirmed the protective effect of current smoking on the development of UC, lower rate of relapse, and reduced need for colectomy in current smokers [51, 52]. On the other hand, cessation of smoking is associated with significantly increased risk of developing UC within 2–5 years of smoking cessation and remained persistently elevated over 20 years [53]. However, contrary to its effect on UC, smoking increases the risk of developing CD twofold [53, 54]. The mechanisms of smoking for the differential effect on UC and CD remain unknown.

Diet is the most commonly reported environmental factors triggering the IBD development and relapses by patients [55]. "Western" diet, which is high in fat and protein but low in fruits and vegetables, is associated with the increased risk of IBD. An extensive systemic literature review has shown that high intakes of total fats, total polyunsaturated fatty acids, omega-6 fatty acids, and meat were associated with an increased risk of UC, and high vegetable intake was associated with a decreased risk of UC [56]. Recent research advances have unraveled the important role of diet and food constituents in regulating gut microbiota and mucosal immunity which directly or indirectly contribute to the pathogenesis of IBD [57].

Clinical Features

The main clinical presentation of UC is diarrhea, often associated with blood [58]. The symptoms are related to the severity and extent of the mucosal disease. The onset of UC is usually insidious, and the symptoms are gradually progressive for weeks or even months. Patients with active disease also complain of rectal bleeding, urgency, crampy abdominal pain, tenesmus, and mucopurulent exudates. Patients with active proctitis only usually present with rectal bleeding, urgency, and tenesmus, and some may occasionally present with severe constipation accompanied with frequent discharge of blood and mucus. Patients may also have systemic symptoms including fever, fatigue, tachycardia, nausea, vomiting, malnutrition, and weight loss. Majority of patients present with mild or moderate symptoms, but a severe attack can occur in about 15% of patients with UC. The acute and severe complications of UC include severe bleeding, fulminant colitis, toxic megacolon, and perforation. The long-term complications are strictures and risk for dysplasia and cancer. The strictures, which are due to repeated episodes of inflammation and muscle hypertrophy, can occur in approximately 10% of cases. The strictures most frequently develop in the rectosigmoid colon and may cause symptoms of obstruction. The risk of developing colorectal carcinoma in patients with UC begins to increase 8–10 years after the initial onset of UC, and the extent and duration of disease are the two most important risk factors for the carcinoma [59]. Extraintestinal involvement can occur in about 10–25% of patients with UC in their lifetime. The common extraintestinal manifestations are anemia, inflammatory arthropathy, metabolic bone disease, erythema nodosum, pyoderma gangrenosum, episcleritis, uveitis, and hepatobiliary disease especially primary sclerosing cholangitis (PSC).

Classifications

There are several clinical classifications for UC according to the disease extent and severity and other factors which are important in determining the treatment modality and frequency of surveillance. The Montreal classification system has been widely accepted (Table 15.1) [60]. The mucosal inflammation in UC generally starts in the rectum and extends proximally, in an uninterrupted pattern, involving part of or the entire colon. Therefore, the disease can be classified as proctitis, left-sided colitis (distal UC), and extensive colitis (pancolitis) accordingly. However, some patients with proctitis or left-sided colitis may have a cecal patch of inflammation and rectal sparing [61].

The severity of UC is classified into remission, mild, moderate, and severe, based on the frequency and severity of diarrhea, the presence of systemic symptoms, and laboratory abnormalities (Table 15.1). The Mayo scoring system is

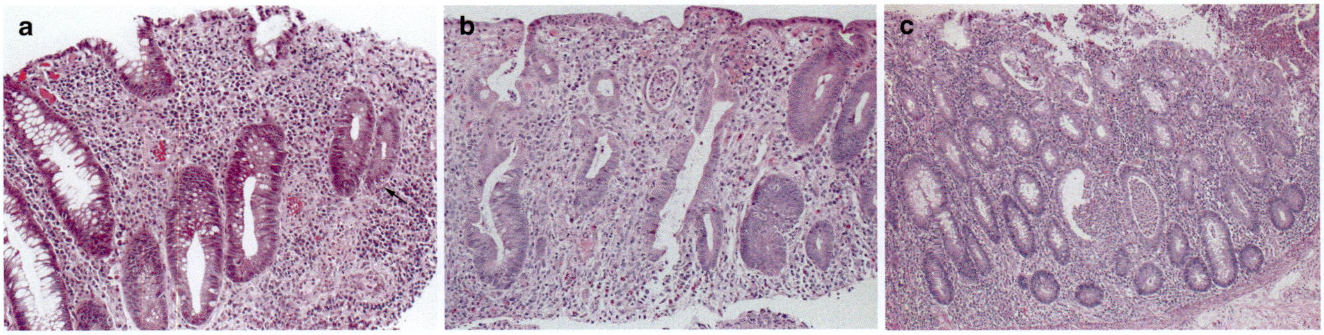

Fig. 15.3 Active inflammation in ulcerative colitis. (**a**) Mild activity, with neutrophils in lamina propria and epithelium (cryptitis, arrow). (**b**) Moderate activity, with occasional crypt abscesses. (**c**) Severe activity, with many crypt abscesses and marked epithelial damage and ulceration

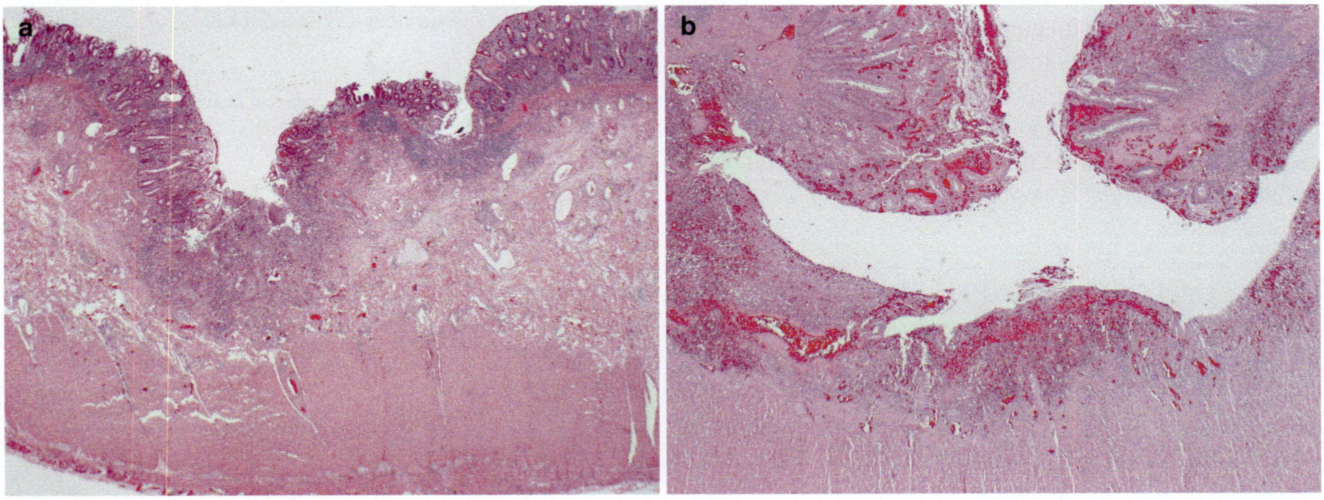

Fig. 15.4 Ulceration. (**a**) Ulcers can be superficial, limited in mucosa, or extend into submucosa. (**b**) Deep ulcers associated with granulation tissue and inflammation

epithelium (cryptitis), and crypt lumina (crypt abscesses) (Fig. 15.3). Neutrophil infiltration causes degeneration and damage of surface epithelium and the top part of crypts leading to mucin and goblet cell depletion, loss of cells, and erosion (Fig. 15.3), and ulcerations are resulted from more severe and extensive mucosal injury and loss of crypt structures. The ulcers are superficial, accompanying with inflamed granulation tissue and reactive/regenerative epithelial changes (Fig. 15.4). In severe cases, fibrinopurulent exudates, focal transmural inflammation, and deep penetrating ulcers may occur. The active colitis is usually diffuse and distributes continuously from the rectum to proximal colon. The degree of active inflammation and mucosal injury can be variable in affected segments. Medical treatment also affects the histological findings. It is not uncommon to see uneven disease distribution with alternative of active colitis and inactive colitis from different parts of the colon, especially on biopsy samples, and changing diagnosis to CD should not be considered under this circumstance (Fig. 15.5).

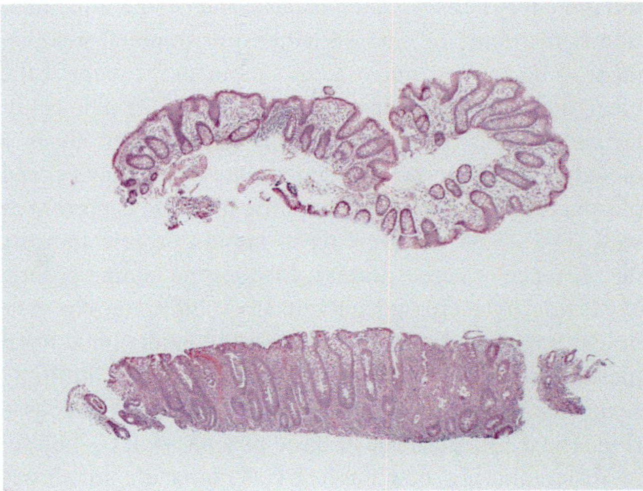

Fig. 15.5 Uneven disease distribution. In this case of treated ulcerative colitis, the biopsy reveals different disease distribution, with one piece showing active chronic colitis (lower) and one unremarkable colonic mucosa (upper)

Neutrophils in lamina propria are intermixed with other inflammatory cells including plasma cells and eosinophils. Sometimes neutrophil margination in the mucosal capillaries may mimic lamina propria infiltration. Bowel preparation may also cause neutrophils present in lamina propria. Therefore, cryptitis and crypt abscesses are more reliable features indicating active disease. Of note, the colonic epithelium overlying lymphoid aggregates and crypts within or immediately adjacent to lymphoid aggregates may contain scattered intraepithelial neutrophils, which is a normal physiologic phenomenon and should not be interpreted as active inflammation. The mimickers of crypt abscesses are withered crypt and eosinophilic crypt abscess. The withered crypt is frequently seen in infectious or ischemic colitis, which is characterized by crypt dilation lined by flattened epithelium, mucin depletion, and luminal accumulation of neutrophils and cell debris. The eosinophilic crypt abscess is a relatively nonspecific histologic finding. Microscopic examination under higher power to identify bilobulated nuclei and dense eosinophilic, granular cytoplasm is necessary to rule out crypt abscesses.

Chronic colitis Chronicity is imperative for diagnosing UC. The earliest features indicating chronic changes are increased lamina propria inflammation and basal plasmacytosis (Fig. 15.6), which can be observed within 2 weeks after the onset of UC [93], while the mucosal and crypt architecture is still preserved. The increased lamina propria inflammation is described as transmucosal because (1) normal colonic mucosa contain much less inflammatory cells in lower third, but the cellularity of lamina propria in UC is markedly increased and filled with inflammatory cells from top to base, and (2) the inflammation is restricted in mucosa with no or minimal involvement of muscularis mucosae or submucosa, except at the ulcer sites and in fulminant colitis (Fig. 15.7). The cellular components of lamina propria inflammation are in a mixed nature but predominantly are lymphocytes and plasma cells. Increased eosinophilic infiltrate is present as well (Fig. 15.8). Neutrophils in lamina propria indicate the presence of active disease. Besides the lamina propria expansion by increased inflammatory infiltrate, one particular important feature of chronic inflammation is basal plasmacytosis, in which the dense plasma cell infiltrate separates the base of crypts from muscularis mucosae (Fig. 15.6). The presence of basal plasmacytosis is helpful in differentiating new-onset UC from acute infectious colitis, since the normal lamina propria inflammatory pattern which is located in the upper part of the mucosa is still preserved in infectious colitis. Focal or diffuse basal plasmacytosis is present in approximately 60% of first attack IBD including both UC and CD, but only in 6% of infectious colitis [93, 94].

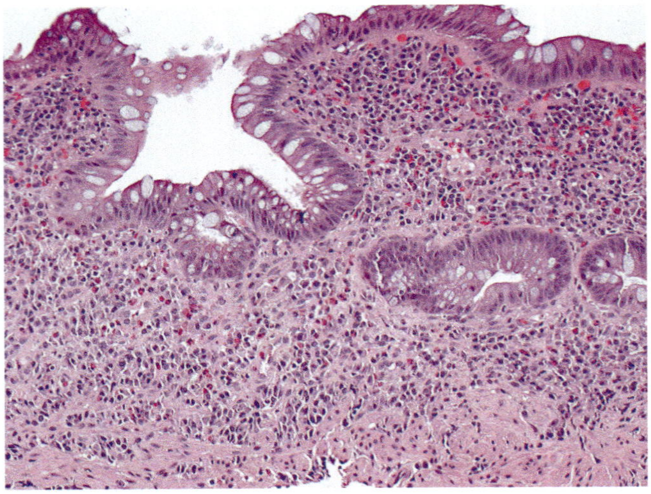

Fig. 15.6 Basal plasmacytosis. Dense plasma cell infiltrate separates the base of crypts from muscularis mucosae in active chronic colitis

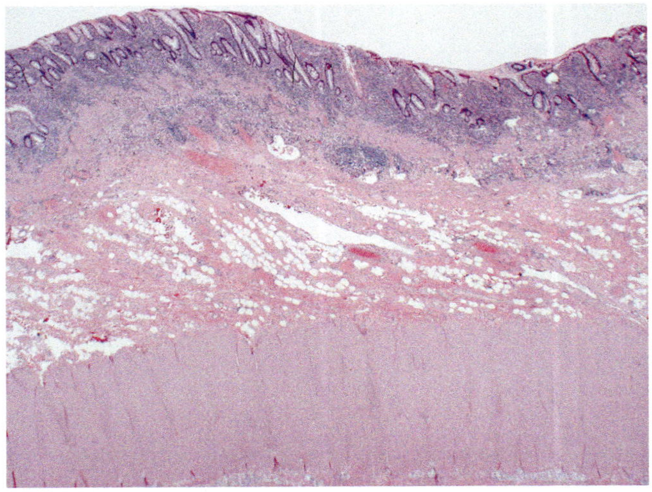

Fig. 15.7 Transmucosal inflammation. The inflammation is mainly limited in mucosa with only focal minimal involvement of muscularis mucosae and superficial submucosa. Note the absence of transmural inflammation and lymphoid aggregates

The crypt and mucosal architectural changes are essential for confirming the chronicity. The crypt distortion refers to the loss of the regular shape, number, and distribution of crypts. The distorted crypts can be dilated, atrophic, branching, budding, irregular, and with significant size and shape variations among each other (Fig. 15.9). At least two bifurcated crypts in a well-oriented section are usually required to consider crypt branching (Fig. 15.10). Crypt atrophy may present as shortened crypt (separation from muscularis mucosae) or deceased density. The distribution of crypts becomes uneven and they are not parallel to each other, with alternative areas of crowded crypts and open lamina propria. Sometimes it is difficult to determine true crypt distortion from artifacts such as due to

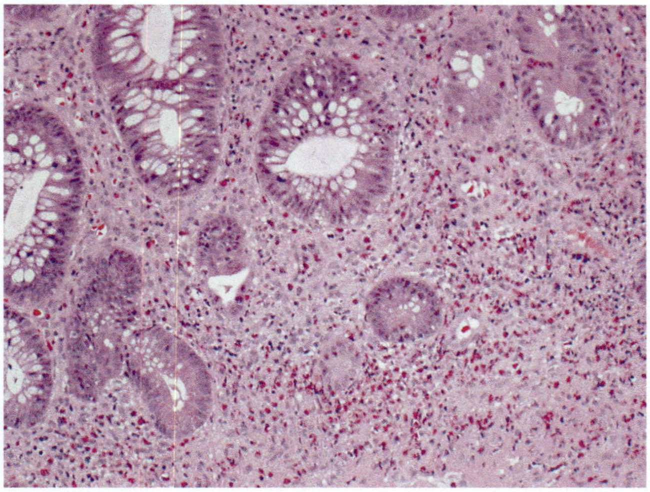

Fig. 15.8 Marked eosinophilic infiltrate can be seen in chronic colitis

poor tissue orientation or tangential cuts. The changes of crypt architecture may be subtle and focal, especially in quiescent inactive chronic colitis (Fig. 15.11). Occasional branched or shortened crypts can be ignored, particularly for those at the rectum, adjacent to a lymphoid aggregate, or at an innominate groove (Fig. 15.12). Although a few studies have proposed criteria for determining crypt distortion in a somewhat quantitative way, these standards are generally not practical [95, 96]. Most of questionable cases can be solved by examining multiple levels or sharing with experienced gastrointestinal pathologist.

The overall mucosal architecture can also be distorted as a result of chronic inflammation, crypt distortion, and regeneration. The luminal border is irregular with mucosal undulation, protrusions, polypoid appearance, or villiform architecture (Fig. 15.13). The villiform architecture can be

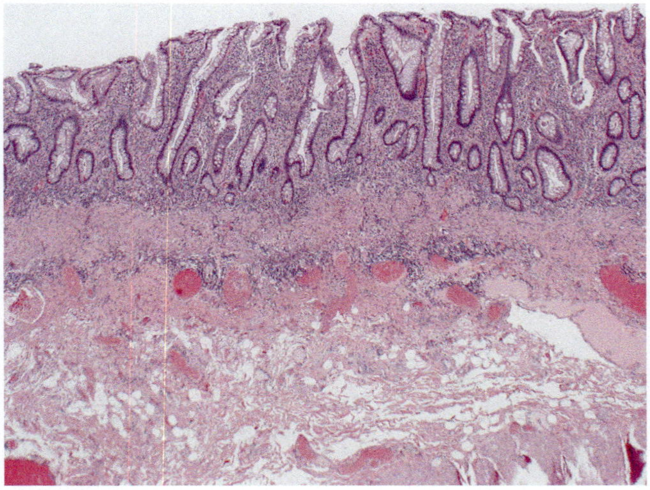

Fig. 15.9 Marked crypt architectural distortion. Irregular-shaped and sized crypts with dilation, branching, and budding

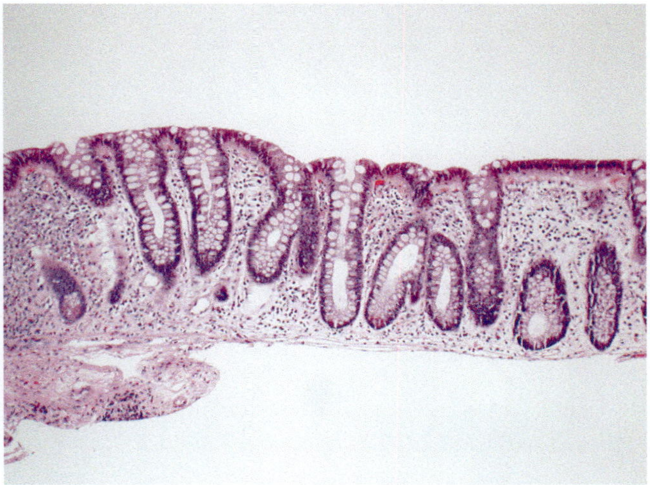

Fig. 15.11 Minimal and subtle crypt architectural changes in inactive chronic colitis

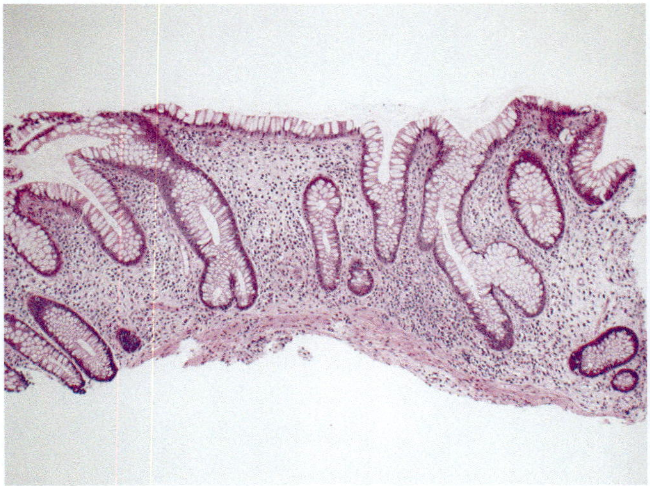

Fig. 15.10 Mild crypt architectural distortion with branching in inactive chronic colitis

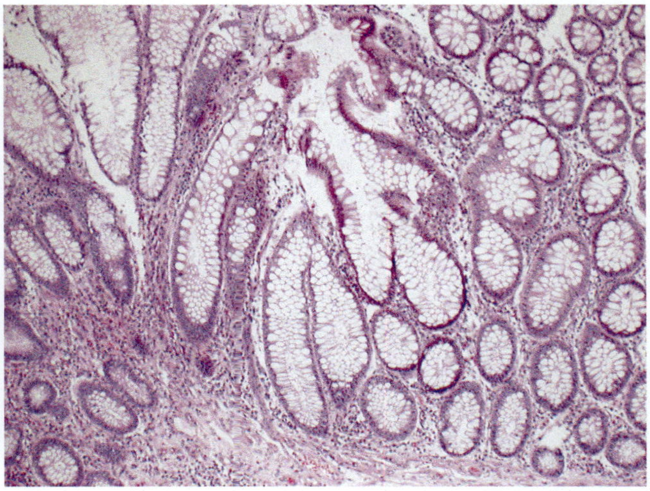

Fig. 15.12 Normal crypt branching in an innominate groove

present in 30% of children and 50% of adults with UC [97], and an extreme example of villiform architecture in colon biopsy may resemble small bowel villi and can be mistakenly read as small bowel biopsy.

Epithelial metaplastic changes are also a marker for chronicity. In normal adults and children, Paneth cells are located within the small bowel and the proximal colon, and the number of Paneth cells is gradually decreasing from the cecum to transverse colon, and they are absent in the left colon (descending, sigmoid, and rectum). Paneth cell metaplasia refers to the presence of Paneth cells in segments where they are not normally found, i.e., the left colon, which is due to chronic epithelial injury and is a sign of longstanding colitis (Fig. 15.14a). The Paneth cell metaplasia is most frequently seen in both UC and CD, which correlates with the disease duration [98, 99], but Paneth cell metaplasia is not entirely specific for IBD. In non-IBD setting, Paneth cell metaplasia may be occasionally seen in diverticular disease, collagenous colitis, polypoid lesions, or neonate enterocolitis. In addition, an increased number of Paneth cells, named Paneth cell hyperplasia, have also been observed in IBD (Fig. 15.14b). One study showed that the numbers of Paneth cells in the proximal colon in IBD cases were 5–10/10 crypts, which were significantly higher than the normal controls (<2/10 crypts) [100]. However, this feature is less widely used. Pseudopyloric metaplasia is another important epithelial damage marker for chronicity. Although it is most commonly seen in the terminal ileum in CD, rare cases of chronic colitis may be manifested with focal or diffuse pseudopyloric metaplasia (Fig. 15.15). Detection of aberrant gastric or small intestinal mucin expression by histo-

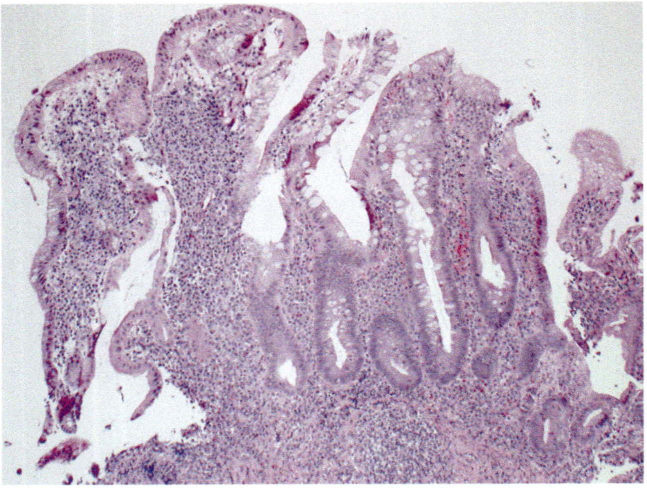

Fig. 15.13 Marked mucosal architectural distortion with polypoid and villiform appearance

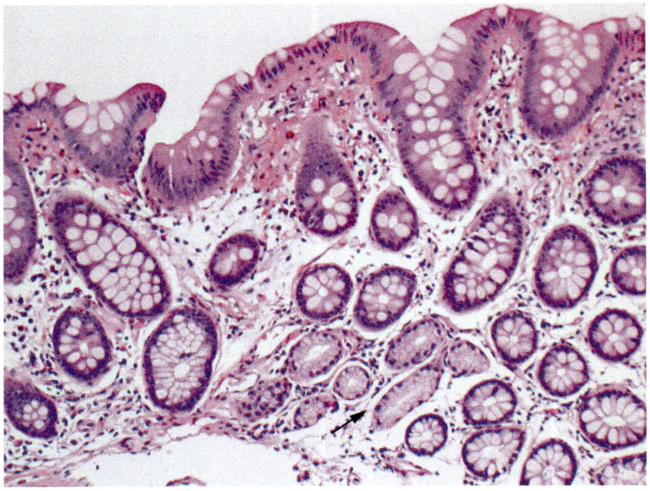

Fig. 15.15 Pseudopyloric metaplasia (arrow) in inactive chronic colitis

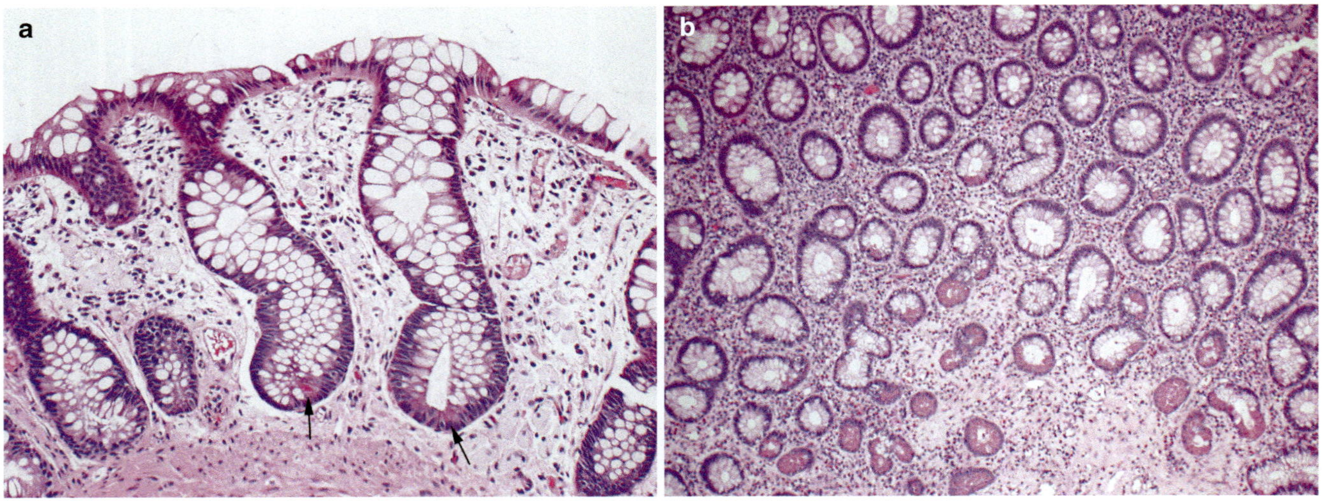

Fig. 15.14 Paneth cell metaplasia. (**a**) Rare Paneth cell metaplasia (arrows) in rectum in quiescent colitis indicates chronicity. (**b**) Paneth cell hyperplasia in right colon in chronic colitis

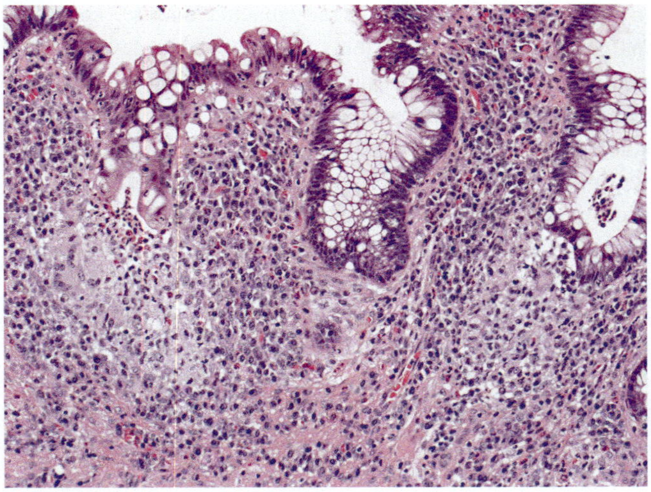

Fig. 15.16 Crypt-rupture granuloma. A loose collection of histiocytes including multinucleated giant cells associated with injured crypts

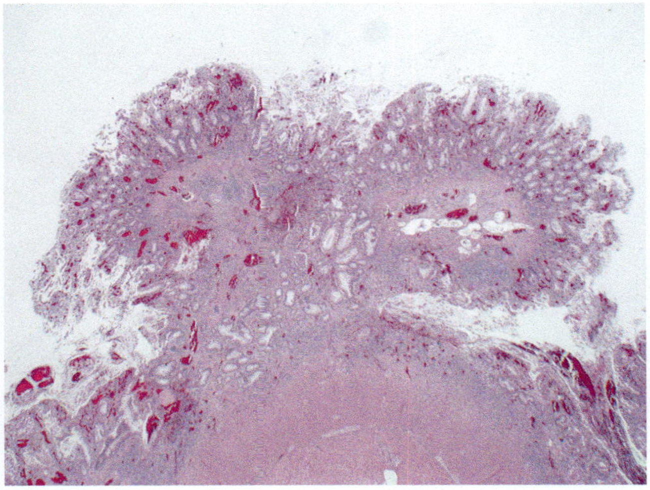

Fig. 15.17 Inflammatory pseudopolyps. Polypoid colonic mucosa containing active chronic inflammation and distorted crypts with ulceration on both sides

chemical or immunostains has been reported in IBD, but their diagnostic value in daily practice has not been established [101, 102].

Granulomas In UC, granulomas associated with crypt rupture or surface epithelial damage are occasionally seen. They are different from the discrete well-formed epithelioid granulomas in CD. There are several terms to describe this type of granulomas, such as cryptolytic lesions, pericryptal granulomas, or ruptured crypt granulomas. They are always associated with a partially injured crypt (if not, examining deeper levels is necessary), loosely surrounded by pale-stained histiocytes and lymphocytes, with rare giant cells and neutrophils (Fig. 15.16). However, ruptured crypt granulomas are not reliable for the discrimination between UC and CD, since they can occur in CD as well, and some cases with suspected IBD and these granulomas identified in initial colorectal biopsies could subsequently develop CD [103, 104].

Inflammatory pseudopolyps Inflammatory pseudopolyps are frequently seen in IBD, but they can also occur in other settings such as ischemic or infectious colitis. They are also morphologically similar to juvenile-type inflammatory polyps, but the proper clinical context can distinguish between inflammatory pseudopolyps in IBD and those syndromic inflammatory polyps. Inflammatory pseudopolyps are related to inflammatory injury and ulceration of colonic mucosa and arise from intervening nonulcerated epithelium with inflammation and regenerative hyperplasia. Microscopically, inflammatory pseudopolyps are characterized by polypoid colonic mucosa with surface erosion, inflamed and edematous lamina propria, and distorted mucosal architecture (Fig. 15.17). The crypts are dilated, branched, or hyperplastic. Cryptitis and crypt abscesses are often present. The epithelium usually shows reactive/regenerative atypia, and it can be difficult to rule out true dysplasia in severe cases. Identifying surface maturation and lack of significant nuclear variations would favor a reactive process, especially with marked inflammation in the background. Some inflammatory pseudopolyps may be entirely composed of granulation tissue. In inactive disease, the presence of inflammatory pseudopolyps may serve as a clue of chronicity, and the polyps can present as a fingerlike mucosal projection with essentially no inflammation.

Although most of the inflammatory pseudopolyps are small, rarely can some become larger (usually >2 cm) and are known as giant inflammatory pseudopolyps. They can cause bowel obstruction or intussusceptions. The giant inflammatory pseudopolyps may also mimic a neoplasm, especially when coexistence with colitis cystica profunda resulting from repeated inflammatory and mechanical injuries. The permeating crypts and mucin-filled cysts in submucosa and muscular layers resemble infiltrating glands and can be misdiagnosed as invasive adenocarcinoma (Fig. 15.18) [105]. Another rare form of inflammatory pseudopolyps is termed as filiform polyps, which is characterized by long wormlike mucosal projections covered with unremarkable or inflamed mucosa containing vessels, smooth muscle fibers, and submucosal tissue as a core [106]. Filiform polyposis is referred to cases bearing a large number of such polyps (Fig. 15.2b). The filiform polyp ranges 0.5–3 cm long and 0.5 cm in diameter. Filiform polyposis is not unique to IBD, and it has been described in intestinal tuberculosis or idiopathic setting [107].

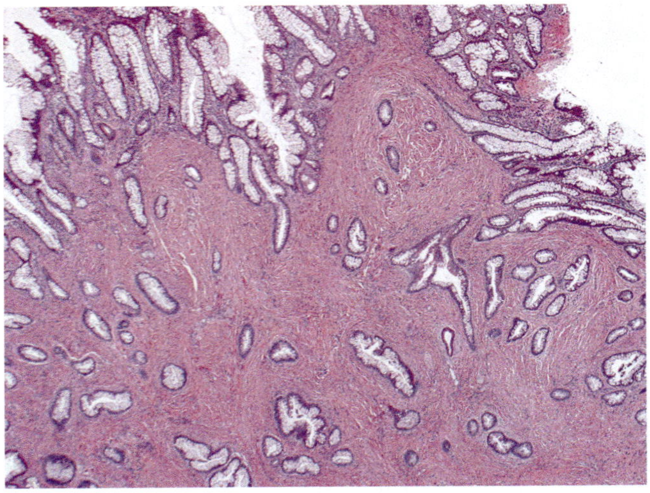

Fig. 15.18 Colitis cystica profunda associated with a giant inflammatory pseudopolyp in ulcerative colitis. The permeating crypts and glands in submucosa mimic invasive adenocarcinoma

Other histologic findings Since the inflammatory changes in UC are limited in mucosa or only with minimal involvement of muscularis mucosae and superficial submucosa in most cases, histologic changes of other layers of colonic wall are not as significant as in CD. Hypertrophy of muscularis mucosae and submucosa fibrosis may be focally present. In severe and longstanding cases, the colonic wall may become thickened and fibrotic which can lead to shortening of the entire colon. Neuronal hypertrophy and hyperplasia is not prominent in UC which can be used as a feature to distinguish CD [108].

Treatment-related changes Topical and systemic medical treatments can affect the histology in UC. The signs of active disease, mucosal injury, and neutrophilic infiltrate can diminish substantially within 4 weeks and eventually disappear in remission phase. The chronic changes can also be resolved but take longer time, including deceasing lamina propria inflammatory cell infiltrate and normalization of crypt and mucosal architectural alterations. In many cases, the disease distribution becomes discontinuous and heterogeneous, which may make a differential diagnosis between UC and CD difficult. Therefore, knowing the treatment history and its effect in histology are important in this setting [109].

Historical grade of disease activity The histological disease activity can be used to evaluate disease severity, disease progression, and treatment efficacy and predict relapse. The disease activity parallels the progressive increase of neutrophil infiltration from lamina propria to crypts and then to apparent epithelial injury. This histologic degree of neutrophil infiltration is also correlated with endoscopic severity and systemic inflammatory indices, such as serum CRP levels [110], although microscopic evidence of activity may persist in some cases with endoscopically inactive disease. There are many histologic score systems that have been developed to grade activity in UC, but none has been formally validated, and the reproducibility of these systems has not been well studied [111]. The modified Riley scoring [112] and Geboes scoring systems [113] were partially validated (Table 15.3), and a recent study showed a significant correlation between the endoscopic and histological grades [114]. However, these score systems are mainly developed for research and assessing clinical trials, and they are relatively complicated and not very practical for daily practice and general pathologists. In our practice, a 4-tier system is used to grade both biopsy and resection specimens [115, 116]:

- Inactive chronic colitis: presence of chronicity, absent or slightly increased inflammatory cells in lamina propria, but no neutrophils
- Mild active chronic colitis: presence of chronicity, increased inflammatory cells in lamina propria with scant neutrophils, and cryptitis
- Moderate active chronic colitis: presence of chronicity, increased inflammatory cells in lamina propria with many neutrophils, cryptitis, crypt abscesses, and focal erosion/ulceration
- Severe active chronic colitis: marked architectural changes, numerous neutrophils with abundant cryptitis and crypt abscesses, extensive glandular destruction and ulceration

Minimal active chronic colitis is occasionally reported for cases with only few neutrophils in lamina propria and rare cryptitis identified within the background mucosa predominantly showing inactive chronic colitis. Of note, the presence of ulceration in biopsy does not necessarily indicate severe disease activity. This finding needs to be combined with overall mucosal destruction and inflammation for adequate grading. Focal or isolated ulceration can be seen in mild and moderate active chronic colitis.

Differential Diagnosis

There are no histologic features specific to UC. The establishment of a diagnosis of UC cannot be based on histology alone, especially on mucosal biopsy, but careful histologic assessment can provide valuable information to help solve diagnostic problems. The differential diagnosis of UC includes a variety of other inflammatory disorders of the colon, but CD remains as the most critical one.

Crohn's Disease

The clinicopathological differences between these two subtypes of IBD are summarized in Table 15.4. From the aspect

Table 15.3 The Geboes and modified Riley scoring systems for histological activity of ulcerative colitis

Geboes scoring system	
Subscore	Features
Grade 0	Architectural changes
0.0	No abnormality
0.1	Mild abnormality
0.2	Mild or moderate diffuse or multifocal abnormalities
0.3	Severe diffuse or multifocal abnormalities
Grade 1	Chronic inflammatory infiltrate
1.0	No increase
1.1	Mild but unequivocal increase
1.2	Moderate increase
1.3	Marked increase
Grade 2A	Lamina propria eosinophils
2A.0	No increase
2A.1	Mild but unequivocal increase
2A.2	Moderate increase
2A.3	Marked increase
Grade 2B	Lamina propria neutrophils
2B.0	No increase
2B.1	Mild but unequivocal increase
2B.2	Moderate increase
2B.3	Marked increase
Grade 3	Neutrophils in epithelium
3.0	None
3.1	<5% crypts involved
3.2	<50% crypts involved
3.3	>50% crypts involved
Grade 4	Crypt destruction
4.0	None
4.1	Probable—local excess of neutrophils in part of crypt
4.2	Probable—marked attenuation
4.3	Unequivocal crypt destruction
Grade 5	Erosion or ulceration
5.0	None
5.1	Recovering epithelium + adjacent inflammation
5.2	Probable erosion 2 focally stripped
5.3	Unequivocal erosion
5.4	Ulcer or granulation tissue

Modified Riley scoring system	
Activity	Features
None Mild Moderate Severe	0: Neutrophils in epithelium = none (3.0) 1: Neutrophils in epithelium = <25% crypts involved (3.1 or 3.2A) 2: Neutrophils in epithelium = ≥25% to ≤75% crypts involved (3.2B or 3.3A) 3: Neutrophils in epithelium = >75% crypts involved (3.3B) 4: Lamina propria neutrophils = mild but unequivocal increase (2B.1) 5: Lamina propria neutrophils = moderate increase (2B.2) 6: Lamina propria neutrophils = marked increase (2B.3) 7: Erosion or ulceration = present (5.1 or 5.2 or 5.3 or 5.4)

Table 15.4 Different pathological features between ulcerative colitis and Crohn's disease

	Ulcerative colitis	Crohn's disease
Macroscopic features	Diffuse and continuous Rectal involvement, no ileal (except backwash ileitis), rare upper GI involvement More severe in distal colon Rare strictures/stenosis No wrapping fat Mild wall thickening No sinus tract, fistula, or abscesses	Segmental and skip areas Entire GI tract involvement, mainly in the ileum and colon, variable rectal involvement, perianal disease Variable disease activity Strictures/stenosis Wrapping fat Marked wall thickening Sinus tract, fistula, or abscesses
Microscopic features	Transmucosal inflammation with chronicity, no transmural inflammation and lymphoid aggregates No deep or fissuring ulcers Minimal mural changes Occasional crypt-rupture granulomas	Transmucosal inflammation with chronicity, transmural inflammation and lymphoid aggregates Deep and fissuring ulcers Mural changes Epithelioid granulomas, unrelated to crypt damage

of pathology, on surgical specimens, the gross and microscopic findings of continuous and diffuse active chronic colitis involving the rectum and a variable length of proximal colon, without transmural inflammation and lymphoid aggregates, epithelioid granulomas, deep or fissuring ulcers, fistulas, and involvement of terminal ileum, would favor UC over CD. To distinct UC and CD based on endoscopic mucosal biopsy is difficult, unless unequivocal features of CD can be identified, such as epithelioid granulomas, ileal involvement, segmental disease in the first set biopsies in non-treated patients, or perianal lesions. At the same time, other possibilities are needed to be ruled out clinically. Several issues that may cause confusion are crypt ruptured granulomas, patchiness of the disease, backwash ileitis, and so-called superficial Crohn's colitis or UC-like Crohn's colitis (UC-like CD).

Granulomas in UC are associated with crypt rupture or surface epithelial damage (Fig. 15.16). They are loosely formed by histiocytes and lymphocytes surrounding injured crypts. On the other hand, granulomas in CD are discrete well-formed epithelioid granulomas that are not associated with crypt rupture. The histiocytes in granulomas of CD contain light eosinophilic cytoplasm which gives them a pinkish color (Fig. 15.19), while the crypt ruptured granulomas are more likely pale stained. Patchy distribution of UC includes rectal sparing, patchy cecum, appendiceal orifice, or ascending colon involvement associated with left-sided colitis or treatment-related uneven healing colitis. They are not true "skip lesions" of CD. Although aphthous ulcers are more frequently seen in CD, they are also present in UC. Be aware of these untypical features in UC which is important to avoid misclassification of IBD. If the initial biopsies before medical treatment or colectomy show active chronic colitis starting from the rectum and continuously extending to proximal colon, without granulomas or ileum involvement, the diagnosis of UC is favored. On resected UC specimens, grossly unremarkable regions including the spared rectum may still show microscopic evidence of active chronic colitis and should not be considered as skip lesions as well. Backwash ileitis in UC is frequently seen, especially for those with pancolitis and severe right-sided colitis. The ileal mucosa shows mild neutrophilic infiltration in lamina propria and surface epithelium with no or minimal epithelial injury, but features of Crohn's ileitis including epithelioid granulomas and apparent chronic changes such as villous architectural distortion or pseudopyloric metaplasia are absent. "Superficial Crohn's colitis" or "UC-like CD" is considered as a subgroup of CD which is characterized by inflammation restricted in mucosa or superficial submucosa with no mural involvement such as deep or fissuring ulcers or transmural lymphoid aggregates, but with other diagnostic features of CD such as segmental disease, ileal involvement, creeping fat, skip lesions, granulomas, and perianal disease or fistulas [117, 118]. Other features including active appendicitis, prominent lamina propria neutrophils, and increased and prominent lymphoid aggregates in mucosa and submucosa may also support a diagnosis of CD [118].

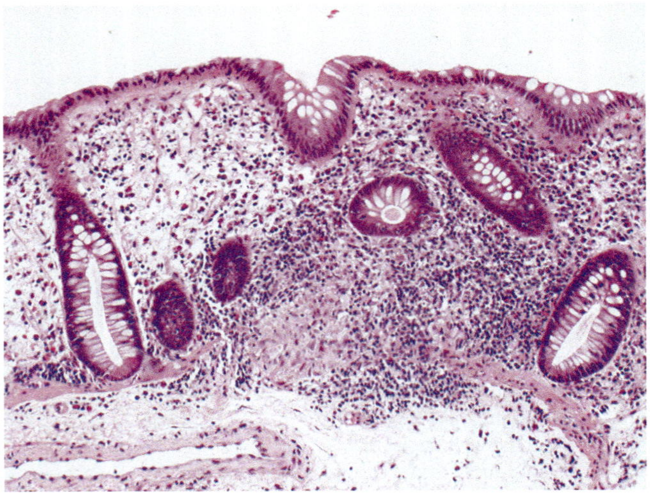

Fig. 15.19 Mucosal epithelioid granuloma in Crohn's disease. The granuloma is composed of compact histiocytes with eosinophilic cytoplasm and not associated with crypt injury

Infectious Colitis

Correlation with serology or stool cultures is required to rule out infectious colitis for the initial diagnosis of IBD since most microorganisms that cause infectious colitis are not identifiable on histology. Most cases of infectious colitis, including self-limited acute colitis, demonstrate a histological pattern of focal or diffuse acute colitis with normal mucosal architecture, characterized by prominent mucosal inflammation, cryptitis, and crypt abscesses, and a variable degree of epithelial injury, ranging from focal crypt loss and erosion to extensive mucosal necrosis and ulceration. Although infectious colitis shows increased cellularity in lamina propria, the gradient of gradually decreased inflammatory infiltrate from the upper to lower part of mucosa is relatively preserved (Fig. 15.20a). In contrast, the lamina propria inflammation in UC does not show this pattern, especially for plasma cells, which densely infiltrate at the base of mucosa known as basal plasmacytosis, a very useful feature to distinguish early stage of UC from infectious colitis. Less commonly, infection can become chronic and persistent leading to a pattern of chronic colitis (Fig. 15.20b), especially in immunocompromised patients. Only a few types of pathogens may be identified on histology, such as cytomegalovirus (CMV), *Entamoeba histolytica*, *Mycobacterium tuberculosis*, or some fungal infections. The differential diagnosis would be relied on clinical history and infectious disease workup.

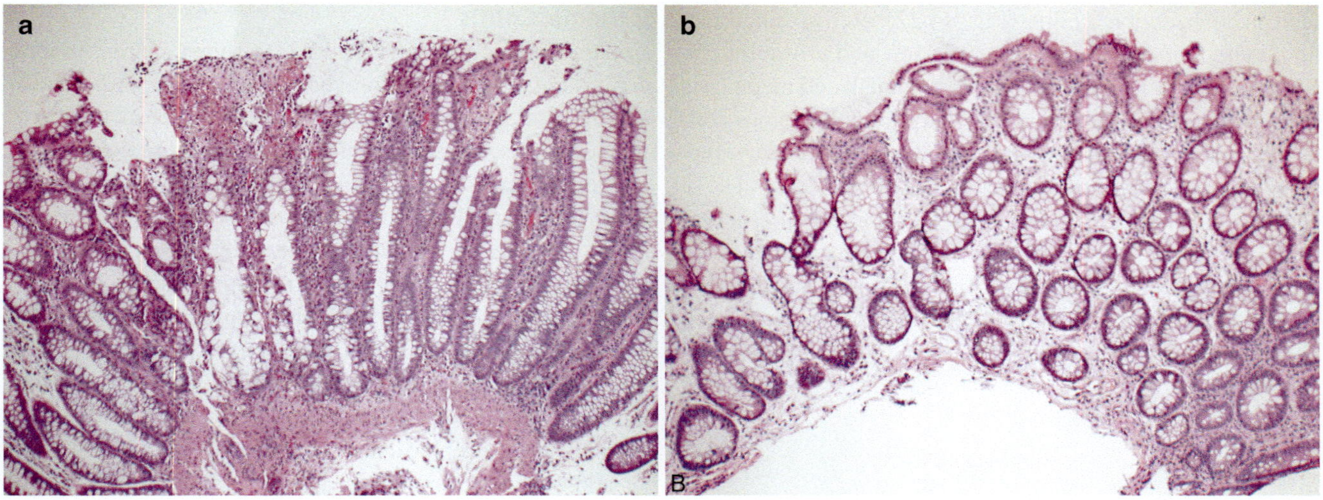

Fig. 15.20 Infectious colitis. (**a**) Acute infectious colitis. Colonic mucosa shows reactive changes with focal acute colitis, normal mucosal architecture, erosion, and no basal plasmacytosis. (**b**) Chronic *Clostridium difficile* colitis showing crypt architectural changes

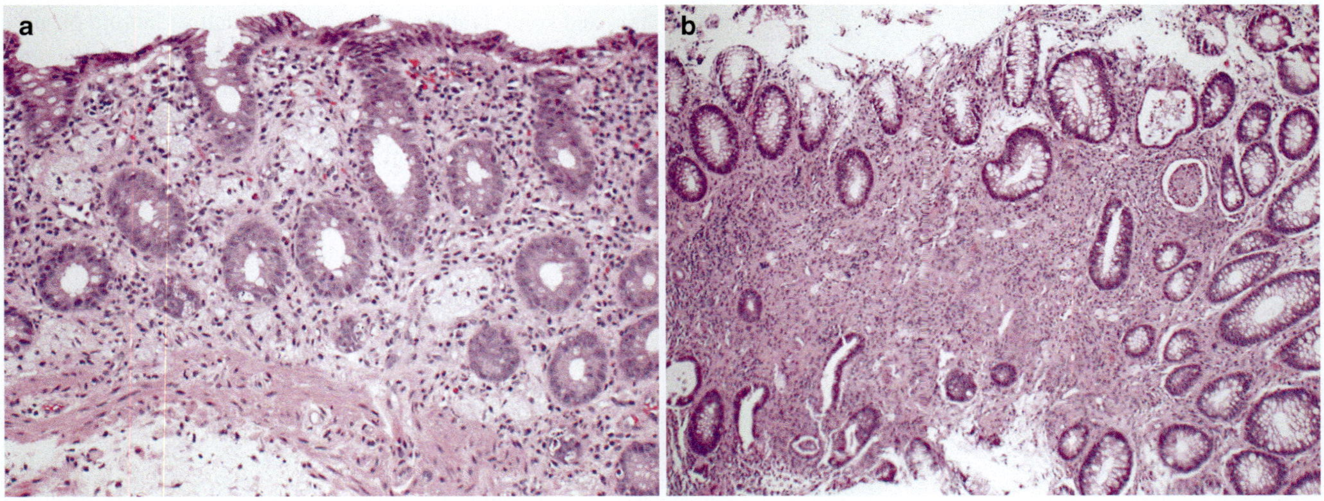

Fig. 15.21 Drug-induced colitis. (**a**) Mycophenolate-induced colitis, characterized by apoptosis, lamina propria inflammation, minimal crypt architectural change, and atrophic crypts. (**b**) Ipilimumab (anti-CTLA-4 monoclonal antibody)-induced colitis, showing crypt dropout, withered crypts, crypt architectural change, and occasional apoptosis

Drug-Induced Colitis

Drug-induced colonic injury can be manifested as active chronic colitis. Apparently, the correct diagnosis needs to correlate with patients' medication history and its relationship to the onset of the colitis and response to medication cessation. NSAIDs are among the most commonly used drugs that can cause gastrointestinal injury. NSAIDs can cause mucosal inflammation, ulceration, and nonspecific colitis. NSAIDs are also associated with increased risk of new onset of IBD, subsequent flares, and higher disease activity [119]. Mycophenolate-associated colonic injury may have IBD-like features, although the majority of mycophenolate-induced colitis show graft-versus-host disease-like changes [120, 121]. Prominent apoptosis, dilated and withered crypts, discontinuous crypt architectural changes, and ischemic changes would favor mycophenolate-induced colitis (Fig. 15.21a). Immunotherapy agents, such as anti-PD-L1 or anti-CTLA4 antibodies, can cause active colitis with apoptosis and crypt atrophy/dropout, but some may also show chronicity mimicking IBD (Fig. 15.21b) [122].

Microscopic Colitis

The diagnosis of microscopic colitis, either collagenous colitis or lymphocytic colitis, is usually straightforward based on the normal endoscopic findings and characteristic microscopic features. However, focal IBD-like changes can be seen in microscopic colitis (Fig. 15.22). Active inflammation, including cryptitis, crypt abscesses, and erosion/ulceration, can occur in over 30% of cases. Paneth cell metaplasia in left colon was observed in up to 44% of collagenous colitis and 14% of lymphocytic colitis patients. Focal crypt architectural changes were present in <10% of cases [123]. On the other hand, features of microscopic colitis, such as focal thickening of subepithelial collagen bands, may be occasionally seen in IBD [124]. Rare IBD cases may initially present as microscopic colitis [125]. Be aware of these IBD-like changes in microscopic colitis which will avoid confusion in daily practice.

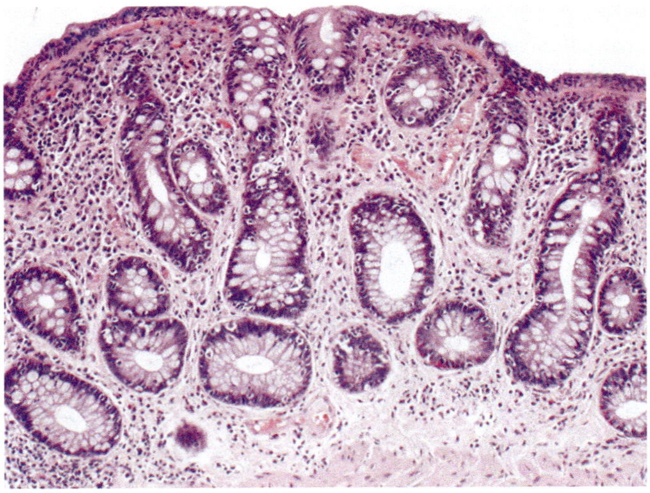

Fig. 15.22 IBD-like changes in microscopic colitis. There is mild crypt architectural distortion in this lymphocytic colitis

Ischemic Colitis

Acute ischemic colitis (Fig. 15.23a) shows lamina propria congestion, edema, inflammation, hemorrhage, and superficial mucosal necrosis, but features of early IBD such as cryptitis, crypt abscesses, basal plasmacytosis, or irregular crypts are not present. Of note, ischemic changes may be present in some fulminant IBD cases. Chronic mucosal injury secondary to ischemia may produce a pattern of active chronic colitis. The features of chronicity in chronic ischemic colitis mimicking UC include crypt architectural distortion, Paneth cell metaplasia in left colon, and active chronic inflammation. But there are other findings which favor chronic ischemia over UC, which are less degree of lamina propria inflammation, atrophic and/or regenerative epithelium, fibrosis and hyalinization in lamina propria, and identification of microthrombi in the adjacent mucosa (Fig. 12.23b).

Autoimmune Enteropathy

The colon can be involved in 60–80% autoimmune enteropathy, and some features resemble UC such as lamina propria expansion by lymphoplasmacytic infiltrate, cryptitis, and crypt abscesses. Crypt architectural distortion and Paneth cell metaplasia can be seen in about 10% of cases. However, other findings, including increased intraepithelial lymphocytes, apoptosis, atrophic crypts with crypt dropout, absence or diminishing goblet cells and/or Paneth cells, would argue against UC (Fig. 15.24) [126, 127].

Diverticular Disease-Associated Colitis

All histological features of IBD can be seen in diverticular disease-associated colitis (DDAC) (Fig. 15.25) [128]. UC-like and CD-like patterns have been described in DDAC

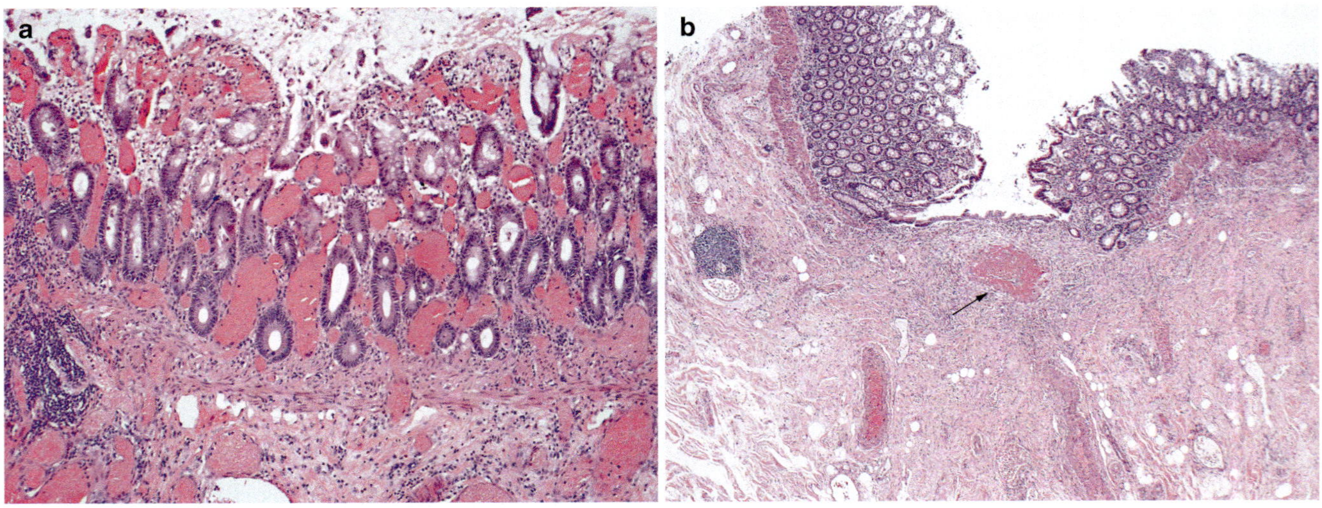

Fig. 15.23 Ischemic colitis. (**a**) Acute ischemic colitis. Note the lamina propria edema, congestion, hemorrhage, and surface epithelial and crypt injury, but no architectural changes or basal plasmacytosis. (**b**) Chronic ischemic colitis. Colonic mucosa with ulceration and minimal inflammation and crypt architectural changes. Note the fibrin thrombus in the submucosa vessel (arrow)

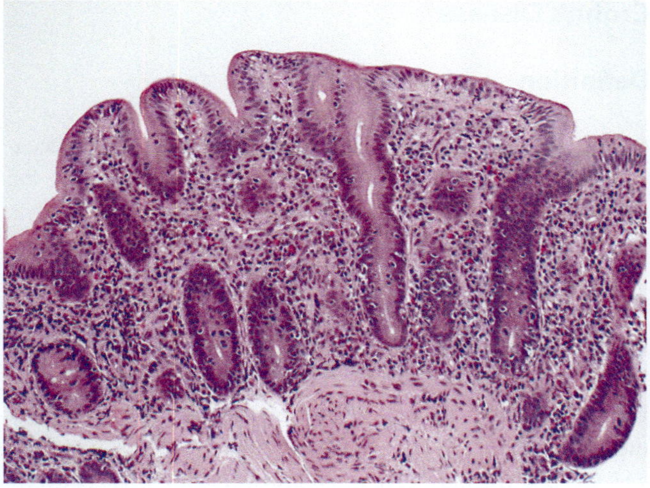

Fig. 15.24 Autoimmune colitis. Although there is lamina propria inflammation and crypt architectural changes, the marked intraepithelial lymphocytosis and absence of goblet cells are diagnostic of autoimmune colitis

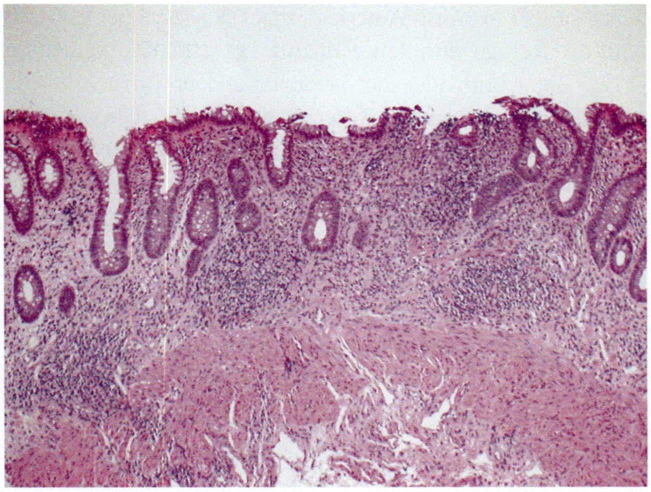

Fig. 15.25 Diverticular disease-associated colitis. It is essentially indistinguishable from inflammatory bowel disease based on the mucosal biopsy, which shows mild active chronic colitis with no specific features

[129]. DDAC and UC can also coexist in elder patients. The diagnosis requires endoscopic findings of diverticulosis and the disease distribution confined to segments involved by diverticular disease. DDAC most commonly involves the sigmoid colon with rectal sparing, an important feature to distinguish UC from DDAC.

Diversion Colitis

Diversion colitis can show a variety of mucosal abnormalities mimicking UC, which includes diffuse inflammatory infiltrate in lamina propria, prominent lymphoid follicles, crypt architectural distortion, crypt atrophy, and aphthous or non-aphthous ulcers (Fig. 15.26). If there is no prior history of IBD, the histological changes are certainly due to diversion. However, in patients with pre-existing IBD, it is difficult to separate diversion colitis from IBD or to determine possible coexistence of both conditions. The presence of prominent lymphoid follicles would favor more for diversion colitis.

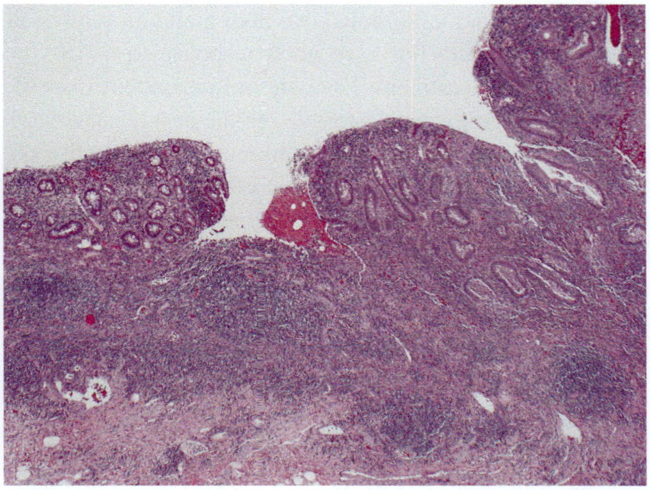

Fig. 15.26 Diversion colitis. Diffuse inflammation with aphthous ulcers. The presence of prominent lymphoid follicles and aggregates favors diversion colitis

Treatment and Prognosis

The goals of UC treatment are to induce remission, control flares, and maintain steroid-free clinical remission [130, 131]. The treatment strategy is based on the disease severity, distribution, and patterns. The management of mild to moderate UC and severe UC is different. The new strategies, including early intervention, more frequent monitoring, and treat-to-target, have been introduced in reducing disease progression (reducing corticosteroid use, disability, bowel damage, hospitalization, and surgeries) [132]. The treat-to-target in UC has switched the goal from clinical remission to endoscopic remission, since 20% of patients with clinical remission still have significant endoscopic disease activity [133]. The medical management of UC mainly includes four types of medications: aminosalicylates, corticosteroids, immunomodulators, and biologics. Aminosalicylates contain 5-aminosalicylate acid (5-ASA), including sulfasalazine, mesalamine, olsalazine, and balsalazide. Topical and/or oral 5-ASA is effective in inducing remission of mild to moderately active UC and in preventing flares [134]. Corticosteroids can be given topically, orally, or intravenously, which are used as the initial treatment for severe UC, in controlling flares in moderate to severe UC, and in those intolerant or refractory to 5-ASA. Immunomodulators, such as azathioprine, mercaptopurine, cyclosporine, and tacrolimus, can help maintain remission in patients who do not have good response to 5-ASA or corticosteroids treatment, have steroid-dependent disease, or are intolerant to corticosteroids. In the past decade, various biologics targeting specific immunological pathways have shown promising therapeutic effect for UC. Several biologic agents have received FDA approval for treating IBD: anti-TNF alpha agents (infliximab, adalimumab, golimumab, and certolizumab pegol), anti-integrin agents (natalizumab and vedolizumab), and anti-IL-12 and IL-23 (ustekinumab). Clinical trials have found that these biologics can result in more clinical responses, clinical remissions, and mucosal healings than placebo for induction therapy [135, 136]. The combination with immunomodulators may have a more beneficial effect on clinical outcomes. More agents are under investigation and may become available soon as treatment options for UC.

Although UC is primarily treated medically, surgical management may be required in some patients, and it is estimated that approximately 20–30% of patients with advanced UC would eventually require a surgical resection. The indications for emergent surgeries include colonic perforation, life-threatening gastrointestinal hemorrhage, toxic megacolon, and acute fulminant colitis refractory to medical treatment. Elective surgery using continence-preserving procedures such as the ileal pouch-anal anastomosis (IPAA) is indicated for those who become refractory to medical therapy, develop severe complications, or have increased cancer risk. Strictures can develop in about 5% of UC cases that may cause obstructive symptoms. Of note, strictures in UC patients are strongly associated with malignancy. A large retrospective study showed that near one-fourth of strictures in UC were malignant, and most of them were located proximal to splenic flexure [137].

UC is considered as a lifelong disease, and its course is unpredictable, which can range from an indolent course with prolonged periods of remission to aggressive and devastating disease. Higher Mayo severity and endoscopic scores, corticosteroid use, younger age at diagnosis, and presence of PSC at time of diagnosis are associated with progression of the disease's extension and poor prognosis. About 70–80% of UC patients experience at least one relapse which occurs more frequently in those with younger age, female gender, initial ESR <30 mm, no smoking, and early relapse (within 1 year after initial diagnosis). The UC patients may have two- to threefold higher risk of developing colorectal cancer, especially for those with concomitant PSC. However, recent studies have shown declining risk of cancer in UC, probably due to improvements in therapy and surveillance [138]. The overall mortality rate of UC is also declining in the modern era, and it is not higher than that of general population [139].

Crohn's Disease

Definition

Crohn's disease is an idiopathic chronic, transmural, and occasionally granulomatous inflammatory disorder involving the entire gastrointestinal tract from the mouth to perianal area, but most commonly affecting the distal small bowel and colon.

Epidemiology

Like UC, the incidence of CD is also steadily increasing after the World War II, and the increased rate has stabilized now [8, 11]. CD and UC may have equal prevalence in North America [140]. For example, in Olmsted County, Minnesota, the prevalence of CD was 28 cases per 100,000 in 1965, increasing to 90.5 per 100,000 in 1980 and 246.7 per 100,000 in 2011 [141]. In the same study, the adjusted prevalence of UC was 286.3 per 100,000 persons [141]. The overall reported annual incidence of CD in North America ranges 3.1–20.2 per 100,000 with an average prevalence of 201 per 100,000 population [142]. But worldwide, the incidence and prevalence of CD vary significantly among different geographic regions, environment, immigrant population, and ethnic groups. Higher incidence of CD occurs in Ashkenazi Jews, in urban population, and in northern countries [143]. Although CD is considered infrequent in Eastern world, increasing incidence of CD has been reported in eastern Asia, which was reported to be 0.54 per 100,000 in the Asia-Pacific IBD study recently [12].

CD demonstrates a slight difference between men and women, with a slight female predominance, and female children may have more severe disease than male children. CD can affect people in any age, but it is rarely diagnosed in early childhood. Like UC, a bimodal peak in incidence is also observed in CD, with the first peak occurring between the ages of 15 and 29 years and a second smaller peak occurring between the ages of 55 and 59 years [144]. Patients diagnosed at age ≥60 years are more likely to have isolated colonic disease and are less likely to develop complicated CD than patients diagnosed at younger ages [145].

Etiology and Pathogenesis

CD is also believed to be caused by chronic unrestrained inflammatory process due to dysfunctional innate and adaptive immune responses which are triggered by environmental factors in susceptible individuals.

Genetic Factors

The role of genetic in CD has been confirmed by large studies of concordance in twins and familial aggregation [146, 147].

CARD15 (caspase recruitment domain family member 15, formerly known as *NOD2*) is the first gene identified to be associated with CD [148]. There are three mutations found within the region of *CARD15* encoding a leucine-rich repeat which is responsible for bacterial recognition, and they are Arg702Trp, Gly908Arg, and the frameshift 1007fs. At least one of these mutations is present in 25–35% of patients with CD [149]. Patients with heterogeneous *CARD15* mutation have 2–4 times increased risk of developing CD, whereas those with homogeneous alleles have 20–40-fold increased risk [150]. The *IL23R* gene involves in the differentiation of Th_{17} cells and leads to dysregulated IL-17 secretion in CD [151]. Mutations in *SLC22A4* and *SLC22A5*, which encode the organic cation transporters OCTN1 and OCTN2, have been associated with CD [152]. Two haplotypes of *DLG5* gene, which encodes a scaffolding protein that helps to maintain epithelial integrity, were found to be associated with *CARD15* mutations in patients with CD or combined CD and UC [153]. Rare polymorphisms of *PPARγ* gene, a nuclear receptor inhibiting NFκB activity, are associated with CD [154]. Like UC, *MDR1* variants are also associated with CD [155]. Genome-wide association studies and meta-analyses have identified more than 200 susceptibility loci for CD and many new genes and pathways in the pathogenesis of CD, such as genes related to autophagy (*ATG16L1* and *IRGM*), innate immune system (*TLR4, CARD9, IL23R, STAT3*), and adaptive immune system (*HLA, TNFSF15, IRF5, PTPN22*) [156].

Immunologic Factors and Intestinal Microbiota

The role of the interaction between dysbiotic intestinal microbiota and dysregulated immune responses in the pathogenesis of IBD has been introduced in the previous section. However, there are differences in the pathways and effector cells between CD and UC. CD has been considered to be predominately driven by Th_1 and Th_{17} response, while UC has been considered as a Th_2-mediated disease [32, 33]. The Th_1 cells produce IFN-γ and IL-12, and this pathway is complicated by the discovery of an additional Th_{17} pathway which involves IL-6, IL-17, TGF-beta, and IL-23. It has been shown that bacterial colonization stimulates IL-23 expression by ileal dendritic cells, and the levels of both IL-23 and IL-17 are increased in CD [157, 158]. The IL-12–IFN-γ and IL-23–IL-17 pathways seem to be mutually exclusive because IFN-γ can suppresses IL-17 production and vice versa. The dysfunctional immune response has resulted from an imbalance between the effector T cells and Treg.

The innate immune responses are deficient at multiple levels in CD. Intestinal dysbiosis and concomitant changes of the intestinal luminal milieu and environment damage the intestinal epithelial barrier leading to increased epithelial permeability and translocation of antigens into lamina propria. Cells involved in innate immune responses are activated, and the expression of most proinflammatory cytokines and chemokines is upregulated in both CD and UC, but Th_1- and Th_{17}-related cytokines involved in innate immunity (e.g., IL-12, IL-23, and IL-27) are selectively activated in CD. The inflammatory response is elicited, maintained, and enhanced by ineffective phagocytosis, bacterial clearance, and impairment of adaptive immune responses [159].

The dysbiosis in CD and UC is different [160]. It is greater in CD than in UC, with a lower microbial diversity, a more altered microbiome composition, and a more unstable microbial community. CD is associated with a loss of more beneficial microorganisms than a gain of more pathogenic ones. The beneficial microorganisms include those involved in butyrate production such as *Faecalibacterium, Christensenellaceae, Methanobrevibacter*, and *Oscillospira*. Patients with CD have a decrease in *Faecalibacterium*, while this genus is not missing in patients with UC [160, 161].

Environmental Factors

The exact mechanisms of how environmental factors influence the development of IBD are still unknown. The hypothesis includes triggering immune responses or directly injuring intestinal epithelial lining. Currently, besides smoking, no other specific environmental factors or infections have been clearly linked to the onset of CD. Smoking is the strongest risk factor and has a paradoxical effect in CD and UC. Active or ex-smokers are at a higher risk to develop CD [53, 54], while many studies have confirmed the protective effect of current smoking on the development of UC, lower rate of relapse, and reduced need for colectomy in current smokers [51, 52]. A Western diet high in fat and carbohydrates and low in fiber and fruit has been shown to be associated with the rising incidence of CD [162]. Vitamin D deficiency has also been found in association with CD, but it is unclear whether this is an underlying cause or a consequence of malabsorption of CD [163]. The other potential risk factors associated with the onset of CD are breastfeeding, hygiene, stress, appendectomy, seasonal variation, and medications such as antibiotics, NSAIDs, and oral contraceptives [164].

Clinical Features

Over 60% of patients have colonic involvement, 20% with colon involvement only, and about 50% with involvement of both the ileum and colon. As with other sites of disease, the clinical presentation of colonic CD is highly variable between patients. Patients with Crohn's colitis typically present with cramping abdominal pain and diarrhea. In comparison to small bowel involvement, bloody diarrhea is more common in patients with Crohn's colitis. Similar to small bowel CD, the transmural inflammation leads to the development of sinus tracts that can penetrate and develop into an abscess, a perforation, or a fistula. A free perforation is rare in patients with CD. The common site of colonic fistulas involves the redundant loop of the sigmoid colon and the terminal ileum. However, fistulas can arise between any segments of visceral inflammation. As such, patients may present with primary colonic fistulas that typically involve the vagina or the bladder. Stricture formation in colonic CD is similar to that seen in the small bowel, which gives patients bowel obstructive symptoms. Of note, malignant strictures can occur in up to 7% in patients with CD. Therefore, endoscopic biopsy to rule out a malignancy is imperative when a colonic stricture is identified. A small subset of patients may develop severe complications such as life-threatening hemorrhage, fulminant colitis, or toxic colitis requiring emergent surgery. Patients may present with systemic symptoms such as weight loss, low fever, unexplained anemia, and growth failure in children. The extraintestinal manifestations are common in patients with Crohn's colitis. The musculoskeletal system is most commonly involved. Perianal fistulas are present in up to 10% of patients at the time of diagnosis, and it may be the presenting complaint in some cases.

Classification

Disease classification can provide useful information in determining the features, phenotypes, and treatment and in predicting the behavior and prognosis of CD. The Montreal classification for CD which was derived from the Vienna classification has been widely adopted [60]. Both systems use age of onset (A), disease location (L), and disease behavior (B) as the predominant parameters and are listed in Table 15.5.

Table 15.5 Vienna and Montreal classification for Crohn's disease

	Vienna classification	Montreal classification
Age at diagnosis (year)	A1: <40	A1: <16
	A2: >40	A2: 17–40
		A3: >40
Location	L1: ileal	L1: ileal
	L2: colonic	L2: colonic
	L3: ileocolonic	L3: ileocolonic
	L4: upper	L4: isolated upper disease[a]
Behavior	B1: non-stricturing, non-penetrating	B1: non-stricturing, non-penetrating
	B2: stricturing	B2: stricturing
	B3: penetrating	B3: penetrating
		P: perianal disease modifier[b]

[a]L4 can be added to L1–L3 when concomitant upper gastrointestinal disease is present

[b]P can be added to B1–B3 when concomitant perianal disease is present

CD can be classified according to the clinical disease activity as mild, moderate, and severe disease using a Crohn's Disease Activity Index (CDAI), which consists of eight factors: number of liquid or soft stools/day, abdominal pain, general well-being, number of complications, opiates for diarrhea, abdominal mass, deviation from normal hematocrit, and % deviation from standard weight [165]. The CDAI is the sum of each after adjustment with a weighting factor which gives a score ranging 0–600. The disease activity is usually arbitrarily labeled as mild for CDAI scores of 150–219, moderate for scores 220–450, and severe for scores >450. But some consider a score >300 is severe and >450 is extremely severe. Remission is accepted as a CDAI <150. Response is defined as a decrease in CDAI ≥100 points, but some studies used a lesser end point with a reduction in CDAI.

CD can also be divided into localized or extensive disease. The localized CD refers to those with affecting <30 cm in extent, while extensive CD indicates intestinal CD affecting >100 cm in extent whatever the location. Although this is arbitrary and there is a gray zone (disease between 30 and 100 cm), the recognition of extensive disease reflects the severer and greater inflammatory burden in clinical management.

According to the response to therapy, CD can be classified as steroid-refractory or steroid-dependent as well. Steroid-refractory CD is defined as that patients who have active disease despite prednisolone up to 0.75 mg/kg/day for a period of 4 weeks, while steroid-dependent disease refers to patients who are either unable to reduce steroid below the equivalent of 10 mg/day within 3 months without recurrent active disease or have a relapse within 3 months of stopping steroids.

Laboratory Findings

Serological studies in CD often reveal anemia due to iron deficiency or vitamin B12 deficiency. ESR and CRP can be used to monitor disease activity and treatment response, to predict the course of the disease, and to subclassify patients. High CRP levels are indicative of active disease, and a decrease in CRP is indicative of treatment response. The tests of multiple antibodies against ASCA, pANCA, CBir1, or OmpC have a limited role in diagnosing CD and differentiating CD from UC. Stool should be tested for enteric pathogens, parasites, and *Clostridium difficile* (*C. difficile*) toxin. Fecal biomarkers (calprotectin and lactoferrin) can provide valuable information in diagnosing and monitoring CD. Fecal calprotectin is a sensitive marker predicting relapse, but its role is limited if the disease is restricted to the small bowel.

Radiological Findings

Plain radiograph is not widely used nowadays, but it can still detect bowel dilatation, obstruction, bowel perforation, or bowel wall thickening. Ultrasound has a limited role in evaluating colonic involvement because it is difficult to visualize the colonic flexures, rectum, and anal region, but it is useful in assessing perianal disease. CT and MRI are similar in sensitivity for active inflammation, but MRE has become an increasingly important tool for the lack of ionizing radiation and an ability to evaluate both mural and extramural involvement. The diagnostic features include fat halo sign or fibro-fatty proliferation, vascular engorgement or comb sign, bowel wall enhancement and thickening, strictures and stenosis, fistulae, and mesenteric/intra-abdominal abscesses, and perianal disease [166, 167]. The main features that distinguish CD from UC are small bowel and perianal involvement, skip lesions, thicker colonic wall, irregular serosal surface, mesenteric creeping fat, and abscesses.

Endoscopic Findings

Ileocolonoscopy with multiple biopsy specimens is essential for diagnosing CD. Endoscopic evaluation may identify aphthous or deep ulcers, skip areas, polypoid mucosal changes with a cobblestone appearance in a discontinuous distribution, inflammatory pseudopolyps, strictures, and fistulae (Fig. 15.27). Crohn's colitis may be endoscopically indistinguishable from UC, but CD typically has skip areas, spares the rectum, and is most severe in the cecum and right colon.

Disease activity Endoscopic scores are commonly used in the clinical trials to measure the efficacy of various drugs on inducing and maintaining mucosal healing. The two most commonly used scoring systems in CD patients without bowel resection are Crohn's Disease Index of Severity (CDEIS) and Simple Endoscopic Score for Crohn's Disease (SES-CD). The CDEIS scores CD activity in five bowel segments (terminal ileum, right colon, transverse, left colon and sigmoid, and rectum), considering specific mucosal lesions such as ulcers and stenosis, and percentage of ulcerated or affected surface [168]. The SES-CD simplifies the CDEIS which includes four variables in five segments of the bowel: ulcer size, the extent of ulcerated surface, the extent of affected surface, and stenosis [169]. However, the main limitation of the endoscopic mucosal activity is that it does not reflect transmural damage and other complications such as fistulas and abscesses. Although both systems are validated with good intra- and interobserver agreement, the correlation between endoscopic and clinical disease activity is not ideal. The SES-CD is preferred because it is simpler to use, reliable, and reproducible and shows a moderate correlation with histological index [170].

Endoscopic mucosal healing Similar to UC, mucosal healing has become the therapeutic goal in CD, and mucosal healing assessed by endoscopy is also useful in evaluating and guiding response to therapy. However, endoscopic mucosal healing does not necessarily coincide with histological healing. The mucosal architectural changes and inflammation can persist after treatment with significant improvement of endoscopic mucosal inflammation scores. Therefore, it is suggested that histological healing should be considered the final target. But the definition and standard of mucosal histological healing have not been established yet.

Endoscopic tissue biopsy Histologic evaluation of biopsy tissue is important in initial diagnosis, disease follow-up, and surveillance. Biopsy from terminal ileum is necessary. Samples from at least four colonic sites and the rectum, with a minimum of two biopsies from each site, are recommended.

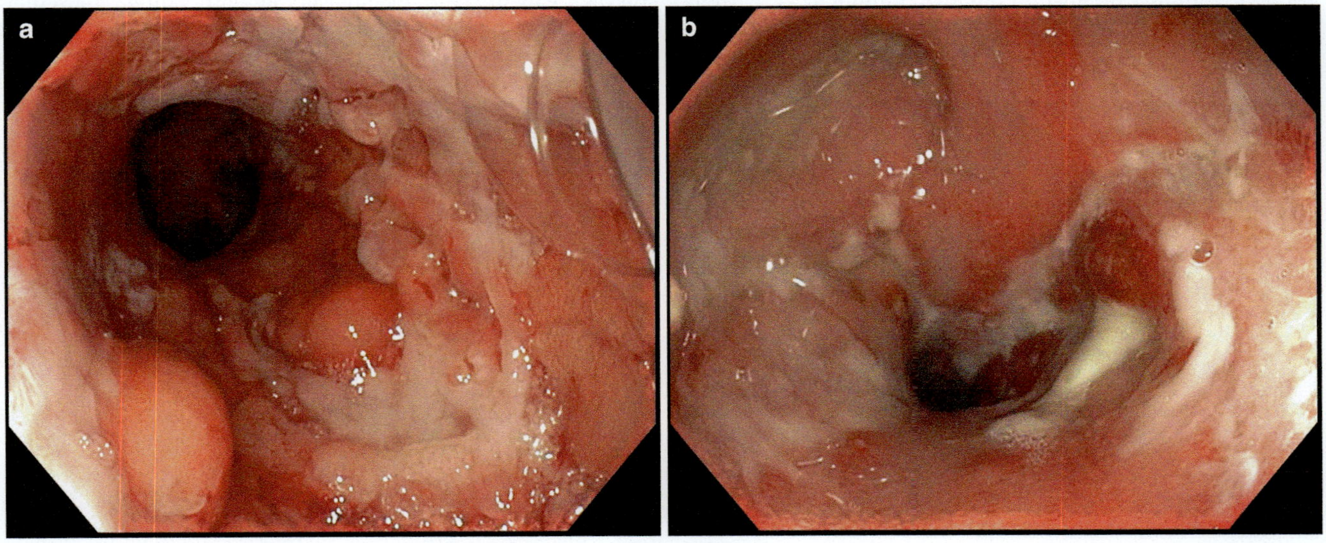

Fig. 15.27 Endoscopic features of Crohn's colitis. (**a**) Severely active Crohn's disease shows cobblestone mucosa with marked edema, erythema, friability, and deep ulceration. (**b**) Colonic stricture in Crohn's colitis

The specimens should be obtained from both diseased and normal-appearing mucosa. More samples may be required for surveillance of dysplasia, such as every 10 cm in the colon and every 5 cm in the rectum, and any suspicious lesions. For example, endoscopic biopsy to rule out a malignancy is imperative when a colonic stricture is identified. Biopsy specimens from different locations should be separately labeled.

Pathological Features

Gross Findings

Crohn's colitis shows similar gross features to those in small bowel CD (Fig. 15.28a, b), which can help to distinguish CD from UC. However, the isolated Crohn's colitis is less likely to form strictures or stenosis, more likely to have subtotal, total, or left-side colitis, compared to patients with ileocolonic CD who show predominantly right-side involvement [117]. The mucosal surface shows variable changes in different disease stage and severity. The earliest mucosal change in CD is small punched-out shallow aphthous ulcers. They can range from tiny ulcers that are difficult to be found to small well-demarcated ulcer with white base, usually 1–3 mm. With disease progressing, the aphthous ulcers become bigger and coalesce to develop longitudinal, linear, and serpiginous ulcers, along the bowel axis. The patchy intervening intact mucosa with edema and submucosal damage between these ulcers gives a classic "cobblestoned" gross appearance. Deep fissures develop in mucosal folds and penetrate into or through muscularis propria, leading to sinus tracts or fistulas. Strictures are common findings. The patchy distribution pattern and sharply delineated injured areas surrounded by normal mucosa, known as skip areas, are unique in CD. Even in extensive colonic involvement, small areas of mucosa with normal appearance are still present. The rectum is usually spared in CD, and the disease is more severe in proximal colon. Inflammatory pseudopolyps are often present.

The colonic wall is rigid and thickened, with a segmental stricture or multiple short strictures. The transition from normal appearing bowel to the affected segment is abrupt. The thickened wall shows hypertrophy of muscular layers and submucosal fibrosis. Wrapping fat, or creeping fat, refers to overgrowth of subserosal and mesenteric adipose tissue extending from the mesenteric attachment to cover part of colonic wall with loss of the bowel-mesentery angle (Fig. 15.28a). Although it is less frequently seen in colonic CD, it is considered as a hallmark in CD. The serosa may also appear granular, congestive, or fibrotic. The affected bowel loop often adheres to another segment of bowel or other organs, with or without fistula formation. Perforation is rare in Crohn's colitis, which typically occurs in right colon. Abscess cavities can be found within the bowel wall or mesentery. Many patients with Crohn's colitis also have perianal involvement, including skin tags, deep ulcers or fissures, sinus tracts or fistulas, abscesses, and strictures. Careful gross examination is necessary to detect these complications. Sections are usually taken every 5 cm or 10 cm including the margins and unaffected areas, in addition to other lesional areas such as strictures, fistulas, and polypoid or mass lesions. Sections from terminal ileum are required if available.

Microscopic Findings

The microscopic diagnostic features of CD in the colon are similar to those in small bowel, including transmural inflammation and lymphoid aggregates, mucosal active chronic inflammation, deep or fissuring ulceration, mucosal architectural distortion, epithelioid granulomas, pseudopyloric metaplasia, Paneth cell metaplasia in left colon, muscular hypertrophy, and some stromal changes such as fibrosis, neu-

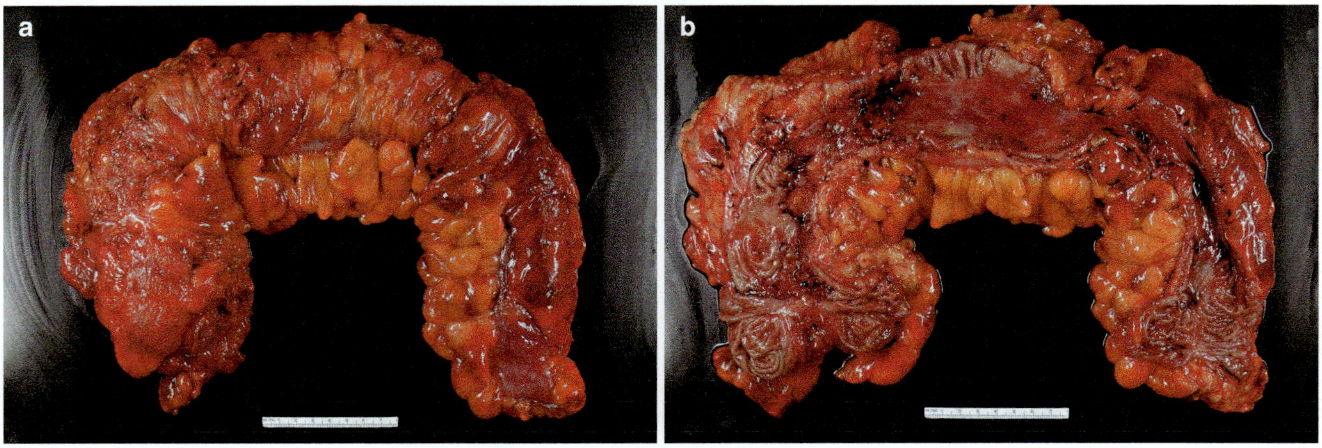

Fig. 15.28 Gross features of Crohn's colitis. (**a**) Wrapping fat and congested serosa. (**b**) Opened specimen shows uneven distribution of the disease (skip lesions), cobblestone mucosa, deep and serpiginous ulcers, and strictures

ral hyperplasia, or vasculitis. The distribution of these changes is patchy or segmental. CD limited to the colon may show less numbers of these key morphological features [171]. Of note, distinguishing CD versus UC is not practical based on mucosal biopsy alone, even with the presence of granulomas.

Granulomas Epithelioid non-necrotizing granuloma is a key feature of CD, although it is not entirely specific. Granulomas can be detected in approximately 50% of resection specimens and 30% of biopsy samples. The frequency of detection of granulomas increases with increasing numbers of submitted sections or biopsy samples and by examining multiple serial sections. They are more frequently seen in the colon than in small bowel. The granulomas in CD are usually small and with less well-defined outlines (Fig. 15.29a, b). The epithelioid histiocytes in the granulomas have abundant eosinophilic cytoplasm which gives the granulomas an eosinophilic color and makes it easier to be identified. Multinucleated giant cells can be present. Necrosis is absent. The granulomas can be found throughout the intestinal wall, but they are more often situated in mucosa, submucosa, subserosa, and ulcer areas, in both unaffected and inflamed regions. The granulomas can also be found in mesenteric lymph nodes in CD. But if the granulomas are only present in lymph nodes, other possibilities have to be considered besides CD. On the other hand, if the granulomas are in the mucosa and associated with crypt rupture (cryptolytic or ruptured crypt granulomas), they are not reliable for considering a diagnosis of CD, as they can occur in many other disorders including UC and infectious colitis [104]. Microgranulomas or poorly formed granulomas, composed of small clusters of loosely arranged histiocytes (typically less than 20 cells), are also frequently seen in CD (Fig. 15.29c). Sometimes, small germinal centers, crushed small vessels with plumped endothelial cells, or tangential cuts at the peripheral of glands can mimic granulomas. Examining deeper cuts can be helpful in this setting. Isolated giant cells can be occasionally seen [172], but their significance is uncertain since they can be found in UC as well, especially those located at the base of crypts.

Mucosal changes The mucosal changes in Crohn's colitis are indistinguishable from those in UC, which basically represent active chronic colitis, with or without non-necrotizing granulomas. The mucosal inflammation in CD is in a discontinuous fashion, often with rectal sparing, which can be helpful in the differential diagnosis, but it is not reliable as UC can also present with patchy distribution such as a cecal or peri-appendiceal patch or treatment-related uneven healing.

The active colitis or disease activity in CD refers to neutrophilic infiltration and epithelial injury. The degree of active inflammation and mucosal injury can be variable in affected segments (Fig. 15.30a, b). The lamina propria is expanded with increased inflammatory infiltrate including neutrophils and eosinophils. Focal cryptitis and crypt abscesses are present. The inflammation causes degeneration and damage of surface epithelium, mucin and goblet cell depletion, and erosion. Alphthous ulcers are commonly seen, more frequently in proximal colon, characterized by small foci of surface neutrophilic infiltrate and erosion, often associated with an underlying lymphoid aggregate/follicle (Fig. 15.31). The mucosa adjacent to the ulcers may be normal or only show mild reactive changes. Alphthous ulcers are not unique for CD, as they can be found in about 20% colectomy specimens in UC [173]. With disease progression, the alphthous ulcers become bigger and deeper, which gives them a knifelike appearance, but ulcers with broad base can occur in CD (Fig. 15.32).

The chronicity in CD is the same with UC, which has been described in detail in the above section, including transmucosal inflammation, basal plasmacytosis or basal lymphoid aggregates, crypt and mucosal architectural distortion, Paneth cell metaplasia in left colon, and pseudopyloric metaplasia (Fig. 15.33). Although determination of chronicity is imperative for diagnosing IBD, it is not helpful in differentiating between CD and UC or among other causes of chronic mucosal injuries.

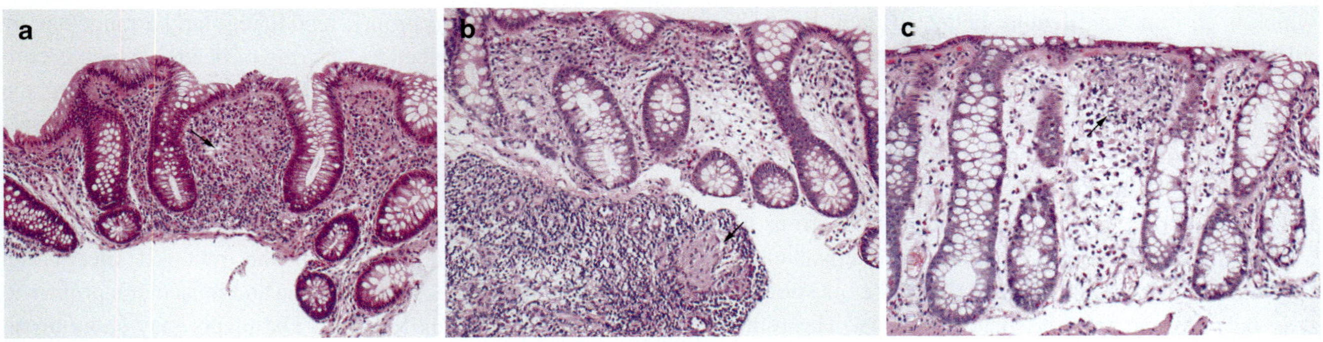

Fig. 15.29 Granulomas. (**a**) Typical small mucosal epithelioid granuloma with less well-defined outlines in Crohn's disease (arrow). (**b**) A similar small epithelioid granuloma identified in submucosa (arrow). (**c**) Poorly formed or microgranuloma in Crohn's disease (arrow)

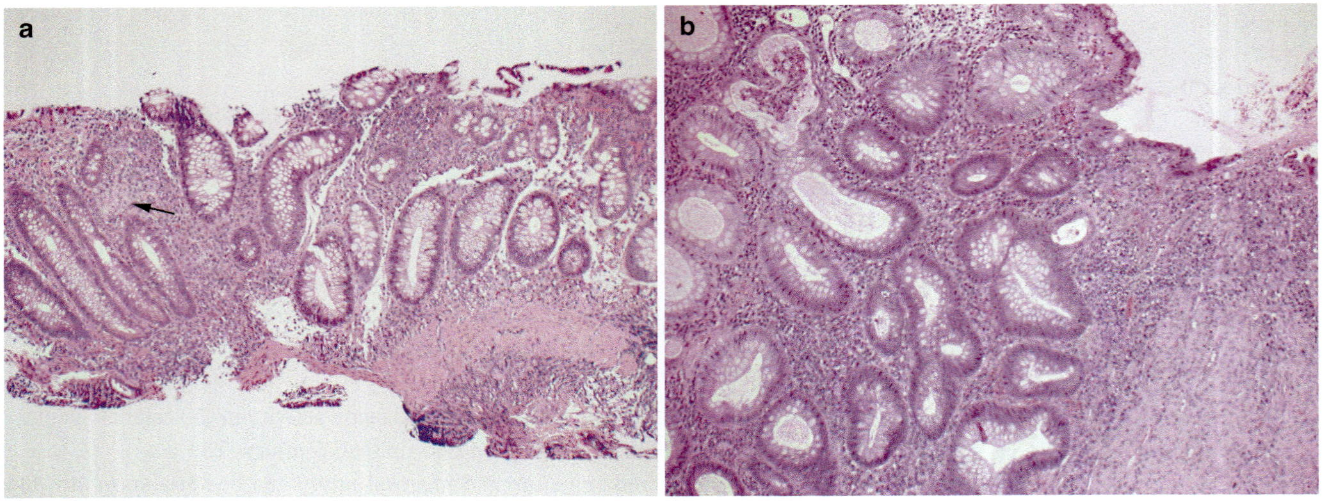

Fig. 15.30 Active chronic colitis of Crohn's colitis. (**a**) Mild active chronic colitis, with mild lamina propria inflammation, mild crypt architectural changes, focal cryptitis, epithelial injury, and a poorly formed granuloma (arrow). (**b**) Moderate to severe active chronic colitis, with crypt abscesses and focal ulceration

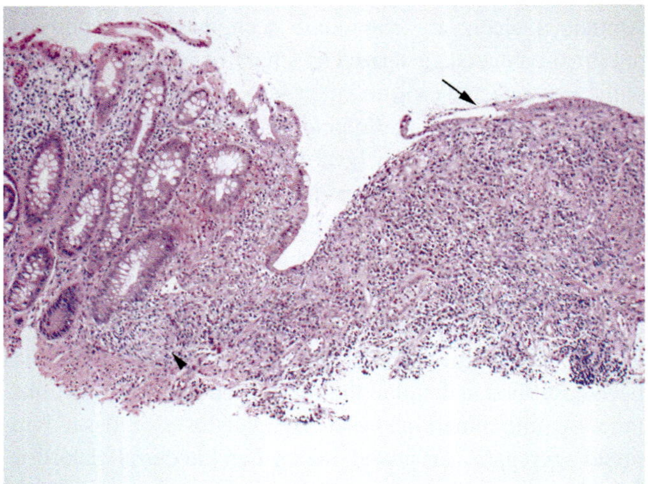

Fig. 15.31 Alphthous ulcer in Crohn's colitis. Surface epithelial neutrophilic infiltrate and erosion on the top of a lymphoid aggregate (arrow). The adjacent colonic mucosa shows mild active chronic colitis with a poorly formed granuloma (arrowhead)

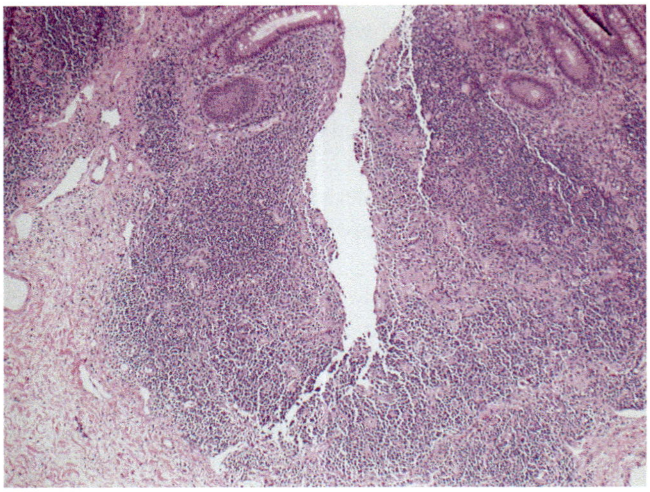

Fig. 15.32 Deep mucosal ulceration with a knifelike appearance, associated with active and chronic inflammation

Mural changes CD involves all layers of colonic wall, which is an important feature being different from UC, but this can only be assessed on resection specimens. Although the active chronic inflammation is predominantly in mucosa, it is not restricted in mucosa as it is in UC. The mononuclear cells and eosinophils can be seen throughout the intestinal wall, known as transmural inflammation. The density of inflammation is typically reduced gradually from mucosa toward the deeper levels. Of note, the diagnostic value of transmural inflammation for CD should be questioned when it is only present in areas beneath ulcers. The transmural inflammation is also manifested as transmural lymphoid aggregates, i.e., lymphoid aggregates with or without germinal centers present in all layers. In particular, the lymphoid aggregates in subserosal space, sometimes in submucosa, along the muscularis propria tend to regularly arrange one by one, a pattern described as "a string of beads," which is considered as a hallmark of CD (Fig. 15.34). Oftentimes, the string of beads is only composed by a few lymphoid aggregates, and the lymphoid aggregates are also loosely formed. These findings may be overlooked by pathologists so that one of the most important diagnostic features of CD may be missed. Besides inflammation, the mucosal ulcers can deepen and extend into submucosa and muscularis propria to form deep ulcers and fissures. The ulcers may show broad base, but more often present as knifelike deep ulcers/fissures, associated with active and chronic inflammation, granulation tissue, and fibrosis (Fig. 15.34).

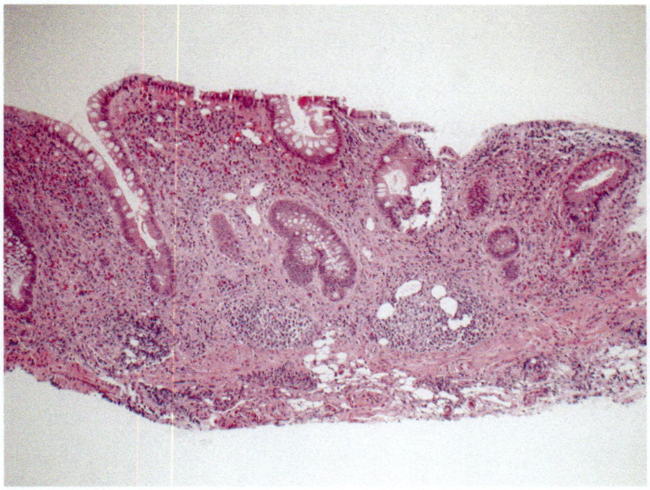

Fig. 15.33 Mucosal chronicity in Crohn's disease. This colon biopsy shows transmucosal inflammation, basal plasmacytosis and lymphoid aggregates, crypt and mucosal architectural distortion

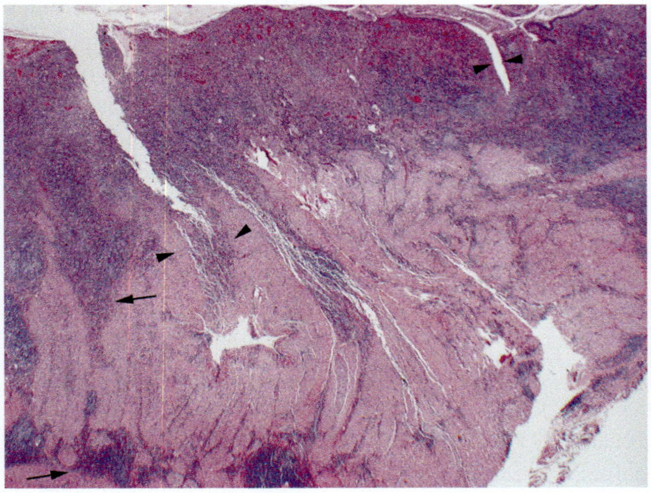

Fig. 15.34 Transmural inflammation and lymphoid aggregates with "a string of beads" pattern along the muscularis propria (arrows). Fissuring ulcers in mucosa (right arrowheads) and extending into muscle layer (left arrowheads)

The colonic wall is much thicker in CD than in UC, especially at the stricture sites. The wall thickening is due to fibrosis and hypertrophy of muscular layers (Fig. 15.35). Indeed, the fibrostenotic change is a major pathological event leading to CD-related complications and mortality. The fibrosis is transmural, but it is more prominent in submucosa, and it can be associated with hypertrophy of muscularis mucosae to obliterate the submucosa, known as obliterative muscularization of submucosa [174]. The muscularis propria is also thickened, especially the inner layer, showing significant hypertrophy with deposition of collagen. The hyperplasia of subserosal fat and mesenteric fat, corresponding to fat wrapping grossly, may also contribute to the strictures, and the extent of fat wrapping is correlated significantly with the degree of active chronic inflammation and extent of transmural lymphoid aggregates. Other histological abnormalities that have been observed in mesentery in CD include fibrosis, perivascular and perineuronal chronic inflammation, thickened lymphatic vessels, and small-sized adipocytes [175].

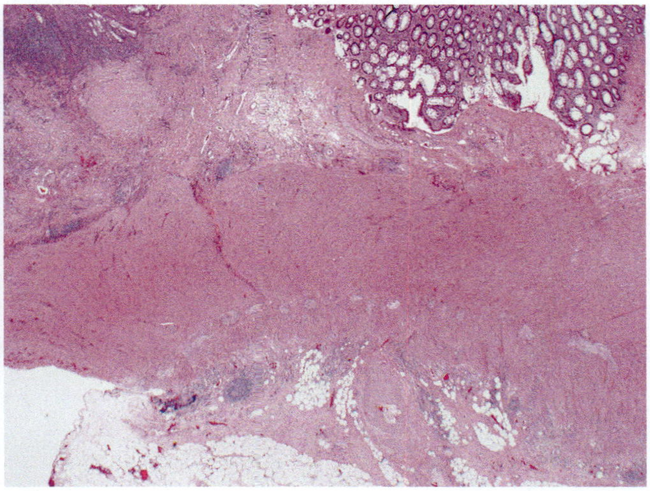

Fig. 15.35 Mural changes in Crohn's colitis. The colonic wall is thickened with fibrosis and hypertrophy of muscular layers. Note the obliterative muscularization of submucosa

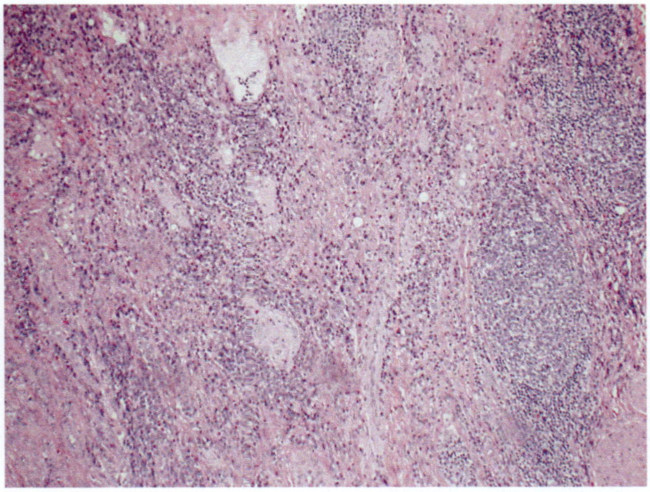

Fig. 15.36 Neural changes. There are increased numbers of nerve fibers and ganglion cells in submucosa, intermixed with dense mononuclear cell infiltrate and lymphoid aggregates

Neural changes Neural changes are common in CD, but they are not specific. There are patchy hypertrophy and hyperplasia of nerve fibers in submucosa and muscularis propria, with increased number of neurons, ganglion cells, and interstitial cells of Cajal (Fig. 15.36). These abnormalities are absent in uninvolved regions and can be used as a diagnostic feature for CD [108, 176].

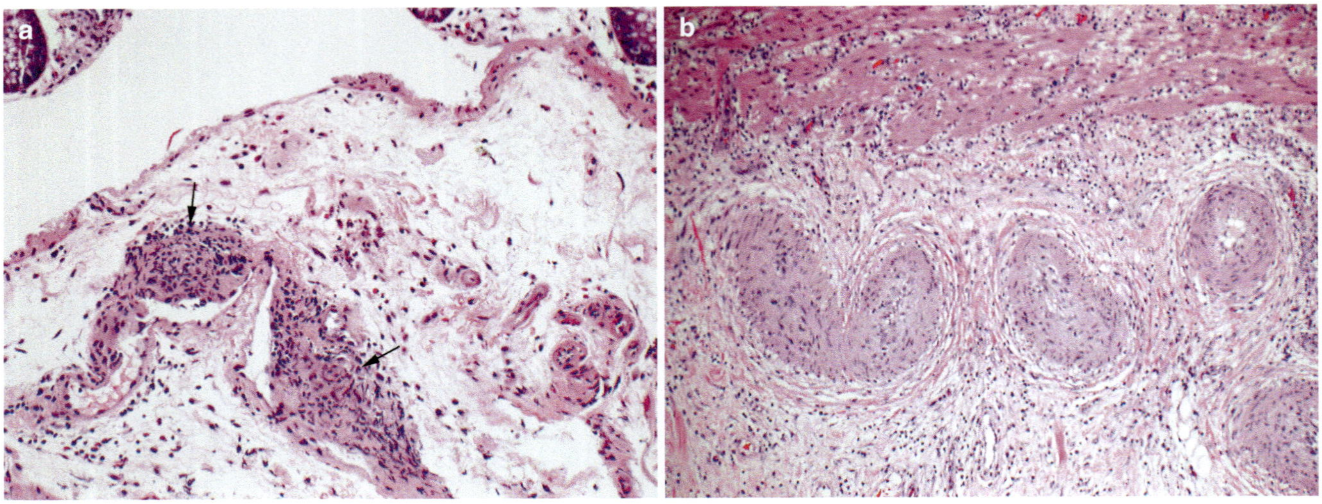

Fig. 15.37 Vascular changes. (**a**) Granulomatous inflammation (arrows) at perivascular area in submucosa. (**b**) Perivascular and intramural fibrosis, intimal proliferation, and obliterative changes

Vascular changes Granulomas associated with both arteries and veins are occasionally seen in CD. However, the granulomas are usually located at perivascular area without direct involvement of vessel wall and lumen (Fig. 15.37a). This is believed to represent a secondary phenomenon due to granulomas involving lymphatic vessels adjacent to blood vessels. Granulomatous vasculitis can occur in a small subset of patients with CD, which is also considered as a secondary change. Other abnormalities include perivascular and intramural inflammatory infiltrate, intimal proliferation, fibrosis of the vessel wall, or obliterative lesions (Fig. 15.37b) [177, 178].

Histological grade of disease activity There are no standard score systems for histologic assessment of disease activity in CD. Some score systems have been developed, but they are not validated and are mainly used for clinical trials, such as Colonic and Ileal Global Histologic Disease Activity Score which incorporates the number of segmental biopsy specimens affected with histological features including epithelial damage, architectural distortion, inflammatory infiltrate in lamina propria and epithelium, and presence of erosions/ulcers and granulomas [179]. We use the same classification system and criteria as being used in UC for evaluating disease activity of CD, i.e., inactive, mild, moderate, and severe activity. Of note, these methods only evaluate the mucosal activity which cannot reflect the transmural changes and discontinuous nature of the disease. In saying that, the microscopic assessment of disease activity in CD is difficult, and the correlation with clinical and endoscopic disease activity is weak.

Ulcerative colitis-like Crohn's disease (superficial Crohn's colitis) Approximately 15% of Crohn's colitis may show UC-like features, either with or without ileal involvement, known as UC-like CD or superficial Crohn's colitis [117, 118, 180], but others argue that superficial Crohn's colitis is rare because the lack of evidence of transmural changes is just due to inadequate sampling. UC-like CD commonly occurs in patients between 20 and 30 years old, which is significantly younger than patients with non-UC-like CD or true UC. It is defined as disease limited to the colonic mucosa or superficial submucosa without mural involvement. Apparently, this diagnosis can only be made on resection specimens, and some patients carry a preoperative diagnosis of UC and undergo an IPAA and then subsequently develop CD because of pouch failure or perianal disease. UC-like CD is different from indeterminate colitis (IC) because (1) UC-like CD is not associated with fulminant colitis, (2) careful gross and microscopic examination can reveal diagnostic features to classify the disease as CD, and (3) diagnosis of CD can be confirmed by involvement of other sites such as small bowel.

Grossly, the mural changes such as fissuring ulcers, sinus tracts, fistulas, strictures, or stenosis are absent; however, creeping fat may be present. The mucosa shows segmental or diffuse involvement, with a cobblestone appearance, ulceration, and pseudopolyps. Microscopically, there are no transmural inflammation and transmural lymphoid aggregates. The disease is more severe in proximal colon. The inflammation predominantly involves mucosa with extension to muscularis mucosae and superficial submucosa. The mucosa shows active chronic colitis, with alphthous ulcers or deep ulcers, but no deep fissuring ulcers. Prominent lamina propria neutrophils and lymphoid aggregates are present, which are helpful features for the diagnosis (Fig. 15.38). Granulomas can be seen in 40% of cases. Other findings such as muscularis mucosae and neural hypertrophy, perivascular lymphoid aggregates, submucosal fibrosis, pseudopyloric metaplasia, Paneth cell metaplasia in left colon, or mild serositis can be seen.

Treatment-related changes The histological changes to therapy in CD are less well studied. A few reports have focused on the effect of biological treatment and found improvement in the mucosal inflammation, but mucosal architectural changes persisted [181], similar to the treatment-related changes in UC. Histological healing may become a potential treatment target because several studies have suggested that it is likely to provide more valuable information for improving patient outcomes and reducing disease-related complications, even though the histological standard of assessing mucosal healing has not been well established yet. Most studies suggest that histologic mucosal healing should indicate completely normal mucosa, or absence of mucosal inflammation and epithelial injury, with residual crypt architectural distortion and/or atrophy. Little is known about the mural changes after medical treatment. Microscopic examination of extracellular matrix on biopsy samples may serve as a biomarker for intestinal fibrosis and predict response of anti-TNF therapy [182]. Anti-fibrotic therapies to prevent and even reverse fibrosis are under development [183].

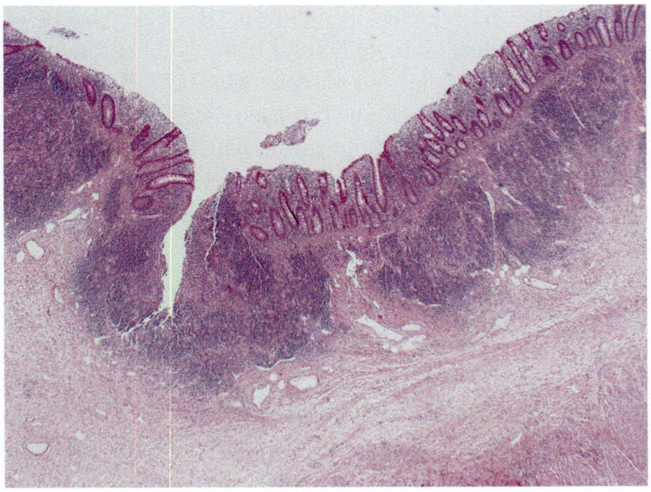

Fig. 15.38 Superficial Crohn's colitis. There is transmucosal inflammation and mucosal knifelike ulcer. The lymphoid aggregates/follicles locate at mucosal and superficial submucosa but not transmurally. This case is supported by involvement of terminal ileum

Colonic mucosal changes in CD without colonic involvement Biopsy of colonic mucosa is routinely performed during ileocolonoscopy when evaluating small bowel CD or undergoing surveillance for dysplasia, even with no clinical and endoscopic evidence of colonic involvement. Majority of the biopsy samples show normal colonic mucosa, but some cases may not be entirely normal. The colonic mucosa can show nonspecific reactive changes, such as increased numbers of mononuclear cells in the lamina propria and proliferative crypts, but there is no neutrophilic infiltrate or crypt architecture distortion (Fig. 15.39a). Focal active colitis (FAC) is occasionally seen in CD [184], which is characterized by a single focus of cryptitis or multiple separate foci of cryptitis in different pieces of tissue accompanied with increased inflammation in lamina propria, but no features of chronic changes (Fig. 15.39b). FAC is a relatedly nonspecific finding that can be seen in normal colon due to bowel preparation effect, irritable bowel syndrome, ischemia, infection, or drug such as antibiotic or NSAIDs-induced injury [185]. However, there is a higher incidence for pediatric patients with FAC to develop CD [186]. Isolated small granulomas may also present within morphologically normal mucosa (Fig. 15.39c). If the granulomas are found at a distance from crypts, they are strongly associated with a diagnosis of CD [104].

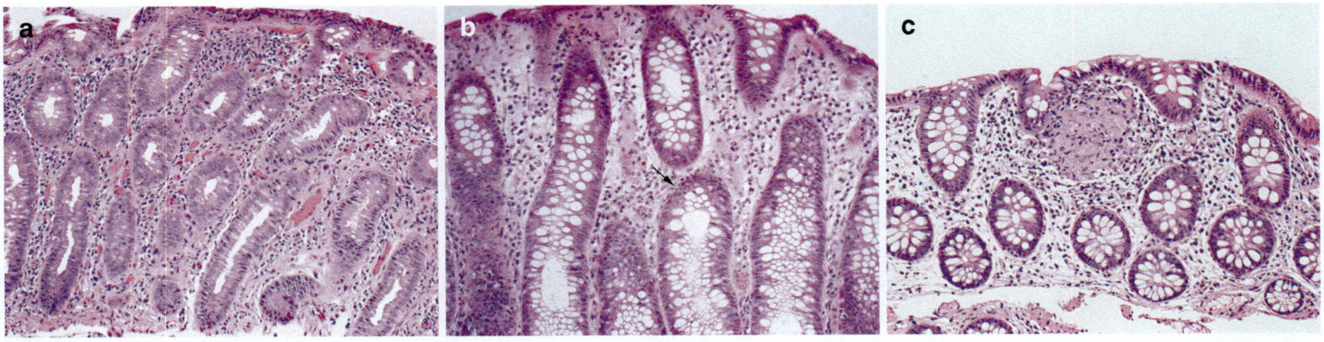

Fig. 15.39 Colonic mucosal changes in Crohn's disease without colonic involvement. (**a**) Reactive colonic mucosa with increased numbers of mononuclear cells in the lamina propria and proliferative crypts, but there is no neutrophilic infiltrate or crypt architecture distortion. (**b**) Focal active colitis. A single focus of cryptitis (arrow) within reactive colonic mucosa with no chronic changes. (**c**) An isolated small granuloma within morphologically normal colonic mucosa

Differential Diagnosis

The diagnosis of CD requires combination of clinical, endoscopic, radiological, and pathological assessment. The pathological diagnosis of CD can be well established in the majority of cases on resection specimens. However, on biopsy samples, the colonic mucosal changes in CD are those of active chronic colitis, with or without non-necrotizing granulomas, which are essentially indistinguishable from those in UC. A specific diagnosis of CD can be given on biopsy only when a case with an established diagnosis of CD or unequivocal evidence such as non-necrotizing granulomas with a proper clinical setting. The main differential diagnoses of colonic CD include UC, infections, granulomatous inflammation, chronic ischemia, DDAC, and Behçet disease. The different features of CD (including superficial Crohn's colitis) from UC have been discussed in the previous section. Differentiating CD from infectious colitis is similar to those in UC as well (also see previous section).

Granulomatous Inflammation

Although the presence of granulomas is a key feature of CD, it is not entirely specific. If the granulomas are associated with crypt injury, they are even less reliable. There are many conditions that can have granulomas in colonic mucosa, including infection (*Mycobacterium tuberculosis*, *Yersinia*, fungal, chlamydial, and parasitic), sarcoidosis, foreign bodies, chronic granulomatous disease, diversion colitis, cord colitis syndrome, and granulomatosis with polyangiitis. Granulomas in infectious colitis typically show necrosis, especially intestinal tuberculosis. Granulomas in tuberculosis are large, multiple, confluent, and with central caseating necrosis, in association with marked active chronic inflammation, mucosal damage, multinucleated giant cells, and ulceration (Fig. 15.40a). However, the granulomas can become hyalinized and calcified, and there is no necrosis in older cases. The diagnosis of tuberculosis is based on identifying acid-fast bacilli on special stains such as Ziehl–Neelsen stain (Fig. 15.40b). The organisms are usually located in necrotic areas or within macrophages. Acid-fast bacilli may only be identified in less than 30% of biopsies. Real-time PCR test is used in conjunction with histological examination, with a moderate sensitivity of 40–75%. Bacterial culture of biopsy tissue is the gold standard, but it takes 3–8 weeks to provide conclusive results [187, 188]. The epithelioid granulomas in sarcoidosis are more compact and well-formed than those in CD. In addition, the mucosa in sarcoidosis does not show the typical active chronic inflammatory changes of CD. In chronic granulomatous disease, the granulomas can be found in nearly 50% of colon biopsies, and they are microgranulomas with no necrosis. The mucosa also shows active chronic colitis. The significant eosinophilia and presence of pigmented macrophages in all levels of intestinal wall are helpful features for distinguishing chronic granulomatous disease from CD (Fig. 15.41) [189]. Cord colitis syndrome has been described in patients after cord blood stem cell transplant, which is manifested as active chronic colitis often with granulomas (Fig. 15.42). It may mimic IBD. However, the typical chronic changes in IBD such as basal plasmacytosis and significant crypt architectural distortion are not prominent in cord colitis syndrome. Mild surface epithelial injury and increased apoptosis are common findings in cord colitis syndrome [190, 191].

Diverticular Disease-Associated Colitis

Distinguishing CD from DDAC is even more difficult, because of segmental distribution and many CD-like histologic features in DDAC, such as transmural inflammation and lymphoid aggregates, fissuring ulcers, fibrosis, granulomas, and even granulomatous vasculitis (Fig. 15.25; also see Fig. 16.11b in Chap. 16) [129, 192–195]. In addi-

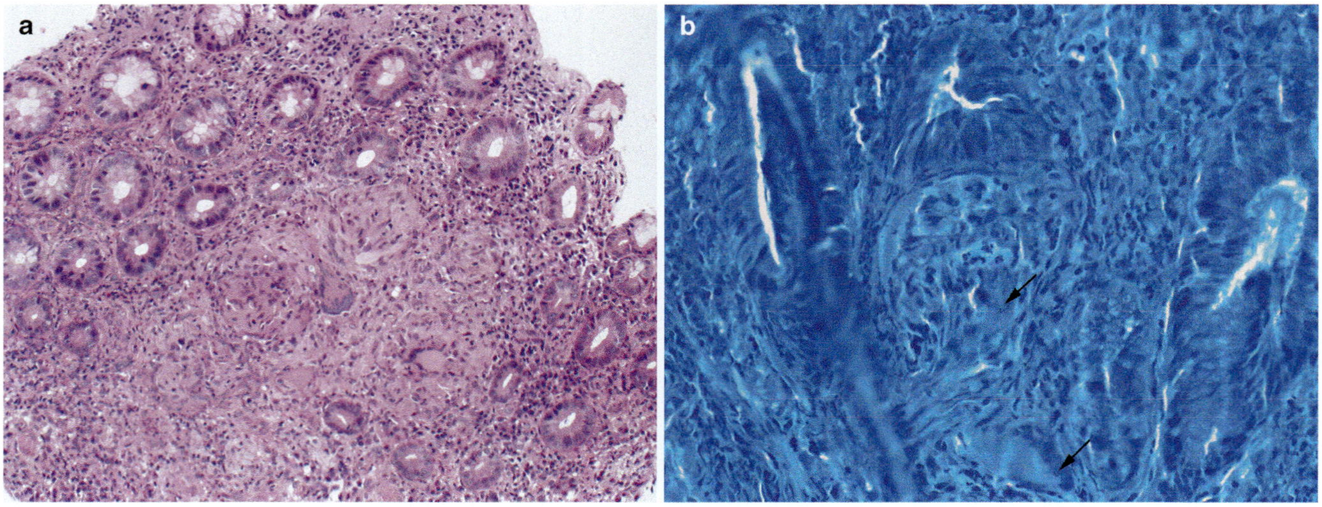

Fig. 15.40 Granulomas in tuberculosis. (**a**) Large, multiple, and confluent with focal necrosis and multinucleated giant cells. (**b**) Identifying acid-fast bacilli (arrows) on Ziehl–Neelsen stain

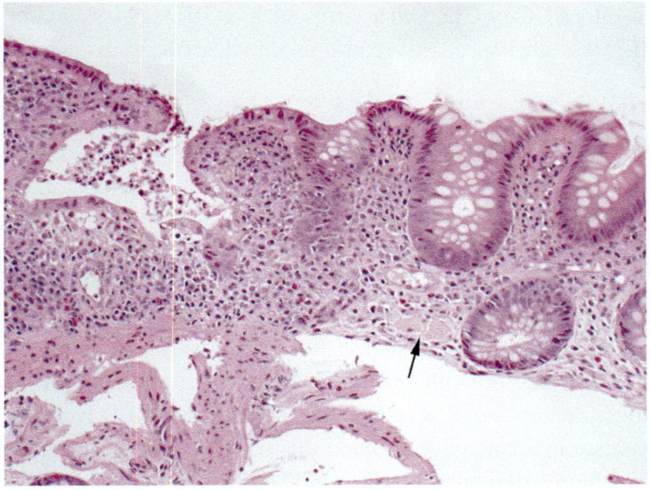

Fig. 15.41 Chronic granulomatous disease. The mucosa shows active chronic colitis with eosinophilia and pigmented macrophages (arrow)

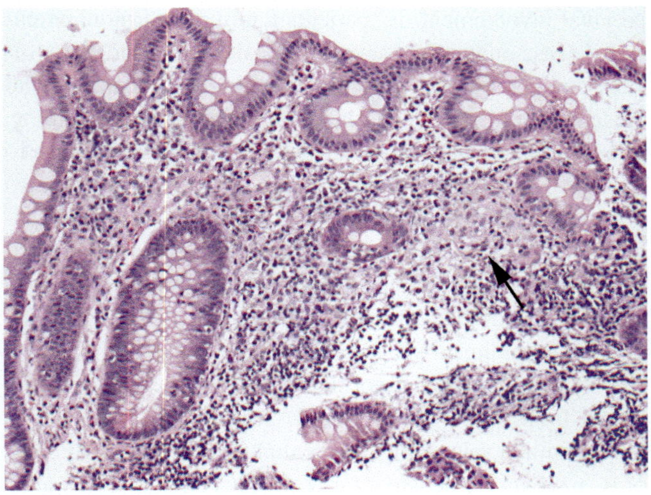

Fig. 15.42 Cord colitis syndrome. In this case, there is mild chronic colitis with a poorly formed granuloma (arrow), rare apoptosis, and lamina propria inflammation, but the crypt architectural change is not prominent

tion, DDAC and CD can also coexist in elder patients. The diagnosis requires endoscopic findings of diverticulosis and the disease distribution confined to segments involved by diverticular disease. Evidence of other site involvement and CD-like inflammatory changes in regions distant from diverticula favors CD over DDAC.

Behçet Disease

The differential diagnosis between CD and Behçet disease is mainly based on clinical findings because of many overlap features between them [196]. Ileocecal area is the most common location of intestinal Behçet disease. There are discrete single or multiple ulcers with crater formation. The mucosal changes are nonspecific. There are transmural inflammation and lymphoid aggregates in Behçet disease as well, but granulomas are absent (Fig 15.43a). The finding of necrotizing lymphocytic vasculitis in small veins and venules, with perivenulitis, intimal thickening, and thrombosis, can help the diagnosis, although they are not pathognomonic for Behçet disease (Fig. 15.43b).

Treatment and Prognosis

Medical therapy is the mainstay of treatment for patients with colonic CD. The use of 5-ASA is controversial because of the uncertainty of benefit in several studies of 5-ASA drugs in patients with colonic CD. Sulfasalazine can be used for the patient with mild to moderate symptoms, but it is not currently recommended because of a high incidence of side effects. Mesalazine has little effect in active colonic CD, but it can be topically used as an adjunctive therapy for left-sided colonic CD. Oral antibiotics can help for the induction or maintenance of remission in active colonic CD. Steroids remain as the first-line therapy, with immunomodulators as steroid-sparing agents for those who have relapsed. For

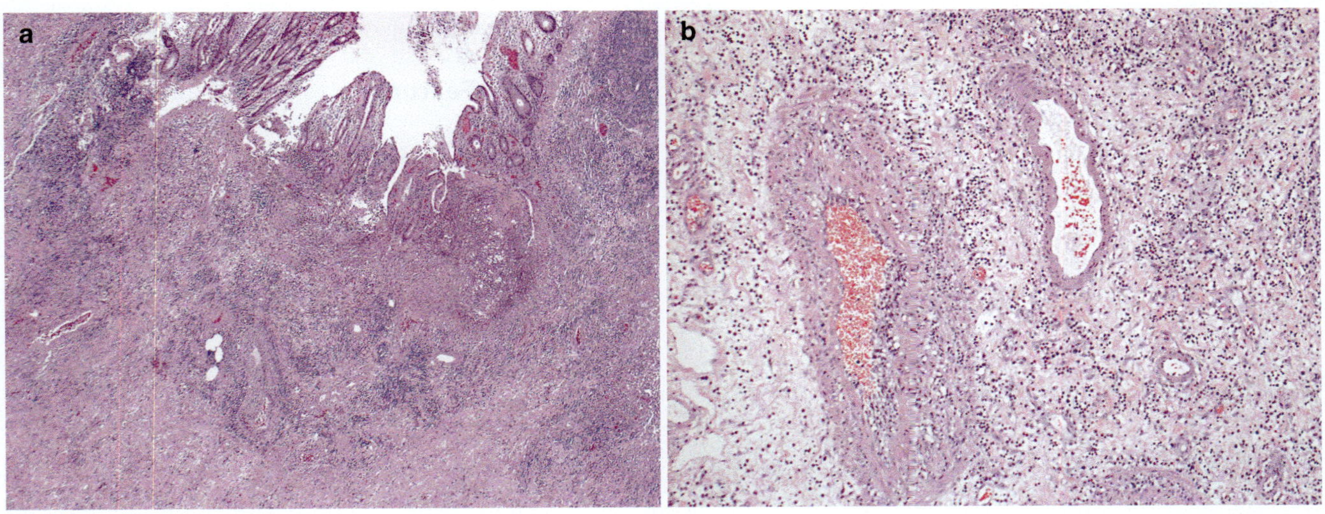

Fig. 15.43 Behçet disease. (**a**) The colon shows mucosal active chronic inflammation, transmural inflammation, scattered lymphoid aggregates, and discrete ulcer. (**b**) Focal necrotizing lymphocytic vasculitis involving small veins with perivenulitis, intimal thickening, and no granulomas, supporting the diagnosis of Behçet disease

steroid-refractory or steroid-dependent patients, anti-TNF therapy should be used if activity is demonstrated [197]. Nutritional therapy has a role in support for the malnourished patients and can help to induce and maintain remission.

Unlike UC, surgery is not curative for Crohn's colitis because of recurrence and involvement in other sites. The purposes of surgery are to provide palliation for the complications (stricture, fistula, and refractory diarrhea) or to manage emergent complications (perforation, fulminant colitis, and bleeding). Total proctocolectomy with an end ileostomy remains the gold standard for patients with Crohn colitis, but the recurrent rate can still be as high as 30% [198]. Total colectomy with an ileorectal anastomosis is possible for young patients with minimal rectal disease. Subtotal colectomy with an ileostomy is an option in emergency or in patients who are severely debilitated. Segmental or limited colonic resection is controversial in colonic CD. The advantage of this procedure is to avoid a stoma and to preserve the function. On the other hand, frequent recurrence which requires further surgeries and interventions is the main disadvantage. Properly selecting patients to balance between bowel function and likelihood of recurrence is crucial. At last, IPAA is contraindicated in patients with CD due to the high recurrence rates. Most patients with CD who undergo IPAA are diagnosed postoperatively. However, IPAA may be considered in highly selected patients who understand the risk and have no evidence of perianal or small bowel disease [199].

Like UC, CD is a chronic and lifelong disease with no known cure. The disease course varies significantly among different people ranging from being benign and experiencing just one episode to very severe and having continuous symptoms. The goals of treatment are to achieve and maintain remission to allow patients to function as normally as possible. About 10–20% of patients have long-term remission after the first flare. But up to 70% of patients will require a second surgery by 10 years after the initial resection. The recurrence rate is nearly 70%. The concept of remission is also evolving. Patients with CDAI <150 is considered as clinical remission, but other criteria including biological (CRP <10 mg/l), endoscopic, radiological, and histological remissions are increasingly required to define remission. Most patients with CD live a normal lifespan. There is a small increase in the risk of colorectal carcinoma in patients with long-standing CD [200]. Other malignancies have also been reported in CD, such as malignant lymphomas, which are likely related to immunosuppressants or biological agents [201].

Indeterminate Colitis

Definition

Indeterminate colitis (IC) is referred to as a small proportion of IBD patients with no unequivocal features to be subclassified as either UC or CD. Other terms such as IBD unclassified or IBD not other specified are also used to describe such cases.

Clinical Features

Approximately 5% of IBD cases with colon involvement may be diagnosed with IC, and the diagnosis rate can be up to 20% in pediatric IBD patients [202, 203]. IC is not a specific clinical entity. It was initially used by pathologists to give an interim diagnosis for those with overlapped UC and CD features or with insufficient clinical, radiologic, serologic, endoscopic, and pathologic information. Over the years, clinicians have adopted this term to describe patients in whom a diagnosis of UC or CD cannot be made based on standard clinical testing. Besides abdominal pain and diarrhea, the other UC- or CD-related clinical presentations are widely variable, such as rectal bleeding, rectal sparing, or perianal involvement. IC patients tend to have more extensive disease and a more severe clinical course, and a significant number of IC cases are diagnosed in patients who present with fulminant colitis and undergo urgent colectomy. The extraintestinal manifestations in IC are also similar to those in UC and CD. Colonoscopic findings in IC are also nonspecific. More importantly, endoscopic evidence of disease involving terminal ileum and upper gastrointestinal tract has been observed in UC, which is not reliable to distinguish UC and CD, especially in children [204, 205]. The radiologic findings in IC may show features of both UC and CD, but mesenteric abnormalities, abscesses, and fistula would favor CD over UC [206]. Serological markers may play a limited role in the differential diagnosis. Nearly 50% of IC patients are negative for both ASCA and pANCA antibodies, and majority of these cases remain indeterminate during their follow-up, while ASCA+/pANCA− can predict CD in 80% and ASCA−/pANCA+ can predict UC in 64% of patients with IC [74].

Pathological Features

By definition, the gross and microscopic examination on colectomy specimens of IC shows histological changes of IBD, but the distinction between UC and CD cannot be made due to overlapping features or absence of unequivocal findings to reach a definitive diagnosis. Macroscopically, the colon shows extensive severe colitis, but some cases demonstrate relative rectal sparing, and the others have a discontinuous disease pattern with extensive intermittent ulceration (Fig. 15.44). Both gross patterns would favor CD over UC, but microscopic examination of the spared rectum and unulcerated areas often shows mild abnormalities [207]. Microscopically, the uncertainty is mainly stemmed from the presence of fulminant colitis and findings of CD-like changes in a background of active chronic colitis, including skip lesions, transmural inflammation and lymphoid aggregates, fissuring ulceration, granulomas, and involvement of terminal ileum (Fig. 15.45a). In IC presented as fulminant colitis, besides extensive mucosal inflammation, ulceration, and necrosis, nonspecific or suppurative transmural inflammation can be present (Fig. 15.45b). The nonspecific transmural inflammation is usually beneath ulceration, with scattered mononuclear cells in submucosa and muscularis propria, a feature that can also be seen in both CD and UC. Furthermore, the surviving mucosa may only show mild inflammation without significant architectural distortion and depletion of goblet cell population, resembling skip lesions in CD. Transmural lymphoid aggregates can occasionally be seen in IC, which are typically focal and loosely formed. Multiple deep fissures in IC are common that have been descried as v-shaped clefts or "knifelike" fissures [207, 208]. The fissures are usually present in ulcerated areas and can penetrate up to the inner layer of muscularis propria. The fissures are sharply demarcated and covered by inflammatory cells. The adjacent surviving mucosa, however, may not show apparent changes of active chronic colitis. The typical deep fissures in CD, which are usually single, in non-ulcerated area, narrow, and deep into the muscle, can be present in about 10% IC. The fissuring ulcers in UC are typically superficial. However, even if these different features of fissures are well described, it is not always possible to separate them, and none of them is considered as disease-specific. Granulomas are usually absent in IC. The presence of well-formed epithelioid granulomas is strongly suggestive of CD. Small mucosal granulomas associated with inflamed or ruptured crypts can be seen in IC which have little value in differential diagnosis [209]. Careful examination of terminal ileum is critical in this setting. Microscopic evidence of active chronic ileitis, especially in those without significant ileocecal involvement and/or disease extension beyond a few centimeters in the terminal ileum, would favor CD. In the inactive phase of IBD, the histological changes may be minimal, and a specific diagnosis of either UC or CD may be impossible.

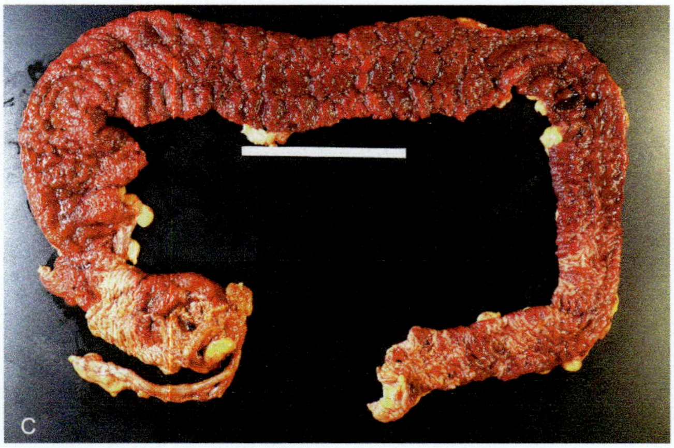

Fig. 15.44 Indeterminate colitis. The total colectomy specimen shows continuous involvement by severe active chronic colitis in most part, but patchy relatively normal appearing mucosa in the rectum (right end) and cecum (left end) that resembles "skip lesion" is present

The diagnosis of IC should not be made when evaluating endoscopic biopsy. The distinction of UC and CD is certainly impossible based on colonic mucosal biopsy, unless well-formed granulomas that are not associated with inflamed or ruptured crypts, epithelial damage, or foreign bodies, or definitive evidence of ileum involvement, can be identified for diagnosing CD. The superficial biopsy

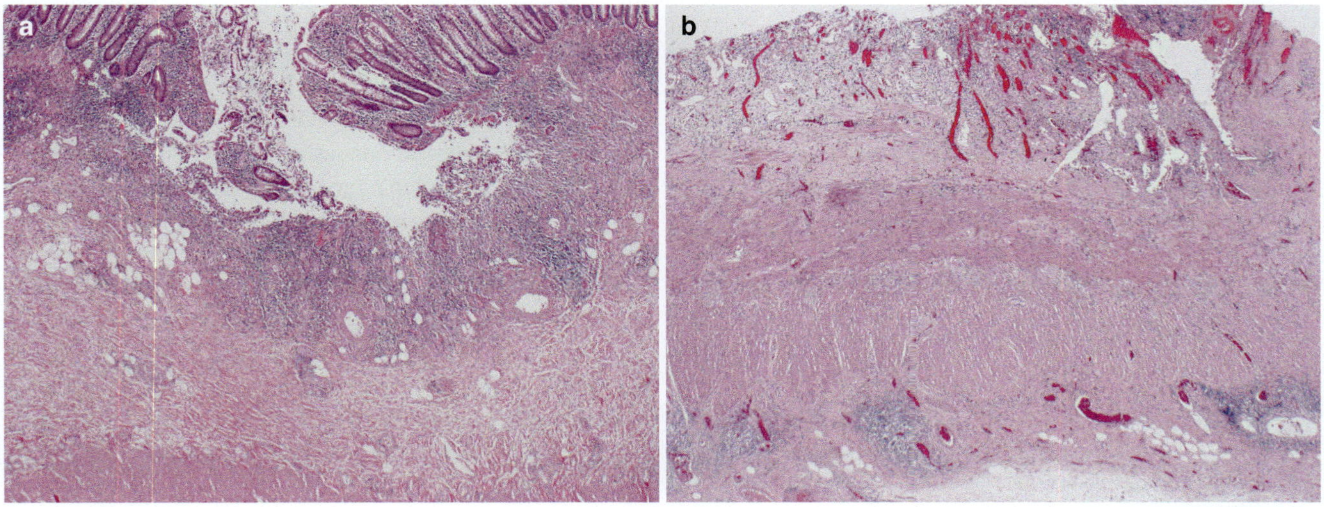

Fig. 15.45 Indeterminate colitis, showing overlap features of ulcerative colitis and Crohn's disease. (**a**) Active chronic colitis with ulceration. The inflammation and ulcer appear deep in submucosa with scattered lymphoid aggregates and submucosal fibrosis, but there are no granulomas or transmural inflammation. (**b**) Fulminant colitis with mucosal necrosis. Although there is no transmural inflammation, a few lymphoid aggregates are identified in the subserosal space

cannot reflect the depth of inflammation and the type of ulceration. The disease extent cannot be accurately determined due to uneven disease distribution, sampling issues, and treatment effect. On the other hand, in untreated patients who are not in fulminant phase, the preoperative biopsy may provide some information for the subclassification. In conjunction with endoscopic and radiologic findings, pathologists can suggest to favor UC or CD based upon the findings in biopsy.

Differential Diagnosis

Although an idea that IC is a third entity independent of IBD has been challenged because some IC patients remain indeterminate in the disease course, there are no sufficient data to support that IC is a unique type of colitis. Therefore, the first step in the differential diagnosis is to exclude other non-IBD colitis, mainly including infectious colitis, ischemic colitis, drug-induced injury, radiation colitis, or DDAC, which have been discussed somewhere else in this book. In the context of differentiating IC versus UC/CD, pathologists should be aware of the unusual features causing the confusion and diagnostic pitfalls leading to a false diagnosis of IC [210]. The common confounding factors that may lead to failure in subclassification are listed in Table 15.6. Insufficient histologic examination, failure in recognizing key diagnostic features of CD, and unawareness of unusual histologic features by pathologists are common reasons for misclassification. Even in fulminant colitis, comprehensive histological evaluation can accurately classify UC or CD in nearly 90% of cases [211]. On the other hand, there is significant disagreement in the pathological diagnosis of IBD, even among specialized gastrointestinal pathologists [212]. A second review may help confirm the diagnosis.

Table 15.6 Common confounding factors leading to a diagnosis of indeterminate colitis

Insufficient clinical, radiologic, endoscopic, and pathologic data
Failure in identifying diagnostic features for UC or CD
Fulminant colitis
Quiescent or inactive IBD with minimal histological changes
Early IBD
Treatment effect
IBD with superimposed conditions: CMV, ischemic, DDAC, or drug
UC with CD-like features: Rectal sparing, patchiness of disease, discontinuous pattern, backwash ileitis, granulomas, transmural inflammation, aphthous or fissuring ulcers, or upper GI involvement
CD with UC-like features: Colon involvement only, UC-like pancolitis, superficial CD, absence of granulomas

Treatment and Prognosis

Since the diagnosis of IC is typically made postoperatively, medical treatment of IC has not been established. Infliximab, tacrolimus, and 6-thioguanines have been tested, but it was difficult to determine the efficacy because there were a very small number of IC patients in the study group and many of them were subsequently diagnosed with UC or CD [213, 214]. The surgical procedure in most IC patients is a total proctocolectomy and IPAA. This procedure is a choice for patients for UC but not for CD, due to a higher rate of pouch failure in CD. The role of IPAA in IC patients is still controversial because of variations among different studies in terms of patient population and inclusion criteria. The average rate of pouch failure in IC is about 20%, which sits between patients with UC (10%) and those with CD (30–60%) [215]. However, if the CD patients were excluded in the studies, then the rates were similar between IC and UC [216–218].

Fulminant Colitis

Definition

Fulminant colitis is a clinical term of severe acute colitis with toxic symptoms and signs such as fever, distended and tender abdomen, severe bloody diarrhea, tachycardia, hypotension, and sepsis [219, 220]. Fulminant colitis usually refers to the most severe form of UC, but can also occur in Crohn's colitis, infectious colitis, ischemic colitis, or radiation colitis.

Clinical Features

Fulminant colitis is present in 5–20% of IBD patients [210, 220, 221]. Fulminant colitis occurs more commonly as the first manifestation of IBD and is less common in patients with a known history of chronic IBD [210]. A small subset of patients with fulminant colitis can have multiple organ dysfunction [222]. Marked dilatation (>6 cm in diameter) of the colon (toxic megacolon), most obvious in transverse colon but may also affect the entire colon, is frequently present in fulminant colitis [223]. A plain X-ray of the abdomen is usually diagnostic in patients with toxic megacolon. The incidence of toxic megacolon is about 1–10% in patients with UC and 2.3–6.3% in patients with CD [224–226]. The exact incidence of toxic megacolon in pediatric IBD in not known but is around 1–5% [223, 227].

Pathological Features

Diffuse mucosal ulcerations, inflammatory pseudopolyps, and fissuring ulcers are commonly present in fulmi-

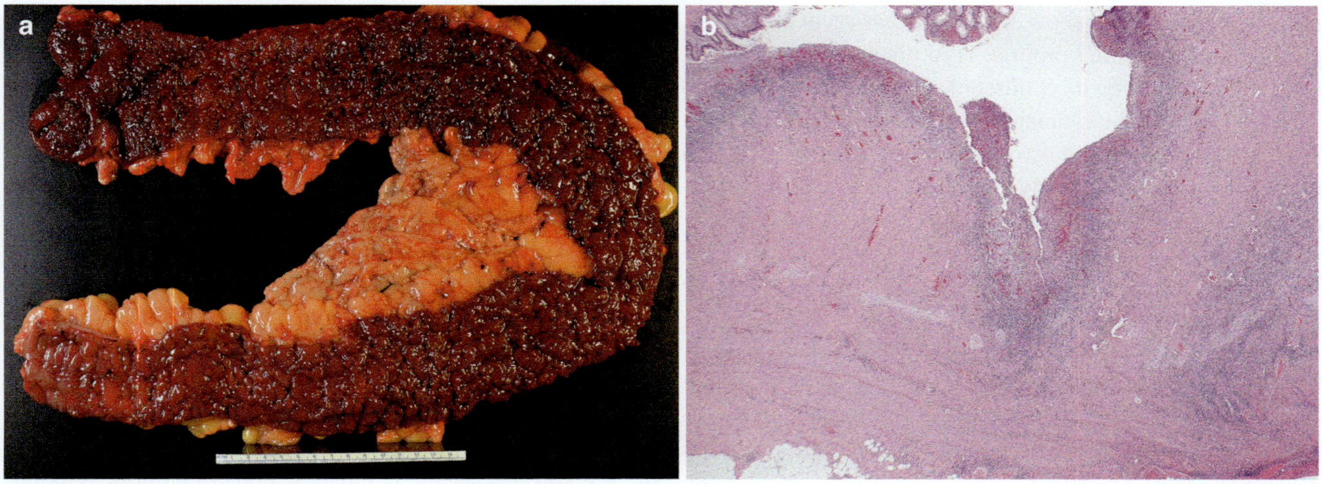

Fig. 15.46 Fulminant colitis. (**a**) Grossly, the colon shows marked dilation with mucosal ulceration, hemorrhage, and necrosis. (**b**) Microscopically, fissuring ulcer extending into the muscularis propria is present

nant colitis (Fig. 15.46a, b). In a clinicopathological study of colectomy specimens from 67 patients with fulminant colitis by Swan et al., 40 had UC, 16 had CD, and 11 had IC [211]. Non-necrotizing granulomas and transmural lymphoid aggregates are specific for the diagnosis of the fulminant CD. Fissuring ulcer and transmural non-aggregated inflammation are not specific for CD and can be present in fulminant UC [211, 228]. Patients with fulminant UC and fissuring ulcer have a higher risk of developing pouchitis after IPAA as compared to patients with non-fulminant UC patients [228]. Deep colonic ulceration is frequently present in megacolon, and perforation with subserosal fistula tracts resulting from deep ulceration can also occur [223].

Differential Diagnosis

Fulminant colitis can occur in UC or CD with superimposed infections of CMV and *Clostridium difficile*, or IBD mimics such as due to ischemic colitis, diverticular disease, radiation-induced injury, infections (*Clostridium difficile, Salmonella, Shigella, Campylobacter*, CMV, rotavirus, *Aspergillus*, and *Entamoeba*), and drug-induced injury [219, 221].

Treatment and Prognosis

The initial therapy for fulminant IBD and IBD-related toxic megacolon is intravenous steroids, and colectomy is reserved for patients not responding to medical treatment [219, 221].

IBD in Children

Approximately 7–20% of patients with IBD are diagnosed in their childhood, and the incidence varies with the studied populations and is highest among children younger than 15 years old [16, 229]. The study from Canadian providence of Ontario showed that pediatric IBD incidence increased from 9.4 per 100,000 children in 1994 to 13.2 per 100,000 children in 2009, and the increase was more frequently among children <10 years old [230]. The increase of pediatric IBD is mainly due to the increase in the diagnosis of pediatric CD, and the incidence of UC remains unchanged in the past few decades [230–232]. In general, UC is more common than CD in the preschool age group, and CD is more common than UC in the older children [233, 234]. There are also several studies showing that CD is more common than UC in pediatric population [230, 232]. Patients with pediatric IBD have more frequent family history of IBD (34%) than adult IBD (19.6%) [235]. Genetic predisposition to pediatric IBD has been identified including five new loci on 16p11 near the cytokine gene IL-27, 22q12, 10q22, 2q37, and 2q37 [236]. Distinct homozygous mutations in genes *IL10RA* and *IL10RB*, encoding the IL10R1 and IL10R2 protein, respectively, have been identified in patients with early-onset IBD [237].

Pediatric UC frequently have patchiness of histological features of chronicity (21%) and relative/absolute rectal sparing (25%) at initial presentation [238]. The initial rectal biopsy from patients with pediatric UC are less likely to show mucosal architectural distortion (32%) than adult UC (58%) and may be mistaken for acute self-limited disease [97]; however, other studies have demonstrated that histological features of chronicity are present in 98–100% of rectal biopsies in patients with pediatric UC [239, 240]. Colonic mucosal biopsies also show significant less crypt branching, plasma cells in lamina propria, cryptitis and crypt abscess, and epithelial injury in children ≤10 years of age than in adult UC [239]. Granulomatous inflammation in the duodenum and stomach can also present in pediatric UC with upper gastrointestinal involvement and should not be misdiagnosed as CD [241].

Pediatric Ulcerative Colitis

The incidence of pediatric UC ranges from 1 to 4 per 100,000/year in most North American and European regions and accounts for 15–20% of all UC patients [242]. In comparison to adult UC, patients with pediatric UC are more frequently presented with pancolitis (60–80%) which is twice often than adults, more frequent hospitalization for an acute severe exacerbation (25–30% over 3–4 years), and often underwent colectomy for medically refractory UC (up to 30–40% in 10-year follow-up) [229, 235, 242]. Children without diagnosis of pancolitis at initial presentation commonly have progression of disease to involve the entire colon during the follow-ups [229, 235]. The most common presentation symptoms for pediatric UC are bloody diarrhea and weight loss or lack of weight gain.

Treatment of pediatric UC is different from adult UC due to more often extensive disease and more aggressive disease course [243]. It is recommended virtually all pediatric UC should be treated with some maintenance therapy, and the 5-ASA requirement and dosing are often higher in children. A consensus guidelines for management of pediatric UC and acute severe UC from the European Crohn's and Colitis Organization (ECCO) and European Society for Pediatric Gastroenterology, Hepatology, and Nutrition (ESPGHAN) have been updated in 2018 [244, 245]. Colectomy is indicated in fulminant UC unresponsive to medical treatment, severe colitis complicated by toxic megacolon and/or perforation, and development of precancerous changes in pediatric UC. Rare colorectal cancers have been reported in pediatric UC patients [231, 246].

Pediatric Crohn's Disease

The reported incidence is around 4.8 per 100,000/year [232]. In pediatric CD, involvement of ileocolonic region is the most common pattern, followed by disease limited to the colon, and isolated terminal ileal disease is uncommon occurring in <10% of children [235, 247]. CD with involvement proximal to the terminal ileum in particular the duodenum and stomach occurs in more than half of the patients with pediatric CD [235]. Abdominal pain, diarrhea, and weight loss are the most common presentations for pediatric CD. Extraintestinal manifestations including skin manifestations, peripheral arthritis, uveitis, and axial arthropathies occur in 23% of patients at initial diagnosis and in 48% of patients during follow-up of pediatric CD [247].

In children and adolescents who have not finished their growth, exclusive eternal nutrition (EEN) is the induction therapy of first choice due to its excellent safety profile, which is preferable over corticosteroids to induce remission based on the consensus guidelines of ECCO/ESPHGHAN on the medical management of pediatric CD [248]. The majorities of pediatric CD require immunomodulatory-based maintenance therapy [248]. Like adult CD, surgical resection remains palliative and aims to control consequence of stricture and penetrating inflammatory complications of the disease while preserving as much as bowel length as possible [249]. The reported cumulative risk of surgery in pediatric CD is 20% at 3 years and 34% at 5 years [247].

IBD-Associated Disorders and Complications

Patients with UC have a 2.4-fold increased risk of developing colorectal cancer (CRC) [250], and PSC occurs in 3–25% of UC patients [66, 67]. The risk of CRC begins to increase 8–10 years after initial diagnosis of UC and requires colonoscopic surveillance [251]; and the probability of CRC in UC patients increases with the disease duration at 1–2% per year after 10 years, 1.6% at 10 years after, 8.3% at 20 years after, and 18.4% at 30 years after the initial diagnosis of UC [252, 253]. In patients with UC, anatomic extent of disease (patients with pancolitis at higher risk than left-sided and proctocolitis), younger age at onset of disease, longer duration of disease, PSC, and family history of CRC are associated with increased risk of CRC [251]. The CRCs in patients of UC are believed to occur through a stepwise progress from inflammation to dysplasia and carcinoma. Dysplasia is the best and most reliable marker of increased risk of CRC in UC patients [254, 255]. In patients with CD, the risk of CRC is similar to patients with UC [200, 253].

Dysplasia

Definition

Dysplasia (intraepithelial neoplasia) is defined as histologically unequivocal neoplastic alteration of colonic epithelium confined to basement membrane [254].

Clinical Features

The incidence of dysplasia in UC is difficult to estimate with an estimated 5% incidence 10 years after and 25% incidence 20 years after initial diagnosis of UC [202]. Dysplasia is present in more than 90% of UC patients with CRC, and can occur in any part of IBD colon but often at the location of cancer, and can occur as isolated focus, multiple foci, or rarely diffusely [202, 255–257]. In Crohn's colitis patients, the estimated 25-year risk of dysplasia ranges from 12% to 25% [258, 259].

Endoscopic surveillance biopsy It has been recommended in 2010 that at least 32 random biopsy specimens from all segment of the colon (covering <0.1% of the colonic surface area) should be taken during endoscopic surveillance for UC patients [253]. However, 32 random biopsies only provide 80% confidence to detect dysplasia involving ≥5% of the colon, and a more number of biopsies will be required for a higher confidence of detection rate [260].

Endoscopic features of dysplasia Dysplasia can occur as visible nodular lesion or without a lesion being visible (invisible dysplasia). The term "dysplasia-associated lesion or mass" (DALM) was first introduced by Blackstone et al. to describe that 7 of 12 UC patients with lesion or mass had CRC [261]. The term "adenoma-like polyp" has been used to describe polypoid dysplasia with a well-defined stalk similar to sporadic adenoma occurring in a colitic region of the colon in contrast to the flat dysplasia detected within the random biopsy from grossly unremarkable colonic mucosa [255]. However, recent studies of chromoendoscopy or high-definition white light indicate that invisible dysplasia accounts only 10% of patients diagnosed with dysplasia; and the majority (90%) of dysplasia is visible [7, 262]. In the recent SCENIC international consensus statement on the surveillance and management of dysplasia in IBD, it has been recommended that the terms DALM, adenoma-like, and non-adenoma-like should be abandoned [7]. A modified terminology from Paris classification [263] has been proposed to report finding on colonoscopic surveillance of patients with IBD. Dysplasia is separated into visible or invisible dysplasia. Visible dysplasia includes polypoid (pedunculated or sessile) (Fig. 15.47a–c) and nonpolypoid (superficial elevated, flat, depressed) with general descriptors for the presence or absence of ulceration and the status of border (distinct or indistinct) [7]. Endoscopically resectable lesion is defined as that (1) distinct margins of the lesion can be identified, (2) the lesion appears to be completely removed on visual inspection after endoscopic resection, (3) histological examination of the resected specimen is consistent with complete removal, and (4) biopsy specimens taken from mucosa immediately adjacent to the resection site are free of dysplasia [7].

Pathological Features

Histologically, dysplasia in IBD is classified as three categories: negative for dysplasia, indefinite for dysplasia, and positive for dysplasia (low and high grade), as proposed by Riddell et al. in 1983 [254] irrespective of the endoscopic features. The Vienna classification using "noninvasive low-grade or high-grade neoplasia" instead of low-grade or high-grade dysplasia has been proposed in 2000 [264] and is more commonly used in European countries and Japan but not in the United States.

Negative for dysplasia Colonic epithelium with reactive epithelial changes and epithelial atypia such as variation in the size and shape of cells and mostly with maturation of surface epithelium, which can be attributed to an inflammatory reaction or regenerative activity, should be classified as negative for dysplasia.

Indefinite for dysplasia Epithelial atypia such as nuclear stratification, enlargement, hyperchromasia, and absence of goblet cells mimicking low-grade dysplasia during active disease with active inflammation, ulceration, or tissue artifacts that is difficult to distinguish between reactive epithelial changes and dysplasia can be put into this category (Fig. 15.48).

Low-grade dysplasia Colonic crypts show villous or tubular configuration with epithelial atypia such as nuclear

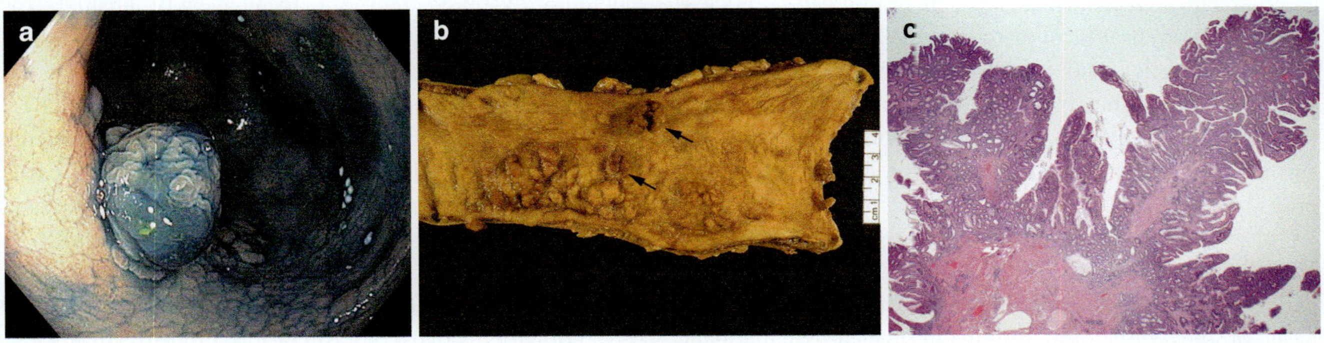

Fig. 15.47 Polypoid dysplasia. (**a**) Surveillance chromoendoscopy shows a polypoid lesion. (**b**) Multiple polypoid lesions (arrows) are present in a total colectomy for ulcerative colitis. (**c**) Histologically, the polyp shows low-grade dysplasia

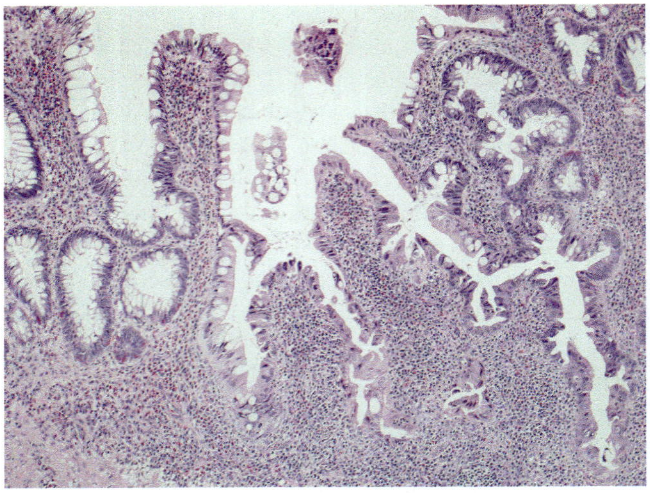

Fig. 15.48 Ulcerative colitis with indefinite for dysplasia. The colonic mucosa shows epithelial atypia with nuclear stratification and hyperchromasia predominantly involving colonic crypts in a background of mild active chronic inflammation

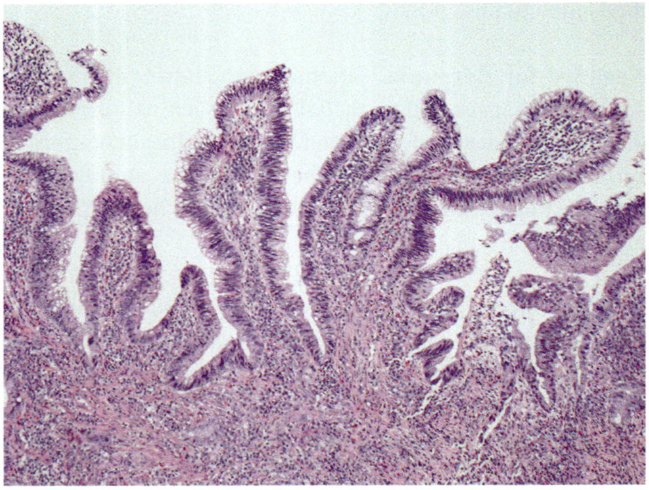

Fig. 15.49 Ulcerative colitis with low-grade dysplasia. Colonic crypts show villous or tubular configuration with nuclear enlargement, hyperchromasia, pleomorphism, and nuclear stratification (confined largely to the basal half of the cells)

enlargement, hyperchromasia, pleomorphism, nuclear crowding with stratification (confined largely to the basal half of the cells), and inverted (dystrophic) goblet cells, which is not attributable to inflammation or regeneration (Fig. 15.49). The dysplasia typically involves both crypt and surface epithelium, but rarely dysplasia can involve crypts only.

High-grade dysplasia Severe epithelial atypia such as nuclear stratification extending to the superficial (luminal) parts of the epithelium, prominent nuclear enlargement, hyperchromasia, pleomorphism, loss of nuclear polarity, and back-to-back or cribriforming architectural alteration may

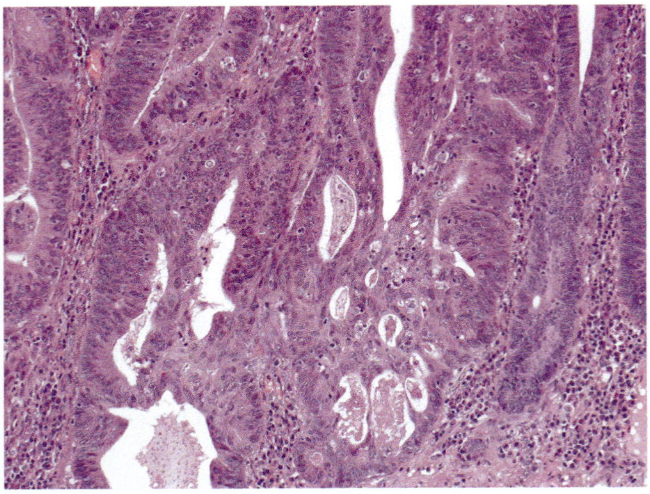

Fig. 15.50 Ulcerative colitis with high-grade dysplasia. The colonic crypts show nuclear stratification extending to the surface, nuclear enlargement, hyperchromasia, pleomorphism, loss of nuclear polarity, and focal cribriforming architectural alteration

also be present (Fig. 15.50). In each biopsy specimen, the presence of the highest grade of dysplasia determines the overall grade of the dysplasia.

There is significant interobserver variability in the interpretation of dysplasia for IBD in biopsy specimens. In general negative for dysplasia and high-grade dysplasia categories have fair level of agreement; and agreement on the indefinite and low-grade dysplasia categories is poor [265, 266]. Due to the significant interobserver variability in the diagnosis of dysplasia in IBD, molecular and non-molecular markers such as Ki-67, p53, sucrase-isomaltase, GLUT1, α-methylacyl-CoA racemase (AMACR), and sialyl-Tn antigen (STn) have been used as adjunct methods to aid in detecting dysplasia [253]. p53 is overexpressed in 33–67% of patients with dysplasia and in 83–95% of CRC in UC patients; however, p53 is also overexpressed in a small proportion of regenerating, non-dysplastic cases [267]. AMACR is expressed in low-grade dysplasia (96%), high-grade dysplasia (80%), and adenocarcinoma (71%), and only 14% of indefinite dysplasia foci are focal weakly positive for AMACR [268].

Treatment and Prognosis

There are only a few follow-up studies for UC patients with diagnosis of indefinite for dysplasia; and 2 of 7 cases progressed to advanced neoplasia (1 high-grade dysplasia and 1 CRC) after a mean 46.8 months of follow-up [269]. In another study of IBD patients (66 of 77 were UC patients) with diagnosis of indefinite for dysplasia, 23.7% (6/22) of patients had dysplasia (1 low-grade dysplasia and 5 high-grade dysplasia) on the surgical resection within 6 months of diagnosis of indefinite for dysplasia; and

25.2% (18/71) developed dysplasia (10 low-grade dysplasia and 5 high-grade dysplasia) and CRCs (3 cases) after a mean 98.6 months of follow-up [270]. The reported rates of CRC in resected dysplastic lesions (mainly low-grade dysplasia) ranged from 2% to 13% [7, 271–274]. Another recent reported rate from a systemic review of 10 studies for CRC developing in UC patients with resected polypoid dysplasia was 2.4% with an annualized incidence of 0.5% [275]. No studies regarding the natural history or incidence for CRC in resected nonpolypoid dysplasia in UC patients are available. After complete removal of endoscopically resectable polypoid dysplastic lesions, surveillance colonoscopy is recommended rather than colectomy; and for endoscopically resectable nonpolypoid dysplastic lesions, surveillance colonoscopy is suggested rather than colectomy [7].

In the past colectomy has been performed more frequently when invisible high-grade dysplasia is identified because of the associated higher risk of CRC. The rates of CRC developing after diagnosis of invisible dysplasia range from 3% to 9% [256, 273, 274]. A systemic review of 20 surveillance studies found that 18 of 81 (22%) UC patients with invisible low-grade dysplasia who undergo colectomy had CRC [276]. The reported rates of CRC in patients with invisible high-grade dysplasia undergoing colectomy ranged from 45% to 67% [7]. Currently, for patients with endoscopically invisible dysplasia (confirmed by a gastrointestinal pathologist), referral is suggested to an endoscopist with expertise in IBD surveillance using chromoendoscopy with high-definition colonoscopy to better identify any visible dysplastic lesions in the same region of the colon with invisible dysplasia for subsequent decisions regarding surveillance colonoscopy versus colectomy [7].

Mucinous Dysplasia and Serrated Change/Polyp

Mucinous dysplasia and serrated change/polyp are two morphological patterns distinct from the conventional dysplasia occurring in the setting of IBD.

Mucinous Dysplasia

An unusual dysplasia demonstrates a villous growth pattern with elongated and distended mucinous epithelium containing small, hyperchromatic, and basally located nuclei with mild cytological atypia (Fig. 15.51a, b) [171, 277, 278]. Mucinous dysplasia has also been termed as "villous dysplasia" or "villous hypermucinous mucosa" [277, 278]. The natural history of IBD patients with mucinous dysplasia is unknown. In the study by Rubio et al., mucinous dysplasia was present in 70% (14 of 20) patients of UC with CRC, but none in 20 UC patients without CRC [277]. *K-ras* mutation was more frequently present in mucinous dysplasia (61%) than in the conventional low-grade dysplasia (4%) [278].

Serrated Change/Polyp

Serrated epithelial change and serrated polyp including hyperplastic polyp (HPP), sessile serrated adenoma/polyp (SSA/P), traditional serrated adenoma (TSA), and serrated polyposis can occur in patients with IBD.

Serrated epithelial change A histological feature can be seen in patients with long-standing IBD. Serrated epithelial change is characterized by the presence of serrated epithelium throughout the entire crypt and distorted crypt architecture with crypts no longer extending down the muscularis mucosae (Fig. 15.52) [279, 280]. It has been previously described as

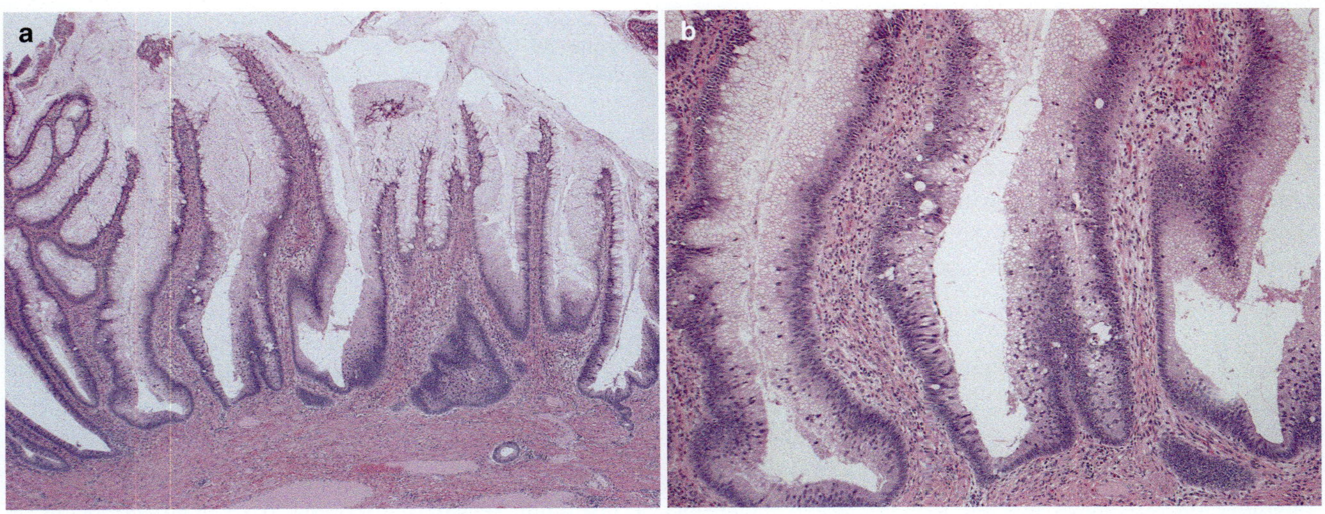

Fig. 15.51 Mucinous dysplasia (**a**) At low power view, there is prominent villous growth pattern with elongated and distended mucinous epithelium containing small, hyperchromatic, and basally located nuclei. (**b**) The mucinous epitheliums present at the base of the crypt show nuclear stratification with mild cytological atypia

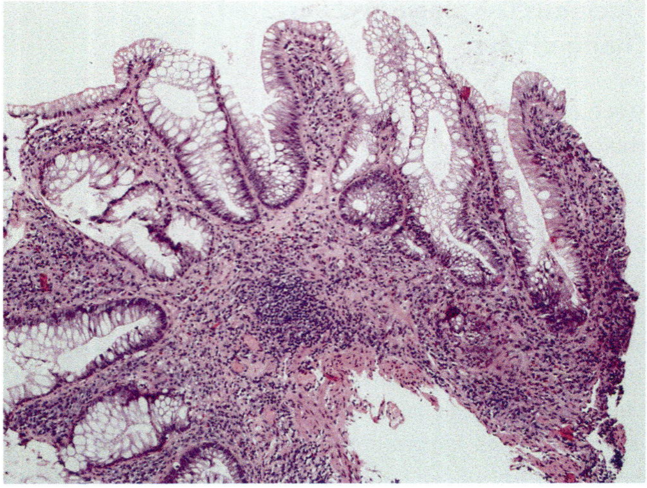

Fig. 15.52 Serrated epithelial change. Colonic mucosa shows distorted crypt architecture and serrated change throughout the entire crypt with crypts no longer reaching muscularis mucosae

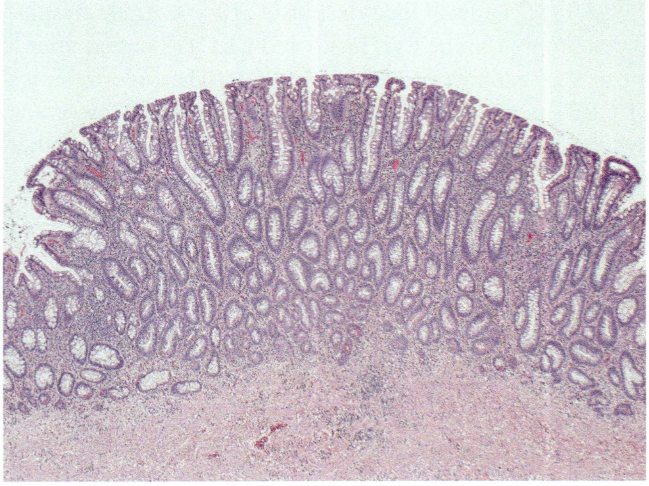

Fig. 15.53 Hyperplastic polyp. A polypoid lesion has morphological feature of hyperplastic polyp in background of inactive chronic ulcerative colitis

"hyperplastic-like mucosal change" in patients with CD [281]. The incidence of serrated epithelial change is around 10/1000 IBD patients [280]. Serrated epithelial change is typically found on flat mucosa, and when visualized serrated epithelial change is flat or nodular mucosa with a discrete polyp [282]. The presence of serrated epithelial change may increase the risk of CRC in IBD patients [282]. In a study of 79 IBD patients with serrated epithelial change by Johnson et al., the presence of serrated epithelial change was associated with other high-risk clinical features for developing CRC such as extensive disease, long-standing disease duration, and PSC [280]. Parian et al. studied 187 patients with serrated epithelial change, in which 21% had synchronous or metachronous dysplasia or CRC, and the rate of developing high-grade dysplasia or CRC was 17 per 1000 patient-years [279].

Hyperplastic polyp HPP present in IBD patients has similar histological features of sporadic HPP (Fig. 15.53). One study showed that HPP was frequently found in 97% of 115 IBD (65 UC and 50 CD) patients [283]. Synchronous multifocal visible dysplasia was present in 12% of IBD patients with HPP [284]. IBD patients with HPP have a very low risk of developing conventional dysplasia or CRC [283]. The HPPs associated with UC show similar genetic alterations to the sporadic HPPs [285].

Serrated polyp The overall prevalence of serrated polyp identified in IBD patients was 1.2% (78 of 6602); and within the 79 serrated polyps, 35 were negative for dysplasia (morphologically equivalent to SSA/P) (Fig. 15.54), 18 were indefinite for dysplasia, and 25 had low-grade dysplasia resembling TSA (Fig. 15.55) [286]. In another study the incidence of SSA/P was 1.39% and TSA was 0.31% in IBD patients [287].

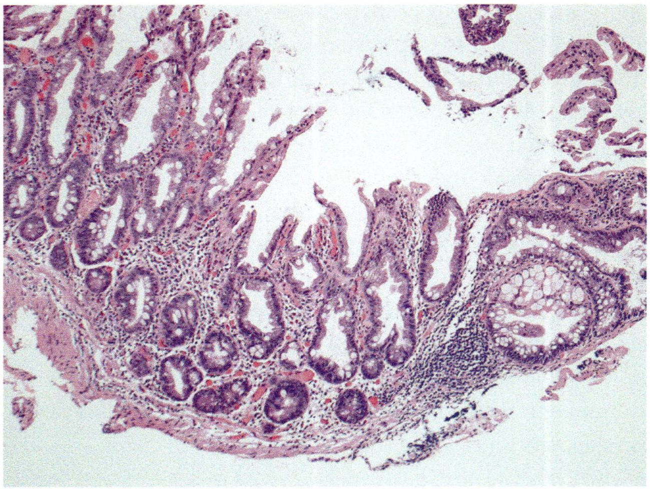

Fig. 15.54 Serrated polyp negative for dysplasia (sessile serrated adenoma/polyp). A serrated polyp shows crypt architecture distortion without epithelial dysplasia, resembling sessile serrated adenoma/polyp

Sessile serrated adenoma/polyp SSA/P tends to occur in females and in the proximal colon and has *BRAF* mutations [286, 287]. Synchronous dysplasia is present in 11–44% of SSA/P [284, 286]. Advanced neoplasia with high-grade dysplasia developed in 4% (1 of 27) of IBD patients with SSA/P during follow-up [286]. Metachronous visible conventional dysplasia was present in 5 of 13 IBD patients with SSA/P after a mean of 2.1 years after the initial diagnosis of SSA/P; and metachronous SSA/P developed in 3 of these 13 patients during follow-up [284].

Traditional serrated adenoma TSA tends to occur in male, in the distal colon, and has *K-ras* mutations [286]. Synchronous dysplasia is present in 76% of TSA [286]. Advanced neoplasia developed in 19% (4 of 27, 3 with high-grade dysplasia and 1 with CRC) of IBD patients with TSA during follow-up [286].

Serrated polyposis There have been 7 reported IBD patients (4 UC and 3 CD) with serrated polyposis [288, 289]. Histologically the polyposis consists of a mixture of HPP and SSA/P and occasional adenomas; and two of these patients had CRC [288, 289].

Superimposed Infection

CMV and *C. difficile* are the two most common superimposed infections occurring in IBD.

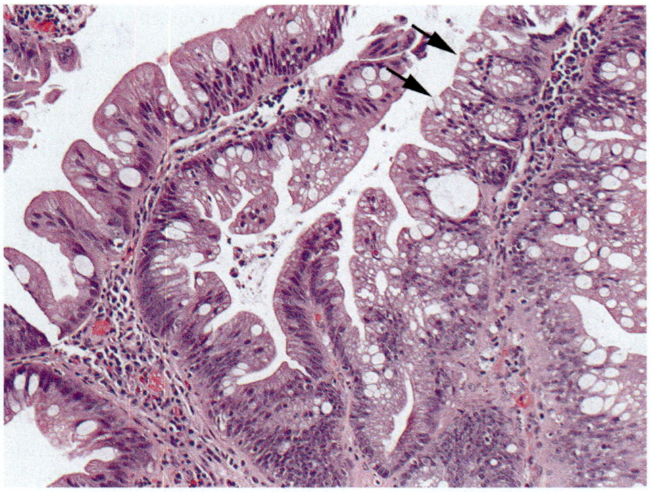

Fig. 15.55 Serrated polyp with dysplasia (traditional serrated adenoma). A serrated polyp shows ectopic crypt foci (arrows), eosinophilic cytoplasm, and low-grade dysplasia

CMV Infection

CMV reactivation is common in both adult and pediatric patients with severe or steroid-refractory UC [290–294]. CMV infection in colonic mucosa has been reported in 5–36% of steroid-refractory UC [291] and in 25% of colectomy for severe colitis [292]. Inflammation in the colon and long-term immunosuppressive therapy can reactivate latent CMV infection in patients with IBD. Local inflammation leads to secretion of proinflammatory cytokines including TNF-α, resulting in activation of CMV replication and migration of CMV-infected monocytes and macrophages in the inflamed tissue and propagating infection [295]. CMV disease is rare in CD, and this may be attributed to different cytokine profiles observed between UC and CD [296, 297].

The clinical presentation of CMV colitis may mimic UC flares and includes abdominal pain, diarrhea, and rectal bleeding. The risk factors for developing CMV reactivation include medically refractory IBD, endoscopic ulcers, and treatment with corticosteroids or immunomodulators but not anti-TNF-α [298]. Refractory disease, treatment with immunomodulators, and age older than 30 years are the independent risk factors associated with CMV disease [299].

Documentation of CMV in the colonic tissues by H&E section, immunohistochemistry, and PCR test for CMV DNA is the gold standard for diagnosis of CMV reactivation in patients with UC. There is no clinical role of measuring CMV antibodies unless CMV viremia is suspected. In the reactivation of CMV, IgG antibody levels do not change, and an increase of IgM antibody titers does not always occur [296]. The characteristic histological features of CMV inclusions are stromal cells larger than normal with intranuclear inclusions surrounded by clear cytoplasm and granular cytoplasmic inclusions (Fig. 15.56a, b). The sensitivity of detect-

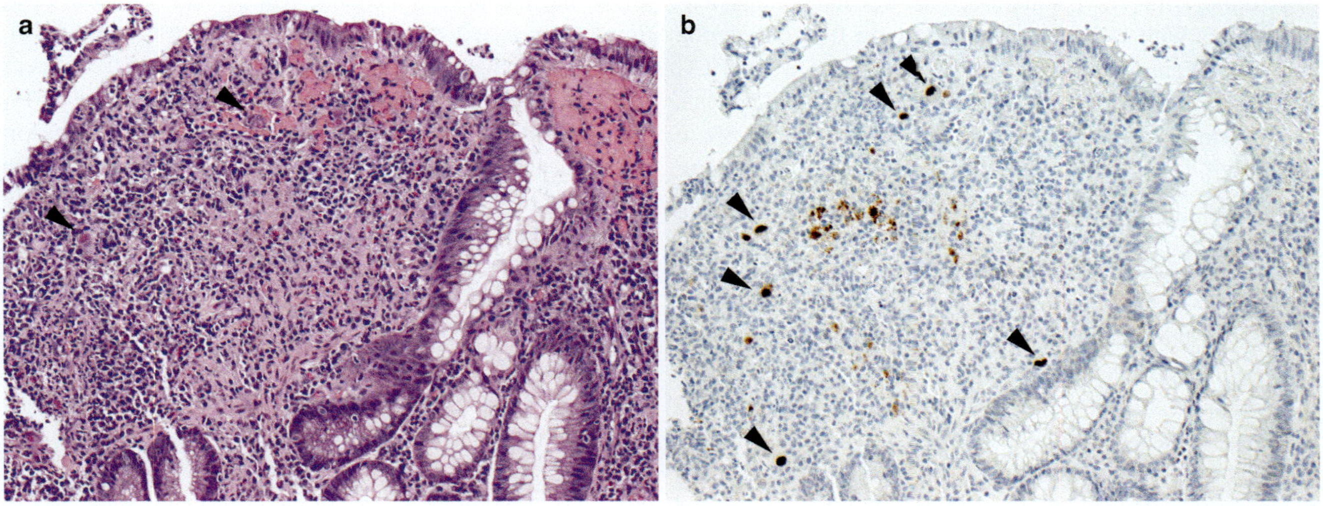

Fig. 15.56 Ulcerative colitis with CMV infection. (**a**) Multiple CMV inclusions (arrowheads) are present within the stromal cells in colonic mucosa with active ulcerative colitis. (**b**) Immunohistochemical stain for CMC highlights the CMV inclusions (arrowheads)

ing CMV viral inclusions on H&E sections can be as low as 10–87% and resulting false negative, and the sensitivity can increase to 78–93% by using immunohistochemistry with antibody to CMV early antigen [300]. Qualitative and quantitative PCR for CMV DNA from colonic tissue has high specificity (93–98.7%) as well as high sensitivity (92–96.7%) [300]. There is no established histological quantitative method for measuring CMV viral load in colonic biopsies from IBD patients. The CMV viral load can be separated into high (≥5 inclusions in a single tissue fragment) and low density (<5 inclusions in a single tissue fragment) based on the number of viral inclusions identified by immunohistochemistry in colonic tissue fragment [301].

The clinical outcome for UC patients with CMV reactivation appears to be worse than the patients without CMV activation, but it is not entirely clear whether CMV is a contributor or bystander [300]. The reactivated CMV infection can disappear without antiviral therapy [302]. Intravenous ganciclovir is the first line of treatment for CMV infection, and the reported remission rates following antiviral therapy were 71–86% [296, 300]. Patients with IBD and high density of CMV inclusions in the colonic biopsies can benefit from antiviral therapy, and they are less likely to require colectomy within 1 year of diagnosis, as compared to patients with low density of CMV inclusions and only showing modest improvement after antiviral therapy [301].

Clostridium difficile Infection

C. difficile is a gram-positive spore-forming anaerobic bacterium and can cause a highly transmissible disease through the fecal-oral route. *C. difficile* exotoxins can cause a spectrum of disease from mild to severe acute colitis, pseudomembranous colitis, and toxic megacolon [303]. Patients with IBD have a 4.8-fold increased risk of *C. difficile* infection as compared to non-IBD patients [304]. The incidence of *C. difficile* infection is increased in both adult and pediatric patients with UC and CD and is more frequent among pediatric patients. The incidence of *C. difficile* in adult UC inpatients ranges from 2.8% to 11.1%, in adult CD patients from 1% to 7.7%, and in pediatric IBD patients from 7.8% to 69% [305]. Recurrent *C. difficile* infection is also more common (32%) in IBD patients than non-IBD patients (24%) [306].

Reductions of gut microbial diversity and increase in proinflammatory species have been identified in patients with IBD, and this dysbiosis may play a role in increasing the risk of *C. difficile* infection in IBD patients [307]. The risk factors of developing *C. difficile* infection in IBD patients include IBD disease itself, recent hospitalization, and genetic and immunological factors such as an IL-4-associated single nucleotide polymorphism (rs2243250) and impaired ability to sustain and generate strong toxin-specific antibody and B-cell response [305]. *C. difficile* infection occurs more frequently in IBD patients with CMV reactivation (17.6%) as compared to IBD patients without CMV activation (8.3%) and is associated with poor outcomes [308]. Use of antibiotic, ongoing steroid, biological, or immunological therapy does not appear to increase the risk of *C. difficile* infection in IBD patients [305].

Asymptomatic carriers of toxigenic *C. difficile* can occur in IBD patients and have been reported in 8.2% of adult and 17% of pediatric IBD outpatients [305]. It is recommended testing for *C. difficile* infection for all acute flare in IBD inpatients with diarrhea [309]. In contrast to the non-IBD patients, the presence of pseudomembranes on colonoscopy is infrequent and is only present in 0–13% of IBD patients with *C. difficile* infection [310, 311]. The colonic biopsies demonstrate microscopic foci of pseudomembranes in only 44% of UC patient with *C. difficile* infection [312].

IBD outpatients with non-severe *C. difficile* infection can be treated with metronidazole, and IBD inpatients regardless of disease severity should be treated with vancomycin-containing regimen as the first-line therapy [303, 313]. *C. difficile* infection in IBD patients is associated with increased morbidity including increased length of hospitalization, excess mortality, subsequent escalation of medical treatment for IBD, and urgent colectomy [305]. Fecal microbiota transplant can be used to treat recurrent *C. difficile* infection in IBD patients [314].

Other Bacterial Infections

Campylobacter species including *C. curvus, C. concisus, C. sputorum,* and *C. jejuni* have been identified in 5% of UC patients [315]. *Edwardsiella tarda* can cause gastroenteritis and has been isolated from UC patients with relapse [316, 317].

Rectal Cuff Inflammation (Cuffitis)

Persisting columnar epithelium can be present in the anal canal in 20% resected pouch even after mucosectomy [318]. Inflammation within the retained rectal cuff (cuffitis) can occur in 13–15% of UC patients after ileoanal anastomosis [319, 320]. Dysplasia can develop within the retained rectal cuff in UC patients, and the reported incidence ranges from 0% to 3.3% [321–324]. Adenocarcinomas have also been rarely reported in the retained rectal cuff in UC patients [325, 326].

References

1. Wilks S. Morbid appearances in the intestine of Miss Bankes. Lond Med Gaz. 1859;2:264.
2. Colombel JF, Mahadevan U. Inflammatory bowel disease 2017: innovations and changing paradigms. Gastroenterology. 2017;152(2):309–12. https://doi.org/10.1053/j.gastro.2016.12.004.
3. Regueiro M, Rodemann J, Kip KE, Saul M, Swoger J, Baidoo L, et al. Physician assessment of ulcerative colitis activity correlates

poorly with endoscopic disease activity. Inflamm Bowel Dis. 2011;17(4):1008–14. https://doi.org/10.1002/ibd.21445.
4. Korelitz BI, Sultan K, Kothari M, Arapos L, Schneider J, Panagopoulos G. Histological healing favors lower risk of colon carcinoma in extensive ulcerative colitis. World J Gastroenterol. 2014;20(17):4980–6. https://doi.org/10.3748/wjg.v20.i17.4980.
5. Rutter M, Saunders B, Wilkinson K, Rumbles S, Schofield G, Kamm M, et al. Severity of inflammation is a risk factor for colorectal neoplasia in ulcerative colitis. Gastroenterology. 2004;126(2):451–9.
6. Gupta RB, Harpaz N, Itzkowitz S, Hossain S, Matula S, Kornbluth A, et al. Histologic inflammation is a risk factor for progression to colorectal neoplasia in ulcerative colitis: a cohort study. Gastroenterology. 2007;133(4):1099–105; quiz 340–1. https://doi.org/10.1053/j.gastro.2007.08.001.
7. Laine L, Kaltenbach T, Barkun A, McQuaid KR, Subramanian V, Soetikno R, et al. SCENIC international consensus statement on surveillance and management of dysplasia in inflammatory bowel disease. Gastroenterology. 2015;148(3):639–51. e28. https://doi.org/10.1053/j.gastro.2015.01.031.
8. Kaplan GG, Ng SC. Understanding and preventing the global increase of inflammatory bowel disease. Gastroenterology. 2017;152(2):313–21 e2. https://doi.org/10.1053/j.gastro.2016.10.020.
9. Benchimol EI, Manuel DG, Guttmann A, Nguyen GC, Mojaverian N, Quach P, et al. Changing age demographics of inflammatory bowel disease in Ontario, Canada: a population-based cohort study of epidemiology trends. Inflamm Bowel Dis. 2014;20(10):1761–9. https://doi.org/10.1097/MIB.0000000000000103.
10. Leddin D, Tamim H, Levy AR. Decreasing incidence of inflammatory bowel disease in eastern Canada: a population database study. BMC Gastroenterol. 2014;14:140. https://doi.org/10.1186/1471-230X-14-140.
11. Molodecky NA, Soon IS, Rabi DM, Ghali WA, Ferris M, Chernoff G, et al. Increasing incidence and prevalence of the inflammatory bowel diseases with time, based on systematic review. Gastroenterology. 2012;142(1):46–54 e42; quiz e30. https://doi.org/10.1053/j.gastro.2011.10.001.
12. Ng SC, Tang W, Ching JY, Wong M, Chow CM, Hui AJ, et al. Incidence and phenotype of inflammatory bowel disease based on results from the Asia-pacific Crohn's and colitis epidemiology study. Gastroenterology. 2013;145(1):158–65 e2. https://doi.org/10.1053/j.gastro.2013.04.007.
13. Victoria CR, Sassak LY, Nunes HR. Incidence and prevalence rates of inflammatory bowel diseases, in midwestern of Sao Paulo State. Brazil Arq Gastroenterol. 2009;46(1):20–5.
14. Edwards CN, Griffith SG, Hennis AJ, Hambleton IR. Inflammatory bowel disease: incidence, prevalence, and disease characteristics in Barbados, West Indies. Inflamm Bowel Dis. 2008;14(10):1419–24. https://doi.org/10.1002/ibd.20495.
15. Benchimol EI, Mack DR, Guttmann A, Nguyen GC, To T, Mojaverian N, et al. Inflammatory bowel disease in immigrants to Canada and their children: a population-based cohort study. Am J Gastroenterol. 2015;110(4):553–63. https://doi.org/10.1038/ajg.2015.52.
16. Cosnes J, Gower-Rousseau C, Seksik P, Cortot A. Epidemiology and natural history of inflammatory bowel diseases. Gastroenterology. 2011;140(6):1785–94. https://doi.org/10.1053/j.gastro.2011.01.055.
17. Takahashi H, Matsui T, Hisabe T, Hirai F, Takatsu N, Tsurumi K, et al. Second peak in the distribution of age at onset of ulcerative colitis in relation to smoking cessation. J Gastroenterol Hepatol. 2014;29(8):1603–8. https://doi.org/10.1111/jgh.12616.
18. Johnston RD, Logan RF. What is the peak age for onset of IBD? Inflamm Bowel Dis. 2008;14 Suppl 2:S4–5. https://doi.org/10.1002/ibd.20545.
19. Halme L, Paavola-Sakki P, Turunen U, Lappalainen M, Farkkila M, Kontula K. Family and twin studies in inflammatory bowel disease. World J Gastroenterol. 2006;12(23):3668–72.
20. Moller FT, Andersen V, Wohlfahrt J, Jess T. Familial risk of inflammatory bowel disease: a population-based cohort study 1977–2011. Am J Gastroenterol. 2015;110(4):564–71. https://doi.org/10.1038/ajg.2015.50.
21. Bernstein CN, Rawsthorne P, Cheang M, Blanchard JF. A population-based case control study of potential risk factors for IBD. Am J Gastroenterol. 2006;101(5):993–1002. https://doi.org/10.1111/j.1572-0241.2006.00381.x.
22. Gordon H, Trier Moller F, Andersen V, Harbord M. Heritability in inflammatory bowel disease: from the first twin study to genome-wide association studies. Inflamm Bowel Dis. 2015;21(6):1428–34. https://doi.org/10.1097/MIB.0000000000000393.
23. Liu JZ, van Sommeren S, Huang H, Ng SC, Alberts R, Takahashi A, et al. Association analyses identify 38 susceptibility loci for inflammatory bowel disease and highlight shared genetic risk across populations. Nat Genet. 2015;47(9):979–86. https://doi.org/10.1038/ng.3359.
24. Jostins L, Ripke S, Weersma RK, Duerr RH, McGovern DP, Hui KY, et al. Host-microbe interactions have shaped the genetic architecture of inflammatory bowel disease. Nature. 2012;491(7422):119–24. https://doi.org/10.1038/nature11582.
25. Parkes M, Barmada MM, Satsangi J, Weeks DE, Jewell DP, Duerr RH. The IBD2 locus shows linkage heterogeneity between ulcerative colitis and Crohn disease. Am J Hum Genet. 2000;67(6):1605–10. https://doi.org/10.1086/316905.
26. Consortium UIG, Barrett JC, Lee JC, Lees CW, Prescott NJ, Anderson CA, et al. Genome-wide association study of ulcerative colitis identifies three new susceptibility loci, including the HNF4A region. Nat Genet. 2009;41(12):1330–4. https://doi.org/10.1038/ng.483.
27. Schwab M, Schaeffeler E, Marx C, Fromm MF, Kaskas B, Metzler J, et al. Association between the C3435T MDR1 gene polymorphism and susceptibility for ulcerative colitis. Gastroenterology. 2003;124(1):26–33. https://doi.org/10.1053/gast.2003.50010.
28. Stokkers PC, Reitsma PH, Tytgat GN, van Deventer SJ. HLA-DR and -DQ phenotypes in inflammatory bowel disease: a meta-analysis. Gut. 1999;45(3):395–401.
29. Ahmad T, Marshall SE, Jewell D. Genetics of inflammatory bowel disease: the role of the HLA complex. World J Gastroenterol. 2006;12(23):3628–35.
30. Sartor RB, Wu GD. Roles for intestinal bacteria, viruses, and fungi in pathogenesis of inflammatory bowel diseases and therapeutic approaches. Gastroenterology. 2017;152(2):327–39. e4. https://doi.org/10.1053/j.gastro.2016.10.012.
31. de Souza HS, Fiocchi C. Immunopathogenesis of IBD: current state of the art. Nat Rev Gastroenterol Hepatol. 2016;13(1):13–27. https://doi.org/10.1038/nrgastro.2015.186.
32. Heller F, Florian P, Bojarski C, Richter J, Christ M, Hillenbrand B, et al. Interleukin-13 is the key effector Th2 cytokine in ulcerative colitis that affects epithelial tight junctions, apoptosis, and cell restitution. Gastroenterology. 2005;129(2):550–64. https://doi.org/10.1016/j.gastro.2005.05.002.
33. Di Sabatino A, Biancheri P, Rovedatti L, MacDonald TT, Corazza GR. New pathogenic paradigms in inflammatory bowel disease. Inflamm Bowel Dis. 2012;18(2):368–71. https://doi.org/10.1002/ibd.21735.
34. Geremia A, Jewell DP. The IL-23/IL-17 pathway in inflammatory bowel disease. Expert Rev Gastroenterol Hepatol. 2012;6(2):223–37. https://doi.org/10.1586/egh.11.107.
35. Sarra M, Monteleone I, Stolfi C, Fantini MC, Sileri P, Sica G, et al. Interferon-gamma-expressing cells are a major source of interleukin-21 in inflammatory bowel diseases. Inflamm Bowel Dis. 2010;16(8):1332–9. https://doi.org/10.1002/ibd.21238.

36. Fantini MC, Becker C, Tubbe I, Nikolaev A, Lehr HA, Galle P, et al. Transforming growth factor beta induced FoxP3+ regulatory T cells suppress Th1 mediated experimental colitis. Gut. 2006;55(5):671–80. https://doi.org/10.1136/gut.2005.072801.
37. Singh B, Read S, Asseman C, Malmstrom V, Mottet C, Stephens LA, et al. Control of intestinal inflammation by regulatory T cells. Immunol Rev. 2001;182:190–200.
38. Shen L, Su L, Turner JR. Mechanisms and functional implications of intestinal barrier defects. Dig Dis. 2009;27(4):443–9. https://doi.org/10.1159/000233282.
39. Anderson CA, Boucher G, Lees CW, Franke A, D'Amato M, Taylor KD, et al. Meta-analysis identifies 29 additional ulcerative colitis risk loci, increasing the number of confirmed associations to 47. Nat Genet. 2011;43(3):246–52. https://doi.org/10.1038/ng.764.
40. Wehkamp J, Harder J, Weichenthal M, Schwab M, Schaffeler E, Schlee M, et al. NOD2 (CARD15) mutations in Crohn's disease are associated with diminished mucosal alpha-defensin expression. Gut. 2004;53(11):1658–64. https://doi.org/10.1136/gut.2003.032805.
41. Duerr RH, Taylor KD, Brant SR, Rioux JD, Silverberg MS, Daly MJ, et al. A genome-wide association study identifies IL23R as an inflammatory bowel disease gene. Science. 2006;314(5804):1461–3. https://doi.org/10.1126/science.1135245.
42. Bernink JH, Peters CP, Munneke M, te Velde AA, Meijer SL, Weijer K, et al. Human type 1 innate lymphoid cells accumulate in inflamed mucosal tissues. Nat Immunol. 2013;14(3):221–9. https://doi.org/10.1038/ni.2534.
43. Andoh A, Sakata S, Koizumi Y, Mitsuyama K, Fujiyama Y, Benno Y. Terminal restriction fragment length polymorphism analysis of the diversity of fecal microbiota in patients with ulcerative colitis. Inflamm Bowel Dis. 2007;13(8):955–62. https://doi.org/10.1002/ibd.20151.
44. Chu H, Khosravi A, Kusumawardhani IP, Kwon AH, Vasconcelos AC, Cunha LD, et al. Gene-microbiota interactions contribute to the pathogenesis of inflammatory bowel disease. Science. 2016;352(6289):1116–20. https://doi.org/10.1126/science.aad9948.
45. Nishida A, Inoue R, Inatomi O, Bamba S, Naito Y, Andoh A. Gut microbiota in the pathogenesis of inflammatory bowel disease. Clin J Gastroenterol. 2018;11(1):1–10. https://doi.org/10.1007/s12328-017-0813-5.
46. Lakatos PL. Environmental factors affecting inflammatory bowel disease: have we made progress? Dig Dis. 2009;27(3):215–25. https://doi.org/10.1159/000228553.
47. Williams CN. Does the incidence of IBD increase when persons move from a low- to a high-risk area? Inflamm Bowel Dis. 2008;14 Suppl 2:S41–2. https://doi.org/10.1002/ibd.20562.
48. Wang YF, Ou-Yang Q, Xia B, Liu LN, Gu F, Zhou KF, et al. Multicenter case-control study of the risk factors for ulcerative colitis in China. World J Gastroenterol. 2013;19(11):1827–33. https://doi.org/10.3748/wjg.v19.i11.1827.
49. Nie JY, Zhao Q. Beverage consumption and risk of ulcerative colitis: systematic review and meta-analysis of epidemiological studies. Medicine (Baltimore). 2017;96(49):e9070. https://doi.org/10.1097/MD.0000000000009070.
50. Ananthakrishnan AN. Environmental triggers for inflammatory bowel disease. Curr Gastroenterol Rep. 2013;15(1):302. https://doi.org/10.1007/s11894-012-0302-4.
51. Cosnes J. Tobacco and IBD: relevance in the understanding of disease mechanisms and clinical practice. Best Pract Res Clin Gastroenterol. 2004;18(3):481–96. https://doi.org/10.1016/j.bpg.2003.12.003.
52. Odes HS, Fich A, Reif S, Halak A, Lavy A, Keter D, et al. Effects of current cigarette smoking on clinical course of Crohn's disease and ulcerative colitis. Dig Dis Sci. 2001;46(8):1717–21.
53. Higuchi LM, Khalili H, Chan AT, Richter JM, Bousvaros A, Fuchs CS. A prospective study of cigarette smoking and the risk of inflammatory bowel disease in women. Am J Gastroenterol. 2012;107(9):1399–406. https://doi.org/10.1038/ajg.2012.196.
54. Birrenbach T, Bocker U. Inflammatory bowel disease and smoking: a review of epidemiology, pathophysiology, and therapeutic implications. Inflamm Bowel Dis. 2004;10(6):848–59.
55. Zallot C, Quilliot D, Chevaux JB, Peyrin-Biroulet C, Gueant-Rodriguez RM, Freling E, et al. Dietary beliefs and behavior among inflammatory bowel disease patients. Inflamm Bowel Dis. 2013;19(1):66–72. https://doi.org/10.1002/ibd.22965.
56. Hou JK, Abraham B, El-Serag H. Dietary intake and risk of developing inflammatory bowel disease: a systematic review of the literature. Am J Gastroenterol. 2011;106(4):563–73. https://doi.org/10.1038/ajg.2011.44.
57. Rapozo DC, Bernardazzi C, de Souza HS. Diet and microbiota in inflammatory bowel disease: the gut in disharmony. World J Gastroenterol. 2017;23(12):2124–40. https://doi.org/10.3748/wjg.v23.i12.2124.
58. Magro F, Gionchetti P, Eliakim R, Ardizzone S, Armuzzi A, Barreiro-de Acosta M, et al. Third European Evidence-based Consensus on Diagnosis and Management of Ulcerative Colitis. Part 1: Definitions, Diagnosis, Extra-intestinal Manifestations, Pregnancy, Cancer Surveillance, Surgery, and Ileo-anal Pouch Disorders. J Crohns Colitis. 2017;11(6):649–70. https://doi.org/10.1093/ecco-jcc/jjx008.
59. Lutgens MW, van Oijen MG, van der Heijden GJ, Vleggaar FP, Siersema PD, Oldenburg B. Declining risk of colorectal cancer in inflammatory bowel disease: an updated meta-analysis of population-based cohort studies. Inflamm Bowel Dis. 2013;19(4):789–99. https://doi.org/10.1097/MIB.0b013e31828029c0.
60. Satsangi J, Silverberg MS, Vermeire S, Colombel JF. The Montreal classification of inflammatory bowel disease: controversies, consensus, and implications. Gut. 2006;55(6):749–53. https://doi.org/10.1136/gut.2005.082909.
61. D'Haens G, Geboes K, Peeters M, Baert F, Ectors N, Rutgeerts P. Patchy cecal inflammation associated with distal ulcerative colitis: a prospective endoscopic study. Am J Gastroenterol. 1997;92(8):1275–9.
62. Schroeder KW, Tremaine WJ, Ilstrup DM. Coated oral 5-aminosalicylic acid therapy for mildly to moderately active ulcerative colitis. A randomized study. N Engl J Med. 1987;317(26):1625–9. https://doi.org/10.1056/NEJM198712243172603.
63. Lewis JD, Chuai S, Nessel L, Lichtenstein GR, Aberra FN, Ellenberg JH. Use of the noninvasive components of the Mayo score to assess clinical response in ulcerative colitis. Inflamm Bowel Dis. 2008;14(12):1660–6. https://doi.org/10.1002/ibd.20520.
64. Turner D, Seow CH, Greenberg GR, Griffiths AM, Silverberg MS, Steinhart AH. A systematic prospective comparison of noninvasive disease activity indices in ulcerative colitis. Clin Gastroenterol Hepatol. 2009;7(10):1081–8. https://doi.org/10.1016/j.cgh.2009.06.024.
65. Duricova D, Burisch J, Jess T, Gower-Rousseau C, Lakatos PL, EpiCom E. Age-related differences in presentation and course of inflammatory bowel disease: an update on the population-based literature. J Crohns Colitis. 2014;8(11):1351–61. https://doi.org/10.1016/j.crohns.2014.05.006.
66. Olsson R, Danielsson A, Jarnerot G, Lindstrom E, Loof L, Rolny P, et al. Prevalence of primary sclerosing cholangitis in patients with ulcerative colitis. Gastroenterology. 1991;100(5 Pt 1):1319–23.
67. Saubermann LJ, Deneau M, Falcone RA, Murray KF, Ali S, Kohli R, et al. Hepatic issues and complications associated with inflammatory bowel disease: a clinical report from the NASPGHAN

inflammatory bowel disease and hepatology committees. J Pediatr Gastroenterol Nutr. 2017;64(4):639–52. https://doi.org/10.1097/mpg.0000000000001492.
68. Jorgensen KK, Grzyb K, Lundin KE, Clausen OP, Aamodt G, Schrumpf E, et al. Inflammatory bowel disease in patients with primary sclerosing cholangitis: clinical characterization in liver transplanted and nontransplanted patients. Inflamm Bowel Dis. 2012;18(3):536–45. https://doi.org/10.1002/ibd.21699.
69. Torres J, Pineton de Chambrun G, Itzkowitz S, Sachar DB, Colombel JF. Review article: colorectal neoplasia in patients with primary sclerosing cholangitis and inflammatory bowel disease. Aliment Pharmacol Ther. 2011;34(5):497–508. https://doi.org/10.1111/j.1365-2036.2011.04753.x.
70. Prantera C, Davoli M, Lorenzetti R, Pallone F, Marcheggiano A, Iannoni C, et al. Clinical and laboratory indicators of extent of ulcerative colitis. Serum C-reactive protein helps the most. J Clin Gastroenterol. 1988;10(1):41–5.
71. Turner D, Mack DR, Hyams J, LeLeiko N, Otley A, Markowitz J, et al. C-reactive protein (CRP), erythrocyte sedimentation rate (ESR) or both? A systematic evaluation in pediatric ulcerative colitis. J Crohns Colitis. 2011;5(5):423–9. https://doi.org/10.1016/j.crohns.2011.05.003.
72. Cioffi M, Rosa AD, Serao R, Picone I, Vietri MT. Laboratory markers in ulcerative colitis: current insights and future advances. World J Gastrointest Pathophysiol. 2015;6(1):13–22. https://doi.org/10.4291/wjgp.v6.i1.13.
73. Mitsuyama K, Niwa M, Takedatsu H, Yamasaki H, Kuwaki K, Yoshioka S, et al. Antibody markers in the diagnosis of inflammatory bowel disease. World J Gastroenterol. 2016;22(3):1304–10. https://doi.org/10.3748/wjg.v22.i3.1304.
74. Joossens S, Reinisch W, Vermeire S, Sendid B, Poulain D, Peeters M, et al. The value of serologic markers in indeterminate colitis: a prospective follow-up study. Gastroenterology. 2002;122(5):1242–7.
75. von Roon AC, Karamountzos L, Purkayastha S, Reese GE, Darzi AW, Teare JP, et al. Diagnostic precision of fecal calprotectin for inflammatory bowel disease and colorectal malignancy. Am J Gastroenterol. 2007;102(4):803–13. https://doi.org/10.1111/j.1572-0241.2007.01126.x.
76. Gisbert JP, McNicholl AG, Gomollon F. Questions and answers on the role of fecal lactoferrin as a biological marker in inflammatory bowel disease. Inflamm Bowel Dis. 2009;15(11):1746–54. https://doi.org/10.1002/ibd.20920.
77. Bunn SK, Bisset WM, Main MJ, Gray ES, Olson S, Golden BE. Fecal calprotectin: validation as a noninvasive measure of bowel inflammation in childhood inflammatory bowel disease. J Pediatr Gastroenterol Nutr. 2001;33(1):14–22.
78. Schoepfer AM, Beglinger C, Straumann A, Safroneeva E, Romero Y, Armstrong D, et al. Fecal calprotectin more accurately reflects endoscopic activity of ulcerative colitis than the Lichtiger index, C-reactive protein, platelets, hemoglobin, and blood leukocytes. Inflamm Bowel Dis. 2013;19(2):332–41. https://doi.org/10.1097/MIB.0b013e3182810066.
79. Kilcoyne A, Kaplan JL, Gee MS. Inflammatory bowel disease imaging: current practice and future directions. World J Gastroenterol. 2016;22(3):917–32. https://doi.org/10.3748/wjg.v22.i3.917.
80. Deepak P, Bruining DH. Radiographical evaluation of ulcerative colitis. Gastroenterol Rep (Oxf). 2014;2(3):169–77. https://doi.org/10.1093/gastro/gou026.
81. Duigenan S, Gee MS. Imaging of pediatric patients with inflammatory bowel disease. AJR Am J Roentgenol. 2012;199(4):907–15. https://doi.org/10.2214/AJR.11.7966.
82. Jacobs JE, Birnbaum BA. CT of inflammatory disease of the colon. Semin Ultrasound CT MR. 1995;16(2):91–101.
83. Rimola J, Rodriguez S, Garcia-Bosch O, Ricart E, Pages M, Pellise M, et al. Role of 3.0-T MR colonography in the evaluation of inflammatory bowel disease. Radiographics. 2009;29(3):701–19. https://doi.org/10.1148/rg.293085115.
84. Travis SP, Schnell D, Krzeski P, Abreu MT, Altman DG, Colombel JF, et al. Developing an instrument to assess the endoscopic severity of ulcerative colitis: the Ulcerative Colitis Endoscopic Index of Severity (UCEIS). Gut. 2012;61(4):535–42. https://doi.org/10.1136/gutjnl-2011-300486.
85. Travis SP, Schnell D, Krzeski P, Abreu MT, Altman DG, Colombel JF, et al. Reliability and initial validation of the ulcerative colitis endoscopic index of severity. Gastroenterology. 2013;145(5):987–95. https://doi.org/10.1053/j.gastro.2013.07.024.
86. Langholz E. Ulcerative colitis. An epidemiological study based on a regional inception cohort, with special reference to disease course and prognosis. Dan Med Bull. 1999;46(5):400–15.
87. Leighton JA, Shen B, Baron TH, Adler DG, Davila R, Egan JV, et al. ASGE guideline: endoscopy in the diagnosis and treatment of inflammatory bowel disease. Gastrointest Endosc. 2006;63(4):558–65. https://doi.org/10.1016/j.gie.2006.02.005.
88. D'Haens G, Sandborn WJ, Feagan BG, Geboes K, Hanauer SB, Irvine EJ, et al. A review of activity indices and efficacy end points for clinical trials of medical therapy in adults with ulcerative colitis. Gastroenterology. 2007;132(2):763–86. https://doi.org/10.1053/j.gastro.2006.12.038.
89. Kim B, Barnett JL, Kleer CG, Appelman HD. Endoscopic and histological patchiness in treated ulcerative colitis. Am J Gastroenterol. 1999;94(11):3258–62. https://doi.org/10.1111/j.1572-0241.1999.01533.x.
90. Joo M, Odze RD. Rectal sparing and skip lesions in ulcerative colitis: a comparative study of endoscopic and histologic findings in patients who underwent proctocolectomy. Am J Surg Pathol. 2010;34(5):689–96. https://doi.org/10.1097/PAS.0b013e3181db84cd.
91. Mutinga ML, Odze RD, Wang HH, Hornick JL, Farraye FA. The clinical significance of right-sided colonic inflammation in patients with left-sided chronic ulcerative colitis. Inflamm Bowel Dis. 2004;10(3):215–9.
92. Anzai H, Hata K, Kishikawa J, Ishii H, Yasuda K, Otani K, et al. Appendiceal orifice inflammation is associated with proximal extension of disease in patients with ulcerative colitis. Color Dis. 2016;18(8):O278–82 https://doi.org/10.1111/codi.13435.
93. Schumacher G, Kollberg B, Sandstedt B. A prospective study of first attacks of inflammatory bowel disease and infectious colitis. Histologic course during the 1st year after presentation. Scand J Gastroenterol. 1994;29(4):318–32.
94. Surawicz CM, Haggitt RC, Husseman M, McFarland LV. Mucosal biopsy diagnosis of colitis: acute self-limited colitis and idiopathic inflammatory bowel disease. Gastroenterology. 1994;107(3):755–63.
95. Jenkins D, Balsitis M, Gallivan S, Dixon MF, Gilmour HM, Shepherd NA, et al. Guidelines for the initial biopsy diagnosis of suspected chronic idiopathic inflammatory bowel disease. The British Society of Gastroenterology Initiative. J Clin Pathol. 1997;50(2):93–105.
96. Tanaka M, Riddell RH, Saito H, Soma Y, Hidaka H, Kudo H. Morphologic criteria applicable to biopsy specimens for effective distinction of inflammatory bowel disease from other forms of colitis and of Crohn's disease from ulcerative colitis. Scand J Gastroenterol. 1999;34(1):55–67.
97. Washington K, Greenson JK, Montgomery E, Shyr Y, Crissinger KD, Polk DB, et al. Histopathology of ulcerative colitis in initial rectal biopsy in children. Am J Surg Pathol. 2002;26(11):1441–9.
98. Tanaka M, Saito H, Kusumi T, Fukuda S, Shimoyama T, Sasaki Y, et al. Spatial distribution and histogenesis of colorectal Paneth

cell metaplasia in idiopathic inflammatory bowel disease. J Gastroenterol Hepatol. 2001;16(12):1353–9.
99. Symonds DA. Paneth cell metaplasia in diseases of the colon and rectum. Arch Pathol. 1974;97(6):343–7.
100. Simmonds N, Furman M, Karanika E, Phillips A, Bates AW. Paneth cell metaplasia in newly diagnosed inflammatory bowel disease in children. BMC Gastroenterol. 2014;14:93. https://doi.org/10.1186/1471-230X-14-93.
101. Shaoul R, Okada Y, Cutz E, Marcon MA. Colonic expression of MUC2, MUC5AC, and TFF1 in inflammatory bowel disease in children. J Pediatr Gastroenterol Nutr. 2004;38(5):488–93.
102. Borralho P, Vieira A, Freitas J, Chaves P, Soares J. Aberrant gastric apomucin expression in ulcerative colitis and associated neoplasia. J Crohns Colitis. 2007;1(1):35–40. https://doi.org/10.1016/j.crohns.2007.06.006.
103. Lee FD, Maguire C, Obeidat W, Russell RI. Importance of cryptolytic lesions and pericryptal granulomas in inflammatory bowel disease. J Clin Pathol. 1997;50(2):148–52.
104. Mahadeva U, Martin JP, Patel NK, Price AB. Granulomatous ulcerative colitis: a re-appraisal of the mucosal granuloma in the distinction of Crohn's disease from ulcerative colitis. Histopathology. 2002;41(1):50–5.
105. Cecinato P, Scaioli E, Leonardi F, Liverani E, Cardamone C, Rosati G, et al. A rare case of giant pseudopolyp and colitis cystica profunda coexistence in an ulcerative colitis patient. Rev Esp Enferm Dig. 2014;106(4):297–8.
106. Appelman H, Threatt BA, Ernest C, Lindernauer SM, Blamey W. Filiform polyposis of the colon: an unusual sequel of ulcerative colitis. Am J Clin Pathol. 1974;62:145–6.
107. Boulagnon C, Jazeron JF, Diaz-Cives A, Ehrhard F, Bouche O, Diebold MD. Filiform polyposis: a benign entity? Case report and literature review. Pathol Res Pract. 2014;210(3):189–93. https://doi.org/10.1016/j.prp.2013.11.001.
108. Geboes K, Collins S. Structural abnormalities of the nervous system in Crohn's disease and ulcerative colitis. Neurogastroenterol Motil. 1998;10(3):189–202.
109. Geboes K. Pathology of inflammatory bowel diseases (IBD): variability with time and treatment. Color Dis. 2001;3(1):2–12.
110. Rosenberg L, Nanda KS, Zenlea T, Gifford A, Lawlor GO, Falchuk KR, et al. Histologic markers of inflammation in patients with ulcerative colitis in clinical remission. Clin Gastroenterol Hepatol. 2013;11(8):991–6. https://doi.org/10.1016/j.cgh.2013.02.030.
111. Mosli MH, Feagan BG, Sandborn WJ, D'Haens G, Behling C, Kaplan K, et al. Histologic evaluation of ulcerative colitis: a systematic review of disease activity indices. Inflamm Bowel Dis. 2014;20(3):564–75. https://doi.org/10.1097/01.MIB.0000437986.00190.71.
112. Feagan BG, Greenberg GR, Wild G, Fedorak RN, Pare P, McDonald JW, et al. Treatment of ulcerative colitis with a humanized antibody to the alpha4beta7 integrin. N Engl J Med. 2005;352(24):2499–507. https://doi.org/10.1056/NEJMoa042982.
113. Geboes K, Riddell R, Ost A, Jensfelt B, Persson T, Lofberg R. A reproducible grading scale for histological assessment of inflammation in ulcerative colitis. Gut. 2000;47(3):404–9.
114. Lemmens B, Arijs I, Van Assche G, Sagaert X, Geboes K, Ferrante M, et al. Correlation between the endoscopic and histologic score in assessing the activity of ulcerative colitis. Inflamm Bowel Dis. 2013;19(6):1194–201. https://doi.org/10.1097/MIB.0b013e318280e75f.
115. Sandborn WJ, Tremaine WJ, Schroeder KW, Steiner BL, Batts KP, Lawson GM. Cyclosporine enemas for treatment-resistant, mildly to moderately active, left-sided ulcerative colitis. Am J Gastroenterol. 1993;88(5):640–5.
116. Gramlich T, Petras RE. Pathology of inflammatory bowel disease. Semin Pediatr Surg. 2007;16(3):154–63. https://doi.org/10.1053/j.sempedsurg.2007.04.005.
117. Soucy G, Wang HH, Farraye FA, Schmidt JF, Farris AB, Lauwers GY, et al. Clinical and pathological analysis of colonic Crohn's disease, including a subgroup with ulcerative colitis-like features. Mod Pathol. 2012;25(2):295–307. https://doi.org/10.1038/modpathol.2011.120.
118. James SD, Wise PE, Zuluaga-Toro T, Schwartz DA, Washington MK, Shi C. Identification of pathologic features associated with "ulcerative colitis-like" Crohn's disease. World J Gastroenterol. 2014;20(36):13139–45. https://doi.org/10.3748/wjg.v20.i36.13139.
119. Klein A, Eliakim R. Non steroidal anti-inflammatory drugs and inflammatory bowel disease. Pharmaceuticals (Basel). 2010;3(4):1084–92. https://doi.org/10.3390/ph3041084.
120. Papadimitriou JC, Cangro CB, Lustberg A, Khaled A, Nogueira J, Wiland A, et al. Histologic features of mycophenolate mofetil-related colitis: a graft-versus-host disease-like pattern. Int J Surg Pathol. 2003;11(4):295–302. https://doi.org/10.1177/106689690301100406.
121. Parfitt JR, Jayakumar S, Driman DK. Mycophenolate mofetil-related gastrointestinal mucosal injury: variable injury patterns, including graft-versus-host disease-like changes. Am J Surg Pathol. 2008;32(9):1367–72.
122. Chen JH, Pezhouh MK, Lauwers GY, Masia R. Histopathologic features of colitis due to immunotherapy with anti-PD-1 antibodies. Am J Surg Pathol. 2017;41(5):643–54. https://doi.org/10.1097/PAS.0000000000000829.
123. Ayata G, Ithamukkala S, Sapp H, Shaz BH, Brien TP, Wang HH, et al. Prevalence and significance of inflammatory bowel disease-like morphologic features in collagenous and lymphocytic colitis. Am J Surg Pathol. 2002;26(11):1414–23.
124. Wang HH, Owings DV, Antonioli DA, Goldman H. Increased subepithelial collagen deposition is not specific for collagenous colitis. Mod Pathol. 1988;1(5):329–35.
125. Giardiello FM, Jackson FW, Lazenby AJ. Metachronous occurrence of collagenous colitis and ulcerative colitis. Gut. 1991;32(4):447–9.
126. Akram S, Murray JA, Pardi DS, Alexander GL, Schaffner JA, Russo PA, et al. Adult autoimmune enteropathy: Mayo Clinic Rochester experience. Clin Gastroenterol Hepatol. 2007;5(11):1282–90; quiz 45. https://doi.org/10.1016/j.cgh.2007.05.013.
127. Masia R, Peyton S, Lauwers GY, Brown I. Gastrointestinal biopsy findings of autoimmune enteropathy: a review of 25 cases. Am J Surg Pathol. 2014;38(10):1319–29. https://doi.org/10.1097/PAS.0000000000000317.
128. Schembri J, Bonello J, Christodoulou DK, Katsanos KH, Ellul P. Segmental colitis associated with diverticulosis: is it the coexistence of colonic diverticulosis and inflammatory bowel disease? Ann Gastroenterol. 2017;30(3):257–61. https://doi.org/10.20524/aog.2017.0126.
129. Tursi A, Elisei W, Brandimarte G, Giorgetti GM, Lecca PG, Di Cesare L, et al. The endoscopic spectrum of segmental colitis associated with diverticulosis. Color Dis. 2010;12(5):464–70. https://doi.org/10.1111/j.1463-1318.2009.01969.x.
130. Ho EY, Cominelli F, Katz J. Ulcerative colitis: what is the optimal treatment goal and how do we achieve it? Curr Treat Options Gastroenterol. 2015;13(1):130–42. https://doi.org/10.1007/s11938-014-0044-5.
131. Harbord M, Eliakim R, Bettenworth D, Karmiris K, Katsanos K, Kopylov U, et al. Third European Evidence-based Consensus on Diagnosis and Management of Ulcerative Colitis. Part 2: Current Management. J Crohns Colitis. 2017;11(7):769–84. https://doi.org/10.1093/ecco-jcc/jjx009.
132. Colombel JF, Narula N, Peyrin-Biroulet L. Management strategies to improve outcomes of patients with inflammatory bowel diseases. Gastroenterology. 2017;152(2):351–61 e5. https://doi.org/10.1053/j.gastro.2016.09.046.

133. Baars JE, Nuij VJ, Oldenburg B, Kuipers EJ, van der Woude CJ. Majority of patients with inflammatory bowel disease in clinical remission have mucosal inflammation. Inflamm Bowel Dis. 2012;18(9):1634–40. https://doi.org/10.1002/ibd.21925.
134. Ford AC, Achkar JP, Khan KJ, Kane SV, Talley NJ, Marshall JK, et al. Efficacy of 5-aminosalicylates in ulcerative colitis: systematic review and meta-analysis. Am J Gastroenterol. 2011;106(4):601–16. https://doi.org/10.1038/ajg.2011.67.
135. Danese S, Fiorino G, Peyrin-Biroulet L, Lucenteforte E, Virgili G, Moja L, et al. Biological agents for moderately to severely active ulcerative colitis: a systematic review and network meta-analysis. Ann Intern Med. 2014;160(10):704–11. https://doi.org/10.7326/M13-2403.
136. Stidham RW, Lee TC, Higgins PD, Deshpande AR, Sussman DA, Singal AG, et al. Systematic review with network meta-analysis: the efficacy of anti-tumour necrosis factor-alpha agents for the treatment of ulcerative colitis. Aliment Pharmacol Ther. 2014;39(7):660–71. https://doi.org/10.1111/apt.12644.
137. Gumaste V, Sachar DB, Greenstein AJ. Benign and malignant colorectal strictures in ulcerative colitis. Gut. 1992;33(7):938–41.
138. Castano-Milla C, Chaparro M, Gisbert JP. Systematic review with meta-analysis: the declining risk of colorectal cancer in ulcerative colitis. Aliment Pharmacol Ther. 2014;39(7):645–59. https://doi.org/10.1111/apt.12651.
139. Selinger CP, Leong RW. Mortality from inflammatory bowel diseases. Inflamm Bowel Dis. 2012;18(8):1566–72. https://doi.org/10.1002/ibd.22871.
140. Malik TA. Inflammatory bowel disease: historical perspective, epidemiology, and risk factors. Surg Clin North Am. 2015;95(6):1105–22, v. https://doi.org/10.1016/j.suc.2015.07.006.
141. Shivashankar R, Tremaine WJ, Harmsen WS, Loftus EV Jr. Incidence and prevalence of Crohn's disease and ulcerative colitis in Olmsted County, Minnesota from 1970 through 2010. Clin Gastroenterol Hepatol. 2017;15(6):857–63. https://doi.org/10.1016/j.cgh.2016.10.039.
142. Kappelman MD, Rifas-Shiman SL, Kleinman K, Ollendorf D, Bousvaros A, Grand RJ, et al. The prevalence and geographic distribution of Crohn's disease and ulcerative colitis in the United States. Clin Gastroenterol Hepatol. 2007;5(12):1424–9. https://doi.org/10.1016/j.cgh.2007.07.012.
143. Ananthakrishnan AN. Epidemiology and risk factors for IBD. Nat Rev Gastroenterol Hepatol. 2015;12(4):205–17. https://doi.org/10.1038/nrgastro.2015.34.
144. Lapidus A, Bernell O, Hellers G, Persson PG, Lofberg R. Incidence of Crohn's disease in Stockholm County 1955–1989. Gut. 1997;41(4):480–6.
145. Heresbach D, Alexandre JL, Bretagne JF, Cruchant E, Dabadie A, Dartois-Hoguin M, et al. Crohn's disease in the over-60 age group: a population based study. Eur J Gastroenterol Hepatol. 2004;16(7):657–64.
146. Spehlmann ME, Begun AZ, Burghardt J, Lepage P, Raedler A, Schreiber S. Epidemiology of inflammatory bowel disease in a German twin cohort: results of a nationwide study. Inflamm Bowel Dis. 2008;14(7):968–76. https://doi.org/10.1002/ibd.20380.
147. Bengtson MB, Solberg C, Aamodt G, Sauar J, Jahnsen J, Moum B, et al. Familial aggregation in Crohn's disease and ulcerative colitis in a Norwegian population-based cohort followed for ten years. J Crohns Colitis. 2009;3(2):92–9. https://doi.org/10.1016/j.crohns.2008.11.002.
148. Hugot JP, Chamaillard M, Zouali H, Lesage S, Cezard JP, Belaiche J, et al. Association of NOD2 leucine-rich repeat variants with susceptibility to Crohn's disease. Nature. 2001;411(6837):599–603. https://doi.org/10.1038/35079107.
149. Newman B, Siminovitch KA. Recent advances in the genetics of inflammatory bowel disease. Curr Opin Gastroenterol. 2005;21(4):401–7.
150. Vermeire S. NOD2/CARD15: relevance in clinical practice. Best Pract Res Clin Gastroenterol. 2004;18(3):569–75. https://doi.org/10.1016/j.bpg.2003.12.008.
151. Brand S. Crohn's disease: Th1, Th17 or both? The change of a paradigm: new immunological and genetic insights implicate Th17 cells in the pathogenesis of Crohn's disease. Gut. 2009;58(8):1152–67. https://doi.org/10.1136/gut.2008.163667.
152. Peltekova VD, Wintle RF, Rubin LA, Amos CI, Huang Q, Gu X, et al. Functional variants of OCTN cation transporter genes are associated with Crohn disease. Nat Genet. 2004;36(5):471–5. https://doi.org/10.1038/ng1339.
153. Stoll M, Corneliussen B, Costello CM, Waetzig GH, Mellgard B, Koch WA, et al. Genetic variation in DLG5 is associated with inflammatory bowel disease. Nat Genet. 2004;36(5):476–80. https://doi.org/10.1038/ng1345.
154. Sugawara K, Olson TS, Moskaluk CA, Stevens BK, Hoang S, Kozaiwa K, et al. Linkage to peroxisome proliferator-activated receptor-gamma in SAMP1/YitFc mice and in human Crohn's disease. Gastroenterology. 2005;128(2):351–60.
155. Brant SR, Panhuysen CI, Nicolae D, Reddy DM, Bonen DK, Karaliukas R, et al. MDR1 Ala893 polymorphism is associated with inflammatory bowel disease. Am J Hum Genet. 2003;73(6):1282–92. https://doi.org/10.1086/379927.
156. Liu JZ, Anderson CA. Genetic studies of Crohn's disease: past, present and future. Best Pract Res Clin Gastroenterol. 2014;28(3):373–86. https://doi.org/10.1016/j.bpg.2014.04.009.
157. Becker C, Wirtz S, Blessing M, Pirhonen J, Strand D, Bechthold O, et al. Constitutive p40 promoter activation and IL-23 production in the terminal ileum mediated by dendritic cells. J Clin Invest. 2003;112(5):693–706. https://doi.org/10.1172/JCI17464.
158. Schmidt C, Giese T, Ludwig B, Mueller-Molaian I, Marth T, Zeuzem S, et al. Expression of interleukin-12-related cytokine transcripts in inflammatory bowel disease: elevated interleukin-23p19 and interleukin-27p28 in Crohn's disease but not in ulcerative colitis. Inflamm Bowel Dis. 2005;11(1):16–23.
159. Haag LM, Siegmund B. Intestinal microbiota and the innate immune system—a crosstalk in Crohn's disease pathogenesis. Front Immunol. 2015;6:489. https://doi.org/10.3389/fimmu.2015.00489.
160. Pascal V, Pozuelo M, Borruel N, Casellas F, Campos D, Santiago A, et al. A microbial signature for Crohn's disease. Gut. 2017;66(5):813–22. https://doi.org/10.1136/gutjnl-2016-313235.
161. Joossens M, Huys G, Cnockaert M, De Preter V, Verbeke K, Rutgeerts P, et al. Dysbiosis of the faecal microbiota in patients with Crohn's disease and their unaffected relatives. Gut. 2011;60(5):631–7. https://doi.org/10.1136/gut.2010.223263.
162. Loftus EV Jr. Clinical epidemiology of inflammatory bowel disease: incidence, prevalence, and environmental influences. Gastroenterology. 2004;126(6):1504–17.
163. Jorgensen SP, Hvas CL, Agnholt J, Christensen LA, Heickendorff L, Dahlerup JF. Active Crohn's disease is associated with low vitamin D levels. J Crohns Colitis. 2013;7(10):e407–13. https://doi.org/10.1016/j.crohns.2013.01.012.
164. Dam AN, Berg AM, Farraye FA. Environmental influences on the onset and clinical course of Crohn's disease-part 1: an overview of external risk factors. Gastroenterol Hepatol. 2013;9(11):711–7.
165. Best WR, Becktel JM, Singleton JW, Kern F Jr. Development of a Crohn's disease activity index. National Cooperative Crohn's Disease Study Gastroenterology. 1976;70(3):439–44.
166. Rimola J, Ordas I, Rodriguez S, Garcia-Bosch O, Aceituno M, Llach J, et al. Magnetic resonance imaging for evaluation of Crohn's disease: validation of parameters of severity and quantitative index of activity. Inflamm Bowel Dis. 2011;17(8):1759–68. https://doi.org/10.1002/ibd.21551.
167. Andersen K, Vogt C, Blondin D, Beck A, Heinen W, Aurich V, et al. Multi-detector CT-colonography in inflammatory bowel

disease: prospective analysis of CT-findings to high-resolution video colonoscopy. Eur J Radiol. 2006;58(1):140–6. https://doi.org/10.1016/j.ejrad.2005.11.004.
168. Mary JY, Modigliani R. Development and validation of an endoscopic index of the severity for Crohn's disease: a prospective multicentre study. Groupe d'Etudes Therapeutiques des Affections Inflammatoires du Tube Digestif (GETAID). Gut. 1989;30(7):983–9.
169. Daperno M, D'Haens G, Van Assche G, Baert F, Bulois P, Maunoury V, et al. Development and validation of a new, simplified endoscopic activity score for Crohn's disease: the SES-CD. Gastrointest Endosc. 2004;60(4):505–12.
170. Kucharski M, Karczewski J, Mankowska-Wierzbicka D, Karmelita-Katulska K, Kaczmarek E, Iwanik K, et al. Usefulness of endoscopic indices in determination of disease activity in patients with Crohn's disease. Gastroenterol Res Pract. 2016;2016:7896478. https://doi.org/10.1155/2016/7896478.
171. Rubio CA, Befrits R, Jaramillo E, Nesi G, Amorosi A. Villous and serrated adenomatous growth bordering carcinomas in inflammatory bowel disease. Anticancer Res. 2000;20(6c):4761–4.
172. Heresbach D, Alexandre JL, Branger B, Bretagne JF, Cruchant E, Dabadie A, et al. Frequency and significance of granulomas in a cohort of incident cases of Crohn's disease. Gut. 2005;54(2):215–22. https://doi.org/10.1136/gut.2004.041715.
173. Yantiss RK, Sapp HL, Farraye FA, El-Zammar O, O'Brien MJ, Fruin AB, et al. Histologic predictors of pouchitis in patients with chronic ulcerative colitis. Am J Surg Pathol. 2004;28(8):999–1006.
174. Koukoulis G, Ke Y, Henley JD, Cummings OW. Obliterative muscularization of the small bowel submucosa in Crohn disease: a possible mechanism of small bowel obstruction. Arch Pathol Lab Med. 2001;125(10):1331–4. https://doi.org/10.1043/0003-9985(2001)125<1331:OMOTSB>2.0.CO;2.
175. Borley NR, Mortensen NJ, Jewell DP, Warren BF. The relationship between inflammatory and serosal connective tissue changes in ileal Crohn's disease: evidence for a possible causative link. J Pathol. 2000;190(2):196–202. https://doi.org/10.1002/(SICI)1096-9896(200002)190:2<196::AID-PATH513>3.0.CO;2-5.
176. Villanacci V, Bassotti G, Nascimbeni R, Antonelli E, Cadei M, Fisogni S, et al. Enteric nervous system abnormalities in inflammatory bowel diseases. Neurogastroenterol Motil. 2008;20(9):1009–16. https://doi.org/10.1111/j.1365-2982.2008.01146.x.
177. Mooney EE, Walker J, Hourihane DO. Relation of granulomas to lymphatic vessels in Crohn's disease. J Clin Pathol. 1995;48(4):335–8.
178. Matson AP, Van Kruiningen HJ, West AB, Cartun RW, Colombel JF, Cortot A. The relationship of granulomas to blood vessels in intestinal Crohn's disease. Mod Pathol. 1995;8(6):680–5.
179. D'Haens GR, Geboes K, Peeters M, Baert F, Penninckx F, Rutgeerts P. Early lesions of recurrent Crohn's disease caused by infusion of intestinal contents in excluded ileum. Gastroenterology. 1998;114(2):262–7.
180. McQuillan A, Appelman HD. Superficial Crohn's disease: a study of 10 patients. Surg Pathol. 1989;2:231–9.
181. Geboes K, Rutgeerts P, Opdenakker G, Olson A, Patel K, Wagner CL, et al. Endoscopic and histologic evidence of persistent mucosal healing and correlation with clinical improvement following sustained infliximab treatment for Crohn's disease. Curr Med Res Opin. 2005;21(11):1741–54. https://doi.org/10.1185/030079905X65457.
182. de Bruyn JR, Becker MA, Steenkamer J, Wildenberg ME, Meijer SL, Buskens CJ, et al. Intestinal fibrosis is associated with lack of response to infliximab therapy in Crohn's disease. PLoS One. 2018;13(1):e0190999. https://doi.org/10.1371/journal.pone.0190999.
183. Rieder F, Fiocchi C, Rogler G. Mechanisms, management, and treatment of fibrosis in patients with inflammatory bowel diseases. Gastroenterology. 2017;152(2):340–50 e6. https://doi.org/10.1053/j.gastro.2016.09.047.
184. Volk EE, Shapiro BD, Easley KA, Goldblum JR. The clinical significance of a biopsy-based diagnosis of focal active colitis: a clinicopathologic study of 31 cases. Mod Pathol. 1998;11(8):789–94.
185. Greenson JK, Stern RA, Carpenter SL, Barnett JL. The clinical significance of focal active colitis. Hum Pathol. 1997;28(6):729–33.
186. Xin W, Brown PI, Greenson JK. The clinical significance of focal active colitis in pediatric patients. Am J Surg Pathol. 2003;27(8):1134–8.
187. Gan HT, Chen YQ, Ouyang Q, Bu H, Yang XY. Differentiation between intestinal tuberculosis and Crohn's disease in endoscopic biopsy specimens by polymerase chain reaction. Am J Gastroenterol. 2002;97(6):1446–51. https://doi.org/10.1111/j.1572-0241.2002.05686.x.
188. Tandon HD, Prakash A. Pathology of intestinal tuberculosis and its distinction from Crohn's disease. Gut. 1972;13(4):260–9.
189. Alimchandani M, Lai JP, Aung PP, Khangura S, Kamal N, Gallin JI, et al. Gastrointestinal histopathology in chronic granulomatous disease: a study of 87 patients. Am J Surg Pathol. 2013;37(9):1365–72. https://doi.org/10.1097/PAS.0b013e318297427d.
190. Gupta NK, Masia R. Cord colitis syndrome: a cause of granulomatous inflammation in the upper and lower gastrointestinal tract. Am J Surg Pathol. 2013;37(7):1109–13. https://doi.org/10.1097/PAS.0b013e31828a827a.
191. Herrera AF, Soriano G, Bellizzi AM, Hornick JL, Ho VT, Ballen KK, et al. Cord colitis syndrome in cord-blood stem-cell transplantation. N Engl J Med. 2011;365(9):815–24. https://doi.org/10.1056/NEJMoa1104959.
192. McCue J, Coppen MJ, Rasbridge SA, Lock MR. Coexistent Crohn's disease and sigmoid diverticulosis. Postgrad Med J. 1989;65(767):636–9.
193. Peppercorn MA. The overlap of inflammatory bowel disease and diverticular disease. J Clin Gastroenterol. 2004;38(5 Suppl 1):S8–10.
194. Burroughs SH, Bowrey DJ, Morris-Stiff GJ, Williams GT. Granulomatous inflammation in sigmoid diverticulitis: two diseases or one? Histopathology. 1998;33(4):349–53.
195. Goldstein NS, Leon-Armin C, Mani A. Crohn's colitis-like changes in sigmoid diverticulitis specimens is usually an idiosyncratic inflammatory response to the diverticulosis rather than Crohn's colitis. Am J Surg Pathol. 2000;24(5):668–75.
196. Yazisiz V. Similarities and differences between Behcet's disease and Crohn's disease. World J Gastrointest Pathophysiol. 2014;5(3):228–38. https://doi.org/10.4291/wjgp.v5.i3.228.
197. Gomollon F, Dignass A, Annese V, Tilg H, Van Assche G, Lindsay JO, et al. 3rd European Evidence-based Consensus on the Diagnosis and Management of Crohn's Disease 2016: Part 1: Diagnosis and Medical Management. J Crohns Colitis. 2017;11(1):3–25. https://doi.org/10.1093/ecco-jcc/jjw168.
198. Amiot A, Gornet JM, Baudry C, Munoz-Bongrand N, Auger M, Simon M, et al. Crohn's disease recurrence after total proctocolectomy with definitive ileostomy. Dig Liver Dis. 2011;43(9):698–702. https://doi.org/10.1016/j.dld.2011.02.017.
199. Martel P, Betton PO, Gallot D, Malafosse M. Crohn's colitis: experience with segmental resections; results in a series of 84 patients. J Am Coll Surg. 2002;194(4):448–53.
200. Canavan C, Abrams KR, Mayberry J. Meta-analysis: colorectal and small bowel cancer risk in patients with Crohn's disease. Aliment Pharmacol Ther. 2006;23(8):1097–104. https://doi.org/10.1111/j.1365-2036.2006.02854.x.
201. Bickston SJ, Lichtenstein GR, Arseneau KO, Cohen RB, Cominelli F. The relationship between infliximab treatment and lymphoma in Crohn's disease. Gastroenterology. 1999;117(6):1433–7.

202. Odze R. Diagnostic problems and advances in inflammatory bowel disease. Mod Pathol. 2003;16(4):347–58. https://doi.org/10.1097/01.MP.0000064746.82024.D1.
203. Prenzel F, Uhlig HH. Frequency of indeterminate colitis in children and adults with IBD—a metaanalysis. J Crohns Colitis. 2009;3(4):277–81. https://doi.org/10.1016/j.crohns.2009.07.001.
204. Sasaki M, Okada K, Koyama S, Yoshioka U, Inoue H, Fujiyama Y, et al. Ulcerative colitis complicated by gastroduodenal lesions. J Gastroenterol. 1996;31(4):585–9.
205. Valdez R, Appelman HD, Bronner MP, Greenson JK. Diffuse duodenitis associated with ulcerative colitis. Am J Surg Pathol. 2000;24(10):1407–13.
206. Gore RM, Marn CS, Kirby DF, Vogelzang RL, Neiman HL. CT findings in ulcerative, granulomatous, and indeterminate colitis. AJR Am J Roentgenol. 1984;143(2):279–84. https://doi.org/10.2214/ajr.143.2.279.
207. Price AB. Overlap in the spectrum of non-specific inflammatory bowel disease—'colitis indeterminate'. J Clin Pathol. 1978;31(6):567–77.
208. Yantiss RK, Odze RD. Diagnostic difficulties in inflammatory bowel disease pathology. Histopathology. 2006;48(2):116–32. https://doi.org/10.1111/j.1365-2559.2005.02248.x.
209. Martland GT, Shepherd NA. Indeterminate colitis: definition, diagnosis, implications and a plea for nosological sanity. Histopathology. 2007;50(1):83–96. https://doi.org/10.1111/j.1365-2559.2006.02545.x.
210. Odze RD. A contemporary and critical appraisal of 'indeterminate colitis'. Mod Pathol. 2015;28 Suppl 1:S30–46. https://doi.org/10.1038/modpathol.2014.131.
211. Swan NC, Geoghegan JG, O'Donoghue DP, Hyland JM, Sheahan K. Fulminant colitis in inflammatory bowel disease: detailed pathologic and clinical analysis. Dis Colon Rectum. 1998;41(12):1511–5.
212. Farmer M, Petras RE, Hunt LE, Janosky JE, Galandiuk S. The importance of diagnostic accuracy in colonic inflammatory bowel disease. Am J Gastroenterol. 2000;95(11):3184–8. https://doi.org/10.1111/j.1572-0241.2000.03199.x.
213. Gornet JM, Couve S, Hassani Z, Delchier JC, Marteau P, Cosnes J, et al. Infliximab for refractory ulcerative colitis or indeterminate colitis: an open-label multicentre study. Aliment Pharmacol Ther. 2003;18(2):175–81.
214. Teml A, Schwab M, Harrer M, Miehsler W, Schaeffeler E, Dejaco C, et al. A prospective, open-label trial of 6-thioguanine in patients with ulcerative or indeterminate colitis. Scand J Gastroenterol. 2005;40(10):1205–13.
215. McIntyre PB, Pemberton JH, Wolff BG, Dozois RR, Beart RW Jr. Indeterminate colitis. Long-term outcome in patients after ileal pouch-anal anastomosis. Dis Colon Rectum. 1995;38(1):51–4.
216. Yu CS, Pemberton JH, Larson D. Ileal pouch-anal anastomosis in patients with indeterminate colitis: long-term results. Dis Colon Rectum. 2000;43(11):1487–96.
217. Robert ME, Skacel M, Ullman T, Bernstein CN, Easley K, Goldblum JR. Patterns of colonic involvement at initial presentation in ulcerative colitis: a retrospective study of 46 newly diagnosed cases. Am J Clin Pathol. 2004;122(1):94–9. https://doi.org/10.1309/XLXK-J84C-3JCW-3RCH.
218. Pishori T, Dinnewitzer A, Zmora O, Oberwalder M, Hajjar L, Cotman K, et al. Outcome of patients with indeterminate colitis undergoing a double-stapled ileal pouch-anal anastomosis. Dis Colon Rectum. 2004;47(5):717–21. https://doi.org/10.1007/s10350-003-0116-4.
219. Portela F, Lago P. Fulminant colitis. Best Pract Res Clin Gastroenterol. 2013;27(5):771–82. https://doi.org/10.1016/j.bpg.2013.08.011.
220. Silverberg MS, Satsangi J, Ahmad T, Arnott ID, Bernstein CN, Brant SR, et al. Toward an integrated clinical, molecular and serological classification of inflammatory bowel disease: report of a Working Party of the 2005 Montreal World Congress of Gastroenterology. Can J Gastroenterol. 2005;19 Suppl A:5a–36a.
221. Autenrieth DM, Baumgart DC. Toxic megacolon. Inflamm Bowel Dis. 2012;18(3):584–91. https://doi.org/10.1002/ibd.21847.
222. Caprilli R, Latella G, Vernia P, Frieri G. Multiple organ dysfunction in ulcerative colitis. Am J Gastroenterol. 2000;95(5):1258–62. https://doi.org/10.1111/j.1572-0241.2000.02019.x.
223. Fazio VW. Toxic megacolon in ulcerative colitis and Crohn's colitis. Clin Gastroenterol. 1980;9(2):389–407.
224. Greenstein AJ, Sachar DB, Gibas A, Schrag D, Heimann T, Janowitz HD, et al. Outcome of toxic dilatation in ulcerative and Crohn's colitis. J Clin Gastroenterol. 1985;7(2):137–43.
225. Latella G, Vernia P, Viscido A, Frieri G, Cadau G, Cocco A, et al. GI distension in severe ulcerative colitis. Am J Gastroenterol. 2002;97(5):1169–75. https://doi.org/10.1111/j.1572-0241.2002.05691.x.
226. Grieco MB, Bordan DL, Geiss AC, Beil AR Jr. Toxic megacolon complicating Crohn's colitis. Ann Surg. 1980;191(1):75–80.
227. Siow VS, Bhatt R, Mollen KP. Management of acute severe ulcerative colitis in children. Semin Pediatr Surg. 2017;26(6):367–72. https://doi.org/10.1053/j.sempedsurg.2017.10.006.
228. Yantiss RK, Farraye FA, O'Brien MJ, Fruin AB, Stucchi AF, Becker JM, et al. Prognostic significance of superficial fissuring ulceration in patients with severe "indeterminate" colitis. Am J Surg Pathol. 2006;30(2):165–70.
229. Gower-Rousseau C, Dauchet L, Vernier-Massouille G, Tilloy E, Brazier F, Merle V, et al. The natural history of pediatric ulcerative colitis: a population-based cohort study. Am J Gastroenterol. 2009;104(8):2080–8. https://doi.org/10.1038/ajg.2009.177.
230. Benchimol EI, Mack DR, Nguyen GC, Snapper SB, Li W, Mojaverian N, et al. Incidence, outcomes, and health services burden of very early onset inflammatory bowel disease. Gastroenterology. 2014;147(4):803–13.e7; quiz e14–5. https://doi.org/10.1053/j.gastro.2014.06.023.
231. Jakobsen C, Paerregaard A, Munkholm P, Wewer V. Paediatric inflammatory bowel disease during a 44-year period in Copenhagen County: occurrence, course and prognosis—a population-based study from the Danish Crohn Colitis Database. Eur J Gastroenterol Hepatol. 2009;21(11):1291–301. https://doi.org/10.1097/MEG.0b013e32832a4ed6.
232. Henderson P, Hansen R, Cameron FL, Gerasimidis K, Rogers P, Bisset WM, et al. Rising incidence of pediatric inflammatory bowel disease in Scotland. Inflamm Bowel Dis. 2012;18(6):999–1005. https://doi.org/10.1002/ibd.21797.
233. Day AS, Ledder C, Leach ST, Lemberg DA. Crohn's and colitis in children and adolescents. World J Gastroenterol. 2012;18(41):5862–9. https://doi.org/10.3748/wjg.v18.i41.5862.
234. Aloi M, Lionetti P, Barabino A, Guariso G, Costa S, Fontana M, et al. Phenotype and disease course of early-onset pediatric inflammatory bowel disease. Inflamm Bowel Dis. 2014;20(4):597–605. https://doi.org/10.1097/01.mib.0000442921.77945.09.
235. Van Limbergen J, Russell RK, Drummond HE, Aldhous MC, Round NK, Nimmo ER, et al. Definition of phenotypic characteristics of childhood-onset inflammatory bowel disease. Gastroenterology. 2008;135(4):1114–22. https://doi.org/10.1053/j.gastro.2008.06.081.
236. Imielinski M, Baldassano RN, Griffiths A, Russell RK, Annese V, Dubinsky M, et al. Common variants at five new loci associated with early-onset inflammatory bowel disease. Nat Genet. 2009;41(12):1335–40. https://doi.org/10.1038/ng.489.
237. Glocker EO, Kotlarz D, Boztug K, Gertz EM, Schaffer AA, Noyan F, et al. Inflammatory bowel disease and mutations affecting the interleukin-10 receptor. N Engl J Med. 2009;361(21):2033–45. https://doi.org/10.1056/NEJMoa0907206.

238. Glickman JN, Bousvaros A, Farraye FA, Zholudev A, Friedman S, Wang HH, et al. Pediatric patients with untreated ulcerative colitis may present initially with unusual morphologic findings. Am J Surg Pathol. 2004;28(2):190–7.
239. Robert ME, Tang L, Hao LM, Reyes-Mugica M. Patterns of inflammation in mucosal biopsies of ulcerative colitis: perceived differences in pediatric populations are limited to children younger than 10 years. Am J Surg Pathol. 2004;28(2):183–9.
240. Boyle B, Collins MH, Wang Z, Mack D, Griffiths A, Sauer C, et al. Histologic correlates of clinical and endoscopic severity in children newly diagnosed with ulcerative colitis. Am J Surg Pathol. 2017;41(11):1491–8. https://doi.org/10.1097/pas.0000000000000939.
241. Queliza K, Ihekweazu FD, Schady D, Jensen C, Kellermayer R. Granulomatous upper gastrointestinal inflammation in pediatric ulcerative colitis. J Pediatr Gastroenterol Nutr. 2018;66(4):620–3. https://doi.org/10.1097/mpg.0000000000001771.
242. Turner D, Levine A, Escher JC, Griffiths AM, Russell RK, Dignass A, et al. Management of pediatric ulcerative colitis: joint ECCO and ESPGHAN evidence-based consensus guidelines. J Pediatr Gastroenterol Nutr. 2012;55(3):340–61. https://doi.org/10.1097/MPG.0b013e3182662233.
243. Ruemmele FM, Turner D. Differences in the management of pediatric and adult onset ulcerative colitis—lessons from the joint ECCO and ESPGHAN consensus guidelines for the management of pediatric ulcerative colitis. J Crohns Colitis. 2014;8(1):1–4. https://doi.org/10.1016/j.crohns.2013.10.006.
244. Turner D, Ruemmele FM, Orlanski-Meyer E, Griffiths AM, Carpi JM, Bronsky J, et al. Management of paediatric ulcerative colitis, part 1: ambulatory care- an evidence-based guideline from ECCO and ESPGHAN. J Pediatr Gastroenterol Nutr. 2018; https://doi.org/10.1097/mpg.0000000000002035.
245. Turner D, Ruemmele FM, Orlanski-Meyer E, Griffiths AM, Carpi JM, Bronsky J, et al. Management of paediatric ulcerative colitis, part 2: acute severe colitis; an evidence-based consensus guideline from ECCO and ESPGHAN. J Pediatr Gastroenterol Nutr. 2018; https://doi.org/10.1097/mpg.0000000000002036.
246. de Ridder L, Turner D, Wilson DC, Koletzko S, Martin-de-Carpi J, Fagerberg UL, et al. Malignancy and mortality in pediatric patients with inflammatory bowel disease: a multinational study from the porto pediatric IBD group. Inflamm Bowel Dis. 2014;20(2):291–300. https://doi.org/10.1097/01.MIB.0000439066.69340.3c.
247. Vernier-Massouille G, Balde M, Salleron J, Turck D, Dupas JL, Mouterde O, et al. Natural history of pediatric Crohn's disease: a population-based cohort study. Gastroenterology. 2008;135(4):1106–13. https://doi.org/10.1053/j.gastro.2008.06.079.
248. Ruemmele FM, Veres G, Kolho KL, Griffiths A, Levine A, Escher JC, et al. Consensus guidelines of ECCO/ESPGHAN on the medical management of pediatric Crohn's disease. J Crohns Colitis. 2014;8(10):1179–207. https://doi.org/10.1016/j.crohns.2014.04.005.
249. Stewart D. Surgical care of the pediatric Crohn's disease patient. Semin Pediatr Surg. 2017;26(6):373–8. https://doi.org/10.1053/j.sempedsurg.2017.10.007.
250. Jess T, Rungoe C, Peyrin-Biroulet L. Risk of colorectal cancer in patients with ulcerative colitis: a meta-analysis of population-based cohort studies. Clin Gastroenterol Hepatol. 2012;10(6):639–45. https://doi.org/10.1016/j.cgh.2012.01.010.
251. Yashiro M. Ulcerative colitis-associated colorectal cancer. World J Gastroenterol. 2014;20(44):16389–97. https://doi.org/10.3748/wjg.v20.i44.16389.
252. Eaden JA, Abrams KR, Mayberry JF. The risk of colorectal cancer in ulcerative colitis: a meta-analysis. Gut. 2001;48(4):526–35.
253. Farraye FA, Odze RD, Eaden J, Itzkowitz SH. AGA technical review on the diagnosis and management of colorectal neoplasia in inflammatory bowel disease. Gastroenterology. 2010;138(2):746–74, 74.e1–4; quiz e12–3. https://doi.org/10.1053/j.gastro.2009.12.035.
254. Riddell RH, Goldman H, Ransohoff DF, Appelman HD, Fenoglio CM, Haggitt RC, et al. Dysplasia in inflammatory bowel disease: standardized classification with provisional clinical applications. Hum Pathol. 1983;14(11):931–68.
255. Itzkowitz SH, Harpaz N. Diagnosis and management of dysplasia in patients with inflammatory bowel diseases. Gastroenterology. 2004;126(6):1634–48.
256. Ullman T, Croog V, Harpaz N, Sachar D, Itzkowitz S. Progression of flat low-grade dysplasia to advanced neoplasia in patients with ulcerative colitis. Gastroenterology. 2003;125(5):1311–9.
257. Harpaz N, Talbot IC. Colorectal cancer in idiopathic inflammatory bowel disease. Semin Diagn Pathol. 1996;13(4):339–57.
258. Kiran RP, Nisar PJ, Goldblum JR, Fazio VW, Remzi FH, Shen B, et al. Dysplasia associated with Crohn's colitis: segmental colectomy or more extended resection? Ann Surg. 2012;256(2):221–6. https://doi.org/10.1097/SLA.0b013e31825f0709.
259. Friedman S, Rubin PH, Bodian C, Harpaz N, Present DH. Screening and surveillance colonoscopy in chronic Crohn's colitis: results of a surveillance program spanning 25 years. Clin Gastroenterol Hepatol. 2008;6(9):993–8; quiz 53–4. https://doi.org/10.1016/j.cgh.2008.03.019.
260. Awais D, Siegel CA, Higgins PD. Modelling dysplasia detection in ulcerative colitis: clinical implications of surveillance intensity. Gut. 2009;58(11):1498–503. https://doi.org/10.1136/gut.2008.169714.
261. Blackstone MO, Riddell RH, Rogers BH, Levin B. Dysplasia-associated lesion or mass (DALM) detected by colonoscopy in long-standing ulcerative colitis: an indication for colectomy. Gastroenterology. 1981;80(2):366–74.
262. Rutter MD, Saunders BP, Wilkinson KH, Kamm MA, Williams CB, Forbes A. Most dysplasia in ulcerative colitis is visible at colonoscopy. Gastrointest Endosc. 2004;60(3):334–9.
263. The Paris endoscopic classification of superficial neoplastic lesions: esophagus, stomach, and colon: November 30 to December 1, 2002. Gastrointest Endosc. 2003;58(6 Suppl):S3–43.
264. Schlemper RJ, Riddell RH, Kato Y, Borchard F, Cooper HS, Dawsey SM, et al. The Vienna classification of gastrointestinal epithelial neoplasia. Gut. 2000;47(2):251–5.
265. Melville DM, Jass JR, Morson BC, Pollock DJ, Richman PI, Shepherd NA, et al. Observer study of the grading of dysplasia in ulcerative colitis: comparison with clinical outcome. Hum Pathol. 1989;20(10):1008–14.
266. Eaden J, Abrams K, McKay H, Denley H, Mayberry J. Inter-observer variation between general and specialist gastrointestinal pathologists when grading dysplasia in ulcerative colitis. J Pathol. 2001;194(2):152–7. https://doi.org/10.1002/path.876.
267. Magro F, Langner C, Driessen A, Ensari A, Geboes K, Mantzaris GJ, et al. European consensus on the histopathology of inflammatory bowel disease. J Crohns Colitis. 2013;7(10):827–51. https://doi.org/10.1016/j.crohns.2013.06.001.
268. Dorer R, Odze RD. AMACR immunostaining is useful in detecting dysplastic epithelium in Barrett's esophagus, ulcerative colitis, and Crohn's disease. Am J Surg Pathol. 2006;30(7):871–7. https://doi.org/10.1097/01.pas.0000213268.30468.b4.
269. Pekow JR, Hetzel JT, Rothe JA, Hanauer SB, Turner JR, Hart J, et al. Outcome after surveillance of low-grade and indefinite dysplasia in patients with ulcerative colitis. Inflamm Bowel Dis. 2010;16(8):1352–6. https://doi.org/10.1002/ibd.21184.
270. Lai KK, Horvath B, Xie H, Wu X, Lewis BL, Pai RK, et al. Risk for colorectal neoplasia in patients with inflammatory bowel disease and mucosa indefinite for dysplasia. Inflamm Bowel Dis. 2015;21(2):378–84. https://doi.org/10.1097/mib.0000000000000286.

271. Kisiel JB, Loftus EV Jr, Harmsen WS, Zinsmeister AR, Sandborn WJ. Outcome of sporadic adenomas and adenoma-like dysplasia in patients with ulcerative colitis undergoing polypectomy. Inflamm Bowel Dis. 2012;18(2):226–35. https://doi.org/10.1002/ibd.21687.
272. Odze RD, Farraye FA, Hecht JL, Hornick JL. Long-term follow-up after polypectomy treatment for adenoma-like dysplastic lesions in ulcerative colitis. Clin Gastroenterol Hepatol. 2004;2(7):534–41.
273. Goldstone R, Itzkowitz S, Harpaz N, Ullman T. Progression of low-grade dysplasia in ulcerative colitis: effect of colonic location. Gastrointest Endosc. 2011;74(5):1087–93. https://doi.org/10.1016/j.gie.2011.06.028.
274. Navaneethan U, Jegadeesan R, Gutierrez NG, Venkatesh PG, Hammel JP, Shen B, et al. Progression of low-grade dysplasia to advanced neoplasia based on the location and morphology of dysplasia in ulcerative colitis patients with extensive colitis under colonoscopic surveillance. J Crohns Colitis. 2013;7(12):e684–91. https://doi.org/10.1016/j.crohns.2013.06.006.
275. Wanders LK, Dekker E, Pullens B, Bassett P, Travis SP, East JE. Cancer risk after resection of polypoid dysplasia in patients with longstanding ulcerative colitis: a meta-analysis. Clin Gastroenterol Hepatol. 2014;12(5):756–64. https://doi.org/10.1016/j.cgh.2013.07.024.
276. Thomas T, Abrams KA, Robinson RJ, Mayberry JF. Meta-analysis: cancer risk of low-grade dysplasia in chronic ulcerative colitis. Aliment Pharmacol Ther. 2007;25(6):657–68. https://doi.org/10.1111/j.1365-2036.2007.03241.x.
277. Rubio CA, Johansson C, Slezak P, Ohman U, Hammarberg C. Villous dysplasia. An ominous histologic sign in colitic patients. Dis Colon Rectum. 1984;27(5):283–7.
278. Andersen SN, Lovig T, Clausen OP, Bakka A, Fausa O, Rognum TO. Villous, hypermucinous mucosa in long standing ulcerative colitis shows high frequency of K-ras mutations. Gut. 1999;45(5):686–92.
279. Parian A, Koh J, Limketkai BN, Eluri S, Rubin DT, Brant SR, et al. Association between serrated epithelial changes and colorectal dysplasia in inflammatory bowel disease. Gastrointest Endosc. 2016;84(1):87–95.e1. https://doi.org/10.1016/j.gie.2015.12.010.
280. Johnson DH, Khanna S, Smyrk TC, Loftus EV Jr, Anderson KS, Mahoney DW, et al. Detection rate and outcome of colonic serrated epithelial changes in patients with ulcerative colitis or Crohn's colitis. Aliment Pharmacol Ther. 2014;39(12):1408–17. https://doi.org/10.1111/apt.12774.
281. Kilgore SP, Sigel JE, Goldblum JR. Hyperplastic-like mucosal change in Crohn's disease: an unusual form of dysplasia? Mod Pathol. 2000;13(7):797–801. https://doi.org/10.1038/modpathol.3880138.
282. Parian AM, Lazarev MG. Serrated colorectal lesions in patients with inflammatory bowel disease. Gastroenterol Hepatol. 2018;14(1):19–25.
283. Shen J, Gibson JA, Schulte S, Khurana H, Farraye FA, Levine J, et al. Clinical, pathologic, and outcome study of hyperplastic and sessile serrated polyps in inflammatory bowel disease. Hum Pathol. 2015;46(10):1548–56. https://doi.org/10.1016/j.humpath.2015.06.019.
284. Jackson WE, Achkar JP, Macaron C, Lee L, Liu X, Pai RK, et al. The significance of sessile serrated polyps in inflammatory bowel disease. Inflamm Bowel Dis. 2016;22(9):2213–20. https://doi.org/10.1097/mib.0000000000000895.
285. Odze RD, Brien T, Brown CA, Hartman CJ, Wellman A, Fogt F. Molecular alterations in chronic ulcerative colitis-associated and sporadic hyperplastic polyps: a comparative analysis. Am J Gastroenterol. 2002;97(5):1235–42. https://doi.org/10.1111/j.1572-0241.2002.05696.x.
286. Ko HM, Harpaz N, McBride RB, Cui M, Ye F, Zhang D, et al. Serrated colorectal polyps in inflammatory bowel disease. Mod Pathol. 2015;28(12):1584–93. https://doi.org/10.1038/modpathol.2015.111.
287. Lee LH, Iacucci M, Fort Gasia M, Ghosh S, Panaccione R, Urbanski S. Prevalence and anatomic distribution of serrated and adenomatous lesions in patients with inflammatory bowel disease. Can J Gastroenterol Hepatol. 2017;2017:5490803. https://doi.org/10.1155/2017/5490803.
288. Srivastava A, Redston M, Farraye FA, Yantiss RK, Odze RD. Hyperplastic/serrated polyposis in inflammatory bowel disease: a case series of a previously undescribed entity. Am J Surg Pathol. 2008;32(2):296–303. https://doi.org/10.1097/PAS.0b013e318150d51b.
289. Feuerstein JD, Flier SN, Yee EU, Pleskow D, Cheifetz AS. A rare case series of concomitant inflammatory bowel disease, sporadic adenomas, and serrated polyposis syndrome. J Crohns Colitis. 2014;8(12):1735–9. https://doi.org/10.1016/j.crohns.2014.07.001.
290. Maher MM, Nassar MI. Acute cytomegalovirus infection is a risk factor in refractory and complicated inflammatory bowel disease. Dig Dis Sci. 2009;54(11):2456–62. https://doi.org/10.1007/s10620-008-0639-6.
291. Ayre K, Warren BF, Jeffery K, Travis SP. The role of CMV in steroid-resistant ulcerative colitis: a systematic review. J Crohns Colitis. 2009;3(3):141–8. https://doi.org/10.1016/j.crohns.2009.03.002.
292. Kambham N, Vij R, Cartwright CA, Longacre T. Cytomegalovirus infection in steroid-refractory ulcerative colitis: a case-control study. Am J Surg Pathol. 2004;28(3):365–73.
293. Domenech E, Vega R, Ojanguren I, Hernandez A, Garcia-Planella E, Bernal I, et al. Cytomegalovirus infection in ulcerative colitis: a prospective, comparative study on prevalence and diagnostic strategy. Inflamm Bowel Dis. 2008;14(10):1373–9. https://doi.org/10.1002/ibd.20498.
294. Cohen S, Martinez-Vinson C, Aloi M, Turner D, Assa A, de Ridder L, et al. Cytomegalovirus infection in pediatric severe ulcerative colitis-a multicenter study from the pediatric inflammatory bowel disease Porto Group of the European Society of Pediatric Gastroenterology, Hepatology and Nutrition. Pediatr Infect Dis J. 2018;37(3):197–201. https://doi.org/10.1097/inf.0000000000001724.
295. Hommes DW, Sterringa G, van Deventer SJ, Tytgat GN, Weel J. The pathogenicity of cytomegalovirus in inflammatory bowel disease: a systematic review and evidence-based recommendations for future research. Inflamm Bowel Dis. 2004;10(3):245–50.
296. Garrido E, Carrera E, Manzano R, Lopez-Sanroman A. Clinical significance of cytomegalovirus infection in patients with inflammatory bowel disease. World J Gastroenterol. 2013;19(1):17–25. https://doi.org/10.3748/wjg.v19.i1.17.
297. Pillet S, Pozzetto B, Roblin X. Cytomegalovirus and ulcerative colitis: place of antiviral therapy. World J Gastroenterol. 2016;22(6):2030–45 https://doi.org/10.3748/wjg.v22.i6.2030.
298. McCurdy JD, Jones A, Enders FT, Killian JM, Loftus EV Jr, Smyrk TC, et al. A model for identifying cytomegalovirus in patients with inflammatory bowel disease. Clin Gastroenterol Hepatol. 2015;13(1):131–7; quiz e7. https://doi.org/10.1016/j.cgh.2014.05.026.
299. McCurdy JD, Enders FT, Jones A, Killian JM, Loftus EV Jr, Bruining DH, et al. Detection of cytomegalovirus in patients with inflammatory bowel disease: where to biopsy and how many biopsies? Inflamm Bowel Dis. 2015;21(12):2833–8. https://doi.org/10.1097/mib.0000000000000556.
300. Sager K, Alam S, Bond A, Chinnappan L, Probert CS. Review article: cytomegalovirus and inflammatory bowel disease. Aliment Pharmacol Ther. 2015;41(8):725–33. https://doi.org/10.1111/apt.13124.
301. Jones A, McCurdy JD, Loftus EV Jr, Bruining DH, Enders FT, Killian JM, et al. Effects of antiviral therapy for patients with

inflammatory bowel disease and a positive intestinal biopsy for cytomegalovirus. Clin Gastroenterol Hepatol. 2015;13(5):949–55. https://doi.org/10.1016/j.cgh.2014.09.042.
302. Matsuoka K, Iwao Y, Mori T, Sakuraba A, Yajima T, Hisamatsu T, et al. Cytomegalovirus is frequently reactivated and disappears without antiviral agents in ulcerative colitis patients. Am J Gastroenterol. 2007;102(2):331–7. https://doi.org/10.1111/j.1572-0241.2006.00989.x.
303. Surawicz CM, Brandt LJ, Binion DG, Ananthakrishnan AN, Curry SR, Gilligan PH, et al. Guidelines for diagnosis, treatment, and prevention of *Clostridium difficile* infections. Am J Gastroenterol. 2013;108(4):478–98; quiz 99. https://doi.org/10.1038/ajg.2013.4.
304. Singh H, Nugent Z, Yu BN, Lix LM, Targownik LE, Bernstein CN. Higher incidence of *Clostridium difficile* infection among individuals with inflammatory bowel disease. Gastroenterology. 2017;153(2):430–8.e2. https://doi.org/10.1053/j.gastro.2017.04.044.
305. D'Aoust J, Battat R, Bessissow T. Management of inflammatory bowel disease with *Clostridium difficile* infection. World J Gastroenterol. 2017;23(27):4986–5003. https://doi.org/10.3748/wjg.v23.i27.4986.
306. Razik R, Rumman A, Bahreini Z, McGeer A, Nguyen GC. Recurrence of *Clostridium difficile* infection in patients with inflammatory bowel disease: the RECIDIVISM study. Am J Gastroenterol. 2016;111(8):1141–6. https://doi.org/10.1038/ajg.2016.187.
307. Kostic AD, Xavier RJ, Gevers D. The microbiome in inflammatory bowel disease: current status and the future ahead. Gastroenterology. 2014;146(6):1489–99. https://doi.org/10.1053/j.gastro.2014.02.009.
308. McCurdy JD, Enders FT, Khanna S, Bruining DH, Jones A, Killian JM, et al. Increased rates of *Clostridium difficile* infection and poor outcomes in patients with IBD with cytomegalovirus. Inflamm Bowel Dis. 2016;22(11):2688–93. https://doi.org/10.1097/mib.0000000000000939.
309. Bitton A, Buie D, Enns R, Feagan BG, Jones JL, Marshall JK, et al. Treatment of hospitalized adult patients with severe ulcerative colitis: Toronto consensus statements. Am J Gastroenterol. 2012;107(2):179–94; author reply 95. https://doi.org/10.1038/ajg.2011.386.
310. Nomura K, Fujimoto Y, Yamashita M, Morimoto Y, Ohshiro M, Sato K, et al. Absence of pseudomembranes in *Clostridium difficile*-associated diarrhea in patients using immunosuppression agents. Scand J Gastroenterol. 2009;44(1):74–8. https://doi.org/10.1080/00365520802321238.
311. Ben-Horin S, Margalit M, Bossuyt P, Maul J, Shapira Y, Bojic D, et al. Prevalence and clinical impact of endoscopic pseudomembranes in patients with inflammatory bowel disease and *Clostridium difficile* infection. J Crohns Colitis. 2010;4(2):194–8. https://doi.org/10.1016/j.crohns.2009.11.001.
312. Wang T, Matukas L, Streutker CJ. Histologic findings and clinical characteristics in acutely symptomatic ulcerative colitis patients with superimposed *Clostridium difficile* infection. Am J Clin Pathol. 2013;140(6):831–7. https://doi.org/10.1309/ajcp2lbrttjbf3kd.
313. Horton HA, Dezfoli S, Berel D, Hirsch J, Ippoliti A, McGovern D, et al. Antibiotics for treatment of *Clostridium difficile* infection in hospitalized patients with inflammatory bowel disease. Antimicrob Agents Chemother. 2014;58(9):5054–9. https://doi.org/10.1128/aac.02606-13.
314. Fischer M, Kao D, Kelly C, Kuchipudi A, Jafri SM, Blumenkehl M, et al. Fecal microbiota transplantation is safe and efficacious for recurrent or refractory *Clostridium difficile* infection in patients with inflammatory bowel disease. Inflamm Bowel Dis. 2016;22(10):2402–9. https://doi.org/10.1097/mib.0000000000000908.
315. Akar M, Aydin F, Yurci MA, Abay S, Ates I, Deniz K. The possible relationship between Campylobacter spp./Arcobacter spp. and patients with ulcerative colitis. Eur J Gastroenterol Hepatol. 2018;30(5):531–8. https://doi.org/10.1097/meg.0000000000001095.
316. Engel JJ, Martin TL. Edwardsiella tarda as a cause of postdysenteric ulcerative colitis. Int J Color Dis. 2006;21(2):184–5. https://doi.org/10.1007/s00384-004-0688-z.
317. Koido S, Ohkusa T, Kato K, Shimamoto N, Takakura K, Odahara S, et al. Edwardsiella tarda superinfection in relapse of ulcerative colitis. J Clin Gastroenterol. 2014;48(2):191–3. https://doi.org/10.1097/01.mcg.0000437809.46982.df.
318. O'Connell PR, Pemberton JH, Weiland LH, Beart RW Jr, Dozois RR, Wolff BG, et al. Does rectal mucosa regenerate after ileoanal anastomosis? Dis Colon Rectum. 1987;30(1):1–5.
319. Lavery IC, Sirimarco MT, Ziv Y, Fazio VW. Anal canal inflammation after ileal pouch-anal anastomosis. The need for treatment. Dis Colon Rectum. 1995;38(8):803–6.
320. Thompson-Fawcett MW, Mortensen NJ, Warren BF. "Cuffitis" and inflammatory changes in the columnar cuff, anal transitional zone, and ileal reservoir after stapled pouch-anal anastomosis. Dis Colon Rectum. 1999;42(3):348–55.
321. Coull DB, Lee FD, Anderson JH, McKee RF, Finlay IG, Dunlop MG. Long-term cancer risk of the anorectal cuff following restorative proctocolectomy assessed by p53 expression and cuff dysplasia. Color Dis. 2007;9(4):321–7. https://doi.org/10.1111/j.1463-1318.2006.01118.x.
322. Remzi FH, Fazio VW, Delaney CP, Preen M, Ormsby A, Bast J, et al. Dysplasia of the anal transitional zone after ileal pouch-anal anastomosis: results of prospective evaluation after a minimum of ten years. Dis Colon Rectum. 2003;46(1):6–13. https://doi.org/10.1097/01.dcr.0000044727.08281.49.
323. Ziv Y, Fazio VW, Sirimarco MT, Lavery IC, Goldblum JR, Petras RE. Incidence, risk factors, and treatment of dysplasia in the anal transitional zone after ileal pouch-anal anastomosis. Dis Colon Rectum. 1994;37(12):1281–5.
324. O'Riordain MG, Fazio VW, Lavery IC, Remzi F, Fabbri N, Meneu J, et al. Incidence and natural history of dysplasia of the anal transitional zone after ileal pouch-anal anastomosis: results of a five-year to ten-year follow-up. Dis Colon Rectum. 2000;43(12):1660–5.
325. Das P, Johnson MW, Tekkis PP, Nicholls RJ. Risk of dysplasia and adenocarcinoma following restorative proctocolectomy for ulcerative colitis. Color Dis. 2007;9(1):15–27. https://doi.org/10.1111/j.1463-1318.2006.01148.x.
326. Chambers WM, Mc CMNJ. Should ileal pouch-anal anastomosis include mucosectomy? Color Dis. 2007;9(5):384–92. https://doi.org/10.1111/j.1463-1318.2007.01211.x.

Non-inflammatory Bowel Disease Colitis

16

Murli Krishna

Microscopic Colitis

Definition

Microscopic colitis (MC) is a chronic colitis associated with watery non-bloody diarrhea and normal endoscopic findings. It includes two distinct but related morphologic patterns of mucosal inflammation: lymphocytic colitis (LC) and collagenous colitis (CC).

Clinical Features

The etiology of MC is not clearly known, and reported associations include medications, celiac disease, autoimmune/systemic inflammatory diseases, and infections. Proposed mechanisms include an abnormal immune response to a luminal agent, an autoimmune response, and in cases of CC, myofibroblast dysfunction leading to subepithelial collagen deposition [1].

Clinically, MC is characterized by long-standing intermittent watery diarrhea, occurring more commonly in females, with a peak incidence in the seventh decade. LC is more common than CC; however, the latter has a stronger association with female gender. Weight loss, abdominal pain, and protein-losing enteropathy are uncommon [2].

MC is endoscopically characterized by normal-appearing mucosa, and multiple random biopsies are usually obtained in patients with diarrhea. In both entities, the distal colon may be less involved or spared; hence more proximal biopsies are recommended. Increased intraepithelial lymphocytes may also be present in biopsies from terminal ileum. In cases of severe CC, abnormalities such as erythema, granularity, and surface erosion may be seen. Rarely, mucosal friability and decreased elasticity lead to tears or perforation, presumably from barotrauma during the procedure [3].

M. Krishna (✉)
Department of Laboratory Medicine and Pathology, Mayo Clinic, Jacksonville, FL, USA
e-mail: Krishna.Murli@mayo.edu

Pathological Features

Lymphocytic Colitis

The diagnostic histological finding in LC is the presence of increased intraepithelial lymphocytes (IELs) with normal crypt architecture (Fig. 16.1a). IELs are easily recognized by the characteristic round nuclei, high nuclear cytoplasmic ratio, and a surrounding halo. In the colon, IELs are normally present but few and generally accepted to be <5 per 100 epithelial cells. While investigators and guidelines suggest a cutoff value of >20 IELs per 100 epithelial cells, counting of IELs and CD3 immunostain is not necessary if one is familiar with the normal histology. Mild subepithelial collagen deposition is acceptable in LC, usually <10 μm in thickness. If there are foci of well-developed subepithelial collagen in biopsies that otherwise appear to show lymphocytic colitis, a diagnosis of collagenous colitis should be rendered. Additional characteristic findings include surface epithelial injury with decreased goblet cells and increased chronic inflammatory cells in the lamina propria, particularly plasma cells (Fig. 16.1b). In a minority of cases focal and mild active (neutrophilic) crypt inflammation (Fig. 16.1c) and minimal crypt architectural changes with Paneth cell metaplasia in distal colon may be present (Fig. 16.1d). While in such cases the diagnosis of lymphocytic colitis may still be applicable, an associated infectious or drug-related etiology may be considered, especially if there is acute exacerbation of a chronic diarrhea [1, 4, 5].

Some variants of LC have been described. Incomplete LC or paucicellular LC refers to patients with less prominent IELs (10–20 IELs per 100 epithelial cells). Another form of LC is called cryptal LC, in which the increased IELs are localized within the cryptal epithelium with no changes in

L. Zhang et al. (eds.), *Surgical Pathology of Non-neoplastic Gastrointestinal Diseases*,
https://doi.org/10.1007/978-3-030-15573-5_16

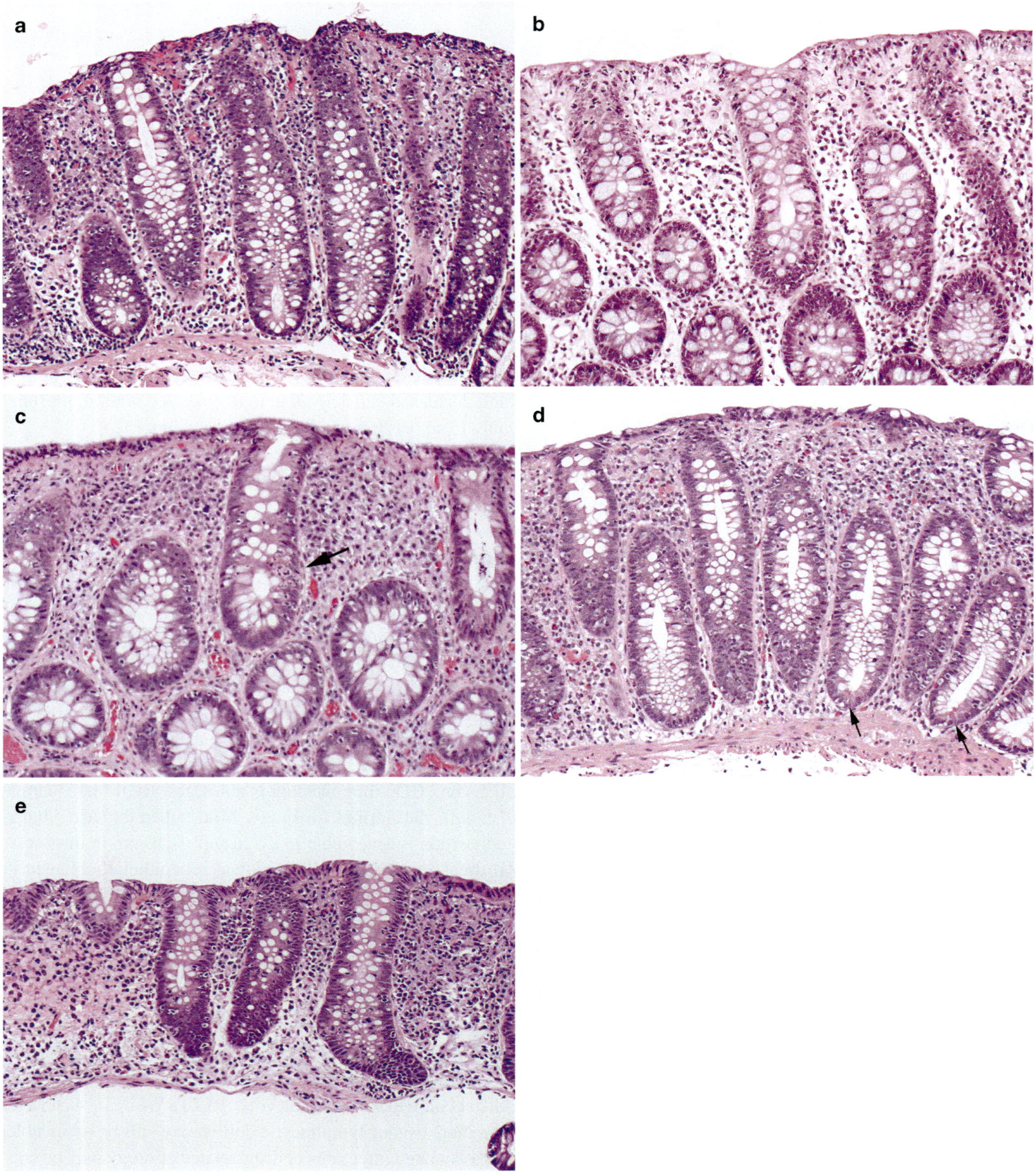

Fig. 16.1 Lymphocytic colitis (LC). (**a**) LC is characterized by prominent intraepithelial lymphocytosis, chronic inflammation in the lamina propria, and preserved crypt architecture. (**b**) The surface epithelium is injured with decreased goblet cells. (**c**) Mild active inflammation with cryptitis (arrow) may be occasionally seen in LC. Slightly thickened subepithelial collagen band is also present in this biopsy. (**d**) Focal Paneth cell metaplasia (arrows) in lymphocytic colitis present in left colon. (**e**) Cryptal LC. Note the increased intraepithelial lymphocytes within the cryptal epithelium, with sparing of the surface epithelium

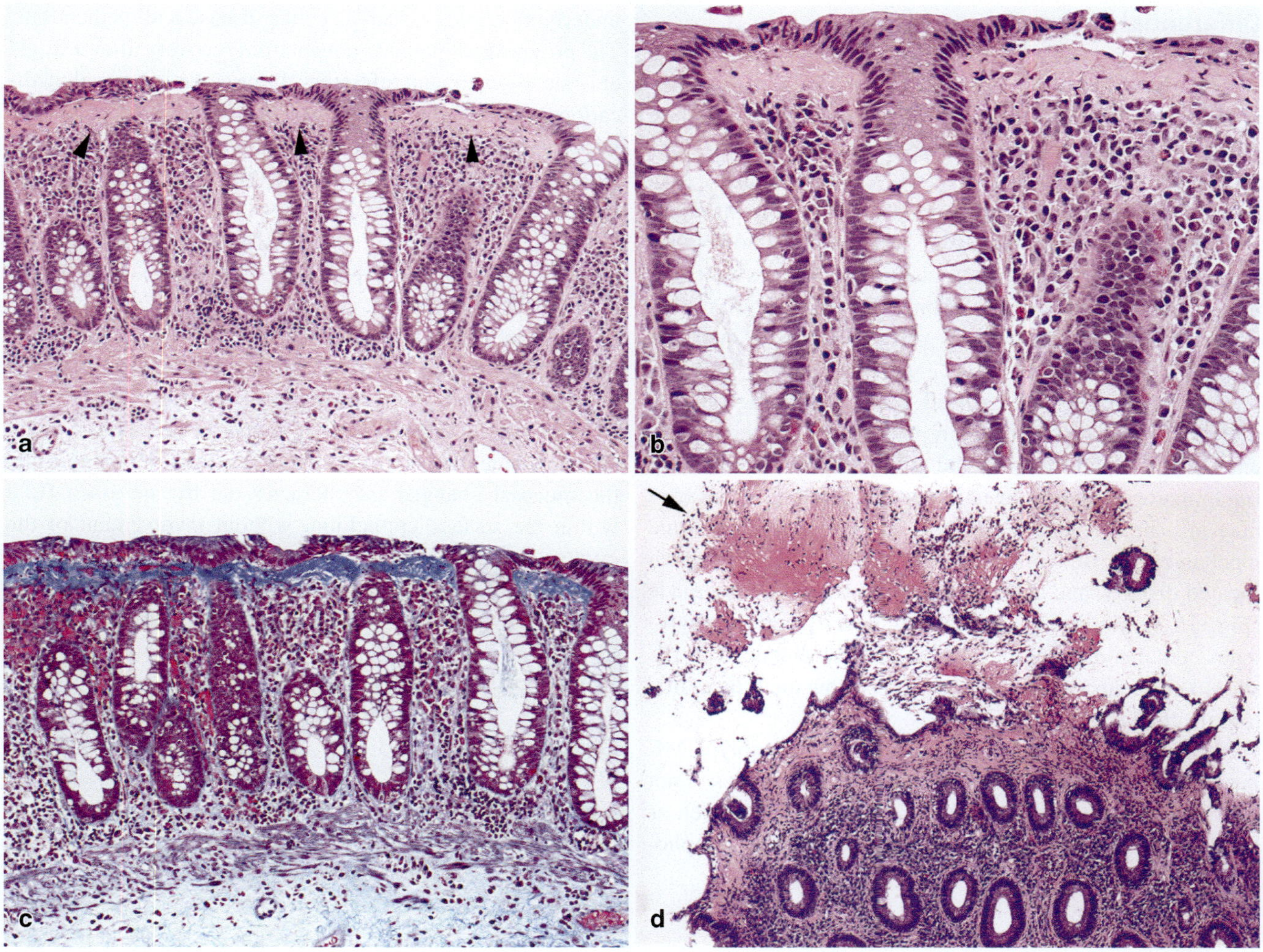

Fig. 16.2 Collagenous colitis (CC). (**a**) CC is characterized by a thickened subepithelial collagen band (arrowheads) and chronic inflammation in the lamina propria. Intraepithelial lymphocytosis may be mild. (**b**) Entrapment of subepithelial capillaries and inflammatory cells within the collagen band, with surface epithelial injury and sloughing. (**c**) Trichrome stain highlights the thickened collagen band. (**d**) "Pseudomembranous collagenous colitis"; pseudomembrane formation (arrow) occurring with collagenous colitis (Courtesy of Dr. Susan Abraham)

surface IELs (Fig. 16.1e). These variants should be considered as a part of the morphologic spectrum of LC [6, 7].

Collagenous Colitis

The diagnostic histological finding in CC is a thickened subepithelial band of collagen, usually associated with damage and loss of surface epithelial cells, and increased chronic inflammatory cells in the lamina propria (Fig. 16.2a). These findings are present in a background of largely preserved crypt architecture. The recommended thickness of the collagen band is >10 μm for diagnosis; however, measurement is usually not necessary. In well-developed cases, the collagen entraps capillaries and inflammatory cells in the lamina propria immediately beneath the surface epithelium (Fig. 16.2b). In equivocal cases a stain for collagen (such as Masson's trichrome or Sirius red) may be helpful in highlighting the collagen band (Fig. 16.2c). Immunohistochemistry for glycoprotein tenascin also delineates the collagen band, but is usually not necessary. In addition to the thickened collagen, intraepithelial lymphocytes may be variably increased. Cryptitis or crypt abscesses may also be present, but are not prominent [1, 4, 5].

The entity reported as "pseudomembraneous collagenous colitis" (Fig. 16.2d) is not well characterized, and possibly results from a pseudomembranous colitis of a different etiology superimposed on pre-existing CC [4, 5, 8].

Differential Diagnosis

The histologic findings of MC are distinctive and generally not confused with other causes of colitis, especially when interpreted in the context of endoscopic and clinical findings. Acute colitis is histologically characterized by predominantly neutrophilic inflammation and no or minimal architectural changes. Idiopathic inflammatory bowel disease shows variable crypt architectural changes of chronicity. Eosinophils may be prominent in MC but should not influence the diagnosis if other findings of MC are present.

Caution should be exercised when evaluating tangentially sectioned biopsies which may give the false appearance of thickened subepithelial collagen. In such cases the inflammatory component is absent. Subepithelial collagen may also be thickened in polyps or in areas with chronic mechanical or ischemic mucosal injury, especially when located distally, and a diagnosis of CC should not be made (Fig. 16.3). Epithelium associated with lymphoid aggregates contains more numerous IELs, and a diagnosis of LC should not be made unless other areas show the typical histologic changes.

While an attempt should be made to further subtype MC into lymphocytic or collagenous type, in some cases it is not possible, and a diagnosis of MC with a descriptor such as "mixed features," "not further classified," "favor lymphocytic," or "favor collagenous" may be acceptable.

Treatment and Prognosis

MC has a relapsing clinical course, and response to treatment depends on managing or eliminating the possible underlying etiology, such as celiac disease and medications. The prognosis of patients ranges from recovery after a single episode to severe and refractory disease. Antidiarrheal medications and topically acting steroids (such as budesonide) are important considerations in the management of these patients. More potent immunosuppression and colectomy may be necessary in refractory cases [2].

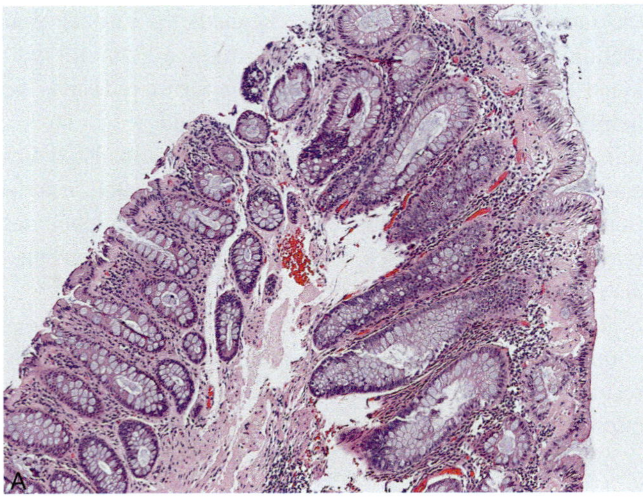

Fig. 16.3 Nonspecific subepithelial collagen thickening in a rectal pseudopolyp

Brainerd Diarrhea

Brainerd diarrhea is a distinct clinicopathologic entity that is thought to result from an infectious etiology, likely viral. Disease clusters have been reported in association with drinking water and consumption of raw milk. Histologically, the mucosal changes are characterized by increased IELs within the surface epithelium, without involvement of the crypts, increased inflammation in the lamina propria, or thickening of subepithelial collagen [9].

Eosinophilic Colitis

Definition

Eosinophilic colitis (EC) is not a well-defined entity and is generally recognized as a condition that is characterized by a predominantly eosinophilic infiltration of the colon. The clinical implication of this diagnosis depends on whether the terminology is used as a primary diagnosis or as a morphologic descriptor for increased eosinophils secondary to a variety of possible causes [10].

Clinical Features

The pathogenesis of eosinophilic gastrointestinal disease is not well defined. In its primary form, it appears to result from a hypersensitivity or allergic reaction. Eosinophilic proctocolitis (also called "allergic proctocolitis") in infants and neonates is a distinct clinicopathologic entity due to allergy to cow's milk or soy protein.

It is important to note that eosinophils may be increased secondarily in a variety of systemic and localized conditions, and a purely morphologic diagnosis of "eosinophilic colitis" should prompt consideration by the pathologist and clinician for a specific underlying condition as a goal for clinical management. Such conditions include parasitic infestation, inflammatory bowel disease, and mast cell disease. Primary EC (or eosinophilic gastrointestinal disease) is thus a clinicopathologic diagnosis used after secondary causes of eosinophilic infiltration are excluded. Some authors prefer using the generic terminology of "intestinal

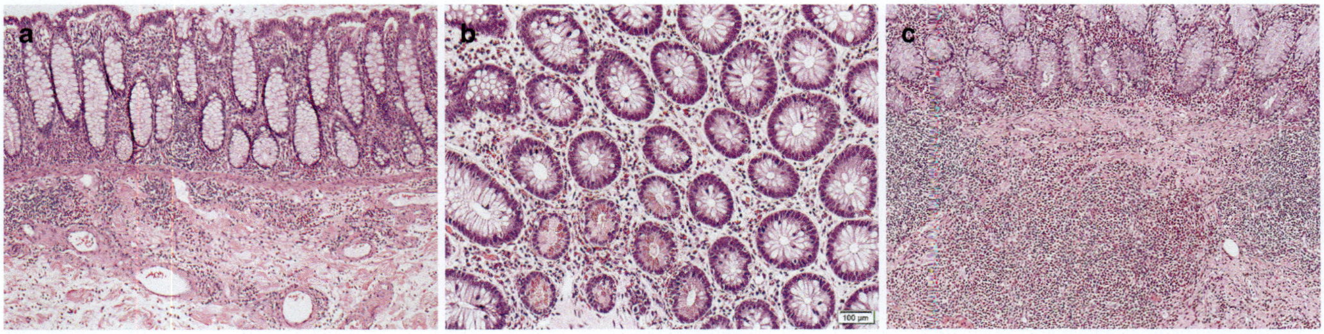

Fig. 16.4 Eosinophilic colitis (EC). (**a**) Colonic mucosa shows increased mucosal and submucosal eosinophils. (**b**) Eosinophilic cryptitis. (**c**) EC occurring in the setting of Churg-Strauss syndrome

eosinophilia" to avoid confusion between a morphologic finding and an etiologic diagnosis, highlighting the need for clinical correlation [11].

Primary EC ("allergic proctocolitis") occurring in infants and neonates is considered by most authors as a distinct entity, and is described below. Among older patients with EC, males and females are equally affected and presenting symptoms include abdominal pain, diarrhea, and rectal bleeding. Eosinophilic gastrointestinal diseases are associated with peripheral eosinophilia in up to 35% of patients. In the serosal form, ascites may be present. Presentation in patients with secondary mucosal eosinophilia will depend on the underlying disease process, but will also likely include gastrointestinal symptoms [12].

Endoscopic findings in EC may be quite variable and nonspecific, and include normal-appearing mucosa, erythema, loss of vascular pattern, nodularity, and ulceration. Changes can be present throughout the colon, but tend to be more pronounced in the ascending colon and rectum. Involvement of the deeper layers may give rise to strictures [13].

Pathologic Features

Eosinophils are normally present in the mucosa of the gastrointestinal tract distal to the esophagus. Due to normal variations, it is impossible to establish thresholds for the diagnosis of eosinophilic gastrointestinal diseases. In the normal colon, the number of eosinophils (and other inflammatory cells) in the lamina propria decreases from proximal to distal, with reported counts ranging from 10 to 70/high-power field (hpf) in the cecum to 1–10/hpf in the rectum. Moreover, eosinophil counts may also show geographic and seasonal variations. For these reasons, determination of increased eosinophils is a subjective evaluation. Although some authors have used a threshold of 20–25 eosinophils/hpf, counting is not recommended routinely [13].

Histologic features that are considered as abnormal include increased eosinophils (subjectively), especially when associated with eosinophilic cryptitis, crypt abscesses, and degranulation. In addition to these findings, eosinophils are also usually present in the muscularis mucosae and submucosa if present in biopsies (Fig. 16.4a–c). Depending on the extent of involvement of the wall, three types of EC are proposed: mucosal, mural, and serosal (Fig. 16.5a, b). As mentioned above, it is important to consider secondary causes of increased eosinophils when performing a histologic evaluation [14, 15].

Differential Diagnosis

EC in its primary form is a diagnosis of exclusion when other causes of increased eosinophils are excluded. Other causes of colonic eosinophilia include parasitic infestation, drugs, mast cell disease, Langerhans cell histiocytosis, vasculitis, idiopathic inflammatory bowel disease, hypereosinophilic syndrome, and eosinophilic leukemia (Table 16.1 and Table 16.2) [14].

Treatment and Prognosis

Management of patients with colonic eosinophilia involves careful consideration for the many possible underlying causes, and treatment should be given accordingly. Primary EC often follows a chronic relapsing clinical course, and treatment is based on the severity of symptoms. Dietary modifications are generally less effective in controlling symptoms in adults. Corticosteroids are often effective, and unless the underlying trigger is controlled, patients may become steroid dependent and develop its side-effects. Other more potent immunomodulatory agents may be considered in severe cases, and surgical management may be necessary in cases with complications [16].

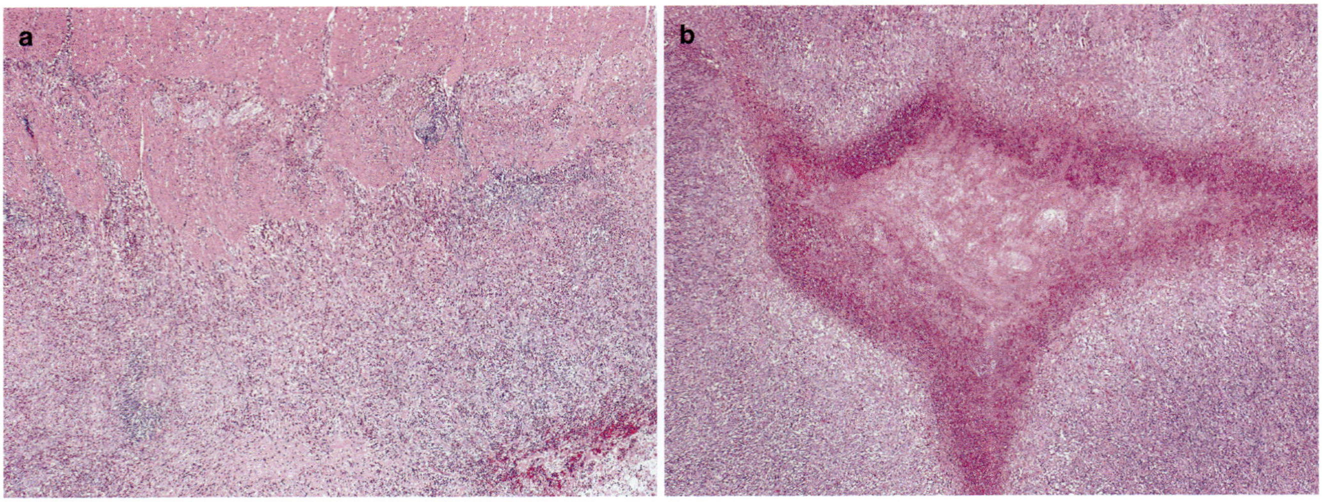

Fig. 16.5 Mural eosinophilic colitis (EC). (**a**) Transmural and subserosal eosinophilic infiltrate. (**b**) An intramural eosinophilic abscess in EC

Table 16.1 Known causes of colonic eosinophilia

Food allergy
Cow milk, soy, eggs, peanuts, seafood
Drugs
Idiopathic inflammatory bowel disease
Parasites
Connective tissue disorders
Vasculitis (Churg-Strauss syndrome)
Hematolymphoid disorders
Systemic mastocytosis

Table 16.2 Clinicopathologic features of (primary) eosinophilic colitis/eosinophilic gastroenteritis

Absence of an underlying disease causing increased eosinophils
Increased eosinophils (subjective assessment)
Eosinophilic cryptitis and crypt abscesses
Eosinophilic degranulation
Eosinophils in mucularis mucosae or deeper layers
Small bowel villous blunting with increased eosinophils

Allergic Proctocolitis

Definition

As mentioned above, the term "allergic proctocolitis" is used to describe a clinicopathologic condition characterized mainly by allergy to cow's milk or soy proteins in infants and neonates. Other proteins (including in breast milk) may also rarely trigger the allergic reaction, hence the preference for a broader clinical terminology of "food protein-induced allergic proctocolitis" or "protein intolerance" [17, 18].

Clinical Features

Affected neonates or infants usually present in the first few months of life. Onset of symptoms is acute or insidious, and relates to the introduction of cow's milk, soy, or other proteins to breast-fed infants, and severity is related to the amount of ingested protein. Symptoms include blood tinged stools, bloody diarrhea, and less often, increased gas, emesis, and abdominal pain. Growth of the child is not affected. Endoscopic findings are limited to the rectosigmoid colon, and include erythema, nodularity, and possibly erosions or ulcers [18].

Pathological Features

Histologically, allergic proctocolitis shows changes predominantly in the rectal mucosa. There is increased eosinophils (generally >60/hpf) with a tendency to localize adjacent to lymphoid follicles. Eosinophilic cryptitis, degranulation, and involvement of muscularis mucosae are commonly present [19].

Treatment and Prognosis

Treatment is focused on elimination of the inciting protein. Infants with proctocolitis develop tolerance to the protein within the first few years, and the long-term prognosis is excellent [17, 20].

Mastocytosis and Mastocytic Colitis

Mastocytosis

Definition

Mastocytosis is a group of disorders characterized by infiltration of neoplastic mast cells in one or more organ systems. This entity is discussed in this chapter because it is an important differential diagnostic consideration for increased mast cells in the colon.

Clinical Features

In 90% of adult patients with mastocytosis there is an activating mutation in the *KIT* gene (D816V), leading to constitutive activation of the receptor and autonomous mast cell proliferation. This mutation occurs less frequently in children. The colon may be involved variably in non-cutaneous forms of mastocytosis, most commonly in indolent systemic mastocytosis [21, 22].

Mastocytosis encompasses multiple clinicopathologic presentations, with the three main categories being (1) cutaneous mastocytosis, (2) systemic mastocytosis, and (3) mast cell sarcoma. In systemic mastocytosis, in addition to the bone marrow, the liver, spleen, lymph nodes, and the gastrointestinal tract are often involved. The gastrointestinal tract is involved in 60–80% of patients, most frequently presenting as abdominal pain and diarrhea. Endoscopic findings are not specific and depend on the extent and density of the mast cell infiltrates. The findings include erythema, edema, mucosal granularity, nodular or polypoid lesions, and ulcers. In some cases the mucosa may appear normal [23, 24].

Pathological Features

Normally, mast cells comprise <5% of the mononuclear cells in the lamina propria, with counts of <15/hpf. Both in normal and reactive or inflammatory conditions, the mast cells are generally mildly increased and dispersed evenly in the lamina propria, without aggregation. Architectural distortion is either absent or mild.

Systemic mastocytosis is diagnosed using criteria defined by the World Health Organization (WHO), including major and minor criteria. The major criteria require the presence of compact clusters of >15 mast cells in extra-cutaneous sites. The neoplastic cells are usually admixed with eosinophils (Fig. 16.6a). On H&E stain, the mast cells are atypical, often with elongated or spindle cell morphology (Fig. 16.6b) and immunohistochemistry for tryptase or CD117 is helpful (Fig.16.6c, d). Other supportive findings include aberrant expression of CD2 and/or CD25 by the mast cells and elevated serum tryptase (Fig. 16.6e) [21]. Isolated atypical enterocolic mast cell aggregates may be occasionally seen in patients with no clinical suspected or established diagnosis of systemic mastocytosis. They are considered as an incidental finding, probably with no clinical significance [25].

Differential Diagnosis

The goal of histologic assessment for mast cell infiltrates in the GI tract should be to distinguish between reactive and neoplastic infiltrates. The clustering, nodular, or sheet-like architecture of the infiltrates and the staining for CD2 or CD25 are important considerations.

Treatment and Prognosis

Treatment of systemic mastocytosis focuses on several approaches. These include avoiding triggers of mast cell degranulation, treatment of acute and chronic mast cell mediator release, and treatment of organ infiltration by mast cells. Symptoms often resulting from mediator release can be controlled with medications such as histamine receptor antagonists, cromolyn, corticosteroids, and anti-anaphylaxis medications. For cytoreductive treatment agents such as interferon, fludarabine cladribine, and tyrosine kinase inhibitors have been used. The overall prognosis for systemic mastocytosis depends on the variant of disease and the degree of organ infiltration by mast cells [26].

Mastocytic Colitis

"Mastocytic enterocolitis" is an entity proposed by Jakate et al. for patients with a clinical picture of diarrhea-predominant irritable bowel syndrome and increased mucosal mast cells (>20 mast cells/hpf). A majority of patients in

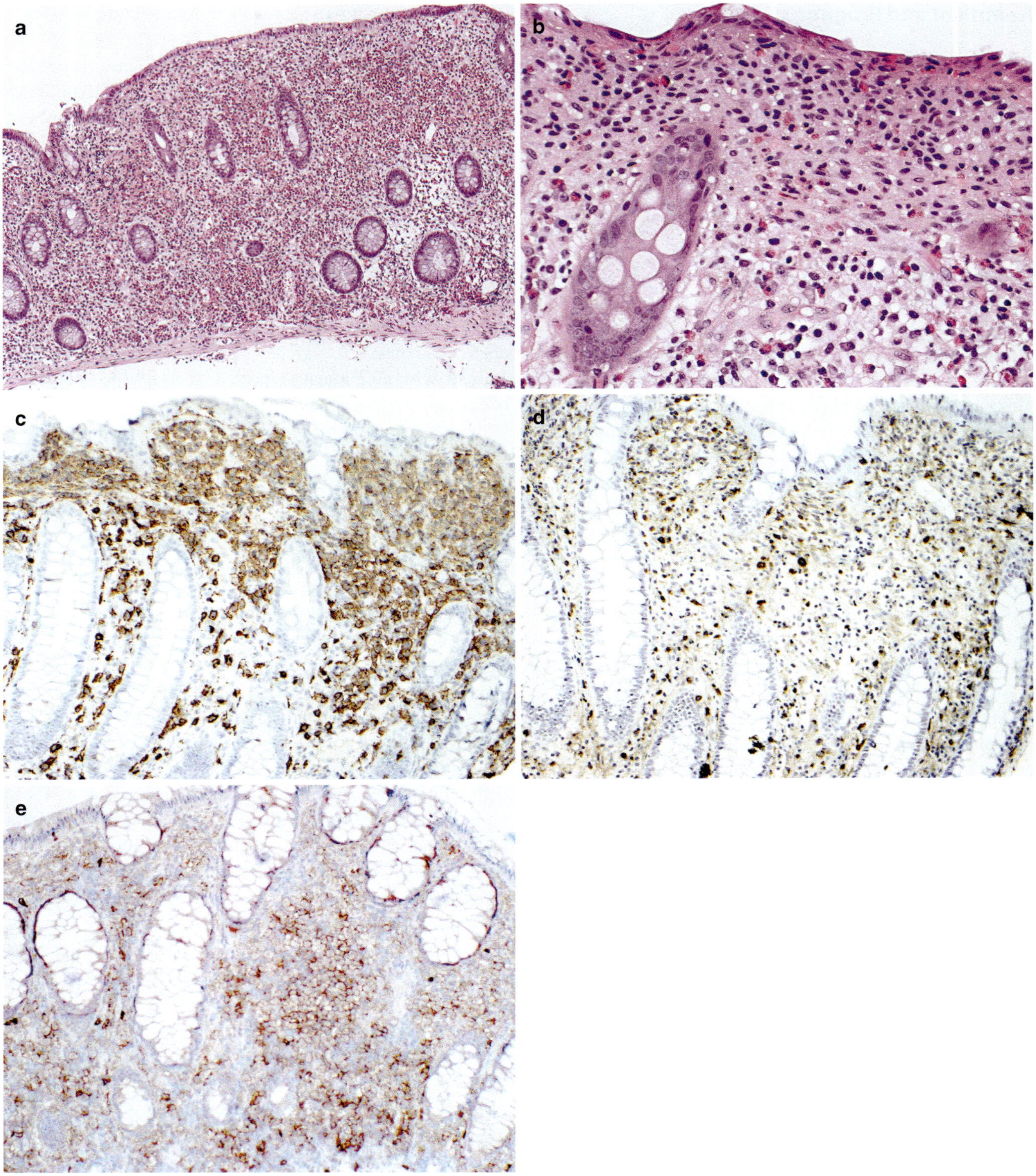

Fig. 16.6 Colonic involvement by systemic mastocytosis. (**a**) The lamina propria is expanded by a mononuclear cell infiltrate and accompanying numerous eosinophils. (**b**) High-power view reveals oval- to spindle-shaped mast cells, which are confirmed by immunostains for CD117 (**c**) and tryptase (**d**). (**e**) Mast cells in systemic mastocytosis are positive for CD25

this study had symptomatic response to antihistaminic H1 blocker treatment. Histologic evaluation for this entity requires the use of mast cell stains. Currently, this diagnosis is not widely accepted and awaits further investigation [27].

Acute Self-limited Colitis

Definition

Acute self-limited colitis (ASLC) is a clinicopathologic diagnosis wherein the biopsies show predominantly neutrophilic inflammation, in the absence of other specific patterns of injury, such as pseudomembrane formation, granulomatous/histiocytic pattern, ischemic/hemorrhagic pattern, or an active chronic colitis pattern [8].

Clinical Features

ASLC is most commonly due to an infection, and the histologic changes result from an acute inflammatory response to the infection and/or mucosal injury. Hence, the terminology is often used interchangeably with "acute infectious colitis." Less commonly, similar changes may occur due to a drug (such as NSAIDs) or even in early evolving phase of idiopathic inflammatory bowel disease (Table 16.3) [28, 29].

Patients present with acute-onset abdominal pain and bloody diarrhea, often with constitutional symptoms such as fever and malaise. Upper gastrointestinal symptoms may also be present. Endoscopic appearance of the colonic mucosa is variable, ranging from erythema, edema, exudates, and erosions or ulcers. The terminal ileum may also be involved [29].

Pathological Features

ASLC is typically characterized by predominantly neutrophilic inflammation in the lamina propria, with cryptitis and/or crypt abscesses, usually involving the upper half of the mucosa, without features of chronicity (Fig. 16.7). Pseudomembranes and aphthous ulcers may be present. In later stages of infection, crypt architectural distortion and larger ulcers may be present raising the differential diagnosis of inflammatory bowel disease [4, 8, 30].

Differential Diagnosis

Differential diagnosis includes other infectious and noninfectious causes of mucosal injury (Table 16.3). Identification of specific infectious agents requires stool examination,

Table 16.3 Common causes of acute self-limited colitis pattern

Infections
Campylobacter jejuni
Salmonella species
Shigella species
Yersinia enterocolitica
Vibrio species
Escherichia coli
Aeromonas species
Clostridium difficile (rarely)
Entamoeba histolytica
Cryptosporidium
Enteric viruses
Medications
NSAIDs
Antibiotics
Chemotherapy

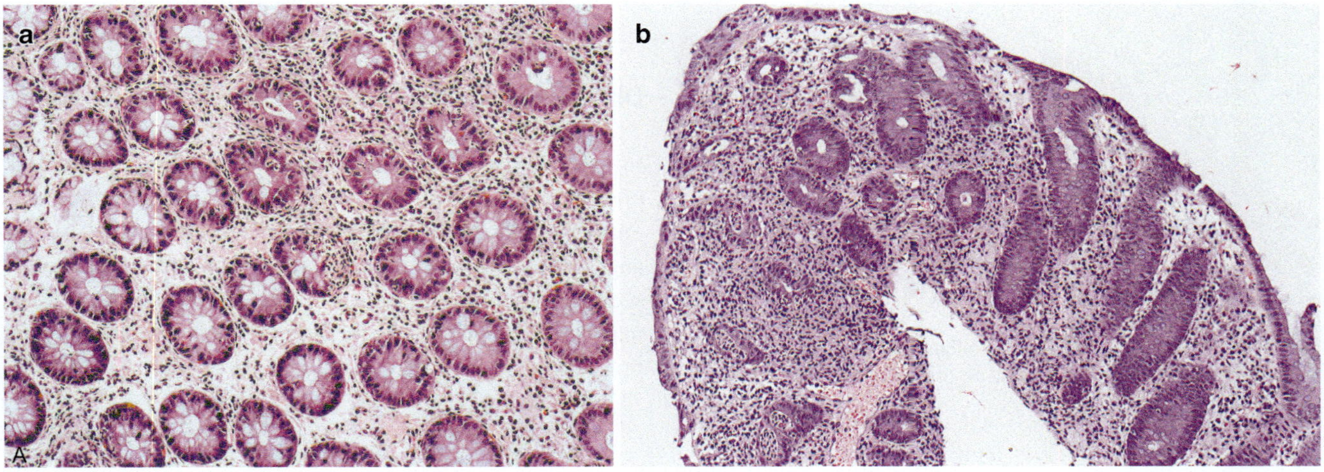

Fig. 16.7 Acute self-limited colitis. (**a**) Acute colitis, consistent with self-limited colitis. There is neutrophilic cryptitis with preserved crypt architecture. (**b**) Acute colitis due to *Salmonella* infection. There is edema, cryptitis, crypt abscesses, and mild crypt architectural changes

including culture. Drug-induced colonic injury can mimic ASLC, and clinical correlation is necessary. Idiopathic inflammatory bowel disease shows the typical architectural distortion and chronic inflammatory changes, including basal plasmacytosis. Acute ischemic colitis may contain neutrophils; however, hemorrhage and necrosis are more prominent [8, 30].

Treatment and Prognosis

Most cases of ASLC resolve after symptomatic treatment, and a pathogen is not commonly identified. Appropriate treatment with antibiotic may be given in severe or progressive cases. Modification of drug therapy may be necessary if the injury is drug-induced.

Focal Active Colitis

Focal active colitis is a descriptive diagnosis that indicates focal neutrophilic inflammation of the mucosa in a background of normal architecture (Fig. 16.8). These foci may not be seen endoscopically, or may be seen as aphthous ulcers. The importance of recognizing this pattern is its weak association with Crohn's disease, particularly in pediatric patients. More commonly, these foci may be due to aggressive bowel preparation, drugs (such as NSAIDs), or infection [31, 32].

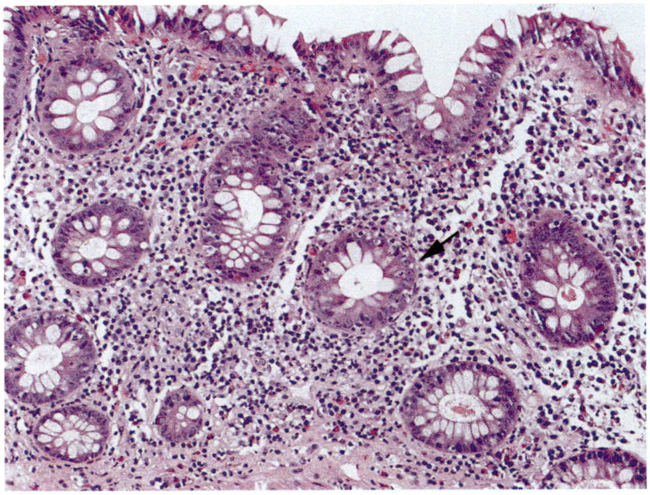

Fig. 16.8 Focal active colitis. The inflammation is characterized by increased plasma cells in the lamina propria and focal cryptitis (arrow)

Radiation Colitis/Proctitis

Definition

Radiation colitis is the injury resulting from exposure to radiation and is a collateral damage occurring in patients treated for cancer.

Clinical Features

The most common clinical setting is treatment for rectal, gynecologic, bladder, or prostate cancers. Acute proctitis is caused by direct DNA damage to the cells in the radiation field, especially the more rapidly proliferative mucosal epithelial cells. Chronic changes result from a combination of mucosal regeneration, fibrosis, and ischemia due to vascular damage and neovascularization [33].

Acute proctitis occurs within days after radiation treatment, with the mucosa showing edema, erythema, and friability. Chronic changes occur after weeks or months and include mucosal atrophy and telangiectasia, ulcers, strictures, fistulas, and adhesions.

Pathological Features

Acute radiation proctitis is characterized by epithelial injury, including increased apoptosis, reactive and degenerative nuclear atypia, and glandular dilatation. Inflammation is generally mild with mostly eosinophils and neutrophils. The lamina propria is congested and edematous (Fig. 16.9a). In chronic radiation proctitis there is mucosal telangiectasia and crypt architectural distortion, atypical stromal cells, stromal fibrosis, and vascular hyalinization (Fig. 16.9b). The mucosal changes may resemble chronic ischemic injury. Mural fibrosis may lead to stricture formation [34].

Differential Diagnosis

In the appropriate clinical context, diagnosis of radiation proctitis is usually not difficult. The vascular changes may mimic those seen with portal hypertensive proctopathy or angiodysplasia. Architectural distortion may mimic that seen in inflammatory bowel disease; however, the inflammatory changes of inflammatory bowel disease are not present [34].

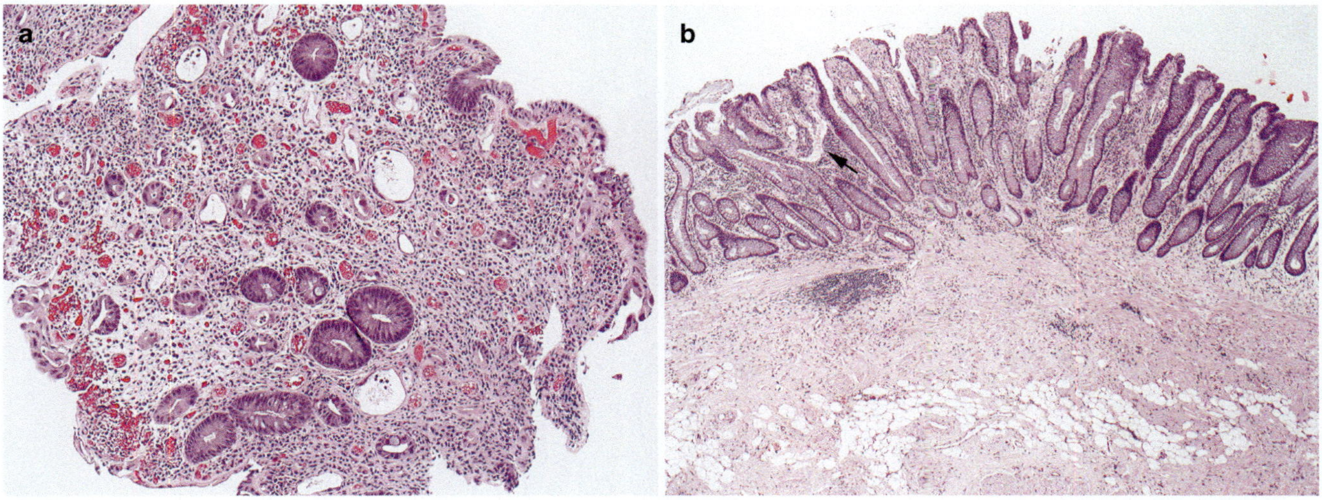

Fig. 16.9 Radiation proctitis. (**a**) Acute radiation proctitis. There is mild inflammation in the lamina propria, atrophy, dilatation and loss of crypts, and scattered crypt epithelial cells with radiation atypia. (**b**) Chronic radiation proctitis. The mucosa shows fibrosis, mild chronic inflammation, ectatic vessels (arrow), and architectural distortion. There is mural fibrosis and lipomatous change in the submucosa

Treatment and Prognosis

Acute radiation proctitis is self-limited and managed with antidiarrheal treatment, hydration, and cessation of radiation exposure. Treatment of chronic radiation proctitis is dependent on the nature of the complications. Mucosal bleeding may be controlled by endoscopic techniques such as laser and radiofrequency ablation. Strictures may be endoscopically dilated. Surgical treatment is utilized for fistulas, strictures, and local reconstruction [35].

Diverticular Disease-Associated Segmental Colitis

Definition

Diverticular disease-associated segmental colitis (DDASC) is a segmental inflammatory process that occurs in the region of colonic diverticula, also clinically referred to as segmental colitis associated with diverticulosis (SCAD). It may be mainly restricted to the mucosa, but when there is involvement of the deeper portions of the diverticula, it is often accompanied by mural or transmural inflammation with fibrosis [36].

Clinical Features

Inflammation limited to the surface mucosa is thought to be caused by long-standing prolapse of the mucosa leading to irritation. Inflammation involving diverticula leads to inflammation, ulceration, and fibrosis in the deeper layers of the wall. The changes are limited to the segment of colon involved by the diverticula [37].

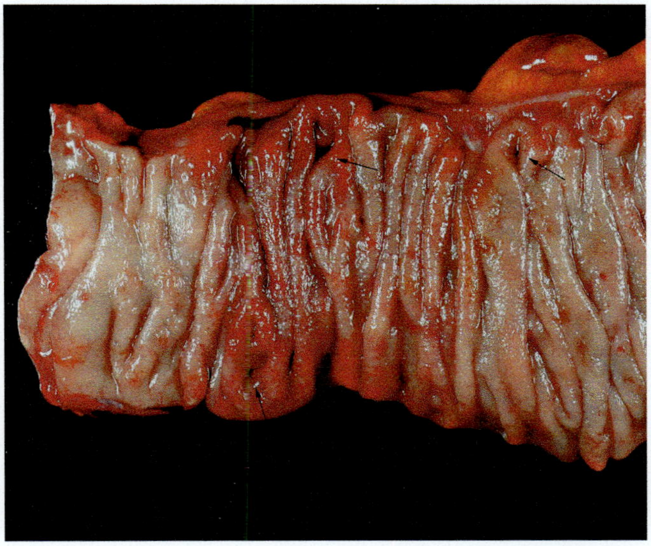

Fig. 16.10 Diverticular disease-associated segmental colitis. There is patchy mucosal edema, congestion, and superficial ulcers. Note the opening of the diverticula (arrows)

DDASC occurs in older patients and often presents with bloody stools, leading to endoscopic evaluation. It occurs in a minority (<5%) of patients with diverticulosis. The colonic mucosa appears inflamed in the descending and sigmoid colon corresponding to a segment of diverticulosis, with erythema or erosions (Fig. 16.10). The rectum and colon proximal to the segment are uninvolved [37, 38].

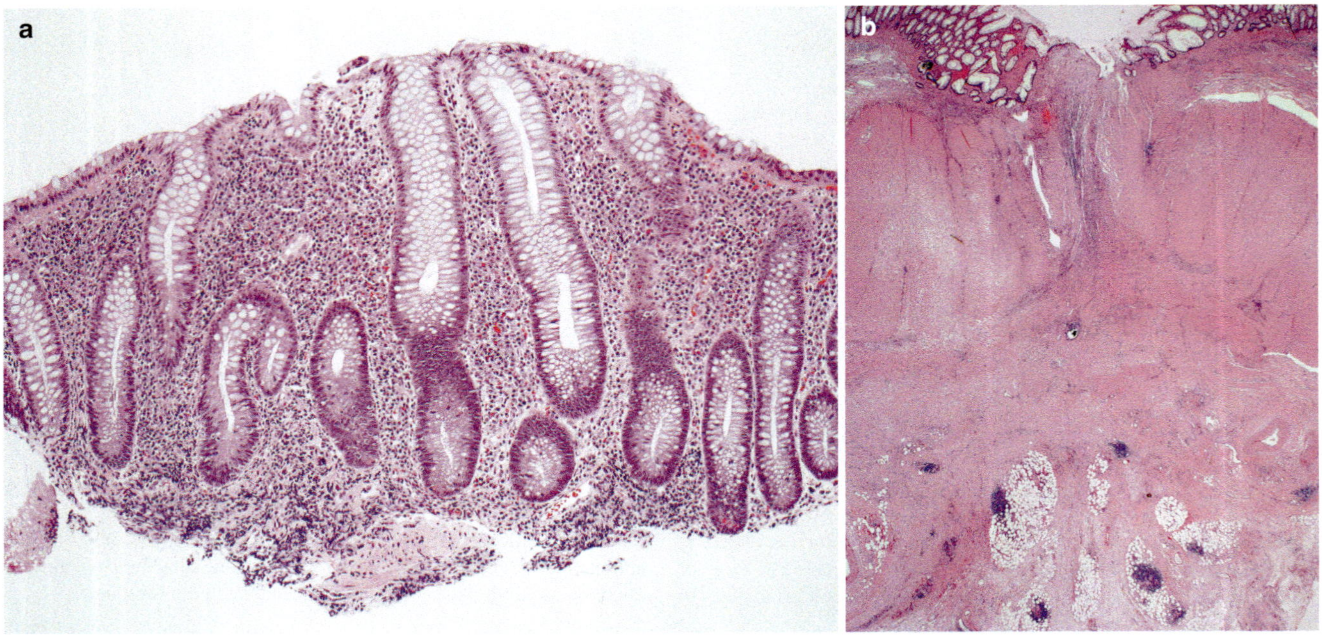

Fig. 16.11 Diverticular disease-associated segmental colitis. (**a**) Mildly active chronic colitis with crypt architectural distortion, resembling idiopathic inflammatory bowel disease. (**b**) Transmural chronic changes mimicking Crohn's disease

Pathological Features

Histologically, the findings in DDASC are variable, ranging from mildly active chronic colitis (Fig. 16.11a) to severely active disease with ulceration. Basal plasmacytosis, lymphoid aggregates, cryptitis, crypt abscesses, and crypt architectural distortion may be present, mimicking idiopathic inflammatory bowel disease. Transmural inflammation and poorly formed or crypt-related granulomas may also be present, raising the possibility of Crohn's disease (Fig. 16.11b) [5, 39].

Differential Diagnosis

The main differential diagnosis of DDASC is inflammatory bowel disease, with the segmental involvement resembling Crohn's disease, especially when there is transmural inflammation and fibrosis. Localization of changes only in the region of diverticulosis would be a strong consideration in the differential diagnosis. In female patients, an uncommon cause of sigmoid stricture with secondary mucosal inflammation is intramural endometriosis [39].

Treatment and Prognosis

Treatment of DDASC follows the treatment of diverticular disease. It includes bowel rest, antibiotics, fiber, and anti-inflammatory medications, with response in a majority of patients. Patients not responding to medical management require surgical resection.

Diversion Colitis

Definition

Diversion colitis (DC) is inflammation of segments of colon or rectum from which the fecal stream has been diverted using a surgical procedure.

Clinical Features

DC is caused by a lack of short chain fatty acids in the excluded segment. These fatty acids are produced by colonic anaerobic bacteria, and are a source of nutrition for the colonocytes. Absence of the fatty acids leads to epithelial injury and inflammation [40].

DC occurs in a specific clinical setting as described above. The diversion may be due to a neoplastic or non-neoplastic process. The procedure may be a colostomy or ileostomy with closure of the distal segment (e.g., Hartmann's procedure). DC occurs in a majority of patients who undergo the procedure; however, only a minority of patients develop symptoms. Patients develop mucoid or bloody discharge with or without abdominal pain, starting

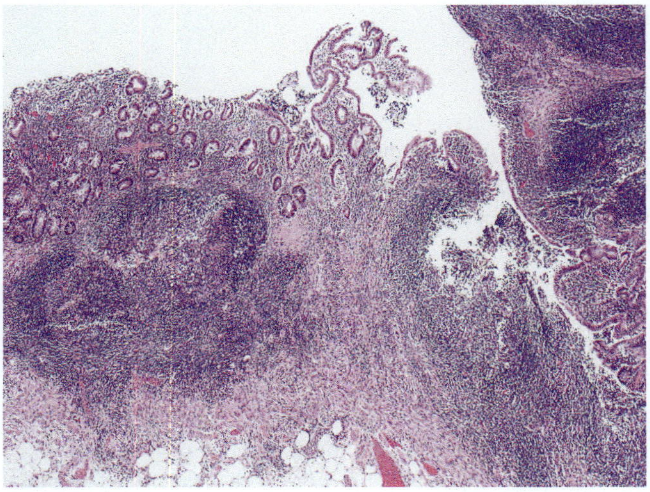

Fig. 16.12 Chronic diversion proctitis in a Hartmann's pouch characterized by prominent lymphoid hyperplasia. There is an associated background change of chronic ulcerative proctitis

a few months after the procedure. Endoscopically, the mucosa shows erythema, edema, nodularity, and aphthous ulcers [41].

Pathological Features

The most characteristic histologic finding is reactive mucosal lymphoid hyperplasia, corresponding to the nodularity seen grossly and endoscopically. Other findings include active chronic mucosal inflammation with cryptitis, crypt abscesses, architectural distortion, and aphthous ulcers (Fig. 16.12) [42].

Differential Diagnosis

Histologic differential diagnosis usually includes inflammatory bowel disease, especially in patients with a known history. In patients with ulcerative colitis initially undergoing abdominal colectomy with creation of a rectal stump (Hartmann pouch), DC may coexist with background ulcerative colitis. In some cases, DC may mimic acute self-limited (infectious) colitis.

Treatment and Prognosis

Most patients with DC are asymptomatic and do not require therapeutic intervention. In patients undergoing re-establishment of fecal stream the inflammatory changes regress. Patients who do not undergo this procedure benefit from short chain fatty acid enemas [40].

Autoimmune Colopathy/Enterocolopathy

Definition

Autoimmune colopathy occurs as part of an enterocolopathy (AIEC) that is considered to occur primarily through an autoimmune mechanism. A majority of patients with autoimmune enteropathy also show involvement of the colon [43].

Clinical Features

The etiology and pathogenesis of AIEC are not clearly defined. A majority of patients have anti-enterocyte antibodies, and many also have an underlying immunodeficiency syndrome. However, it is noted that anti-enterocyte antibodies are not entirely specific to this condition, and may be present with other diseases such as HIV infection, inflammatory bowel disease, or celiac disease. Some patients also have other antibodies, such as anti-goblet cell, anti-parietal cell, and antinuclear antibodies. Inherited disease syndromes associated with AIEC include the immune dysregulation, polyendocrinopathy, and X-linked (IPEX) syndrome and the autoimmune polyendocrinopathy, mucocutaneous candidiasis, and ectodermal dystrophy (APECED) syndrome [44].

Patients with AIEC present with secretory diarrhea, malabsorption, and severe weight loss that is not responsive to gluten-free diet or total parenteral nutrition. Testing for anti-enterocyte antibodies, evaluation for associated clinical conditions, and exclusion of other possible causes are therefore important. A set of diagnostic criteria have been proposed for AIEC. Endoscopic findings in the colon include mucosal erythema, friability, and loss of normal vascular pattern [45].

Pathological Features

Histologically, the colonic mucosa shows variable mixed inflammation and architectural changes, including lymphoplasmacytic inflammation, neutrophilic cryptitis, crypt abscesses, and increased intraepithelial lymphocytes, the latter especially in crypt bases. Apoptotic bodies are easily seen, and in cases with anti-goblet cell antibodies, there may be decrease or loss of goblet cells, endocrine cells, and Paneth cells (Fig. 16.13). In the small bowel, there is a malabsorption pattern with severe blunting of villi [44].

Differential Diagnosis

Patients with AIEC commonly have both upper and lower endoscopies due to their clinical presentation. The small

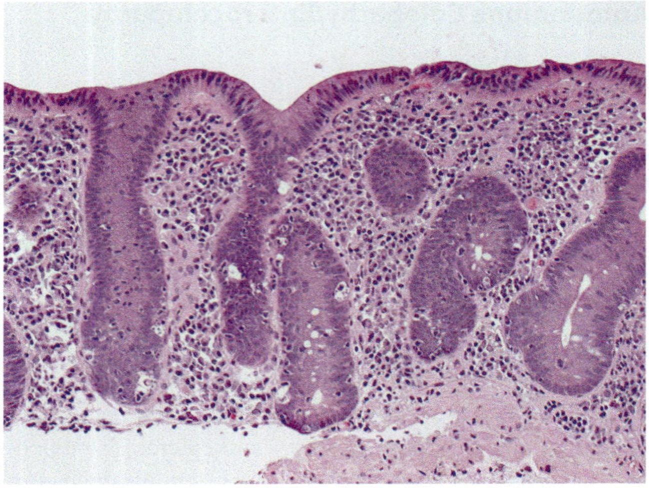

Fig. 16.13 Autoimmune colopathy. The colonic mucosa shows lymphoplasmacytic inflammation, mildly increased intraepithelial lymphocytes, and apoptotic bodies. Note the absence of goblet cells and Paneth cells

bowel biopsies usually show striking changes of a malabsorption pattern with diagnostic considerations including celiac disease, tropical sprue, bacterial overgrowth, olmesartan-associated enteropathy, and autoimmune enteropathy. Colonic biopsies should be interpreted in conjunction with changes in the small bowel, if biopsies from the latter are also available. If evaluated in isolation, the colon biopsies may resemble other more common forms of injury [44].

Treatment and Prognosis

Immunosuppression is the main approach to treat for patients with AIEC, in addition to nutritional management including total parenteral nutrition [46, 47].

Malakoplakia

Definition

Malakoplakia is a rare disorder characterized by a predominantly histiocytic inflammation containing Michaelis-Gutmann bodies.

Clinical Features

The disorder is thought to result from a defect in macrophage function resulting in the inability to digest microorganisms in lysozomes. The most common organisms are gram negative bacteria, especially *E. coli*. The lysozomes contain variably digested bacteria that become concentrically encrusted with calcium, phosphate, and iron to form the diagnostic Michaelis-Gutmann bodies [48].

Malakoplakia most commonly involves the genitourinary tract. Within the gastrointestinal tract, the left colon is the most common site. Underlying immunodeficiency may be present and a minority of patients have colonic adenocarcinoma. Outside of the urinary tract where there is a female predominance, malakoplakia has no age, gender, or racial predilection. Patients generally present with diarrhea, fever, and abdominal pain, without obstruction. Endoscopically, the most common finding is the presence of tan-yellow mucosal plaques or nodules. Multinodular, polypoid, or mass lesions may also be present [49].

Pathological Features

Histologically, there is a diffuse infiltrate of histiocytes with eosinophilic granular cytoplasm, admixed with neutrophils. Variable numbers of these histiocytes contain the Michaelis-Gutmann bodies (Figs. 16.14a, b). These structures are round

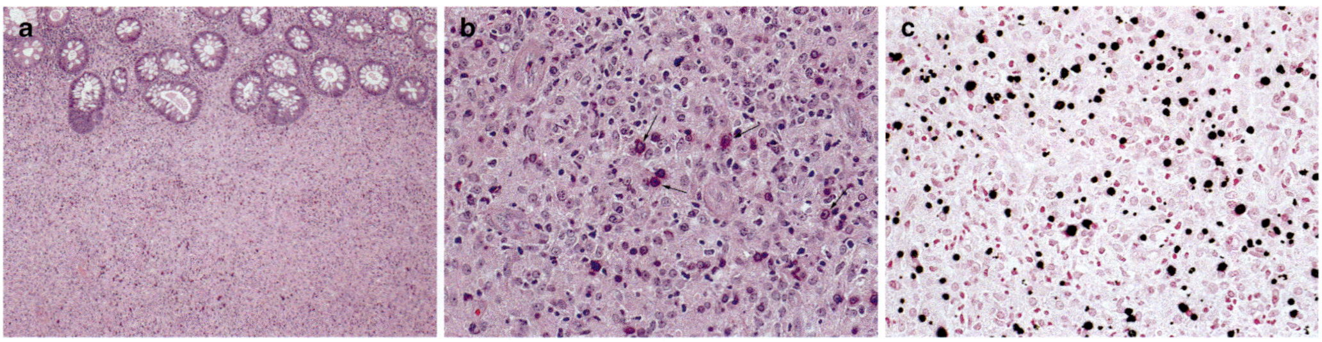

Fig. 16.14 Malakoplakia. (**a**) Dense histiocytic infiltrate admixed with other inflammatory cells, including neutrophils. (**b**) The histiocytes contain abundant eosinophilic cytoplasm with many Michaelis-Gutmann bodies (arrows), the latter a characteristic finding in malakoplakia. (**c**) The Michaelis-Gutmann bodies are highlighted with a von Kossa stain

lamellated concretions, which can be highlighted with a von Kossa stain for calcium (Fig. 16.14c) [49].

Differential Diagnosis

The differential diagnosis of malakoplakia includes other conditions (infectious and noninfectious) that contain abundant histiocytes. Infectious diseases include mycobacterial and fungal infections as well as Whipple's disease. Noninfectious conditions include storage diseases and xanthogranulomatous reactions. The latter may resemble malakoplakia, but the Michaelis-Gutmann bodies are absent. Mucosal xanthomas are usually small and not likely to be confused with malakoplakia.

Treatment and Prognosis

Given the role of bacteria in the pathogenesis of malakoplakia, antibiotic treatment has been used, with varying success. Surgical resection of the involved segment may be performed if clinically indicated [49, 50].

Cord Colitis Syndrome

Cord colitis syndrome (CCS) is a persistent diarrheal illness occurring after cord blood hematopoietic stem cell transplantation, in the absence of graft-versus-host disease or other causes. In the patients originally reported by Herrera et al., the syndrome developed between 3 and 10 months after transplantation. Typical changes of mucosal injury are seen endoscopically, including erythema, edema, and ulcerations. Although often diagnosed in the colon, other areas of the gastrointestinal tract may also be involved. The etiology is suspected to be an infectious agent; however, a causative microorganism has not been definitely identified [51, 52].

Histologically, CCS is characterized by a chronic active colitis including granulomatous inflammation in a majority of patients (see Fig. 15.42 in Chap. 15). There is neutrophilic infiltrates within the lamina propria and crypts, mild architectural distortion, and Paneth cell metaplasia in the left colon. Fewer apoptosis are generally seen for the degree of mucosal injury compared to graft-versus-host disease. Granulomas may be well-formed or loose aggregates of histiocytes. It is important that the clinicopathologic evaluation includes microbiologic testing and special stains to exclude other identifiable infectious causes for the changes [51].

Patients with CCS improve after treatment with antibiotics such as fluoroquinolone and metronidazole; however, recurrence is common after discontinuation of treatment [51].

Colitis in Systemic Diseases

Graft-Versus-Host Disease

Definition

Graft-versus-host disease (GVHD) is an immunologic reaction in which the donor T lymphocytes attack the host tissues.

Clinical Features

GVHD is dependent on multiple variables, including antigenic (mostly HLA) mismatch between the donor and the recipient, previous sensitization, and prophylaxis. It has been proposed that tissue damage due to conditioning treatment and subsequent activation and clonal expansion of donor T cells against host antigens underlies acute GVHD. In chronic GVHD the persistence of the donor T cell clones, in addition to possible autoimmune phenomenon, leads to ongoing tissue damage. Prophylactic immunosuppressive treatment and depletion of donor lymphocytes may decrease the onset and intensity of GVHD [53].

GVHD was historically classified into acute or chronic depending on the time of onset and clinical presentation: acute if occurring within 100 days after transplantation and chronic if occurring after 100 days. However, overlap exists between these arbitrary definitions, and a more recent guideline addresses this by recommending the following categories: (1) classic acute GVHD (≤100 days); (2) persistent, recurrent, or late acute GVHD (>100 days); (3) classic chronic GVHD (any time with features of chronic GVHD); and (4) overlap syndrome (any time, with features of both acute and chronic) [54].

The gastrointestinal tract is the second most common site of involvement after the skin. Patients with gastrointestinal involvement present with nausea, vomiting, diarrhea, hematochezia, and abdominal pain. Typical endoscopic findings include an "orange peel" appearance, spotty redness, sloughing, and larger mucosal defects. Rectosigmoid biopsies have the highest diagnostic yield; however, sampling of the upper GI tract may also be done, where the best yield is in duodenal biopsies [55].

Pathological Features

Histologically, the most diagnostic feature of GVHD in mucosal biopsies is the presence of increased apoptosis in the epithelial cells, most easily recognized in the proliferative zones of the mucosa. In the colon, apoptosis is seen in the crypt epithelium. Presence of crypt apoptosis without crypt destruction is the earliest stage of the disease. More severe injury is characterized by dilatation and loss of crypts, cryptitis, and crypt abscesses, followed by ulceration (Fig. 16.15a, b). The National Institutes of Health Pathology Working Group recommends three categories for reporting: (1) negative for GVHD, (2) possible GVHD, and (3) likely

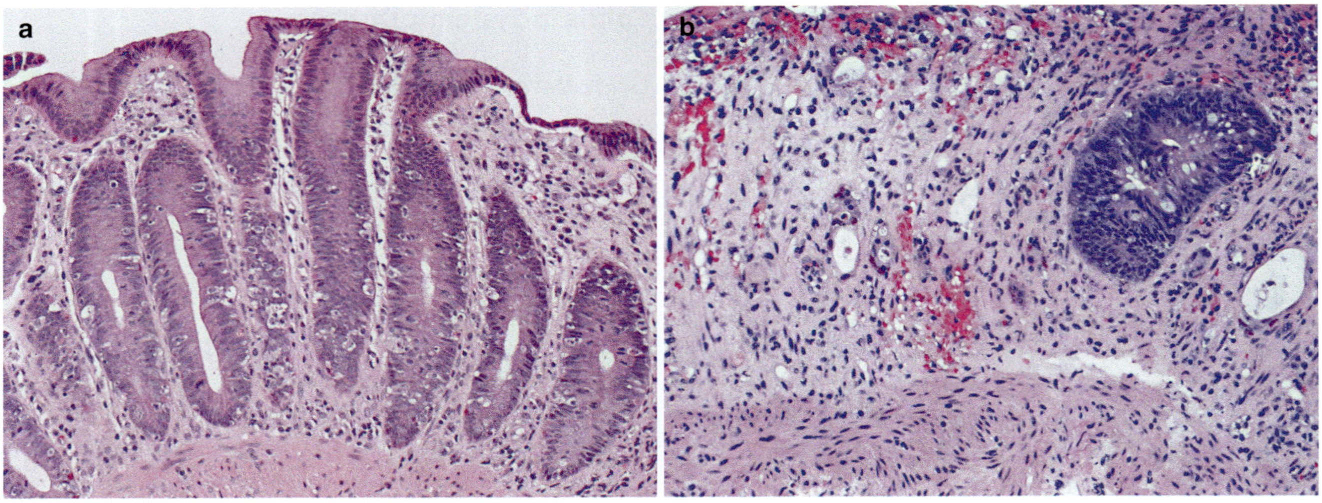

Fig. 16.15 Graft-versus-host disease (GVHD). (**a**) GVHD with numerous crypt apoptosis. (**b**) GVHD with prominent crypt loss and surface erosion

GVHD. However, no single universally accepted classification is currently used [54].

There is no universally accepted grading scheme for acute GVHD either. The most commonly used grading system for colonic GVHD was described by Lerner:

- Grade 1: scattered isolated crypt apoptosis without crypt loss
- Grade 2: crypt apoptosis with individual crypt loss
- Grade 3: loss of two or more contiguous crypts
- Grade 4: extensive crypt loss with mucosal denudation

Differential Diagnosis

The histologic differential diagnosis of GVHD includes other causes of colitis, especially infections (such as cytomegalovirus) and drug toxicity. Immunohistochemistry for cytomegalovirus should be considered in this setting. A majority of patients with clinically suspected GVHD have supportive findings on biopsies. It is also possible that GVHD may coexist with other etiologies for colitis.

Treatment and Prognosis

The mainstay of first-line treatment is immunosuppression with corticosteroids, with sustained response in <50% of patients with acute GVHD, and 40–50% with chronic GVHD. Second-line treatments include other immunosuppressive agents, as well as more recently, the use of targeted therapies. Despite treatment chronic GVHD remains a major cause of morbidity and mortality, either directly or due to complications related to its treatment [53].

Sarcoidosis

Sarcoidosis is a chronic granulomatous disorder of unknown etiology, involving the lungs in 90% of the cases. Approximately 50% of patients with lung disease also have extra-pulmonary involvement, and the gastrointestinal tract is involved in <5% of these cases. Gastrointestinal sarcoidosis is most common in the stomach, and the anorectum and colon are less frequently involved. Sarcoidosis is more common in the African-American population and women [56].

Clinical manifestations of gastrointestinal sarcoidosis include abdominal pain, weight loss, protein-losing enteropathy, symptoms of obstruction, and bleeding. Endoscopic findings depend on the extent of involvement, and include normal-appearing mucosa, erythema, diffuse thickening, nodularity, and ulceration [56].

Histologically, sarcoidosis shows non-necrotizing granulomas, either isolated or confluent, with or without ulceration (Fig. 16.16). Differential diagnosis of sarcoidosis typically includes other causes of granulomatous disease, the foremost being Crohn's disease and infections. A helpful clinical clue to the diagnosis is a history of sarcoidosis if present. At the minimum, acid fast and fungal stains should be performed in these cases, and on repeat endoscopy tissue culture studies should be considered [57].

Corticosteroids are the first line of treatment for patients with sarcoidosis, and in progressive disease, other agents such as methotrexate may also be considered [56].

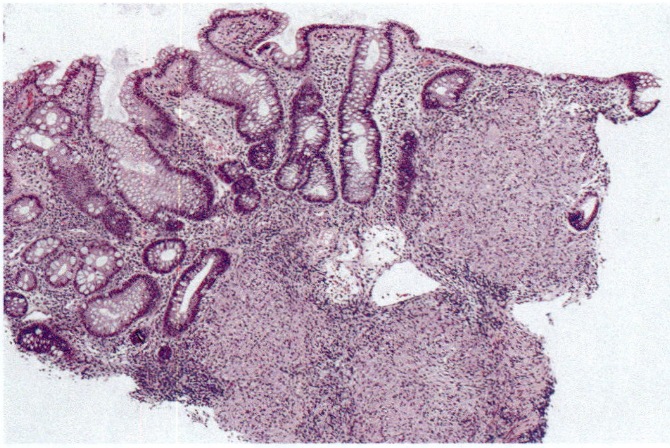

Fig. 16.16 Rectal involvement by sarcoidosis. Patient had a history of sarcoidosis and stains were negative for microorganisms. There are multiple well-formed, non-necrotizing, and confluent granulomas, associated with mucosal injury

Behçet Disease

Behçet disease is a systemic vasculitic disorder affecting multiple organs. The disease is typically characterized by oral ulcers and variable involvement of other sites including genitalia, eyes, skin, joints, central nervous system, and the gastrointestinal tract. A positive pathergy test may be present, in which there is an exaggerated response to minor skin injury. The disease is more common in the Middle East and Asian regions ("Silk Road Disease"), and is rare in Western countries. Gastrointestinal involvement has been reported in 3–26% of patients with Behçet disease, and is more common in children compared to adults [58].

Symptoms associated with gastrointestinal Behçet disease include abdominal pain, hematochezia, diarrhea, nausea, and vomiting. The disease most commonly involves the terminal ileum and right colon. Other gastrointestinal sites may also be involved. The ulcers are typically aphthoid or larger, the latter characteristically punched out, single or multiple, round or ovoid. The ulcers are more commonly located on the anti-mesenteric border, a feature of distinction with Crohn's disease [59].

Histologically, the earliest abnormality is focal active colitis, corresponding to the aphthous lesion. These foci enlarge to become well-defined ulcers, which may be deep and associated with transmural inflammation and lymphoid aggregates. The adjacent mucosa is inflamed and regenerative, but the remaining background mucosa is essentially normal. Ischemic mucosal changes are typically not seen. Stricture, perforation, and fistula may occur. The vasculitis affects the submucosal and subserosal vessels, and mostly involves veins (see Fig. 15.43 in Chap. 15). The vasculitis is characterized by intramural mononuclear cells and neutrophils. Veins in other sites may also be involved (such as cutaneous thrombophlebitis) [60].

The differential diagnosis of Behçet disease includes other causes of ulcers, such as Crohn's disease and NSAID-induced ulcers. Currently, the favored treatment of Behçet disease is by the TNF-alpha inhibitor infliximab, replacing the older agents. Surgical treatment is indicated in cases with complications, and recurrent disease around the anastomosis is common [59].

Chronic Granulomatous Disease

Chronic granulomatous disease (CGD) is an inherited immune deficiency disorder that affects the NADPH oxidase system of the phagocytes. The NADPH oxidase system produces superoxides that have an important role in killing intracellular microorganisms. Multiple gene mutations are implicated, the most common being the CYBB mutation with an X-linked recessive inheritance pattern. Other mutations are autosomal recessive. The frequency of CGD in the United States is 1 in 200,000, and a majority of patients are diagnosed before the age of 5 years. The disease reduces the life expectancy to 25–35 years [61].

The gastrointestinal tract is involved in the vast majority of patients, with the colon being most frequently involved. Endoscopic findings include those of an active chronic colitis, with skip lesions and anorectal involvement, including formation of strictures. Histologically, there is presence of pigmented (lipofuscin-laden) macrophages (see Fig. 15.41 in Chap. 15), granulomas, and active chronic colitis. Acid and fungal stains are usually negative for microorganisms [62].

Therapeutic options for CGD include aggressive antimicrobial prophylaxis and treatment, interferon gamma injections, and stem cell transplantation. Gene therapy remains in the trial stage and may become a therapeutic option in the future [63].

Common Variable Immunodeficiency

Common variable immunodeficiency (CVID) syndrome (also called adult-onset hypogammaglobulinemia) is the second most common immunodeficiency syndrome after IgA deficiency and the most common symptomatic immunodeficiency

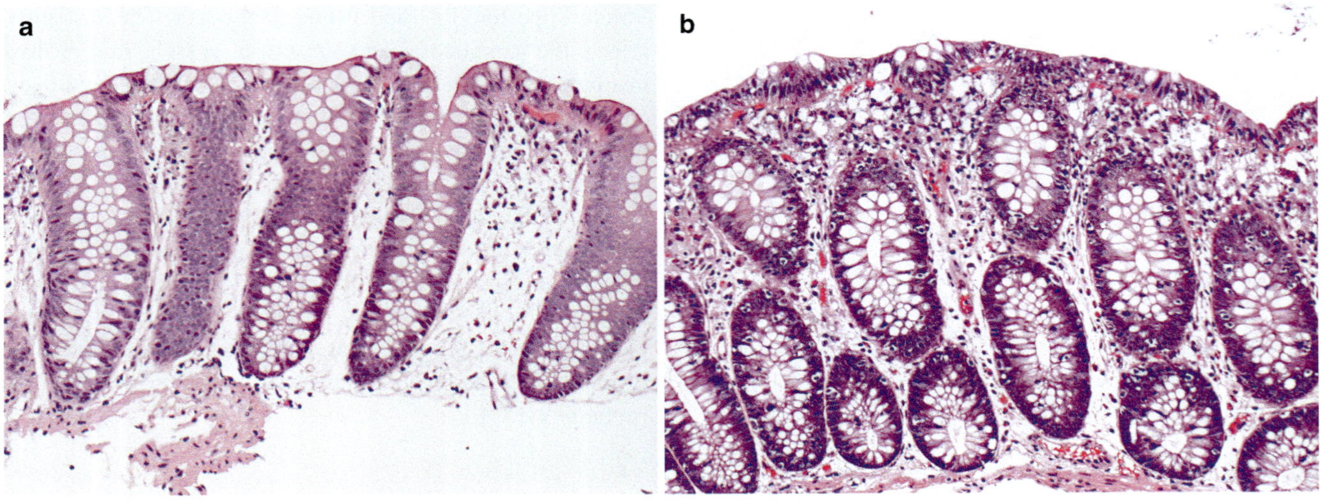

Fig. 16.17 Common variable immunodeficiency. (**a**) Unremarkable colonic mucosa with essentially no plasma cells in the lamina propria. (**b**) Lymphocytic colitis pattern but with apoptosis and absence of plasma cells in the lamina propria

in adults. It is a disorder of B lymphocyte development resulting in a defect in immunoglobulin production. Mutations implicated in the disease are known in approximately 10% of cases [64].

The clinical presentation in CVID is broad with involvement of multiple organs. Gastrointestinal tract is the second most commonly involved organ (after the respiratory tract), with infectious complications occurring in 10–40% cases. Symptoms of CVID include bloating, abdominal pain, and diarrhea. Endoscopic abnormalities may be seen both in the upper and lower tracts, such as changes of gastritis, small bowel villous atrophy, and colitis [64, 65].

Histologically, in approximately two thirds of the patients, there is a decrease in plasma cells in the lamina propria; in the remaining patients, the plasma cells may appear adequate in number but are hypofunctional. In the colon the mucosal abnormalities are quite variable, including changes resembling quiescent or active inflammatory bowel disease, increased apoptosis, granulomas, infections, microscopic colitis, or nodular lymphoid hyperplasia (Fig. 16.17a, b). The changes are therefore not specific and should be interpreted in the clinical context. CVID is also associated with an increased risk for malignancies [66].

The mainstay of preventative management for CVID is lifelong immunoglobulin replacement, in conjunction with antimicrobial prophylaxis. Other treatments may be necessary depending on the specific clinical situation [64].

References

1. Langner C, Aust D, Ensari A, Villanacci V, Becheanu G, Miehlke S, et al. Histology of microscopic colitis-review with a practical approach for pathologists. Histopathology. 2015;66(5):613–26.
2. Storr MA. Microscopic colitis: epidemiology, pathophysiology, diagnosis and current management—An update. ISRN Gastroenterol. 2013;2013(18):1–12.
3. Cruz-Correa M, Milligan F, Giardiello FM, Bayless TM, Torbenson M, Yardley JH, et al. Collagenous colitis with mucosal tears on endoscopic insufflation: a unique presentation. Gut. 2002;51(4):600.
4. Patil DT, Odze RD. Biopsy diagnosis of colitis: an algorithmic approach. Virchows Arch. 2018;472(1):67–80.
5. Choi EK, Appelman HD. Chronic colitis in biopsy samples: is it inflammatory bowel disease or something else? Surg Pathol Clin. 2017;10(4):841–61.
6. Goldstein NS, Bhanot P. Paucicellular and asymptomatic lymphocytic colitis: expanding the clinicopathologic spectrum of lymphocytic colitis. Am J Clin Pathol. 2004;122(3):405–11.
7. Guagnozzi D, Landolfi S, Vicario M. Towards a new paradigm of microscopic colitis: Incomplete and variant forms. World J Gastroenterol. 2016;22(38):8459–71.
8. Jessurun J. The differential diagnosis of acute colitis: clues to a specific diagnosis. Surg Pathol Clin. 2017;10(4): 863–885.12.
9. Osterholm MT, MacDonald KL, White KE, Wells JG, Spika JS, Potter ME, et al. An outbreak of a newly recognized chronic diarrhea syndrome associated with raw milk consumption. JAMA. 1986;256(4):484–90.
10. Díaz Del Arco C, Taxonera C, Olivares D, Fernández Aceñero MJ. Eosinophilic colitis: case series and literature review. Pathol Res Pract. 2018;214(1):100–4.
11. Hurrell JM, Genta RM, Melton SD. Histopathologic diagnosis of eosinophilic conditions in the gastrointestinal tract. Adv Anat Pathol. 2011;18(5):335–48.
12. Okpara N, Aswad B, Baffy G. Eosinophilic colitis. World J Gastroenterol. 2009;15(24):2975–9.
13. Gaertner WB, Macdonald JE, Kwaan MR, Shepela C, Madoff R, Jessurun J, Melton GB. Eosinophilic colitis: University of Minnesota experience and literature review. Gastroenterol Res Pract. 2011;2011:857508. https://doi.org/10.1155/2011/857508.
14. McCarthy AJ, Sheahan K. Classification of eosinophilic disorders of the small and large intestine. Virchows Arch. 2018;472(1):15–28.
15. Conner JR, Kirsch R. The pathology and causes of tissue eosinophilia in the gastrointestinal tract. Histopathology. 2017;71(2):177–99.

16. Zhang M, Li Y. Eosinophilic gastroenteritis: a state-of-the-art review. J Gastroenterol Hepatol. 2017;32(1):64–72.
17. Nowak-Węgrzyn A. Food protein-induced enterocolitis syndrome and allergic proctocolitis. Allergy Asthma Proc. 2015;36(3):172.
18. Koksal BT, Barıs Z, Ozcay F, Yilmaz OO. Single and multiple food allergies in infants with proctocolitis. Allergol Immunopathol (Madr). 2018;46(1):3–8.
19. Winter HS, Antonioli DA, Fukagawa N, Marcial M, Goldman H. Allergy-related proctocolitis in infants: diagnostic usefulness of rectal biopsy. Mod Pathol. 1990;3(1):5.
20. Bischoff SC. Food allergy and eosinophilic gastroenteritis and colitis. Curr Opin Allergy Clin Immunol. 2010;10(3):238–45.
21. Magliacane D, Parente R, Triggiani M. Current concepts on diagnosis and treatment of mastocytosis. Transl Med UniSa. 2014;8:65–74.
22. Valent P, Akin C, Metcalfe DD. Mastocytosis: 2016 Updated WHO classification and novel emerging treatment concepts. Blood. 2017;129(11):1420–7.
23. Ramsay DB, Stephen S, Borum M, Voltaggio L, Doman DB. Mast cells in gastrointestinal disease. Gastroenterol Hepatol (NY). 2010;6(12):772–7.
24. Kochi S, Nakamura S, Oshiro Y, Kurahara K, Kawasaki K, Yaita H, Fuchigami T. Endoscopic findings of indolent systemic mastocytosis involving the colon. Endoscopy. 2014;46 Suppl 1 UCTN:E678–9. https://doi.org/10.1055/s-0034–1390916.
25. Johncilla M, Jessurun J, Brown I, Hornick JL, Bellizzi AM, Shia J, Yantiss RK. Are enterocolic mucosal mast cell aggregates clinically relevant in patients without suspected or established systemic mastocytosis? Am J Surg Pathol. 2018;42(10):1390–5.
26. Vaes M, Benghiat FS, Hermine O. Targeted treatment options in mastocytosis. Front Med (Lausanne). 2017;4:110.
27. Jakate S, Demeo M, John R, Tobin M, Keshavarzian A. Mastocytic enterocolitis: increased mucosal mast cells in chronic intractable diarrhea. Arch Pathol Lab Med. 2006;130(3):362–7.
28. Lamps LW. Infective disorders of the gastrointestinal tract. Histopathology. 2007;50(1):55–63.
29. Meuwissen SG, Vandenbroucke-Grauls CM, Geboes K. Spectrum of acute self-limiting colitis: role of the clinician and pathologist. Ital J Gastroenterol Hepatol. 1999;31(8):807–16.
30. Kumar NB, Nostrant TT, Appelman HD. The histopathologic spectrum of acute self-limited colitis (acute infectious-type colitis). Am J Surg Pathol. 1982;6(6):523–9.
31. Greenson JK, Stern RA, Carpenter SL, Barnett JL. The clinical significance of focal active colitis. Hum Pathol. 1997;28(6):729–33.
32. Shetty S, Anjarwalla SM, Gupta J, Foy CJ, Shaw IS, Valori RM, Shepherd NA. Focal active colitis: a prospective study of clinicopathological correlations in 90 patients. Histopathology. 2011;59(5):850–6.
33. Grodsky MB, Sidani SM. Radiation proctopathy. Clin Colon Rectal Surg. 2015;28(2):103–11.
34. Fajardo LF. The pathology of ionizing radiation as defined by morphologic patterns. Acta Oncol. 2005;44(1):13–22.
35. Hauer-Jensen M, Wang J, Boerma M, Fu Q, Denham JW. Radiation damage to the gastrointestinal tract: mechanisms, diagnosis, and management. Curr Opin Support Palliat Care. 2007;1(1):23–9.
36. Freeman HJ. Segmental colitis associated diverticulosis syndrome. World J Gastroenterol. 2016;22(36):8067–9.
37. Koutroubakis IE, Antoniou P, Tzardi M, Kouroumalis EA. The spectrum of segmental colitis associated with diverticulosis. Int J Color Dis. 2005;20(1):28–32.
38. Tursi A, Elisei W, Brandimarte G, Giorgetti GM, Lecca PG, Di Cesare L, et al. The endoscopic spectrum of segmental colitis associated with diverticulosis. Color Dis. 2010;12(5):464–70.
39. Lamps LW, Knapple WL. Diverticular disease-associated segmental colitis. Clin Gastroenterol Hepatol. 2007;5(1):27–31.
40. Kabir SI, Kabir SA, Richards R, Ahmed J, MacFie J. Pathophysiology, clinical presentation and management of diversion colitis: a review of current literature. Int J Surg. 2014;12(10):1088–92.
41. Tominaga K, Kamimura K, Takahashi K, Yokoyama J, Yamagiwa S, Terai S. Diversion colitis and pouchitis: a mini-review. World J Gastroenterol. 2018;24(16):1734–47.
42. Yeong M, Bethwaite PB, Prasad J, Isbister WH. Lymphoid follicular hyperplasia—a distinctive feature of diversion colitis. Histopathology. 1991;19(1):55–61.
43. Masia R, Peyton S, Lauwers GY, Brown I. Gastrointestinal biopsy findings of autoimmune enteropathy: a review of 25 cases. Am J Surg Pathol. 2014;38(10):1319–29.
44. Greenson JK. The biopsy pathology of non-coeliac enteropathy. Histopathology. 2015;66(1):29–36.
45. Akram S, Murray JA, Pardi DS, et al. Adult autoimmune enteropathy: Mayo Clinic Rochester experience. Clin Gastroenterol Hepatol. 2007;5:1282–90.
46. Gupta NK, Yilmaz O, Fisher M, Yajnik V. Abatacept: a new treatment option for refractory adult autoimmune enteropathy. J Clin Gastroenterol. 2014;48:55–8.
47. Montalto M, D'Onofrio F, Santoro L, Gallo A, Gasbarrini A, Gasbarrini G. Autoimmune enteropathy in children and adults. Scand J Gastroenterol. 2009;44:1029–36.
48. Lou TY, Teplitz C. Malakoplakia: pathogenesis and ultrastructural morphogenesis. A problem of altered macrophage (phagolysosomal) response. Hum Pathol. 1974;5(2):191–207.
49. Yousef GM, Naghibi B, Hamodat MM. Malakoplakia outside the urinary tract. Arch Pathol Lab Med. 2007;131(2):297–300.
50. Sato H, Tsukamoto T, Mizuno Y, Ichikawa T, Kotani Y, Honda K, Hatta K, Kuroda M. Endoscopic mucosal resection of a rectal malakoplakia in a healthy adult. Dig Endosc. 2014;26(6):749–51.
51. Herrera AF, Soriano G, Bellizzi AM, Hornick JL, Ho VT, Ballen KK, et al. Cord colitis syndrome in cord-blood stem-cell transplantation. N Engl J Med. 2011;365:815–24.
52. Gupta NK, Masia R. Cord colitis syndrome: a cause of granulomatous inflammation in the upper and lower gastrointestinal tract. Am J Surg Pathol. 2013;37(7):1109–13.
53. Garnett C, Apperley JF, Pavlů J. Treatment and management of graft-versus-host disease: improving response and survival. Ther Adv Hematol. 2013;4(6):366–78.
54. Salomao M, Dorritie K, Mapara MY MY, Sepulveda A. Histopathology of graft-vs-host disease of gastrointestinal tract and liver: An update. Am J Clin Pathol. 2016;145(5):591–603.
55. Endo K, Fujishima F, Kuroha M, Moroi R, Motoyuki Onodera M, et al. Effective and less invasive diagnostic strategy for gastrointestinal GVHD. Endosc Int Open. 2018;6(3):E281–91.
56. Vahid B, Spodik M, Braun KN, Ghazi LJ, Esmaili A. Sarcoidosis of gastrointestinal tract: a rare disease. Dig Dis Sci. 2007;52(12):3316–20.
57. Stemboroski L, Gaye B, Makary R, Monteiro C, Eid E. Isolated gastrointestinal sarcoidosis involving multiple gastrointestinal sites presenting as chronic diarrhea. ACG Case Rep J. 2016;3(4):e198.
58. Zeidan MJ, Saadoun D, Garrido M, Klatzmann D, Six A, Cacoub P. Behçet's disease physiopathology: a contemporary review. Auto Immun Highlights. 2016;7(1):4. https://doi.org/10.1007/s13317-016-0074-1.
59. Skef W, Hamilton MJ, Arayssi T. Gastrointestinal Behçet's disease: a review. World J Gastroenterol. 2015;21(13):3801–12.
60. Kara T, Düşmez AD. Pathologic features of Behçet's disease in the tubular gut. Pathol Res Int. 2012;2012:216254. https://doi.org/10.1155/2012/216254.
61. Winkelstein JA, Marino MC, Johnston RB Jr, Boyle J, Curnutte J, Gallin JI, et al. Chronic granulomatous disease. Report on

a national registry of 368 patients. Medicine (Baltimore). 2000;79(3):155–69.
62. Alimchandani M, Lai JP, Aung PP, Khangura S, Kamal N, Gallin JI, et al. Gastrointestinal histopathology in chronic granulomatous disease: a study of 87 patients. Am J Surg Pathol. 2013;37(9):1365–72.
63. Arnold DE, Heimall JR. A review of chronic granulomatous disease. Adv Ther. 2017;34(12):2543–57.
64. Chiriaco M, Salfa I, Di Matteo G, Rossi P, Finocchi A. Chronic granulomatous disease: clinical, molecular, and therapeutic aspects. Pediatr Allergy Immunol. 2016;27(3): 242–53.
65. Khangura SK, Kamal N, Ho N, Quezado M, Zhao X, Marciano B, et al. Gastrointestinal features of chronic granulomatous disease found during endoscopy. Clin Gastroenterol Hepatol. 2016;14(3):395–402.
66. Daniels JA, Lederman HM, Maitra A, Montgomery EA. Gastrointestinal tract pathology in patients with common variable immunodeficiency (CVID): a clinicopathologic study and review. Am J Surg Pathol. 2007;31(12):1800–12.

Infectious Disorders of the Colon

17

Bobbi S. Pritt

Introduction

Infectious colitis is a significant cause of morbidity and mortality worldwide. Diarrhea, defined by the World Health Organization (WHO) as the "passage of a 3 or more loose or liquid stools per day, or more frequently than is normal for the individual" [1], represents one of the most common manifestations of infectious colitis and may be disabling or life-threatening. The WHO estimates that there are 1.7 billion cases of childhood diarrheal disease and 525,000 childhood deaths each year, making diarrhea a leading cause of death and malnutrition in children under the age of 5 years [1]. In the United States, the Centers for Disease Control and Prevention (CDC) estimates that 47.8 million cases of acute diarrheal illness occur each year, resulting in nearly $150 million of expenses to the American healthcare system [2, 3].

Diarrheal illnesses are caused by a broad spectrum of bacteria, viruses, fungi, and parasites, many of which are transmitted through consumption of contaminated food or water [4]. The CDC identified four bacteria (*Salmonella enterica* [multiple serotypes], *Clostridium perfringens*, *Campylobacter* spp., and *Staphylococcus aureus*) and one virus (norovirus) as the most common pathogens causing foodborne illness in the United States [5]. Norovirus also enters the top 5 causes of outbreaks in the United States associated with drinking or recreational water, along with *Giardia duodenalis* (a small intestinal parasite), two enteropathogenic bacteria (*Shigella* spp. and *Campylobacter* spp.), and the parasite *Cryptosporidium* spp. [6]. Other enteric pathogens are associated with significant disease in certain populations such as members of the *Mycobacterium avium* complex in profoundly immunocompromised hosts and helminth (worm) infections in patients living in resource-limited settings with poor sanitation [4]. One category of helminth infections—the soil-transmitted helminth infections—is classified by the WHO as a neglected tropical disease and is estimated to affect 1.5 billion people worldwide (one-fifth of the world's population) [7].

In addition to diarrhea, other common manifestations of infectious colitis include anemia due to microscopic blood loss or frank hematochezia, abdominal pain, weight loss, nausea, and vomiting. The length and type of symptoms are important considerations for guiding laboratory evaluation and treatment. The American College of Gastroenterologists (ACG) recommends that laboratory stool studies be considered for cases of moderate to severe disease and for symptoms exceeding 7 days, so that the causative agent can be identified and directed therapy begun [4, 8]. Testing may also be indicated for patients at increased risk of severe disease such as immunocompromised hosts, the elderly, and neonates [9]. Laboratory testing in cases of mild illness of 7 or fewer days duration is not generally indicated since the infection is likely to be self-limited and not require pathogen-specific therapy [10]. Microbiologic testing may include conventional stool (and occasionally blood) culture, ova and parasite exam, and singleplex and multiplex nucleic acid amplification tests (NAATs), some of which can simultaneously detect bacterial, viral, and parasitic pathogens [9]. Testing for fecal leukocytes or their associated markers (e.g., fecal lactoferrin) may also be useful for assessing the type of enteric pathogen; a positive test is consistent with invasive microbial infection but can also be positive in noninfectious conditions such as idiopathic inflammatory bowel disease (IBD).

Biopsy is not generally performed for cases of acute gastroenteritis, but may be obtained in cases of persistent, chronic, or relapsing diarrhea and unexplained intestinal symptoms. Thus, the surgical pathologist may have the opportunity to evaluate the tissue and assess whether the findings are consistent with an infectious process or are more likely due to a noninfectious inflammatory process such as

B. S. Pritt (✉)
Department of Laboratory Medicine and Pathology, Mayo Clinic, Rochester, MN, USA
e-mail: pritt.bobbi@mayo.edu

L. Zhang et al. (eds.), *Surgical Pathology of Non-neoplastic Gastrointestinal Diseases*,
https://doi.org/10.1007/978-3-030-15573-5_17

IBD. If the findings are consistent with an infectious etiology, then the pathologist should attempt to identify the specific agent when possible. Some pathogens produce distinct pathologic features characteristic or suggestive of a specific organism or group of organisms (e.g., viral inclusions, pseudomembranes, or flask-shaped ulcers), allowing for generation of a specific diagnosis. Other pathogens, however, cause minimal to no histologic changes or result in nonspecific inflammatory changes (e.g., focal active colitis), thus limiting the pathologist's ability to provide a definitive diagnosis [11–15]. This chapter focuses on the primary bacteria, fungi, viruses, and parasites that infect the colon.

Bacterial Infections

Introduction

Bacteria are a primary cause of infectious colitis worldwide. Infection is most often acquired through ingestion of contaminated food or water, with *Campylobacter* spp., non-typhoidal *Salmonella* spp., *Shigella* spp., and several pathotypes of *Escherichia coli* being the most common culprits—both within the United States and in travelers [5, 6, 16]. Additional pathogens such as *Salmonella typhi* and *Vibrio cholerae* are not common in the United States but are prevalent in regions of the world with poor sanitation. Other bacteria have a universal distribution, but only cause disease in specific hosts or under certain circumstances. For example, *Clostridioides* (formerly *Clostridium*) *difficile* causes infection predominantly in individuals whose gut flora has been altered by exposure to antibiotics [17], while members of the *Mycobacterium avium* complex cause intestinal disease in profoundly immunocompromised hosts [4, 18]. Bacteria cause intestinal disease through a number of mechanisms such as mucosal invasion and toxin production [15]. In some cases, invasive bacteria spread to the blood, mesenteric lymph nodes, or other extraintestinal sites [15]. Bacterial colitis is usually self-limited with patients having full resolution of symptoms in 10–14 days [15]. Therefore patients who undergo colonoscopy with biopsy are typically those with unusual or prolonged symptoms, or those who do not respond to standard therapy [12, 14]. Many bacterial pathogens cause overlapping histologic patterns so that it is often not possible to definitively identify the specific bacterium. However, the pathologist can narrow the differential diagnosis by recognizing characteristic histologic patterns associated with various bacterial enteropathogens. The most commonly observed histologic patterns are listed in Table 17.1 [13–15, 19, 20]. It is important to note that the histopathologic changes associated with some organisms may overlap with those of IBD or ischemic colitis [13]. There may also be overlap between the histologic patterns, with some organisms having more than one pattern [13]. The most common bacterial pathogens of the colon and their associated histologic pattern and clinical manifestations are shown in Table 17.1 as well. This chapter will focus on the organisms for which the colon is the primary site of infection and the accompanying histopathologic features are well described. Organisms for which there is a lack of information regarding the associated pathologic features such as *Plesiomonas* species and some *E. coli* pathotypes are not included in this chapter. Bacteria that may infect the colon but predominantly infect other regions of the gastrointestinal tract are discussed in other chapters of this book, such as *Mycobacteria* spp. (Chap. 11), *Actinomyces* spp. (Chap. 19), *Rhodococcus equi* (Chap. 19), *Chlamydia trachomatis* serovars L1, L2, and L3 (lymphogranuloma venereum; Chap. 20), and *Treponema pallidum* (Chap. 20).

Table 17.1 Common bacterial infections of the colon by primary histologic pattern[a]

Histologic pattern	Organism (disease)	Predominant clinical manifestations	Primary histopathologic features
Minimal or no inflammatory changes	*Bradyspira* spp. (intestinal spirochetosis)	Usually asymptomatic; may be associated with watery diarrhea	"Fuzzy" basophilic mat of densely packed spirochetes at the brush border; highlighted with silver impregnation methods and commercially available *T. pallidum* IHC
	EAEC	Nausea, vomiting, abdominal pain, watery diarrhea; chronic diarrhea in AIDS patients	Gram-negative bacteria adherent to the luminal surface; minimal to no inflammation
	EPEC	Fever, mucoid diarrhea; infants and AIDS patients.	Similar to EAEC
	Neisseria gonorrhoeae (gonorrheal proctitis)	Often asymptomatic; may be associated with mucopurulent discharge, tenesmus, and pruritus	Cryptitis, rarely ulcers; usually extending <10 cm from anal verge
	Vibrio spp.	Mild to severe, profuse watery diarrhea ("rice water" stools), rapid dehydration, shock	Normal mucosa or slight increase in neutrophils in the lamina propria

Table 17.1 (continued)

Histologic pattern	Organism (disease)	Predominant clinical manifestations	Primary histopathologic features
Acute self-limited colitis	*Aeromonas* spp.	Nausea, vomiting, bloody diarrhea, abdominal pain	Ulceration, focal, mild architectural distortion
	Campylobacter spp. (campylobacteriosis)	Fever, abdominal pain, usually bloody diarrhea, malaise, relapsing disease common	Usually no significant crypt distortion; occasionally mild architectural distortion
	Non-typhoidal *Salmonella* (salmonellosis)	Nausea, vomiting, fever, watery or bloody diarrhea	Marked architectural distortion may be present
	Shigella spp. (shigellosis)	Fever, abdominal pain, watery or bloody diarrhea, intestinal perforation, HUS, rarely chronic disease	Marked architectural distortion may be present, occasional pseudomembranes
	Treponema pallidum (syphilis)	Usually asymptomatic; ulceration, anal bleeding, discharge, pain with defection	Dense lymphoplasmacytic infiltrate, cryptitis; rarely granulomatous inflammation; obliterative endarteritis. See Chap. 20
Diffuse histiocytic inflammation	Members of the *Mycobacterium avium* complex (MAC)	Usually immunocompromised hosts (e.g., MAC in patients with AIDS)	Diffuse infiltrates of foamy histiocytes in lamina propria; histiocytes contain many acid fast bacilli. See Chap. 11
	Rhodococcus equi (malakoplakia)	Usually immunocompromised hosts; pulmonary disease predominates, but extrapulmonary disease may involve the GI tract	Malakoplakia with cytoplasmic mineralized bodies (Michaelis-Gutmann bodies) within histiocytes. See Chap. 16, Non-IBD Colitis
Predominantly granulomatous inflammation	*Actinomyces* spp. (Actinomycosis)	Fever, abdominal pain, weight loss; occasionally palpable mass; rarely perianal fistula	Mixed suppurative and granulomatous inflammation, abscesses, actinomycotic granules +/− Splendore-Hoeppli reaction; occasional dense fibrotic reaction. See Chap. 19
	Mycobacterium tuberculosis (tuberculosis)	Chronic disease with fever, night sweats, abdominal pain, weight loss, diarrhea, constipation, palpable mass	Cecum and ascending colon most commonly involved; caseating mycobacteria highlighted with acid fast stains. See Chap. 11
	Yersinia enterocolitica, *Y. pseudotuberculosis* (yersiniosis)	Fever, abdominal pain, watery diarrhea, acute appendicitis, rarely chronic disease	Cryptitis, mixed suppurative and granulomatous inflammation, lymphoid hyperplasia, lymphoid aggregates, mucosal ulceration, mesenteric lymph node involvement
Predominantly lymphohistiocytic inflammation	*Chlamydia trachomatis* L1–L3 serovars (LGV)	Anorectal pain, mucopurulent discharge, and tenesmus	Ulcers, diffuse follicular lymphohistiocytic infiltrates, architectural distortion. See Chap. 20
	Salmonella Typhi/ Paratyphi (typhoid fever)	Fever, abdominal pain, watery or bloody diarrhea, headache, rash, constipation, leukopenia	Diffuse histiocytic inflammation, ulcers over hyperplastic Peyer patches, architectural distortion, rare granulomas
Ischemic	EHEC	Bloody diarrhea (predominantly), severe abdominal cramps, mild/no fever, obstruction (due to edema), massive hemorrhage, HUS, TTP	Hemorrhage, acute inflammation, marked edema, crypt withering, mucosal necrosis, and microthrombi within small blood vessels Occasional pseudomembranes
Pseudomembrane formation	*Clostridioides difficile*	Fever, abdominal pain, watery diarrhea, may progress to fulminant colitis and toxic megacolon, rarely bloody diarrhea	Rarely full-thickness mucosal necrosis. Acute colitis without pseudomembranes occasionally seen
Necrotizing enterocolitis	*Clostridioides septicum*, *C. perfringens*	Fever, abdominal pain and distension, gastrointestinal hemorrhage, perforation	Hemorrhage, submucosal edema, necrosis, pneumatosis, pseudomembranes, large Gram-positive bacilli

Abbreviations: *AIDS* acquired immune deficiency syndrome, *EAEC* enteroaggregative *Escherichia coli*, *EHEC* enterohemorrhagic *E. coli*, *EPEC* enteropathogenic *E. coli*, *HUS* hemolytic uremic syndrome, *IHC* immunohistochemical stain, *LGV* lymphogranuloma venereum, *NTM* non-tuberculous mycobacteria, *TTP* thrombotic thrombocytopenic purpura

[a]Some pathogens may occasionally demonstrate more than one histologic pattern

Minimal or No Inflammatory Changes Cases of bacterial infection with this pattern have a normal-appearing mucosa or exhibit only minimal inflammatory changes such as increased inflammatory cells in the lamina propria. This pattern may be seen with the enteroaggregative and enteropathogenic *Escherichia coli*, *Neisseria* species, *Staphylococcus aureus*, toxigenic *Vibrio cholerae* O1, and *Bradyspira* spp., the causative agents of intestinal spirochetosis [12, 13, 21]. Enteric viruses can also cause little to no inflammatory changes [13].

Acute Infectious-Type Colitis Pattern (AITC) This common pattern of bacterial colitis, also known as the acute self-limited colitis pattern, may be seen with a number of bacterial enteropathogens, including several members of the *Enterobacteriaceae* (*Aeromonas* spp., *Campylobacter* spp., non-typhoidal *Salmonella*, and *Shigella* spp.,) and *Treponema pallidum* [12, 13]. The AITC pattern may also occasionally be seen with *Clostridioides difficile* infection and enteroinvasive *E. coli*, although the features of the latter are not well described [12, 14, 15]. As the name implies, symptoms are usually self-resolving. The primary histopathologic picture is that of cryptitis in a background of preserved crypt architecture (Fig. 17.1) [15]. Mucosal edema, crypt abscess, crypt rupture, neutrophil infiltrate in the lamina propria, mucosal erosions, and small granulomas usually associated with crypt rupture may also be seen [14, 15]. Thrombosis is not usually present, thus differentiating this form of neutrophil-rich colitis from ischemic pattern infectious colitis (see below). Inflammatory changes are most prominent in the mid to upper regions of the crypts. There may also be an increased number of lymphocytes in the lamina propria, but a basal plasmacytosis should not be present [22, 23]. The lack of crypt distortion and basal plasmacytosis is helpful for distinguishing acute infectious colitis from IBD; however, the presence of crypt distortion does not rule out infection since some bacterial pathogens may also cause crypt architectural changes (see below). Biopsies of resolving acute infectious-type colitis may demonstrate residual surface damage and increased intraepithelial lymphocytes which should not be confused with lymphocytic colitis. Focal cryptitis may also be seen in the resolving stage of AITC [22]. Correlation with the clinical picture is usually sufficient for differentiating these conditions.

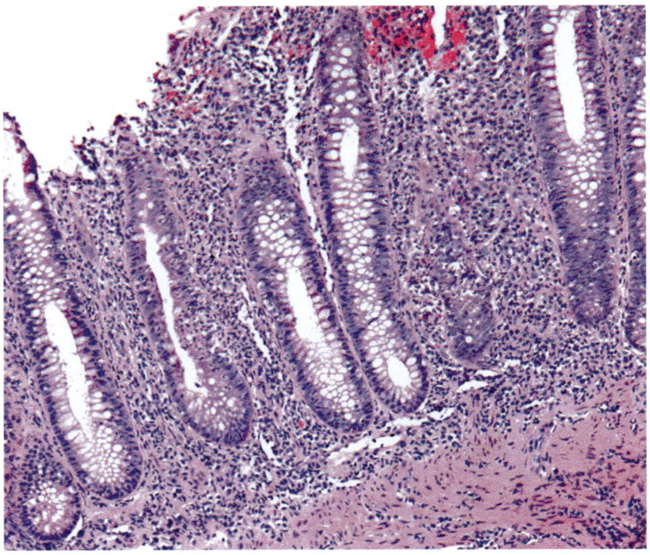

Fig. 17.1 Acute infectious-type colitis pattern, demonstrating cryptitis, crypt abscess, erosion, and neutrophils in the lamina propria. The crypt architecture is preserved. Accompanying laboratory testing detected *Campylobacter jejuni*. (Courtesy of Dr. Laura Lamps)

Architectural Distortion As mentioned above, some bacteria that are associated with the AITC pattern can cause significant architectural distortion, thus mimicking the findings of IBD. *Salmonella* (non-typhoidal and typhoidal serotypes) and *Shigella* spp., specifically, may cause pronounced architectural distortion, whereas *Aeromonas* spp. and *Campylobacter* spp. generally cause milder distortion [12]. Again, the lack of basal plasmacytosis is helpful for distinguishing an infectious etiology from IBD [12].

Diffuse Histiocytic Pattern This pattern is characterized by a diffuse, dense, infiltrate of histiocytes with abundant eosinophilic or foamy cytoplasm within the lamina propria [20, 24]. The infiltrate may significantly expand the lamina propria and cause associated crypt distortion. In some cases, epithelial injury may also be seen [20]. Well-formed granulomas are not usually present [24]. The primary bacteria associated with this pattern in the colon are *Rhodococcus equi* (causing malakoplakia) and non-tuberculosis *Mycobacteria* spp. (e.g., members of the *Mycobacterium avium* complex) [12]. Less commonly, the Whipple disease bacterium, *Tropheryma whipplei*, may involve the colon and impart a similar appearance. These entities are described further in other chapters in the text. When this histiocytic pattern is seen, other causes of lamina propria infiltrates such as pigmented infiltrates (e.g., melanosis), fat accumulation (xanthoma), mucin accumulation (muciphages), malakoplakia, and neoplastic conditions should be considered [20]. *Histoplasma capsulatum* can cause a similar infiltrate in the intestine (see below).

Predominantly Granulomatous Inflammation Pattern The presence of granulomas within the mucosa may be seen with a variety of entities including IBD, drug reaction, foreign body reaction, and infection [20]. The most common bacteria causing this pattern are *Yersinia* spp. and *Mycobacterium tuberculosis*. Both may cause pathologic features that overlap with those of IBD, including chronic active colitis with crypt distortion, patchy disease of the

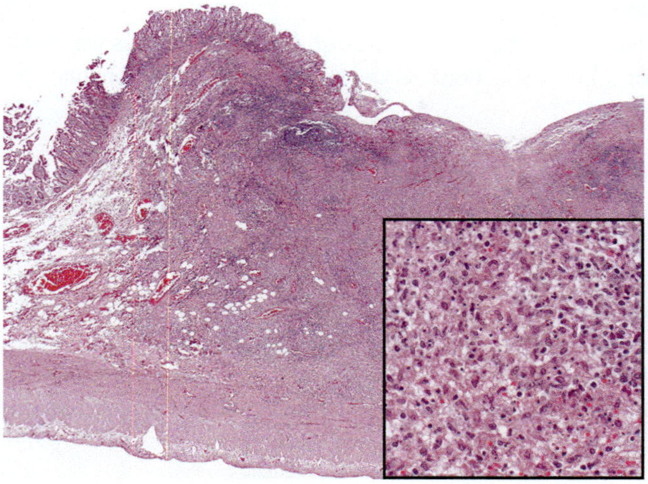

Fig. 17.2 Predominantly lymphohistiocytic inflammation pattern in a case of typhoid fever. An eosinophilic infiltrate within the submucosa is seen at low magnification associated with lymphoid aggregates and a large overlying ulcer. Higher magnification (inset) reveals the infiltrate to be composed of intermixed histiocytes and lymphocytes, with a dearth of neutrophils

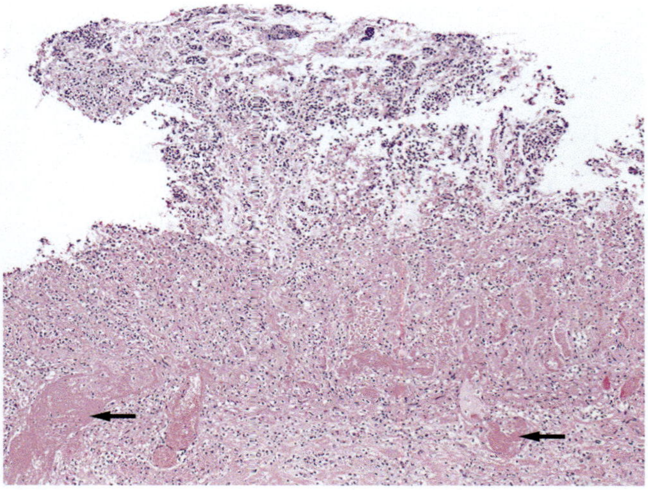

Fig. 17.3 Ischemic pattern of infectious colitis due to *Clostridioides difficile* colitis. Note that there is full-thickness mucosal necrosis and many of the small blood vessels in the submucosa contain microthrombi (arrows). A characteristic "mushroom-shaped" exudate (pseudomembrane) is also seen

colon and ileum, and involvement of multiple sites; thus tuberculosis and *Yersinia* infection should be considered in all cases of granulomatous colitis [20]. Other bacteria associated with a granulomatous pattern are *Actinomyces* spp. (with mixed suppurative inflammation), other *Mycobacterium* spp., and, rarely, *Treponema pallidum*, the causative agent of syphilis [12].

Predominantly Lymphohistiocytic Inflammation Pattern This pattern is characterized by a histiocytic infiltrate with prominent lymphocytes/lymphoid follicles (Fig. 17.2). Neutrophils are not prominent, and granulomas are rare. Significant crypt distortion may be seen. The primary organisms associated with this infectious pattern are *Chlamydia trachomatis*, L1–L3 serovars (lymphogranuloma venereum [LGV]), and *Salmonella enterica* serotypes Typhi and Paratyphi [12]. This pattern may also be seen in the resolving stage of AITC [20].

Ischemic Pattern The main histologic findings of this pattern are superficial mucosal necrosis, frequent hemorrhage, capillary fibrosis, and sloughing of the mucosal layer, occasionally forming a pseudomembrane. Microthrombi may be seen within small blood vessels. Enterohemorrhagic *Escherichia coli*, *Clostridium perfringens*, and *Clostridioides difficile* are the primary associated bacteria (Fig. 17.3). Infections with this pattern can be very challenging to differentiate from noninfectious causes of acute ischemia based on histologic features alone, and thus clinical correlation and microbiology testing are necessary [20]. Of note, the vasotrophic fungi can cause a similar histologic pattern [13].

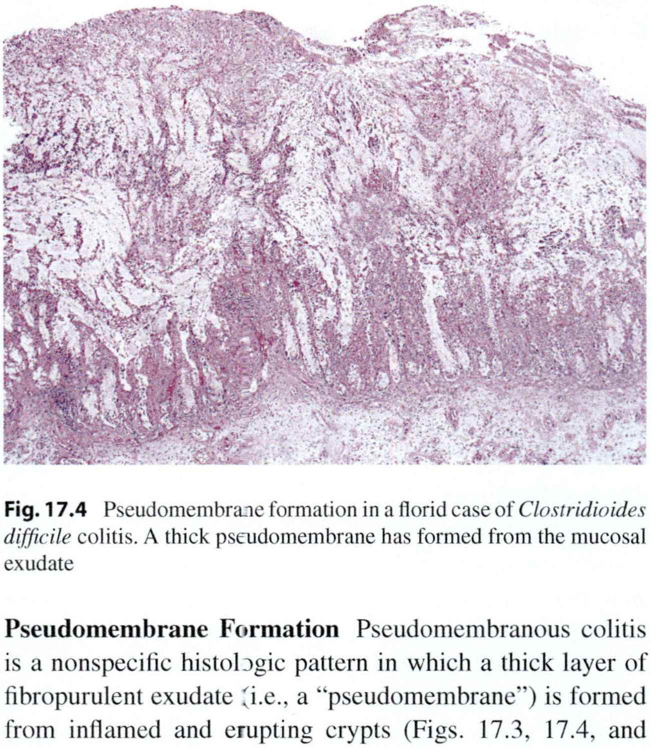

Fig. 17.4 Pseudomembrane formation in a florid case of *Clostridioides difficile* colitis. A thick pseudomembrane has formed from the mucosal exudate

Pseudomembrane Formation Pseudomembranous colitis is a nonspecific histologic pattern in which a thick layer of fibropurulent exudate (i.e., a "pseudomembrane") is formed from inflamed and erupting crypts (Figs. 17.3, 17.4, and 17.5) [25]. *Clostridioides difficile* is the primary causative agent, but *Clostridium ramosum*, Enterohemorrhagic *Escherichia coli*, occasionally *Shigella* spp., non-typhoidal *Salmonella*, *Klebsiella oxytoca*, *Staphylococcus aureus*, *Plesiomonas shigelloides*, and even some viruses (e.g., cytomegalovirus) and parasites (e.g., *Entamoeba histolytica*, *Schistosoma mansoni*, *Strongyloides stercoralis*) can also cause pseudomembrane formation [25]. Noninfectious conditions such as certain medications, illicit drugs, chemicals,

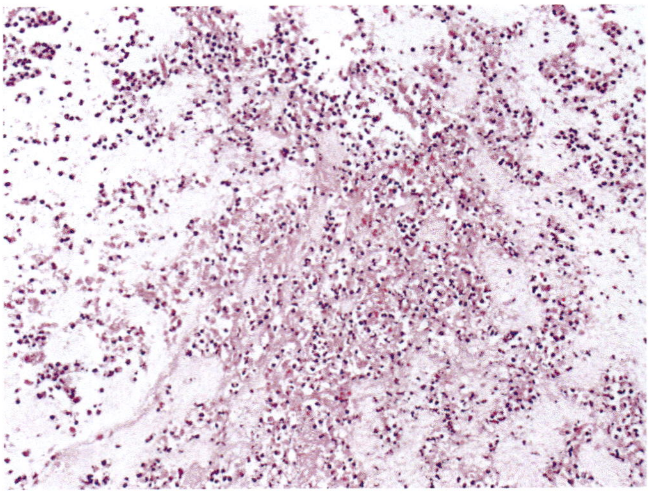

Fig. 17.5 Higher magnification of the exudative pseudomembranous layer from Fig. 17.4, demonstrating its composition of abundant mucus, neutrophils, and necrotic debris

and inflammatory conditions including IBD may also be associated with pseudomembrane formation, thus requiring careful correlation with clinical features and other laboratory test results [25].

Aeromonas Species

Definition

Aeromonas spp. are Gram-negative bacilli in the family *Enterobacteriaceae*. They have only recently been recognized as a cause of gastroenteritis, although this role is still controversial [26]. The most commonly implicated species are *A. hydrophila* and *A. sobria.* Infection is thought to be acquired through ingestion of fecally contaminated food and water [12].

Clinical Features

Most patients experience a mild, self-limited illness with nausea, vomiting, diarrhea, and cramping abdominal pain. A minority of patients (15–25%), however, experience more severe illness with dysentery and fecal leukocytes. Some may experience chronic symptoms over months to years which may clinically mimic IBD [12]. Treatment is not indicated for most infections, but can be useful in severe or chronic cases [12].

Pathological Features

Gross Findings

By endoscopy, the bowel may appear edematous with erosions, friability, exudates, and loss of the typical vascular pattern [12]. Cases are commonly segmental and thus mimic IBD. Pancolitis has also been noted [12].

Microscopic Findings

The histopathologic features of *Aeromonas* colitis are those of AITC [12]. Focal crypt architectural distortion may be seen [12].

Differential Diagnosis

As with other causes of AITC, microbiology studies are needed to identify the etiologic agent and may also be helpful for differentiating infectious causes from IBD—particular in subacute or chronic cases of *Aeromonas* gastroenteritis. Ischemic colitis may also enter the differential diagnosis based on the gross findings. However, microscopic features of ischemia such as mucosal necrosis and crypt withering are not seen with *Aeromonas* infection.

Campylobacter Species (Campylobacteriosis)

Definition

Campylobacter species are curved Gram-negative rods in the family *Enterobacteriaceae* and are one of the most common causes of diarrhea worldwide [5, 6, 16, 27]. In the United States alone, the bacterium is estimated to cause 1.3 million illnesses each year [27]. *Campylobacter jejuni* causes an estimated 90% of human infections, with other species such as *C. coli* and *C. fetus* making up the remaining 10% [27]. Infection is usually associated with consumption of contaminated food (e.g., undercooked poultry) and water. Infection is a nationally notifiable disease in the United States [28].

Clinical Features

All ages may be infected, but infants, children, and young adults are most likely to experience symptomatic infection [12]. Patients commonly present with diarrhea (usually bloody), fever, abdominal pain, and occasionally nausea and vomiting [12, 27]. The incubation period is 2–4 days, and most patients have a resolution of symptoms in 2–5 days from illness onset [27]. Fecal leukocytes are usually present. Relapse is frequent, and severe, chronic, and even disseminated infections may be seen, particularly in HIV-positive patients [27]. Importantly, infection is associated with Guillain-Barré syndrome, reactive arthropathy, Henoch-Schönlein purpura, and exacerbations of pre-existing IBD. Treatment is generally supportive with fluid and electrolyte replacement; antibiotics may be considered for patients with manifestations of, or risk factors for, severe disease [27].

Pathological Features

Gross Findings

By endoscopy, the mucosa may appear friable with associated hemorrhage, inflammatory exudate, and erythema [12]. Ulcers may also be present.

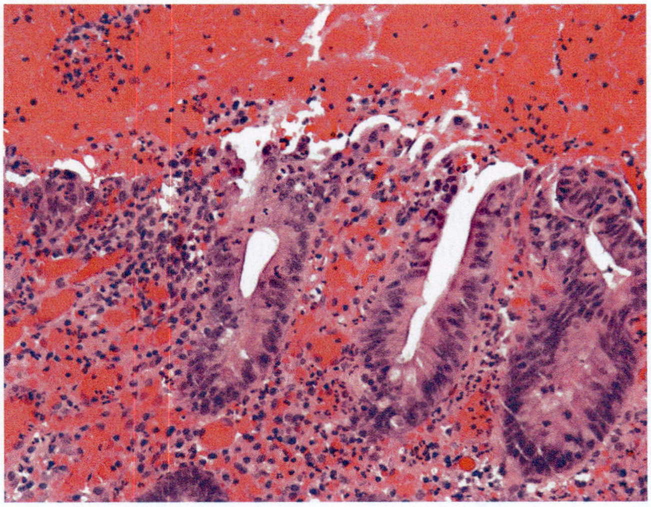

Fig. 17.6 Acute infectious type colitis with pronounced hemorrhage due to *Campylobacter* sp. (Courtesy of Dr. Laura Lamps)

Microscopic Findings

The histopathologic features of *Campylobacter* colitis are those of AITC (Fig. 17.1) [12]. Pronounced hemorrhage (Fig. 17.6) or focal crypt architectural distortion may also be seen.

Differential Diagnosis

As with other causes of AITC, microbiology studies are needed to identify the etiologic agent, and may also be helpful for differentiating infectious causes from IBD when crypt distortion is present [12].

Escherichia coli

Definition

Escherichia coli is a Gram-negative bacillus in the family *Enterobacteriaceae*. It is an important component of the normal bowel flora, being the most common member of the aerobic bacteria [11, 29]. While most *E. coli* are nonpathogenic, some specific *E. coli* types are capable of causing diarrheal disease through adherence, invasion, and/or production of enterotoxins. There are six pathotypes of diarrheagenic *E. coli*: enteroaggregative, enterohemorrhagic, enteroinvasive, enteropathogenic, enterotoxigenic, and diffusely adherent *E. coli* (EAEC, EHEC, EIEC, EPEC, ETEC, and DAEC, respectively) [29]. Of these, EHEC is most commonly encountered in pathology preparations [12] and will be the focus of this section. EHEC is acquired through ingestion of contaminated food and water. Commonly implicated foods include undercooked hamburger, unpasteurized milk, and produce [29]. Infection may also be passed from person to person through the fecal-oral route [29]. Disease is due primarily to the production of a cytotoxin similar to that produced by *Shigella* spp. (i.e., shiga toxin); however, in contrast to shigellosis, EHEC (also known as shiga toxin-producing *E. coli* [STEC]) does not invade the intestinal mucosa [29]. The CDC estimates that 265,000 cases of EHEC occur in the United States each year, of which the serogroup O157:H7 causes approximately 36% of infections [29].

Clinical Features

After an incubation period of 3–5 days, patients classically present with diarrhea (usually bloody) and severe abdominal pain. Notably, fever is mild or absent, and fecal leukocytes are only seen in one-third of cases [13, 29]. Most patients fully recover in 5–7 days, but 5–10% of infected individuals develop hemolytic-uremic syndrome (HUS) [29]. Young children and the elderly are at the greatest risk for HUS [29]. Antibiotics should not be given for EHEC infection since it increases the risk of HUS [29].

Pathological Features

Gross Findings

By endoscopy, patients with EHEC have severe colonic edema and hemorrhage [13]. Purulent exudate, erosions, and ulcerations are also common [12]. Significant edema can cause intestinal obstruction. The right colon is more commonly affected than the left [12].

Microscopic Findings

EHEC is characterized by an ischemic pattern of colitis, with significant hemorrhage, acute inflammation, marked edema of the lamina propria and submucosa, crypt withering, mucosal necrosis, lamina propria hyalinization, and microthrombi within small blood vessels [12]. Occasionally pseudomembranes are observed. The histologic appearance of intestinal biopsies from patients with EPEC and EAEC is unremarkable, although Gram-negative bacilli may occasionally be seen at the mucosal surface [12]. Degenerated epithelial cells and neutrophils may also be seen at the mucosal surface. Intestinal biopsies from patients with ETEC and EIEC are seldom examined by biopsy, and therefore the pathology has not been well described [12]. Based on the known pathophysiology of infection, the histologic appearance of ETEC is thought to be similar to that of EAEC with minimal accompanying inflammatory reaction. Similarly, EIEC pathology is thought to be similar to that of *Shigella* spp. [12].

Differential Diagnosis

The primary differential diagnoses of EHEC infection are ischemic colitis, IBD, and *Clostridioides difficile* colitis [12, 13]. Microbiology testing is necessary for identifying the etiologic agent; it is important to notify the microbiology laboratory when EHEC is suspected so that appropriate testing can be performed.

Salmonella Species (Non-typhoid Salmonellosis, Typhoid Fever)

Definition

Salmonella species are Gram-negative bacilli in the family *Enterobacteriaceae*. *Salmonella enterica* is the primary human pathogen and is classified into typhoidal and non-typhoidal serotypes based on the composition of several antigens [30]. *Salmonella enterica* serotypes Typhi and Paratyphi cause typhoid (enteric) fever, while several *Salmonella enterica* non-typhoidal serotypes including serotypes Typhimurium, Enteritidis, Newport, and Javiana are responsible for non-typhoidal salmonellosis (gastroenteritis) [31, 32]. For simplicity, *Salmonella* is commonly designated only its serotype (e.g., *S.* Typhi, *S.* Enteritidis). Both typhoidal and non-typhoidal serotypes are transmitted through the fecal-oral route, usually via contaminated food and water, and are important causes of food-associated illness and traveler's diarrhea [32]. Sexual transmission among men who have sex with men (MSM) has also been reported. The CDC estimates that non-typhoidal *Salmonella* serotypes are responsible for 1.2 million cases each year, with 23,000 associated hospitalizations and 450 deaths [32]. Foods implicated in recent outbreaks in the United States include raw turkey, chicken, pasta salad, shell eggs, raw sprouts, and precut melon and Kellogg's® Honey Smacks® cereal [32]. Recent cases have also been associated with live backyard poultry, pet guinea pig, and pet turtle contact [32]. Infection is most common in June, July, and August. Patients at increased risk of infection are children under 5 years of age, immunocompromised individuals, non-breast fed infants, and individuals with achlorhydria [32]. Unlike non-typhoidal *Salmonella* serotypes, typhoidal serotypes do not have an animal reservoir. *Salmonella* gastroenteritis (a.k.a. salmonellosis) and typhoid fever are both nationally notifiable diseases in the United States [28].

Clinical Features

Salmonellosis is characterized by watery to bloody diarrhea, abdominal pain, nausea, vomiting, and fever [32]. Patients typically develop symptoms 12–72 hours after infection and experience symptoms for 4–7 days [32]. Most individuals recover without specific treatment, but some experience severe symptoms, including dehydration requiring hospitalization, toxic megacolon, and extraintestinal disease [32]. Supportive therapy without antimicrobial agents is the mainstay for patients with mild-to-moderate intestinal infection, whereas antimicrobials are reserved for patients with severe disease, patients at risk for severe disease (e.g., immunocompromised hosts, infants, and the elderly), and patients with extraintestinal infection [32].

Typhoid fever differs from salmonellosis in having a longer incubation period (6–30 days), more insidious onset, and initial occurrence of systemic rather than intestinal symptoms [31]. Patients usually present with rising fever, headache, malaise, abdominal pain, and a transient truncal rash ("rose spots"). Hepatosplenomegaly and leukopenia are common [31]. Diarrhea usually begins in the second or third week of infection and may progress from watery to bloody. Constipation may also occur. Severe gastrointestinal bleeding and intestinal perforation are well-described complications [31]. Symptoms can last for a month if untreated [31]. Definitive diagnosis is by culture of blood or, less commonly, bone marrow. Antibiotic therapy is recommended to shorten the course and decrease the risk of death [31]. A vaccine is available for high-risk individuals, but it is not 100% effective in preventing infection.

Pathological Features

Gross Findings

In salmonellosis, the findings are similar to other causes of acute self-limited bacterial colitis, with mucosal erythema, exudates, and ulceration [12, 13]. In contrast, typhoid fever has more distinctive findings, with thickened mucosa and scattered nodules corresponding to hyperplastic Peyer's patches [12]. Ulcers are commonly present; aphthoid ulcers characteristically overlie nodular Peyer's patches and may progress to discoid ulcers, linear ulcers, and associated necrosis. In some instances, the mucosa may appear grossly normal [12]. Suppurative mesenteric lymphadenitis may also be seen. Toxic megacolon and perforation may occur in severe cases [13]. Any level of the gastrointestinal tract can be affected in typhoid fever, but the right colon, ileum, and appendix are preferentially involved due to the abundance of lymphoid tissue [13].

Microscopic Findings

The histopathologic picture of salmonellosis is that of AITC (Fig. 17.7) [13]. Severe cases may demonstrate a fibrinous exudate, crypt architectural distortion, and mucus depletion [12, 13]. The histopathologic features of typhoid fever mirror the gross manifestations, with hyperplastic Peyer's patches and overlying ulceration [12, 13]. The lesions initially begin with acute inflammation of the mucosa overlying the Peyer's patches and may have an AITC pattern. Over time, the infiltrate is replaced with histiocytes along with smaller numbers of lymphocytes and plasma cells (Fig. 17.2). There is a dearth of neutrophils in mature lesions. These cells infiltrate and obliterate the lymphoid follicles and surrounding submucosa, followed by necrosis and ulceration of the overlying mucosa (Fig. 17.8) [12, 13]. Overtime, the ulcers may become very deep, extending to, and sometimes through, the muscularis propria [12]. Significant crypt architectural distortion is common, mimicking the histologic features of IBD [13].

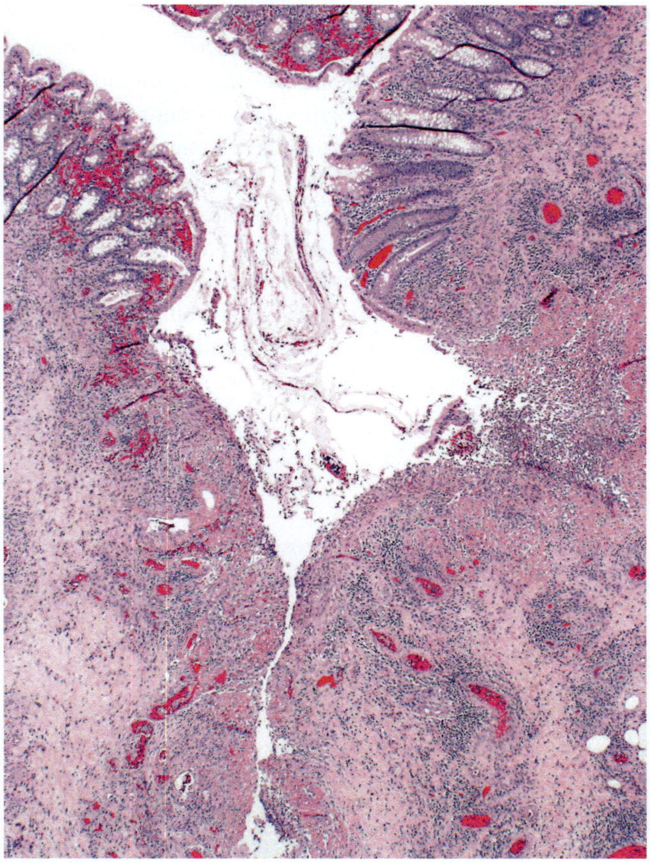

Fig. 17.7 Non-typhoidal salmonellosis with acute colitis and ulceration. As is common with this infection, no significant crypt architectural distortion is present. (Courtesy of Dr. Laura Lamps)

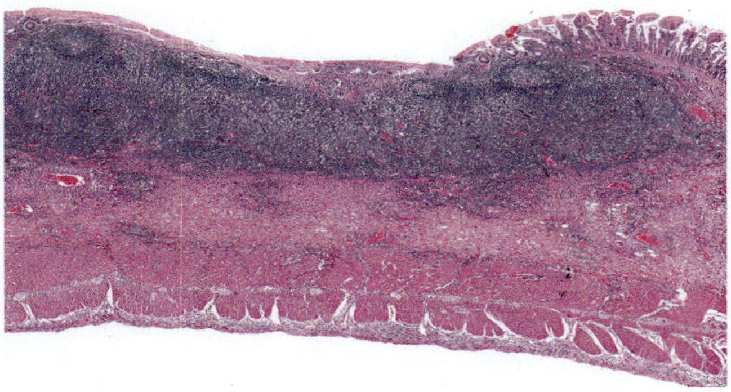

Fig. 17.8 Large aphthous ulcer of typhoid fever overlying a hyperplastic Peyer's patch

Differential Diagnosis

As with all causes of AITC, microbiology studies are required to definitively identify the causative bacterium in cases of non-typhoidal and typhoidal disease. Depending on the degree of architectural distortion, IBD may also be in the differential diagnosis [13].

Shigella Spp. (Shigellosis)

Definition

Shigella spp. are Gram-negative bacilli in the family *Enterobacteriaceae*. There are four *Shigella* species, of which *Shigella dysenteriae* is considered the most virulent [33]. *Shigella dysenteriae* and *S. boydii* are found primarily in resource-limited countries, whereas *S. sonnei* and *S. flexneri* are more commonly reported in resource-rich settings such as the United States [12]. They are one of the most causes of gastroenteritis in the United States and worldwide [5, 6, 16]. In the United States alone, there are an estimated 500,000 infections each year, making it the third most common cause of gastrointestinal infection after *Salmonella* and *Campylobacter* species [33]. Infection is a nationally notifiable disease in the United States [28].

Clinical Features

Patients of all ages can be infected, although children under the age of 6 years, MSM, and malnourished/debilitated patients are most commonly affected [33]. After an incubation period of 1–2 days, patients commonly present with fever, malaise, and abdominal pain, followed by the onset of watery diarrhea and, later, bloody diarrhea with mucus [33]. The volume of stool is relatively low, and therefore dehydration from shigellosis is uncommon [33]. Symptoms generally last 5–7 days, although it may take several months for stool consistency and frequency to return to normal [33]. Well-described complications include toxic megacolon, sepsis, perforation, post-infectious (reactive) arthritis, HUS, seizures (usually in children), and Reiter syndrome [12, 33]. Treatment is supportive with fluid and electrolyte replacement. Antibiotics are generally reserved for patients with manifestations of, or risk factors for, severe disease [33].

Pathological Features

Gross Findings

By endoscopy, the mucosa is edematous and may be hemorrhagic [12]. Ulcers may also be present. Occasionally pseudomembranes may be present. The large bowel is most commonly involved (left > right), but the ileum may also be affected. The distribution of gross pathologic findings is usually continuous in early disease but may later become patchy as infection resolves [12, 13].

Microscopic Findings

The histopathologic features of *Shigella* colitis are those of AITC [12]. As infection progresses, increased mucosal inflammation and crypt architectural changes may occur [12, 13]. Pseudomembrane formation may occasionally be seen (Fig. 17.9) [12].

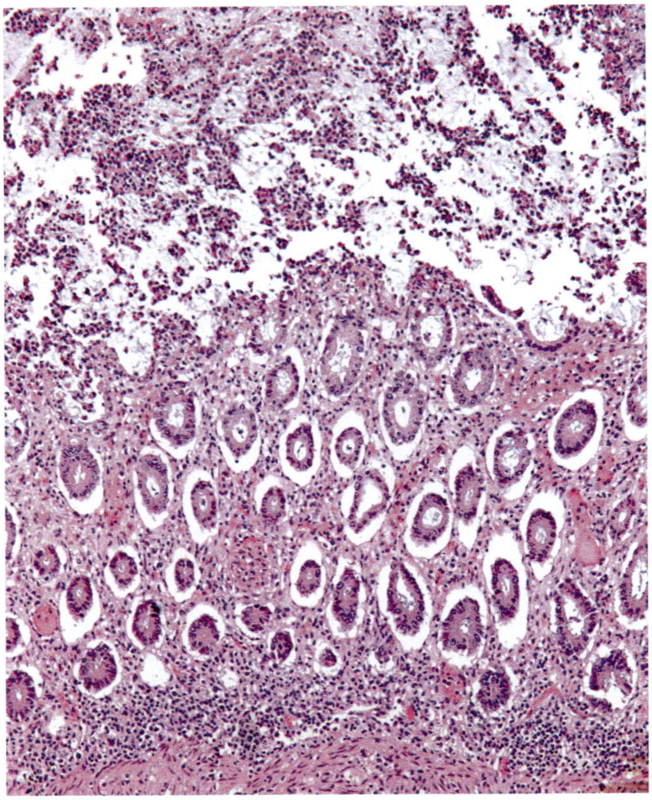

Fig. 17.9 Shigellosis demonstrating the acute infectious-type colitis pattern and pseudomembrane formation. (Courtesy of Dr. Laura Lamps)

Differential Diagnosis

Grossly, the contiguous involvement of the ileum and right bowel may resemble ulcerative colitis, whereas the patchy distribution during resolving disease mimics Crohn's disease. Differentiating shigellosis from IBD may be more difficult when significant crypt architectural distortion is present. *Clostridioides difficile* infection may also enter the differential diagnosis when pseudomembranes are present. As with other causes of AITC and pseudomembranous colitis, microbiology stool studies are needed to identify the etiologic agent and may be helpful for differentiating infectious causes from IBD [12].

Yersinia Species (Yersiniosis)

Definition

Yersinia are Gram-negative coccobacilli in the family *Enterobacteriaceae* [34]. *Yersinia enterocolitica* is the primary cause of human gastrointestinal disease, with *Y. pseudotuberculosis* causing a smaller number of cases. Transmission is usually through ingestion of contaminated food and water, including undercooked pork and unpasteurized dairy products. *Yersinia enterocolitica* is estimated to cause 117,000 illnesses each year in the United States, with an associated 640 hospitalizations and 35 deaths [34].

Clinical Features

After an incubation period of 4–7 days, patients commonly present with abdominal pain and diarrhea (often bloody). In adults and older children, right-sided abdominal pain and fever may be the predominant clinical features and may be confused with appendicitis [34]. Infection usually lasts 1–3 weeks, but cases of chronic yersiniosis have been well described. Immunocompromised hosts, patients with various debilitating conditions, and patients with iron overload are at increased risk of severe disease [12]. Treatment is usually supportive, but antimicrobial therapy is indicated for patients with manifestations of, or risk factors for, severe disease [34].

Pathological Features

Gross Findings

By endoscopy, the bowel mucosa appears thickened and edematous with nodules overlying Peyer's patches [12]. Linear and aphthoid ulcers may be present.

Microscopic Findings

Both species have similar histopathologic features, including suppurative, granulomatous, and mixed patterns of inflammation, lymphoid hyperplasia, mucosal ulceration, and cryptitis [12]. Granulomas are usually epithelioid with prominent lymphoid cuffs and associated giant cells [12]. The granulomas of *Y. pseudotuberculosis* may be suppurative with central stellate microabscesses. Lymphoid hyperplasia is commonly seen with both bacteria and may include with transmural lymphoid aggregates mimicking Crohn's disease [12].

Differential Diagnosis

The primary differential diagnosis is other granulomatous processes including tuberculosis [12]. Acid fast stains are useful for detecting *Mycobacteria* spp. When lymphoid hyperplasia predominates, then typhoid fever also enters the differential [12]. The overall pathologic picture may also resemble Crohn's disease. In comparison to yersiniosis, Crohn's disease is more likely to have features chronicity including crypt architectural distortion, prominent neural hyperplasia, and thickening of the muscularis mucosae [12]. Correlation with clinical features and results of stool microbiology tests are required for definitive diagnosis.

Clostridioides difficile

Definition

Clostridioides (formerly *Clostridium*) *difficile*, or simply, "*C. dif*" is a large, spore-forming, anaerobic, Gram-positive bacillus capable of producing two enterotoxins (toxins A and B) [12, 17, 35]. Disease with this bacterium most commonly occurs when broad-spectrum antibiotics disrupt the normal colonic flora, allowing *C. difficile* to multiply and produce enterotoxins. While infection was initially associated with health-care settings, community-acquired cases involving a hypervirulent strain, BI/NAP1/027, are now well described [35]. This BI/NAP1/027 strain produces an additional toxin (binary toxin) in addition to toxins A and B and is highly resistant to the fluoroquinolones [36]. *C. difficile* spores are highly resistant to heat, acid, and antibiotics and may be present in large numbers in the environment, particularly in health-care settings [17]. Asymptomatic children and adults may also harbor this bacterium and serve as disease reservoirs [35]. The CDC estimates that nearly 500,000 cases of *C. difficile* colitis occurred in 2011 [36].

Clinical Features

Patients with *C. difficile* colitis may have a spectrum of manifestations ranging from mild diarrhea, to pseudomembranous colitis, to fulminant, life-threatening infection [12]. Watery diarrhea is a predominant feature of all forms and is commonly accompanied by abdominal pain, fever, and cramping [12]. Occasionally bloody diarrhea is seen [12]. Manifestations of severe infection include perforation and toxic megacolon [12]. Although pseudomembranes are characteristic for infection, they are not always present, particularly in immunocompromised hosts [35]. Vancomycin is the mainstay for treatment of *C. difficile* colitis, but the rate of relapse is high (≥20%), requiring repeated therapy or fecal microbial transplantation [17].

Pathological Features

Gross Findings

By endoscopy and in resected specimens, classic pseudomembranous disease manifests as scattered to confluent, white-yellow-green plaques (Fig. 17.10) that increase in number when progressing from the proximal to distal colon [25, 35]. The plaques bleed when the pseudomembrane is scraped off [12].

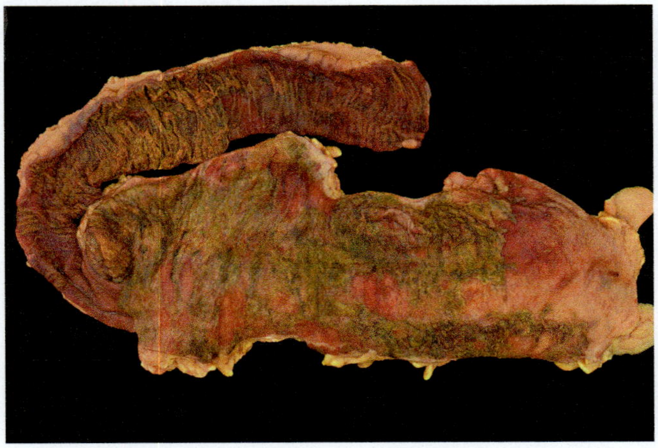

Fig. 17.10 Portion of large and small bowel coated with adherent yellow-green pseudomembranes in a fatal case of *Clostridioides difficile* infection. (Image courtesy of Dr. Aishwarya Ravindran and Dr. Joseph Maleszewski)

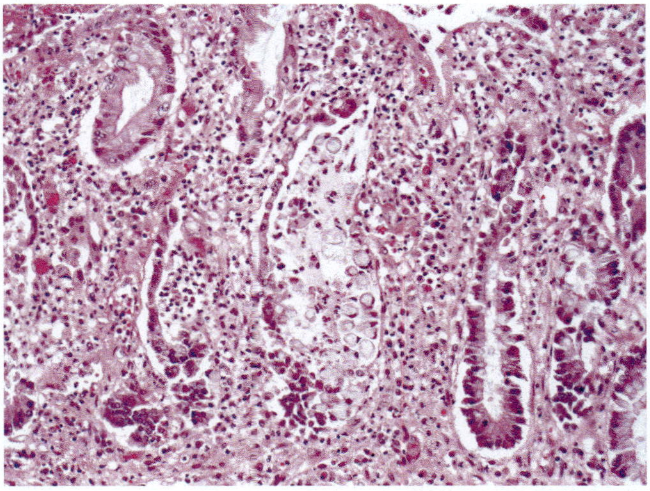

Fig. 17.11 Case of *Clostridioides difficile* infection with dilated, attenuated crypts containing neutrophils and degenerated goblet cells mimicking signet ring cells These sloughed and inflammatory cells are released into the lumen to create the pseudomembrane

Microscopic Findings

Features of *C. difficile* colitis may vary from a mild acute colitis to a florid ischemic pattern with full-thickness necrosis of the bowel wall [35]. In pseudomembranous disease, the crypts are dilated with degenerated epithelial cells, necrotic debris, and acute inflammatory cells (Fig. 17.11) which "explodes" into the lumen to form a "mushroom" or "volcano" lesion (Fig. 17.3). These lesions coalesce to form a thick mucopurulent exudate (pseudomembrane) (Fig. 17.4). The pseudomembrane is composed of abundant mucus, fibrin, neutrophils, and necrotic debris (Fig. 17.5) [35].

Differential Diagnosis

The differential diagnosis of *C. difficile* colitis includes other causes of pseudomembrane formation, including infectious and noninfectious etiologies [35]. Careful examination of histopathologic features, along with correlation with clinical presentation and stool microbiology tests, is essential for differentiating infectious from noninfectious causes such as colon ischemia and IBD [12].

Bradyspira Species (Intestinal Spirochetosis)

Definition

Intestinal spirochetosis is a condition characterized by a dense mat of spirochetes at the luminal surface of the colonic and appendiceal mucosa [12]. It is a relatively common finding, being detected in 2–7% of rectal biopsies in the North America and Europe and 11–34% in resource-limited settings. MSM (men who have sex with men) and HIV-infected individuals have the highest rate of infection (up to 54%) [11, 12]. The associated spirochetes are in the genus

Bradyspira and include *B. aalborgi* and *B. pilosicoli*. Organisms are thought to be acquired through ingestion of contaminated food or water [12].

Clinical Features

The pathogenicity and associated clinical features of *Bradyspira* infection are controversial. While a variety of clinical features, such as chronic watery diarrhea and abdominal pain, have been associated with intestinal spirochetosis, this condition is also seen in asymptomatic individuals [12]. Determining the associated pathology is particularly challenging in immunocompromised patients who often have concomitant infections. Regardless, some individuals experience symptom resolution with antimicrobial therapy, thus suggesting that intestinal spirochetosis can cause intestinal symptoms [12].

Pathological Features

Gross Findings

Macroscopic pathologic features are usually mild or absent [12].

Microscopic Findings

The sigmoid colon, rectum, and appendix are most commonly involved [35]. The terminal ileum may also be involved. The predominant feature of intestinal spirochetosis is the presence of a dense basophilic "fuzzy" layer of spirochetes at the luminal mucosal border (Figs. 17.12 and 17.13) [12]. Invasion is not present, and the underlying mucosa has little to no changes. The spirochetes can be highlighted using silver impregnation methods such as the Warthin-Starry and Steiner stains (Figs. 17.12 and 17.13) [12]. They also stain with periodic acid-Schiff (PAS), Giemsa, Alcian blue (pH 2.5), and Fontana-Masson [12, 35]. By transmission electron microscopy, the spirochetes can be seen embedded within invaginations of the enterocyte membrane [35].

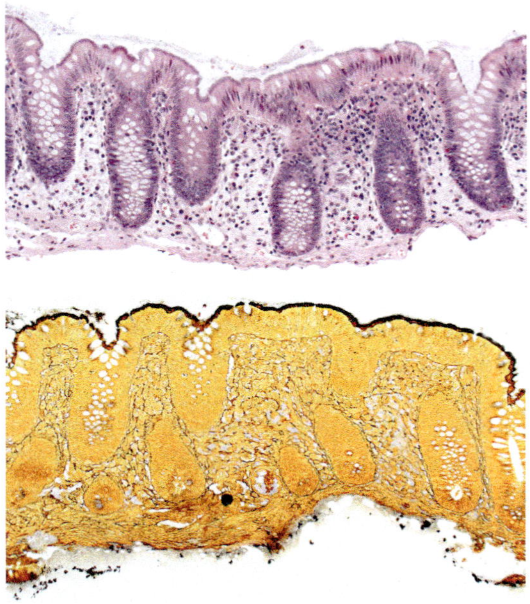

Fig. 17.12 Intestinal spirochetosis. The primary histologic feature is a dense fuzzy basophilic layer of embedded spirochetes at the luminal mucosal border (top). The spirochetes are highlighted using a silver impregnation method (bottom)

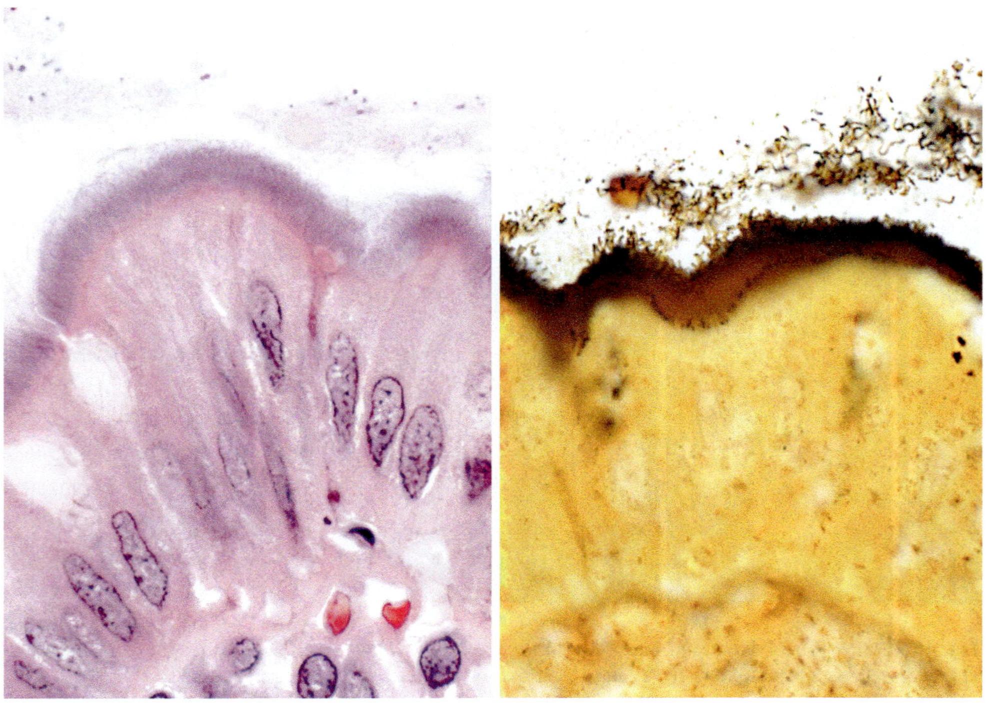

Fig. 17.13 Intestinal spirochetosis. High magnification (100× with oil immersion) allows for visualization of the numerous spirochetes embedded at the mucosal brush border (left, H&E; right, Steiner stain). The shape of the spirochetes can be best appreciated in the detached organisms above the brush border using the Steiner stain

Immunohistochemical Features

There is significant cross-reactivity between the antigens of *Bradyspira* spp. and *Treponema pallidum*, and thus commercially available immunohistochemical (IHC) stains can be used to highlight the spirochetes of intestinal spirochetosis. While *T. pallidum* IHC staining is seldom necessary for diagnosis, it is important to note the antigenic cross-reactivity so that positive staining of luminal spirochetes is not erroneously used to make a diagnosis of syphilis.

Differential Diagnosis

The primary differential diagnosis of intestinal spirochetosis is normal or mildly inflamed colonic mucosa in which the brush border is prominently stained. In general, the microvilli of the brush border are shorter than spirochetes and more eosinophilic. When in doubt, histochemical or immunohistochemical stains as mentioned above can be used to assess for the presence of luminal spirochetes.

Fungal Infections

Both yeasts and filamentous fungi may infect the lower intestinal tract and are a particular risk for immunocompromised patients such as organ transplant recipients, patients receiving immunosuppressive chemotherapy, and individuals with AIDS [14]. Intestinal involvement is often a component of disseminated disease and may be the initial presenting manifestation of infection. Clinical manifestations overlap significantly among the various fungi and commonly include nausea, vomiting, watery to bloody diarrhea, abdominal pain, and fever [14]. The pathologist may play an important role in detecting the infection and identifying the presumptive pathogen based on characteristic morphologic features (Table 17.2) [37, 38]. It is often possible to positively definitively identify candidiasis (see Chap. 5, section on esophageal infection), mucormycosis, and the endemic dimorphic fungi based on morphologic features alone [14]. Similarly, the hyaline (non-pigmented), narrow, regularly septate fungi (e.g., *Aspergillus*, *Fusarium*) can usually be differentiated from the *Mucorales*; however, there is significant overlap in morphologic features among the hyaline regularly septate hyphae, and therefore fungal culture or, less commonly, NAAT is required for definitive identification [14, 37]. Identification of the infecting genus is necessary as antifungal therapy may differ based on the involved organism, and therefore culture, or broad-range fungal sequencing, should be performed [14, 38]. Of note, several of the endemic dimorphic fungi may involve the gastrointestinal tract (e.g., *Histoplasma capsulatum*, *Coccidioides immitis/C. posadasii*, *Paracoccidioides brasiliensis*). Of these, *H. capsulatum* is the most likely to involve the gut and is discussed in further detail below.

Aspergillus Species (Aspergillosis)

Definition

Aspergillus is a genus of ubiquitous non-pigmented (hyaline) environmental fungi capable of causing human disease in select circumstances. Disease in immunocompetent hosts

Table 17.2 Common fungal infections of the colon[a]

Fungus (disease)	Predominant clinical manifestations	Primary histopathologic features
Aspergillus spp. (aspergillosis)	Usually immunocompromised hosts; fever, vomiting, abdominal pain, diarrhea, GI bleeding; occasionally mass lesion; most patients have concurrent lung involvement	Invasive aspergillosis characterized by nodular infarct with angioinvasion and surrounding zone of ischemic necrosis, minimal inflammation to marked neutrophilic response depending on state of the host immune system; narrow septate hyphae, classically with acute angle branching, extending from infarcted tissue in radial or parallel arrays
Candida spp. (candidiasis)	Similar to *Aspergillus*; often component of disseminated disease	Mucosal erosions/ulcers, neutrophil infiltrates and abscess formation, necrosis; rare granuloma formation. Inflammation may be minimal in profoundly immunocompromised hosts. Yeasts, pseudohyphae and/or hyphae invading mucosa, submucosa, and/or muscular layer. Angioinvasion and perforation may occur. See Chap. 5
Cryptococcus spp. (cryptococcosis)	Usually immunocompromised hosts; component of disseminated disease. Abdominal pain, distension	Ulcers, nodules, suppurative necrotizing inflammatory response, and inflammation may be minimal in profoundly immunocompromised hosts. Variably sized (2–20 μm), round, intra- and extra-cellular yeasts with non-staining halo (capsule); narrow-based budding. Capsule is highlighted with mucin stains
Histoplasma capsulatum (histoplasmosis)	Usually immunocompromised hosts but rarely immunocompetent hosts; component of disseminated disease; fever, abdominal pain	Ulcers, nodules, diffuse lymphohistiocytic infiltrates in the mucosa and submucosa; small (2–5 μm) ovoid yeasts within histiocytes; yeasts exhibit narrow-based budding (best seen with GMS or PAS); pseudocapsule (non-staining halo around yeasts) on H&E
Mucorales (mucormycosis)	Usually immunocompromised hosts; similar to *Aspergillus*	Nodular infarction with angioinvasion similar to *Aspergillus*; hyphae are pauciseptate, irregular with narrow and broad forms, thin walls that easily collapse (crumpled cellophane appearance), random branching at various angles

[a]Not all inclusive

is uncommon and typically limited to allergic manifestations, as well as fungal ball and minimally invasive disease in patients with pre-existing pulmonary disease. In comparison, disease in immunocompromised hosts can be a medical emergency leading to rapidly life-threatening disease and requiring urgent treatment. *Aspergillus fumigatus* and *A. flavus* are the most common pathogens, but several other species including *A. niger*, *A. terreus*, *A. versicolor*, and *A. nidans* may also cause human disease [39]. Infection is acquired almost exclusively through inhalation of microscopic airborne spores, leading to primary infection of the respiratory tract, with the potential for subsequent hematogenous dissemination to other organs in immunocompromised hosts [40]. Extrapulmonary involvement has been reported in 25–60% of cases of invasive aspergillosis and is seen almost entirely in the context of primary pulmonary infection [40]. Only rarely has primary intestinal apergillosis been reported, presumably from ingestion of infectious spores [40].

Clinical Features

Invasive aspergillosis of the small or large intestine is seen almost exclusively in immunocompromised hosts, and most have clinical or radiologic features of concomitant pulmonary disease [14, 39, 40]. Common intestinal symptoms are fever, vomiting, abdominal pain, diarrhea, and gastrointestinal bleeding [14]. First-line therapy of invasive disease is voriconazole [39].

Pathological Features

Gross Findings

Any level of the gastrointestinal tract can be involved. The mucosa is commonly erythematous, edematous, and ulcerated [14]. Occasionally an inflammatory mass (aspergilloma) may be seen. Transmural infarction is common, as is formation of characteristic "target lesions" with central necrosis and surrounding hemorrhage [14].

Microscopic Findings

Aspergillus is highly angioinvasive, resulting in nodular infarcts and surrounding ischemic necrosis. Narrow (3–12 μm diameter), regularly septate hyphae, classically with acute angle, dichotomous branching, are typically seen extending from infarcted tissue in radial or parallel arrays and readily crossing tissue planes (Fig. 17.14) [14, 37]. The hyphae may be seen on H&E but are best highlighted with GMS and PAS fungal stains. Depending on the extent of immune compromise, the associated host response may range from minimal inflammation to marked neutrophilic infiltrates [14].

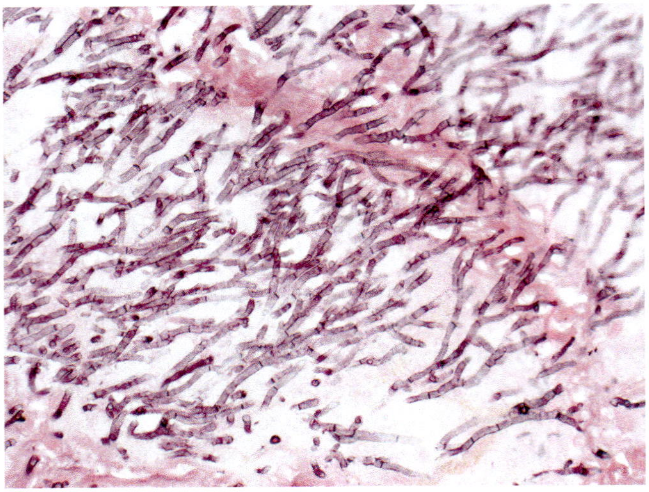

Fig. 17.14 Invasive aspergillosis. GMS stain (40×; pink counterstain) highlights the numerous narrow, regularly septate, hyphae with acute angle branching extending in parallel arrays across tissue planes. While characteristic for *Aspergillus* spp., hyphae with this appearance cannot be reliably differentiated from similar non-pigmented regular septate hyphae such as those of *Fusarium* species

Differential Diagnosis

Several hyaline molds, such as *Fusarium*, *Paecilomyces*, and *Scedosporium*, have a nearly identical histologic appearance to that of *Aspergillus*, so that definitive identification cannot be made from tissue morphology alone [37, 38]. The only exception to this is when *Aspergillus* fruiting heads are seen in tissue: a rare occurrence that is typically seen when the infection is contiguous with an airspace. Given the limitations of morphologic identification, a suggested pathology report is "Narrow, regularly septate hyphae with acute angle branching. Differential diagnosis includes *Aspergillus* sp. Culture is required for definitive identification."

Mucorales (Mucormycosis)

Definition

The *Mucorales* is an order within the *Zygomycetes* comprising multiple genera that cause human mucormycosis (formerly zygomycosis) [37, 39]. Like *Aspergillus*, the mucorales are ubiquitous environmental fungi that rarely cause disease in immunocompetent hosts but can cause serious, life-threatening disease in immunocompromised hosts [39]. *Rhizopus* spp. are the most common cause of mucormycosis, but several other genera including *Mucor*, *Rhizomucor*, and *Lichtheimia* also cause disease [37]. There are five main forms of mucormycosis: rhinocerebral, pulmonary, cutaneous, gastrointestinal, and disseminated [39]. Gastrointestinal mucormycosis is an uncommon form of infection seen primarily in premature infants and malnourished individuals that is thought to result from ingestion of fungal spores [39]. Disseminated mucormycosis may also involve the gastrointestinal tract and is seen in the setting of severe immune compromise and concomitant pulmonary infection [39].

Clinical Features

Patients with gastrointestinal involvement commonly present with nausea, vomiting, abdominal pain, and, occasionally, gastrointestinal bleeding [39]. In neonates, the presentation may resemble that of necrotizing enterocolitis. Treatment is usually with lipid formulations of amphotericin B [39]. The mucorales do not respond to voriconazole, an agent commonly used for prophylaxis and treatment of aspergillosis.

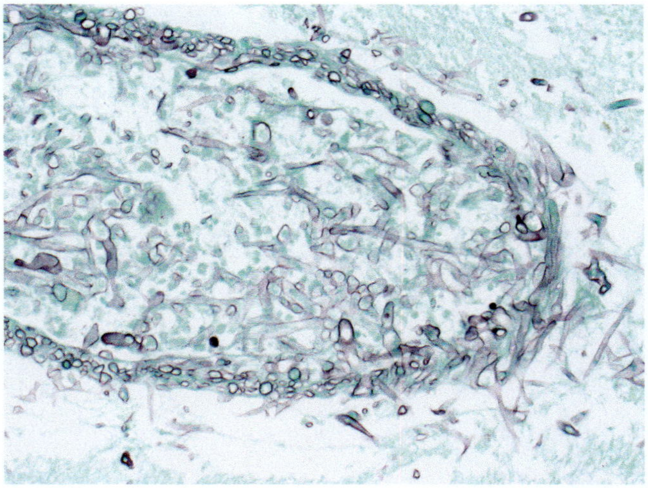

Fig. 17.16 Mucormycosis with angioinvasion of a large blood vessel (GMS stain)

Pathological Features

Gross Findings

Any level of the gastrointestinal tract can be involved. The gross findings are similar to those of aspergillosis, with ulceration and infarction being common findings. Ulcers may be large with irregular, rolled edges, mimicking malignancy [14].

Microscopic Findings

As with aspergillosis, nodular infarction with angioinvasion (Figs. 17.15 and 17.16) is a characteristic microscopic finding [14]. However, the hyphae differ from those of *Aspergillus* spp. by being pauciseptate, with irregular diameters ranging from 5 to 20 μm [37]. The hyphal walls are very thin and easily collapse during histologic processing, giving the appearance of "crumpled cellophane" (Fig. 17.15) [14, 37]. Branching occurs at various angles including acute and right angles [14, 38]. The hyphae are usually visible with H&E, particularly in areas of necrosis, and may be highlighted using GMS and PAS, although staining may be pale [37].

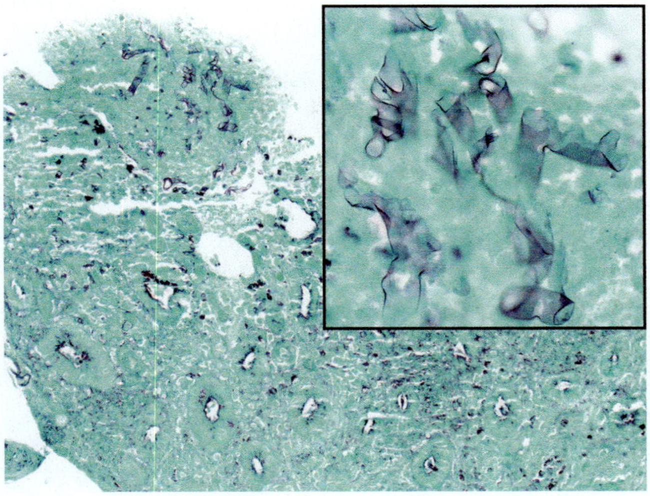

Fig. 17.15 Intestinal mucormycosis. GMS stain demonstrates foci of invasive hyphae with associated necrosis. On high magnification (inset 100×), the thin and partially collapsed walls with "crumpled cellophane" appearance, irregular branching pattern, and paucity of visible septae are easily appreciated

Differential Diagnosis

The *Mucorales* can often be differentiated from the uniformly narrow, regularly septate molds such as *Aspergillus* by their broad, irregular, crumpled, pauciseptate hyphae [37]. A rare entity that must also be considered in the differential diagnosis is gastrointestinal basidiobolomycosis caused by *Basidiobolus ranarum*, a fungus in the order of *Entomophthorales* [41]. The *Entomophthorales* are closely related to the *Mucorales*, both being members of the *Zygomycetes*; however, they have very different pathogenic potentials. Basidiobolomycosis is a chronic infection seen primarily in immunocompetent patients. The hyphae are indistinguishable from those of the mucorales but are found in the setting of intense granulomatous inflammation with prominent eosinophils, neutrophils, granulation tissue, and fibrosis (Fig. 17.17) [37]. The hyphae are commonly seen with peripheral Splendore-Hoeppli reaction (Fig. 17.18).

Cryptococcus Species (Cryptococcosis)

Definition

Cryptococcus is a ubiquitous environmental fungus capable of causing human disease in select circumstances [39]. The two most common species are *Cryptococcus neoformans* and

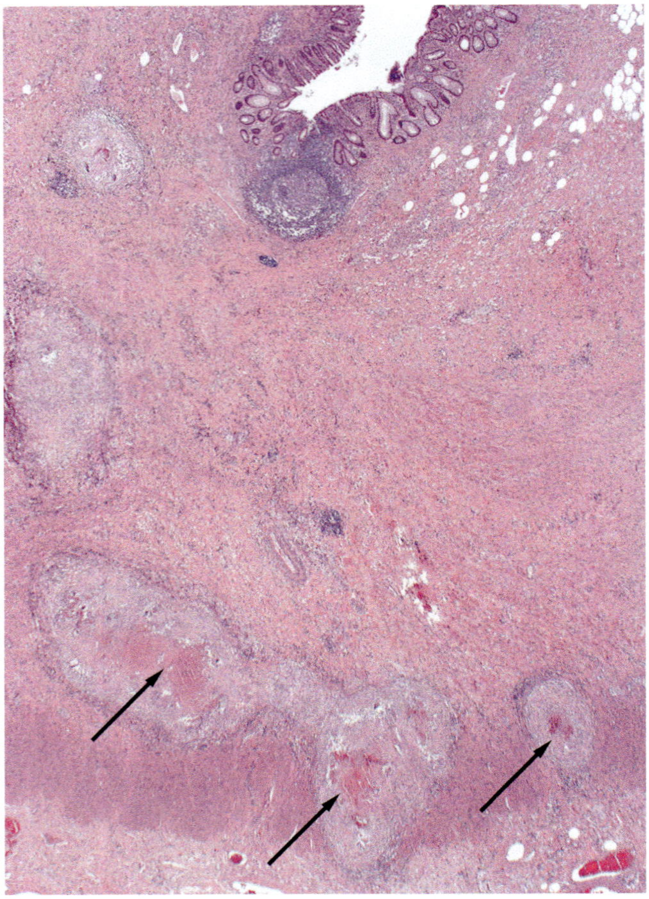

Fig. 17.17 Basidiobolomycosis due to *Basidiobolus ranarum*, a fungus closely related to the *Mucorales*. Unlike mucormycosis, infection is seen in immunocompetent hosts and is associated with a pronounced granulomatous response. Hyphae are present within granulomas (arrows) surrounded by Splendore-Hoeppli phenomenon

C. gattii. *C. neoformans* is found throughout the world and causes disease primarily in immunocompromised hosts; it is a saprophytic organism, commonly associated with pigeons. In comparison, *C. gattii* is found in the tropics, subtropics, and Pacific Northwest, associated with eucalyptus trees, and may infect immunocompromised and immunocompetent hosts [39]. Infection is acquired through inhalation of fungal spores, resulting in a primary respiratory infection in susceptible individuals [39]. The fungus can disseminate from the lungs to other organs and has a predilection for the central nervous system. Gastrointestinal involvement occurs almost exclusively in immunocompromised hosts and is due to dissemination from a primary respiratory source; however, rare cases of gastrointestinal involvement in immunocompetent hosts and cases of primary intestinal cryptococcosis have been reported [42]. Both *C. neoformans* and *C. gattii* can cause disseminated disease [39].

Clinical Features

Most patients will have clinical or radiographic evidence of pulmonary and central nervous system involvement [14]. Symptoms of intestinal involvement include abdominal pain and distension. Treatment varies with the severity of disease; severe extra-pulmonary disease is treated with liposomal amphotericin B plus flucytosine [43].

Pathological Features

Gross Findings

Any level of the gastrointestinal tract can be involved. The mucosa may appear normal or exhibit ulcers and nodules, occasionally with an accompanying thick white exudate [14].

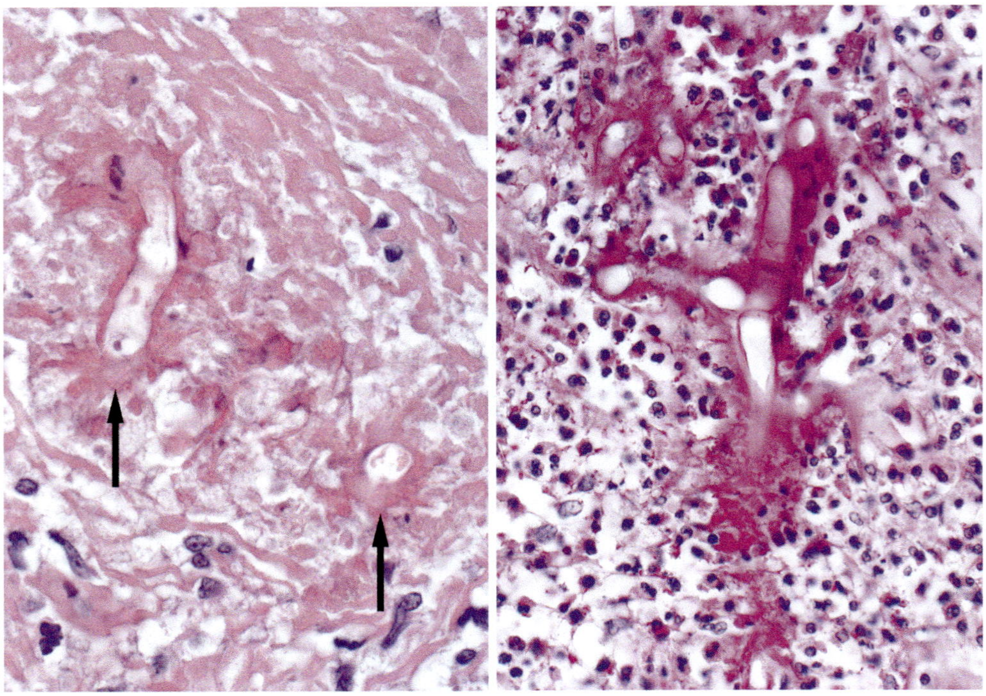

Fig. 17.18 Higher magnification of the case of basidiobolomycosis shown in Fig. 17.17, demonstrating the Splendore-Hoeppli reaction around hyphae (arrows; left panel). The hyphal walls are highlighted with PAS stain (right panel)

Microscopic Findings

The diagnostic feature of intestinal cryptococcosis due to *C. neoformans* or *C. gattii* is the presence of variably sized (2–20 μm), round, intra- and extra-cellular yeasts within the mucosa and/or submucosa (Fig. 17.19) [14, 37, 38]. The two species are morphologically identical. The yeasts typically have a non-staining halo corresponding to the presence of a mucopolysaccharide capsule and are divided by narrow-based budding. Rare pseudohyphae may also be seen [38]. The associated inflammatory response is generally suppurative and necrotizing, although inflammation may be absent or minimal in profoundly immunocompromised hosts [14, 37, 38]. In patients with some degree of native immunity, a granulomatous response may be seen with occasional formation of a mass lesion (cryptococcoma). The yeast capsule stains deeply with mucin stains such as mucicarmine (Fig. 17.20) and Alcian blue. The cell wall may also be highlighted using Fontana-Masson, although this varies widely by the stain formulation being used, and may stain other similar-appearing yeasts [38].

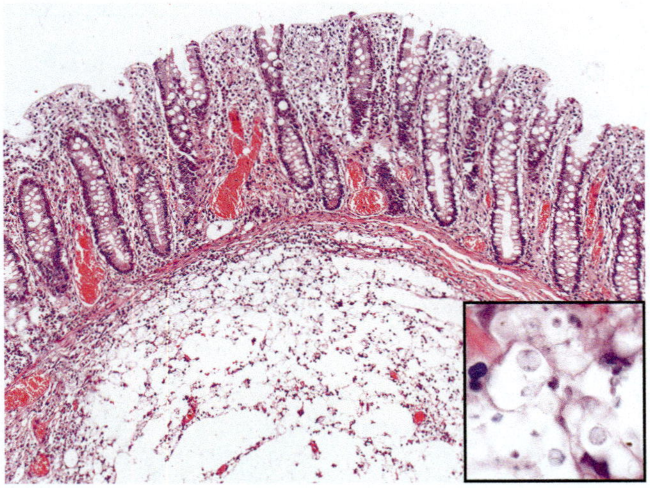

Fig. 17.19 Intestinal cryptococcosis involving the mucosa and submucosa. Variably sized faintly staining basophilic yeasts are apparent on H&E (inset 100×) with a notable clear halo corresponding with the mucopolysaccharide capsule. Note the lack of an associated immune response in this profoundly immunocompromised patient

Differential Diagnosis

The yeasts of *Cryptococcus* spp. can usually be differentiated from other yeasts by their variable size, capsule, and narrow-based budding. Other yeasts that infect humans do not have a true capsule, and thus its presence is diagnostic for *Cryptococcus.* It is important to note that the cell wall of *Blastomyces dermatitidis* may be faintly mucicarmine positive and should not be interpreted as evidence of a capsule. Features useful for differentiating *B. dermatitidis* from *Cryptococcus* spp. are its uniformly large size (8–15 μm diameters) and thick refractile cell wall. *Histoplasma capsulatum* may also be in the differential diagnosis, particularly

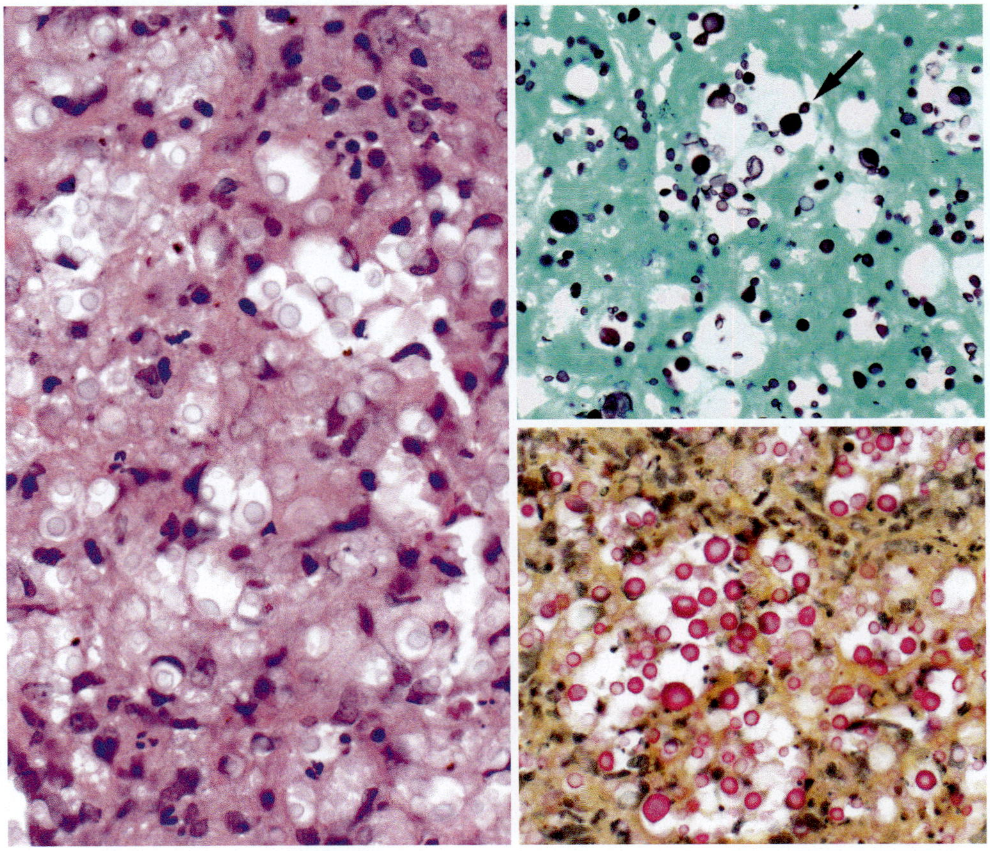

Fig. 17.20 Staining patterns of *Cryptococcus* spp. on H&E (left), GMS (upper right), and mucicarmine (lower right) using the 40× objective. Note the size variability and presence of a narrow-based bud (arrow)

when only small forms are seen but is more likely oval rather than round and lacks a capsule (see below). Occasional cases of capsular-deficient cryptococcosis have been noted, but the cell wall may still stain with Fontana-Masson [37].

Histoplasma capsulatum (Histoplasmosis)

Definition

Histoplasma capsulatum is a saprophytic fungus with a near-worldwide distribution [39]. *H. capsulatum* var. *capsulatum* is found in close association with river valleys in all continents except Antarctica, while *H. capsulatum* var. *duboisii* is found in Africa [39]. It is a thermally dimorphic fungus, growing as a mold in the environment (25 °C), predominantly in soil enriched with bird or bat droppings, and as a yeast in humans (36 °C). Infection is acquired primarily through inhalation of microscopic airborne microconidia, resulting in a primary pulmonary infection with the potential for dissemination to other organs. Gastrointestinal tract involvement is seen in 70 to 90% of cases with disseminated infection [14, 44]. Most patients are profoundly immunocompromised, but intestinal histoplasmosis can less commonly occur in immunocompetent patients such as young children and the elderly [14, 44]. This section will focus on *H. capsulatum* var. *capsulatum*, the most common cause of intestinal histoplasmosis.

Clinical Features

Most patients will have clinical or radiographic evidence of pulmonary and disseminated disease [14]. Common manifestations of gastrointestinal involvement include fever and abdominal pain [14].

Pathological Features

Gross Findings

Any level of the gastrointestinal tract can be involved. The mucosa may appear normal or ulcerated and nodular [14]. Occasionally a mass lesion (histoplasmoma) may be seen [14].

Microscopic Findings

The diagnostic feature of intestinal histoplasmosis is the presence of small (2–5 μm), ovoid yeasts within histiocytes in the mucosa and submucosa (Figs. 17.21 and 17.22). The histiocytic expansion may be pronounced and associated with nodules and ulcers of the involved mucosa, particularly overlying Peyer's patches [14]. The associated immune response is predominantly lymphoplasmacytic, although may occasionally include formation of discrete granulomas. In profoundly immunocompromised hosts, there may be little to no associated inflammation. The yeasts may be extremely difficult to see on H&E but can occasionally appear as small intracellular objects with a narrow surrounding clear zone or halo (Figs. 17.21 and 17.23). The halo (pseudocapsule) results from the poorly stained cell wall rather than the presence of a true capsule as seen with *Cryptococcus* spp. [38]. The yeasts exhibit narrow-based budding, which is best seen with GMS or PAS (Fig. 17.22).

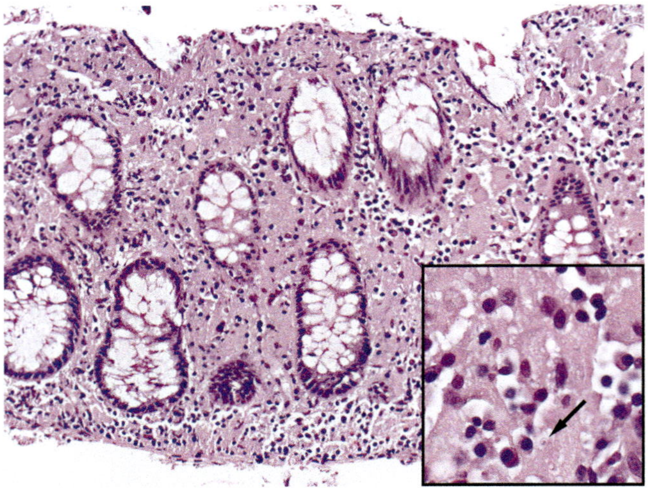

Fig. 17.21 Intestinal histoplasmosis with a diffuse histiocytic mucosal infiltrate. Yeasts are difficult to see on H&E, with only rare forms present (inset)

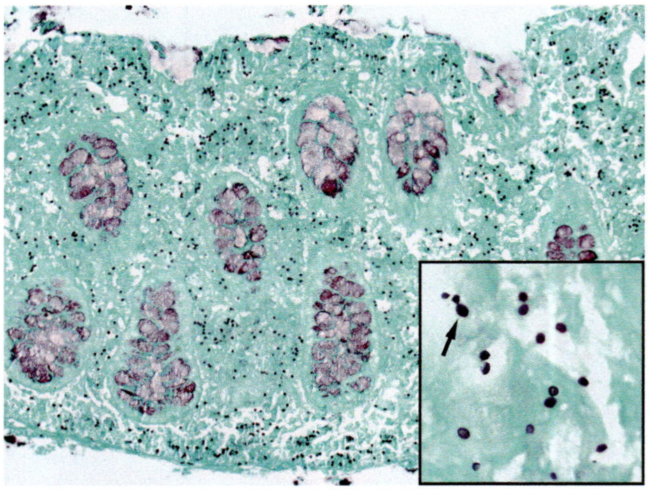

Fig. 17.22 GMS staining of the case of intestinal histoplasmosis shown in Fig. 17.21. Note that numerous small oval-shaped yeasts are seen within the histiocytic infiltrate. Occasional dividing forms with narrow-based budding forms are seen (inset, arrow)

Differential Diagnosis

The overall histologic picture of intestinal histoplasmosis is similar to that of other diffuse histiocytic processes such as malakoplakia and *Mycobacterium avium* complex infection. The presence of small intracellular yeasts allows these processes to be excluded and narrows the differential to other yeast infections. The morphology of *H. capsulatum* is similar to that of *Cryptococcus* spp. (see above) but with uniformly small rather than variably sized forms. Unlike *Cryptococcus* spp., *H. capsulatum* also lacks a capsule. Other small yeasts that may enter the differential include *Talaromyces* (formerly *Penicillium*) *marneffei* (patients from Southeast Asia) and *Candida glabrata*. *T. marneffei* can be differentiated by its mean of reproduction; it divides by transverse septae rather than budding. *C. glabrata* is more difficult to differentiate but causes a suppurative rather than histiocytic inflammatory reaction and is more easily visible on H&E. The morphologic appearance of *C. glabrata* is otherwise identical to that of *H. capsulatum*, requiring culture or NAAT to differentiate them [38].

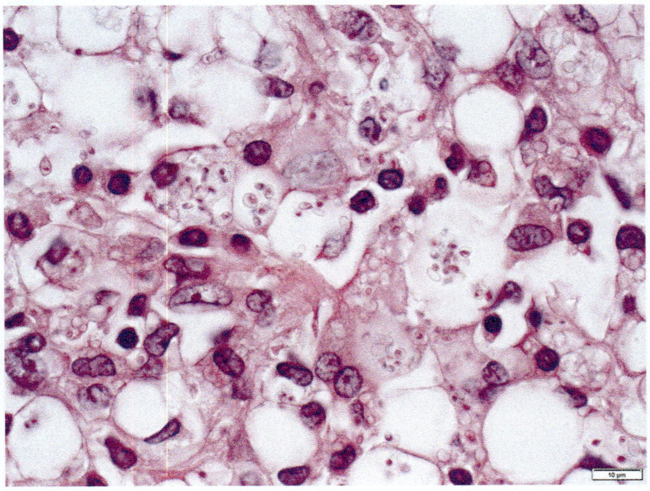

Fig. 17.23 Florid intestinal histoplasmosis with numerous yeasts visible with routine H&E staining. This patient presented with intestinal perforation due to transmural histoplasmosis

Viral Infections

A large variety of viruses may infect the colon, and most are capable of infecting other regions of the intestinal tract as well [11, 14, 45]. The associated clinical and pathologic features depend primarily on the specific virus and the immune status of the host (Table 17.3). This section will focus on cytomegalovirus (CMV) and human immunodeficiency virus (HIV); the reader is referred to other chapters in the text for a discussion on adenovirus (Chap. 11) and herpes simplex virus (HSV; Chaps. 5 and 20).

Cytomegalovirus (CMV Colitis)

Definition

CMV is a member of the Herpesviridae, found worldwide and capable of infecting a wide range of epithelial, endothelial, and mesenchymal cells [45]. An estimated 50 to 80% of the general population have been infected by age 35. Like other herpesviruses, the virus remains latent following primary infection and may reactivate in response to various environmental factors or when the host becomes immunocompromised. CMV colitis most commonly occurs in the setting of reactivated disease and may occur in both immunocompetent and immunocompromised hosts [14, 46]. It poses the greatest risk to immunocompromised patients such as those with AIDS and those receiving immunosuppressive medications (e.g., cancer chemotherapy, treatment of IBD, transplant recipients) [46].

Clinical Features

Symptoms may vary with the patient's immune status. Infection in immunocompetent patients is generally

Table 17.3 Common viral infections of the colon[a]

Virus (abbreviation)	Infected cell type	Predominant clinical manifestations	Primary histopathologic features
Adenovirus	Epithelial cells	Diarrhea, fever, abdominal pain, weight loss, GI bleeding	Mucosal ulceration, epithelial cell degeneration, neutrophil infiltrate. Intra-nuclear inclusions commonly in surface epithelium but also crypts; see Chap. 11
Cytomegalovirus (CMV)	Primarily endothelial and stromal cells; also epithelial cells	Primarily immunocompromised patients; diarrhea (bloody or non-bloody), fever, abdominal pain, weight loss	Mucosal ulcers, cryptitis, mixed inflammation with neutrophils, enlarged cells with nuclear (Cowdry A) and cytoplasmic inclusions. Inclusions are usually deep in the ulcer base
Herpes simplex virus (HSV)	Epithelial cells	Anorectal pain and discharge, inguinal adenopathy, perianal vesicles, diarrhea, abdominal pain, fever	Mucosal ulcers with neutrophil infiltrate; characteristic viral cytopathic changes in epithelial cells at ulcer edges and sloughed exudate: multinucleated cells with molded nuclei and marginated chromatin; smudgy or Cowdry type A intra-nuclear inclusion. See Chaps. 5 and 20
Human immunodeficiency virus (HIV)	Macrophages within the lamina propria	Acquired immunodeficiency syndrome (AIDS) enteropathy: chronic diarrhea, weight loss	Mucosal atrophy, increased apoptosis in epithelium, fewer mitotic figures than expected for degree of mucosal injury

[a]Not all inclusive

characterized by self-limited diarrhea, fever, abdominal pain, and weight loss, although patients with underlying IBD may experience more severe disease [14]. Immunocompromised patients such as those with AIDS and transplant recipients are also at risk for more severe disease [14]. Rare complications include toxic megacolon, perforation, and segmental bowel ischemia [14]. Specific anti-viral treatment is not usually indicated in immunocompetent patients but is commonly used in patients at risk for severe disease [45, 46].

Pathological Features

Gross Findings

Common gross manifestations include ulcers, hemorrhage, obstructive mass lesions, and pseudomembranes [14, 46]. Ulcers may be single or multiple, superficial, or deep and are often well demarcated with a "punched-out" appearance. Occasionally, cobblestone-like confluent ulcers may be seen, mimicking the ulcers of Crohn's disease [14, 46].

Microscopic Findings

The histologic features vary considerably from minimal changes (Figs. 17.24 and 17.25) to frank necrosis, abscess formation, ulceration, and occasional pseudomembrane formation (Figs. 17.26, 17.27, 17.28, and 17.29) [14, 46]. Nonspecific cryptitis is a common finding, along with a mixed inflammatory infiltrate in the lamina propria, mucosa ulceration, crypt abscess, and a large number of apoptotic enterocytes [14]. The most helpful microscopic feature is the presence of infected cells with characteristic cytopathic effect. Inclusions are seen primarily in endothelial and stromal cells in the colon and only rarely in epithelial cells. Infected cells are enlarged as indicated by the viruses name (cyto-MEGALO-virus), being up to four times larger than uninfected cells, and have both intra-cytoplasmic and intra-nuclear inclusions [45]. The intra-nuclear inclusion is characteristically described as a Cowdry type A or "owl's eye" inclusion, with a large eosinophilic viral inclusion, peripheral clearing ("halo"), and condensed host chromatin along the nuclear membrane (Figs. 17.25, 17.27, and 17.29). Of note, the halo is an artifact of fixation and is not seen in air-dried preparations [45]. The intra-cytoplasmic inclusions are indistinct, eosinophilic to basophilic, and may be positive using PAS (Fig. 17.30) and GMS stains [45]. Interestingly, the intra-nuclear inclusion is negative with these stains.

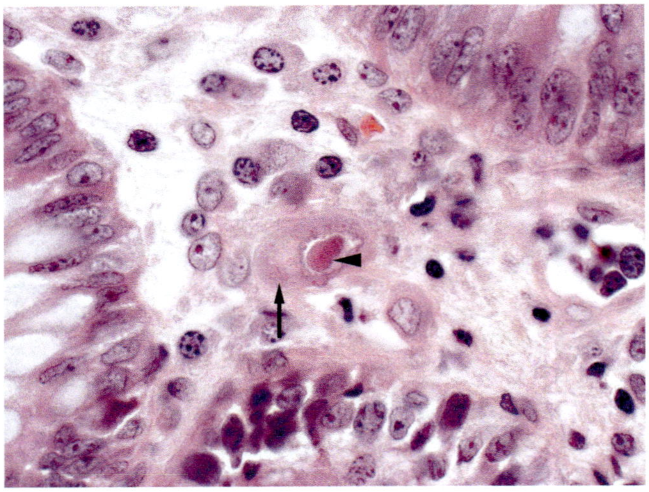

Fig. 17.25 Higher powered view demonstrating an enlarged endothelial cell with finely granular intra-cytoplasmic inclusions (arrow) and a large intra-nuclear inclusion (arrowhead) with peripheral clearing, characteristic of cytomegalovirus infection

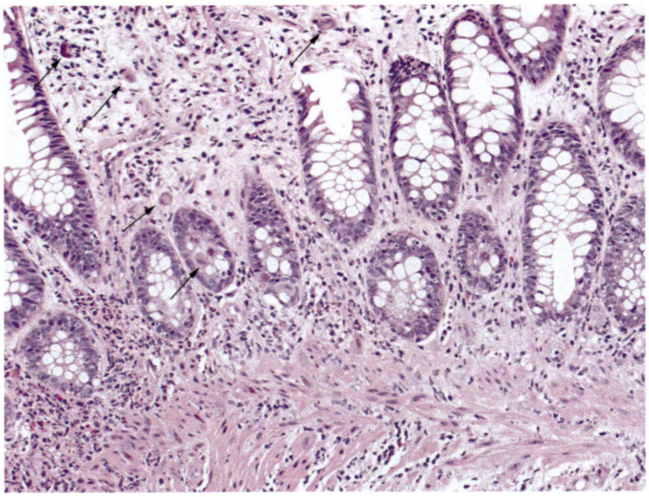

Fig. 17.24 Cytomegalovirus (CMV) infection with minimal associated inflammation and increased apoptotic cells. Occasional endothelial cells, stromal cells, and epithelial cells demonstrate characteristic CMV cytopathic effect (arrows)

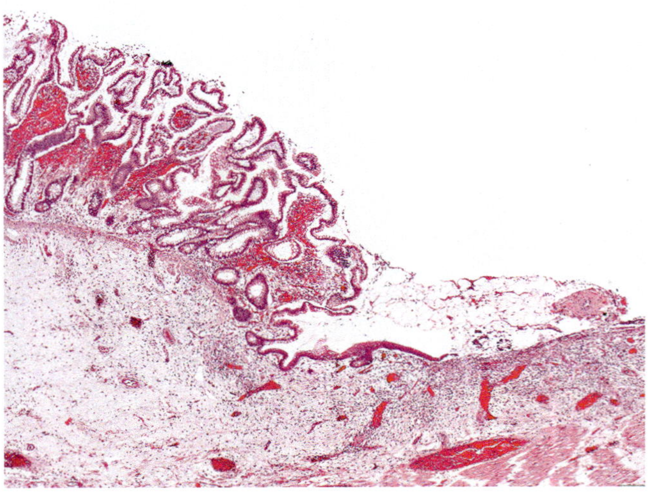

Fig. 17.26 Cytomegalovirus infection of the small bowel with a large ulcer

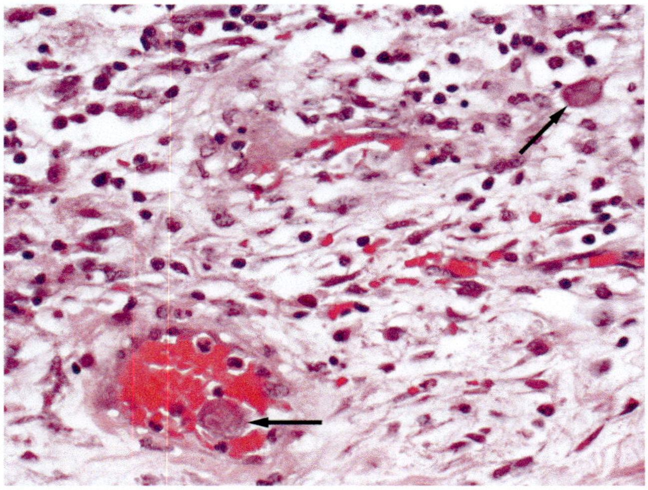

Fig. 17.27 Higher magnification of the case shown in Fig. 17.26 demonstrating cytomegalovirus-infected endothelia and stromal cells with characteristic cytopathic effect (arrows)

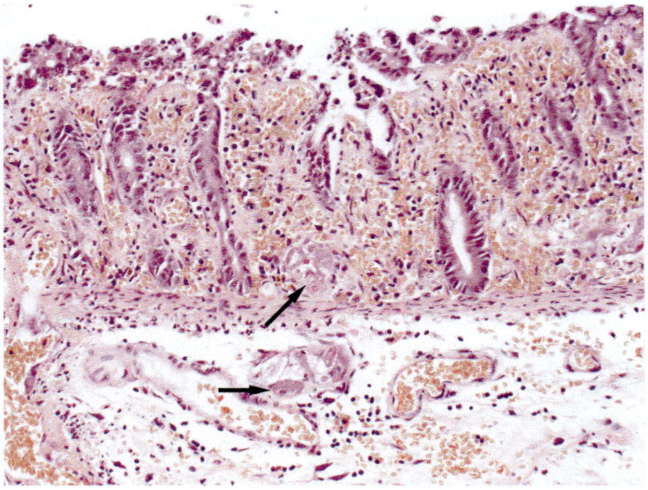

Fig. 17.29 A different region of the case shown in Fig. 17.28 demonstrates endothelial and epithelial cells with characteristic cytopathic effect of cytomegalovirus (arrows)

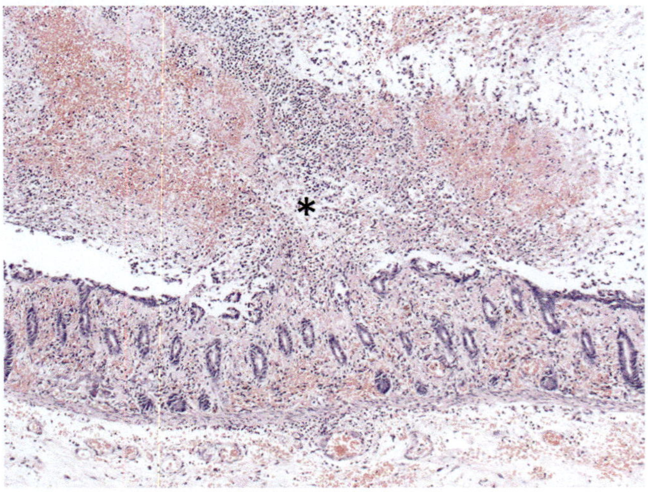

Fig. 17.28 Cytomegalovirus colitis with pseudomembrane formation (asterisk)

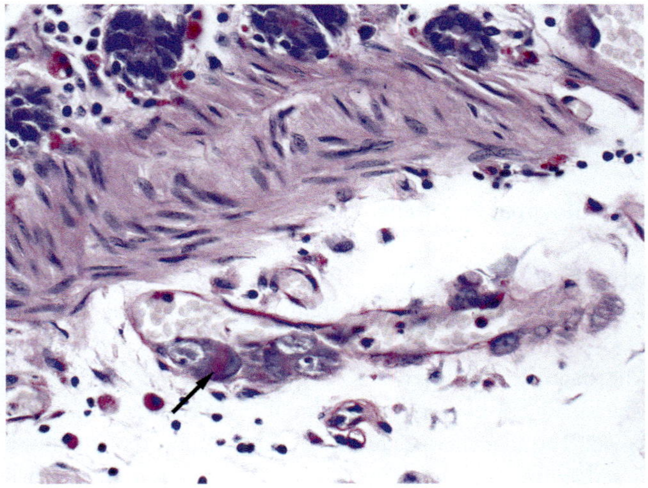

Fig. 17.30 Cytomegalovirus infected endothelial cell (arrow) with positively staining intra-cytoplasmic including by PAS. Note that the intra-nuclear inclusion has not stained with this method

Immunohistochemical Features

Commercial IHC stains for CMV are widely available and particularly useful for detection of rare infected cells and confirmation of the infecting virus when the morphology is atypical [45]. Asymptomatic CMV reaction may occur in immunocompromised patients, and therefore positive IHC or in situ hybridization staining for CMV must be correlated with the clinical picture [45].

Differential Diagnosis

While the owl's eye inclusion is characteristic of CMV infection, this appearance may be seen with other viral intranuclear inclusions such as those of adenovirus, HSV, and varicella-zoster virus (VZV). However, these other viruses lack the overall cellular enlargement and intracytoplasmic inclusions found in CMV-infected cells [45]. CMV IHC or NAAT may be useful in challenging cases. When intracytoplasmic inclusions are strongly positive for PAS or GMS, they must be differentiated from intracellular yeasts.

Human Immunodeficiency Virus (HIV Enterocolopathy)

Definition

HIV-1 and HIV-2 are two closely related retroviruses in the *Lentivirus* genus [45]. Together they are responsible for one of the most significant public health threats worldwide. HIV-1 is the most common virus, being estimated to infect more than

35 million individuals worldwide, whereas HIV-2 infection is found primarily in West Africa. HIV infection is nationally notifiable in the United States. The CDC estimates that 1.1 million persons ages 13 and older were HIV positive by the end of 2015, of which an estimated 15% had not yet been diagnosed [28]. Unlike most other viral infections, most of the morbidity and mortality associated with HIV is due to host immunosuppression from infection of CD4+ T lymphocytes, dendritic cells, and macrophages [45]. However, certain manifestations such as HIV enterocolopathy may be due to the specific actions of the virus itself, or a secondary autoimmune reaction to the virus [14]. HIV enterocolopathy is generally defined by a spectrum of morphologic changes seen in the intestine of HIV-infected individuals with chronic diarrhea, in which no other cause of the patient's symptoms has been found [14]. This condition may be found during all stages of HIV infection, from acute disease to AIDS [47]. The actual cause of diarrhea in these individuals is unknown, and some believe that HIV enterocolopathy does not represent a specific disease entity [47]. Treatment is supportive.

Clinical Features

By definition, patients have diarrhea and may also experience malabsorption and weight loss.

Pathological Features

Gross Findings

By colonoscopy, the bowel usually appears normal.

Microscopic Findings

The small bowel is more commonly affected than the large bowel. The characteristic histologic features are similar to those of mild graft versus host disease (GVHD) with increased enterocyte apoptosis and fewer mitotic figures than expected for the degree of mucosal injury present (Figs. 17.31 and 17.32).

Immunohistochemical Features

IHCs for the HIV p24 antigen are commercially available and may be useful for identifying viral antigen expression in gut lymphoid tissue (Fig. 17.33).

Differential Diagnosis

The primary differential diagnosis is GVHD and drug-related injury, including antiretroviral agents [14, 47]. Clinical correlation and p24 immunostaining can be useful in resolving this differential [14].

Parasitic Infections

A number of protozoan and helminthic parasites may infect the colon. While many of the protozoa are commensal organisms that are not associated with human disease, *Entamoeba*

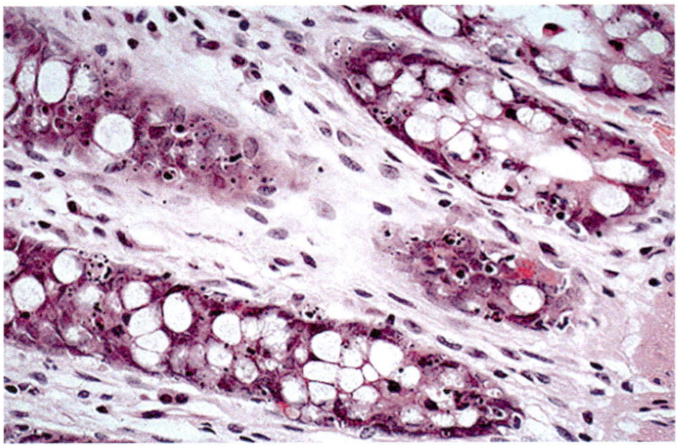

Fig. 17.32 Higher magnification of the case shown in Fig. 17.31 demonstrates the increased number of apoptotic bodies within enterocytes. No mitotic figures are apparent, despite the degree of apoptosis. (Image courtesy of Dr. Sebastian Lucas)

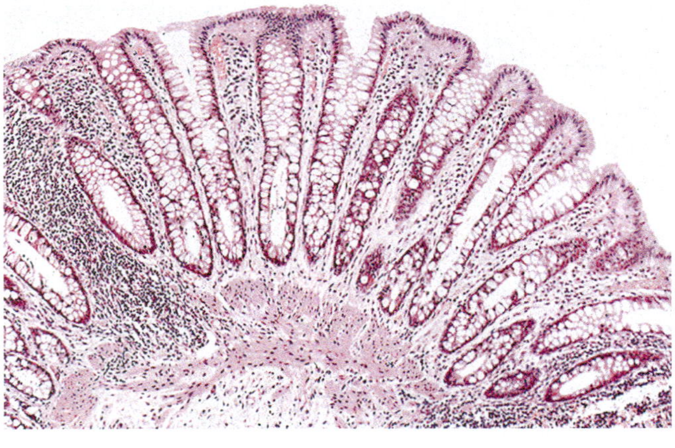

Fig. 17.31 HIV enterocolopathy demonstrating preserved colonic architecture and normal number of inflammatory cells in the lamina propria. (Image courtesy of Dr. Sebastian Lucas)

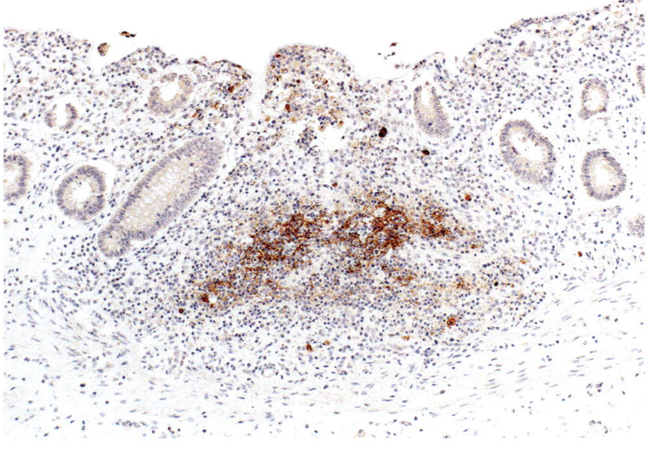

Fig. 17.33 HIV-1 p24 immunostaining of the lower anorectal margin demonstrating scattered positive cells within the lymphoid aggregate. (Image courtesy of Dr. Sebastian Lucas)

Table 17.4 Common protozoal infections of the colon[a]

Protozoan (disease)	Predominant clinical manifestations	Primary histopathologic features
Cryptosporidium spp. (cryptosporidiosis)	Profuse, foul-smelling cholera-like watery diarrhea, nausea, vomiting, abdominal cramps, low-grade fever, weight loss, weakness, myalgia. Prolonged symptoms in immunocompromised hosts, with increased incidence of extraintestinal disease	Variable involvement of the duodenum, small intestine, and colon (see Chap. 11). Parasite developmental forms present at the brush border as small (1–4.5 μm diameter) basophilic objects; may have accompanying increased number of acute inflammatory cells, enterocyte necrosis and sloughing, dilated colonic crypts with decreased goblet cells and increased mitotic figures. More severe pathology in immunocompromised hosts
Entamoeba histolytica (amebiasis)	Many asymptomatic. Symptoms include watery to bloody diarrhea, fever, dysentery, extraintestinal dissemination	Flask-shaped ulcers, trophozoites (12–35 μm greatest dimension) with small round nuclei, peripheral chromatin, and central karyosome; ingested erythrocytes in the cytoplasm. Organisms are periodic acid Schiff reaction positive and commonly seen at the invading edge of the ulcer with surrounding clearing
Balantidioides coli (balantiosis)	Occasionally asymptomatic; when present, symptoms resemble those of amebiasis with diarrhea, dysentery, extraintestinal spread	Flask-shaped ulcers, large (50–200 μm greatest dimension) ovoid trophozoites with circumferential cilia and kidney bean-shaped macronucleus at the periphery of the ulcer rather than in the necrotic center

[a]Not all inclusive; prevalence varies by geographic location and exposure history

Table 17.5 Common helminthic infections of the colon[a]

Helminth (disease)	Predominant clinical manifestations	Primary histopathologic features
Enterobius vermicularis (enterobiasis, pinworm infection)	Many are asymptomatic. Nocturnal anal pruritus is the most common symptom	Usually an incidental finding in the appendix (see Chap. 19). Rarely cause minute ulcers; entrapped worms and eggs can elicit a granulomatous response
Schistosoma spp. (schistosomiasis)	Varies with stage of infection; intestinal involvement usually associated with diarrhea and abdominal pain	Characteristic large eggs, each containing a larva (miracidium), throughout the bowel wall with surrounding granulomatous inflammation; occasionally Splendore-Hoeppli reaction. Also inflammatory polyps, bilharziomas (inflammatory mass containing numerous eggs)
Trichuris trichiura (trichuriasis, whipworm infection)	Most are asymptomatic. Diarrhea, abdominal pain, and tenesmus with heavy infections; rarely intussusception and rectal prolapse	Cecum most heavily infected; slender anterior end of the worm is embedded in the mucosa, while the larger posterior (containing eggs in gravid females) is in the lumen. A prominent bacillary and stichosome are commonly seen. Usually no to mild inflammation; heavy infections with dilated crypts, edema, and increased numbers of chronic inflammatory cells in the mucosa

[a]Not all inclusive; prevalence varies by geographic location and exposure history

histolytica and *Balantidioides coli* are known pathogens that can cause severe, invasive disease [48]. Many helminthic infections cause subclinical or mild infections; however, they are all capable of causing symptomatic disease under the right circumstances. The severity of disease manifestations is often directly proportional to the worm burden [48, 49]. Tables 17.4 and 17.5 list the protozoa and helminths that can infect the colon, with the most clinically significant of these described in greater detail below. Cryptosporidiosis, cyclosporiasis, and cystoisosporiasis can involve the colon, but most commonly involve the small intestine and are discussed in greater detail in Chap. 11. Similarly, *Enterobius vermicularis* (pinworm) is covered in Chap. 19, whereas *Strongyloides stercoralis* and the anisakids are discussed in Chap. 11. The reader is referred to several excellent atlases of parasitic infectious diseases, including those published by Orihel and Ash [50] and the Armed Forces Institute of Pathology [51, 52], as well as to the CDC DPDx website [49] and a recent review of laboratory diagnostics for parasitic diseases of the gastrointestinal tract [53]. The CDC DPDx offers a rapid free telediagnostic service for histopathology and microbiology slides suspected of containing a parasite.

Entamoeba histolytica (Amebiasis)

Definition

Entamoeba histolytica is a protozoan parasite that causes intestinal and extraintestinal amebiasis [49]. Infection occurs primarily in resource-limited settings but is also seen in travelers, institutionalized patients, and MSM [49]. Transmission is via ingestion of environmentally resistant cysts in contaminated food or water [49]. Sexual transmission and spread via fomites has also been reported [49].

Clinical Features

Entamoeba histolytica infection has a broad spectrum of manifestations including asymptomatic colonization, mild colitis, dysentery, formation of an inflammatory mass (ameboma), and dissemination to extraintestinal sites [49]. Approximately 10–20% of infected individuals develop symptoms [49]. Symptoms are produced when the amebae invade the bowel wall and may include abdominal pain, watery or bloody diarrhea, anorexia, malaise, and fulminating dysentery [49, 54]. When invading amebae enter the portal blood supply, they may disseminate to the liver, or less commonly, other organs [49]. Treatment varies with the stage of infection; for symptomatic patients, a luminal amebicide is used in conjunction with an antiparasitic drug with systemic penetration [49].

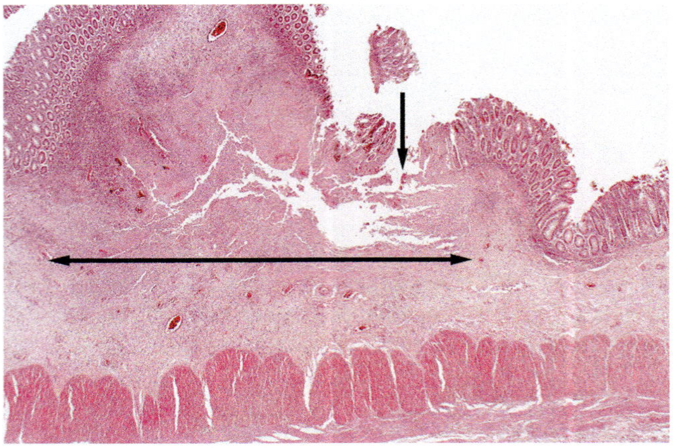

Fig. 17.34 *Entamoeba histolytica* infection (amebiasis) with the formation of a characteristic "flask-shaped" ulcer, in which the base is broader than the apex (arrows)

Pathological Features

Gross Findings

The primary gross feature is discreet or coalesced ulcers with heaped undermined borders and a central gray-white necrotic exudate [54]. Amebic ulcers usually have a focal distribution, with the cecum being the most commonly involved site; however, other regions of the colon can be affected [54]. Amebomas appear as well-defined, firm expansions of the colon wall and may be associated with a circumferential (i.e., "napkin ring") constriction [54].

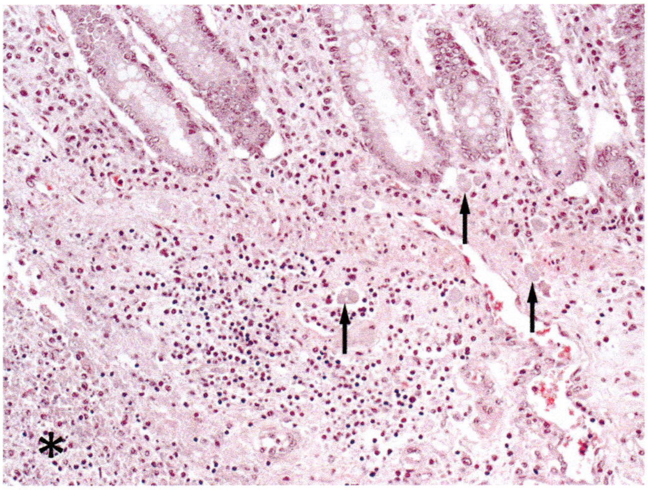

Fig. 17.35 Trophozoites of *Entamoeba histolytica* (arrows) are best identified at the leading edge of the ulcer in the submucosa, away from the ulcer bed (asterisk). They often are surrounded by a clear zone which facilitates their identification

Microscopic Findings

The definitive histopathologic feature of amebiasis is the presence of *E. histolytica* invading the bowel wall [54]. Only trophozoites are seen in tissue; the cyst forms seen in stool are not present [49]. Although other *Entamoeba* species, including the morphologically identical *E. dispar*, can be found in human stool specimens, only *E. histolytica* is capable of invasion, and thus the presence of amebic trophozoites within tissue is diagnostic for amebiasis [49]. Infection begins as a small region of mucosal necrosis at the site of invasion [54]. After invading through the mucosa, the trophozoites invade laterally into the submucosa, forming an ulcer with a base that is broader than its apex, giving it a so-called flask-shaped (Fig. 17.34) [54]. The ulcer crater contains cellular debris, fibrin, and trophozoites, although the latter may be difficult to identify. Trophozoites are best seen at the advancing edge of the ulcer in the submucosa and are commonly surrounded by a clear zone which facilitates their identification (Fig. 17.35) [54]. The associated inflammatory response is usually composed of mononuclear cells. Amebomas are comprised of granulation tissue, fibrosis, and chronic inflammatory cells (Fig. 17.36). Trophozoites are typically clustered in the submucosa near regions of ulceration [54].

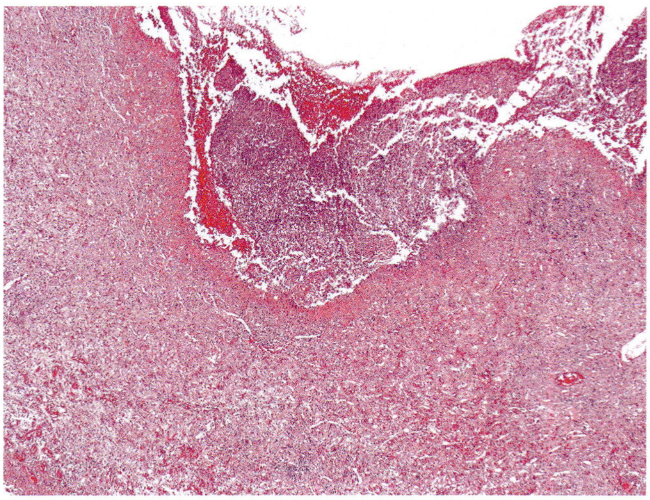

Fig. 17.36 Ameboma of *Entamoeba histolytica*, comprised of granulation tissue, fibrosis, and chronic inflammatory cells

E. histolytica trophozoites typically measure 10–35 μm in greatest dimension in tissue sections and have an ameboid appearance with pseudopod cytoplasmic projects, a dense vacuolated cytoplasm, and a single round nucleus measuring approximately 4–5 μm in diameter (Fig. 17.37). Ingested

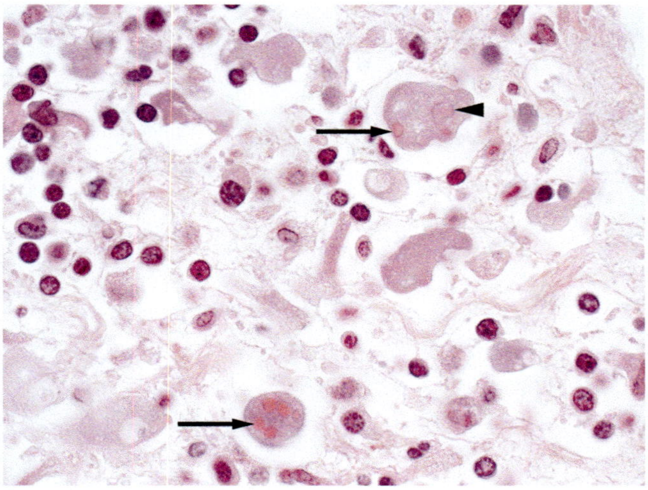

Fig. 17.37 High magnification of the case shown in Fig. 17.36 demonstrating several *Entamoeba histolytica* trophozoites admixed with lymphocytes and plasma cells. The trophozoites have a surrounding clear zone, round nucleus with peripheral condensed chromatin and central karyosome (arrowhead), and some contain ingested erythrocytes in their cytoplasm (arrows)

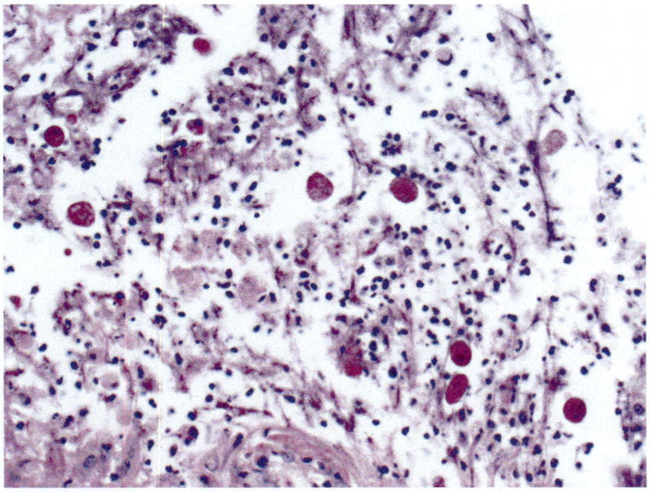

Fig. 17.38 *Entamoeba histolytica* trophozoites highlighted with PAS staining

erythrocytes are occasionally seen in the trophozoite cytoplasm. The nucleus has a characteristic chromatin pattern, with peripheral chromatin lining the nuclear membrane, and a centrally placed karyosome (nucleolus-like structure) [54]. Unlike stool specimens, the central karyosome is often not seen in tissue due to the plane of sectioning. Amebic trophozoites contain abundant glycogen in their cytoplasm and are readily highlighted by PAS stain (Fig. 17.38).

Differential Diagnosis

The primary differential diagnosis of *E. histolytica* trophozoites in tissue sections is large host cells such as histiocytes and ganglion cells [54]. Macrophage cytoplasm may also stain strongly PAS and should not be confused with amebae. Fortunately, the unique characteristics of the amebic nucleus allow for ready differentiation of amebae from host cells in most cases [54].

Balantidioides coli (Balantiosis)

Definition

Balantidioides (formerly *Balantidium*, a.k.a. *Neobalantidium*) *coli* is the largest protozoan parasite to infect humans, and the only ciliate [49]. It causes a disease called neobalantidiasis (formerly balantidiasis) which has similar clinical and pathologic features to amebiasis [55]. Pigs are a natural host of *B. coli*, and therefore human infection is most commonly found in pig-raising regions of the world [49]. Transmission is via the fecal oral route, with occasional human-to-human transmission in the presence of poor hygiene [55].

Clinical Features

Infection may be asymptomatic in the absence of invasion. When present, symptoms mimic those of intestinal amebiasis, with watery or bloody diarrhea, dysentery, and extraintestinal involvement [55]. Treatment is with one of several antibiotics [49].

Pathological Features

Gross Findings

The colon and appendix are most commonly involved, with the ileum being a less common site of infection [55]. The gross findings in the colon are essentially identical to those of amebiasis, with ulcer formation. Extraintestinal diseases may involve the liver, vagina, bladder, ureter, and lung [55].

Microscopic Findings

The histopathologic features of balantiosis are essentially the same as those of amebiasis, including formation of flask-shaped ulcers (Fig. 17.39). The definitive histopathologic feature of neobalantidiasis is the presence of *B. coli* invading the bowel wall [55]. They are most commonly seen at the periphery of the ulcer rather than in the necrotic center (Figs. 17.39 and 17.40) [55]. Cysts are not seen in tissue sections [49]. The trophozoites are very large (50–200 μm), ovoid, and covered with circumferential cilia (Fig. 17.41). They have a large kidney-shaped macronucleus.

Differential Diagnosis

Given their distinctive morphologic features, including large size and cilia, the trophozoites are rarely mistaken for host cells. When present in peritoneal fluid (e.g., due to bowel perforation), they must be differentiated from the significantly smaller ciliated host cells [55].

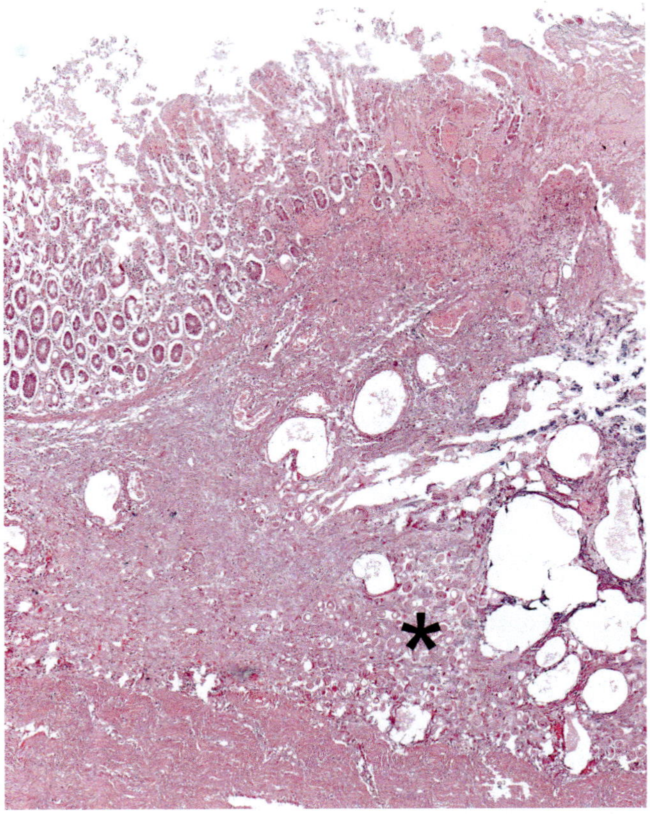

Fig. 17.39 *Balantidioides coli* trophozoites at the expanding edge of an ulcer within the submucosa (asterisk)

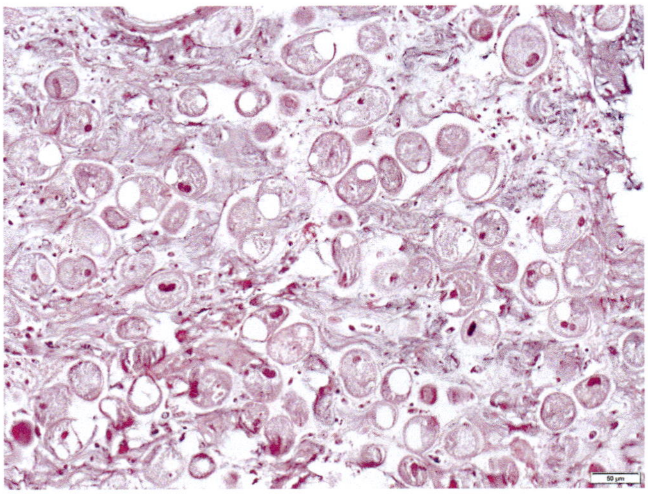

Fig. 17.40 Higher magnification of the *Balantidioides coli* trophozoites from the case shown in Fig. 17.39 demonstrates their ovoid shape and large basophilic macronucleus

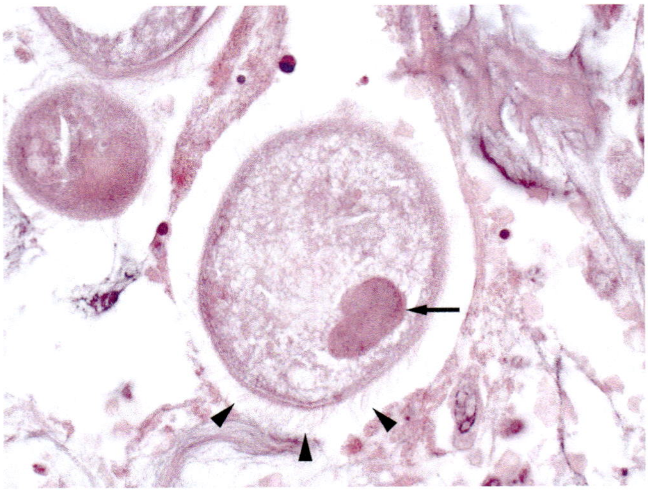

Fig. 17.41 *Balantidioides coli* trophozoite with circumferential cilia (arrowheads) and a large kidney bean-shaped macronucleus (arrow)

Trichuris trichiura (Trichuriasis, Whipworm Infection)

Definition

Trichuris trichiura is an intestinal nematode (roundworm) transmitted through ingestion of infectious eggs in fecally contaminated soil, produce, and water [49]. It is one of several "soil-transmitted helminths" recognized by the WHO as a neglected tropical infection [7]. Combined, the soil transmitted helminths are estimated to infect 1.5 billion individuals worldwide [7]. Following ingestion of the egg, the larva hatches in the small intestine and matures into an adult. The adult worm takes up residence in the colon where it embeds its slender anterior end into the mucosa and feeds on host tissue secretions. Male and female worms mate, and the female releases fertilized eggs into the intestinal lumen which are shed in the stool. The eggs must mature in the soil before becoming infectious to humans, and thus trichuriasis can be prevented through proper disposal and treatment of human feces. As expected, trichuriasis is uncommon in resource-rich settings with adequate sanitation facilities, such as the United States and Europe [56].

Clinical Features

Most infections are light and asymptomatic, with the prevalence of symptoms increasing with the worm burden [49, 56]. In heavy infections, symptoms include mucoid, occasionally blood-streaked diarrhea, abdominal pain, and tenesmus. Rectal prolapse and intussusception can result from severe and prolonged tenesmus [49, 56]. Treatment is with albendazole or a related agent [49].

Pathological Features

Gross Findings

Trichuris trichiura adult worms may be discovered on routine screening colonoscopy and removed intact for pathologic examination. They are usually found in highest number in the cecum but may also be found throughout the colon and in the appendix [56]. Worms are tan-white with a smooth outer cuticle and an overall "whip-like" shape with one end (the anterior) being significantly more slender than the other [49]. On endoscopy, the slender anterior end can be seen embedded in the intestinal mucosa, while the larger posterior hangs free in the lumen (Fig. 17.42). Mature female worms are 3.5–5 cm long and have a straight tail, whereas males are slightly shorter and have a curved tail (Fig. 17.42) [56]. Removal of the worm during colonoscopy commonly produces small petechiae [56]. In heavy infections, the mucosa may be erythematous, edematous, friable, and even frankly hemorrhagic [56].

Microscopic Findings

As discussed above, *T. trichiura* has a unique placement in the colon, with the slender anterior end embedded in the superficial mucosa and the broader posterior end hanging free [56]. Thus it is common to see cross sections of a narrow anterior end (100–150 μm in diameters) within the mucosa, with significantly larger cross sections (400–700 μm in diameters) of the broader posterior in the lumen (Fig. 17.43). When the worm is a gravid female, characteristic eggs measuring 50–55 μm long by 20–25 μm wide with bipolar mucoid plugs may be seen within the uterus (Fig. 17.44). As with all helminth eggs in tissue, narrowing the condenser will allow the features of the eggs to be more easily seen. The associated host inflammatory response is generally mild, with increased numbers of chronic inflammatory cells and eosinophils in the mucosa. Increased mitotic activity may also be observed in nearby crypt epithelial cells [56]. Like other nematodes, *T. trichiura* has a thick eosinophilic acellular cuticle ("skin") with underlying well-developed musculature, a full gastrointestinal tract, and either male or female reproductive organs. In addition to these general diagnostic morphologic features, *T. trichiura* has specific features that allow for its definitive identification. First, its placement within the colon is characteristic; no other worm of this size has this arrangement in the

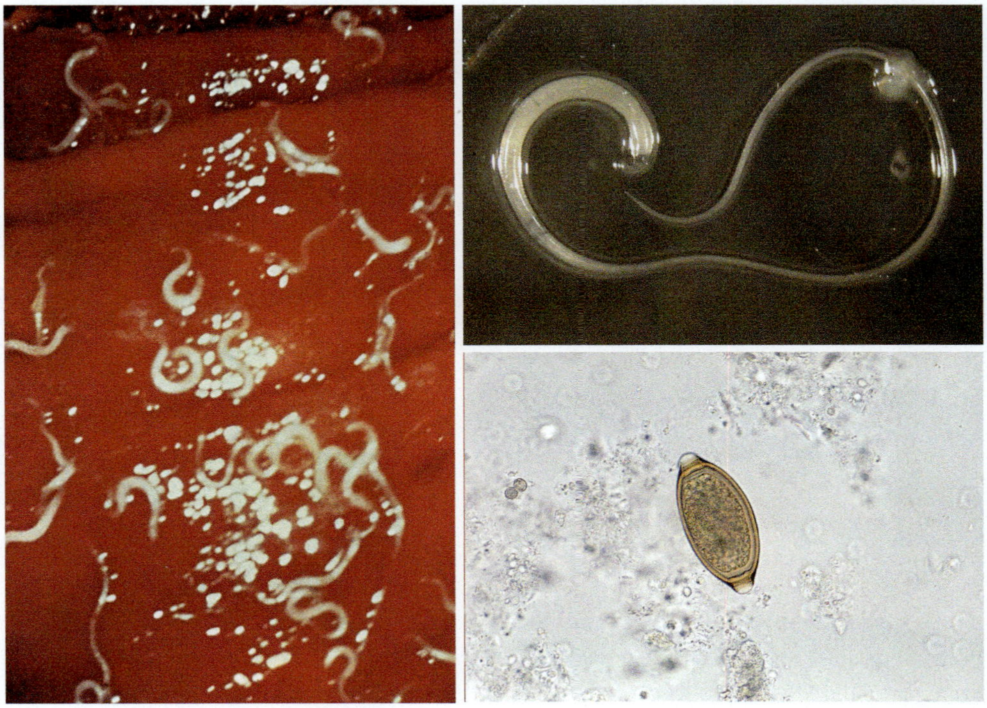

Fig. 17.42 *Trichuris trichiura* seen on endoscopy (left) and following removal (upper right). The adult worm has a long slender anterior end and broad posterior, giving it a "whip" shape; females have a straight tail (shown), while males have a tightly curled tail. The anterior end of the worm is embedded into the intestinal mucosa, while the broad end hangs free in the lumen, facilitating mating and release of eggs into the stool. The eggs of *T. trichiura* are 50–55 μm long by 20–25 μm wide and have bipolar mucoid plugs (bottom right)

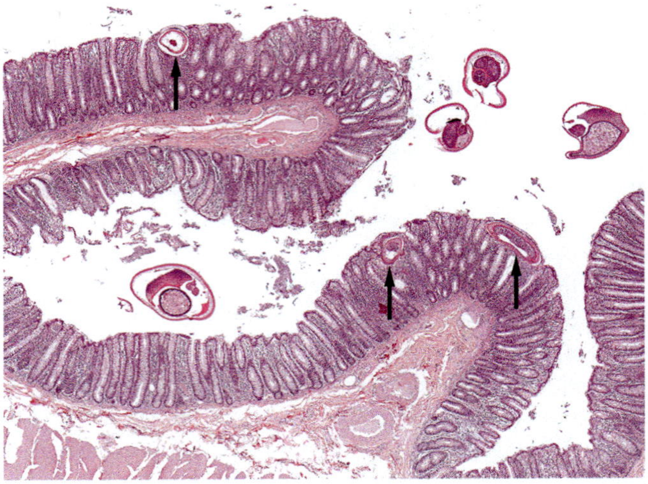

Fig. 17.43 *Trichuris trichiura* adults in an intestinal biopsy. The slender anterior end of the adult worms is threaded through the mucosa (arrows), while the broader posterior hangs freely in the lumen. At least two adults are seen in this biopsy

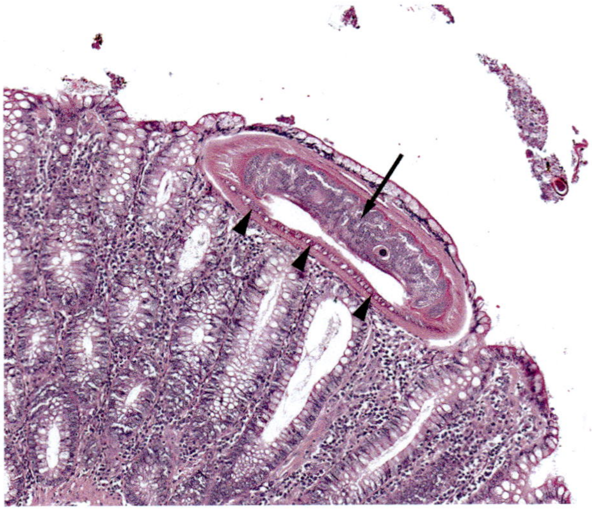

Fig. 17.45 Higher magnification of the anterior portion of an adult *Trichuris trichiura* from Fig. 17.44 demonstrating the stichosome (arrow) and bacillary band (arrowheads). These features, in conjunction with the size of the worm and its placement in the mucosa, are diagnostic for *T. trichuris*

Fig. 17.44 Higher magnification of the case shown in Fig. 17.44 demonstrating a gravid female *Trichuris trichiura* with intrauterine eggs (left). The characteristic features of the eggs can be appreciated, including the bipolar plugs (arrows). Narrowing the condenser (bottom, right) from the normal view (top, right) serves to improve the contrast of the eggs and facilitates their identification

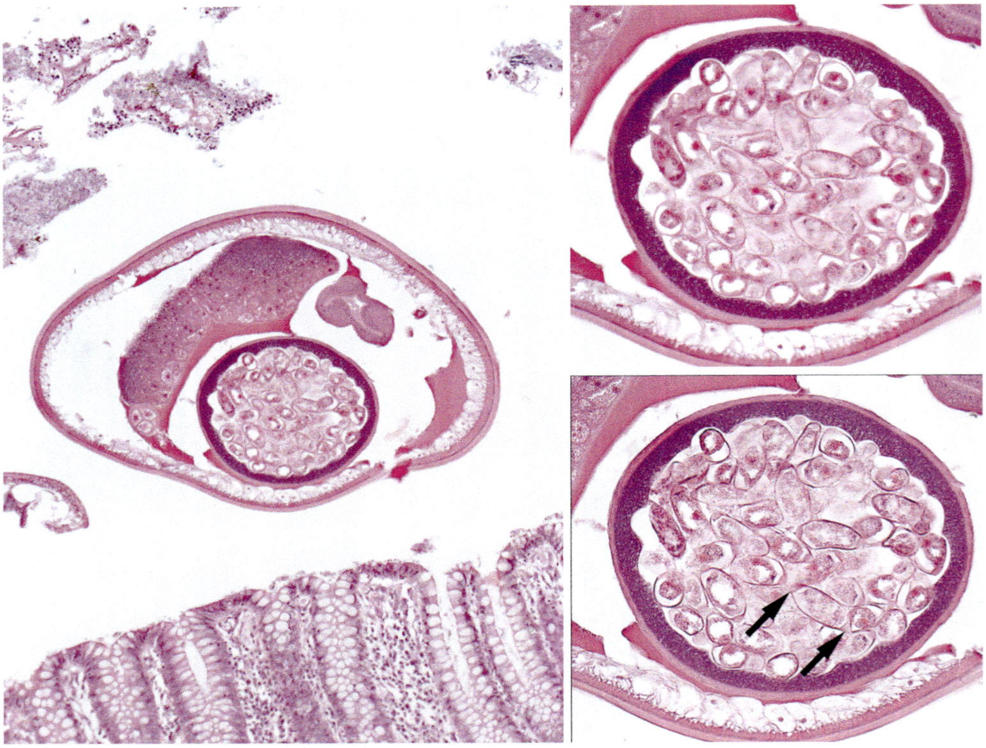

human intestinal tract. However, this placement is not always seen, particularly when the worm is removed during colonoscopy and submitted for histologic sectioning. Fortunately, the presence of other morphologic features—the stichosome (long chain of large basophilic glandular cells), bacillary band (narrow band of basophilic cells), and, if present, intrauterine eggs (Figs. 17.44 and 17.45)—also allows for definitive identification [56].

Differential Diagnosis

The morphologic features of adult *T. trichiura* are diagnostic for trichuriasis [56]. Foreign matter such as vegetable (food) material may present an occasional convincing helminthic mimic but can be differentiated from true helminths by the lack of a cuticle/tegument, characteristic internal structures, as well as a tendency to exhibit birefringence with polarized light [48].

Schistosoma Species (Schistosomiasis)

Definition

Schistosoma is a genus of parasitic trematodes (flukes) that reside in the blood vessels of its host [49]. There are six primary *Schistosoma* species that infect humans, of which five cause intestinal disease: *S. mansoni*, *S. japonicum*, *S. intercalatum*, *S. mekongi*, and *S. guineensis* [48, 49]. *S. mansoni* and *S. japonicum* are responsible for the majority of cases of intestinal schistosomiasis [57]. Schistosomiasis is categorized as a neglected tropical infection by the WHO, with an estimated 206.4 million people at risk worldwide [7]. It is found in the tropics and subtropics worldwide, including parts of the Mediterranean, although most patients at risk of disease live in Africa [7, 48, 49]. Humans become infected when cercariae-microscopic free-swimming forms of the parasite directly penetrate intact skin when an individual is in contact with infested water [49]. Following penetration of the skin, the cercariae enter the bloodstream and migrate to the lungs and then the liver. The worms reach maturity in the liver and form male-female pairs (Fig. 17.46) before traveling to their final destination in the mesenteric venules. The schistosomes are slender flat worms with separate male and female sexes. The female resides within a longitudinal groove in the body of the male, leaving only periodically to lay eggs into the vessel and surrounding tissue. The eggs have characteristic shapes which readily allow for their identification in stool specimens (Fig. 17.46). The eggs of *S. mansoni* eggs are 114–180 μm long by 45–70 μm wide and have a large lateral spine, while the eggs of *S. intercalatum* and *S. guineensis* resemble those of *S. haematobium* with a terminal spine and length of approximately 200 μm [49]. The eggs of *S. japonicum* and *S. mekongi* are smaller (50–100 μm long) and have a small inconspicuous spine. An estimated 50% of the eggs migrate through the intestinal wall, aided by the host inflammatory response to the eggs, and are shed in the feces [57]. The remaining portion of the eggs remain in bowel wall or are passively carried to the liver, resulting in significant damage to the affected tissues [49]. Eggs that are shed in stool will hatch when in contact with fresh water and release a free-swimming ciliated miracidium larva, which can then infect a suitable snail host. After undergoing several life cycle stages in the snail, cercariae are eventually released into the water to infect the next host, thus completing the life cycle [49].

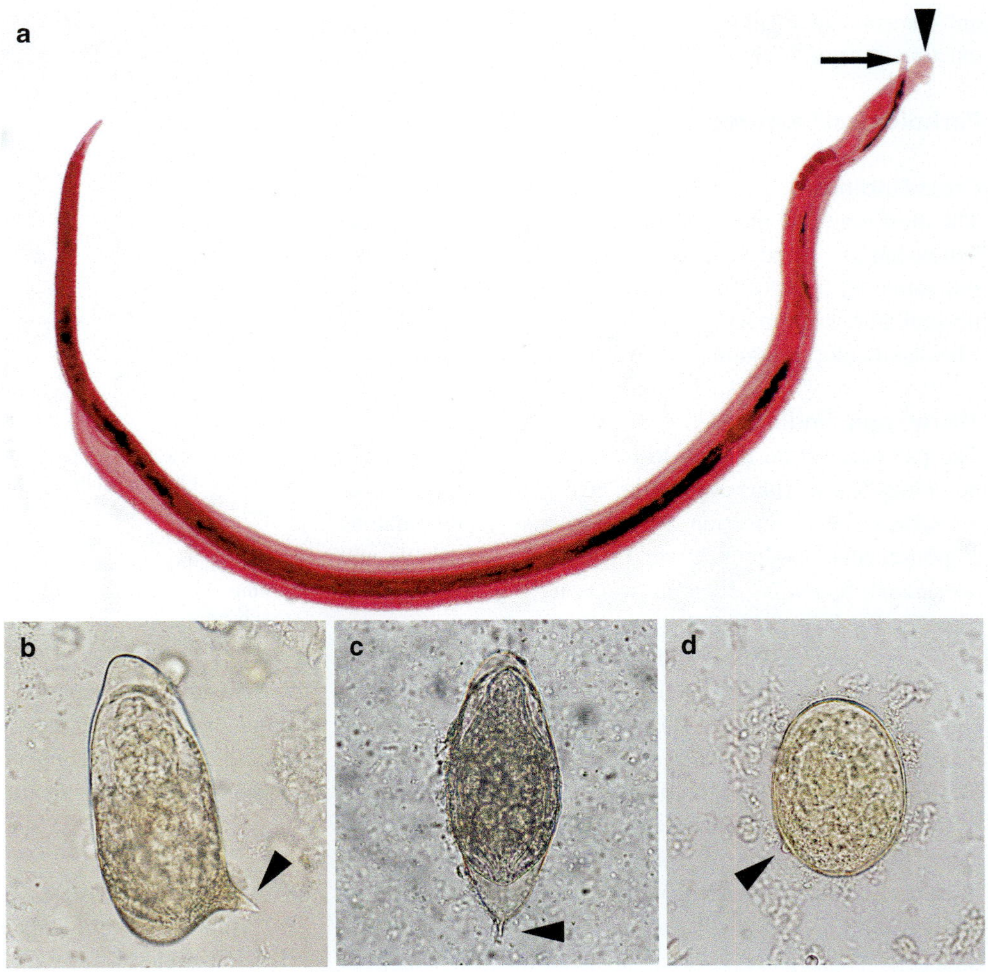

Fig. 17.46 *Schistosoma mansoni* adult pair (**a**; carmine stain). Note that the slender female resides within a longitudinal groove of the male; the arrow and arrowhead point to the anterior ends of the female and male, respectively. The eggs of *Schistosoma* spp. are large and have characteristic spines; shown are the eggs of *S. mansoni* (**b**), *S. haematobium* (**c**), and *S. japonicum* (**d**), with arrowheads denoting their spines

Clinical Features

The clinical presentation varies with the stage of infection [57]. There may be a transient pruritic maculopapular rash at the site of cercariae penetration (cercarial dermatitis), particularly in previously exposed individuals [57]. Two to four weeks later, the patient may experience transient fever, wheezing, cough, hives, dysentery, hepatosplenomegaly, diffuse lymphadenopathy, pulmonary infiltrates, and peripheral eosinophilia due to an immune response to the worms and later the eggs (acute schistosomiasis or Katayama fever) [57]. While these manifestations may be troublesome, the most serious symptoms occur during the chronic phase of infection in which intestinal and liver damage occurs from retained eggs and the associated host immune response [57]. Patients with light infections may be asymptomatic, but over time, particularly in heavy infections, patients may develop abdominal pain, bloody diarrhea, and weight loss [14]. Anemia may occur with continued blood loss, and protein-losing enteropathy has been described. In severe cases, intestinal obstruction, intussusception, perforation, rectal prolapse, perianal abscesses, and fistulas may occur [14]. Patients with substantial liver involvement may experience varices and portal colopathy and other manifestations of cirrhosis [14]. Treatment of chronic schistosomiasis is with the anti-parasitic agent, praziquantel, although it will not reverse existing scarring [49].

Pathological Features

Gross Findings

The most common intestinal findings are petechial mucosal hemorrhages, mucosal granularity, punctate ulcers, and inflammatory polyposis [14]. On occasional, a large discreet fibroinflammatory mass (bilharzioma) may be formed [57]. The distal colon is commonly involved.

Microscopic Findings

The pathognomonic finding in intestinal schistosomiasis is numerous *Schistosoma* eggs in the mucosa, submucosa, and/or serosa, in conjunction with a robust granulomatous response, eosinophilic infiltrate (Figs. 17.47 and 17.48), and occasional Splendore-Hoeppli reaction (Fig. 17.49) [57]. The eggs are large (100–200 μm in greatest dimension, varying by species) and thin-walled and, in recent or active disease, contain a visible miracidium within. Some *Schistosoma* spp. eggs have a prominent spine which allows for identification to the species level (Figs. 17.47 and 17.48) [48, 49]. However, there is often significant distortion of the egg wall in tissue sections, and thus the presence or absence of characteristic spines must be interpreted with caution (Fig. 17.48). An ova and parasite exam provides the best morphology for species identification and can be recommended as a follow-up test [57]. In remote disease, only calcified eggs with little to no inflammatory reaction may be seen. Segmental colonic fibrosis is a rare complication of intestinal schistosomiasis [57]. In resected colon specimens, adults may rarely be observed within the venous plexus of the vascular stalk (Fig. 17.50) [57].

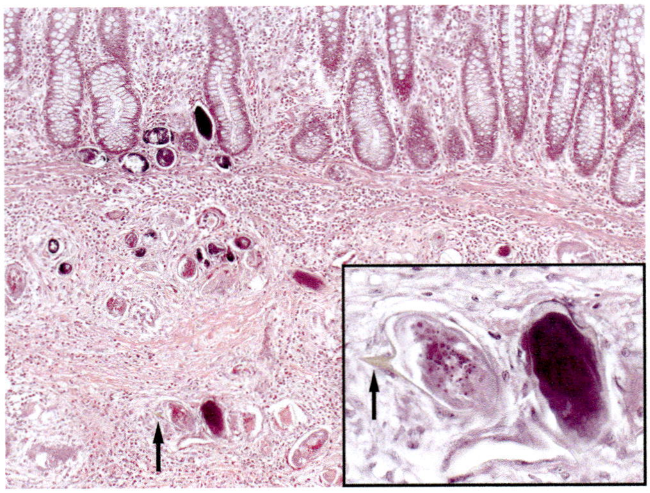

Fig. 17.47 *Schistosoma mansoni* eggs within the mucosa and submucosa of a colon biopsy, with associated granulomatous host response. Eggs are seen in different stages, with some being fully calcified and others having a visible miracidium within (inset). A well-defined lateral spine (arrows) is seen on one egg, allowing an identification of *S. mansoni* to be made from the histopathologic findings

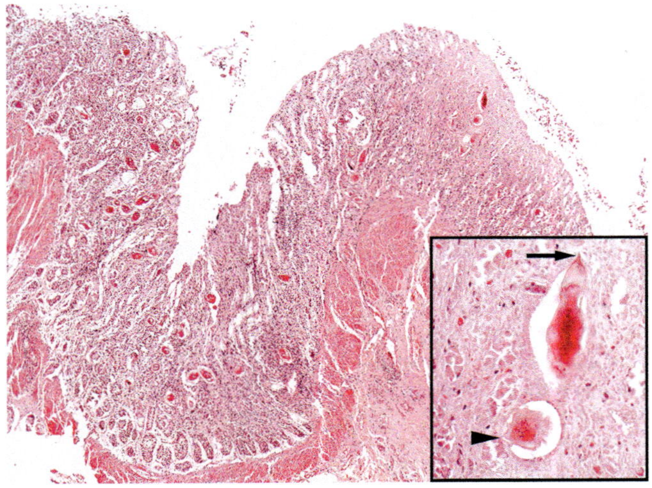

Fig. 17.48 Intestinal biopsy containing numerous *Schistosoma* eggs in the mucosa. Occasional eggs demonstrate a well-defined terminal spine (arrow), allowing for identification of *S. intercalatum/S. guineensis*. Caution must be exercised when searching for egg spines since the egg wall morphology is commonly distorted during histologic processing, resulting in production of numerous folds and protruberances (arrowhead)

Differential Diagnosis

The primary differential diagnosis of intestinal schistosomiasis is other causes of granulomas in the bowel, particularly

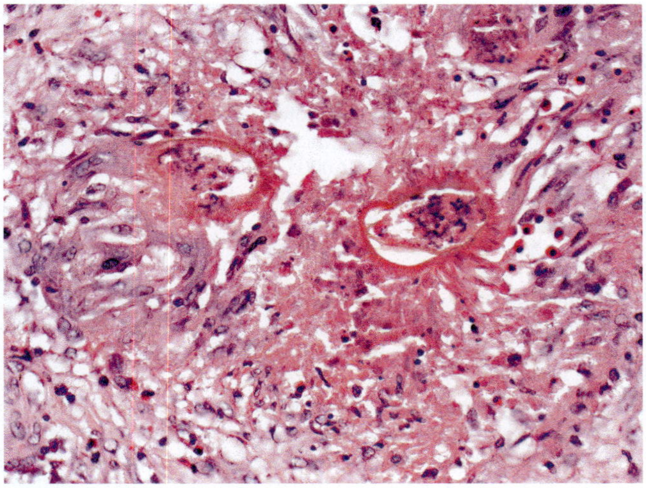

Fig. 17.49 *Schistosoma* sp. eggs within a granuloma with prominent Splendore-Hoeppli phenomenon. Note the numerous eosinophils in the accompanying inflammatory infiltrate

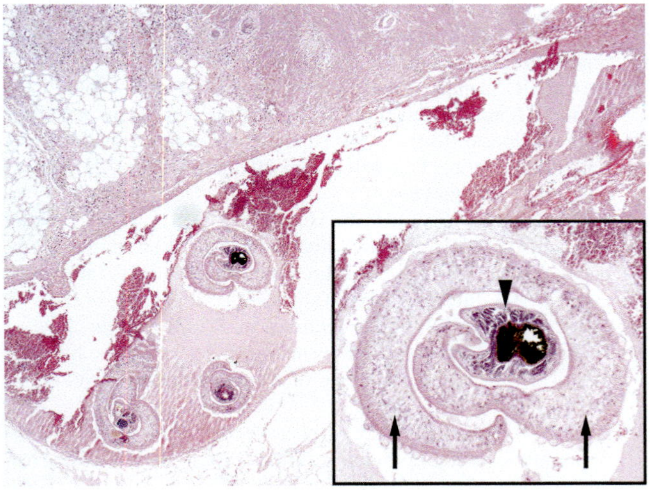

Fig. 17.50 *Schistosoma* sp. adults within a mesenteric venule (inset) with the larger male (arrows) and female (arrow head) seen in cross section. The black pigment is hemozoin formed as a waste product from digestion of the host's hemoglobin

when definitive eggs are not seen. Foreign bodies and large calcified bodies may occasionally resemble eggs, requiring careful clinical and histopathologic correlation. *Schistosoma* is the primary worm to deposit eggs in the large bowel; however, rarely eggs from other helminths may become embedded in the bowel wall, such as those of *Enterobius vermicularis* and *Ascaris lumbricoides*. In these cases, the size and morphologic features of the eggs can be used easily to provide a definitive identification. When the egg morphology is not clear, a series of ova and parasite (O&P) exams can be performed [57]. The O&P exam is also the preferred method for identifying the causative *Schistosoma* species in cases of intestinal schistosomiasis, although this is not required for treatment [49].

References

1. World Health Organization. Diarrhoea. World Health Organization, Geneva, Switzerland. 2018. http://www.who.int/topics/diarrhoea/en/. 29 July 2018.
2. Scallan E, Griffin PM, Angulo FJ, Tauxe RV, Hoekstra RM. Foodborne illness acquired in the United States—unspecified agents. Emerg Infect Dis. 2011;17(1):16–22. https://doi.org/10.3201/eid1701.091101p2.
3. Scallan E, Hoekstra RM, Angulo FJ, Tauxe RV, Widdowson MA, Roy SL, et al. Foodborne illness acquired in the United States—major pathogens. Emerg Infect Dis. 2011;17(1):7–15. https://doi.org/10.3201/eid1701.P11101.
4. Shane AL, Mody RK, Crump JA, Tarr PI, Steiner TS, Kotloff K, et al. 2017 infectious diseases society of America clinical practice guidelines for the diagnosis and management of infectious diarrhea. Clin Infect Dis. 2017;65(12):e45–80. https://doi.org/10.1093/cid/cix669.
5. Centers for Disease Control and Prevention. Estimates of foodborne illness in the United States. Centers for Disease Control and Prevention, Atlanta, GA. 2016. https://www.cdc.gov/foodborneburden/index.html. 29 July 2018.
6. Centers for Disease Control and Prevention. Healthy water. Centers for Disease Control and Prevention, Atlanta, GA. 2016. https://www.cdc.gov/healthywater/. 29 July 2018.
7. World Health Organization. Neglected tropical diseases. World Health Organization, Geneva, Switzerland. 2018. http://www.who.int/neglected_diseases/en/. 29 July 2018.
8. Riddle MS, DuPont HL, Connor BA. ACG clinical guideline: diagnosis, treatment, and prevention of acute diarrheal infections in adults. Am J Gastroenterol. 2016;111(5):602–22. https://doi.org/10.1038/ajg.2016.126.
9. Ramanan P, Bryson AL, Binnicker MJ, Pritt BS, Patel R. Syndromic panel-based testing in clinical microbiology. Clin Microbiol Rev. 2018;31(1) https://doi.org/10.1128/CMR.00024–17.
10. DuPont HL. Acute infectious diarrhea in immunocompetent adults. N Engl J Med. 2014;370(16):1532–40. https://doi.org/10.1056/NEJMra1301069.
11. Lauwers GY, Mino-Kenudson M, Kradin RL. Infections of the gastrointestinal tract. In: Kradin RL, editor. Diagnostic pathology of infectious disease. 2nd ed. Atlanta, GA: Elsevier; 2018. p. 232–71.
12. Lamps LW. Bacterial gastrointestinal infections. In: Procop GW, Pritt BS, editors. Pathology of infectious diseases. Atlanta, GA: Elsevier; 2015. p. 297–325.
13. Lamps LW. Update on infectious enterocolitides and the diseases that they mimic. Histopathology. 2015;66(1):3–14. https://doi.org/10.1111/his.12582.
14. Lamps LW. Infectious diseases of the colon. In: Iacobuzio-Donahue CA, Montgomery EA, editors. Gastrointestinal and liver pathology. 2nd ed. Atlanta, GA: Elsevier; 2012. p. 297–351.
15. Cerilli LA, Greenson JK. The differential diagnosis of colitis in endoscopic biopsy specimens: a review article. Arch Pathol Lab Med. 2012;136(8):854–64. https://doi.org/10.5858/arpa.2012–0205-RA.
16. Centers for Disease Control and Prevention. The pretravel consultation, self-treatable conditions: travelers' diarrhea. Centers for Disease Control and Prevention, Atlanta, GA. 2017. https://wwwnc.cdc.gov/travel/yellowbook/2018/the-pre-travel-consultation/travelers-diarrhea. 31 July 2018.
17. Leffler DA, Lamont JT. Clostridium difficile Infection. N Engl J Med. 2015;373(3):287–8. https://doi.org/10.1056/NEJMc1506004.
18. Centers for Disease Control and Prevention. AIDSinfo: guidelines for prevention and treatment of opportunistic infections in HIV-infected adults and adolescents. Centers for Disease Control and Prevention, Atlanta, GA. 2018. https://aidsinfo.nih.gov/contentfiles/lvguidelines/adult_oi.pdf. 12 Aug 2018.

19. Jessurun J. The differential diagnosis of acute colitis: clues to a specific diagnosis. Surg Pathol Clin. 2017;10(4):863–85. https://doi.org/10.1016/j.path.2017.07.008.
20. Patil DT, Odze RD. Biopsy diagnosis of colitis: an algorithmic approach. Virchows Arch. 2018;472(1):67–80. https://doi.org/10.1007/s00428-017-2274-0.
21. Esteve M, Salas A, Fernandez-Banares F, Lloreta J, Marine M, Gonzalez CI, et al. Intestinal spirochetosis and chronic watery diarrhea: clinical and histological response to treatment and long-term follow up. J Gastroenterol Hepatol. 2006;21(8):1326–33. https://doi.org/10.1111/j.1440-1746.2006.04150.x.
22. Nostrant TT, Kumar NB, Appelman HD. Histopathology differentiates acute self-limited colitis from ulcerative colitis. Gastroenterology. 1987;92:318–28.
23. Kumar NB, Nostrant TT, Appelman HD. The histopathologic spectrum of acute self-limited colitis (acute infectious-type colitis). Am J Surg Pathol. 1982;6(6):523–9.
24. Pritt BS, Mathison BA, Milner DA, Procop GW, Schuetz AN. Introduction to infectious diseases pathology. In: Pritt BS, editor. Atlas of fundamental infectious diseases histopathology: a guide for daily practice. Chicago, IL: College of American Pathologists Press; 2018. p. 1–18.
25. Tang DM, Urrunaga NH, Von Rosenvinge EC. Pseudomembranous colitis: not always *Clostridium difficile*. Cleve Clin J Med. 2016;83(5):361–6.
26. Janda JM, Abbott SL. The genus *Aeromonas*: taxonomy, pathogenicity, and infection. Clin Microbiol Rev. 2010;23(1):35–73.
27. Centers for Disease Control and Prevention. Campylobacter (campylobacteriosis). Centers for Disease Control and Prevention, Atlanta, GA. 2017. https://www.cdc.gov/campylobacter/index.html. 2 Sept 2018.
28. Centers for Disease Control and Prevention. 2018 national notifiable infectious diseases. Centers for Disease Control and Prevention, Atlanta, GA. 2018. https://wwwn.cdc.gov/nndss/conditions/notifiable/2018/infectious-diseases/. 13 Aug 2018.
29. Centers for Disease Control and Prevention. *E. coli* (*Escherichia coli*). Centers for Disease Control and Prevention, Atlanta, GA. 2018. https://www.cdc.gov/ecoli/index.html. 3 Sept 2018.
30. Buchan BW, Faron ML, Humphries RM, Dekker J, Ledeboer NA. Escherichia, shigella, and salmonella. In: Carroll KC, Pfaller MA, Landry ML, AJ MA, Patel R, Richter SS, et al., editors. Manual of clinical microbiology. Washington, DC: ASM Press; 2019. p. In Press.
31. Centers for Disease Control and Prevention. Infectious diseases related to travel: typhoid & paratyphoid fever. In: Yellow Book. Centers for Disease Control and Prevention, Atlanta, GA. 2017. https://wwwnc.cdc.gov/travel/yellowbook/2018/infectious-diseases-related-to-travel/typhoid-paratyphoid-fever. 31 July 2018.
32. Centers for Disease Control and Prevention. Salmonella. Centers for Disease Control and Prevention, Atlanta, GA. 2018. https://www.cdc.gov/salmonella/index.html. 30 July 2018.
33. Centers for Disease Control and Prevention. *Shigella*—Shigellosis. Centers for Disease Control and Prevention, Atlanta, GA. 2018. https://www.cdc.gov/shigella/index.html. 2 Sept 2018.
34. Centers for Disease Control and Prevention. *Yersinia enterocolitica* (Yersiniosis). Centers for Disease Control and Prevention, Atlanta, GA. 2016. https://www.cdc.gov/yersinia/index.html. 3 Sept 2018.
35. Schuetz AN, Pritt BS. Bacterial infections. In: Pritt BS, editor. Atlas of fundamental infectious diseases histopathology: a guide for daily practice. Chicago, IL: College of American Pathologists Press; 2018. p. 19–90.
36. Centers for Disease Control and Prevention. Healthcare-associated infections. Centers for Disease Control and Prevention, Atlanta, GA. 2015. https://www.cdc.gov/hai/organisms/cdiff/cdiff_clinicians.html. 3 Sept 2018.
37. Guarner J, Brandt ME. Histopathologic diagnosis of fungal infections in the 21st century. Clin Microbiol Rev. 2011;24(2):247–80. https://doi.org/10.1128/CMR.00053-10.
38. Procop GW, Pritt BS. Fungal infections. In: Pritt BS, editor. Atlas of fundamental infectious diseases histopathology: a guide for daily practice. Chicago, IL: College of American Pathologists Press; 2018. p. 91–148.
39. Centers for Disease Control and Prevention. Fungal diseases. Centers for Disease Control and Prevention, Atlanta, GA. 2018. https://www.cdc.gov/fungal/diseases/mucormycosis/index.html. 8 Sept 2018.
40. Eggimann P, Chevrolet JC, Starobinski M, Majno P, Totsch M, Chapuis B, et al. Primary invasive aspergillosis of the digestive tract: report of two cases and review of the literature. Infection. 2006;34(6):333–8. https://doi.org/10.1007/s15010-006-5660-0.
41. Geramizadeh B, Heidari M, Shekarkhar G. Gastrointestinal basidiobolomycosis, a rare and under-diagnosed fungal infection in immunocompetent hosts: a review article. Iran J Med Sci. 2015;40(2):90–7.
42. Melato M, Gorji N. Primary intestinal cryptococcosis mimicking adenomatous polyp in an HIV-negative patient. Am J Gastroenterol. 1998;93(9):1592–3. https://doi.org/10.1111/j.1572-0241.1998.00492.x.
43. Perfect JR, Dismukes WE, Dromer F, Goldman DL, Graybill JR, Hamill RJ, et al. Clinical practice guidelines for the management of cryptococcal disease: 2010 update by the infectious diseases society of america. Clin Infect Dis. 2010;50(3):291–322. https://doi.org/10.1086/649858.
44. Yang B, Lu L, Li D, Liu L, Huang L, Chen L, et al. Colonic involvement in disseminated histoplasmosis of an immunocompetent adult: case report and literature review. BMC Infect Dis. 2013;13:143. https://doi.org/10.1186/1471-2334-13-143.
45. Milner DA, Pritt BS. Viral infections. In: Pritt BS, editor. Atlas of fundamental infectious diseases histopathology: a guide for daily practice. Chicago, IL: College of American Pathologists Press; 2018. p. 149–92.
46. Baniak N, Kanthan R. Cytomegalovirus colitis: an uncommon mimicker of common colitides. Arch Pathol Lab Med. 2016;140(8):854–8. https://doi.org/10.5858/arpa.2015-0176-RS.
47. Dikman AE, Schonfeld E, Srisarajivakul NC, Poles MA. Human immunodeficiency virus-associated diarrhea: still an issue in the era of antiretroviral therapy. Dig Dis Sci. 2015;60(8):2236–45. https://doi.org/10.1007/s10620-015-3615-y.
48. Mathison BA, Pritt BS. Parasitic infections. In: Pritt BS, editor. Atlas of fundamental infectious diseases histopathology: a guide for daily practice. Chicago, IL: College of American Pathologists Press; 2018. p. 193–288.
49. Centers for Disease Control and Prevention. DPDx—Laboratory Identification of Parasites of Public Health Concern. Centers for Disease Control and Prevention, Atlanta, GA. 2018. https://www.cdc.gov/dpdx/index.html. 1 Sept 2018.
50. Orihel TC, Ash LR. Parasites in human tissues. American Society for Clinical Pathology: Chicago, IL; 1995.
51. Meyers WM, Firpo A, Wear DJ. Topics on the pathology of protozoan and invasive arthropod diseases. Armed Forces Institute of Pathology: Washington, DC; 2011.
52. Meyers WM, Neafie RC, Marty AM, Wear DJ. Pathology of infectious diseases. Armed Forces Institute of Pathology: Washington, DC; 2000.

53. Garcia LS, Arrowood M, Kokoskin E, Paltridge GP, Pillai DR, Procop GW, et al. Laboratory diagnosis of parasites from the gastrointestinal tract. Clin Microbiol Rev. 2017;31(1): e00025–17.
54. Klassen-Fischer MK, Wear DJ, Neafie RC. Amebiasis. In: Meyers WM, Firpo A, Wear DJ, editors. Topics on the pathology of protozoan and invasive arthropod diseases. Washington, DC: Armed Forces Institute of Pathology; 2011. p. 1–15.
55. Neafie RC, Andersen EM, Klassen-Fischer MK. Balantidiasis. In: Meyers WM, Firpo A, Wear DJ, editors. Topics on the pathology of protozoan and invasive arthropod diseases. Washington, DC: Armed Forces Institute of Pathology; 2011. p. 1–15.
56. Marty AM, Neafie RC. Trichuriasis. In: Meyers WM, Neafie RC, Marty AM, Wear DJ, editors. Pathology of infectious diseases. Washington, DC: Armed Forces Institute of Pathology; 2000. p. 461–70.
57. Cheever AW, Neafie RC. Schistosomiasis. In: Meyers WM, Neafie RC, Marty AM, Wear DJ, editors. Pathology of infectious diseases. Washington, DC: Armed Forces Institute of Pathology; 2000. p. 23–48.

18 Drug-Induced Injury, Vascular, Congenital, Motility, Polyps, and Miscellaneous Disorders

Vishal S. Chandan

Drug-Induced Injury

Every year multiple new medications are approved for clinical use, and many of them can cause clinically significant injury to the colon. However, there are certain characteristic injury patterns that should prompt consideration for drug-induced injury to the colon. The intent here is to provide a practical guide for surgical pathologists to recognize the histological features and differential diagnosis of drug-induced injury to the colon. Of note, most drugs cause nonspecific patterns of injury that can show considerable overlap with histological changes caused by other drugs, infections, or autoimmune diseases. The type and severity of these changes also depend on a number of factors such as the dose of the medication, drug interactions, mechanism of action, and the patients' underlying health. Definitive confirmation of a drug as a cause for injury to the colon would ultimately require correlation with the clinical findings and cessation of the suspected drug resulting in resolution of symptoms.

Non-steroidal Anti-inflammatory Drugs (NSAIDs)

NSAIDs are one of the most commonly used medications in the world.

Gastrointestinal tract bleeding is the most common side effect [1]. NSAIDs are also an important cause of mucosal injury to the colon [2]. Risk factors for NSAIDs-related injuries include concurrent steroid use, alcohol, smoking, age over 60 years, and prior NSAIDs-related injury [3, 4]. Erosions and ulcers are commonly seen within the first few months of NSAIDs use, and they most commonly involve the ileocecal region or proximal colon (Fig. 18.1), while strictures usually develop with long-term use [5]. NSAIDs-related injury to the colon may resemble lymphocytic colitis or collagenous colitis, although the degree of intraepithelial lymphocytosis and subepithelial collagen deposition may be patchier and less prominent [6–8]. NSAIDs-related injury to the colon may also show regenerative crypts and lamina propria fibrosis, somewhat resembling ischemic colitis. Other findings include increased eosinophils, pyloric metaplasia, focal cryptitis, pseudomembranous colitis, and increased crypt apoptosis [9, 10]. NSAIDs can also cause diaphragm disease of the colon [11, 12]. NSAIDs have also been reported to cause chronic colitis that can be morphologically indistinguishable from inflammatory bowel disease [13].

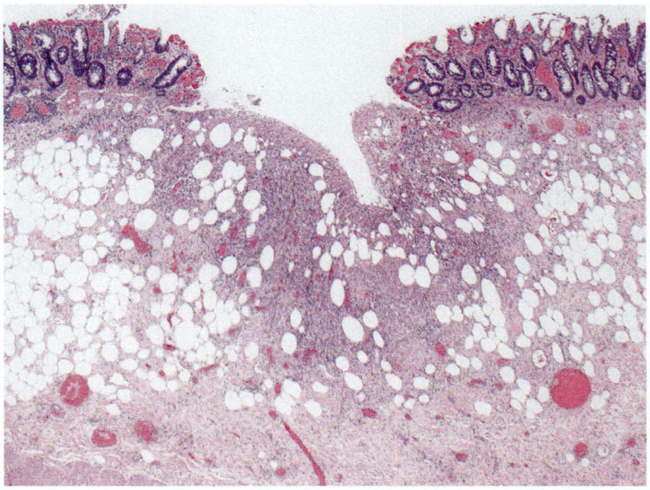

Fig. 18.1 NSAIDs-related colonic injury. Focal ulceration due to chronic NSAIDs use is present in resected colon

Mycophenolate

Mycophenolate is an antiproliferative agent used in solid organ and stem cell transplant patients. It is a well-known

V. S. Chandan (✉)
Department of Pathology, University of California – Irvine, Irvine, CA, USA
e-mail: vchandan@uci.edu

L. Zhang et al. (eds.), *Surgical Pathology of Non-neoplastic Gastrointestinal Diseases*, https://doi.org/10.1007/978-3-030-15573-5_18

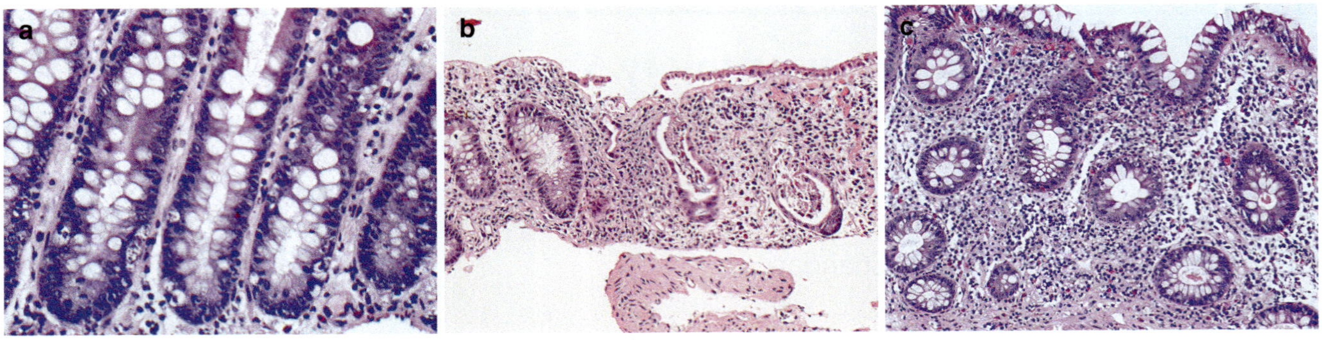

Fig. 18.2 Mycophenolate-induced colonic injury. (**a**) Colonic mucosa shows prominent crypt apoptosis. (**b**) Colonic mucosa shows occasional crypt apoptosis, dilated crypts with attenuated epithelial cells and epithelial necrosis, architectural distortion, and crypt loss resemble acute graft-versus-host disease. (**c**) Focal cryptitis-like pattern

cause of clinically significant gastrointestinal mucosal injury. The presenting symptoms may include diarrhea, vomiting, nausea, dyspepsia, and melena. The histological features within the colon resemble acute graft-versus-host disease and include prominent crypt apoptosis (Fig. 18.2a), dilated crypts lined by attenuated epithelial cells, architectural distortion, crypt loss with lamina propria edema, and increased inflammatory cells (Fig. 18.2b) [14–16]. Histological clues that favor mycophenolate-induced colitis over acute graft-versus-host disease may include increased eosinophils (>15 lamina propria eosinophils per 10 high-power fields), absence of endocrine cell clusters, and lack of apoptotic microabscesses [17]. A subset of patients may also show normal or near normal morphology, inflammatory bowel disease-like changes, ischemia-like, and self-limited colitis-like changes (Fig. 18.2c) [16]. An increased awareness of the histological spectrum of changes associated with mycophenolate within the colon may be useful to avoid diagnostic errors by the pathologist.

Sodium Polystyrene Sulfonate (Kayexalate)

Kayexalate is a cation-exchange resin used in treatment of hyperkalemia. The resin exchanges the potassium present in the colon for its sodium. The Kayexalate itself is now believed to be toxic to the colonic mucosa [18]. Risk factors for Kayexalate injury include renal disease, transplant, and postoperative state. Erosions, pseudomembranes, ulcers, and mucosal to transmural necrosis with perforation can develop within the colon (Fig.18.3a, b) [19–21]. The histology is usually not entirely specific as it can show mucosal ischemic-type changes with erosions, ulcerations, and necrosis. However, the presence of characteristic Kayexalate crystals overlying the necrotic or ulcerated tissue can be diagnostic, if identified on histology. Kayexalate crystals are rhomboid or triangular in shape and deeply basophilic on hematoxylin and eosin (H&E) stain (Figs. 18.3c, d). They also can be highlighted on PAS-D (the crystals are magenta color), Diff-Quik, and acid-fast stains (the crystals are black). They exhibit a distinctive internal mosaic pattern that resembles fish scales. These crystals are refractile but do not polarize. The differential is cholestyramine (a bile acid binding resin) and sevelamer. The crystals of cholestyramine are also basophilic and angulated, but they can be distinguished from Kayexalate by their greater opacity and lack of a mosaic pattern.

Sevelamer

Sevelamer carbonate is an anion exchange resin which is a phosphate binder. It is used in patients with chronic renal failure to treat hyperphosphatemia. It has been associated with colonic mucosal injury, but its exact etiological role remains unclear as it may just be an innocent bystander [22]. Patients may present with hematochezia [23]. Associated mucosal findings can include crypt distortion, Paneth cell metaplasia, cryptitis, mucosal prolapse type changes, and inflammatory polyp (Fig. 18.4a) [22]. Rare cases of sevelamer-induced colitis presenting as a pseudotumor and sigmoid colon diverticula perforation associated with sevelamer have also been reported [24, 25]. On the H&E stain, the crystals of sevelamer appear broad, curved, and irregularly spaced. Like Kayexalate, they also show fish scale pattern. However, they also show a characteristic two-toned color imparted by bright pink linear accentuations with a rusty yellow background (Fig. 18.4b). However, some crystals embedded in an area of ulcer, necrosis, or ischemia may acquire a deep eosinophilic or rusty brown color. On the PAS-D stain, the sevelamer crystals acquire a violet color. These crystals are exclusively identified in patients with chronic kidney disease and this is an important clue toward their diagnosis.

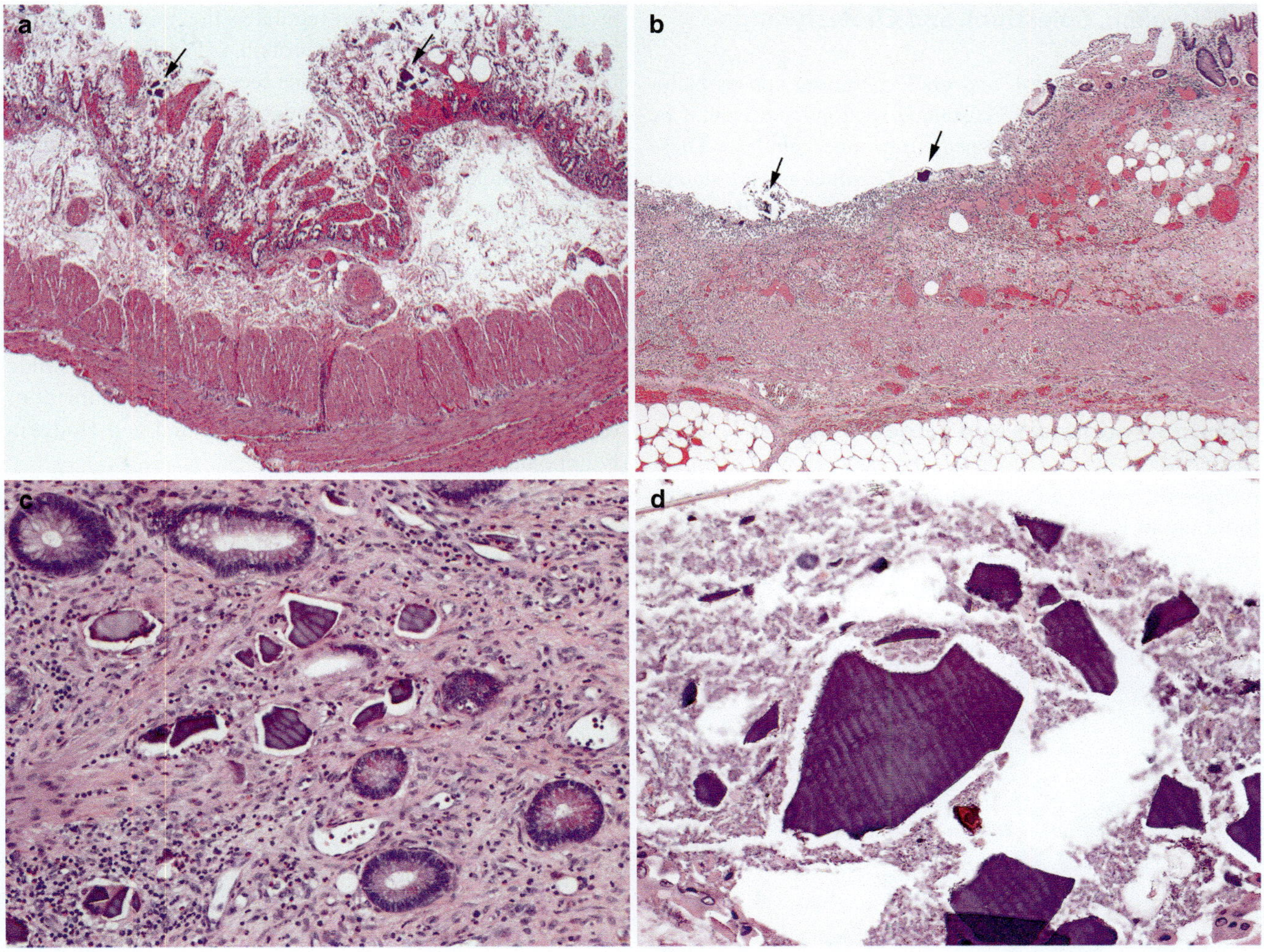

Fig. 18.3 Kayexalate-induced ischemic injury. (**a**) Early ischemic-type injury with epithelial necrosis, hemorrhage, and luminal Kayexalate crystals (arrows) is present in resected colon. (**b**) Colonic ulceration with transmural necrosis and luminal adherent with Kayexalate crystals (arrows) is present in another resected colon. (**c**) Kayexalate crystals are embedded within the lamina propria in colonic mucosa adjacent to ulceration. (**d**) High-power view of Kayexalate crystals show rhomboid or triangular in shape and deeply basophilic with characteristic fish scale appearance on H&E stain

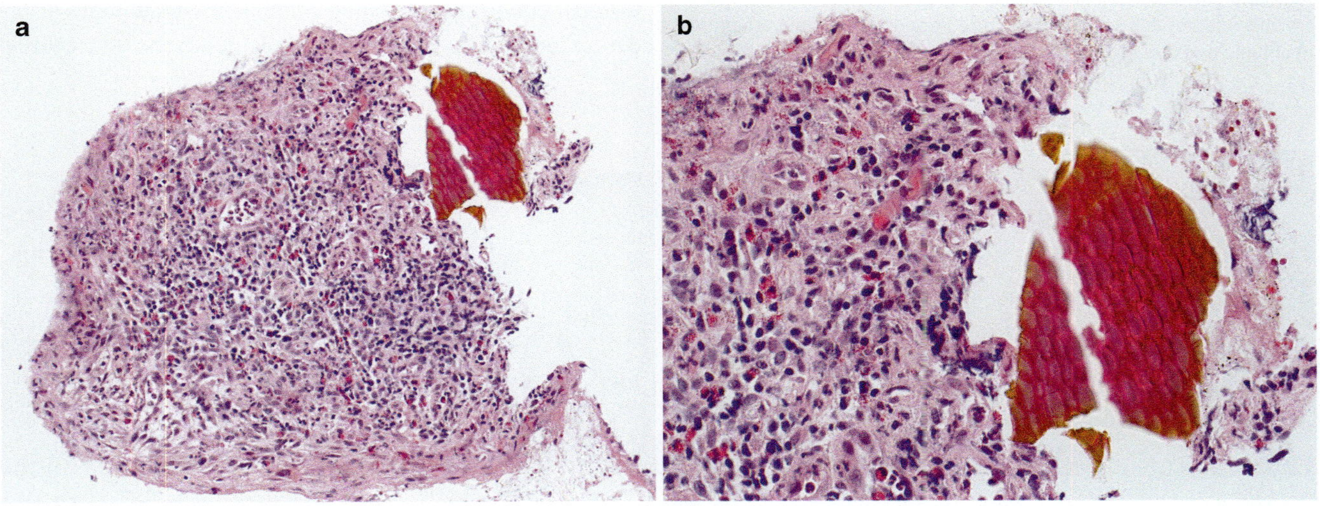

Fig. 18.4 Sevelamer carbonate. (**a**) Sevelamer crystal is present in a biopsy from colonic ulcer. (**b**) High-power view of Sevelamer crystal show fish scale appearance and a characteristic two-toned color imparted by bright pink linear accentuations with a rusty yellow background

Colesevelam, Colestipol, and Cholestyramine

Colesevelam, colestipol, and cholestyramine appear histologically identical on H&E-stained sections and cannot be morphologically distinguished from one another. These crystals lack the internal fish scale-like ridges and are stained dark brown, magenta, or orange depending on the tissue thickness and staining conditions (Fig. 18.5) [26]. They are believed to be innocent bystanders that probably lack the ability to cause significant direct mucosal injury to the gastrointestinal tract [26].

Immunomodulators and Targeted Agents

Immunotherapy is an emerging entity in cancer treatment. Ipilimumab is a monoclonal antibody that works to activate the immune system by targeting cytotoxic T-lymphocyte-associated antigen-4-blocking (CTLA-4), a protein receptor that downregulates the immune system [27]. Programmed cell death protein 1 (PD-1 or CD279) is found on T cells as a cell surface receptor and functions as an immune checkpoint to prevent cytotoxic T cell activation by self-antigens [28]. Some tumors show high levels of its ligand (PD-L1), blunting the immune response against them [29]. PD-1 and PDL-1 inhibitors (such as pembrolizumab, nivolumab, and atezolizumab) have proved successful in prolonging survival for patients with metastatic melanoma, lung carcinoma, renal cell carcinoma, mismatch repair-deficient colorectal carcinoma, and urothelial carcinoma. Idelalisib (a phosphoinositide 3-kinase inhibitor) was recently approved for treatment of relapsed chronic lymphocytic leukemia and non-Hodgkin lymphoma.

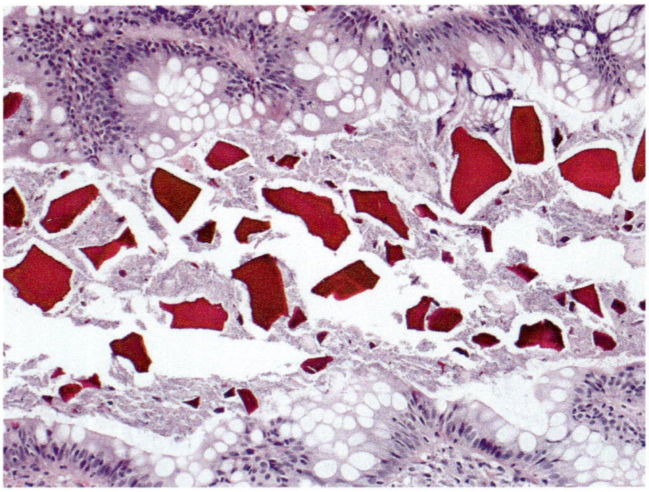

Fig. 18.5 Cholestyramine crystals. Multiple magenta-colored luminal crystals without fish scale-like fracture lines on H&E stain are present in colonic mucosal biopsy

Diarrhea is usually the most common adverse event. Endoscopy examination may show exudates, granularity, loss of vascularity, and ulcerations [30]. Rarely may patients also develop colonic perforation as a fatal complication [31]. All immunomodulators produce fairly similar histological changes within the colonic mucosa, consisting of increased crypt apoptosis with neutrophilic inflammation (Fig. 18.6a) and intraepithelial lymphocytosis (Fig. 18.6b) [32, 33]. Patients receiving these drugs for longer periods may develop architectural distortion, increased chronic inflammation, and basal plasmacytosis, resembling inflammatory bowel disease-type changes (Fig. 18.6c) [32, 34–36]. Awareness of these histological features is important to distinguish them from potential mimickers, such as graft-versus-host disease, autoimmune enteropathy, cytomegalovirus/infectious colitis, and inflammatory bowel disease.

Colchicine

Colchicine is an alkaloid used for treatment of gout and other medical conditions including immune/rheumatologic disorders. Common side effects of colchicine include nausea,

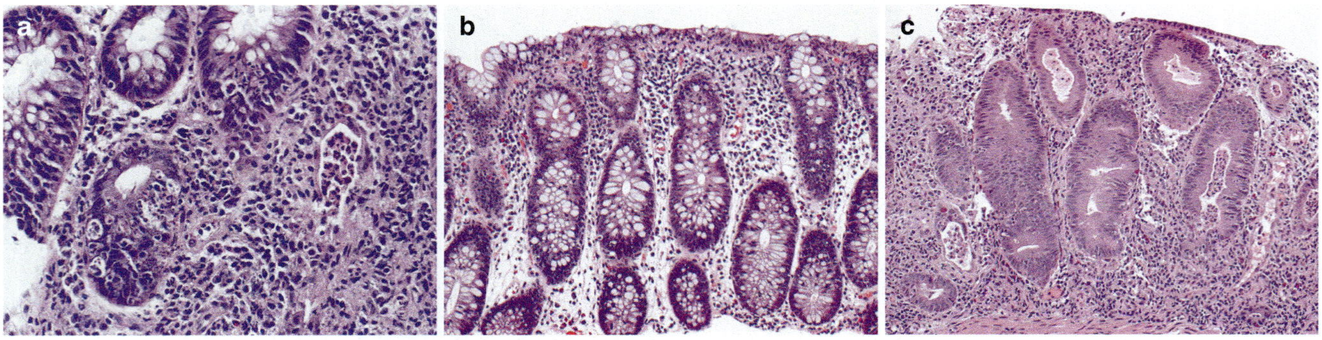

Fig. 18.6 PDL-1 inhibitor-induced colonic injury. (**a**) GVHD-like pattern with increased crypt apoptosis with neutrophilic inflammation and focal crypt dropout. (**b**) Lymphocytic colitis-like pattern with intraepithelial lymphocytosis. (**c**) Inflammatory bowel disease-like pattern with cryptitis, crypt abscess, increased chronic inflammation, and basal plasmacytosis

vomiting, diarrhea, and abdominal pain. The most noticeable feature of colchicine toxicity is mitotic arrest in metaphase with absent mitotic spindles and bizarre chromatin patterns, especially ring mitosis [37]. The morphological features also include metaphase mitoses (ring mitosis) and loss of epithelial polarity (Fig. 18.7). These histological changes are usually not seen in patients taking colchicine without clinical evidence of toxicity. Hence when these changes are identified by the pathologist, it is important to reconcile with the patient's medication list, since if colchicine is the offending agent, then the patient is probably toxic. Of note, even therapeutic doses of colchicine may rarely cause ring mitosis, especially in colorectal polyps [38]. The histological findings of colchicine toxicity regress on cessation of the drug.

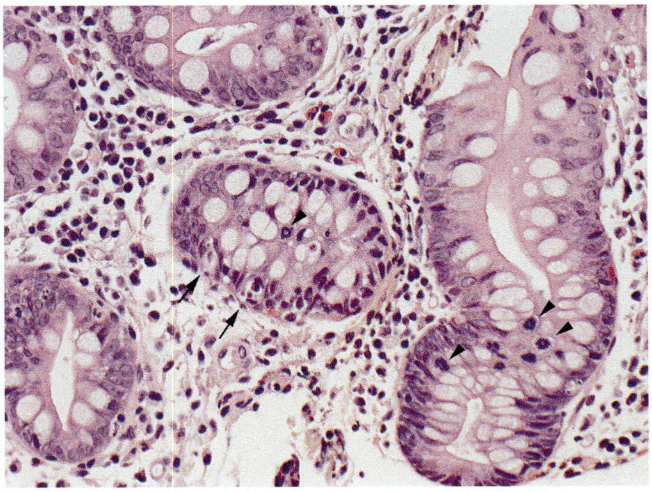

Fig. 18.7 Colchicine toxicity. Colonic mucosa shows numerous ring mitosis (arrowheads), increased crypt apoptosis (arrows), and reactive epithelial change

Pancreatic Enzyme Supplements (Fibrosing Colonopathy)

This is a distinct entity first described in the 1990s in patients with cystic fibrosis who developed colonic strictures while they were taking high-dose pancreatic enzymes [39–42]. It is most commonly seen in children between the ages of 1 and 15 years. Occasional cases have also been described in adults even in the absence of pancreatic enzyme supplementation [43, 44]. Almost all patients have a history of high-dose pancreatic enzyme therapy for 1–2 years before the clinical diagnosis. The presenting symptoms are abdominal pain, nausea, and vomiting. However, some patients may also develop diarrhea, ascites, and weight loss. The pathogenesis of this entity is poorly understood. However, it is postulated that the entrapped enzyme pellets impacted within the thick fecal material cause pressure necrosis of the mucosa. Direct toxicity of the pancreatic enzymes to the epithelium may also play a role.

It commonly affects the right and transverse colon (Fig. 18.8a) [39]. The sigmoid colon and rectum are usually spared. However, there have been rare cases involving the entire colon [45, 46]. The mucosal surface shows cobblestoning and patchy erosions (Fig. 18.8b). Segmental thickening of the colonic wall is often a characteristic finding of this entity. On histology, the mucosa shows patchy cryptitis and crypt abscesses with architectural distortion. The lamina propria and submucosa show dense fibrosis (Fig. 18.8c, d). The submucosa often shows keloid-like bands of collagen (Fig. 18.8e). In some cases, the fibrosis may extend to involve the muscularis propria. Most cases also show a prominent infiltrate composed of eosinophils and mast cells involving the entire bowel wall. The eosinophils can range from 25 to 160 per high-power field.

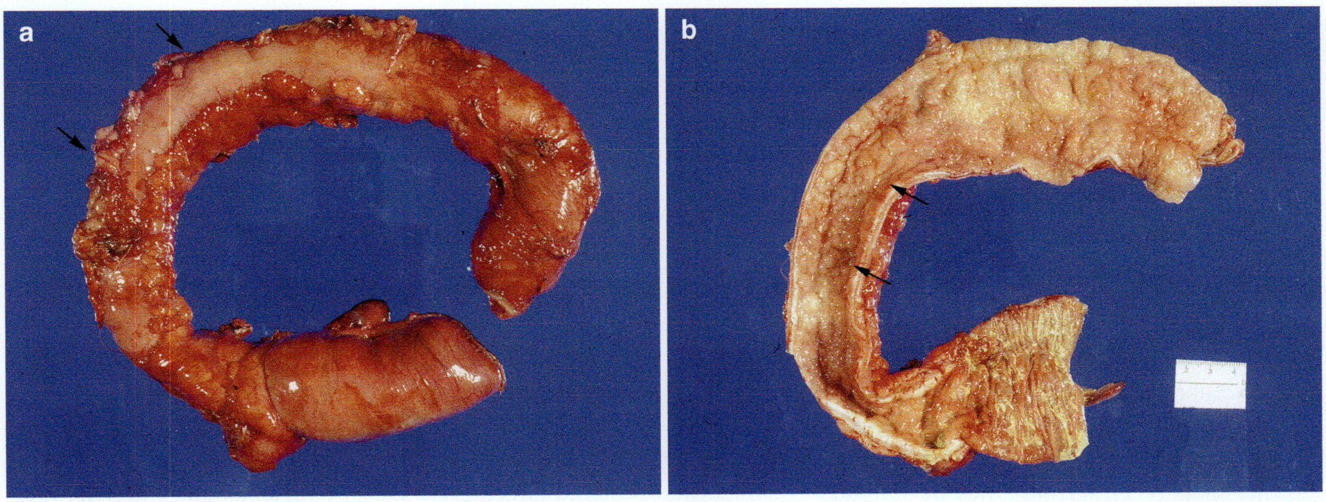

Fig. 18.8 Fibrosing colonopathy. (**a**) The resected colon from a cystic fibrosis patient shows segmental thickening of the colonic wall with strictures (arrows). (**b**) The mucosal surface shows cobblestoning (arrows) and erosions within the segment with stricture. (**c**) Histological section from the strictured segment shows thickened submucosa with dense fibrosis. (**d**) Trichrome stain shows prominent submucosal fibrosis. (**e**) The submucosa shows keloid-like bands of collagen

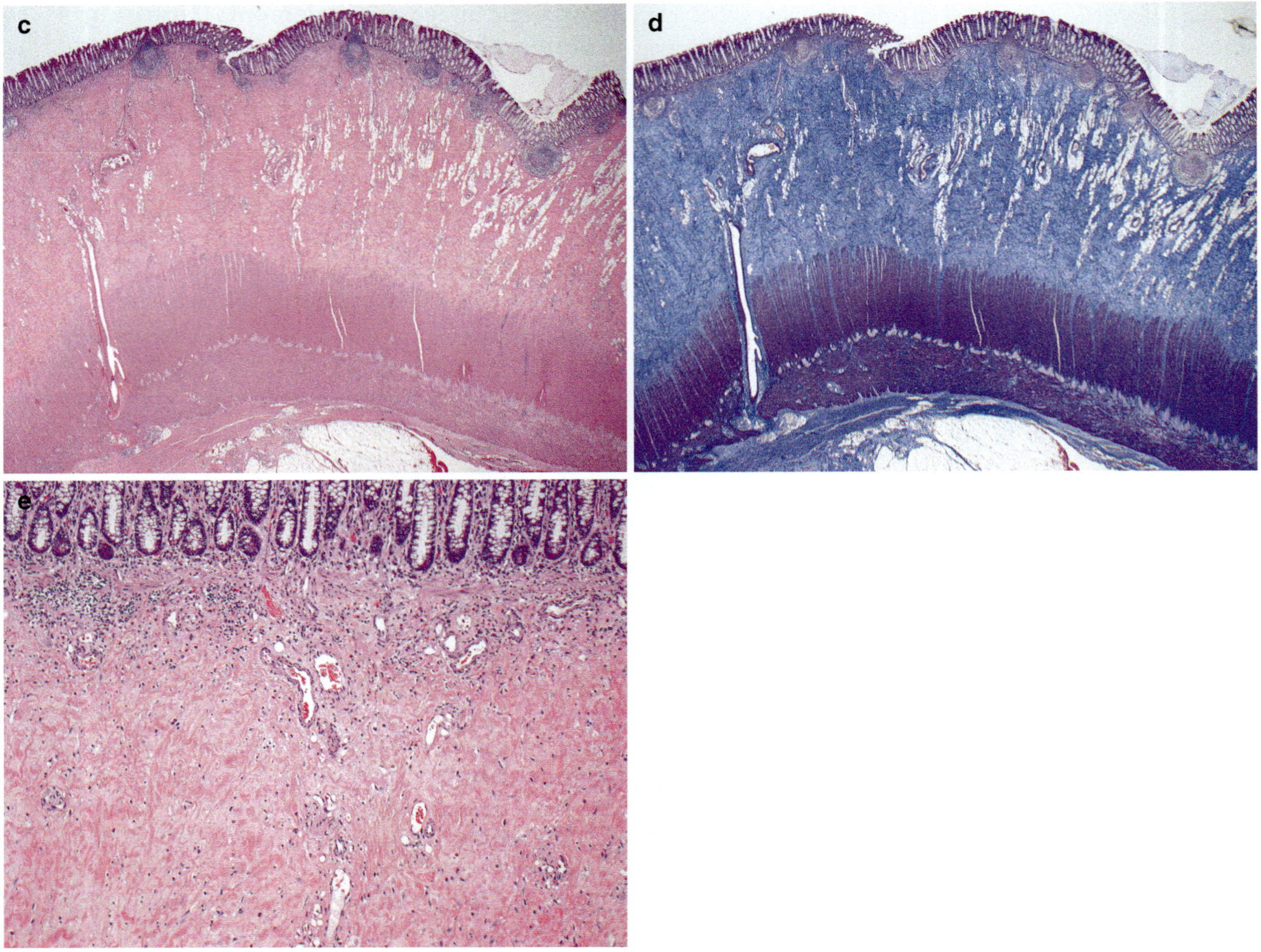

Fig. 18.8 (continued)

Due to the presence of strictures and involvement of the right colon, Crohn's disease is in the differential. However, the presence of prominent fibrosis involving the lamina propria and submucosa as well as absence of transmural inflammation and granulomas is usually helpful in differentiating fibrosing colonopathy from Crohn's disease. Due to the presence of fibrosis, scleroderma also comes within the differential. However, scleroderma typically shows degenerative changes within the muscle fibers, thickened blood vessels, and serosal fibrosis. Amyloidosis may also come into the differential and the use of Congo red stain should be helpful. Advanced stages of hollow visceral myopathy can show extensive fibrous replacement of the muscularis propria and can morphologically resemble fibrosing colonopathy. The patient's history of cystic fibrosis and high-dose pancreatic enzyme therapy is the only way to definitely distinguish between both these disorders. Fibrosing colonopathy is usually treated by surgical resection of the involved bowel segment.

Oral Contraceptive

The use of oral contraceptive pills has been associated with increased risk of thrombosis and subsequent ischemia of the small bowel and colon [47–49]. Hence, a diagnosis of ischemic colitis in a young female should always raise a consideration for drug as a potential etiology, particularly oral contraceptive agents. Sometimes the ischemic changes become reversible after conservative management and discontinuation of the oral contraceptive agents [47].

Clofazimine

Clofazimine is a drug used to treat leprosy and other mycobacterial infections. Patients with clofazimine toxicity present with abdominal pain, bowel obstruction, perforation, and abdominal lymphadenopathy. Histologically they show intra-abdominal accumulations of crystallized drug within histiocytes of the abdominal lymph nodes and bowel wall [50]. Lewis et al.[51] have also reported crystal-storing histiocytosis due to massive accumulation of Charcot-Leyden crystals presenting as numerous colonic polyps in an elderly woman with eosinophilic colitis who was on clofazimine.

Antimicrobial Drugs and Antibiotics

Antibiotic-associated colitis has been considered to be synonymous with pseudomembranous colitis due to *C. difficile*. It has been associated with drugs such as penicillin, clindamycin, trimethoprim sulfamethoxazole, and cephalosporin [52]. Proton pump inhibitors have also been associated with community-acquired *C. difficile* colitis [53].

Enemas, Laxatives, and Oral Bowel Preparation Agents

Sodium phosphate bowel preparation solutions have been associated with focal active colitis, aphthous ulcers, and mildly increased crypt apoptosis (see also Chap. 2, section "Bowel Preparation Effect" and Fig. 2.13) [54]. Anthraquinones and other laxatives induce apoptosis within the colonic epithelium, resulting in melanosis coli. However, most patients with melanosis coli are diagnosed incidentally when undergoing endoscopy for other reasons. The pigment in melanosis coli is ceroid and contains melanin and glycoconjugates, derived from processing of apoptotic epithelial cells into lipofuscin and anthranoids [55].

Heavy Metals

Gold salt therapy is the most common cause of heavy metal-induced enterocolitis [56]. Majority of patients with gold salt toxicity are women with rheumatoid arthritis. The presence of HLA DRB10404 allele increases the risk of gold-induced enterocolitis [57]. The injury results from either direct mucosal toxicity or an immune-mediated hypersensitivity reaction. Gold salts may also increase the risk of cytomegalovirus infection. The symptoms of gold-induced enterocolitis usually start within a few weeks of starting the treatment. The patients present with nausea, vomiting, diarrhea, fever, proteinuria, and hypogammaglobulinemia. Rarely, they may also experience perforation, megacolon, and death [58, 59]. The colon may show hemorrhage, edema, and mural thickening [58, 59]. Usually segmental colitis is seen with erosions, ulcerations, and diffuse acute and chronic inflammation. There may also be a prominent eosinophilic infiltrate. Some features may simulate inflammatory bowel disease, although the glandular architecture is more or less preserved. Rare cases may also show pseudomembrane formation [60].

Chemotherapy

Many chemotherapeutic agents cause gastrointestinal side effects such as nausea and diarrhea. Paclitaxel has been associated with colonic perforation [61]. Chemotherapeutic agents can also cause ischemia, pseudomembranous colitis, and the development of opportunistic infections such as candida, herpes, and cytomegalovirus. Methotrexate can rarely cause toxic megacolon and malabsorption [62]. 5-FU has been associated with loss of nuclear polarity, increased apoptosis, nuclear pyknosis, and karyorrhexis within the colonic mucosa resulting in mucosal necrosis and erosion [63, 64].

Neutropenic enterocolitis is a syndrome associated with chemotherapeutic drugs where the colon exhibits severe necrotizing colitis with marked edema, vasculitis, and hemorrhage with epithelial necrosis in the setting of neutropenia (see also Chap. 14, section "Neutropenic Enterocolitis" and Fig. 14.28) [65–68]. Typically, neutropenic colitis begins 7–10 days after initiation of chemotherapy. The patients present with fever, abdominal pain, nausea, vomiting, and diarrhea. The mucosa becomes ulcerated (Fig. 18.9a, b) and a pseudomembrane composed of fibrin and necrotic cellular debris may also develop (Fig. 18.9c). Prominent crypt apoptosis, focal crypt dropout, and glandular

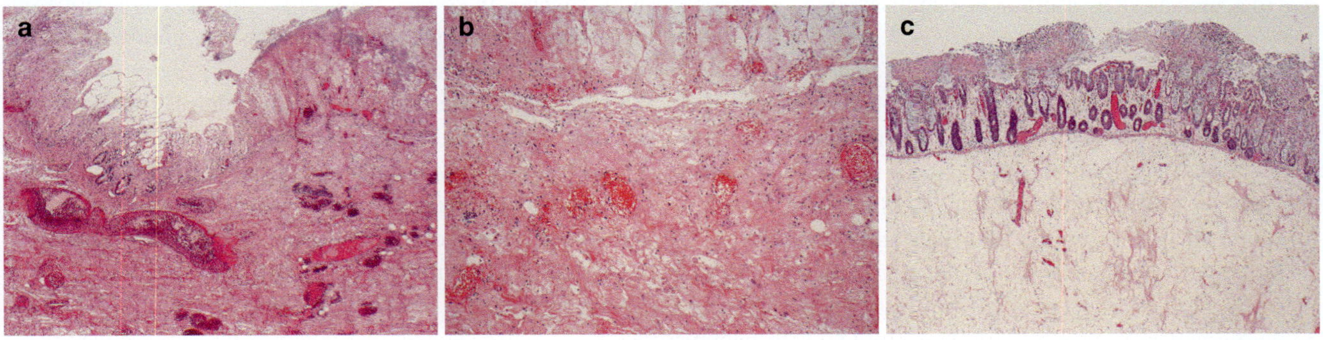

Fig. 18.9 Neutropenic colitis. (**a**) Mucosal hemorrhage and necrosis is present in the resected colon in a patient with leukemia and treated with chemotherapy. (**b**) Higher-power view from the necrotic areas shows striking paucity of acute inflammatory cells including neutrophils. (**c**) Pseudomembrane formation composed of fibrin and necrotic cellular debris but no significant neutrophilic infiltrates and prominent submucosal edema in another resected colon with neutropenic colitis

regeneration are also often seen. Despite the degree of mucosal damage, there is striking paucity of acute inflammatory cells including neutrophils (Fig. 18.9b). It is the absence of neutrophils in the presence of significant cell injury that allows a diagnosis of neutropenic enterocolitis to be made on histology.

Chemical Colitis (Glutaraldehyde)

Chemical disinfectants such as glutaraldehyde which are used to clean endoscopy instruments can also be toxic to the colonic mucosa. They can be retained in the endoscope due to inadequate flushing after disinfection [69–71]. The patient usually experiences abdominal pain and bloody diarrhea within a few hours to a couple of days after the endoscopy [72]. The colon may show edema, erosions, ulceration, or mucosal necrosis. The histology resembles ischemic colitis or injury due to toxin-producing bacteria. Mucin depletion and increased eosinophils may also be seen.

Ischemia and Other Vascular Disorders

The term ischemia is generic and it includes a number of conditions that cause decreased blood flow and oxygen supply to the colon with or without concomitant increase in demand for oxygen. The diagnosis of ischemic injury to the colon should be made after appropriate correlation with the clinical, endoscopic, and radiological findings. The pathologist should make an attempt to identify a possible etiology as this could help in treatment of the underlying cause. Ischemic colitis is the most common form of ischemic injury of the gastrointestinal tract with an annual incidence of 15–17 per 100,000 [73–75]. It accounts for 1 of every 2000 hospital admissions [76].

Acute Ischemic Colitis

Definition

Acute ischemic colitis is characterized by injury to the colon due to acute vascular insufficiency and ischemia.

Clinical Features

Patients with cardiac disease and older than 60 years are at significant risk for ischemic colitis. It is more commonly seen in females, although males may present at significantly younger age compared to females [77, 78]. Patients typically present with abdominal pain, diarrhea, and hematochezia.

A number of conditions can cause ischemic colitis and they can be basically classified into two main categories: occlusive and nonocclusive causes (Table18.1). In patients with atherosclerotic vascular disease, thromboembolism is the most common cause of acute ischemic colitis. Irrespective of the initial etiological event, the compromise of the mesenteric blood flow induces a varying degree of ischemic injury to the colon. The severity of the ischemia determines the extent and viability of the colon and its treatment options as well as the final prognosis.

Table 18.1 Predisposing conditions and causes for ischemic colitis

Occlusive causes	Nonocclusive causes
Arterial	*Hypoperfusion*
Thrombosis or embolization of mesenteric arteries	Heart failure
Vasculitis	*Shock*
Polyarteritis nodosa	Anaphylaxis
Churg-Strauss	Hemodialysis
Henoch-Schonlein purpura	Pancreatitis
Wegener's granulomatosis	*Drugs*
Kawasaki disease	Antihypertensives
Small vessel disease	Cocaine
Diabetes mellitus	Danazol
Amyloidosis	Digitalis
Radiation	Estrogen
Infections	NSAIDsSimvastatin
Cytomegalovirus	Stimulant laxatives
E. coli O157:H7	Tegaserod
Hypercoagulable states	*Mechanical*
Protein C, S, and Z or factor III deficiency	Adhesions
Anticardiolipin syndrome	Volvulus
Factor V Leiden mutation	Diverticulitis
Iatrogenic/surgical	Strangulated hernia
Cardiopulmonary bypass	Tumors
Aortoiliac reconstruction	*Others*
Colectomy	Long-distance running
Barium enema	
Colonoscopy	
Others	
Trauma	
Portal hypertension	
Lymphocytic phlebitis	

History plays a pivotal role in accurate diagnosis of ischemic colitis, especially if the patient has predisposing factors such as thrombotic disorders, aortic surgery, and dehydration. The accurate and early diagnosis of ischemic colitis needs collaboration of diverse specialties and the utilization of many diagnostic tools [79, 80]. X-rays remain a useful tool, as they can help in ruling out other potential diagnoses such as bowel obstruction. Ultrasound, and in particular color Doppler sonography, is sensitive in detection of early structural changes in colonic wall caused by ischemia. However, colonoscopy has been regarded as the new gold standard for diagnosis of ischemic colitis [79, 81, 82]. Early endoscopic findings include hemorrhagic purple nodules. These may disappear in a couple of days or lead to formation of ulcers. Other findings may include petechiae, edema, easily friable mucosa, and pseudomembranes. In severe cases, the mucosa can appear dusky, cyanotic, or even black. CT with intravenous and oral contrast media is also considered as a test of choice by some for diagnosis of ischemic colitis [73, 83].

Pathological Features

The gross features of ischemic colitis are the same irrespective of the etiology. The splenic flexure and the sigmoid colon are the two most commonly involved areas (the so-called watershed areas) as they are highly prone to ischemic damage. Ischemic injury is usually localized and segmental in nature.

In the early stages, the bowel wall appears pale and edematous with congestion, hemorrhage, and mucosal sloughing (Fig. 18.10). Later the serosa becomes dusky and dark red. The mucosa becomes necrotic and ulcerated and pseudomembranes may also be seen. In advanced stages, transmural necrosis, pneumatosis intestinalis, and perforation may develop. Chronic or recurrent bouts of ischemic injury may lead to fibrosis and strictures. The mesenteric vessels should be examined for presence of thrombi, emboli, or atherosclerosis.

In early stages, histological changes may be patchy in nature. They may show separation and loss of surface epithelium. Lamina propria shows edema, hemorrhage, and dilated vessels (Fig.18.11a). Crypt dropout, mucosal necrosis, and ulceration develop later. The lamina propria would eventually show fibrin deposition (Fig. 18.11b). Acute inflammation in

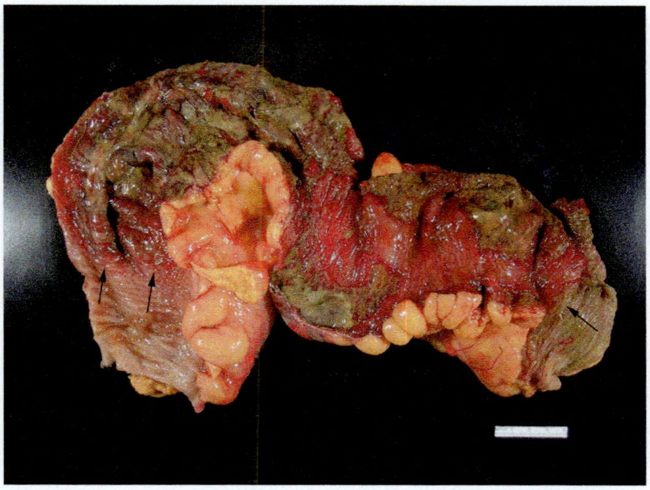

Fig. 18.10 Ischemic colitis. A resected colon shows segmental mucosal congestion, hemorrhage, and mucosal sloughing with well demarcated boundary (arrows), from adjacent nonischemic bowel

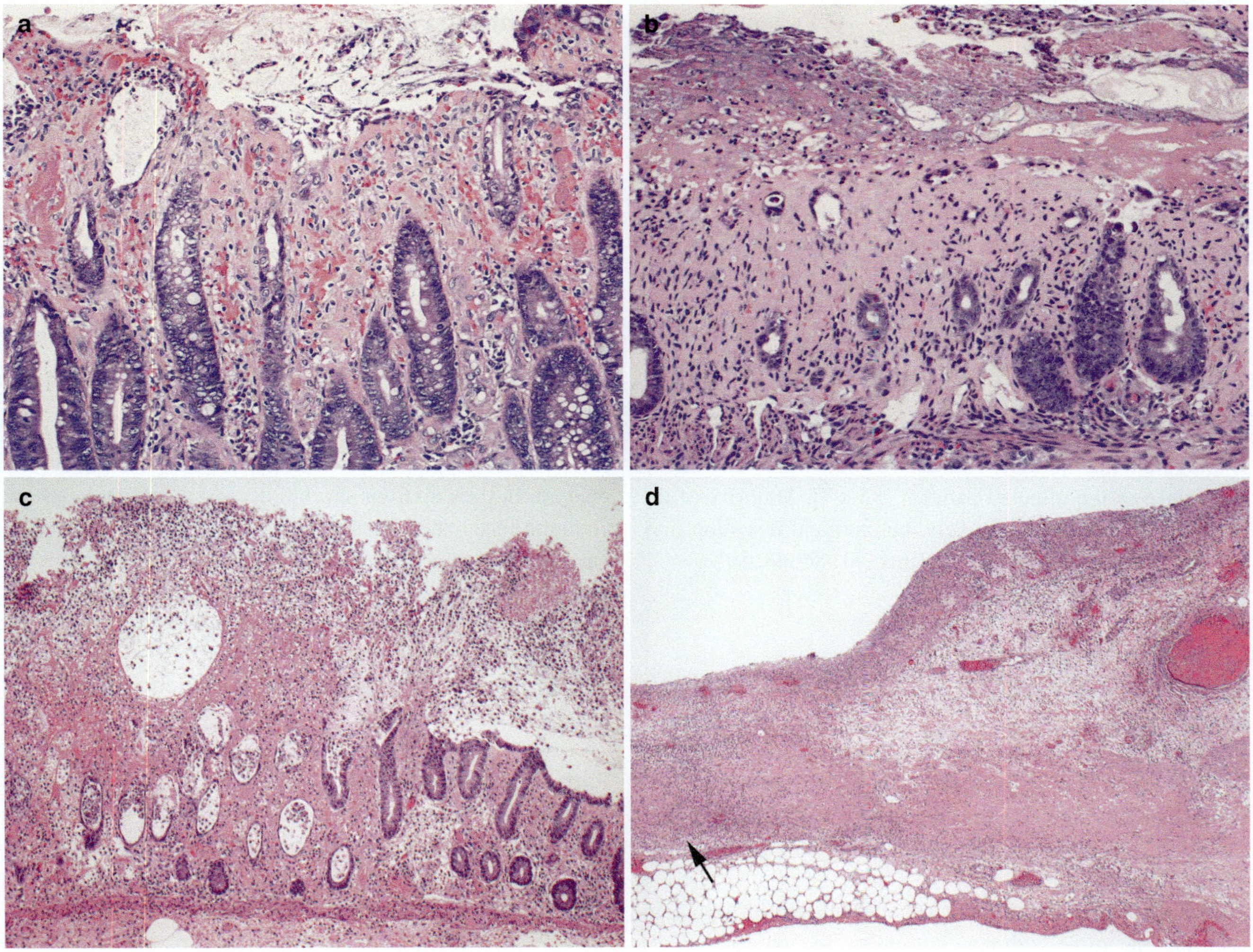

Fig. 18.11 Ischemic colitis. (**a**) Colonic mucosa shows loss of surface epithelium, lamina propria edema, hemorrhage, and dilated vessels in early stage of ischemic colitis. (**b**) Ischemic injury with crypt dropout, mucosal necrosis, and mild fibrosis in lamina propria. (**c**) Ischemic injury with pseudomembrane formation. (**d**) Extensive ulceration with necrosis of muscular layer (arrow) in severe ischemic colitis

the lamina propria and cryptitis may also be seen. Eventually, the crypts may fill with mucus and inflammatory cells, leading to pseudomembrane formation (Fig. 18.11c). After the initial ischemic damage, the acute inflammatory cells phase out and are replaced by chronic inflammatory cells such as lymphocytes, plasma cells, and macrophages. The macrophages remove the red blood cells from areas of hemorrhage forming hemosiderin-laden macrophages. Hence, these hemosiderin-containing macrophages can be an important diagnostic feature of ischemia. Fibrin and granulation tissue replace areas of ulceration. In severe cases, necrosis of muscular layer or transmural necrosis can occur (Fig. 18.11d).

The pathologist should try to determine the cause of ischemia, although in most cases it is not obvious. The intestinal and mesenteric vessels should be evaluated for occlusive etiologies or other unusual causes such as fungal vasculitis, parasitic infestations, or viral infection.

Differential Diagnosis

Crohn's disease may come in the differential as ischemic colitis can often be segmental and show a patchy distribution. However, the presence of coexisting systemic ischemic diseases, occlusive vascular changes, and glandular ghosts, with absence of rectal involvement, granulomas, and transmural lymphoid aggregates, should help in the differential diagnosis.

Pseudomembranous colitis may also be in the differential. However, in pseudomembranous colitis, there are minimal crypt atrophy and no hyalinization of lamina propria, and the histological changes are diffuse with pseudomembranes distributed along the length of the colon. Stool studies are usually positive for *C. difficile*.

Treatment and Prognosis

Ischemic colitis may ultimately lead to bowel perforation, peritonitis, persistent bleeding, and intestinal strictures [84]. If untreated, the mortality rate can be high, especially due to the nature of the affected patients [85–87]. Majority of the cases are treated conservatively, but surgical resection may be needed in around 20% of patients [81, 84, 88, 89].

Chronic Ischemic Colitis

Definition

Chronic ischemic colitis is a gradually developing intestinal ischemia from chronic mesenteric vascular insufficiency and severe anoxia, without complete cessation of the blood supply.

Clinical Features

Postprandial abdominal pain and intermittent bloody diarrhea are the most common presenting symptoms and are mainly seen in females older than 60 years [90].

Pathological Features

Grossly the mucosa may show foci of atrophy, granularity, and pseudopolyps similar to segmental active chronic colitis. In addition, erosions, hemorrhage, and edema may also be seen. The left colon is more frequently involved and the rectum is usually spared.

On microscopy, there may be architectural distortion, Paneth cell metaplasia, endocrine cell hyperplasia, and regenerative activity mimicking active chronic colitis seen in inflammatory bowel disease. A subset of cases may also show basal lymphoplasmacytosis. Lamina propria may also show hyalinization, hemosiderin deposition, congestion, and hemorrhage. Fibrosis causing fibrotic thickening of the bowel wall and strictures may also be seen.

Differential Diagnosis

Inflammatory bowel disease, especially Crohn's disease, can be distinguished from chronic ischemic colitis by the presence of transmural inflammation and non-necrotizing granulomas within the bowel wall away from the areas of ulceration and necrosis.

Treatment and Prognosis

Most patients are treated with surgical resection of the involved bowel segment. However, some ischemic strictures can be treated by endoscopic dilatations [90, 91].

Mass-Forming Ischemic Colitis

Definition

Mass-forming ischemic colitis is an unusual variant of ischemic colitis that can present as a mass lesion mimicking malignancy clinically [92].

Clinical Features

Mass-forming ischemic colitis is usually seen in the elderly who are in their sixth or seventh decade of life and is more common in females. Presenting symptoms include abdominal pain, hematochezia, and diarrhea. It most commonly involves the right colon. The endoscopic appearance is usually suggestive of a malignancy as a polypoid or fungating mass is seen obstructing the colonic lumen (Fig. 18.12a) [92, 93]. There may also be marked ulceration or stricturing lesions on endoscopy.

Pathological Features

Histology of the mucosal biopsies or sections obtained from the lesion shows classical features of acute ischemic colitis (Fig. 18.12b). On resection specimens, marked edema involving the submucosa and the muscularis propria is usually seen. It is presumed that this edema is responsible for the polypoid and multinodular elevations of the mucosa.

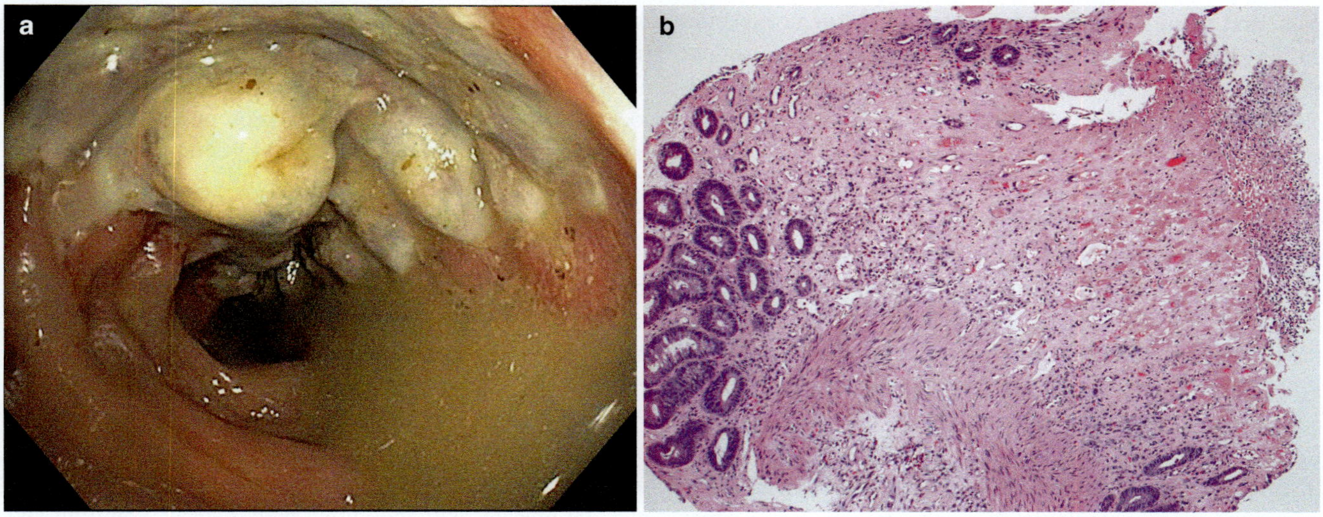

Fig. 18.12 Mass-forming ischemic colitis. (**a**) A polypoid or fungating mass is seen obstructing the colonic lumen. (**b**) Colonic mucosal biopsy from the polypoid mass shows ischemic-type injury

Hence, the finding of ischemic colitis in the setting of a mass lesion within the colon that is suspicious for carcinoma, particularly if located in the cecum or right colon, in an elderly woman with known risk factors for ischemic colitis, should raise consideration for mass-forming ischemic colitis.

Differential Diagnosis

The distinction from a neoplastic condition can be challenging. However, an acute onset of symptoms, discordance between colonoscopic and imaging findings, and biopsy findings of ischemic colitis without dysplasia or malignancy from a well-sampled mass lesion are important clues for this entity.

Treatment and Prognosis

Mass-forming ischemic colitis is usually treated conservatively including intravenous fluid and nutrition support as well as broad-spectrum antibiotics. The majority of patients show complete resolution or significant reduction on size of the mass lesion [92].

Vasculitis

Many types of vasculitis affect the colon, although they are rare. The diagnosis usually involves a combination of clinical features, radiological findings, and serologic tests. Mucosal biopsies are usually good for small vessel vasculitis, while medium vessel vasculitis is seen in resection specimens mainly performed for ischemic colitis. Only the salient features of primary vasculitis involving the colon will be discussed here.

Colon in Systemic Vasculitis

Medium vessel vasculitis such as polyarteritis nodosa (PAN) and Kawasaki disease involves the main visceral arteries such as celiac and mesenteric arteries. They are considered within the spectrum of necrotizing vasculitis. Small vessel vasculitis such as granulomatosis with polyangiitis (GPA, formerly known as Wegener's granulomatosis), eosinophilic granulomatosis with polyangiitis (EGPA, previously known as Churg-Strauss syndrome), and Henoch-Schonlein purpura (HSP) causes necrotizing or leukocytoclastic injury to the capillaries and venules.

Polyarteritis Nodosa

PAN usually involves the celiac and mesenteric arteries. It is commonly associated with hepatitis B infection with a less common association with hepatitis C and HIV infection [94–96]. The term "nodosa" is derived from the nodularity of the blood vessels which in turn is related to pseudoaneurysms. Transmural fibrinoid necrosis of the arteries is its histological characteristic. Early stages of the disease show neutrophilic infiltrate, while in the later stages, chronic inflammatory cells such as lymphocytes, monocytes, and macrophages are usually seen (see also Chap. 14, section "Polyarteritis Nodosa" and Fig. 14.11).

Kawasaki Disease

Kawasaki disease is usually seen in children less than 5 years of age. Patients usually have cervical lymphadenopathy, bilateral conjunctivitis, swollen lips, fever, rashes on the palms and soles, and a strawberry tongue [97]. This disease typically involves the coronary arteries, which show necrotizing vasculitis and may develop aneurysms, thrombosis, or rupture. Patients may also present with diarrhea, abdominal pain, and vomiting [98]. Biopsy usually shows nonspecific colitis and ischemic changes [99]. Kawasaki disease should be considered as a possibility in any child presenting with abdominal symptoms and prolonged fever of unknown cause.

Granulomatosis with Polyangiitis

GPA is an antineutrophil cytoplasmic antibody (ANCA)-positive necrotizing granulomatous vasculitis that can involve the mesenteric arteries resulting in ischemic injury to the bowel (see also Chap. 14, section "Granulomatosis with Polyangiitis"). Patients can present with bloody diarrhea and colonoscopy may show pancolitis with ulcers [100, 101]. Rarely, it can mimic ulcerative colitis [102]. The histological findings may show mixed inflammation, ischemic changes with necrotizing granulomatous vasculitis, and granulomas (Fig. 18.13). The granulomas are typically necrotizing with palisading by epithelioid histiocytes. Multinucleated giant cells are also commonly seen in the areas of necrosis or vasculitis. Due to the presence of granulomatous inflammation, infectious causes should be excluded.

Eosinophilic Granulomatosis with Polyangiitis (Churg-Strauss Syndrome)

EGPA is an allergic small vessel vasculitis which is associated with granulomatous inflammation of the respiratory tract, asthma, peripheral eosinophilia, and eosinophil-rich necrotizing vasculitis. Patients are usually ANCA positive. Patients present with abdominal pain, bleeding, and even intestinal perforation [103]. Histological findings may show transmural inflammation with prominence of eosinophils, as well as small- and medium-sized vessel vasculitis with necrotizing granulomas [104]. There can be multifocal distributed transmural vasculitis showing all stages of activity in small- and medium-sized arteries and veins located in the submucosa, muscularis propria, and subserosal layers of the colon (see also Chap. 14, section "Eosinophilic Granulomatosis with Polyangiitis (Churg-Strauss Syndrome)" and Fig. 14.13).

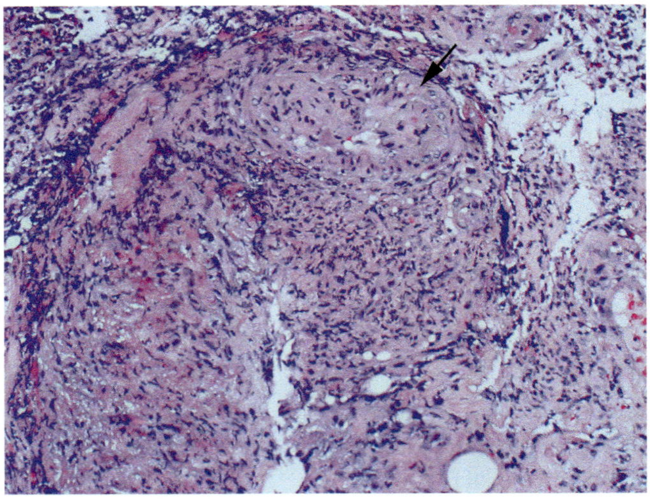

Fig. 18.13 Granulomatosis with polyangiitis (Wegener's granulomatosis). Necrotizing vasculitis with neutrophilic infiltration, necrotizing granulomas is present in submucosal vein. The artery (arrow) is relatively spared with necrotizing inflammation

Henoch-Schonlein Purpura

HSP is a self-limited, systemic, small vessel vasculitis associated with IgA deposition. Hence, it is also known IgA vasculitis (see also Chap. 14, section "Henoch-Schönlein Purpura" and Fig. 14.12). It is usually seen in children with only rare cases reported in adults. About two-thirds of the patients with HSP have gastrointestinal tract involvement and can present with abdominal pain, nausea, vomiting and gastrointestinal bleeding [105–107]. Endoscopy may show colonic ulcers especially within the rectum. The classic histological finding of HSP is leukocytoclastic vasculitis, but vasculitis may be infrequently seen on gastrointestinal biopsies. The most common histologic finding in the gastrointestinal tract is lamina propria hemorrhage with fibrin deposition and red cell sludging with nuclear debris (Fig. 18.14a) [108]. Acute colitis or proctitis characterized by cryptitis and crypt abscesses may also be seen [108]. The small vessels may show fibrinoid necrosis with neutrophilic and mononuclear infiltrates in the vascular wall (Fig. 18.14b). Fibrin thrombi may also be seen. Some cases may clinically mimic inflammatory bowel disease [107, 109].

Enterocolic Lymphocytic Phlebitis

Definition

Enterocolic lymphocytic phlebitis (ELP) is a rare isolated intestinal phlebitis of unknown etiology.

Clinical Features

ELP is usually seen in patients in the sixth decade of life and affects both men and women almost equally [110]. The term ELP is synonymous with mesenteric inflammatory veno-occlusive disease [111–113], intramural mesenteric vasculitis [114], isolated granulomatous phlebitis [115], lymphocytic venulitis [116], and necrotizing and giant cell granulomatous phlebitis [117].

Patients commonly present with acute abdominal pain, nausea and vomiting, diarrhea, and/or rectal bleeding. There are no specific endoscopic or imaging findings that would indicate a diagnosis of ELP. The exact etiology of this disease is unknown. However, there has been some reported association with a few drugs such as hydroxyethyl rutoside (Venoruton), a phlebotonic drug used in Europe for varicose veins and antiandrogen drug flutamide [118, 119]. Recently, ELP has also been suggested to be a part of IgG4 related disease [120, 121].

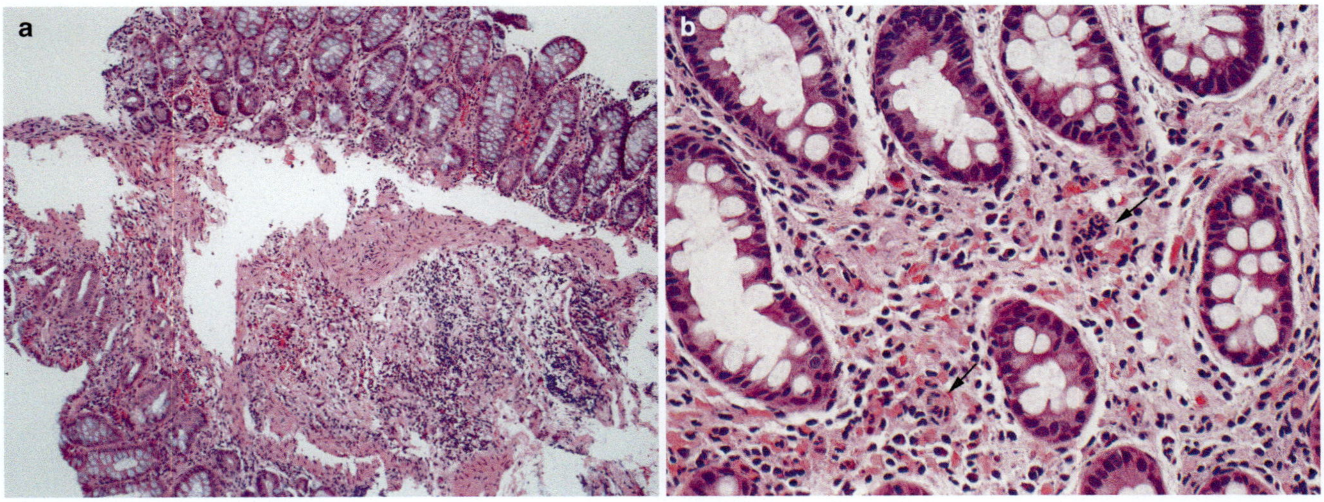

Fig. 18.14 Henoch-Schonlein purpura. (**a**) Colonic mucosa biopsy shows lamina propria hemorrhage with focal fibrin deposition and red cell sludging with nuclear debris in submucosa. (**b**) The capillaries in lamina propria show vasculitis with neutrophilic and mononuclear infiltrates in the vascular wall (arrows)

Pathological Features

The right colon is the most commonly involved site. Gross examination may show intestinal infarction, thickening of the bowel wall, ulceration, or even a mass-like lesion [110].

One of the main histological characteristics of ELP is the typical vascular changes. The veins show prominent lymphocytic phlebitis affecting veins of all sizes, including intramural venules and small veins of the intestine as well as large mesenteric veins (Fig. 18.15a). The involved vessels are often located in the bowel wall, particularly in the submucosa. The arteries are invariably uninvolved [122, 123]. The lymphocytic phlebitis is characterized by diffuse lymphocytic infiltration of the venous wall and dense perivenular infiltrate forming lymphocytic cuffs of variable thickness. This cuff of small uniform-appearing lymphocytes, with occasional plasma cells and rare eosinophils, is usually concentric.

Immunostain studies have shown a prominence of perivenular CD3-positive T lymphocytes and only occasional B lymphocytes, suggesting lymphocyte-mediated vascular damage [114, 116, 122]. Other types of phlebitis such as necrotizing phlebitis, granulomatous phlebitis, and multinucleated giant cells can also be found in association with lymphocytic phlebitis [115, 122, 124–126]. Endothelial and myointimal hyperplasia with near complete occlusion of vessel lumen may also be seen (Fig. 18.15b). Fresh and/or organized venous thrombi are also a striking histological feature of this entity. Transmural hemorrhagic ischemic infarction may also be seen. In summary, ELP presents as an artery-sparing vasculitis limited to the gastrointestinal tract, with obvious phlebitis in viable and ischemic portions of resected bowel.

Differential Diagnosis

The differential diagnosis includes systemic vasculitis such as systemic lupus erythematosus, Behcet's disease, EGPA, and rheumatoid arthritis. However, these systemic vasculitis disorders usually do not present with isolated colonic manifestations and florid gastrointestinal phlebitis. Moreover, histologically, these conditions primarily involve the arteries but not the veins as seen with ELP.

Treatment and Prognosis

Surgical resection is usually curative and most patients recover completely. The pathological diagnosis of ELP usually requires submucosal vessels, which are difficult to obtain on mucosal biopsies. Often time, endoscopic mucosal biopsies are superficial and may only show features of ischemic colitis. Thus, preoperative diagnosis can be difficult; hence, the diagnosis may be delayed or missed as a venous source of intestinal ischemia is seldom suspected and often overlooked.

Idiopathic Myointimal Hyperplasia of Mesenteric Veins

Definition

Idiopathic myointimal hyperplasia of mesenteric veins (IMHMV) is a rare cause of chronic colonic ischemia caused by noninflammatory obliteration of medium- to large-sized mesenteric and mural veins.

Clinical Features

Most cases occur in young to middle-aged men who present with recurrent, progressively severe abdominal pain and bloody diarrhea [127]. Left colon and rectosigmoid colon are most commonly involved. Endoscopy may show ulceration, mucosal

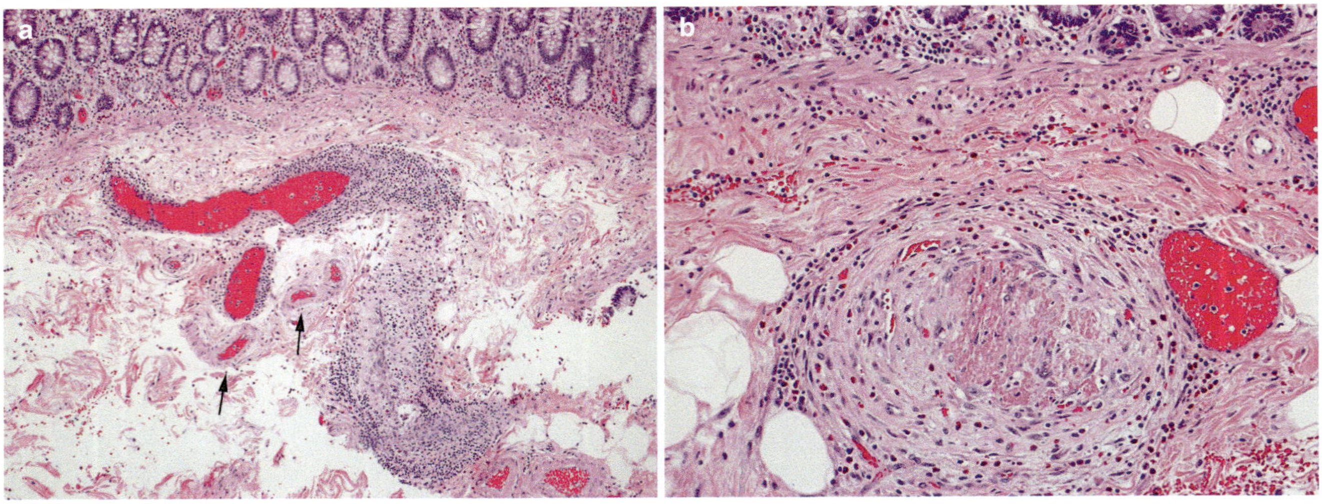

Fig. 18.15 Enterocolic lymphocytic phlebitis. (**a**) Lymphocytic phlebitis with diffuse lymphocytic infiltration of the venous wall and dense perivenular infiltrate in submucosal vein is present in the colon adjacent to ulceration. The submucosal artery (arrows) is not affected. (**b**) Endothelial and myointimal hyperplasia with near complete occlusion of submucosal vein

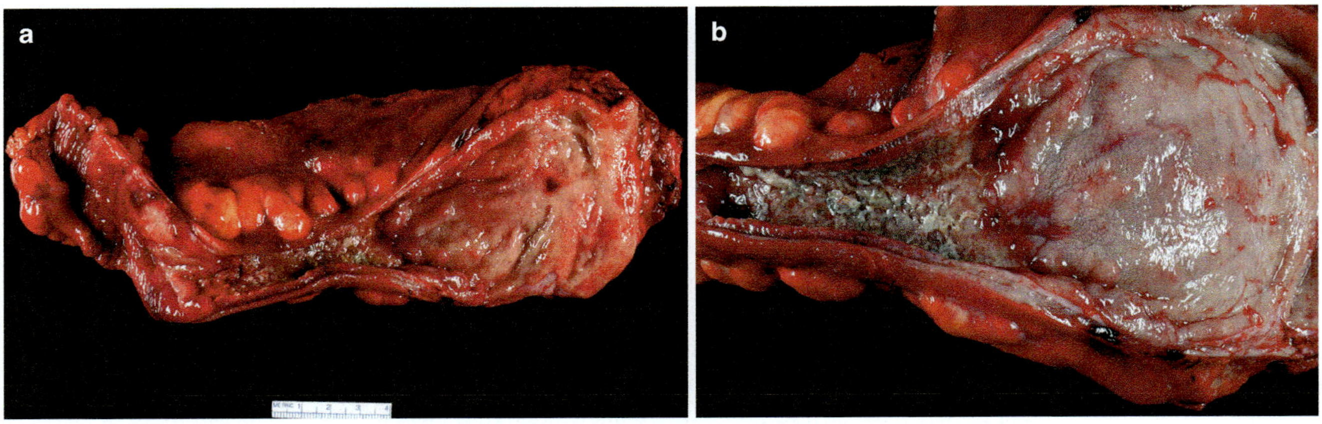

Fig. 18.16 Idiopathic myointimal hyperplasia of mesenteric veins. (**a**) The resected sigmoid colon shows strictures associated with ulcers and thickened pericolonic fat. (**b**) A closer view of colonic mucosa ulceration within the strictured area

erythema, granularity, and cobblestone appearance. These changes may simulate the endoscopic appearance of ischemic colitis and inflammatory bowel disease. This disorder has been postulated to be a result of arteriovenous fistulization [128, 129].

Pathological Features

Resection specimens on gross may show strictures associated with ulcers and serositis with thickened mesenteric fat (Fig. 18.16a, b). The mucosa demonstrates ischemic-type injury (Fig. 18.17a) with pathognomonic histological features seen in the mural blood vessels and are characterized by markedly thickened walls of the veins, causing stenosis and sometimes even occlusion (Fig. 18.17b) without significant inflammatory cell infiltrates in the submucosa and in the subserosa. The thickening is due to concentric proliferation of the smooth muscle cells in the intima and media of small- to medium-sized intramural veins. The arteries are normal; however, the veins can be easily mistaken as arteries due to their enlarged and muscular walls, and an elastin stain can be used to demonstrate the markedly thickened walls of the veins (Fig. 18.17c)[127, 130].

Mucosal biopsies usually show mild ischemic changes. However, a recent study has shown that both resection and biopsy specimens can show distinct vascular changes in the mucosa [127]. They concluded that the presence of arteriolized capillaries with thickened walls and swollen endothelial cells seen scattered between colonic crypts within the mucosa were highly sensitive and specific for this entity. In addition, subendothelial fibrin deposits, brightly eosinophilic thrombi, and perivascular hyalinization were also common and specific features that can help in recognition of IMHMV in biopsy samples [127]. Hence, it would be important for

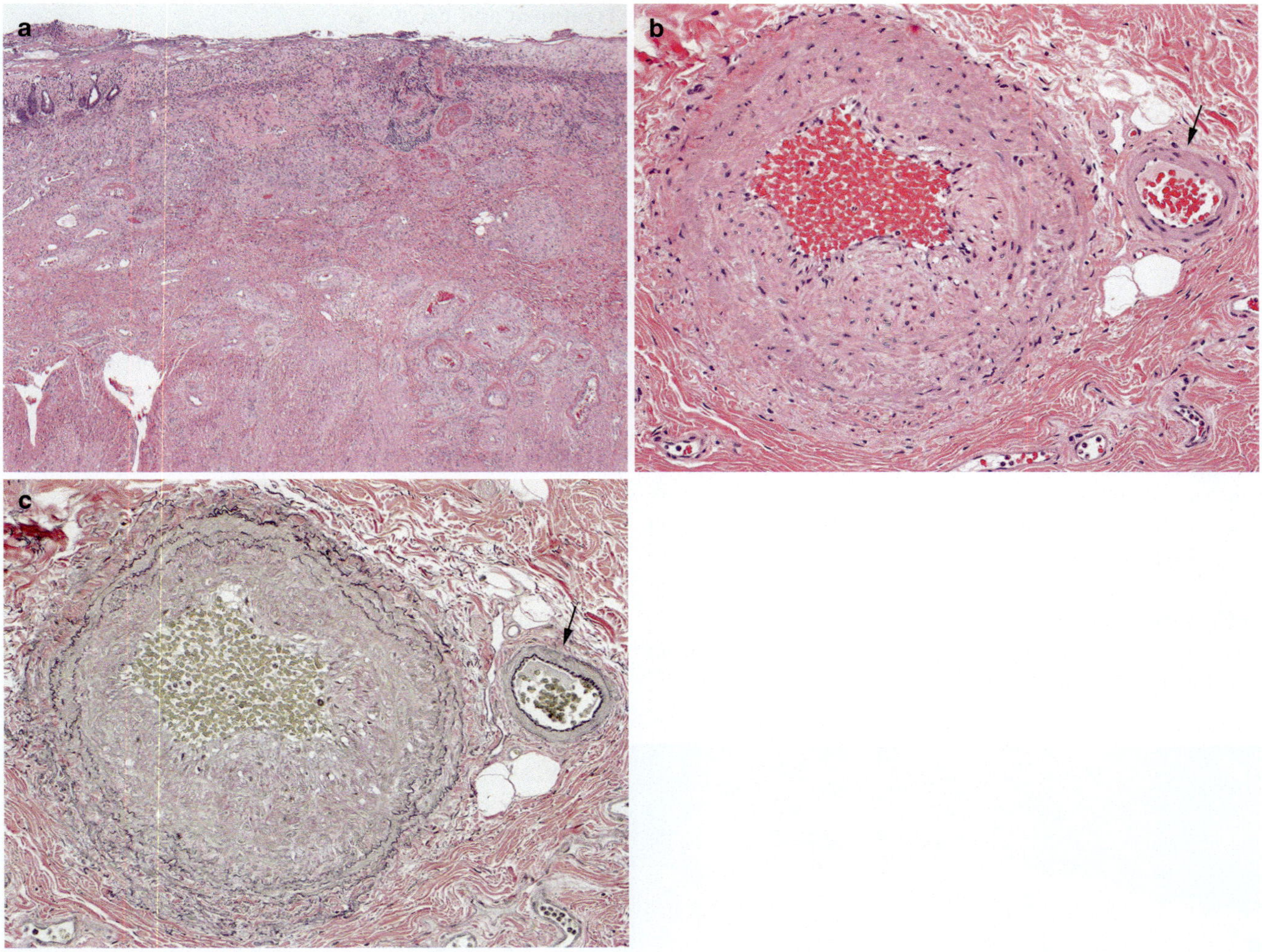

Fig. 18.17 Idiopathic myointimal hyperplasia of mesenteric veins. (**a**) Histological sections from strictured and ulcerated region shown in Fig. 18.16 show ischemic-type injury with ulceration and submucosal veins with prominent thickened wall and hyalinization. (**b**) The subserosal vein also shows thickened wall with concentric proliferation of the smooth muscle cells in the intima and media and is without significant inflammatory cell. The subserosal artery is normal (arrow). (**c**) Thickened subserosal vein and normal artery (arrow) are demonstrated by VVG stain

pathologists to suggest the possibility of IMHMV when these features are encountered in mucosal biopsy specimens from elderly patients with suspected inflammatory bowel disease or ischemic colitis.

Differential Diagnosis

Radiation colopathy can show ischemic and regenerative epithelial changes accompanied by lamina propria hyalinization that is most prominent in the superficial mucosa [131]. Vascular spaces in radiation colopathy are usually ectatic and may contain infrequent fibrin thrombi, but they are not thick-walled. ELP is differentiated from IMHMV by the presence of lymphocytic phlebitis characterized by diffuse lymphocytic infiltration of the venous wall and dense perivenular infiltrate forming lymphocytic cuffs of variable thickness. Moreover, arteriolization and hyalinization of mucosal vessels are not characteristic features of ELP.

Treatment and Prognosis

Resection of the affected segment is usually curative [128].

Arteriovenous Malformation and Angiodysplasia

Arteriovenous Malformation

Definition

Arteriovenous malformation (AVM) is congenital in origin and develops during embryologic or fetal life.

Clinical Features

They are typically present at birth. Hence, they can manifest clinically with bleeding at any age. The bleeding from them can be massive and recurrent [132, 133]. Rarely can patients also present with portal hypertension [134].

AVMs result in direct communication between the arteries and veins. This results in arterial blood flowing directly into the venous system at a much higher pressure than normal. Angiographic studies are useful in outlying the vascular architecture and locating the exact site of the lesion [133].

Pathological Features

AVMs are most commonly seen in the sigmoid colon and rectum (Fig. 18.18a). They are usually seen in the submucosa and subserosa. It consists of a tangled mass of tortuous and variably dilated arteries and veins. The veins undergo "arterialization," developing a thickened muscular wall due to exposure to increased arterial blood pressure. Histologically, they show complex clusters of tortuous, dilated vascular vessels that look intermediate in structure—between an artery and a vein (Fig. 18.18b, c).

Differential Diagnosis

Hemangioma and telangiectasia can be distinguished from AVM by presence of distorted and malformed vessels.

Treatment and Prognosis

Surgical resection of the involved segment is curative.

Angiodysplasia

Definition

Angiodysplasia is usually an acquired condition characterized by the presence of a cluster of abnormally dilated blood vessels in the mucosa and submucosa of the colon.

Clinical Features

It is commonly seen in the elderly and bleeding is usually chronic and recurrent [135]. In a small subset of patients, the bleeding can be massive and life-threatening [136]. The incidence of angiodysplasia increases with age as it is an acquired condition associated with aging. Colon is the most frequent site of angiodysplasia in the gastrointestinal tract [137]. Endoscopy is currently the main tool for diagnosis of angiodysplasia [138].

Pathological Features

It is commonly seen in the right colon but can be seen throughout the length of the colon. They are extremely dif-

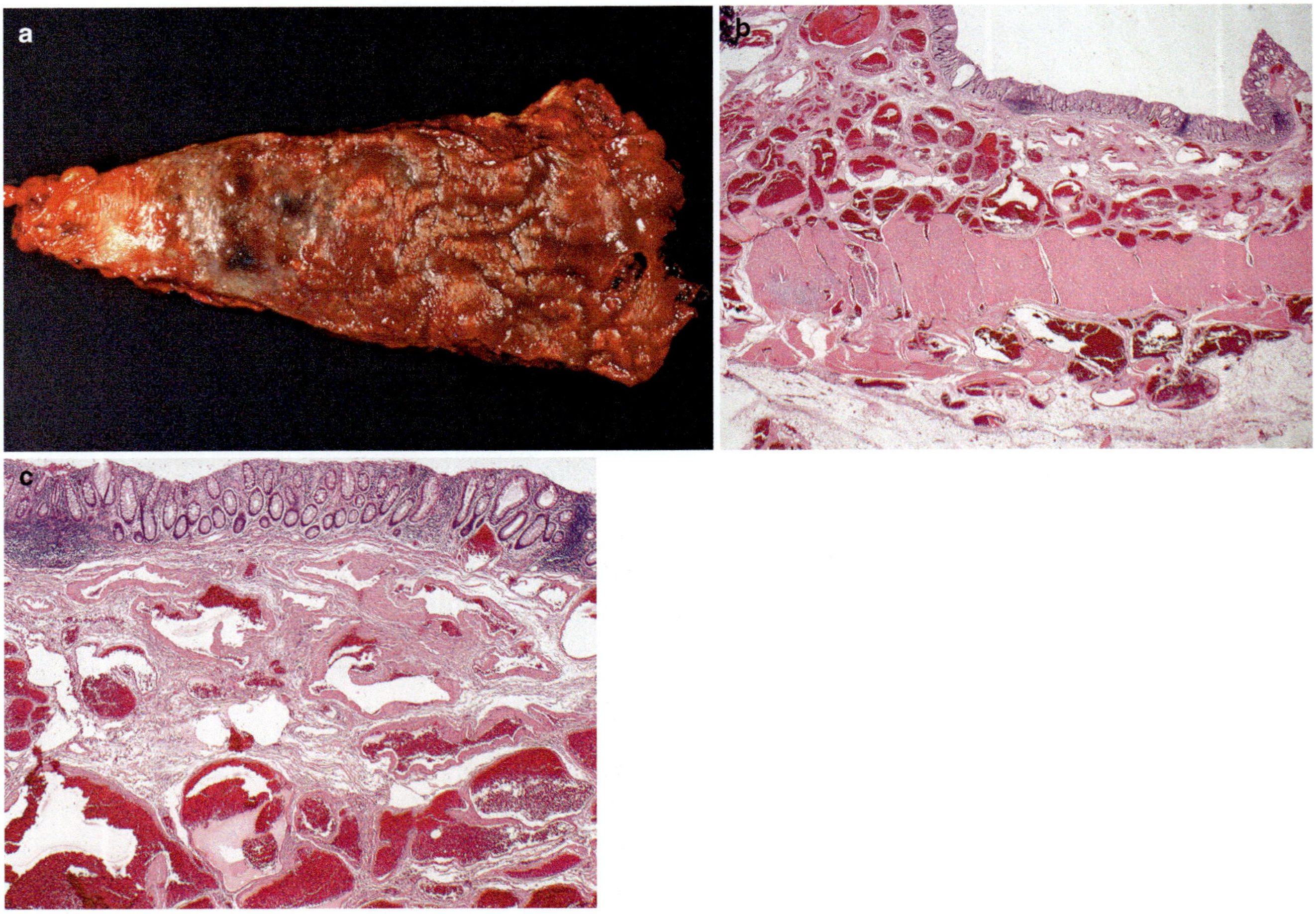

Fig. 18.18 Arteriovenous malformation. (**a**) A gross photo of AVM in resected rectosigmoid colon. The mucosal surface shows dusky mosaic appearance. (**b**) A low-power view of colon section shows complex clusters of tortuous, dilated vascular vessels involving submucosa, muscularis propria, and subserosa. (**c**) A higher-power view of AVM present in submucosa

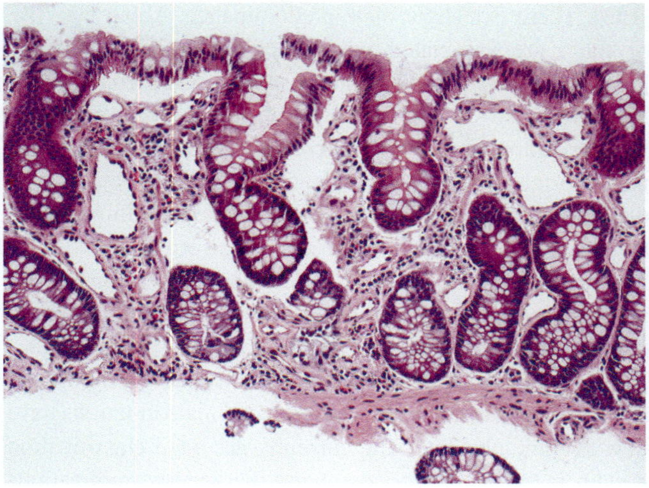

Fig. 18.19 Angiodysplasia. Colonic biopsy from angiodysplasia shows dilated capillaries in the mucosa

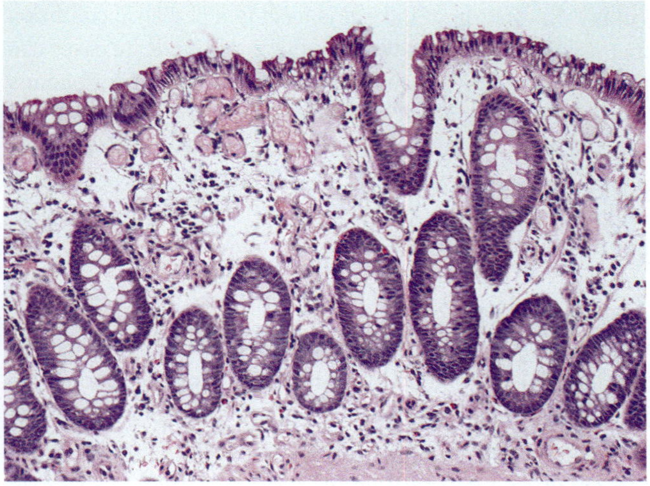

Fig. 18.20 Portal hypertensive colopathy. Rectal biopsy from a patient with cirrhosis and portal hypertension shows dilated capillaries within the lamina propria

ficult to detect on gross examination of the resection specimen. In fresh specimen, they may appear as only a small focus of enhanced vascular markings and erythema. After formalin fixation, these lesions may not be visible on the mucosal surface. Hence, some have used specific injection techniques for their diagnosis on resection specimens [139].

Histologically, angiodysplasias appear as abnormally dilated, distorted, tortuous veins and venules within the submucosa with some associated dilated capillaries in the overlying mucosa (Fig. 18.19). The affected vessels are lined by endothelium with only little or no smooth muscle. The pathological diagnosis of angiodysplasia can be challenging on biopsies, as the main histologic abnormality is usually present in the submucosa, which may not be sampled in endoscopic biopsies.

Differential Diagnosis

Hemangioma can be distinguished from angiodysplasia by the presence of distorted and tortuous vessels.

Treatment and Prognosis

Therapeutic endoscopy and selective embolization are usually able to control the bleeding in most cases. Patients with uncontrolled bleeding may require surgical resection [138].

Portal Hypertensive Colopathy

Definition

Portal hypertensive colopathy is defined as venous and capillary ectasia within the colonic mucosa seen in association with portal hypertension.

Clinical Features

Patients are usually asymptomatic but may present with lower gastrointestinal bleeding and anemia [140]. Endoscopy is diagnostic, and it may show telangiectasia or angiodysplasia-like lesions, erythematous patches, and varices within the colon [141]. The pathogenesis remains poorly understood. Portal hypertension seems to play an important role, and there is an association with a hyperkinetic circulatory state.

Pathological Features

Colonic mucosal capillary ectasia is the main pathological finding in portal hypertensive colopathy [142, 143]. Dilated capillaries are seen within the lamina propria (Fig. 18.20). Mucosal edema with erythema may also be seen.

Treatment and Prognosis

Portal hypertensive colopathy may be treated by laser photocoagulation therapy or transjugular intrahepatic portosystemic shunt placement [140].

Congenital and Acquired Anatomic Disorders

Congenital Disorders

Congenital anomalies of the colon are uncommon and the exact cause of most anomalies is unknown. However, the causes may include chromosomal abnormalities, maternal exposure to infection or drugs, maternal diseases such as diabetes, and single gene defects.

Malrotation

This results from an error of rotation. Complete failure of rotation (non-rotation) results in the colon lying in the left abdomen. Incomplete or mixed rotation results in the cecum placed in the right upper quadrant. Patients are at risk of volvulus. Malrotation of the gut is usually a pediatric condition that usually presents in the first month of life. Rare cases can present in adults as acute bowel obstruction and ischemia [144]. Plain abdominal radiographs are not useful and the investigation of choice is a contrast-enhanced CT scan. All patients, irrespective of age, should undergo surgery as it is impossible to predict the development of catastrophic complications [145].

Atresia and Stenosis

Colonic atresia and stenosis are rare. Colonic atresia has an incidence of 1 in 20,000 live births and comprises about 1.8–15% of intestinal atresias. The colonic stenosis is even rarer [146]. They can be seen in association with Hirschsprung's disease or as a part of multiple gastrointestinal atresia syndrome [147]. Mesenteric vascular accident occurring during the course of fetal development is the most commonly accepted theory for their development. Other proposed theories include failure of recanalization, intestinal perforation, drugs, and environmental factors. The symptoms usually start at birth and present as failure to pass meconium in association with rapidly progressive abdominal distention. The rectum contains mucus with absence of meconium. The preoperative diagnosis can be made with a contrast enema. Surgical excision is usually the treatment of choice. The prognosis is usually good for patients with isolated colonic atresia and stenosis [148].

Duplication

Colonic duplications are uncommon and usually present in the first decade of life as an acute abdomen or bowel obstruction [149]. They are rare in adults [150, 151]. Colonic duplications can be short or involve the entire colon [152]. The clinical presentations may vary, depending on the location and size of the duplication, the presence of gastric mucosa or pancreatic tissue, and the anatomical type. They can be diagnosed during laparotomy for other expected common diseases such as intussusception, gastrointestinal bleed, perforation, and obstruction. An abdominal X-ray, ultrasonography, and CT can be helpful in detecting colonic duplication. Colonoscopy is also a very useful diagnostic tool for this entity. The lining epithelium may consist of intestinal, gastric, or respiratory type epithelium. It may also contain heterotopic tissue such as pancreatic rests. Duplications usually have a thick wall with well-formed muscle layers. Surgical resection is the standard of treatment to avoid possible complications such as obstruction, bleeding, intussusception, perforation, and malignant change.

Anorectal Malformations

Anorectal malformations are uncommon but complex congenital anomalies. They have been reported to have an incidence of approximately 1 in every 4000–5000 live births [153]. There is a slight male predominance. About 60–70% of them are associated with other congenital anomalies [154]. Associated cardiac anomalies can range from 10% to 30% [155]. 30–50% of these patients also have spinal and vertebral anomalies. Tethered cord is the most common spinal abnormality [156, 157]. Trisomy 21 and microdeletion of the chromosome 22q11.2 are the two most common mutations associated with anorectal malformations [158]. Downregulation of the Sonic Hedgehog Homolog (SHH) signaling pathway has also been shown to play a role in the development of anorectal malformations [159].

Previous classification systems that relied on high, low, and intermediate definitions of anorectal malformations have now become obsolete. The currently accepted classification system is based on prognostic and therapeutic implications [160]. In male patients, the five major groups are rectoperineal fistula, rectourethral bulbar fistula, imperforate anus without fistula, rectourethral prostatic fistula, and rectobladder neck fistula. In females, the rectum connects to the vagina instead of ending in the urethra or urinary system. The five major types of female anomalies are rectoperineal fistula, rectovestibular fistula, imperforate anus without fistula, rectovaginal fistula, and cloaca. The most common malformations in males are rectourethral bulbar fistula; while it is the vestibular fistula for females. The second most common anomaly for each sex is the perineal fistula. After ruling out other associated diseases, the treatment of any anorectal malformation is either to perform a colostomy or primary surgical repair of the anomaly.

Diverticular Disease

Definition and Types

Diverticulum is a pouch-like structure projecting outward from the colonic wall. It can be of two broad categories: true and false. A false diverticulum is a protrusion of the submucosa and mucosa into the muscularis propria, while a true diverticulum is a protrusion of all layers of the colonic wall. True diverticula are usually congenital in origin. Diverticulosis is the presence of single or multiple diverticula. Diverticulitis is the inflammation of the diverticula but without involvement of the in-between mucosa.

Clinical Features

Most patients with colonic diverticulosis are asymptomatic. Some patients present with symptoms of diarrhea, constipation, bloating, and passage of mucus and bleeding per rectum. Patients with acute diverticulitis may present with abdominal pain, abdominal tenderness, and fever. Diverticular bleeding is the cause of up to half of all hematochezia [161]. Diverticular disease is uncommon in younger individuals with an incidence of 5% at age of 40 and increasing substantially to over 60% in patients 80 years or older [162]. Right-sided diverticula are more common in Asians, while the left-sided disease is more common in the western hemisphere.

Diverticular disease is caused by a combination of inherent structural alterations within the colonic wall, motility abnormalities, and reduced dietary fiber [163]. The fecal material may obstruct the diverticular sac and cause mucosal ulcer and inflammation. This may lead to prolonged exposure to bacterial flora, which may ultimately lead to diverticulitis. Endoscopy is the most effective in diagnosing colonic diverticular bleeding. CT scan appears to be the test of choice for detection of diverticulitis [164].

Pathological Features

The sigmoid colon is the most common site for diverticular disease (>90%). The entire colon may be involved in about 15% of cases. Grossly, the bowel wall may be thickened and shortened (Fig. 18.21a). The diverticula usually measure around 0.5–1 cm (Fig. 18.21b). There may also be serosal fat wrapping, adhesions, and abscesses (Fig. 18.21c). Erythema and ulceration may be seen around the diverticula. Prolapse-type inflammatory polyps (Fig. 18.21d) may also be seen within the adjacent mucosa.

Microscopy shows flask-shaped mucosal outpouches extending into the muscularis propria and sometimes also into the subserosal adipose tissue (Fig. 18.22a). The mucosa within the diverticulum itself may not show any significant abnormality or may show acute and chronic inflammation, including foci of cryptitis, Paneth cell metaplasia, and mild architectural distortion. Diverticulitis shows acute suppurative inflammation and even peridiverticular abscess formation (Fig. 18.22b). Some cases may also show perforation with fistula formation. In such cases, serositis and fat necrosis may also be seen. Marked peridiverticulitis may form a mass lesion, and these changes may grossly mimic a neoplasm. A small subset of patients with diverticular disease may develop changes similar to Crohn's disease

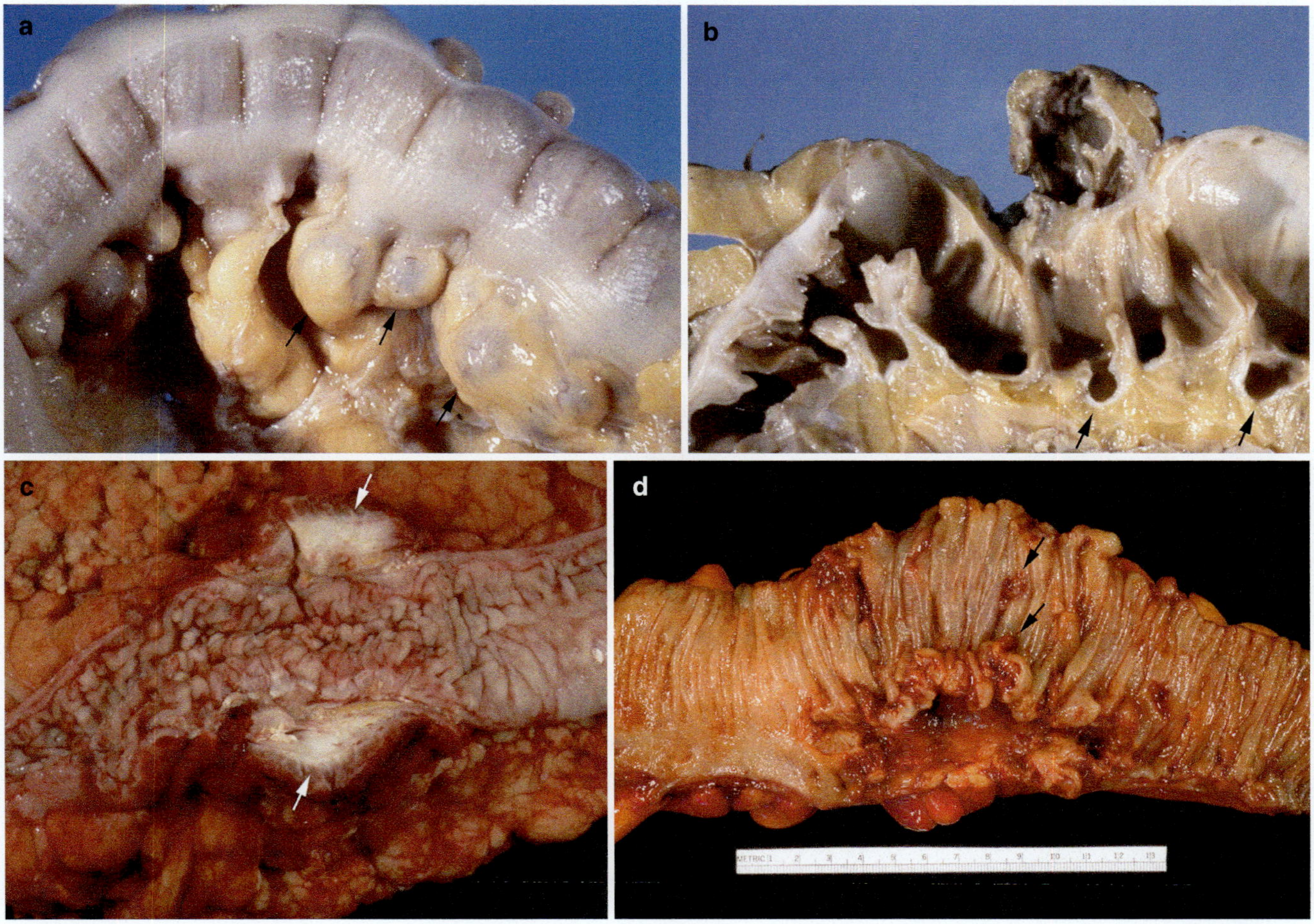

Fig. 18.21 Diverticular disease. (**a**) A gross external view of sigmoid colon shows multiple diverticular outpouches (arrows) in the subserosal fat. (**b**) A cross section of colonic diverticulosis reveals multiple diverticula extending into the subserosal fat (arrows). (**c**) Subserosal abscess (arrows) due to ruptured diverticula is present in diverticular disease. (**d**) Prolapse-type inflammatory polyps (arrows) are present in diverticular disease

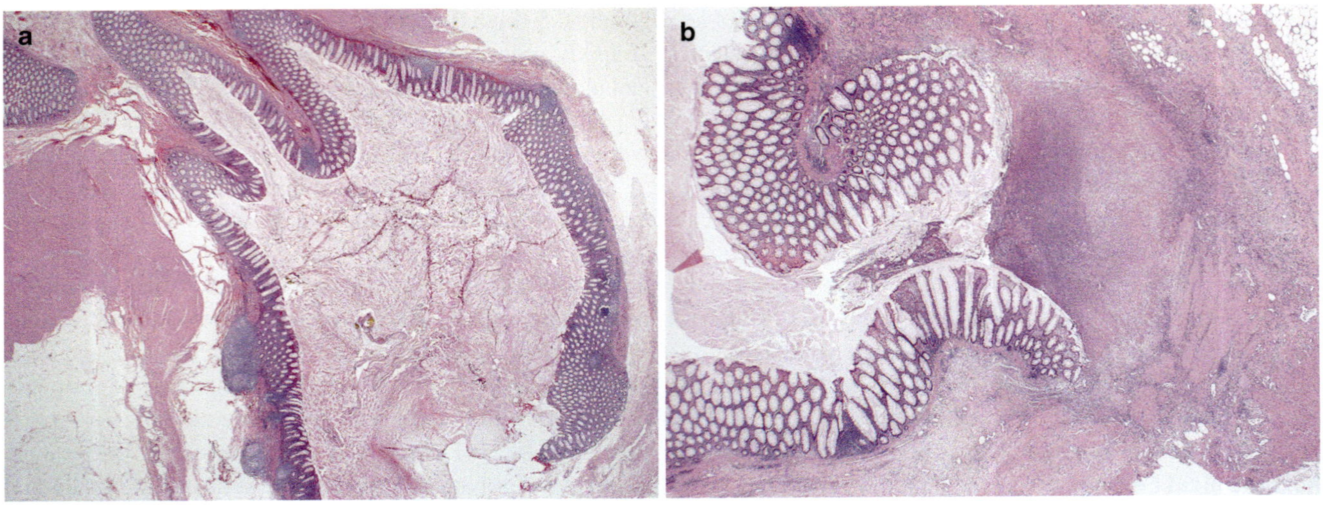

Fig. 18.22 Diverticular disease. (**a**) Histological section of colonic diverticulum extending into the subserosal adipose tissue. (**b**) Diverticulitis with acute suppurative inflammation and peridiverticular abscess formation

("Crohn's-like diverticulitis," see also Chap. 16, section "Diverticular Disease-Associated Segmental Colitis") [165]. Hence, Crohn-like inflammatory response can be a localized reaction to diverticulitis and does not necessarily indicate chronic inflammatory bowel disease.

Differential Diagnosis

Inflammatory bowel disease needs to be distinguished from diverticulosis associated colitis. On resection specimens, this should not pose a major problem as obvious diverticula can be recognized and inflammatory changes can be seen related to the distribution of the diverticula. However, this distinction can be difficult on biopsy specimens as chronic colitis of diverticulosis shows changes similar to chronic inflammatory bowel disease. In such cases correlation with the endoscopic and clinical findings is very important. Inflammation above and below the segment involved by diverticula should suggest infection or inflammatory bowel disease. Terminal ileum or upper gastrointestinal tract involvement favors Crohn's disease.

Treatment and Prognosis

Medical treatment focuses on increasing the bulk of stool in the colon (high-fiber diet) to help decrease the amount of pressure in the colon. Antibiotics are used for treatment of active diverticulitis. Surgical intervention may be needed for severe cases [166].

Intussusception

Definition

Colonic intussusception is defined as invagination of one segment of the colon into an immediately adjacent segment.

Clinical Features

Majority of the cases occur in infants, with a peak incidence between 3 and 5 months of age. It is the most common abdominal emergency in early childhood. The etiology of pediatric intussusception is idiopathic in nearly 90% of cases [167]. Predisposing factors include anatomic variations in the developing gastrointestinal tract such as anterior insertion of the terminal ileum with respect to the cecum, decreased rigidity of the cecum secondary to the absence or underdeveloped taenia coli, intestinal duplication, and malrotation; infections such as adenovirus and rotavirus which cause hypertrophy of the Peyer's patches; and noninfectious etiologies such as celiac disease, Crohn's disease, cystic fibrosis, and intestinal allergies [168–171].

Intussusception is rare in adults, with a mean age of 50 years [167, 172]. However, in adults, up to 90% of cases have an identifiable cause [173, 174]. Benign or malignant neoplasms cause a majority of cases (nearly 60–70% of cases); and the remainder of cases are caused by infections, Crohn's disease, and postoperative adhesions.

Intussusception usually starts with a lead point, such as lymphadenopathy, polyp, or neoplasm, which acts as a focal area of traction that draws the proximal bowel within the peristalsing distal bowel. Symptoms occur due to continued peristaltic contractions of the intussuscepted segment against the obstruction. Continued invagination results in edema, leading to compromised vascular flow to the bowel, resulting in ischemia to the affected segment that, if left untreated, can result in necrosis and perforation.

The clinical presentation varies, but patients usually present with marked abdominal pain and signs of bowel obstruction. It is one of the most common abdominal emergencies in pediatric age group. Children younger than 2 years classically present with acute-onset colicky abdominal pain with excessive irritability and crying. In adults, the clinical presentation of intussusception can be nonspecific. However, most common presenting symptom is abdominal pain, with associated symptoms of nausea, vomiting, obstipation, gastrointestinal bleeding, change in bowel habits, constipation, or bloating. Ultrasound is highly sensitive and specific in diagnosing intussusception, especially in children [175]. In adults, the diagnostic modalities include abdominal X-ray, ultrasound, CT, pre-op colonoscopy, and opaque enema [176].

Pathological Features

Intussusceptions can develop anywhere in the colon, but the hepatic flexure is the most common site. On gross, variable external and internal signs of ischemic injury to the colon (Fig. 18.23a, b) may be seen if the intussusception has not spontaneously resolved. Serosal adhesions may also be seen, especially if the patient has had recurrent bouts of intussusceptions. On microscopy, most intussusceptions show variable degree of ischemic injury which appears similar to ischemic injury due to other causes (Fig. 18.23c). The histological changes may vary depending on whether it is an acute, chronic, or acute on chronic intussusception. In patients with adenovirus infection as an etiology, markedly lymphoid hyperplasia may be seen, and the overlying epithelium may be damaged or even necrotic. Intranuclear viral inclusions which may appear as reddish globules surrounded by halos or purple nuclear smudges may also be seen. Immunostain for adenovirus can be used for confirmation.

Treatment and Prognosis

In children, reduction by ultrasound-guided or fluoroscopic pneumatic or hydrostatic enema is successful in 85–90% of cases [177]. Some intussusceptions reduce spontaneously. They may also be reduced manually during surgery without a resection. Surgical resection is indicated for cases with perforation, infarction, or irreducibility [178]. Most of the time optimal outcomes are achieved.

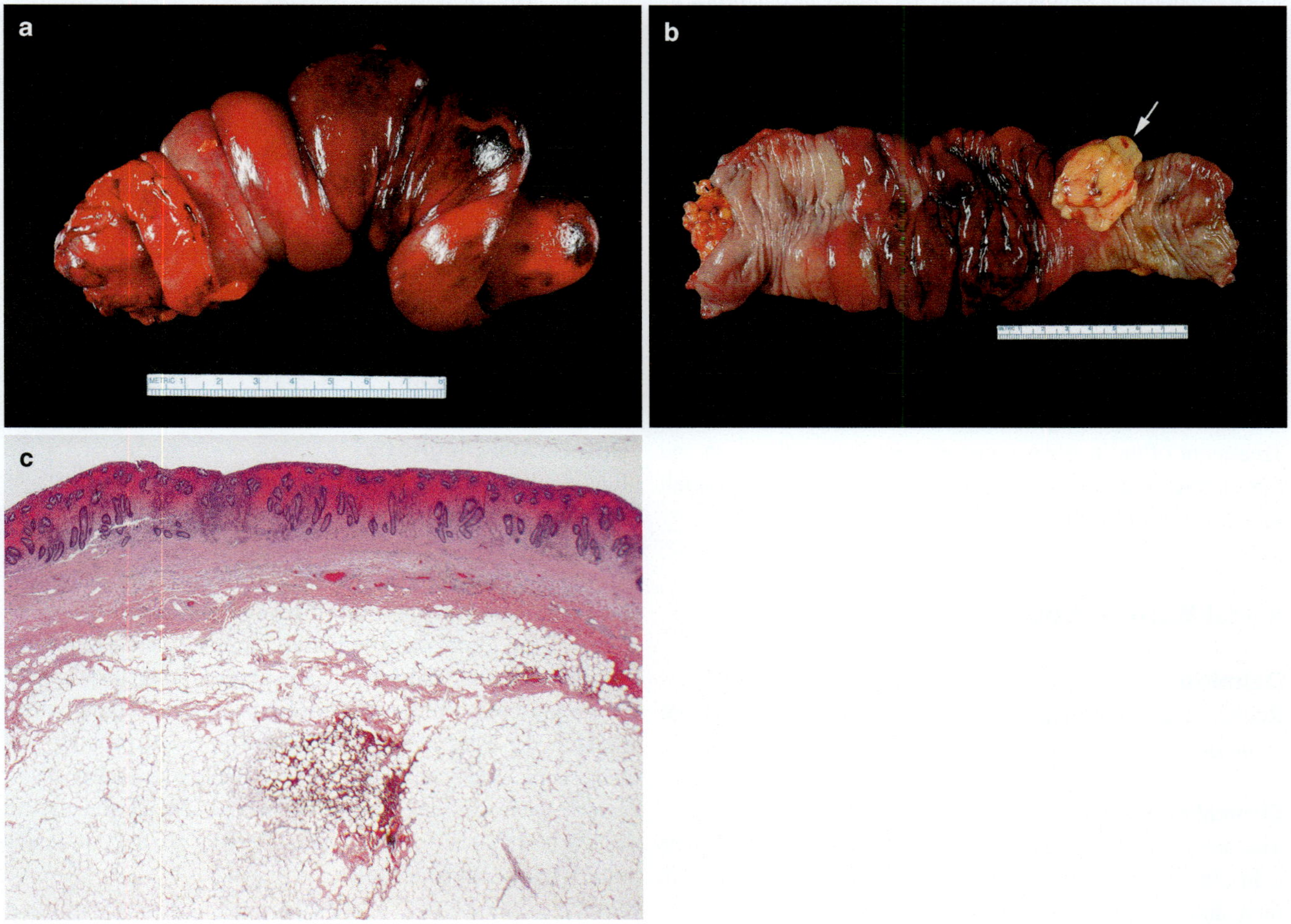

Fig. 18.23 Colonic intussusception. (**a**) An external view of colonic intussusception in rectosigmoid colon due to submucosal lipoma shows dilated colon with dusky serosal surface due to ischemic injury. (**b**) The intussuscepted portion of colon proximal to the lipoma (arrow) shows demarcated dusky mucosa due to ischemia. (**c**) Ischemic-type injury with mucosal congestion and hemorrhage is present in mucosa overlying the submucosal lipoma

Volvulus

Definition

Volvulus involves twisting of the bowel wall around itself or its mesentery.

Clinical Features

The two most common types of colonic volvulus include sigmoid and cecal volvulus [179]. Colonic volvulus is rare in children. Pregnant patients are at an increased risk for colonic volvulus. This is possibly related to the gravid uterus pushing upward on the colon and making it more prone to torsion. High-fiber diets and cultural factors such as consumption of large quantity of food after prolonged fasts have also been shown as predisposing factors for sigmoid volvulus [180].

Clinical presentation may be variable. Patients usually present with abdominal distention, constipation, or nausea and vomiting. Some patients will have recurring episodes which spontaneously resolve. If there is ischemia of the involved segment, the patients may also have severe abdominal pain, peritonitis, and evidence of shock. Abdominal radiographs may be useful in diagnosis, as they may demonstrate a large sigmoid loop in the shape of a "bent inner tube" or "omega loop." Otherwise, abdominal CT is almost always diagnostic [181, 182].

Pathological Features

On gross, the colon may be massively distended with thinning of the intestinal wall. It may also show signs of infarction or ischemia. Pneumatosis coli may also be seen. Histologically, the colon shows variable degree of ischemic changes and necrosis. The bowel wall may show markedly attenuated muscularis mucosae and muscularis propria.

Treatment and Prognosis

Treatment often involves emergent surgical exploration and bowel resection. Prompt diagnosis and treatment is crucial; otherwise bowel ischemia may ensue [183].

Rectal Mucosal Prolapse

Definition

Rectal mucosal prolapse is defined as a protuberance of some or all layers of the rectum through the anus.

Clinical Features

The prevalence of rectal mucosal prolapse is estimated to be 1 in 100,000 people per year [184, 185]. It occurs in both men and women with almost the same frequency; and is commonly seen in the third or fourth decade of life. The term rectal mucosal prolapse includes a number of entities such as solitary rectal ulcer syndrome, proctitis cystica profunda, inflammatory cloacogenic polyp, and rectal intussusception.

The exact cause of this entity is unclear, but chronic and severe constipation appears to play a role. The patients usually present with chronic constipation, which can be associated with straining during defecation, rectal bleeding, tenesmus, mucoid secretion from the rectum, rectal pain, and a sense of incomplete evacuation [186, 187]. Up to a quarter of patients may be asymptomatic [188]. The ulceration is thought to be related to pressure necrosis, ischemia, and mechanical trauma.

Endoscopy shows ulcerated and indurated areas on the anterior or anteriolateral wall of the rectum. There may also be a palpable mass on digital examination raising a consideration for a malignant process. Inflammatory cloacogenic polyps may present as small sessile polyps at the anorectal junction.

Pathological Features

Grossly, the mucosa may appear erythematous and/or ulcerated. Polypoid lesions may also be seen. These changes are usually seen within 15 cm of the anal margin, along the anal margin. The histological features include a spectrum of changes including thickening of the mucosal layer along with crypt architectural distortion, fibromuscular obliteration of the lamina propria, upward extension of muscle fibers from the muscularis mucosae toward the lumen in between the crypts, surface ulceration, hyperplastic and serrated mucosal changes, mild acute and chronic inflammation, and reactive epithelial atypia (Fig. 18.24a–c). The colonic mucosa may also be misplaced in the submucosa and even in the muscularis propria, which is often associated with cystic dilation filled with mucin. This has been referred as colitis or proctitis cystica profunda (Fig. 18.24d) and may cause confusion with an invasive carcinoma.

Differential Diagnosis

Rectal adenocarcinoma is the main differential diagnosis, as rectal mucosal prolapse may present as a raised polypoid or ulcerated lesion with stricture. The disordered growth pattern and regenerative atypia may also suggest a neoplastic process. However, the overall benign and reactive appearance of the glandular epithelium, absence of desmoplastic stromal reaction, and presence of fibromuscular hyperplasia of the muscularis mucosae and lamina propria should help in making the right diagnosis of rectal mucosal prolapse. Of note, sometimes changes similar to rectal mucosal prolapse can be seen overlying a mass lesion, and hence if the clinical concern remains for a neoplastic process, then a repeat biopsy may also be useful.

Treatment and Prognosis

Patients who are asymptomatic or minimally symptomatic can be treated with bulk laxatives and reassurance. Topical therapies such as sucralfate enema, corticosteroids, and sul-

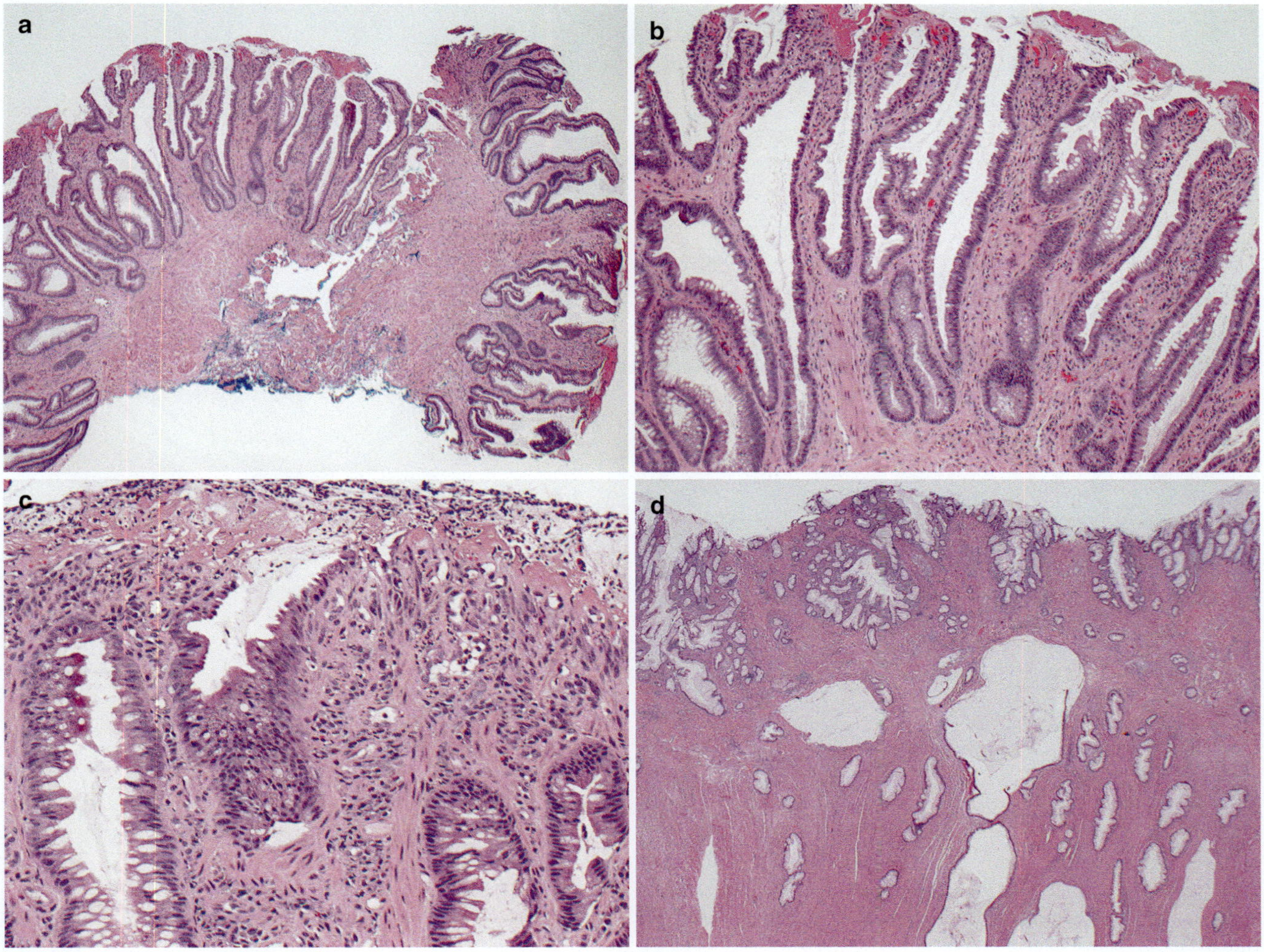

Fig. 18.24 Rectal mucosal prolapse. (**a**) A low-power view of rectal mucosal prolapse shows hyperplastic and reactive serrated crypts, crypt architectural distortion; fibromuscular obliteration of the lamina propria. (**b**) The reactive serrated crypts are separated by upward extension of muscle fibers from the muscularis mucosae. (**c**) Surface erosion, acute and chronic inflammation is present in rectal mucosal prolapse. (**d**) Colitis cystic profunda, characterized by misplaced benign colonic glands in submucosa and muscularis propria with focal cystic change and extravasated mucin, mimicking an invasive adenocarcinoma

fasalazine enemas have been reported to be effective in some cases. Surgical treatment is reserved for patients who suffer from full-thickness rectal mucosal prolapse or for those who are resistant to conservative management [189].

Pneumatosis Coli

Definition

Pneumatosis coli is a condition characterized by air filled spaces within the colonic wall.

Clinical Features

It is more commonly seen in males than females (M:F ratio 3:1) between the ages of 30–50 years [190, 191]. An autopsy series reported an incidence of 0.03% in the general population [192]. Its symptoms are generally nonspecific and many cases are identified incidentally on imaging studies. Although some patients may present with abdominal pain, diarrhea, abdominal distension, and bloody stool [193], the diagnosis of pneumatosis coli is primarily radiologic. A CT scan is the most sensitive imaging modality for detection.

The exact cause for this entity is not known, but there are two main proposed theories. The first is the mechanical theory that suggests that pneumatosis coli results from increased intraluminal pressure that forces air into the bowel wall via mucosal defects [194]. The second is the infectious theory, which postulates that pneumatosis coli results from cysts formed by gas-producing organisms [194, 195]. Finally, a combined hypothesis proposes that pneumatosis coli develops from a synergism of mechanical and infectious processes [194].

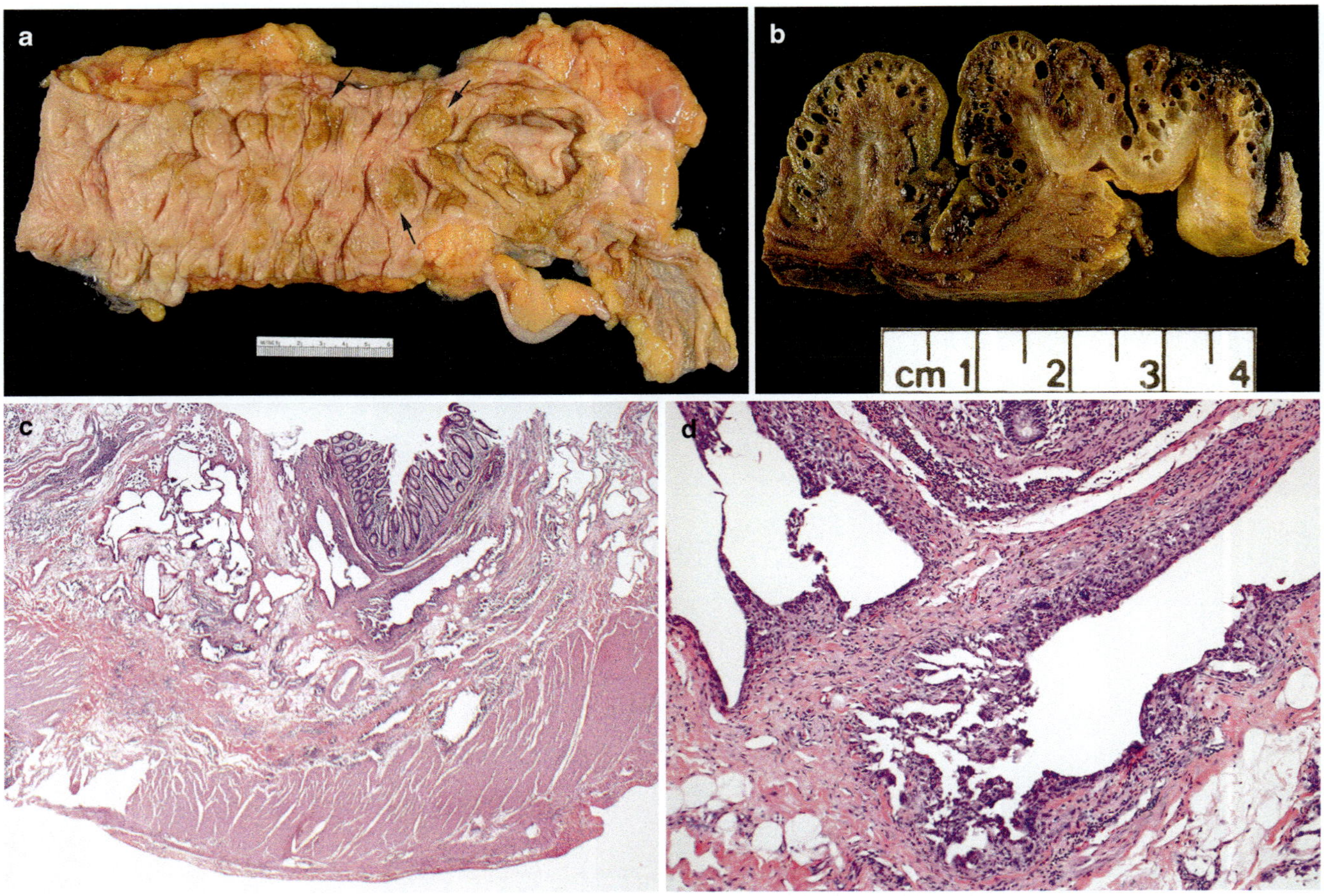

Fig. 18.25 Pneumatosis coli. (**a**) Multiple yellowish mucosal nodules or plaques (arrows) are present in the right colon due to pneumatosis coli. (**b**) Cross section of another case of pneumatosis coli secondary to ischemic bowel disease shows numerous cystic spaces predominantly present in the submucosa. (**c**) Histologically, the gas-filled cysts present in the submucosa are lined by foreign body giant cells and mild chronic inflammation. (**d**) High-power view of air spaces surrounded by foreign body giant cells

A number of conditions have been associated with pneumatosis coli, including infection, ischemia, chronic obstructive pulmonary disease, connective tissue disorders, organ transplantation, leukemia, medications, traumatic diseases secondary to endoscopic or surgical procedures, and intestinal obstruction [192, 196–199].

Pathological Features

On gross examination, the affected segment of colon may show multiple gas-filled spaces (Fig. 18.25a, b). On histology, the gas-filled cysts are lined by foreign body giant cells with mild chronic inflammation (Fig. 18.25c, d).

Differential Diagnosis

Lipoma or mature adipose tissue is the main differential for pneumatosis coli. However, the presence of foreign body giant cells and absence of nuclei within these spaces helps in distinguishing pneumatosis coli from adipocytes. If needed, s100 immunostain can be used, as it will be negative in pneumatosis coli and positive within adipocytes.

Treatment and Prognosis

Patients who are asymptomatic or only mildly symptomatic can be observed closely. For symptomatic patients, nonsurgical treatment modalities include antibiotics, octreotide, metoclopramide, erythromycin, bowel rest, high flow oxygen, and hyperbaric oxygen therapy. Surgical intervention is usually needed in patients with signs of perforation or bowel necrosis [200].

Motility Disorders

Introduction

Normal motility of the colon depends on the proper interaction between smooth muscle, nervous system, interstitial cells of Cajal (ICC), and various neuroendocrine peptides. Bowel dysmotility can result due to abnormalities within or between any of these components. The pathogenesis of many of these disorders is poorly understood. Some of the diseases such as Hirschsprung's disease manifest with distinct clinical features, whereas others have nonspecific clinical features. Of note, many of these disorders have no characteristic pathological features and have absence of standardized diagnostic criteria.

The neuromuscular network of the colon is composed of the muscularis mucosae which is a thin superficial layer of smooth muscle that separates mucosa from the submucosa and the muscularis propria which is the thick outer layer composed of the inner circular and an outer longitudinal layer. The outer longitudinal layer forms the thick localized bands of muscle, known as the tenia coli. The inner circular layer of the muscularis propria at the rectum becomes thickened to form the inner anal sphincter. The external anal sphincter is composed of skeletal muscle and is connected to the skeletal muscle of the pelvic floor.

The neural network is composed of extrinsic and intrinsic neural plexus. The extrinsic nerve supply consists of both the sympathetic and parasympathetic nerve fibers. The sympathetic nerve fibers originate from the prevertebral ganglia, while the parasympathetic fibers arise from the vagus nerve. The intrinsic neural plexus is composed of three plexuses: the submucosal plexus (Meissner's plexus), the deep submucosal plexus (Henle's plexus), and the myenteric plexus (Auerbach's plexus). The myenteric plexus is located between the inner circular and outer longitudinal muscle layers and is the most prominent of them all. It is composed of clusters of ganglion cells connected by a rich network of nerves. The ICC also play a pivotal role in bowel motility. They represent the pacemaker cells of bowel peristalsis. These are difficult to see on the H&E stain and can be highlighted by the CD117 or DOG-1 immunostains. The ICC have a close association with smooth muscle cells and neural plexuses. There is also a distinct ICC plexus in the submucosa.

Neural Disorders

Hirschsprung's Disease

Definition

Hirschsprung's disease is due to congenital absence of ganglion cells (aganglionosis), resulting in bowel dysmotility. Synonyms include aganglionic/congenital megacolon, congenital intestinal aganglionosis, and aganglionosis.

Clinical Features

It is the most common cause of congenital intestinal obstruction. The estimated incidence is 1 in every 5000 live born infants (0.02%) with a striking male predominance (M:F = 4:1) [201, 202]. It occurs in approximately 1% of patients with trisomy 21. 10–15% of patients with Hirschsprung's disease also have associated congenital anomalies like trisomy 21, tetrasomy 9p, and other serious neurologic abnormalities such as congenital central hypoventilation syndrome, neuroblastoma, and neural crest abnormalities [203–205].

Majority of the patients present in the neonatal period. Delayed passage of meconium is the most common form of clinical presentation in newborns. Chronic constipation, abdominal distention, and vomiting may be seen in infants and older children. A small subset of patients may also present as necrotizing enterocolitis or volvulus. However, rare cases have also been described in adults [206].

Failure of appropriate migration and survival of the neural crest-derived ganglion cell precursors within the bowel during embryogenesis is the main pathogenesis for Hirschsprung's disease [207, 208]. A number of genes such as *EDNRB*, *RST*, *EDN3*, *GDNF*, *SOX10*, *ECE1*, *NTN*, *ZEB2*, *PHOX2B*, *NRG1*, *TCF4*, and *KIAA1279* have been associated with pathogenesis of Hirschsprung's disease [209]. The familial forms of long- and short-segment disease are autosomal dominant with incomplete penetrance. The sporadic cases usually have a variable pattern of inheritance.

Pathological Features

On gross, the distal aperistaltic segment appears narrow and the proximal segment is widely dilated due to obstruction. Several forms of Hirschsprung's disease have been defined:

- *Classic Hirschsprung's disease*: The aganglionic segment begins in the distal colon/rectum and extends proximally for a variable distance into the adjoining dilated proximal bowel.
- *Short-segment Hirschsprung's disease*: The aganglionic segment involves several centimeters of the rectum and rectosigmoid colon.
- *Long-segment Hirschsprung's disease*: The entire colon is aganglionic, and it may also extend into the small bowel.
- *Zonal colonic aganglionosis (skip segment Hirschsprung's disease)*: Only a short segment of the colon is aganglionic, and ganglion cells are present both proximal and distal to the aganglionic segment.

On histology, there will be complete lack of ganglion cells in all neural plexuses with associated hypertrophy of the Schwannian nerve fibers. Immunostains such as neuron-specific enolase (NSE), Bcl-2, cathepsin D, protein gene product 9.5 (PGP9.5), and NeuN can be used to highlight the ganglion cells and as an adjunct for diagnosis of Hirschsprung's disease [210–213]. Of note, in routine surgical pathology practice, none of these markers offer significant advantage over thorough examination of H&E-stained sections. The use of acetylcholinesterase (AChE), on fresh frozen tissue to highlight the AChE-positive nerve fibers in the muscularis mucosae and the lamina propria in patients with Hirschsprung's disease, has now fallen out of favor in routine diagnostic surgical pathology. Calretinin immunostain on paraffin-embedded formalin fixed tissue has been shown to be superior to AChE for diagnosis of Hirschsprung's disease [214–216]. In normal colon, calretinin highlights the ganglion cells (nuclear staining) and also shows granular immunoreactivity within the nerve fibers in the lamina propria, muscularis mucosae, and submucosa (Fig. 18.26a, b). In patients with Hirschsprung's disease, there will be complete absence of staining for both ganglion cells and nerve

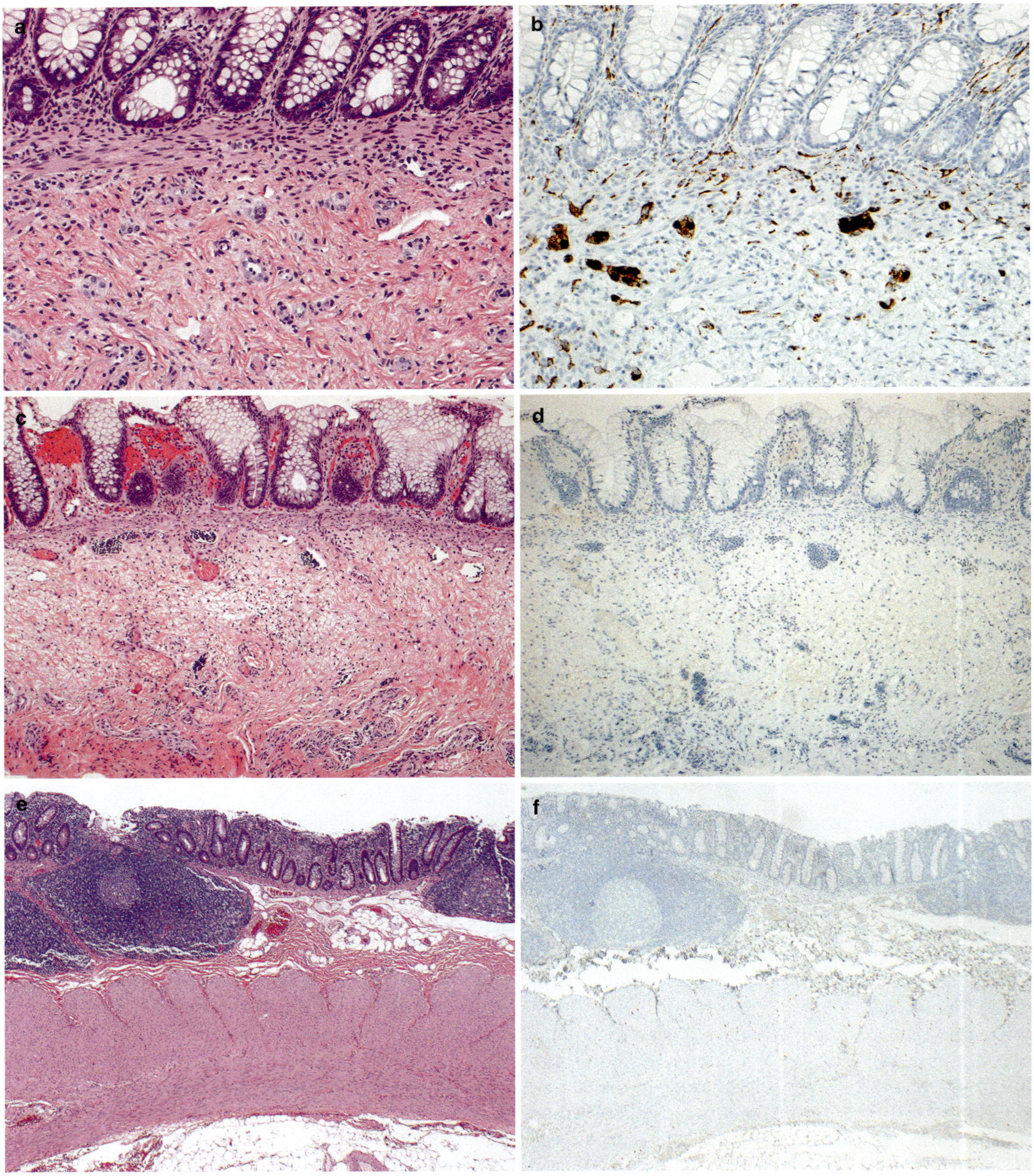

Fig. 18.26 Hirschsprung's disease. (**a**) Normal rectal mucosal biopsy shows presence of clusters of submucosal ganglion cells. (**b**) Calretinin immunostain highlights the submucosal ganglion cells and nerve twigs in mucosa and submucosa. (**c**) No submucosal ganglion cells are present in rectal biopsy from Hirschsprung's disease. (**d**) Calretinin immunostain is complete negative for ganglion cells or nerve twigs. (**e**) Section from aganglionic segment of Hirschsprung's disease shows absence of ganglion cells in submucosa and myenteric plexus. (**f**) Calretinin immunostain is negative for ganglion cells and nerve twigs

fibers (Fig. 18.26c, d). Hence, presence of any staining within the nerve fibers, even in the absence of ganglion cells, excludes the possibility of Hirschsprung's disease [217]. Whereas, a complete absence of staining on the calretinin stain would support a diagnosis of Hirschsprung's disease. Of note, calretinin stain can show positivity in mast cells, but this can be easily differentiated from the staining seen in nerve fibers and should not cause diagnostic problems.

A full-thickness transmural biopsy offers an ideal assessment of the neural plexus (Fig. 18.26e, f), but they require general anesthesia and are associated with risks of stricture and perforation. Hence, rectal suction mucosal biopsies are commonly obtained, used for preoperative diagnosis of Hirschsprung's disease. These biopsies should be obtained at least 2–3 cm above the pectinate (dentate) line, as there may be paucity of ganglion cells within 2 cm from the pectinate line [218]. The biopsies should also be >3 mm in diameter and at least 1/3 of its thickness should be submucosa [218]. More than two biopsies increase adequacy and minimize the false-negatives. The presence of anal squamous mucosa within the biopsy indicates proximity to the pectinate line and its presence should be specifically mentioned in the pathology report. Each laboratory should establish its own protocol for handling these cases, as a diagnosis of Hirschsprung's disease rests on absence of ganglion cells. At Mayo Clinic, we examine multiple serial sections on three slides and also perform a calretinin immunostain on all biopsies submitted for evaluation of Hirschsprung's disease.

Differential Diagnosis

The presence of ganglion cells in patients with clinical features of Hirschsprung's disease remains a diagnostic challenge. The differential diagnosis for these cases includes intestinal neuronal dysplasia (which itself is a controversial entity), meconium ileus, intestinal malformations, hypoganglionosis, and intestinal pseudoobstruction.

Treatment and Prognosis

Treatment usually includes surgical excision of the involved bowel segment and restoration of the bowel continuity. The prognosis in most surgically treated cases is excellent.

Hypoganglionosis

Intestinal hypoganglionosis is very rare and accounts for 3–5% of all classified congenital intestinal innervation disorders [219]. It refers to reduced number of ganglia in the neural plexuses, decreased number of ganglion cells per ganglion, and reduced size of ganglia [220]. The patients most commonly present in infancy or childhood with only a few cases reported in adults [221, 222]. Presenting symptoms include chronic constipation and/or enterocolitis. The histopathological features include hypertrophy of the muscularis mucosae, decrease in the activity of AChE in the lamina propria, and significant reduction in the number of myenteric ganglia (Fig. 18.27) [219]. Hypoganglionosis can be focal, segmental, or diffuse. There are no uniformly accepted criteria for what constitutes hypoganglionosis. It has been suggested that hypertrophic nerves with large gaps between ganglia, in particular when flanked or interrupted by tiny ganglia containing only 1–2 ganglion cells, are suggestive of hypoganglionosis [218]. As occasional cases of colon resections performed for unrelated reasons, patients without any motility issues can show reduced or fewer number of ganglion cells. This questions the validity of evaluating ganglion cell numbers in patients with motility disorders. The treatment and long-term outcome of hypoganglionosis is similar to Hirschsprung's disease.

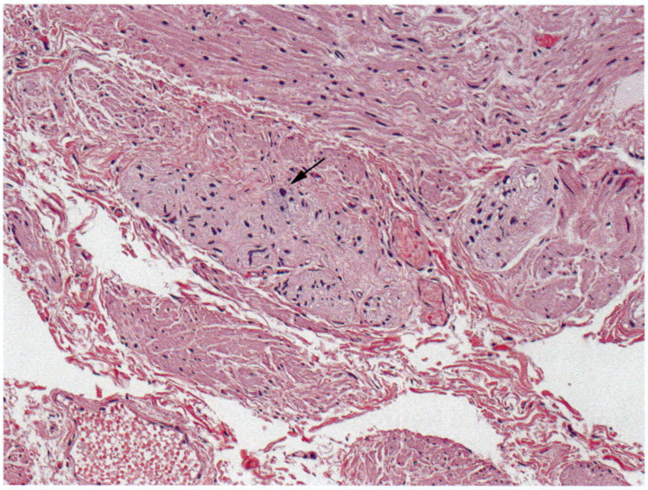

Fig. 18.27 Intestinal hypoganglionosis. A full-thickness transmural biopsy shows significant reduction in the number of ganglions (arrow) in myenteric plexus

Hyperganglionosis

Hyperganglionosis is defined as an increase in number of ganglion cells and neural hyperplasia. It is also known as intestinal neuronal dysplasia (IND). IND-A and IND-B are the two forms hyperganglionosis [223].

IND-A constitutes less than 5% of cases of IND and it is extremely rare. It is usually seen in neonates and infants. The patients present with diarrhea, bloody stools, and intestinal obstruction. Histologically, it is characterized by increased number of ganglion cells in each ganglion (myenteric hyperplasia), sympathetic aplasia, and inflammation within the colon [224]. Surgical excision is usually curative.

IND-B is a controversial entity and considered to be an anomaly of the parasympathetic neural system of the bowel. It is characterized by increased number of large ganglion cells in the submucosal neural plexuses and prominent neural hyperplasia (Fig. 18.28). It constitutes 95% of all IND cases. Patients present with chronic constipation. Current diagnostic criteria are based solely on the proportion of "giant submucosal ganglia," defined as more than eight ganglion cells per ganglion in a 15-μm-thick frozen section stained histochemically with lactate dehydrogenase (LDH) to highlight mature and immature ganglion cells [225]. They require that the biopsy should be obtained at least 8 cm proximal to the pectinate line, a minimum of 25 submucosal ganglia must be analyzed, more than 20% of submucosal ganglia must be giant ganglia, a giant ganglion contains more than eight nerve cell cross sections, and the patient should be older than 1year [225]. Conservative medical therapy with laxatives is the first line of treatment, and surgery is reserved for cases that do not respond to medical treatment. Anal sphincter myomectomy appears to be helpful in some patients, and only rare patients require partial or complete colectomy [226].

Familial Visceral Neuropathies

This group of genetic diseases is rare and characterized by pseudoobstruction, myenteric plexus abnormalities, variable inheritance patterns, and extraintestinal manifestations. On microscopy, the nerves appear vacuolated, and ganglion cells show discrete eosinophilic intranuclear inclusions [227].

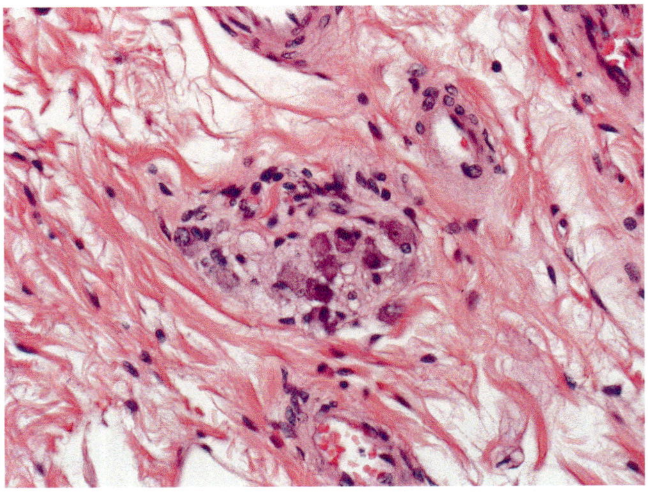

Fig. 18.28 Intestinal neuronal dysplasia (IND-B). The submucosal ganglion shows increased number (>8) of ganglion cells

Muscle Disorders

Both familial and sporadic forms of myopathic forms have been described [228]. The familial form may also involve other organs (such as hepatobiliary tract or genitourinary tract). Smooth muscle degeneration is assumed to be responsible for the underlying disease, although the pathogenesis in most cases is not well understood.

The patients can present in childhood or adulthood. Presenting symptoms include intestinal pseudoobstruction, constipation, abdominal pain, and dysphagia. On gross examination, the involved segment of the colon is often dilated. Ulceration and ischemic injury may be seen in the mucosa [228].

On histology, there would be degeneration and fibrous replacement of the smooth muscle. Degenerative changes such as cytoplasmic vacuoles, variation in the size of the muscle fiber, and fibrosis are seen in the muscularis propria and they may also involve the muscularis mucosae. There may also be thinning of the bowel wall. The fibrosis may be subtle to appreciate on the H&E stain and a trichrome stain is useful in highlighting the fibrosis. Other changes such as variation in the nuclear size, increased mitotic activity, and hyperchromasia may also be seen. The muscle fibers may also show amphophilic inclusions which are PAS negative and most likely represent degenerating smooth muscle fibers [229]. Rare cases of familial visceral myopathy may show alpha-actin cytoplasmic inclusions (Fig. 18.29a, b), and they are best highlighted with the alpha-actin immunostain [230].

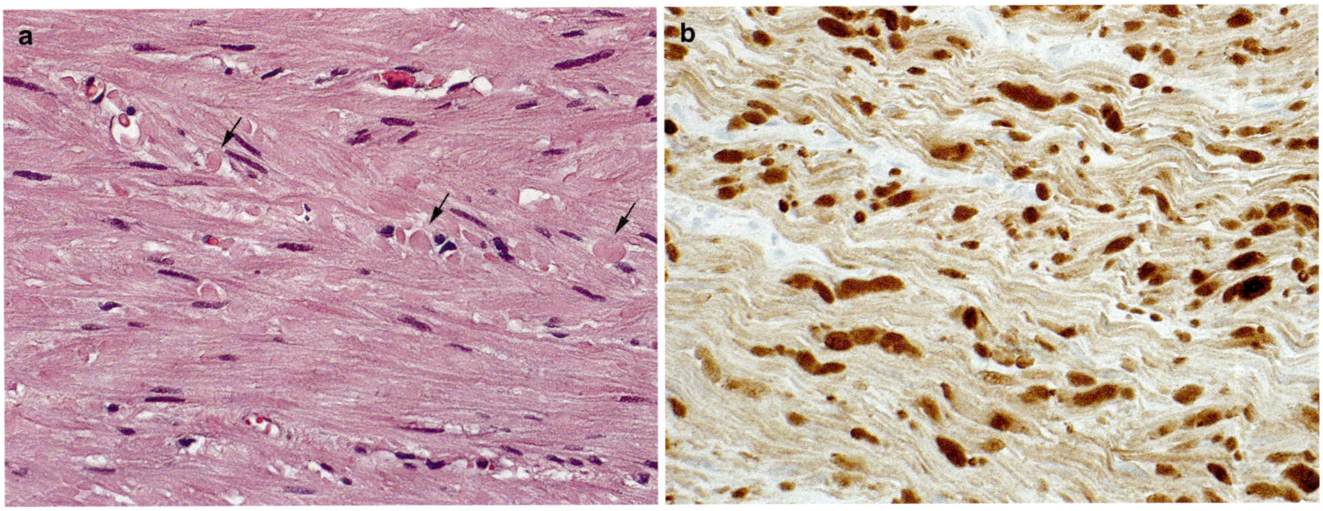

Fig. 18.29 Visceral myopathy. (**a**) Eosinophilic cytoplasmic inclusions (arrows) are present in muscularis propria in a case with familial visceral myopathy.(**b**) Immunostain for smoothelin highlights the cytoplasmic inclusions

The inner circular muscle layer of the muscularis propria may show absence of staining with smooth muscle actin immunostain in cases with deficient smooth muscle alpha actin [231, 232]. Of note, artifactual changes such as cytoplasmic pseudo-inclusions, vacuolation, and thinning of the muscle layers may also be seen in colonic resections. Radiation and chronic ischemia may also cause fibrosis and thinning of the muscularis propria. Measuring the ratio and relative thickness of the circular and longitudinal muscle layers has little practical value, as their thickness varies amongst individuals, method of sectioning, and anatomic location.

Mitochondrial disorders may show both myopathic and neuropathic changes. Some cases may show muscle atrophy and increased number of abnormal-appearing mitochondria in the ganglion cells and muscle cells. Megamitochondria may also be seen in the ganglion cells [233]. However, a subset of them may not show any significant abnormality on H&E-stained sections.

Colonic Pseudoobstruction

Intestinal pseudoobstruction is an uncommon syndrome characterized by acute, recurrent, or chronic symptoms suggestive of obstruction of the large intestine without any radiologic, surgical, or endoscopic evidence of mechanical obstruction. It is caused by disorders causing impairment of intrinsic neuromuscular or extrinsic control of gut motility [228, 234]. The clinical presentation depends on the regions of the gut affected, the time course of the disease, and the presence of any extraintestinal effects.

Acute colonic pseudoobstruction syndrome (also called Ogilvie's syndrome) is often associated with significant extraintestinal illnesses, and its underlying pathophysiology still remains largely unknown. It usually occurs after abdominal surgery or abdominal trauma and the entire bowel becomes paralyzed and distended [234]; and they are usually seen in patients in the sixth decade of life and more common in males. Clinical features closely mimic acute large-bowel obstruction, and the patients may present with colicky abdominal pain, abdominal distention, constipation, nausea, and vomiting. No specific histological features are associated with this condition. Perforation occurs most commonly in the cecum and results from progressive distention and local ischemia. The diagnosis is usually clinical and the treatment is supportive.

Chronic colonic pseudoobstruction is also called colonic inertia or slow-transit constipation. It is manifested mainly by constipation (defined as two or fewer bowel movements per week). It may be caused by extrinsic denervation (e.g., multiple sclerosis, spinal cord injury) or an intrinsic neuropathy (suggested by deficiencies of substance P, calcitonin gene-related peptide [CGRP], and other peptidergic neurotransmitters in the myenteric plexus) [235, 236]. ICC have also been proposed to play a role in the pathophysiologic mechanism of chronic colonic pseudoobstruction [237, 238]. It usually affects children (up to 10 years) and adult women. On gross, the intestinal wall may appear contracted, thickened, and markedly stenotic (Fig. 18.30a). On histology, melanosis coli is a common finding. The myenteric plexus may show decreased neuronal processes, immature neurons, and clusters of variably sized intraganglionic nuclei (Fig. 18.30b) [239–242]. Some patients may also show increase in neuronal supporting tissues highlighted by the S100 immunostain. A subset of patients may also show a significantly lower ratio of thickness of the circular to longitudinal muscle [243]. The smooth muscle cells may show hyaline cytoplasmic inclusions and abnormal staining patterns for muscle markers such as desmin and smoothelin. However, it is very subjective and difficult to quantify muscle hypertrophy or neural hyperplasia and it is also unclear if these changes are primary or secondary in nature. Of all these changes, the reduced number of ICC appears to be the only consistent finding in most cases. The CD117 immunostain may show significantly reduced ICC and enteric neurofilaments in all three layers of the muscularis propria, and this reduction may be most significant in the inner circular muscle layer (Fig. 18.30c). A cutoff value of 7 ICC per high-power field in the inner circular muscle layer has been proposed as a further confirmation to the clinical diagnosis of chronic colonic pseudoobstruction in surgically resected specimens [244]. Surgical intervention is usually the treatment of choice.

Motility Disorders in Systemic Diseases

A number of systemic disorders such as scleroderma, diabetes, and amyloidosis can cause intestinal dysmotility. Patients with scleroderma show collagen replacement of the muscle layer, especially the inner circular layer (Fig. 18.31a, b) [228]. Fibrosis of the muscularis propria can lead to muscle weakness, resulting in diverticula. However, in scleroderma, the disease involvement is predominantly seen in the esophagus. Many patients with diabetes, especially type 1 diabetes, develop diarrhea, constipation, and delayed intestinal transit [245]. These changes are related to visceral neuropathy involving the parasympathetic or sympathetic nervous system and microangiopathy. The colon may show dilatation, markedly thickened muscularis propria, fibrosis within the muscle fibers, and vascular changes including fibrinoid necrosis. Patients with amyloidosis can show amyloid deposition in the muscularis propria (myopathy) or neural plexuses (neuropathy) and may present as intestinal pseudoobstruction [246, 247].

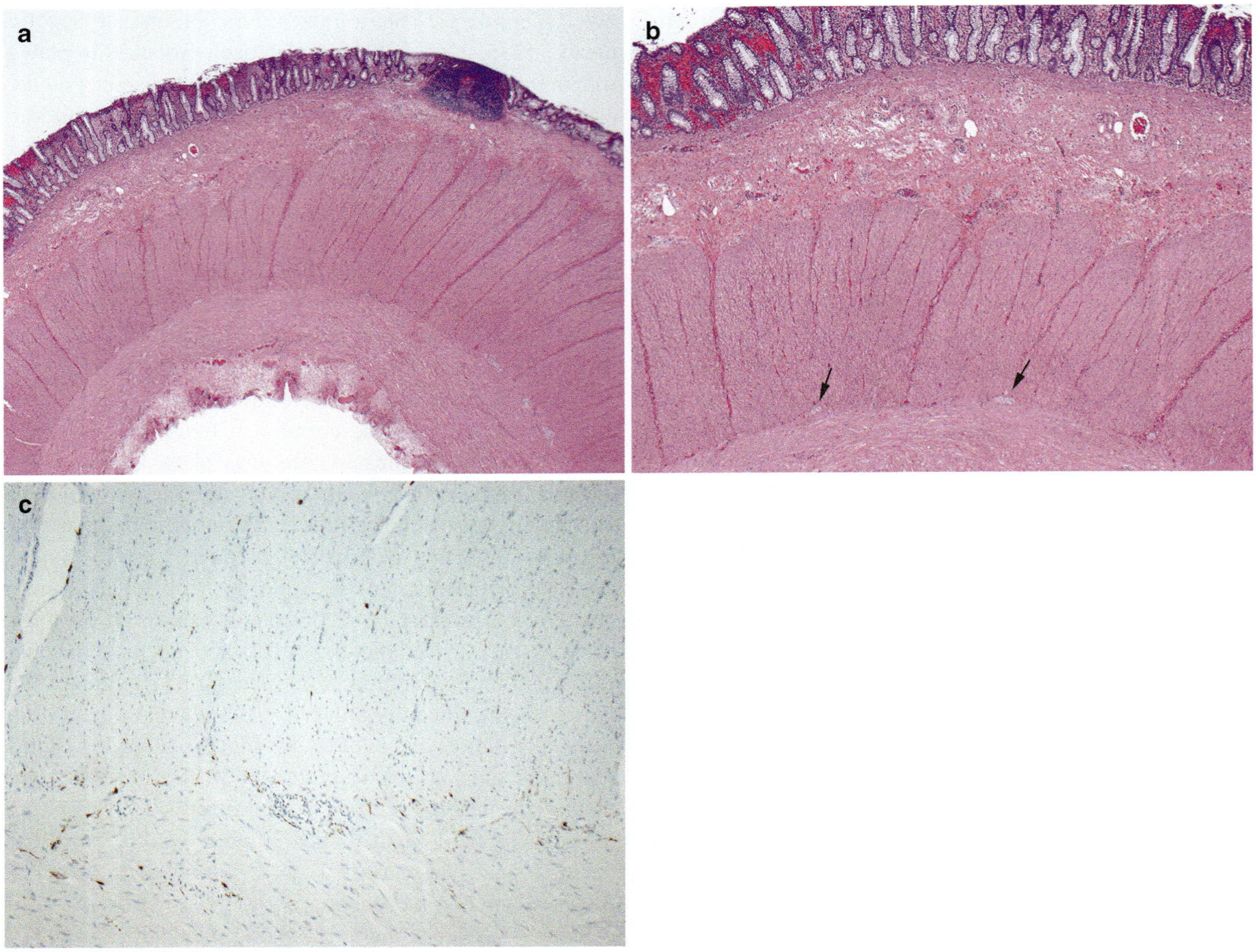

Fig. 18.30 Chronic colonic pseudoobstruction. (**a**) The muscularis propria appears to be hypertrophic in a patient with colonic inertia. (**b**) The myenteric plexuses are small in size (arrows). (**c**) CD117 immunostain shows significantly reduced ICC of the muscularis propria

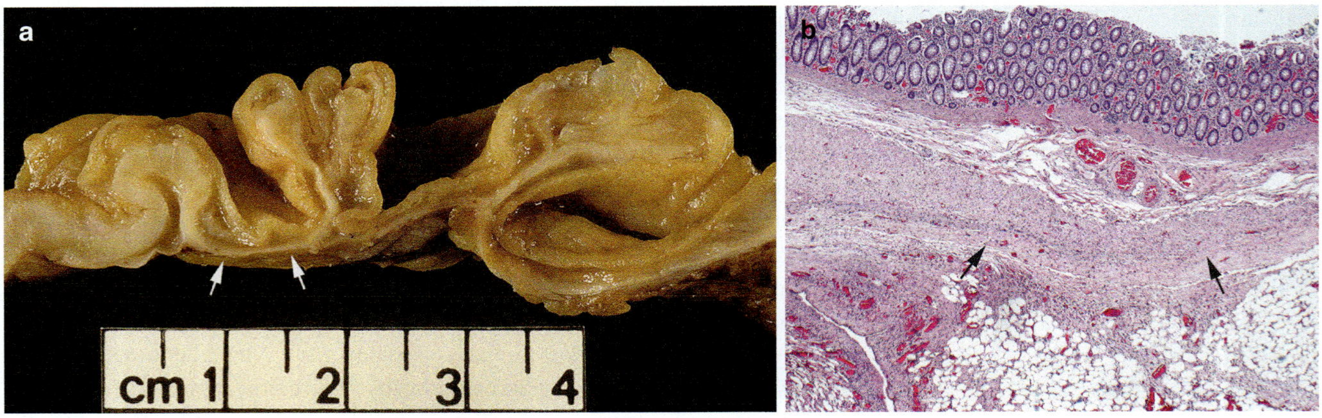

Fig. 18.31 Scleroderma. (**a**) A cross section of colon from a patient with scleroderma shows marked thinning of muscularis propria (arrows) in affected colon. (**b**) Histological section shows marked atrophy of both inner and outer layers of muscularis propria (arrows) in the colon affected by scleroderma

Polypoid Lesions

Colonic polyp is any growth that projects into the intestinal lumen above the mucosal surface. The term polyp by itself has no clinical significance. They vary in size, shape, and nature of behavior. They may be single or multiple, benign or malignant, congenital or acquired, symptomatic or asymptomatic, neoplastic or nonneoplastic, and sessile or pedunculated. Histopathological examination of the polyp remains the gold standard of determining the type of polyp and whether it is neoplastic or nonneoplastic in nature. Macroscopic characterization of a colon polyp is of limited value in determining patient management [248, 249].

Inflammatory Polyp

Inflammatory polyps are mucosal projections composed of a mixture of inflammatory cells, stromal component, and epithelial cells. They are also known as inflammatory pseudopolyps. They usually develop in response to either localized disorders such as infectious colitis or ischemic colitis or could be related to diffuse inflammatory diseases such as inflammatory bowel disease [250–253].

These polyps are usually less than 2 cm in size and they can be sessile or pedunculated. However, a subset of them can grow larger in size and even cause colonic obstruction [252–254]. Filiform polyposis is a distinctive but rare benign nonsyndromic polyposis that is occasionally encountered in the colon of patients with inflammatory bowel disease or rarely outside the setting of inflammatory bowel disease [255, 256]. Filiform polyposis is characterized by one to hundreds, slender, arborizing, vermiform projections in the colon. Inflammatory polyps on histology are composed of a mixture of inflamed lamina propria, architectural distortion of the colonic mucosa with cryptitis and crypt abscesses (Fig. 18.32a). Surface erosions and ulcerations may be seen, and some of these polyps may be composed entirely of inflamed granulation tissue.

The inflamed colonic epithelium can show significant reactive epithelial atypia which can mimic a dysplastic or neoplastic process. However, this reactive epithelial atypia would be usually concentrated at the base of the crypts with adequate surface maturation and this should be helpful in distinguishing it from "true" dysplasia. Of note, rare inflammatory polyps may develop dysplasia [257]. Occasionally, enlarged multinucleated stromal cells may also be seen in inflammatory polyps mimicking a sarcoma (pseudosarcomatous change, Fig. 18.32b) [258].

The inflammatory polyps can be difficult to distinguish from juvenile polyps on histology due to significant morphological overlap between both. This distinction can be done largely on the clinical information.

Inflammatory cap polyp and cap polyposis is a rare condition in which the patient presents with diarrhea or constipation, mucoid stools, and blood in stools [259–261]. Endoscopy shows multiple small sessile or semi-pedunculated polyps usually less than 2 cm within the rectosigmoid colon. Rarely, they may be seen involving the entire colon. Histology shows inflamed lamina propria, dilated distorted colonic crypts, and a distinctive "cap" of inflamed and ulcerated granulation tissue. The mainstay of initial treatment is conservative; however, symptomatic and complicated cases require surgical intervention.

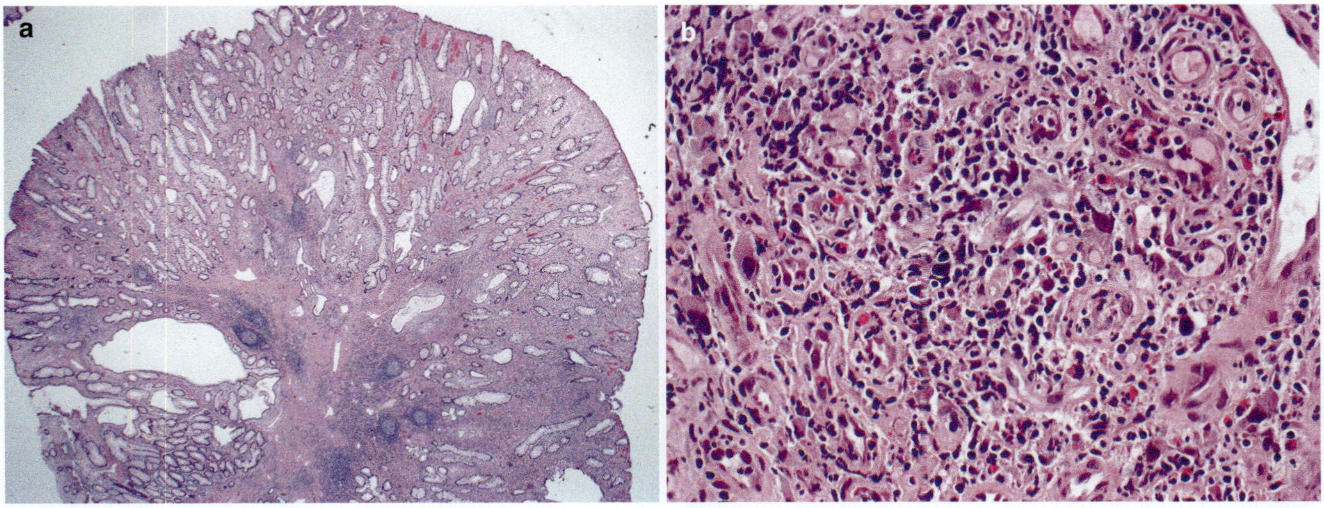

Fig. 18.32 Inflammatory polyp. (**a**) A polypoid colonic mucosa shows cystic dilatation of crypts, inflammation and edema in lamina propria. (**b**) Enlarged hyperchromatic stromal cells (pseudosarcomatous change) within granulation tissue are present in inflammatory polyp

Peutz-Jeghers Polyp (PJP)

The PJPs usually vary in size between 0.5 and 5 cm and they are often pedunculated (Fig. 18.33a). Microscopically, they show a prominent and distinctive arborizing architecture composed of prominent bands of smooth muscle derived from the underlying muscularis mucosae (Fig. 18.33b). The overlying epithelium is composed of normal-appearing colonic epithelium which may show epithelial hyperplasia and overgrowth. The lamina propria typically does not show increased inflammation. The background colonic mucosa is also usually unremarkable. Dysplasia is unusual, but a small subset of these polyps can develop dysplastic change that can progress to carcinoma [262, 263].

A subset of PJPs may show foci of epithelial misplacement or "pseudoinvasion" into the underlying stroma or intestinal wall, simulating invasive adenocarcinoma. However, the lack of a desmoplastic stromal reaction, lack of cytologic atypia, presence of laminal propria around the deep displaced crypts, and hemosiderin deposition should help in making the distinction between "pseudoinvasion" and invasive adenocarcinoma.

Surveillance guidelines for PJP are empiric recommended that upper gastrointestinal endoscopy, video capsule endoscopy, and colonoscopy are recommended first at age 8 years. If polyps are found, the examination should be repeated every 3 years. If none are found, a second baseline examination should be done at age 18 years and then every 3 years thereafter. Treatment involves colonoscopic removal of polyps (probably all those >0.5 or 1 cm in diameter). Clearing of all polyps is preferable. Colectomy is sometimes necessary to control colonic polyps and especially if neoplastic change is found in colonic polyps [264].

Juvenile Polyp

Juvenile polyps of the colon usually measure less than 2 cm in size and can be pedunculated or sessile in nature. Isolated or sporadic juvenile polyps are most commonly seen in the rectosigmoid colon. However, in juvenile polyposis coli, they can be as many as 200 polyps involving the colon (Fig. 18.34a). Microscopically, they show abundant distorted and mucus-filled dilated colonic crypts with excess of lamina propria showing edema and inflammation (Fig. 18.34b, c). The stroma/epithelium ratio is abnormally greater than normal. Only occasional strands of smooth muscle fibers may be seen within the lamina propria. Surface erosions are frequent, causing bleeding and anemia. A subset of patients may also show larger, villiform, and multilobulated polyps which may give a gross appearance of several polyps attached to a single stalk. Ganglioneuromatous proliferations composed of nerve bundle and mature ganglion cells as well as tubular adenomas may also be seen in patients with juvenile polyposis syndrome. Dysplasia may be seen in up to 30% of polyps in patients with juvenile polyposis syndrome, but dysplasia is almost nonexistent in isolated or sporadic juvenile polyps [265, 266].

There are no morphological features that can help separate sporadic/isolated juvenile polyps that are unassociated with a syndrome from syndromic juvenile polyps. The juvenile polyps can mimic inflammatory polyps and may be indistinguishable from pseudopolyps arising in the setting of inflammatory bowel disease.

Patients with sporadic/isolated juvenile polyps have no increased risk for malignancy and hence do not require follow-up [267, 268]. On the other hand, patients with juvenile polyposis syndrome have a 40% risk of developing colorec-

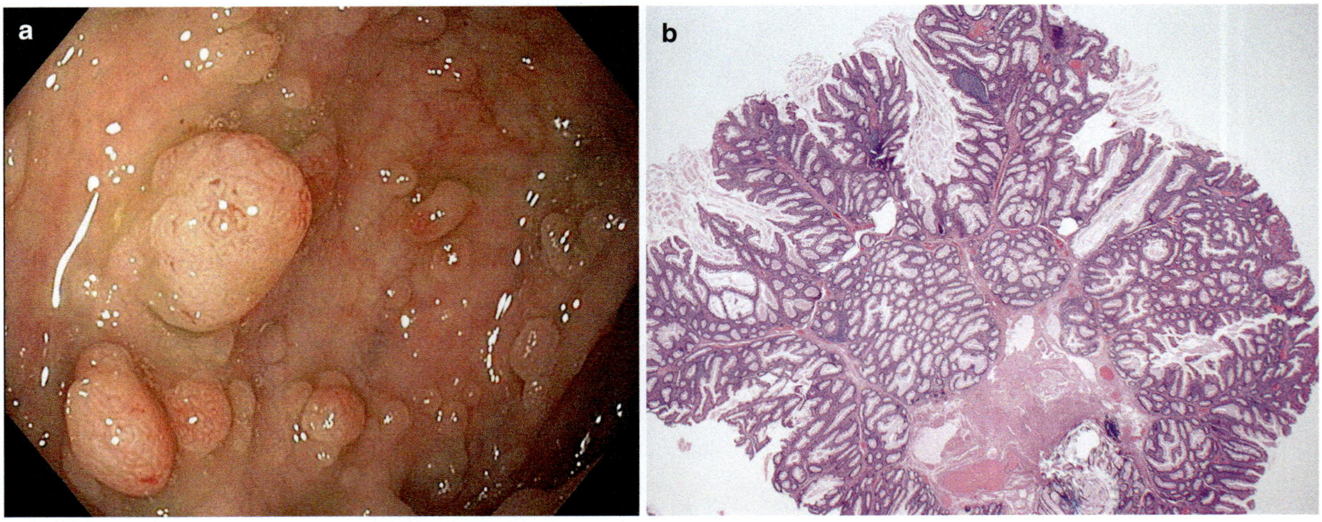

Fig. 18.33 Peutz-Jeghers polyp. (**a**) Colonoscopy shows multiple variable-sized polyps present in the colon in a patient with Peutz-Jeghers syndrome. (**b**) Histological section of a Peutz-Jeghers polyp shows prominent arborizing smooth muscle bands derived from the underlying muscularis mucosae

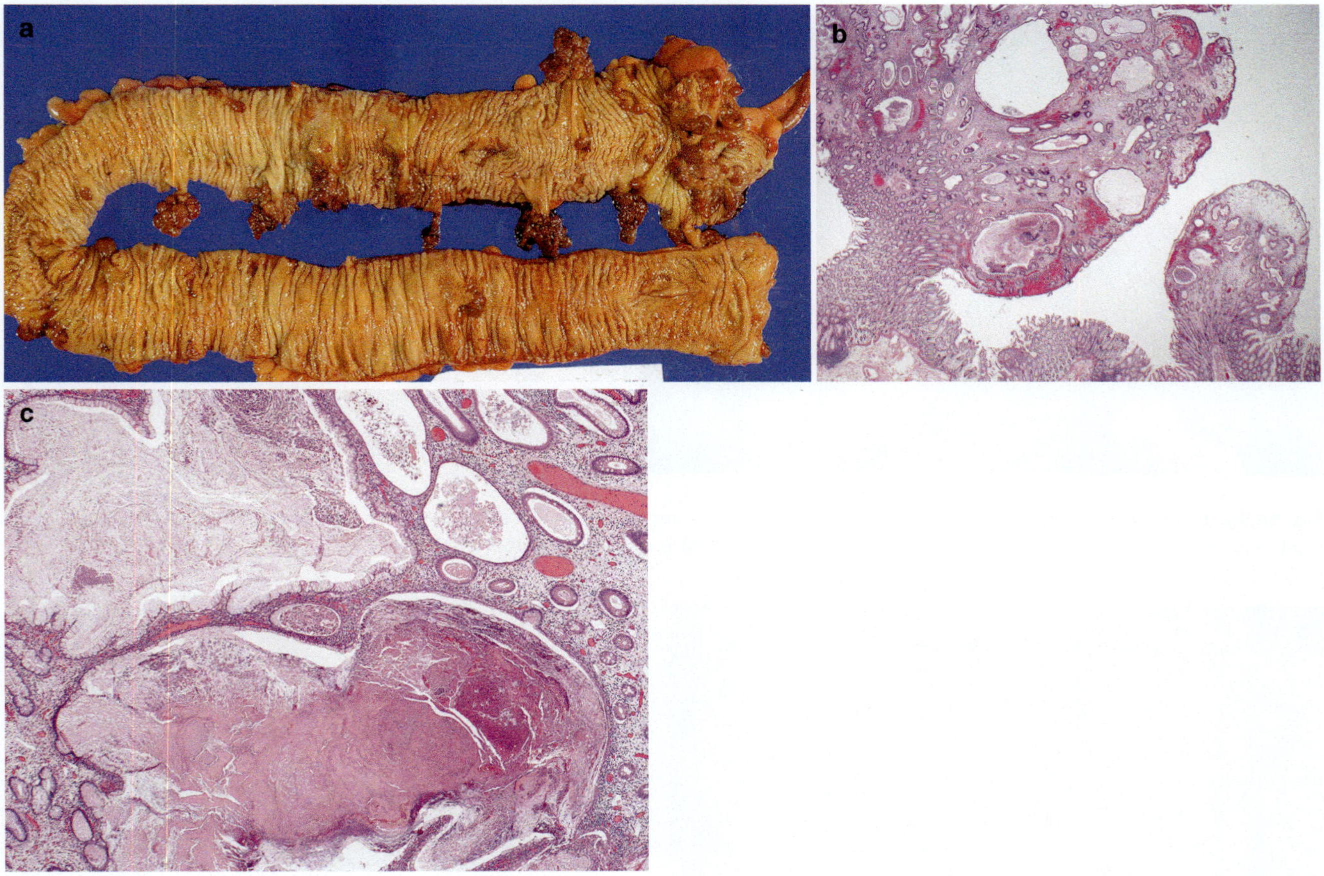

Fig. 18.34 Juvenile polyp. (**a**) A total colectomy specimen shows multiple pedunculated and multilobulated juvenile polyps. (**b**) The juvenile polyps show abundant distorted and dilated colonic glands with prominent lamina propria edema. (**c**) Higher-power view of dilated colonic crypt filled with mucin and inflammatory cells

tal carcinoma [269]. Colonoscopy should be performed annually, beginning at age 12 years or earlier if symptoms occur, especially rectal bleeding. It should be repeated every 1–3 years, depending on polyp burden and polyps ≥5 mm should be removed [264].

Cronkhite-Canada Syndrome (CCS)

The polyposis in CCS involves the entire gastrointestinal tract except the esophagus [270, 271]. The polyps range in size from a few millimeters to 1.5 cm (Fig. 18.35a). On histology, the CCS polyps have a hamartomatous appearance. They show cystically dilated colonic crypts, edematous lamina propria with mild mononuclear inflammation (Fig. 18.35b). A prominent mast cell, eosinophilic, or IgG4-positive plasma cell infiltrate may be seen [270, 272–275]. The CCS polyps are microscopically indistinguishable from colonic juvenile polyps [274]. However, the most important microscopic finding that distinguishes CCS from juvenile polyposis syndrome is the presence of lamina propria edema, gland/crypt architectural distortion, and inflammation in the intervening endoscopically/macroscopically normal-appearing nonpolypoid colonic mucosa. The intervening nonpolypoid mucosa in juvenile polyposis syndrome is normal.

CCS polyps are considered nonneoplastic with controversial malignant potential, although rare cases of adenoma and colorectal carcinoma have been reported [276–279].

Cowden Syndrome

Up to 90% of patients with Cowden syndrome have colorectal polyps [280–282]. Most of the patients are asymptomatic and these polyps are diagnosed at screening colonoscopy. More than half of the patients have more than 50 colonic polyps, usually affecting the entire colon (Fig. 18.36a) [283]. These colon polyps are of hamartomatous type and usually small and sessile. They can be easily overlooked as insignificant benign non-classifiable mesenchymal polyps. They can appear as lesions with relatively preserved or mildly abnormal crypt architecture, lamina propria that shows bland spindle cells arranged in a concentric manner around cross-cut crypts, some adipose tissue, and lymphoid hyperplasia [284].

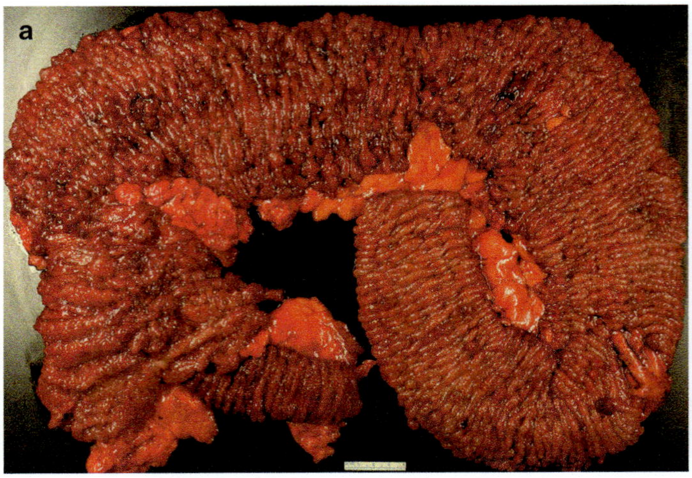

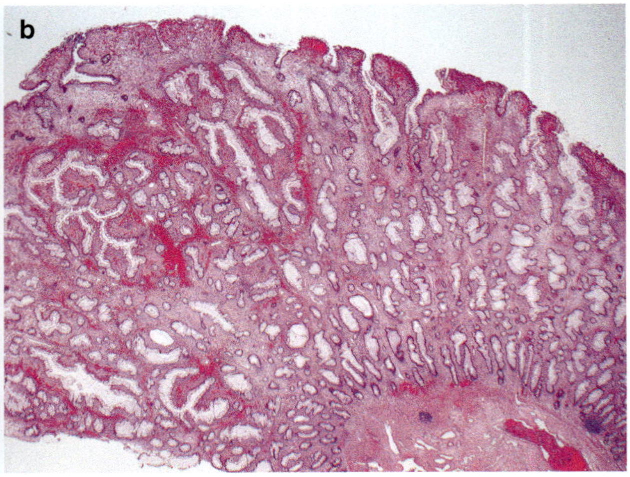

Fig. 18.35 Cronkhite-Canada syndrome.(**a**) Numerous small polyps are present in this total colectomy from a patient with Cronkhite-Canada syndrome. (**b**)The polyp shows cystically dilated colonic crypts and edematous lamina propria

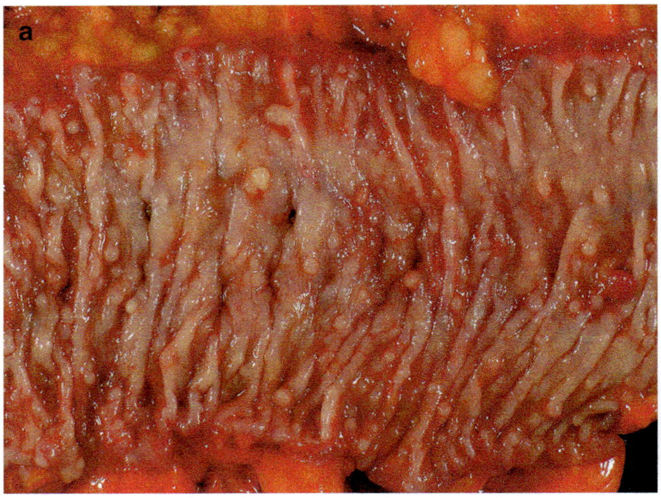

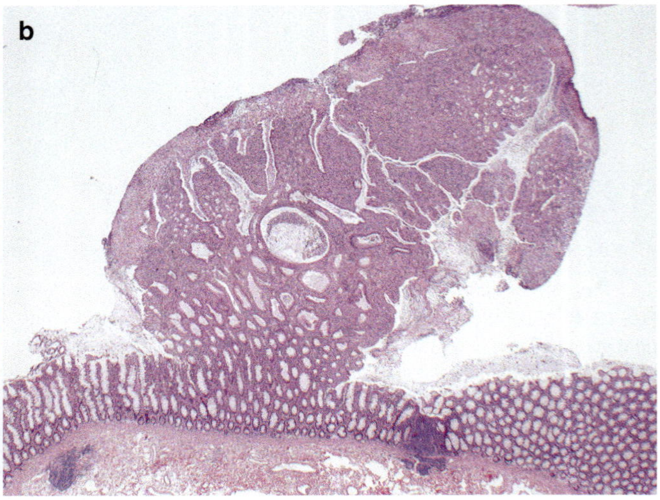

Fig. 18.36 Cowden syndrome. (**a**) Multiple small and sessile polyps in resected colon from a patient with Cowden syndrome. (**b**) Hamartomatous type polyp with cystically dilated colonic crypts and prominent granulation in the lamina propria

Some polyps may resemble juvenile polyps (Fig. 18.36b). Polyps such as ganglioneuroma, lipoma, fibrolipoma, inflammatory polyp, tubular adenoma, and hyperplastic polyp may also be seen in patients with Cowden syndrome [283, 285–288]. A recent study has shown that intramucosal lipomas are an important diagnostic feature of Cowden syndrome [289]. About a third of their patients with intramucosal lipomas (Fig. 18.37) had Cowden syndrome. Hence, increased awareness of this lesion by pathologists should be useful for diagnosis of Cowden syndrome. According to another recent study, the most distinctive features of Cowden syndrome hamartomatous polyps compared with other hamartomatous polyps include colonic predominance, small size, nonexophytic configuration, absence of inflammation in the lamina propria, absence of cystic glands filled with mucin, presence of nerve fibers, smooth muscle, ganglion cells, and adipose tissue in the lamina propria [288].

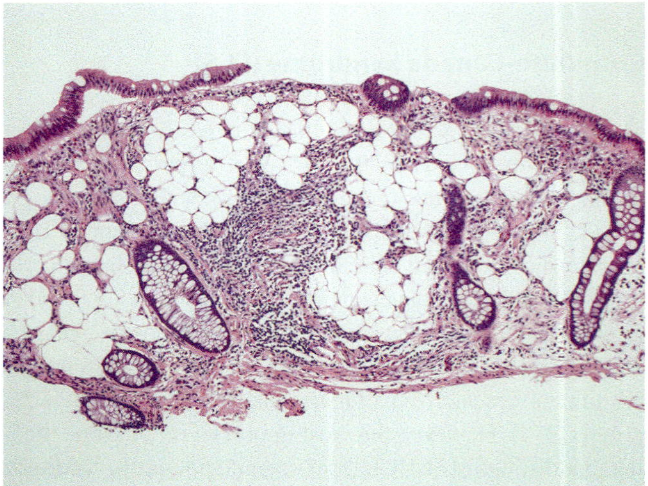

Fig. 18.37 Intramucosal lipoma in Cowden syndrome. The colonic polyp shows aggregates of adipose tissue and lymphoid aggregate between colonic crypts

The lifetime risk for colonic adenocarcinoma in patients with Cowden syndrome with PTEN mutations is 10–15% [282, 290]. Colonoscopy is recommended starting at the age of 15 years and repeated every 2 years [264].

Miscellaneous Disorders

IgG4-Related Disease in Colon

IgG4-related disease is a steroid responsive systemic condition characterized by storiform fibrosis, obliterative phlebitis, and lymphoplasmacytic infiltrate including increased IgG4-positive plasma cells. Most patients also have elevated serum IgG4 levels [291, 292]. Involvement of the colon by IgG4-related disease is extremely rare. Hiyoshi et al. reported a case of a 74-year-old female who underwent right hemicolectomy for a lesion within the ileocecal region [293]. The resected specimen showed subserosal sclerosis and an increased number of IgG4-positive plasma cells (150/HPF) and an elevated IgG4/IgG ratio (50%), leading to a diagnosis of IgG4-related disease. Chetty et al. have reported well-circumscribed sclerosing nodules containing IgG4-positive plasma cells within the colon presenting as mucosal polypoid lesions [294]. Rarely, IgG4-related disease of the colon may mimic Crohn's disease [295].

Melanosis Coli

Melanosis coli is the deposition of lipofuscin pigment in macrophages within the colonic lamina propria. Any segment of the colon can be involved, but it usually affects the proximal colon more often than the left colon (Fig. 18.38a). It is a frequent incidental finding in colonic biopsies. However, melanosis coli usually spares tubular adenomas and hyperplastic polyps as it has been hypothesized that within these lesions the apoptotic fragments remain in the neoplastic epithelium or are lost intraluminally and do not reach the lamina propria [296]. Macrophages filled with brown pigment are seen within the lamina propria (Fig. 18.38b). The pigment can stain with PAS stain. The basic mechanism is related to increased epithelial apoptosis [297]. Damage to the colonic epithelial cells results in increased apoptosis, formation of lysosomal bodies, and ingestion by macrophages which ultimately leads to lipofuscin-containing macrophages. Chronic use of anthraquinone laxative has also been attributed with melanosis coli. Other causes of increased apoptosis, such as NSAIDs and inflammatory bowel disease, are additional etiologies for melanosis coli [297–299].

Endometriosis and Endosalpingiosis

Endometriosis is a presence of endometrial glands and/or stroma outside the uterus. It is typically seen in young to middle-aged women and commonly involves the rectosigmoid colon. The patients are usually asymptomatic, but a subset can present with abdominal pain due to adhesions. It can also manifest as a mass lesion or polyps [300, 301]. Rare cases may also manifest as volvulus or acute colonic obstruction [302, 303]. On gross examination, the foci of endometriosis appear sclerotic with punctate hemorrhagic areas. On microscopy, the endometrial glands are composed of bland longitudinal nuclei with apical cilia, surrounded by stroma composed of bland spindle cells and thin-walled capillaries (Fig. 18.39a). Red blood cells, hemorrhage, and hemosiderin-laden macrophages are often intermingled within the foci of endometriosis. In addition, fibrosis and prominent smooth muscle proliferation

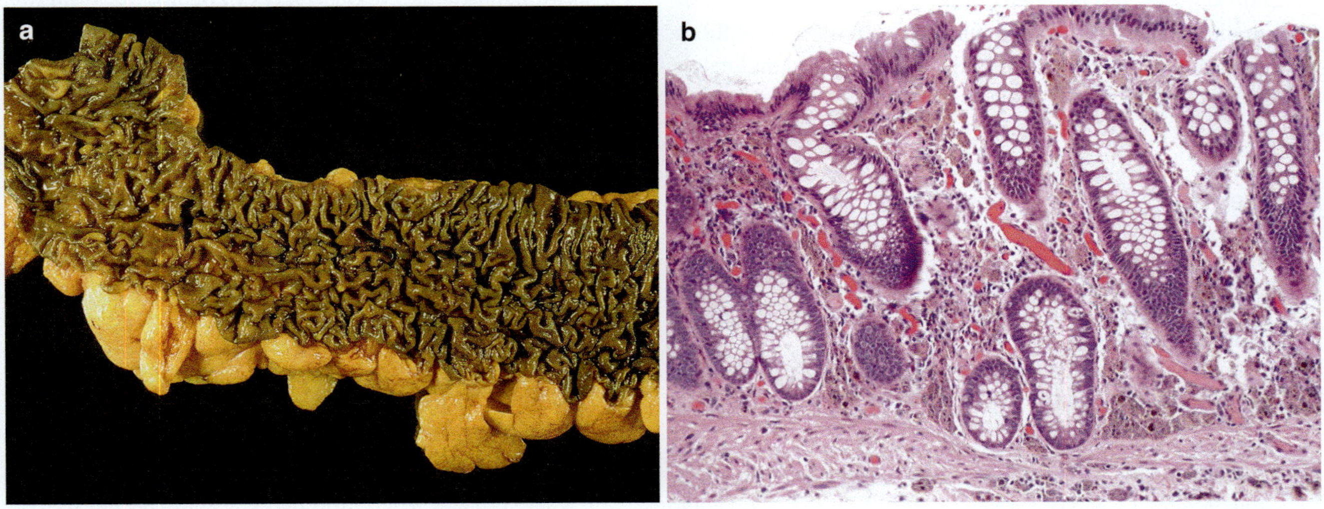

Fig. 18.38 Melanosis coli. (**a**) Melanosis coli is present in this resected proximal colon, the colonic mucosa shows dark brown discoloration. (**b**) Numerous macrophages filled with brown pigments are present in the lamina propria

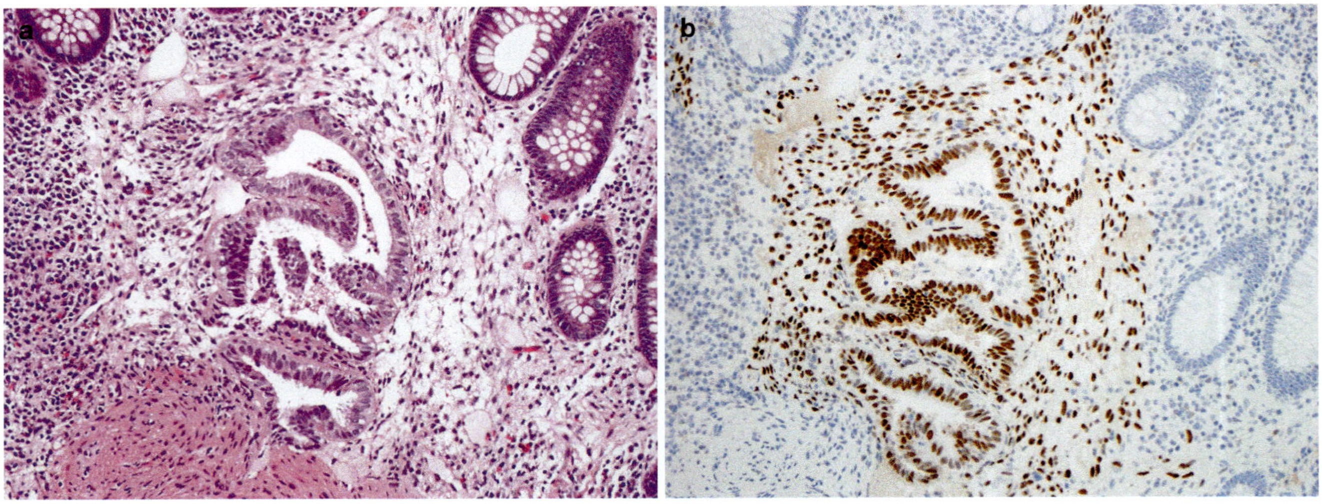

Fig. 18.39 Endometriosis. (**a**) Colonic biopsy shows a focus of endometrial glands composed of bland longitudinal nuclei with apical cilia, surrounded by ovarian-type stroma composed of bland spindle cells. (**b**) Both the endometrial glands and ovarian-type stroma are positive for immunostain for estrogen receptor

may surround the foci of endometriosis. Endometriosis is usually present on the serosal surface, but may also involve the muscularis propria and submucosa. The epithelial cells are positive for estrogen receptor, progesterone receptor, and PAX8 immunostains, while the stroma labels with CD10 (Fig. 18.39b). The differential diagnosis includes invasive adenocarcinoma and this can be really problematic to differentiate on small biopsies or frozen section. The glandular epithelium may show nuclear atypia mimicking an adenocarcinoma, but the presence of hemorrhage, hemosiderin-laden macrophages, and stromal cells should help in establishing the correct diagnosis. Endometriosis is usually treated with hormone therapy and analgesics. Severe cases with extensive adhesions or obstruction may require surgical excision. Of note, rare cases of endometriosis may undergo malignant transformation and have an associated carcinoma [304, 305].

Endosalpingiosis is characterized by the presence of benign glands lined by ciliated tubal-type epithelium without endometrial stroma. It can rarely involve the colon and result in intestinal obstruction [306].

References

1. Pirmohamed M, James S, Meakin S, Green C, Scott AK, Walley TJ, et al. Adverse drug reactions as cause of admission to hospital: prospective analysis of 18 820 patients. Br Med J. 2004;329(7456):15–9.
2. Bjarnason I, Hayllar J, Macpherson ANJ, Russell ANS. Side effects of nonsteroidal anti-inflammatory drugs on the small and large intestine in humans. Gastroenterology. 1993;104(6):1832–47.
3. Jaszewski R. Frequency of gastroduodenal lesions in asymptomatic patients on chronic aspirin or nonsteroidal antiinflammatory drug therapy. J Clin Gastroenterol. 1990;12(1):10–3. https://doi.org/10.1097/00004836-199002000-00004.
4. Carson JL, Strom BL, Morse ML, West SL, Soper KA, Stolley PD, et al. The relative toxicity of the nonsteroidal anti-inflammatory drugs. Arch Intern Med. 1987;147(6):1054–9. https://doi.org/10.1001/archinte.147.6.1054.
5. Allison MC, Howatson AG, Torrance CJ, Lee FD, Russell RI. Gastrointestinal damage associated with the use of nonsteroidal antiinflammatory drugs. N Engl J Med. 1992;327(11):749–54. https://doi.org/10.1056/NEJM199209103271101.
6. Goldstein NS, Cinenza AN. The histopathology of nonsteroidal anti-inflammatory drug-associated colitis. Am J Clin Pathol. 1998;110(5):622–8.
7. Kakar S, Pardi DS, Burgart LJ. Colonic ulcers accompanying collagenous colitis: implication of nonsteroidal anti-inflammatory drugs. Am J Gastroenterol. 2003;98(8):1834–7. https://doi.org/10.1111/j.1572-0241.2003.07579.x.
8. Riddell RH, Tanaka M, Mazzoleni G. Non-steroid anti-inflammatory drugs as a possible cause of collagenous colitis: a case-control study. Gut. 1992;33(5):683–6.
9. Lee FD. Importance of apoptosis in the histopathology of drug related lesions in the large intestine. J Clin Pathol. 1993;46(2):118–22.
10. Shetty S, Anjarwalla SM, Gupta J, Foy CJW, Shaw IS, Valori RM, et al. Focal active colitis: a prospective study of clinicopathological correlations in 90 patients. Histopathology. 2011;59(5):850–6. https://doi.org/10.1111/j.1365-2559.2011.04019.x.
11. Wang YZ, Sun G, Cai FC, Yang YS. Clinical features, diagnosis, and treatment strategies of gastrointestinal diaphragm disease associated with nonsteroidal anti-inflammatory drugs. Gastroenterol Res Pract. 2016;2016:3679741. https://doi.org/10.1155/2016/3679741.
12. Munipalle PC, Little M, Garud T, Henderson D. NSAID-induced diaphragmatic disease of the colon. BMJ Case Rep. 2013;2013:bcr2012008448. https://doi.org/10.1136/bcr-2012-008448.
13. Deshpande V, Hsu M, Kumarasinghe MP, Lauwers GY. The clinical significance of incidental chronic colitis: a study of 17 cases. Am J Surg Pathol. 2010;34(4):463–9. https://doi.org/10.1097/PAS.0b013e3181d0fd76.
14. Parfitt JR, Jayakumar S, Driman DK. Mycophenolate mofetil-related gastrointestinal mucosal injury: variable injury patterns, including graft-versus-host disease-like changes. Am J Surg Pathol. 2008;32(9):1367–72. https://doi.org/10.1097/PAS.0b013e31816bf3fe.

15. Al-Absi AI, Cooke CR, Wall BM, Sylvestre P, Ismail MK, Mya M. Patterns of injury in mycophenolate mofetil-related colitis. Transplant Proc. 2010;42(9):3591–3. https://doi.org/10.1016/j.transproceed.2010.08.066.
16. Selbst MK, Ahrens WA, Robert ME, Friedman A, Proctor DD, Jain D. Spectrum of histologic changes in colonic biopsies in patients treated with mycophenolate mofetil. Mod Pathol. 2009;22(6):737–43. https://doi.org/10.1038/modpathol.2009.44.
17. Star KV, Ho VT, Wang HH, Odze RD. Histologic features in colon biopsies can discriminate mycophenolate from GVHD-induced colitis. Am J Surg Pathol. 2013;37(9):1319–28. https://doi.org/10.1097/PAS.0b013e31829ab1ef.
18. Harel Z, Harel S, Shah PS, Wald R, Perl J, Bell CM. Gastrointestinal adverse events with sodium polystyrene sulfonate (Kayexalate) use: a systematic review. Am J Med. 2013;126(3):264.e9–e24. https://doi.org/10.1016/j.amjmed.2012.08.016.
19. Dunlap RH, Martinez R. Total colectomy for colon perforation after Kayexalate administration: a case report and literature review of a rare complication. J Surg Case Rep. 2016;2016(10):rjw167. https://doi.org/10.1093/jscr/rjw167.
20. Rashid A, Hamilton SR. Necrosis of the gastrointestinal tract in uremic patients as a result of sodium polystyrene sulfonate (Kayexalate) in sorbitol: an underrecognized condition. Am J Surg Pathol. 1997;21(1):60–9. https://doi.org/10.1097/00000478-199701000-00007.
21. Wootton FT, Rhodes DF, Lee WM, Fitts CT. Colonic necrosis with Kayexalate-sorbitol enemas after renal transplantation. Ann Intern Med. 1989;111(11):947–9.
22. Swanson BJ, Limketkai BN, Liu TC, Montgomery E, Nazari K, Park JY, et al. Sevelamer crystals in the gastrointestinal tract (GIT): a new entity associated with mucosal injury. Am J Surg Pathol. 2013;37(11):1686–93. https://doi.org/10.1097/PAS.0b013e3182999d8d.
23. Chintamaneni P, Das R, Kuan SF, Kermanshahi TR, Hashash JG. Hematochezia associated with sevalamer-induced mucosal injury. ACG Case Rep J. 2014;1(3):145–7. https://doi.org/10.14309/crj.2014.32.
24. Yamaguchi T, Ohyama S, Furukawa H, Sato N, Ohnishi I, Kasashima S, et al. Sigmoid colon diverticula perforation associated with sevelamer hydrochloride administration: a case report. Ann Med Surg. 2016;10:57–60. https://doi.org/10.1016/j.amsu.2016.07.020.
25. Okwara C, Choi C, Park JY. Sevelamer-induced colitis presenting as a pseudotumor. Clin Gastroenterol Hepatol. 2015;13(7):A39–40. https://doi.org/10.1016/j.cgh.2015.02.015.
26. Arnold MA, Swanson BJ, Crowder CD, Frankel WL, Lam-Himlin D, Singhi AD, et al. Colesevelam and colestipol: novel medication resins in the gastrointestinal tract. Am J Surg Pathol. 2014;38(11):1530–7. https://doi.org/10.1097/PAS.0000000000000260.
27. Peggs KS, Quezada SA, Korman AJ, Allison JP. Principles and use of anti-CTLA4 antibody in human cancer immunotherapy. Curr Opin Immunol. 2006;18(2):206–13. https://doi.org/10.1016/j.coi.2006.01.011.
28. Keir ME, Butte MJ, Freeman GJ, Sharpe AH. PD-1 and its ligands in tolerance and immunity. Ann Rev Immunol. 2008;26:677–704.
29. McDermott DF, Atkins MB. PD-1 as a potential target in cancer therapy. Cancer Med. 2013;2(5):662–73. https://doi.org/10.1002/cam4.106.
30. Berman D, Parker SM, Siegel J, Chasalow SD, Weber J, Galbraith S, et al. Blockade of cytotoxic T-lymphocyte antigen-4 by ipilimumab results in dysregulation of gastrointestinal immunity in patients with advanced melanoma. Cancer Immun. 2010;10:11.
31. Dilling P, Walczak J, Pikiel P, Kruszewski WJ. Multiple colon perforation as a fatal complication during treatment of metastatic melanoma with ipilimumab-case report. Polski Przegl Chir/Pol J Surg. 2014;86(2):94–6. https://doi.org/10.2478/pjs-2014-0017.
32. Kwak HA, Hart J. The many faces of medication-related injury in the gastrointestinal tract. Surg Pathol Clin. 2017;10(4):887–908. https://doi.org/10.1016/j.path.2017.07.007.
33. Weidner AS, Panarelli NC, Geyer JT, Bhavsar EB, Furman RR, Leonard JP, et al. Idelalisib-associated colitis. Am J Surg Pathol. 2015;39(12):1661–7. https://doi.org/10.1097/PAS.0000000000000522.
34. Verschuren EC, van den Eertwegh AJ, Wonders J, Slangen RM, van Delft F, van Bodegraven A, et al. Clinical, endoscopic, and histologic characteristics of ipilimumab-associated colitis. Clin Gastroenterol Hepatol. 2016;14(6):836–42. https://doi.org/10.1016/j.cgh.2015.12.028.
35. Chen JH, Pezhouh MK, Lauwers GY, Masia R. Histopathologic features of colitis due to immunotherapy with anti-PD-1 antibodies. Am J Surg Pathol. 2017;41(5):643–54. https://doi.org/10.1097/PAS.0000000000000829.
36. Cramer P, Bresalier RS. Gastrointestinal and hepatic complications of immune checkpoint inhibitors. Curr Gastroenterol Rep. 2017;19(1):3. https://doi.org/10.1007/s11894-017-0540-6.
37. Iacobuzio-Donahue CA, Lee EL, Abraham SC, Yardley JH, Wu TT. Colchicine toxicity: distinct morphologic findings in gastrointestinal biopsies. Am J Surg Pathol. 2001;25(8):1067–73. https://doi.org/10.1097/00000478-200108000-00012.
38. Torbenson M, Montgomery EA, Iacobuzio-Donahue C, Yardley JH, Wu TT, Abraham SC. Colchicine effect in a colonic hyperplastic polyp: a lesion mimicking serrated adenoma. Arch Pathol Lab Med. 2002;126(5):615–7.
39. Pawel BR, de Chadarevian JP, Franco ME. The pathology of fibrosing colonopathy of cystic fibrosis: a study of 12 cases and review of the literature. Hum Pathol. 1997;28(4):395–9.
40. Smyth RL, Ashby D, O'Hea U, Burrows E, Lewis P, van Velzen D, et al. Fibrosing colonopathy in cystic fibrosis: results of a case-control study. Lancet. 1995;346(8985):1247–51.
41. Smyth RL. Fibrosing colonopathy in cystic fibrosis. Arch Dis Child. 1996;74(5):464–8.
42. Chaun H. Colonic disorders in adult cystic fibrosis. Can J Gastroenterol. 2001;15(9):586–90.
43. Franzen D, Went P, Buhlmann U. Fibrosing colonopathy in absence of pancreatic enzyme supplementation in one adult patient with cystic fibrosis. Indian J Gastroenterol. 2008;27(3):133–4.
44. Brett AS, Mack EH. Fibrosing colonopathy in adults with cystic fibrosis. AJR Am J Roentgenol. 2008;190(1):W73. https://doi.org/10.2214/AJR.06.1589.
45. Pettei MJ, Leonidas JC, Levine JJ, Gorvoy JD. Pancolonic disease in cystic fibrosis and high-dose pancreatic enzyme therapy. J Pediatr. 1994;125(4):587–9.
46. Knabe N, Zak M, Hansen A, Moesgaard J, Kvist N, Beck B, et al. Extensive pathological changes of the colon in cystic fibrosis and high-strength pancreatic enzymes. Lancet. 1994;343(8907):1230.
47. Ghahremani GG, Meyers MA, Farman J, Port RB. Ischemic disease of the small bowel and colon associated with oral contraceptives. Gastrointest Radiol. 1977;2(3):221–8.
48. Parker WA, Morris ME, Shearer CA. Oral contraceptive-induced ischemic bowel disease. Am J Hosp Pharm. 1979;36(8):1103–7.
49. Schmid R, Cello JP. Ischemic disease of the colon and oral contraceptives. West J Med. 1977;126(5):378–85.
50. Sukpanichnant S, Hargrove NS, Kachintorn U, Manatsathit S, Chanchairujira T, Siritanaratkul N, et al. Clofazimine-induced crystal-storing histiocytosis producing chronic abdominal pain in a leprosy patient. Am J Surg Pathol. 2000;24(1):129–35.
51. Lewis JT, Candelora JN, Hogan RB, Briggs FR, Abraham SC. Crystal-storing histiocytosis due to massive accumulation of charcot-leyden crystals: a unique association producing colonic polyposis in a 78-year-old woman with eosinophilic colitis. Am

J Surg Pathol. 2007;31(3):481–5. https://doi.org/10.1097/01.pas.0000213420.46127.9c.
52. Cappell MS. Colonic toxicity of administered drugs and chemicals. Am J Gastroenterol. 2004;99(6):1175–90. https://doi.org/10.1111/j.1572–0241.2004.30192.x.
53. Dial S, Delaney JAC, Barkun AN, Suissa S. Use of gastric acid-suppressive agents and the risk of community-acquired Clostridium difficile-associated disease. J Am Med Assoc. 2005;294(23):2989–95. https://doi.org/10.1001/jama.294.23.2989.
54. Driman DK, Preiksaitis HG. Colorectal inflammation and increased cell proliferation associated with oral sodium phosphate bowel preparation solution. Hum Pathol. 1998;29(9):972–8. https://doi.org/10.1016/S0046–8177(98)90203–9.
55. Walker NI, Bennett RE, Axelsen RA. Melanosis coli. A consequence of anthraquinone-induced apoptosis of colonic epithelial cells. Am J Pathol. 1988;131(3):465–76.
56. Wong V, Wyatt J, Lewis F, Howdle P. Gold induced enterocolitis complicated by cytomegalovirus infection: a previously unrecognised association. Gut. 1993;34(7):1002–5.
57. Evron E, Brautbar C, Becker S, Fenakel G, Abend Y, Sthoeger Z, et al. Correlation between gold-induced enterocolitis and the presence of the HLA-DRB1*0404 allele. Arthritis Rheum. 1995;38(6):755–9.
58. Eaves R, Hansky J, Wallis P. Gold induced enterocolitis: case report and a review of the literature. Aust NZ J Med. 1982;12(6):617–20.
59. Fam AG, Paton TW, Shamess CJ, Lewis AJ. Fulminant colitis complicating gold therapy. J Rheumatol. 1980;7(4):479–85.
60. Reinhart WH, Kappeler M, Halter F. Severe pseudomembranous and ulcerative colitis during gold therapy. Endoscopy. 1983;15(2):70–1. https://doi.org/10.1055/s-2007–1021470.
61. Rose PG, Piver MS. Intestinal perforation secondary to paclitaxel. Gynecol Oncol. 1995;57(2):270–2. https://doi.org/10.1006/gyno.1995.1140.
62. Atherton LD, Leib ES, Kaye MD. Toxic megacolon associated with methotrexate therapy. Gastroenterology. 1984;86(6):1583–8. https://doi.org/10.1016/S0016–5085(84)80176–6.
63. Floch MH, Hellman L. The effect of five-fluorouracil on rectal mucosa. Gastroenterology. 1965;48(4):430–7. https://doi.org/10.1016/S0016–5085(65)80003–8.
64. Milles SS, Muggia AL, Spiro HM. Colonic histologic changes induced by 5-fluorouracil. Gastroenterology. 1962;43:391–9.
65. Nesher L, Rolston KV. Neutropenic enterocolitis, a growing concern in the era of widespread use of aggressive chemotherapy. Clin Infect Dis. 2013;56(5):711–7. https://doi.org/10.1093/cid/cis998.
66. Avigan D, Richardson P, Elias A, Demetri G, Shapiro M, Schnipper L, et al. Neutropenic enterocolitis as a complication of high dose chemotherapy with stem cell rescue in patients with solid tumors: a case series with a review of the literature. Cancer. 1998;83(3):409–14.
67. Cunningham SC, Fakhry K, Bass BL, Napolitano LM. Neutropenic enterocolitis in adults: case series and review of the literature. Dig Dis Sci. 2005;50(2):215–20.
68. Rodrigues FG, Dasilva G, Wexner SD. Neutropenic enterocolitis. World J Gastroenterol. 2017;23(1):42–7. https://doi.org/10.3748/wjg.v23.i1.42.
69. Dolce P, Gourdeau M, April N, Bernard PM. Outbreak of glutaraldehyde-induced proctocolitis. Am J Infect Control. 1995;23(1):34–9.
70. West AB, Kuan SF, Bennick M, Lagarde S. Glutaraldehyde colitis following endoscopy: clinical and pathological features and investigation of an outbreak. Gastroenterology. 1995;108(4):1250–5.
71. Rozen P, Somjen GJ, Baratz M, Kimel R, Arber N, Gilat T. Endoscope-induced colitis: description, probable cause by glutaraldehyde, and prevention. Gastrointest Endosc. 1994;40(5):547–53.
72. Ahishali E, Uygur-Bayramicli O, Dolapcioglu C, Dabak R, Mengi A, Isik A, et al. Chemical colitis due to glutaraldehyde: case series and review of the literature. Dig Dis Sci. 2009;54(12):2541–5. https://doi.org/10.1007/s10620–008–0630–2.
73. Gilshtein H, Hallon K, Kluger Y. Ischemic colitis caused increased early and delayed mortality. World J Emerg Surg. 2018;13:31. https://doi.org/10.1186/s13017–018–0193–2.
74. Scharff JR, Longo WE, Vartanian SM, Jacobs DL, Bahadursingh AN, Kaminski DL. Ischemic colitis: spectrum of disease and outcome. Surgery. 2003;134(4):624–9; discussion 9–30. https://doi.org/10.1016/S0039.
75. Huguier M, Barrier A, Boelle PY, Houry S, Lacaine F. Ischemic colitis. Am J Surg. 2006;192(5):679–84. https://doi.org/10.1016/j.amjsurg.2005.09.018.
76. Elder K, Lashner BA, Al Solaiman F. Clinical approach to colonic ischemia. Cleve Clin J Med. 2009;76(7):401–9. https://doi.org/10.3949/ccjm.76a.08089.
77. Higgins PD, Davis KJ, Laine L. Systematic review: the epidemiology of ischaemic colitis. Aliment Pharmacol Ther. 2004;19(7):729–38. https://doi.org/10.1111/j.1365–2036.2004.01903.x.
78. Glauser PM, Wermuth P, Cathomas G, Kuhnt E, Kaser SA, Maurer CA. Ischemic colitis: clinical presentation, localization in relation to risk factors, and long-term results. World J Surg. 2011;35(11):2549–54. https://doi.org/10.1007/s00268–011–1205–5.
79. Washington C, Carmichael J. Management of ischemic colitis. Clin Colon Rectal Surg. 2012;25(4):228–35. https://doi.org/10.1055/s-0032–1329534.
80. Feuerstadt P, Brandt LJ. Colon ischemia: recent insights and advances. Curr Gastroenterol Rep. 2010;12(5):383–90. https://doi.org/10.1007/s11894–010–0127-y.
81. Green BT, Tendler DA. Ischemic colitis: a clinical review. South Med J. 2005;98(2):217–22. https://doi.org/10.1097/01.SMJ.0000145399.35851.10.
82. Theodoropoulou A, Koutroubakis IE. Ischemic colitis: clinical practice in diagnosis and treatment. World J Gastroenterol. 2008;14(48):7302–8. https://doi.org/10.3748/wjg.14.7302.
83. Romano S, Romano L, Grassi R. Multidetector row computed tomography findings from ischemia to infarction of the large bowel. Eur J Radiol. 2007;61(3):433–41. https://doi.org/10.1016/j.ejrad.2006.11.002.
84. Netz U, Galandiuk S. The management of ischemic colitis. In: Current surgical therapy; Elsevier, Philadelphia, 2017;171–6.
85. Sun D, Wang C, Yang L, Liu M, Chen F. The predictors of the severity of ischaemic colitis: a systematic review of 2823 patients from 22 studies. Color Dis. 2016;18(10):949–58. https://doi.org/10.1111/codi.13389.
86. Yadav S, Dave M, Edakkanambeth Varayil J, Harmsen WS, Tremaine WJ, Zinsmeister AR, et al. A population-based study of incidence, risk factors, clinical spectrum, and outcomes of ischemic colitis. Clin Gastroenterol Hepatol. 2015;13(4):731–8. https://doi.org/10.1016/j.cgh.2014.07.061.
87. O'Neill S, Yalamarthi S. Systematic review of the management of ischaemic colitis. Color Dis. 2012;14(11):e751–e63. https://doi.org/10.1111/j.1463–1318.2012.03171.x.
88. Brandt LJ, Feuerstadt P, Longstreth GF, Boley SJ. ACG clinical guideline: epidemiology, risk factors, patterns of presentation, diagnosis, and management of colon ischemia (CI). Am J Gastroenterol. 2015;110(1):18–44. https://doi.org/10.1038/ajg.2014.395.
89. Castleberry AW, Turley RS, Hanna JM, Hopkins TJ, Barbas AS, Worni M, et al. A 10-year longitudinal analysis of surgical management for acute ischemic colitis. J Gastrointest Surg. 2013;17(4):784–92. https://doi.org/10.1007/s11605–012–2117-x.
90. Moawad J, Gewertz BL. Chronic mesenteric ischemia. Clinical presentation and diagnosis. Surg Clin North Am. 1997;77(2):357–69.

91. Moawad J, McKinsey JF, Wyble CW, Bassiouny HS, Schwartz LB, Gewertz BL. Current results of surgical therapy for chronic mesenteric ischemia. Arch Surg. 1997;132(6):613–8; discussion 8–9
92. Khor TS, Lauwers GY, Odze RD, Srivastava A. "Mass-forming" variant of ischemic colitis is a distinct entity with predilection for the proximal colon. Am J Surg Pathol. 2015;39(9):1275–81. https://doi.org/10.1097/PAS.0000000000000438.
93. Brandt LJ, Katz HJ, Wolf EL, Mitsudo S, Boley SJ. Simulation of colonic carcinoma by ischemia. Gastroenterology. 1985;88(5):1137–42. https://doi.org/10.1016/S0016-5085(85)80072-X.
94. Mahr A, Guillevin L, Poissonnet M, Aymé S. Prevalences of polyarteritis nodosa, microscopic polyangiitis, Wegener's granulomatosis, and Churg-Strauss syndrome in a French urban multiethnic population in 2000: acapture-recapture estimate. Arthritis Care Res. 2004;51(1):92–9.
95. Gayraud M, Guillevin L, Toumelin PL, Cohen P, Lhote F, Casassus P, et al. Long-term followup of polyarteritis nodosa, microscopic polyangiitis, and Churg-Strauss syndrome: analysis of four prospective trials including 278 patients. Arthritis Rheum. 2001;44(3):666–75. https://doi.org/10.1002/1529-0131(200103)44:3<666::AID-ANR116>3.0.CO;2-A.
96. Trepo C, Guillevin L. Polyarteritis nodosa and extrahepatic manifestations of HBV infection: the case against autoimmune intervention in pathogenesis. J Autoimmun. 2001;16(3):269–74. https://doi.org/10.1006/jaut.2000.0502.
97. Brogan PA, Dillon MJ, Bose A, Burgner D, Shingadia D, Tulloh R, et al. Kawasaki disease: an evidence based approach to diagnosis, treatment, and proposals for future research. Arch Dis Child. 2002;86(4):286–90. https://doi.org/10.1136/adc.86.4.286.
98. Bagrul D, Karadeniz EG, Koca S. Gastrointestinal involvement in Kawasaki disease: a case report. Cardiol Young. 2018;28(8):1070–3. https://doi.org/10.1017/S1047951118000847.
99. Ohnishi Y, Mori K, Inoue M, Satake N, Yano M. A case of Kawasaki disease presenting as sigmoid colitis. J Med Ultrason (2001). 2018;45(2):381–4. https://doi.org/10.1007/s10396-017-0808-3.
100. Sinnott JD, Matthews P, Fletcher S. Colitis: an unusual presentation of Wegener's granulomatosis. BMJ Case Rep. 2013;2013:bcr2012007566. https://doi.org/10.1136/bcr-2012-007566.
101. Qian Q, Cornell L, Chandan V, Hartman R, Caples S. Hemorrhagic colitis as a presenting feature of Wegener granulomatosis. J Gastrointestin Liver Dis. 2010;19(4):445–7.
102. Timmermann S, Perez Bouza A, Junge K, Neumann UP, Binnebosel M. Initial diagnosis of Wegener's granulomatosis mimicking severe ulcerative colitis: a case report. J Med Case Rep. 2013;7:141. https://doi.org/10.1186/1752-1947-7-141.
103. Kim YB, Choi SW, Park IS, Han JY, Hur YS, Chu YC. Churg-Strauss syndrome with perforating ulcers of the colon. J Korean Med Sci. 2000;15(5):585–8. https://doi.org/10.3346/jkms.2000.15.5.585.
104. Memain N, De BM, Guillevin L, Wechsler B, Meyer O. Delayed relapse of Churg-Strauss syndrome manifesting as colon ulcers with mucosal granulomas: 3 cases. J Rheumatol. 2002;29(2):388–91.
105. Calvo-Río V, Loricera J, Mata C, Martín L, Ortiz-Sanjuán F, Alvarez L, et al. Henoch-schönlein purpura in Northern Spain: clinical spectrum of the disease in 417 patients from a single center. Medicine (United States). 2014;93(2):106–13. https://doi.org/10.1097/MD.0000000000000019.
106. Saulsbury FT. Henoch-Schonlein purpura in children: report of 100 patients and review of the literature. Medicine. 1999;78(6):395–409. https://doi.org/10.1097/00005792-199911000-00005.
107. Chang WL, Yang YH, Lin YT, Chiang BL. Gastrointestinal manifestations in Henoch-Schönlein purpura: a review of 261 patients. Acta Paediatr Int J Paediatr. 2004;93(11):1427–31. https://doi.org/10.1080/08035250410020181.
108. Louie CY, Gomez AJ, Sibley RK, Bass D, Longacre TA. Histologic features of gastrointestinal tract biopsies in IgA vasculitis (Henoch-Schonlein purpura). Am J Surg Pathol. 2018;42(4):529–33. https://doi.org/10.1097/PAS.0000000000001036.
109. Esaki M, Matsumoto T, Nakamura S, Kawasaki M, Iwai K, Hirakawa K, et al. GI involvement in Henoch-Schönlein purpura. Gastrointest Endosc. 2002;56(6):920–3. https://doi.org/10.1016/S0016-5107(02)70376-3.
110. Ngo N, Chang F. Enterocolic lymphocytic phlebitis: clinicopathologic features and review of the literature. Arch Pathol Lab Med. 2007;131(7):1130–4.
111. Knauer M, Haid A, Gruber-Mösenbacher U, Wenzl E. Mesenteric inflammatory veno-occlusive disease (MIVOD)—a rare cause of intestinal ischemia. Wien Klin Wochenschr. 2005;117(17):610–4. https://doi.org/10.1007/s00508-005-0416-x.
112. Lavu K, Minocha A. Mesenteric inflammatory veno-occlusive disorder: a rare entity mimicking inflammatory bowel disorder. Gastroenterology. 2003;125(1):236–9. https://doi.org/10.1016/S0016-5085(03)00663-2.
113. Lie JT. Mesenteric inflammatory veno-occlusive disease (MIVOD): an emerging and unsuspected cause of digestive tract ischemia. Vasa—J Vasc Dis. 1997;26(2):91–6.
114. Corsi A, Ribaldi S, Coletti M, Bosman C. Intramural mesenteric venulitis—a new cause of intestinal ischaemia. Virchows Arch. 1995;427(1):65–9. https://doi.org/10.1007/BF00203739.
115. Martinet O, Reis ED, Joseph JM, Saraga E, Gillet M. Isolated granulomatous phlebitis: rare cause of ischemic necrosis of the colon: report of a case. Dis Colon Rectum. 2000;43(11):1601–3. https://doi.org/10.1007/BF02236749.
116. Arora DS, Mahmood T, Wyatt JI. Lymphocytic venulitis: an unusual association with microscopic colitis. J Clin Pathol. 1999;52(4):303–4. https://doi.org/10.1136/jcp.52.4.303.
117. Stevens SMB, Gue S, Finck ES. Necrotizing and giant cell granulomatous phlebitis of caecum and ascending colon. Pathology. 1976;8(3):259–64. https://doi.org/10.3109/00313027609059006.
118. Chergui MH, Vandeperre J, Van Eeckhout P. Enterocolic lymphocytic phlebitis: acase report. Acta Chir Belg. 1997;6:293–6.
119. Wright CL, Čačala S. Enterocolic lymphocytic phlebitis with lymphocytic colitis, lymphocytic appendicitis, and lymphocytic enteritis. Am J Surg Pathol. 2004;28(4):542–7. https://doi.org/10.1097/00000478-200404000-00015.
120. Laco J, Orhalmi J, Bartova J, Zimandlova D. Enterocolic lymphocytic phlebitis as a newly recognized manifestation of IgG4-related disease. Int J Surg Pathol. 2015;23(2):165–9. https://doi.org/10.1177/1066896914539549.
121. Comtesse S, Friemel J, Fankhauser R, Weber A. Enterocolic lymphocytic phlebitis of the cecal pole and appendix vermiformis with increase of IgG4-positive plasma cells. Virchows Arch. 2014;464(1):113–6. https://doi.org/10.1007/s00428-013-1507-0.
122. Saraga E, Bouzourenne H. Enterocolic (lymphocytic) phlebitis: a rare cause of intestinal ischemic necrosis: a series of six patients and review of the literature. Am J Surg Pathol. 2000;24(6):824–9. https://doi.org/10.1097/00000478-200006000-00007.
123. Medlicott SAC, Guggisberg KA, DesCôteaux JG, Beck P. Enterocolic lymphocytic phlebitis: statistical analysis of histology features in viable and ischemic bowel. Int J Surg Pathol. 2006;14(3):200–5. https://doi.org/10.1177/1066896906289995.
124. Abraham SC, Solem CA, Hauser SC, Smyrk TC. Chronic antral ulcer associated with gastroduodenal lymphocytic phlebitis. Am J Surg Pathol. 2004;28(12):1659–63. https://doi.org/10.1097/00000478-200412000-00018.
125. Charron P, Smith J. Mesenteric venulitis in a 71-year-old man after acute appendicitis. Am Surg. 2005;71(7):574–7.

126. De Marco L, Cavazza A, Pastore L, Rossi G, Piana S, Putrino I, et al. Enterocolic phlebitis. A case report and review of the literature. Pathologica. 2003;95(4):203–8.
127. Yantiss RK, Cui I, Panarelli NC, Jessurun J. Idiopathic myointimal hyperplasia of mesenteric veins: an uncommon cause of ischemic colitis with distinct mucosal features. Am J Surg Pathol. 2017;41(12):1657–65. https://doi.org/10.1097/PAS.0000000000000905.
128. Genta RM, Haggitt RC. Idiopathic myointimal hyperplasia of mesenteric veins. Gastroenterology. 1991;101(2):533–9. https://doi.org/10.1016/0016-5085(91)90035-J.
129. Abu-Alfa AK, Ayer U, West AB. Mucosal biopsy findings and venous abnormalities in idiopathic myointimal hyperplasia of the mesenteric veins. Am J Surg Pathol. 1996;20(10):1271–8. https://doi.org/10.1097/00000478-199610000-00014.
130. Kao PC, Vecchio JA, Hyman NH, West AB, Blaszyk H. Idiopathic myointimal hyperplasia of mesenteric veins: a rare mimic of idiopathic inflammatory bowel disease. J Clin Gastroenterol. 2005;39(8):704–8. https://doi.org/10.1097/00004836-200509000-00011.
131. Sarin A, Safar B. Management of radiation proctitis. Gastroenterol Clin N Am. 2013;42(4):913–25. https://doi.org/10.1016/j.gtc.2013.08.004.
132. Haringsma J, Tytgat GN. Chronic intestinal bleeding caused by congenital arteriovenous malformations. Endoscopy. 1988;20(6):330–1. https://doi.org/10.1055/s-2007-1018209.
133. Freud E, Kidron D, Gornish M, Barak R, Golinski D, Zer M. The value of precise preoperative localization of colonic arteriovenous malformation in childhood. Am J Gastroenterol. 1993;88(3):443–6.
134. Manns RA, Vickers CR, Chesner IM, McMaster P, Elias E. Portal hypertension secondary to sigmoid colon arteriovenous malformation. Clin Radiol. 1990;42(3):203–4.
135. Foutch PG. Angiodysplasia of the gastrointestinal tract. Am J Gastroenterol. 1993;88(6):807–18. https://doi.org/10.1111/j.1572-0241.1993.tb03057.x.
136. Almeida N, Figueiredo P, Lopes S, Freire P, Lérias C, Gouveia H, et al. Urgent capsule endoscopy is useful in severe obscure-overt gastrointestinal bleeding: original article. Dig Endosc. 2009;21(2):87–92. https://doi.org/10.1111/j.1443-1661.2009.00838.x.
137. Ueno S, Nakase H, Kasahara K, Uza N, Kitamura H, Inoue S, et al. Clinical features of Japanese patients with colonic angiodysplasia. J Gastroenterol Hepatol(Australia). 2008;23(8 PART2):e363–e6. https://doi.org/10.1111/j.1440-1746.2007.05126.x.
138. Sami SS, Al-Araji SA, Ragunath K. Review article: gastrointestinal angiodysplasia—pathogenesis, diagnosis and management. Aliment Pharmacol Ther. 2014;39(1):15–34. https://doi.org/10.1111/apt.12527.
139. Boley SJ, Sammartano R, Adams A, DiBiase A, Kleinhaus S, Sprayregen S. On the nature and etiology of vascular ectasias of the colon. Degenerative lesions of aging. Gastroenterology. 1977;72(4 Pt 1):650–60.
140. Urrunaga NH, Rockey DC. Portal hypertensive gastropathy and colopathy. Clin Liver Dis. 2014;18(2):389–406. https://doi.org/10.1016/j.cld.2014.01.008.
141. Guimaraes RA, Perazzo H, Machado L, Terra C, Perez RM, Figueiredo FA. Prevalence, variability, and outcomes in portal hypertensive colopathy: a study in patients with cirrhosis and paired controls. Gastrointest Endosc. 2015;82(3):469–76.e2. https://doi.org/10.1016/j.gie.2015.01.036.
142. Naveau S, Bedossa P, Poynard T, Mory B, Chaput JC. Portal hypertensive colopathy—a new entity. Dig Dis Sci. 1991;36(12):1774–81. https://doi.org/10.1007/BF01296624.
143. Kozarek RA, Botoman VA, Bredfeldt JE, Roach JM, Patterson DJ, Ball TJ. Portal colopathy: prospective study of colonoscopy in patients with portal hypertension. Gastroenterology. 1991;101(5):1192–7.
144. Bhatia S, Jain S, Singh CB, Bains L, Kaushik R, Gowda NS. Malrotation of the gut in adults: an often forgotten entity. Cureus. 2018;10(3):e2313. https://doi.org/10.7759/cureus.2313.
145. Zengin A, Ucar BI, Duzgun SA, Bayhan Z, Zeren S, Yaylak F, et al. Adult midgut malrotation presented with acute bowel obstruction and ischemia. Int J Surg Case Rep. 2016;22:5–7. https://doi.org/10.1016/j.ijscr.2016.03.018.
146. Dalla Vecchia LK, Grosfeld JL, West KW, Rescorla FJ, Scherer LR, Engum SA. Intestinal atresia and stenosis: a 25-year experience with 277 cases. Arch Surg. 1998;133(5):490–6; discussion 6–7
147. Amiel J, Lyonnet S. Hirschsprung disease, associated syndromes, and genetics: a review. J Med Genet. 2001;38(11):729–39.
148. Mirza B, Iqbal S, Ijaz L. Colonic atresia and stenosis: our experience. J Neonatal Surg. 2012;1(1):4.
149. Ildstad ST, Tollerud DJ, Weiss RG, Ryan DP, McGowan MA, Martin LW. Duplications of the alimentary tract. Clinical characteristics, preferred treatment, and associated malformations. Ann Surg. 1988;208(2):184–9.
150. Caklili OT, Tuncer I, Colak Y, Kosemetin D, Ceyran AB. Colonic duplication in adulthood presenting with diarrhea. Endoscopy. 2013;45(Suppl 2 UCTN):E430–1. https://doi.org/10.1055/s-0033-1358805.
151. Shah KR, Joshi A. Complete genitourinary and colonic duplication: a rare presentation in an adult patient. J Ultrasound Med. 2006;25(3):407–11.
152. Jung HI, Lee HU, Ahn TS, Lee JE, Lee HY, Mun ST, et al. Complete tubular duplication of colon in an adult: a rare cause of colovaginal fistula. Ann Surg Treat Res. 2016;91(4):207–11. https://doi.org/10.4174/astr.2016.91.4.207.
153. Cuschieri A, Ayme S, Haeusler M, et al. Descriptive epidemiology of isolated anal anomalies: a survey of 4.6 million births in Europe. Am J Med Genet. 2001;103(3):207–15.
154. Herman RS, Teitelbaum DH. Anorectal malformations. Clin Perinatol. 2012;39(2):403–22. https://doi.org/10.1016/j.clp.2012.04.001.
155. Teixeira OH, Malhotra K, Sellers J, Mercer S. Cardiovascular anomalies with imperforate anus. Arch Dis Child. 1983;58(9):747–9.
156. Golonka NR, Haga LJ, Keating RP, Eichelberger MR, Gilbert JC, Hartman GE, et al. Routine MRI evaluation of low imperforate anus reveals unexpected high incidence of tethered spinal cord. J Pediatr Surg. 2002;37(7):966–9; discussion 9
157. Nievelstein RA, Vos A, Valk J, Vermeij-Keers C. Magnetic resonance imaging in children with anorectal malformations: embryologic implications. J Pediatr Surg. 2002;37(8):1138–45.
158. Marcelis C, de Blaauw I, Brunner H. Chromosomal anomalies in the etiology of anorectal malformations: a review. Am J Med Genet A. 2011;155A(11):2692–704. https://doi.org/10.1002/ajmg.a.34253.
159. Zhang J, Zhang ZB, Gao H, Zhang D, Wang WL. Down-regulation of SHH/BMP4 signalling in human anorectal malformations. J Int Med Res. 2009;37(6):1842–50. https://doi.org/10.1177/147323000903700620.
160. Bischoff A, Bealer J, Pena A. Controversies in anorectal malformations. Lancet Child Adolesc Health. 2017;1(4):323–30. https://doi.org/10.1016/S2352-4642(17)30026-3.
161. Wong SK, Ho YH, Leong AP, Seow-Choen F. Clinical behavior of complicated right-sided and left-sided diverticulosis. Dis Colon Rectum. 1997;40(3):344–8.
162. Delvaux M. Diverticular disease of the colon in Europe: epidemiology, impact on citizen health and prevention. Aliment Pharmacol Ther. 2003;18(Suppl 3):71–4.
163. Schieffer KM, Kline BP, Yochum GS, Koltun WA. Pathophysiology of diverticular disease. Expert Rev Gastroenterol Hepatol.

2018;12(7):683–92. https://doi.org/10.1080/17474124.2018.1481746.

164. Lameris W, van Randen A, Bipat S, Bossuyt PM, Boermeester MA, Stoker J. Graded compression ultrasonography and computed tomography in acute colonic diverticulitis: meta-analysis of test accuracy. Eur Radiol. 2008;18(11):2498–511. https://doi.org/10.1007/s00330-008-1018-6.
165. Gledhill A, Dixon MF. Crohn's-like reaction in diverticular disease. Gut. 1998;42(3):392–5. https://doi.org/10.1136/gut.42.3.392.
166. Sinclair A. Diverticular disease of the gastrointestinal tract. Prim Care. 2017;44(4):643–54. https://doi.org/10.1016/j.pop.2017.07.007.
167. Begos DG, Sandor A, Modlin IM. The diagnosis and management of adult intussusception. Am J Surg. 1997;173(2):88–94. https://doi.org/10.1016/S0002-9610(96)00419-9.
168. Schéyé T, Dechelotte P, Tanguy A, Dalens B, Vanneuville G, Chazal J. Anatomical and histological study of the ileocecal valve: possible correlations with the pathogenesis of idiopathic intussusception in infants. Anat Clin. 1983;5(2):83–92. https://doi.org/10.1007/BF01798978.
169. Buettcher M, Baer G, Bonhoeffer J, Schaad UB, Heininger U. Three-year surveillance of intussusception in children in Switzerland. Pediatrics. 2007;120(3):473–80. https://doi.org/10.1542/peds.2007-0035.
170. Rao PL, Kumar V. Waugh's syndrome. Indian J Pediatr. 2005;72(1):86.
171. Al-Momani H. Waugh syndrome: a report of 7 patients and review of the published reports. Ann Saudi Med. 2014;34(6):527–31. https://doi.org/10.5144/0256-4947.2014.527.
172. Eisen LK, Cunningham JD, Aufses AH Jr. Intussusception in adults: institutional review. J Am Coll Surg. 1999;188(4):390–5. https://doi.org/10.1016/S1072-7515(98)00331-7.
173. Azar T, Berger DL. Adult intussusception. Ann Surg. 1997;226(2):134–8. https://doi.org/10.1097/00000658-199708000-00003.
174. Zubaidi A, Al-Saif F, Silverman R. Adult intussusception: a retrospective review. Dis Colon Rectum. 2006;49(10):1546–51. https://doi.org/10.1007/s10350-006-0664-5.
175. Wiersma F, Allema JH, Holscher HC. Ileoileal intussusception in children: ultrasonographic differentiation from ileocolic intussusception. Pediatr Radiol. 2006;36(11):1177–81. https://doi.org/10.1007/s00247-006-0311-2.
176. Guillén-Paredes MP, Campillo-Soto A, Martín-Lorenzo JG, Torralba-Martínez JA, Mengual-Ballester M, Cases-Baldó MJ, et al. Adult intussusception—14 case reports and their outcomes. Rev Esp Enferm Dig. 2010;102(1):32–40. https://doi.org/10.4321/S1130-01082010000100005.
177. Lioubashevsky N, Hiller N, Rozovsky K, Segev L, Simanovsky N. Ileocolic versus small-bowel intussusception in children: can US enable reliable differentiation? Radiology. 2013;269(1):266–71. https://doi.org/10.1148/radiol.13122639.
178. Marsicovetere P, Ivatury SJ, White B, Holubar SD. Intestinal intussusception: etiology, diagnosis, and treatment. Clin Colon Rectal Surg. 2017;30(1):30–9. https://doi.org/10.1055/s-0036-1593429.
179. Halabi WJ, Jafari MD, Kang CY, Nguyen VQ, Carmichael JC, Mills S, et al. Colonic volvulus in the United States: trends, outcomes, and predictors of mortality. Ann Surg. 2014;259(2):293–301. https://doi.org/10.1097/SLA.0b013e31828c88ac.
180. Raveenthiran V, Madiba TE, Atamanalp SS, De U. Volvulus of the sigmoid colon. Colorectal Dis. 2010;12(7 Online):e1–17.
181. Atamanalp SS. Sigmoid volvulus: diagnosis in 938 patients over 45.5 years. Tech Coloproctol. 2013;17(4):419–24. https://doi.org/10.1007/s10151-012-0953-z.
182. MacAri M, Spieler B, Babb J, Pachter HL. Can the location of the CT whirl sign assist in differentiating sigmoid from caecal volvulus? Clin Radiol. 2011;66(2):112–7. https://doi.org/10.1016/j.crad.2010.09.010.
183. Kapadia MR. Volvulus of the small bowel and colon. Clin Colon Rectal Surg. 2017;30(1):40–5. https://doi.org/10.1055/s-0036-1593428.
184. Tjandra JJ, Fazio VW, Church JM, Lavery IC, Oakley JR, Milsom JW. Clinical conundrum of solitary rectal ulcer. Dis Colon Rectum. 1992;35(3):227–34. https://doi.org/10.1007/BF02051012.
185. Burke AP, Sobin LH. Eroded polypoid hyperplasia of the rectosigmoid. Am J Gastroenterol. 1990;85(8):975–80. https://doi.org/10.1111/j.1572-0241.1990.tb06791.x.
186. Martin CJ, Parks TG, Biggart JD. Solitary rectal ulcer syndrome in Northern Ireland, 1971–1980. Br J Surg. 1981;68(10):744–7. https://doi.org/10.1002/bjs.1800681021.
187. Sharara AI, Azar C, Amr SS, Haddad M, Eloubeidi MA. Solitary rectal ulcer syndrome: endoscopic spectrum and review of the literature. Gastrointest Endosc. 2005;62(5):755–62. https://doi.org/10.1016/j.gie.2005.07.016.
188. Borrelli O, De Angelis G. Solitary rectal ulcer syndrome: it's time to think about it. J Pediatr Gastroenterol Nutr. 2012;54(2):167–8. https://doi.org/10.1097/MPG.0b013e318230153e.
189. Forootan M, Darvishi M. Solitary rectal ulcer syndrome: a systematic review. Medicine (Baltimore). 2018;97(18):e0565. https://doi.org/10.1097/MD.0000000000010565.
190. Koss LG. Abdominal gas cysts (pneumatosis cystoides intestinorum hominis); an analysis with a report of a case and a critical review of the literature. AMA Arch Pathol. 1952;53(6):523–49.
191. Jamart J. Pneumatosis cystoides intestinalis. A statistical study of 919 cases. Acta Hepatogastroenterol. 1979;26(5):419–22.
192. Heng Y, Schuffler MD, Haggitt RC, Rohrmann CA. Pneumatosis intestinalis: areview. Am J Gastroenterol. 1995;90(10):1747–58. https://doi.org/10.1111/j.1572-0241.1995.tb08065.x.
193. Liu T, Zhang S, Mao H. Gastrointestinal malignant neoplasms disguised as pneumatosis cystoids intestinalis: a case report and literature review. Medicine (Baltimore). 2017;96(51):e9410. https://doi.org/10.1097/MD.0000000000009410.
194. Rennenberg RJ, Koek GH, Van Hootegem P, Stockbrügger RW. Pneumatosis cystoides intestinalis, four cases of a rare disease. Neth J Med. 2002;60(1):22–5.
195. Forgacs P, Wright PH Wyatt AP. Treatment of intestinal gas cysts by oxygen breathing. Lancet. 1973;1(7803):579–82.
196. Boerner RM, Fried DB, Warshauer DM, Isaacs K. Pneumatosis intestinalis. Two case reports and a retrospective review of the literature from 1985 to 1995. Dig Dis Sci. 1996;41(11):2272–85. https://doi.org/10.1007/BF02071412.
197. St. Peter SD, Abbas MA, Kelly KA. The spectrum of pneumatosis intestinalis. Arch Surg. 2003;138(1):68–75. https://doi.org/10.1001/archsurg.138.1.68.
198. Ho LM, Paulson EK, Thompson WM. Pneumatosis intestinal is in the adult: benign to life-threatening causes. Am J Roentgenol. 2007;188(6):1604–13. https://doi.org/10.2214/AJR.06.1309.
199. Ecker JA, Williams RG, Clay KL. Pneumatosis cystoides intestinalis—bullous emphysema of the intestine: areview of the literature. Am J Gastroenterol. 1971;56(2):125–36. https://doi.org/10.1111/j.1572-0241.1971.tb04186.x.
200. Feuerstein JD, White N, Berzin TM. Pneumatosis intestinalis with a focus on hyperbaric oxygen therapy. Mayo Clin Proc. 2014;89(5):697–703. https://doi.org/10.1016/j.mayocp.2014.01.026.
201. Rescorla FJ, Morrison AM, Engles D, West KW, Grosfeld JL. Hirschsprung's disease. Evaluation of mortality and long-term function in 260 cases. Arch Surg. 1992;127(8):934–41; discussion 41–2
202. Amiel J, Sproat-Emison E, Garcia-Barcelo M, Lantieri F, Burzynski G, Borrego S, et al. Hirschsprung disease, associated

syndromes and genetics: a review. J Med Genet. 2008;45(1):1–14. https://doi.org/10.1136/jmg.2007.053959.
203. Clausen N, Andersson P, Tommerup N. Familial occurrence of neuroblastoma, von Recklinghausen's neurofibromatosis, Hirschsprung's agangliosis and jaw-winking syndrome. Acta Paediatr Scand. 1989;78(5):736–41.
204. Flageole H, Fecteau A, Laberge JM, Guttman FM. Hirschsprung's disease, imperforate anus, and Down's syndrome: a case report. J Pediatr Surg. 1996;31(6):759–60.
205. Melaragno MI, Brunoni D, Patricio FR, Corbani M, Mustacchi Z, dos Santos RC, et al. A patient with tetrasomy 9p, Dandy-Walker cyst and Hirschsprung disease. Ann Genet. 1992;35(2):79–84.
206. Do MY, Myung SJ, Park HJ, Chung JW, Kim IW, Lee SM, et al. Novel classification and pathogenetic analysis of hypoganglionosis and adult-onset Hirschsprung's disease. Dig Dis Sci. 2011;56(6):1818–27. https://doi.org/10.1007/s10620-010-1522-9.
207. Badner JA, Sieber WK, Garver KL, Chakravarti A. A genetic study of Hirschsprung disease. Am J Hum Genet. 1990;46(3):568–80.
208. Puri P, Gosemann JH. Variants of Hirschsprung disease. Semin Pediatr Surg. 2012;21(4):310–8. https://doi.org/10.1053/j.sempedsurg.2012.07.005.
209. Mundt E, Bates MD. Genetics of Hirschsprung disease and anorectal malformations. Semin Pediatr Surg. 2010;19(2):107–17. https://doi.org/10.1053/j.sempedsurg.2009.11.015.
210. Swaminathan M, Kapur RP. Counting myenteric ganglion cells in histologic sections: an empirical approach. Hum Pathol. 2010;41(8):1097–108. https://doi.org/10.1016/j.humpath.2009.12.012.
211. Yang S, Donner LR. Detection of ganglion cells in the colonic plexuses by immunostaining for neuron-specific marker NeuN: an aid for the diagnosis of Hirschsprung disease. Appl Immunohistochem Mol Morphol. 2002;10(3):218–20.
212. Karim S, Hession C, Marconi S, Gang DL, Otis CN. The identification of ganglion cells in Hirschsprung disease by the immunohistochemical detection of ret oncoprotein. Am J Clin Pathol. 2006;126(1):49–54. https://doi.org/10.1309/YG56-BUXH-WURF-JP3E.
213. Park SH, Min H, Chi JG, Park KW, Yang HR, Seo JK. Immunohistochemical studies of pediatric intestinal pseudo-obstruction: bcl2, a valuable biomarker to detect immature enteric ganglion cells. Am J Surg Pathol. 2005;29(8):1017–24.
214. Barshack I, Fridman E, Goldberg I, Chowers Y, Kopolovic J. The loss of calretinin expression indicates aganglionosis in Hirschsprung's disease. J Clin Pathol. 2004;57(7):712–6. https://doi.org/10.1136/jcp.2004.016030.
215. Guinard-Samuel V, Bonnard A, De Lagausie P, Philippe-Chomette P, Alberti C, El Ghoneimi A, et al. Calretinin immunohistochemistry: a simple and efficient tool to diagnose Hirschsprung disease. Mod Pathol. 2009;22(10):1379–84. https://doi.org/10.1038/modpathol.2009.110.
216. Kapur RP, Reed RC, Finn LS, Patterson K, Johanson J, Rutledge JC. Calretinin immunohistochemistry versus acetylcholinesterase histochemistry in the evaluation of suction rectal biopsies for hirschsprung disease. Pediatr Dev Pathol. 2009;12(1):6–15. https://doi.org/10.2350/08-02-0424.1.
217. Gonzalo DH, Plesec T. Hirschsprung disease and use of calretinin in inadequate rectal suction biopsies. Arch Pathol Lab Med. 2013;137(8):1099–102. https://doi.org/10.5858/arpa.2012-0220-OA.
218. Knowles CH, De Giorgio R, Kapur RP, Bruder E, Farrugia G, Geboes K, et al. Gastrointestinal neuromuscular pathology: guidelines for histological techniques and reporting on behalf of the Gastro 2009 International Working Group. Acta Neuropathol. 2009;118(2):271–301. https://doi.org/10.1007/s00401-009-0527-y.
219. Dingemann J, Puri P. Isolated hypoganglionosis: systematic review of a rare intestinal innervation defect. Pediatr Surg Int. 2010;26(11):1111–5. https://doi.org/10.1007/s00383-010-2693-3.
220. Meier-Ruge WA, Brunner LA, Engert J, Heminghaus M, Holschneider AM, Jordan P, et al. A correlative morphometric and clinical investigation of hypoganglionosis of the colon in children. Eur J Pediatr Surg. 1999;9(2):67–74. https://doi.org/10.1055/s-2008-1072216.
221. Qadir I, Salick MM, Barakzai A, Zafar H. Isolated adult hypoganglionosis presenting as sigmoid volvulus: a case report. J Med Case Rep. 2011;5:445. https://doi.org/10.1186/1752-1947-5-445.
222. Aldossary MY, Privitera A, Elzamzami O, Alturki N, Sabr K. A rare case of adult-onset rectosigmoid hypoganglionosis. Am J Case Rep. 2018;19:557–61. https://doi.org/10.12659/AJCR.907109.
223. Milla PJ, Smith VV. Intestinal neuronal dysplasia. J Pediatr Gastroenterol Nutr. 1993;17(4):356–7.
224. Rajalakshmi T, Makhija P, Babu MK, Kini U. Intestinal neuronal dysplasia type A. Indian J Pediatr. 2003;70(10):839–41.
225. Meier-Ruge WA, Bruder E, Kapur RP. Intestinal neuronal dysplasia type B: one giant ganglion is not good enough. Pediatr Dev Pathol. 2006;9(6):444–52. https://doi.org/10.2350/06-06-0109.1.
226. Kapur RP, Reyes-Mugica M. Intestinal neuronal dysplasia type B: an updated review of a problematic diagnosis. Arch Pathol Lab Med. 2019;143(2):235–43. https://doi.org/10.5858/arpa.2017-0524-RA.
227. Barnett JL, McDonnell WM, Appelman HD, Dobbins WO. Familial visceral neuropathy with neuronal intranuclear inclusions: diagnosis by rectal biopsy. Gastroenterology. 1992;102(2):684–91.
228. Krishnamurthy S, Schuffler MD. Pathology of neuromuscular disorders of the small intestine and colon. Gastroenterology. 1987;93(3):610–39.
229. Knowles CH, Nickols CD, Scott SM, Bennett NI, de Oliveira RB, Chimelli L, et al. Smooth muscle inclusion bodies in slow transit constipation. J Pathol. 2001;193(3):390–7. https://doi.org/10.1002/1096-9896(2000)9999:9999<::AID-PATH797>3.0.CO;2-C.
230. Sipponen T, Karikoski R, Nuutinen H, Markkola A, Kaitila I. Three-generation familial visceral myopathy with alpha-actin-positive inclusion bodies in intestinal smooth muscle. J Clin Gastroenterol. 2009;43(5):437–43. https://doi.org/10.1097/MCG.0b013e31817d3f84.
231. Smith VV, Lake BD, Kamm MA, Nicholls RJ. Intestinal pseudo-obstruction with deficient smooth muscle alpha-actin. Histopathology. 1992;21(6):535–42.
232. Knowles CH, Silk DBA, Darzi A, Veress B, Feakins R, Raimundo AH, et al. Deranged smooth muscle α-actin as a biomarker of intestinal pseudo-obstruction: a controlled multinational case series. Gut. 2004;53(11):1583–9. https://doi.org/10.1136/gut.2003.037275.
233. Perez-Atayde AR, Fox V, Teitelbaum JE, Anthony DA, Fadic R, Kalsner L, et al. Mitochondrial neurogastrointestinal encephalomyopathy: diagnosis by rectal biopsy. Am J Surg Pathol. 1998;22(9):1141–7. https://doi.org/10.1097/00000478-199809000-00014.
234. Coulie B, Camilleri M. Intestinal pseudo-obstruction. Annu Rev Med. 1999;50:37–55. https://doi.org/10.1146/annurev.med.50.1.37.
235. Koch TR, Carney JA, Go L, Go VL. Idiopathic chronic constipation is associated with decreased colonic vasoactive intestinal peptide. Gastroenterology. 1988;94(2):300–10.
236. Gittes GK, Kim J, Yu G, de Lorimier AA. Severe constipation with diffuse intestinal myenteric hyperganglionosis. J Pediatr Surg. 1993;28(12):1630–2.
237. He C, Burgart L, Wang L, Pemberton J, Young Fadok T, Szurszewski J, et al. Decreased interstitial cell of Cajal volume in patients with

slow- transit constipation. Gastroenterology. 2000;118(1):14–21. https://doi.org/10.1016/S0016-5085(00)70409-4.
238. Lyford GL, He CL, Soffer E, Hull TL, Strong SA, Senagore AJ, et al. Pan-colonic decrease in interstitial cells of Cajal in patients with slow transit constipation. Gut. 2002;51(4):496–501.
239. Krishnamurthy S, Heng Y, Schuffler MD. Chronic intestinal pseudo-obstruction in infants and children caused by diverse abnormalities of the myenteric plexus. Gastroenterology. 1993;104(5):1398–408.
240. Park HJ, Kamm MA, Abbasi AM, Talbot IC. Immunohistochemical study of the colonic muscle and innervation in idiopathic chronic constipation. Dis Colon Rectum. 1995;38(5):509–13.
241. Wedel T, Roblick UJ, Ott V, Eggers R, Schiedeck TH, Krammer HJ, et al. Oligoneuronal hypoganglionosis in patients with idiopathic slow-transit constipation. Dis Colon Rectum. 2002;45(1):54–62.
242. Wedel T, Spiegler J, Soellner S, Roblick UJ, Schiedeck TH, Bruch HP, et al. Enteric nerves and interstitial cells of Cajal are altered in patients with slow-transit constipation and megacolon. Gastroenterology. 2002;123(5):1459–67.
243. Murray RD, Qualman SJ, Powers P, Caniano DA, McClung HJ, Ulysses B, et al. Rectal myopathy in chronically constipated children. Pediatr Pathol. 1992;12(6):787–98.
244. Wang LM, McNally M, Hyland J, Sheahan K. Assessing interstitial cells of Cajal in slow transit constipation using CD117 is a useful diagnostic test. Am J Surg Pathol. 2008;32(7):980–5. https://doi.org/10.1097/PAS.0b013e318164e469.
245. Valdovinos MA, Camilleri M, Zimmerman BR. Chronic diarrhea in diabetes mellitus: mechanisms and an approach to diagnosis and treatment. Mayo Clin Proc. 1993;68(7):691–702.
246. Tada S, Iida M, Yao T, Kitamoto T, Yao T, Fujishima M. Intestinal pseudo-obstruction in patients with amyloidosis: clinicopathologic differences between chemical types of amyloid protein. Gut. 1993;34(10):1412–7.
247. Liapis K, Michelis FV, Delimpasi S, Karmiris T. Intestinal pseudo-obstruction associated with amyloidosis. Amyloid. 2011;18(2):76–8. https://doi.org/10.3109/13506129.2010.548085 .
248. Keighley MRB, Williams NS. Surgery of the anus, rectum and colon. Philadelphia: WB Saunders; 1993.
249. Gordon PH, Nivatvongs S. Principles and practice of surgery for the colon, rectum and anus. 2nd ed. St. Louis: Quality Medical; 1999.
250. Pidala MJ, Slezak FA, Hlivko TJ. Delayed presentation of an inflammatory polyp following colonic ischemia. Am Surg. 1993;59(5):315–8.
251. De Backer AI, Van Overbeke LN, Mortele KJ, Ros PR, Pelgrims J. Inflammatory pseudopolyposis in a patient with toxic megacolon due to pseudomembranous colitis. JBR-BTR. 2001;84(5):201.
252. Nakano H, Miyachi I, Kitagawa Y, Saito H, Yamauchi M, Horiguchi Y, et al. Crohn's disease associated with giant inflammatory polyposis. Endoscopy. 1987;19(6):246–8. https://doi.org/10.1055/s-2007-1018294.
253. Yada S, Matsumoto T, Kudo T, Hirahashi M, Yao T, Mibu R, et al. Colonic obstruction due to giant inflammatory polyposis in a patient with ulcerative colitis. J Gastroenterol. 2005;40(5):536–9. https://doi.org/10.1007/s00535-004-1580-x.
254. Abou Rached A, Saba J, El Masri L, Nakhoul M, Razzouk C. Obstructive giant inflammatory polyposis: is it related to the severity or the duration of the inflammatory bowel disease? Two Case Reports. Case Rep Gastrointest Med. 2018;2018:3251549. https://doi.org/10.1155/2018/3251549.
255. Hokama A, Nagahama M, Kishimoto K, Fujita J. Colonic stricture with filiform polyposis in Crohn's disease. BMJ Case Rep. 2014;2014:bcr2014204710. https://doi.org/10.1136/bcr-2014-204710.
256. Tsung SH. Filiform polyposis in a patient without inflammatory bowel disease. Ann Clin Lab Sci. 2013;43(1):98–100.
257. Wyse J, Lamoureux E, Gordon PH, Bitton A. Occult dysplasia in a localized giant pseudopolyp in Crohn's colitis: a case report. Can J Gastroenterol. 2009;23(7):477–8.
258. Jessurun J, Paplanus SH, Nagle RB, Hamilton SR, Yardley JH, Tripp M. Pseudosarcomatous changes in inflammatory pseudopolyps of the colon. Arch Pathol Lab Med. 1986;110(9):833–6.
259. De Petris G, Dhungel BM, Chen L, Pasha SF. Inflammatory "cap" polyposis: acase report of a rare nonneoplastic colonic polyposis. Int J Surg Pathol. 2014;22(4):378–82. https://doi.org/10.1177/1066896913501383.
260. Li JH, Leong MY, Phua KB, Low Y, Kader A, Logarajah V, et al. Cap polyposis: a rare cause of rectal bleeding in children. World J Gastroenterol. 2013;19(26):4185–91. https://doi.org/10.3748/wjg.v19.i26.4185.
261. Ng KH, Mathur P, Kumarasinghe MP, Eu KW, Seow-Choen F. Cap polyposis: further experience and review. Dis Colon Rectum. 2004;47(7):1208–15. https://doi.org/10.1007/s10350-004-0561-8.
262. Tsai HL, Lin CH, Cheng YL, Huang CW, Wang JY. Rectal carcinoma in a young female patient with Peutz-Jeghers syndrome: a case report. Med Princ Pract. 2014;23(1):89–91. https://doi.org/10.1159/000351835.
263. Derici H, Peker Y, Tatar F, Cin N, Deniz V. Multiple malign gastrointestinal polyps and rectal carcinoma in a young patient with Peutz-Jeghers syndrome. Int J Color Dis. 2007;22(1):85–6. https://doi.org/10.1007/s00384-005-0001-9.
264. Syngal S, Brand RE, Church JM, Giardiello FM, Hampel HL, Burt RW. ACG clinical guideline: genetic testing and management of hereditary gastrointestinal cancer syndromes. Am J Gastroenterol. 2015;110(2):223–62. https://doi.org/10.1038/ajg.2014.435.
265. Gupta SK, Fitzgerald JF, Croffie JM, Chong SK, Pfefferkorn MC, Davis MM, et al. Experience with juvenile polyps in North American children: the need for pancolonoscopy. Am J Gastroenterol. 2001;96(6):1695–7. https://doi.org/10.1111/j.1572-0241.2001.03860.x.
266. Wu TT, Rezai B, Rashid A, Luce MC, Cayouette MC, Kim C, et al. Genetic alterations and epithelial dysplasia in juvenile polyposis syndrome and sporadic juvenile polyps. Am J Pathol. 1997;150(3):939–47.
267. Kapetanakis AM, Vini D, Plitsis G. Solitary juvenile polyps in children and colon cancer. Hepato-Gastroenterology. 1996;43(12):1530–1.
268. Nugent KP, Talbot IC, Hodgson SV, Phillips RKS. Solitary juvenile polyps: not a marker for subsequent malignancy. Gastroenterology. 1993;105(3):698–700. https://doi.org/10.1016/0016-5085(93)90885-G.
269. Brosens LAA, Van Hattem A, Hylind LM, Iacobuzio-Donahue C, Romans KE, Axilbund J, et al. Risk of colorectal cancer in juvenile polyposis. Gut. 2007;56(7):965–7. https://doi.org/10.1136/gut.2006.116913.
270. Ward EM, Wolfsen HC. Review article: the non-inherited gastrointestinal polyposis syndromes. Aliment Pharmacol Ther. 2002;16(3):333–42. https://doi.org/10.1046/j.1365-2036.2002.01172.x.
271. Daniel ES, Ludwig SL, Lewin KJ, Ruprecht RM, Rajacich GM, Schwabe AD. The Cronkhite-Canada syndrome: an analysis of clinical and pathologic features and therapy in 55 patients. Medicine (United States). 1982;61(5):293–309.
272. Riegert-Johnson DL, Osborn N, Smyrk T, Boardman LA. Cronkhite-Canada syndrome hamartomatous polyps are infiltrated with IgG4 plasma cells [1]. Digestion. 2007;75(2–3):96–7. https://doi.org/10.1159/000102963.
273. Sweetser S, Ahlquist DA, Osborn NK, Sanderson SO, Smyrk TC, Chari ST, et al. Clinicopathologic features and treatment

outcomes in Cronkhite-Canada syndrome: support for autoimmunity. Dig Dis Sci. 2012;57(2):496–502. https://doi.org/10.1007/s10620-011-1874-9.
274. Burke AP, Sobin LH. The pathology of Cronkhite-Canada polyps. A comparison to juvenile polyposis. Am J Surg Pathol. 1989;13(11):940–6. https://doi.org/10.1097/00000478-198911000-00004.
275. Fan RY, Wang XW, Xue LJ, An R, Sheng JQ. Cronkhite-Canada syndrome polyps infiltrated with IgG4-positive plasma cells. World J Clin Cases. 2016;4(8):248–52. https://doi.org/10.12998/wjcc.v4.i8.248.
276. Malhotra R, Sheffield A. Cronkhite-Canada syndrome associated with colon carcinoma and adenomatous changes in C-C polyps. Am J Gastroenterol. 1988;83(7):772–6.
277. Katayama Y, Kimura M, Konn M. Cronkhite-Canada syndrome associated with a rectal cancer and adenomatous changed in colonic polyps. Am J Surg Pathol. 1985;9(1):65–71. https://doi.org/10.1097/00000478-198501000-00011.
278. Jain A, Nanda S, Chakraborty P, Kundra A, Anuradha S, Reddy BSN, et al. Cronkhite-Canada syndrome with adenomatous and carcinomatous transformation of colonic polyp. Indian J Gastroenterol. 2003;22(5):189–90.
279. Rappaport LB, Sperling HV, Stavrides A. Colon cancer in the Cronkhite-Canada syndrome. J Clin Gastroenterol. 1986;8(2):199–202.
280. Eng C. Will the real Cowden syndrome please stand up: revised diagnostic criteria. J Med Genet. 2000;37(11):828–30.
281. Stanich PP, Owens VL, Sweetser S, Khambatta S, Smyrk TC, Richardson RL, et al. Colonic polyposis and neoplasia in Cowden syndrome. Mayo Clin Proc. 2011;86(6):489–92. https://doi.org/10.4065/mcp.2010.0816.
282. Heald B, Mester J, Rybicki L, Orloff MS, Burke CA, Eng C. Frequent gastrointestinal polyps and colorectal adenocarcinomas in a prospective series of PTEN mutation carriers. Gastroenterology. 2010;139(6):1927–33. https://doi.org/10.1053/j.gastro.2010.06.061.
283. Stanich PP, Pilarski R, Rock J, Frankel WL, El-Dika S, Meyer MM. Colonic manifestations of PTEN hamartoma tumor syndrome: case series and systematic review. World J Gastroenterol. 2014;20(7):1833–8. https://doi.org/10.3748/wjg.v20.i7.1833.
284. Borowsky J, Setia N, Lauwers G. Gastrointestinal tract pathology in PTEN hamartoma tumour syndrome: a review of 43 cases. Mod Pathol. 2015;28:149.
285. Chi SG, Kim HJ, Park BJ, Min HJ, Park JH, Kim YW, et al. Mutational abrogation of the PTEN/MMAC1 gene in gastrointestinal polyps in patients with Cowden disease. Gastroenterology. 1998;115(5):1084–9.
286. Ngeow J, Heald B, Rybicki LA, Orloff MS, Chen JL, Liu X, et al. Prevalence of germline PTEN, BMPR1A, SMAD4, STK11, and ENG mutations in patients with moderate-load colorectal polyps. Gastroenterology. 2013;144(7):1402–9, 9.e1–5. https://doi.org/10.1053/j.gastro.2013.02.001.
287. Shaco-Levy R, Jasperson KW, Martin K, Samadder NJ, Burt RW, Ying J, et al. Gastrointestinal polyposis in Cowden syndrome. J Clin Gastroenterol. 2017;51(7):e60–e7. https://doi.org/10.1097/MCG.0000000000000703.
288. Shaco-Levy R, Jasperson KW, Martin K, Samadder NJ, Burt RW, Ying J, et al. Morphologic characterization of hamartomatous gastrointestinal polyps in Cowden syndrome, Peutz-Jeghers syndrome, and juvenile polyposis syndrome. Hum Pathol. 2016;49:39–48. https://doi.org/10.1016/j.humpath.2015.10.002.
289. Caliskan A, Kohlmann WK, Affolter KE, Downs-Kelly E, Kanth P, Bronner MP. Intramucosal lipomas of the colon implicate Cowden syndrome. Mod Pathol. 2018;31(4):643–51. https://doi.org/10.1038/modpathol.2017.161.
290. Tan MH, Mester JL, Ngeow J, Rybicki LA, Orloff MS, Eng C. Lifetime cancer risks in individuals with germline PTEN mutations. Clin Cancer Res. 2012;18(2):400–7. https://doi.org/10.1158/1078-0432.CCR-11-2283.
291. Vasaitis L. IgG4-related disease: a relatively new concept for clinicians. Eur J Intern Med. 2016;27:1–9. https://doi.org/10.1016/j.ejim.2015.09.022.
292. Deshpande V, Zen Y, Chan JKC. Consensus statement on the pathology of IgG4-related disease. Mod Pathol. 2012;139:1–12.
293. Hiyoshi Y, Oki E, Zaitsu Y, Ando K, Ito S, Saeki H, et al. IgG4-related disease of the ileocecal region mimicking malignancy: a case report. Int J Surg Case Rep. 2014;5(10):669–72. https://doi.org/10.1016/j.ijscr.2014.08.003.
294. Chetty R, Serra S, Gauchotte G, Märkl B, Agaimy A. Sclerosing nodular lesions of the gastrointestinal tract containing large numbers of IgG4 plasma cells. Pathology. 2011;43(1):31–5. https://doi.org/10.1097/PAT.0b013e328340e450.
295. Ciccone F, Ciccone A, Di Ruscio M, Vernia F, Cipolloni G, Coletti G, et al. IgG4-related disease mimicking Crohn's disease: acase report and review of literature. Dig Dis Sci. 2018;63(4):1072–86. https://doi.org/10.1007/s10620-018-4950-6.
296. Coyne JD. Melanosis coli in hyperplastic polyps and adenomas. Int J Surg Pathol. 2013;21(3):261–3. https://doi.org/10.1177/1066896912468212.
297. Byers RJ, Marsh P, Parkinson D, Haboubi NY. Melanosis coli is associated with an increase in colonic epithelial apoptosis and not with laxative use. Histopathology. 1997;30(2):160–4.
298. Shemesh E, Bat L, Niv Y, Newmann G. Melanosis coli within an adenomatous polyp. Gastrointest Endosc. 1983;29(4):327–9.
299. Ewing CA, Kalan M, Chucker F, Ozdemirli M. Melanosis coli involving pericolonic lymph nodes associated with the herbal laxative Swiss Kriss: a rare and incidental finding in a patient with colonic adenocarcinoma. Arch Pathol Lab Med. 2004;128(5):565–7. https://doi.org/10.1043/1543-2165(2004)128<565:MCIPLN>2.0.CO;2.
300. Ramai D, Linn S, Murphy T, Reddy M. Transmural polypoid endometriosis of the sigmoid colon. J Gastrointest Surg. 2018;22:2184–6. https://doi.org/10.1007/s11605-018-3762-5.
301. Rana R, Sharma S, Narula H, Madhok B. A case of recto-sigmoid endometriosis mimicking carcinoma. Springerplus. 2016;5:643. https://doi.org/10.1186/s40064-016-2221-6.
302. Baden DN, van de Ven A, Verbeek PC. Endometriosis with an acute colon obstruction: a case report. J Med Case Rep. 2015;9:150. https://doi.org/10.1186/s13256-015-0609-5.
303. Ito D, Kaneko S, Morita K, Seiichiro S, Teruya M, Kaminishi M. Cecal volvulus caused by endometriosis in a young woman. BMC Surg. 2015;15:77. https://doi.org/10.1186/s12893-015-0063-8.
304. Li N, Zhou W, Zhao L, Zhou J. Endometriosis-associated recto-sigmoid cancer: a case report. BMC Cancer. 2018;18(1):905. https://doi.org/10.1186/s12885-018-4797-4.
305. Palla VV, Karaolanis G, Bliona T, Katafigiotis I, Anastasiou I, Hassiakos D. Endometrioid adenocarcinoma arising from colon endometriosis. SAGE Open Med Case Rep. 2017;5:2050313X17745204. https://doi.org/10.1177/2050313X17745204.
306. McCluggage WG, Clements WD. Endosalpingiosis of the colon and appendix. Histopathology. 2001;39(6):645–6.

Part VII

Non-neoplastic Diseases of the Appendix and Anus

19 Non-neoplastic Diseases of Appendix

Samar Said

Acute Appendicitis

Definition

Acute appendicitis is acute inflammation involving vermiform appendix, which is one of the most common causes of acute abdomen in adults and children.

Clinical Features

Acute appendicitis can occur at any age. However, it is much more common in children and young adults. Causes of acute appendicitis include luminal obstruction (by fecalith, undigested food, lymphoid hyperplasia, mucin accumulation, polyp/tumor, or foreign body material) superimposed by bacterial infection, hypersensitivity reaction, and infection. Clinically, patients present with periumbilical abdominal pain that later localizes to the right lower quadrant, mild fever, anorexia, and nausea. Atypical location of the appendix can result in atypical presentation. Mixed aerobic and anaerobic bacteria are often isolated by culture in cases of acute appendicitis. The isolated bacteria might play a secondary role after mucosal injury, and they have been linked to a higher risk of abscess formation [1–4].

Pathological Features

Gross Findings

Grossly, the appendix may appear swollen and erythematous. The serosa appears dull and grey and may show purulent exudate. Grossly normal appendix is seen in early lesions when the inflammation is limited to the mucosa and submucosa. A fecalith can be identified in a third of cases. Perforation from mural necrosis and abscess formation may also be seen on gross examination.

Microscopic Findings

Microscopic examination demonstrates neutrophilic or mixed inflammatory infiltrate with neutrophilic cryptitis, crypt abscesses, and ulceration (Fig. 19.1a–c). The acute inflammation may be restricted to the mucosa in early lesions but later extends to the submucosa and muscularis propria (Fig. 19.1d). In cases where the inflammation is limited to the mucosa, deeper levels might be helpful in revealing the mural inflammation. Progressive transmural inflammation results in serositis and sometimes perforation (Fig. 19.1d). Gangrenous appendicitis is referred to severe cases with mural necrosis and hemorrhage (Fig. 19.1e). Thrombosed vessels and luminal neutrophils can be seen. Luminal neutrophils alone, however, are not sufficient for a diagnosis of acute appendicitis. If appendectomy is not performed in the acute phase, chronic changes will eventually develop and include serosal fibrous adhesions and submucosal fibrosis. In addition, the inflammatory infiltrate becomes more mixed with both acute (neutrophils) and chronic inflammatory cells (lymphocytes, eosinophils, histiocytes, and plasma cells). Granulation tissue with foreign body-type giant cells suggests prior rupture. Mucin extravasation can also be seen [4].

Complications

Complications are usually seen in cases with severe inflammation, cases that are not treated, or cases with delayed treatment due to delayed diagnosis. The major complications are:

1. Perforation: This is the most common complication of acute appendicitis resulting in peritonitis and abscess formation. Young children and elderly patients are at

S. Said (✉)
Department of Laboratory Medicine and Pathology, Mayo Clinic, Rochester, MN, USA
e-mail: said.samar@mayo.edu

L. Zhang et al. (eds.), *Surgical Pathology of Non-neoplastic Gastrointestinal Diseases*,
https://doi.org/10.1007/978-3-030-15573-5_19

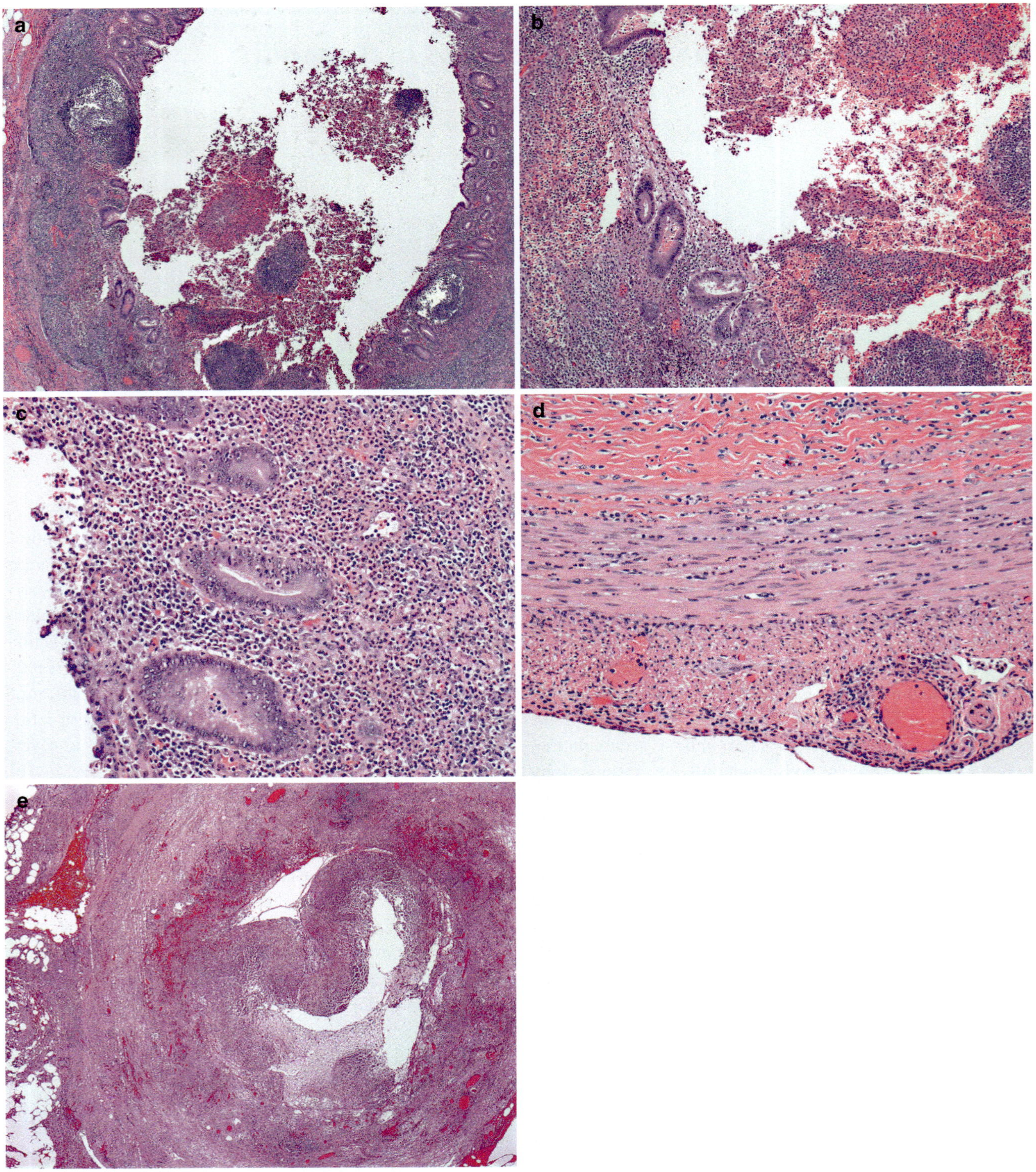

Fig. 19.1 Acute appendicitis. (**a**) Luminal fibrinoinflammatory exudate and mucosal erosion. (**b**) Higher-power picture with similar findings. (**c**) Neutrophilic infiltrate and cryptitis. (**d**) Mural and serosal neutrophilic inflammation. (**e**) Gangrenous appendicitis showing mural necrosis with hemorrhage

increased risk. Perforation rate is also higher in HIV-positive patients [5].

2. Periappendiceal abscesses: This is seen mainly in perforated appendices.
3. Fistula formation: This is usually seen in untreated cases where the inflammation extends outside the appendix and results in fistulation into small bowel, colon, or skin surface.

4. Infertility: This results from obstruction of an adjacent fallopian tube.
5. Pylephlebitis: This results from inflammation of adjacent blood vessels.
6. Stump appendicitis: Stump appendicitis is residual or progressive acute inflammation in the remaining stump of the appendix after appendectomy. It is an uncommon late complication. The diagnosis is usually made late, which increases the incidence of necrosis, gangrene, and perforation in these patients. Microscopic examination reveals findings similar to acute appendicitis with neutrophilic infiltrate and transmural inflammation. Necrosis, perforation, and rarely granulomatous inflammation may be present [6–8].

Differential Diagnosis

Periappendicitis secondary to peritonitis due to other intra-abdominal causes: histologically, the neutrophilic infiltration is limited to the serosa and periappendiceal tissue with fibrin deposition and serosal adhesions without associated mural or mucosal inflammation that are typically seen in acute appendicitis.

Inflammatory bowel disease: chronic changes are seen, and the patients may have a history of inflammatory bowel disease (see below).

Treatment and Prognosis

Appendectomy is the only curative treatment of acute appendicitis. For patients with abscess formation, elective appendectomy after intravenous antibiotic therapy and/or drainage is appropriate. Antibiotic therapy covering Gram-negative and anaerobic organisms also plays an important role in the management; an interval appendectomy can be performed 4–6 weeks later. The complication rate of appendectomy is approximately 10%, and the overall mortality rate is less than 1%, which is mainly due to severe complications rather than to the surgery.

Chronic Appendicitis

Definition

The definition of chronic appendicitis is controversial. It has been used to describe chronic changes and fibrous replacement of the appendix wall after severe, prolonged, or recurrent episodes of acute appendicitis. In general, it is an umbrella diagnosis that includes any type of chronic inflammatory conditions of the appendix other than the classic acute appendicitis. Some forms of chronic appendicitis are described below.

Xanthogranulomatous Appendicitis

This results from progression of untreated acute appendicitis. Foam cells and multinucleated histiocytes are the predominant inflammatory infiltrate (Fig. 19.2a, b). Hemosiderin deposition and luminal obliteration can also be seen [9, 10].

Interval Appendicitis

This term is used when ruptured acute appendicitis is treated with antibiotics and drainage followed by appendectomy 4–8 weeks later. Neutrophilic cryptitis, crypt abscesses,

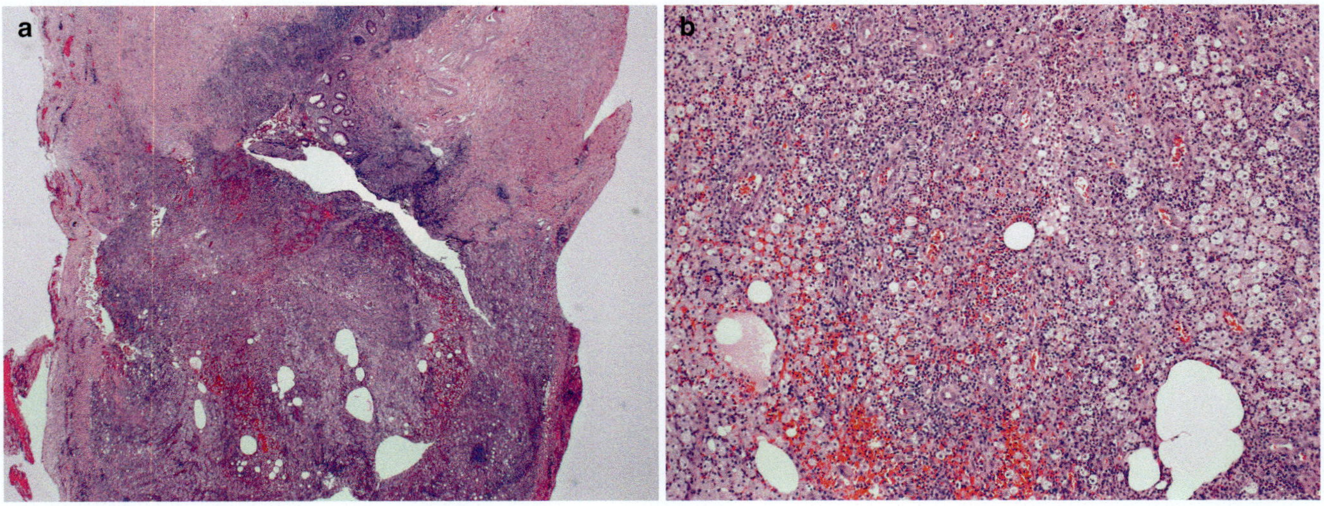

Fig. 19.2 Xanthogranulomatous appendicitis. (**a**) Dense mucosal and mural inflammatory infiltrate. (**b**) The inflammatory infiltrate is composed of mainly histiocytes with some lymphocytes and neutrophils

granulomas, giant cells, crypt distortion, mural fibrosis, and transmural chronic inflammation with lymphoid aggregates can be seen on histologic examination, mimicking Crohn's disease (Fig. 19.3a). Xanthogranulomatous inflammation is seen in at least a third of cases (Fig. 19.3b, c) [9, 11, 12].

Inflammatory Bowel Disease

Ulcerative Colitis

Approximately 50% of patients with ulcerative colitis have appendiceal involvement. This is typically seen in patients with pancolitis; however, it can also occur as a skip lesion in patients with partial colon involvement including cases with rectal only disease. Grossly, mucosal erythema and ulceration may be seen. The histologic findings are similar to those seen in the colon. Neutrophilic cryptitis and crypt abscesses indicate activity. Erosions, ulceration, and suppurative luminal exudate may also be present (Fig. 19.4a). Chronic changes include crypt architectural distortion, lamina propria lymphoplasmacytic infiltrate, basal lymphoplasmacytosis, and Paneth cell hyperplasia (Fig. 19.4b) [13, 14].

Crohn's Disease

Approximately 20% of patients with Crohn's disease have appendiceal involvement. These patients usually have extensive ileocolonic involvement, and rarely the appendicitis might be the first manifestation of disease [15]. The histologic findings are similar to those seen in the colon and include neutrophilic cryptitis, crypt accesses, ulceration, transmural inflammation with lymphoid aggregates, fissures, fistula formation, nonnecrotizing granulomas, and Paneth cell hyperplasia (Fig. 19.5a–c). Occasionally, the granulomas may have focal necrosis. Knowing the patient's history of Crohn's disease is important as idiopathic granulomatous appendicitis has very similar histologic findings [16, 17].

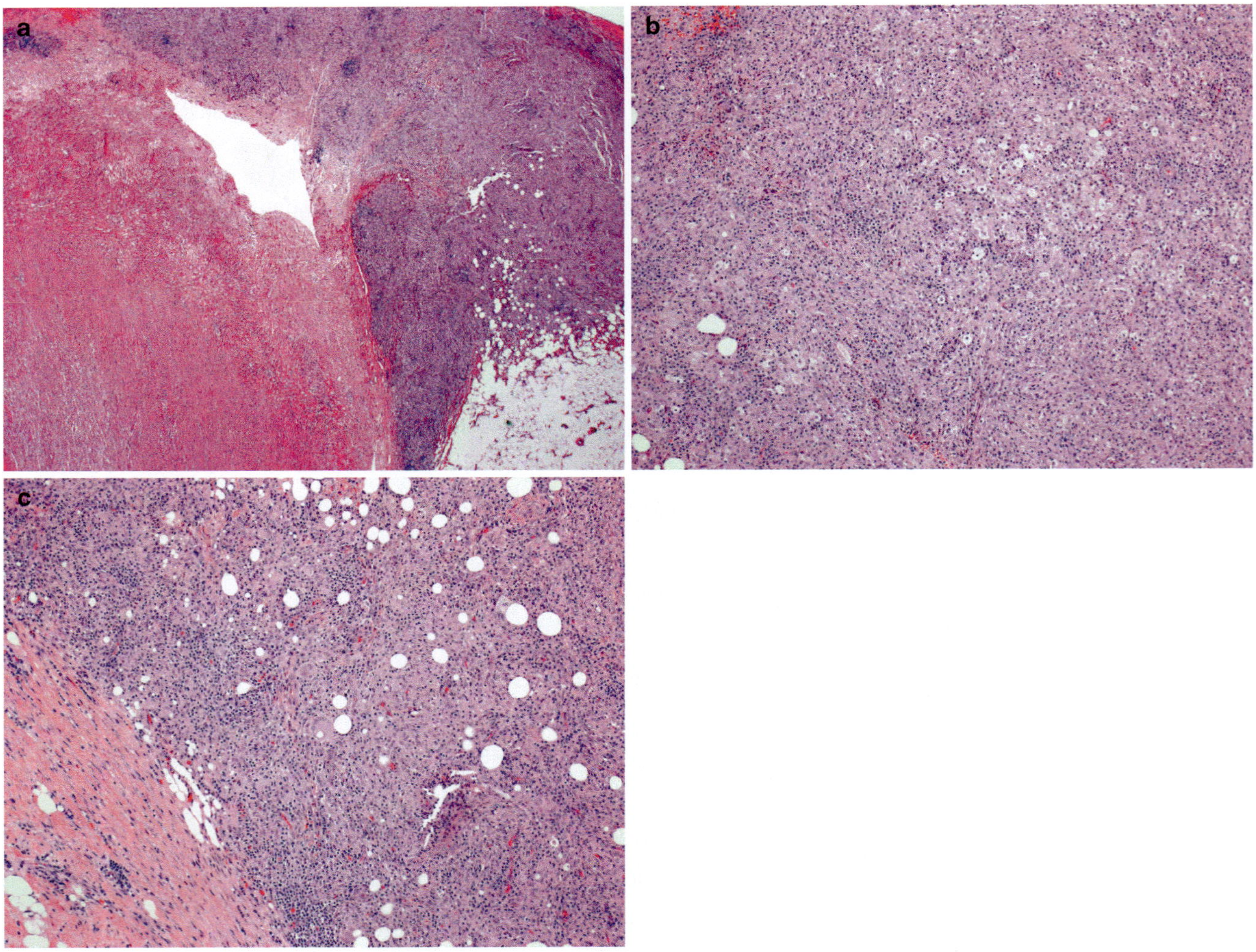

Fig. 19.3 Interval appendicitis from a patient with perforated appendicitis, who was treated with antibiotics and percutaneous drain followed by appendectomy 2 months later. (**a**). Marked appendiceal inflammation. (**b**) The inflammation appears xanthogranulomatous in some areas. (**c**) There are also granulomatous inflammation and giant cells

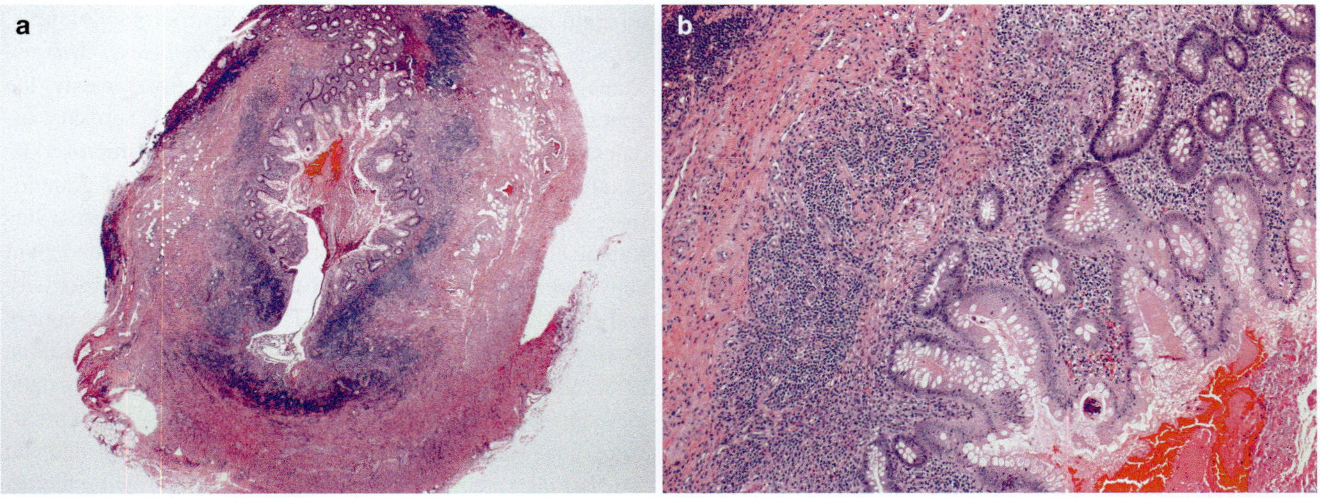

Fig. 19.4 Appendiceal involvement in ulcerative colitis. (**a**) Mucosal inflammation, focal ulceration and architectural distortion. (**b**) Basal lymphoplasmacytosis, crypt architectural distortion, and active chronic inflammation

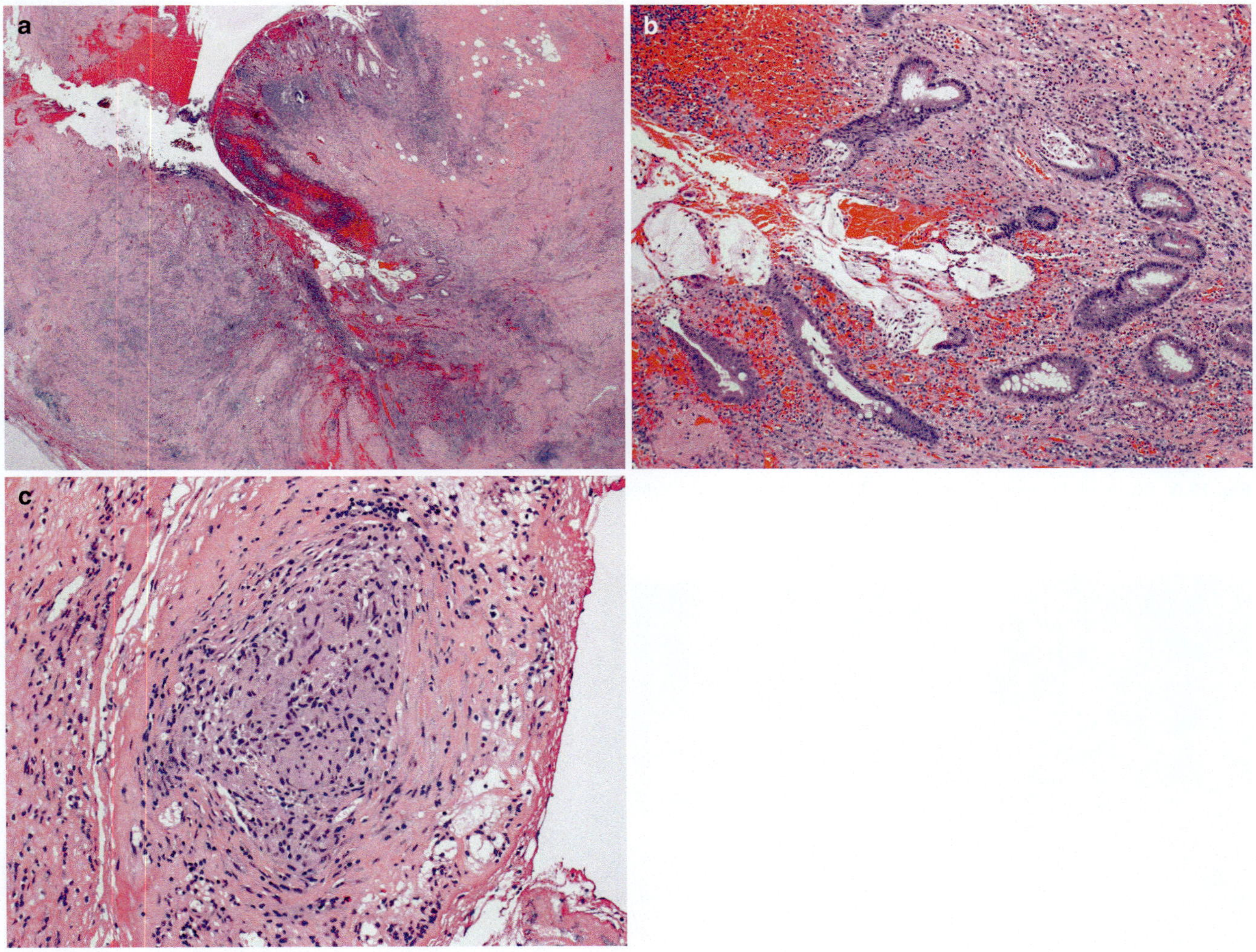

Fig. 19.5 Appendiceal involvement in Crohn's disease. (**a**) Marked mucosal inflammation, knife-like ulceration, architectural distortion, and focal transmural inflammation with lymphoid aggregates. (**b**) Mucosal changes similar to those in colon including cryptitis and crypt branching. (**c**) A subserosal nonnecrotizing granuloma

Eosinophilic Appendicitis

Eosinophilic appendicitis is rare. Histologically, transmural eosinophil-rich inflammation with variable degree of neutrophilic inflammation is seen (Fig. 19.6a, b). The most common cause is parasitic infection such as due to *Strongyloides stercoralis* and *Schistosoma japonicum*. Cases with no identifiable parasites have been reported [1, 18–21].

Granulomatous Appendicitis

Granulomatous appendicitis is uncommon. It can be primary without an identifiable cause (idiopathic granulomatous appendicitis) or secondary to conditions such as sarcoidosis, infection, Crohn's disease, interval appendicitis, and foreign body reaction. Infectious causes include bacteria (*Yersinia*, tuberculosis), parasites (schistosomiasis, strongyloidiasis, parasite ova), and fungi (*Candida*, *Histoplasma*, *Mucor*). Management depends on the underlying cause. Grossly, the appendix might be normal in size or enlarged. Serosal exudates and fibrous adhesion may be present. On microscopic examination, the distinct finding is the presence of granulomas, which are composed of histiocytic aggregates surrounded by lymphocytes with or without multinucleated giant cells and necrosis (Fig. 19.7a, b). Cryptitis, crypt abscesses, and crypt distortion can be seen. The underlying cause cannot usually be determined with certainty based on histology alone and requires correlation with the clinical and laboratory data, although some histologic clues (such as the presence of polarizable material, whether the granulomas are well formed and whether they are necrotizing) might help in narrowing the list of differential diagnosis [11, 14, 22, 23]. Idiopathic granulomatous appendicitis and sarcoidosis are mentioned below.

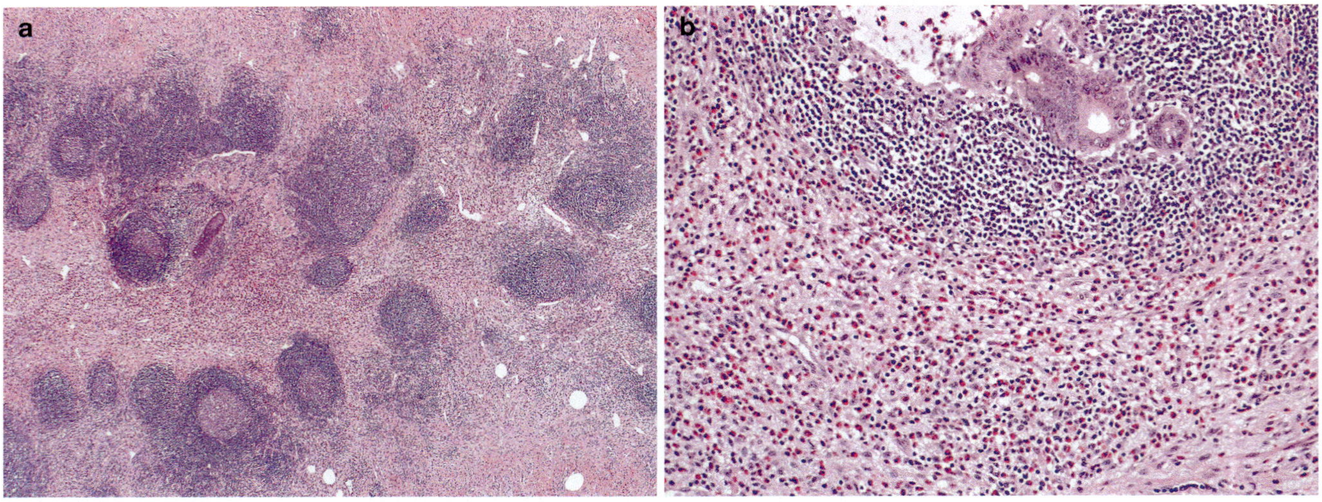

Fig. 19.6 Eosinophilic appendicitis. (**a** and **b**) Dense transmural eosinophilic infiltrate in appendix

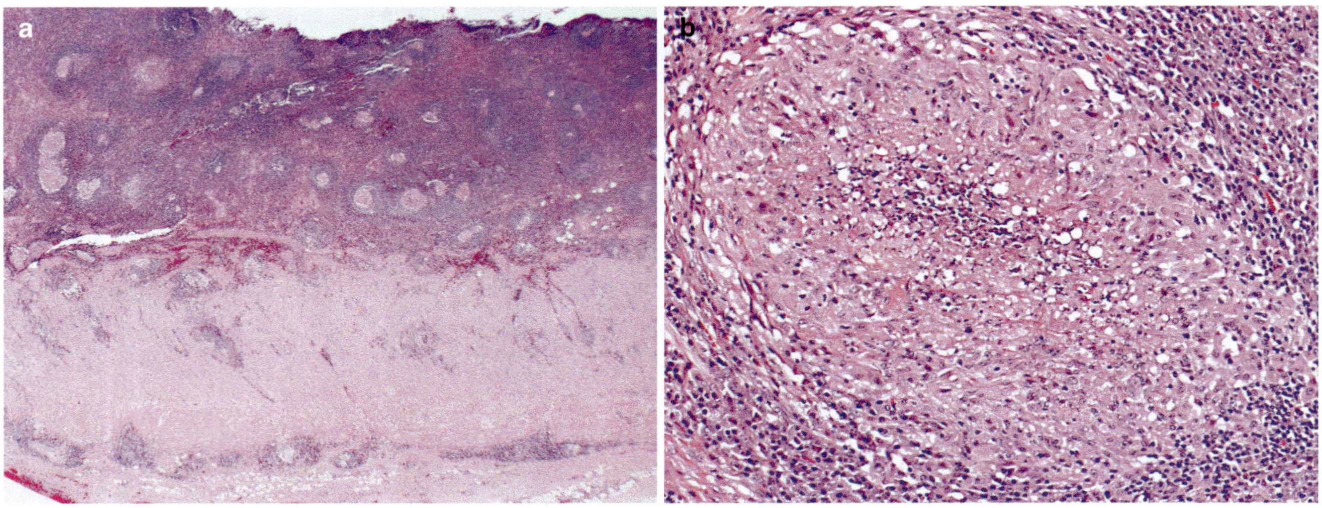

Fig. 19.7 Granulomatous appendicitis. (**a**) Inflammation of the appendiceal wall including multiple granulomas. (**b**) The well-formed granulomas are composed of histiocytic aggregates surrounded by lymphocytes

Idiopathic Granulomatous Appendicitis

Idiopathic granulomatous appendicitis is more common in young adults (average age 29 years). It affects males and females equally. This diagnosis is usually made in patients without a history of Crohn's disease as the histologic findings of the two entities can have significant overlap. Histologically, multiple typically nonnecrotizing granulomas are seen in any layer of the appendiceal wall. Other findings include neutrophilic cryptitis, crypt abscesses, erosions, ulcerations, and chronic changes such as fissures, transmural lymphoid aggregates, and mural fibrosis. The granulomas in idiopathic granulomatous appendicitis are usually more than that seen in Crohn's disease (average 0.3 granulomas per tissue section in Crohn's disease vs. 20 in idiopathic granulomatous appendicitis), while fistulization tends to be more common in Crohn's disease than idiopathic granulomatous appendicitis. Involvement of other bowel sites also favors Crohn's disease. Nevertheless, the histologic findings of the two conditions overlap and this diagnosis should be reserved for non-Crohn's patients. Long-term follow-up might be needed for definitive diagnosis as small percentage of these patients might develop Crohn's disease in the future [24].

Sarcoidosis

Sarcoidosis of the appendix is rare. Histologically, multiple well-formed epithelioid, nonnecrotizing granulomas are present in any layer of the appendix. Neutrophilic cryptitis, fibrosis, and focal necrosis within the granulomas can also be seen. The diagnosis should be made in patients who have clinical evidence of sarcoidosis after exclusion of other causes of granulomatous appendicitis [25–27].

Infectious Appendicitis

This can cause acute or chronic appendicitis. The organisms can be identified on the hematoxylin and eosin (H&E) slides or by immunohistochemical stains, *in situ* hybridization, PCR, or culture [28].

Bacterial Appendicitis

Malakoplakia

This results from incomplete digestion and accumulation of bacteria in histiocytes. Histologically, there is an inflammatory infiltrate composed of mainly histiocytes with eosinophilic cytoplasm and scattered lymphocytes and plasma cells, which results in diffuse or nodular thickening of the mucosa. The characteristic finding is the presence of Michaelis-Gutmann bodies, which are round laminated structures that may have a targetoid appearance and can be highlighted by calcium or iron stains [29].

Yersinia

The two species that are usually involved are *Yersinia enterocolitica* and *Yersinia pseudotuberculosis*. Acute enteritis is seen in young children, whereas terminal ileitis and mesenteric adenitis are seen in older children and young adults. *Yersinia* can cause acute or granulomatous appendicitis. Grossly, the appendix is usually normal. The histologic findings are variable and include unremarkable appendix, mild superficial neutrophilic inflammation only, and suppurative granulomatous inflammation (that have only few B-cells) with large epithelioid granulomas with central microabscesses surrounded by a prominent lymphoid cuff. Lymphoid hyperplasia is typically present and some regional lymph nodes may show granulomatous inflammation with or without neutrophilic inflammation [30, 31].

Actinomyces israelii

It is an uncommon cause of appendicitis. Histologically, acute and chronic inflammation (Fig. 19.8a), abscess formation, fistulas, and perforation may occur. The organisms appear as dark blue long filaments associated with sulfur granules (Fig. 19.8b) [32, 33].

Campylobacter jejuni

It is detected in some cases of acute appendicitis, but it is not clear whether it represents the primary cause of the appendicitis or superimposed infection. Histologically, the findings are similar to those seen in acute appendicitis [34, 35].

Mycobacteria

Isolated infection of the appendix has been reported; however, in the majority of cases, this is associated with tuberculosis infection of the lung and other gastrointestinal sites. Histologically, granulomatous inflammation (usually necrotizing) is typically present (Fig. 19.9a, b), and acid-fast positive bacilli are seen on special stains such as AFB stain. PCR can subtype the organism [21, 36].

Clostridium difficile

This is usually associated with colonic involvement. The characteristic histologic finding is the presence of pseudomembrane formation. Cryptitis, crypt abscesses, and ulceration may also be seen [37, 38].

Spirochetosis

Spirochetosis may rarely affect the appendix. Histologically, no inflammation is typically seen. The organisms are seen on the H&E stain as a hazy band on the surface epithelium which can be highlighted by silver stains like Warthin starry stain. Of note, *Treponema pallidum* immunohistochemical stain will also highlight the organisms due to cross-reaction of the stain with spirochetosis [39].

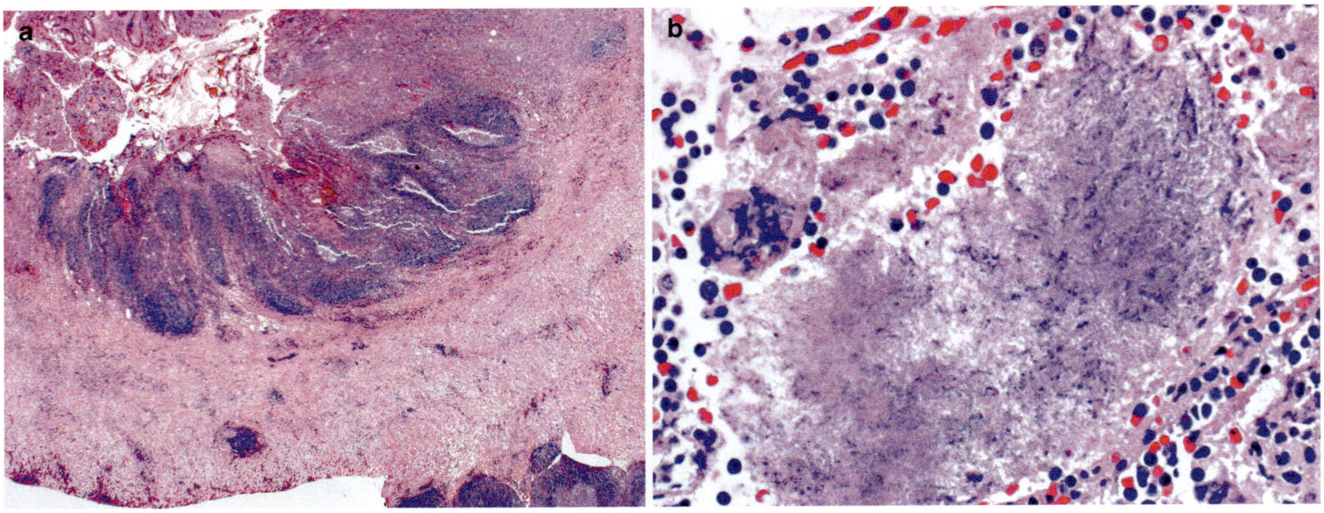

Fig. 19.8 Actinomycosis of the appendix. (**a**) Inflamed appendix with lymphoid hyperplasia. (**b**) The organisms with long filaments appear dark blue (fungal ball) on the H&E

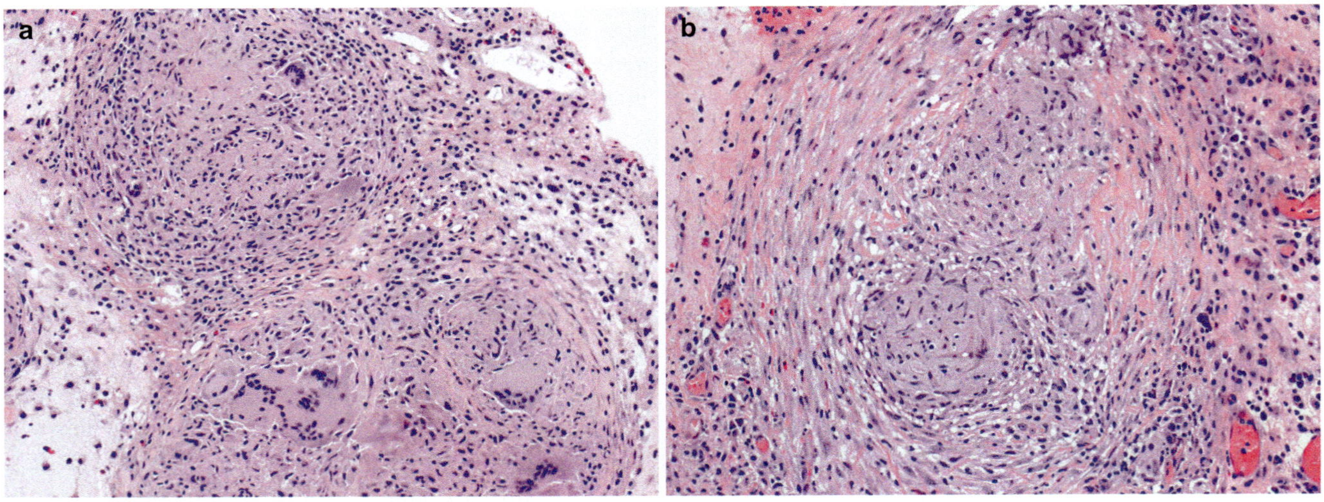

Fig. 19.9 Granulomatous appendicitis due to *Mycobacterium tuberculosis* (confirmed by culture). (**a** and **b**) Multiple confluent granulomas with giant cells. Note the necrosis is not apparent in this case

Viral Appendicitis

Adenovirus

Adenovirus is the most common virus detected in the appendix. Microscopic examination shows prominent lymphoid hyperplasia, viral inclusions, and sometime erosions. The viral inclusions are best seen in the intact epithelium cells with eosinophilic ragged appearance, loss of polarity, and loss of goblet cell mucin at low power. Most of the viral intranuclear inclusions are Cowdry type B bodies which show prominent nuclear smudging. Cowdry type A inclusions, seen as sharply demarcated intranuclear inclusions surrounded by a clear zone or halo, are rarely seen. The lymphoid hyperplasia can result in intussusception especially in infants and young children. Rotavirus and echovirus are other viruses that are implicated in causing intussusception due to lymphoid hyperplasia [40, 41].

Cytomegalovirus (CMV)

CMV infection is usually seen in immunocompromised hosts and can cause acute appendicitis. Histologic features include neutrophilic inflammation, crypt apoptosis, ulceration, and viral cytopathic effects, which are usually seen in the endothelial and stromal cells and less commonly in the epithelial cells. The viral inclusions can be cytoplasmic or both cytoplasmic and intranuclear. CMV immunohistochemical stain can be used to confirm the diagnosis [42, 43].

Epstein-Barr Virus (EBV)

EBV infection is an uncommon cause of acute appendicitis. Histologic features include expansion of the interfollicular area by a polymorphous population of inflammatory cells with scattered transformed lymphocytes and immunoblasts. Superimposed acute neutrophilic appendicitis may occur [44].

Measles Virus

Acute appendicitis may occur in the prodromal or fulminant phases of measles virus infection. Histologic features include lymphoid hyperplasia, multinucleated giant cells (i.e., Warthin-Finkeldey cells), and syncytial epithelial cells. Acute suppurative appendicitis may be seen in the late stages which are thought to be due to luminal obstruction by the lymphoid hyperplasia [45].

Varicella-Zoster Virus (VZV)

VZV is a very rare cause of acute appendicitis. The clinical history might indicate VZV infection, and the presence of viral inclusions histologically should facilitate the diagnosis. The diagnosis is confirmed with VZV immunohistochemical stain or PCR analysis [46, 47].

Fungal Appendicitis

Fungal infection of the appendix usually occurs in the setting of systemic fungal infection that affects mainly immunocompromised patients such as patients with organ transplantation or patients receiving chemotherapy. Fungal infections that can involve the appendix include *Histoplasma capsulatum*, aspergillosis, mucormycosis, and candidiasis. Histologic examination typically shows neutrophilic inflammation, denudation, and degeneration of the epithelial surface. Granulomas can also be seen. The inflammation may be mild despite high volume of organisms. Fungal stains such as GMS and PAS can help highlighting the organisms [48–50].

Parasitic Appendicitis

Enterobius vermicularis (Pinworm)

It is the most common parasite seen in the appendix, especially in temperate climates. It is more common in late childhood and early adolescence (5–15 years old). Pruritus ani might result from the presence of eggs and worms in the stool. The worms are found in the lumen of the appendix (Fig. 19.10a, b) usually without associated inflammation or clinical symptoms. However, parasite ova can cause mucosal inflammation and rarely granulomatous inflammation, and increased eosinophils in the lamina propria can be seen although, the latter is not typical of *Enterobius vermicularis* infection. In addition, mucocele might result from obstruction by large worms. Rarely do the worms invade surrounding tissue which can cause ulceration and marked inflammation composed of eosinophils and neutrophils (Fig. 19.11a, b). Grossly, the worms are white and measure 2–5 mm. Microscopically, the worms have a thick outer cuticle with lateral ala projects. Internal organs or eggs may be visible inside the worm (Fig. 19.10b) [51, 52].

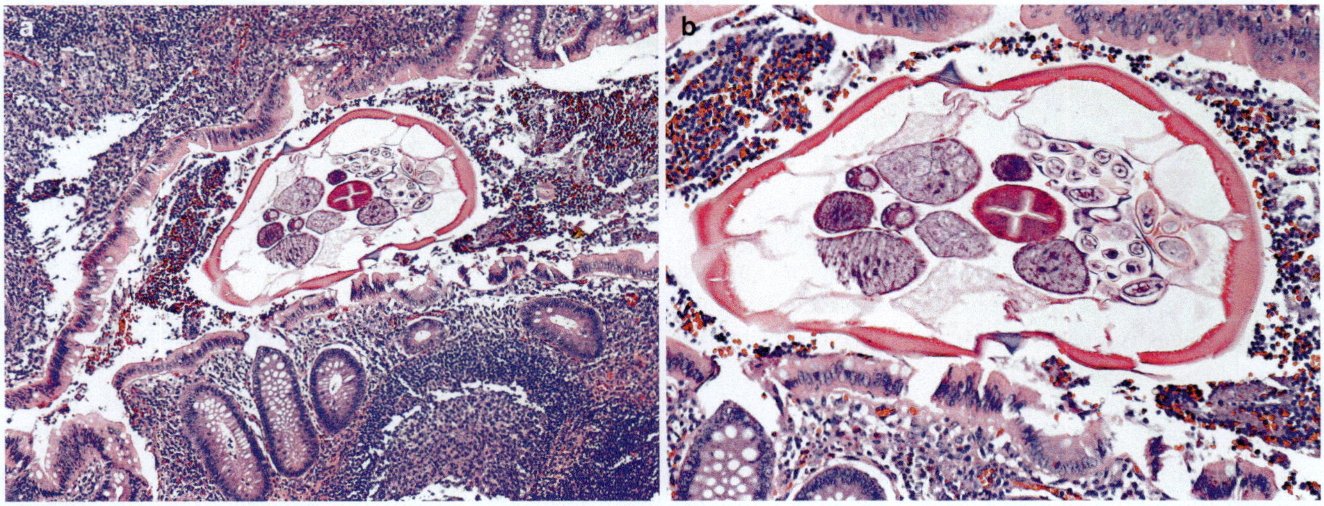

Fig. 19.10 *Enterobius vermicularis*. (**a**) *Enterobius vermicularis* is present in the appendiceal lumen. (**b**) Thick outer cuticle, two lateral ala, and internal organs can be seen

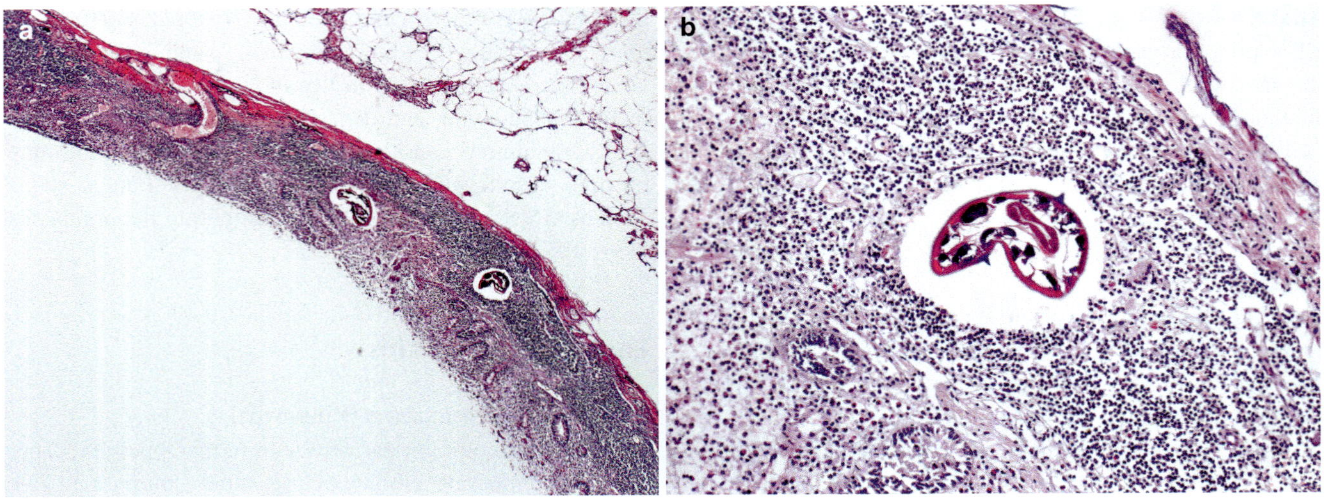

Fig. 19.11 *Enterobius vermicularis*. (**a**) *Enterobius vermicularis* worms are present within the appendiceal wall. (**b**) Higher-power picture showing the worm invading into the tissue, associated with increased inflammation

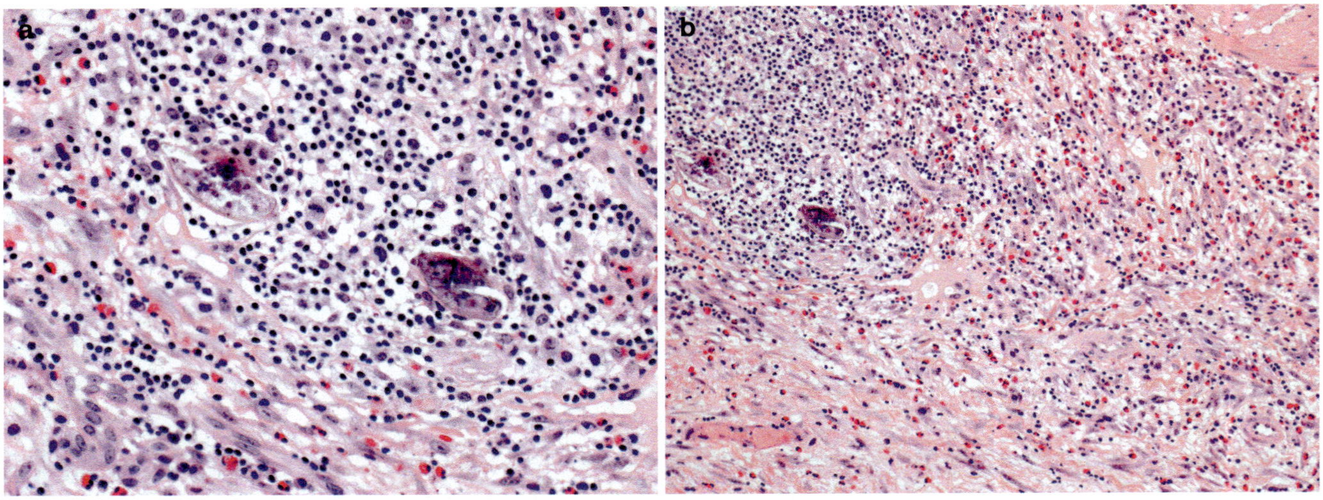

Fig. 19.12 *Schistosoma* of the appendix. (**a**) *Schistosoma* eggs surrounded by inflammation. (**b**) The inflammation is rich in eosinophils

Strongyloides stercoralis

Strongyloides stercoralis causes eosinophilic appendicitis with diffuse eosinophilic infiltrate, abscess formation, and necrosis. Granulomas might also be seen. Examining the stool specimens is a better way to detect the organism than the histologic examination [18, 19].

Schistosoma

Schistosoma causes eosinophilic appendicitis (Fig. 19.12a, b). Granulomas, acute and chronic inflammation, and submucosal fibrosis can also be seen. *Schistosoma* ova can be seen in the mucosa and/or other parts of the wall [20, 53, 54].

Other Organisms Detected in Appendix

Other organisms that can be rarely seen in the appendix include Herpes simplex type 1 (HSV), Human herpes virus 6 (HHV6) [43], *Dientamoeba fragilis*, *Endolimax nana*, Cryptosporidium protozoans [55], *Ascaris lumbricoides*, *Trichuris trichiura* (whipworm) (Fig. 19.13a, b) [56], *Entamoeba histolytica* [57],

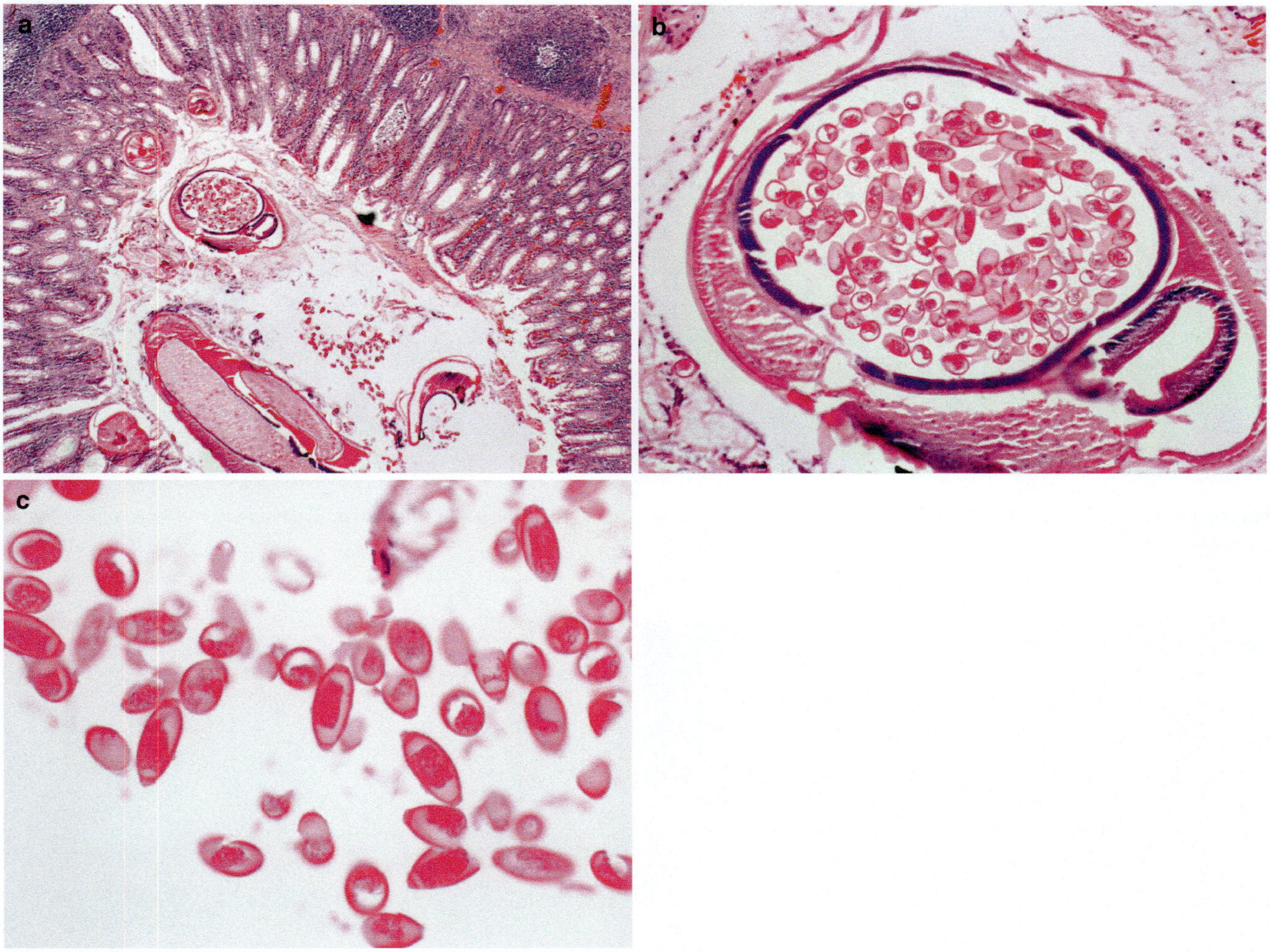

Fig. 19.13 *Trichuris trichiura*. (**a**) The worms are present in the appendiceal lumen and wall. (**b**) A cross-section of a female *Trichuris trichiura* with multiple eggs. (**c**) *Trichuris trichiura* eggs are barrel-shaped and have bipolar protuberances

Helicobacter pylori [58], *Balantidium coli* (Fig. 19.14a, b), and *Raoultella planticola* [59].

Periappendicitis

Periappendicitis occurs in intra-abdominal conditions associated with peritonitis. It is found in 1–5% of appendectomies performed for clinical suspicion of acute appendicitis. Causes include gonococcal and chlamydial salpingitis, yersiniosis, Meckel diverticulitis, intraperitoneal abscess, urologic disorders, colonic neoplasm, infectious colitis, abdominal aortic aneurysm, bacterial peritonitis, and gastrointestinal perforation. Grossly, the appendix has dull grey surface and might be coated with fibrinous exudate. Microscopic examination shows neutrophilic infiltration in the serosa that may extend to the periappendiceal tissue with fibrin deposition and serosal adhesions (Fig. 19.15a, b). The inflammation rarely extends to the muscularis propria, and by definition, mucosal inflammation is absent, a finding that helps in differentiating it from acute appendicitis. Submitting the entire appendix for microscopic examination is recommended to look for mucosal acute inflammation to rule out acute appendicitis. Of note, preoperative mechanical manipulation of the appendix may cause mild diffuse neutrophilic infiltration of the appendix serosa [60]. However, this is usually not associated with fibrin deposition or serosal adhesion [61, 62].

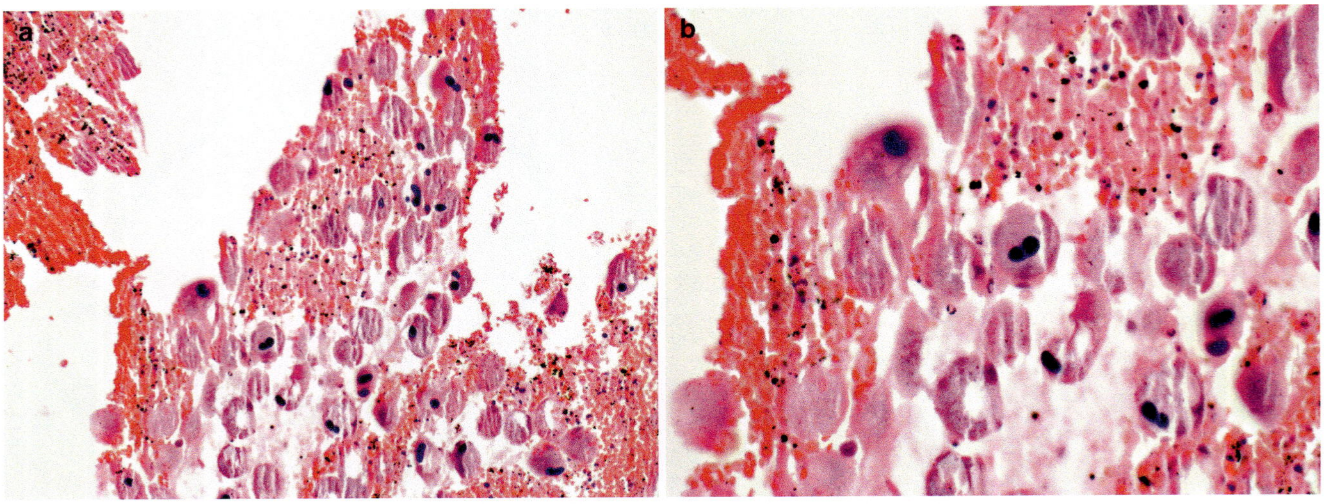

Fig. 19.14 *Balantidium coli*. (**a**) *Balantidium coli* organisms are present in the appendiceal lumen. (**b**) The *Balantidium coli* have long sausage-shaped macronucleus

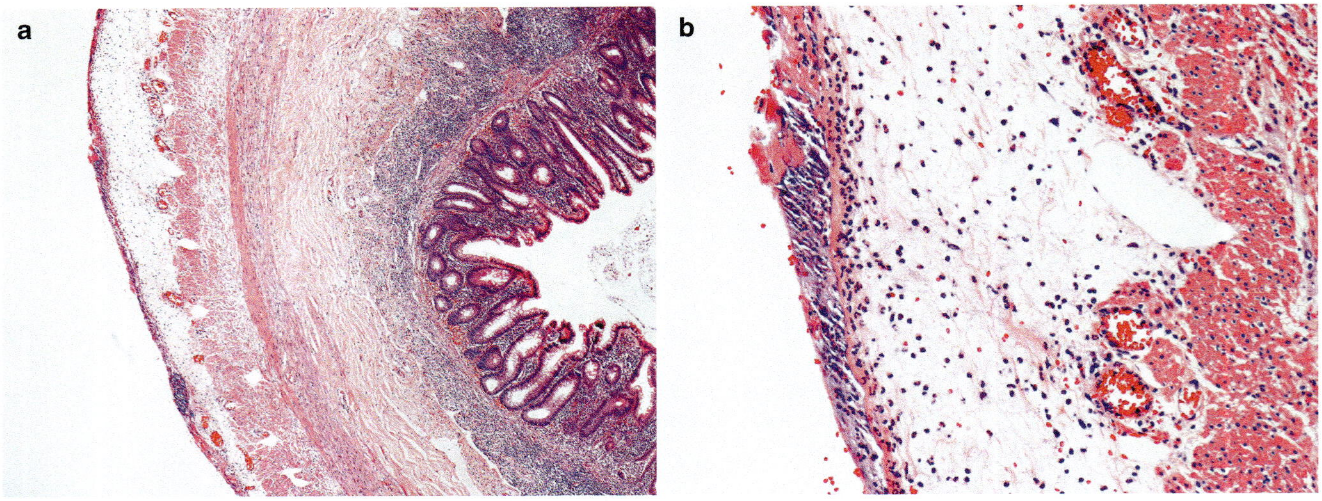

Fig. 19.15 Periappendicitis. (**a**) Inflammation limited to the appendiceal serosa. (**b**) Neutrophilic infiltrate of the serosa

Congenital and Acquired Anatomic Disorders

Atypical Locations

Normally, the appendix is located in the lower right abdomen. However, depending on the position and shape of the cecum that occur during organ development, growth, and rotation, the appendix may have atypical locations. The appendix also has more superior location during pregnancy [63].

Duplication

Duplication of the appendix is rare. There are three types of appendiceal duplication: (1) incomplete duplication (type A) where the two appendices have a common base; (2) complete duplication (type B) where the first appendix presents at the usual location at the confluence of teniae coli and the second appendix present at various location along the colon with only one cecum present; and (3) complete duplication of the cecum with each one having its own appendix (type C) [64].

Absence and Atresia

Agenesis and atresia of the appendix are rare. Congenital absence of the appendix has been associated with other congenital malformation such as congenital diaphragmatic hernia. The possibility of atypical location of the appendix should be excluded. Atresia of the appendix may be associated with atresia of the entire ileocecal region or other sites of the small bowel. Atretic appendix can develop acute appendicitis; however, the diagnosis of atresia should be made after pathologic examination [65, 66].

Septal Formation

Complete or incomplete septal formation within the appendix lumen can occur primarily in children and young adults. This could represent a congenital abnormality or develops secondary to inflammation or ischemia due to thrombosed vessels [67].

Diverticular Disease

Diverticular disease of the appendix is rare, but the incidence is increased in patients with cystic fibrosis due to the thick mucous secretions. Diverticula can be acquired or congenital. Congenital diverticula have muscularis propria in its wall as opposed to the acquired diverticula that lack muscular layer. Most appendiceal diverticula are acquired, developing secondary to increased intraluminal pressure, resulting in mucosal herniation through weak areas of the muscularis propria such as sites of penetration arteries. These are more common in older adult males, usually small (less than 5 mm) and located in the distal third of the appendix (60%) on the mesenteric border. Due to the lack of muscularis propria in its wall, acquired diverticula are more susceptible to perforation especially when inflamed (diverticulitis). Grossly, the diverticula may or may not be seen especially in the presence of severe inflammation and abscess formation. The appendix may appear edematous. The serosa may look dusty and have yellow-tan exudates if perforation occurs. Histologically, acquired diverticula appear as herniation of the appendix epithelium through the muscularis propria (Fig. 19.16a, b). In congenital diverticula, muscularis propria is part of the diverticula wall. Fibrous obliteration, acute inflammation, abscess formation, and perforation may or may not be present. Chronic changes such as muscular hypertrophy, transmural or periappendiceal fibrosis, and lymphoid atrophy may also be present and suggest previous inflammation or rupture. The presence of mucinous extravasation into periappendiceal tissue or serosal surface due to diverticulum rupture can mimic low-grade appendiceal mucinous neoplasm. Rarely, this may be associated with displaced benign epithelium where localized pseudomyxoma peritonei comes to the differential. The absence of dysplasia and malignant glands, the absence of filiform growth pattern and crowded crypts, and the identification of diverticula grossly or microscopically should help in the differential diagnosis; however, deeper sectioning and submitting more tissue may be needed [68–70].

Fibrous Obliteration of the Appendiceal Lumen

Fibrous obliteration of the lumen, also known as neuroma or neural hyperplasia, is a common finding seen in approximately a third of appendectomy specimens. It increases with age, and it is common in appendectomies with ruptured diverticula. It may represent a normal part of aging or a sequela of prior acute appendicitis. The tip of the appendix is usually affected, but the whole appendix may be progressively involved. Grossly, affected areas appear white and narrow. Histologically, the lumen of the appendix is occluded and replaced by spindle cells including fibroblasts, Schwann

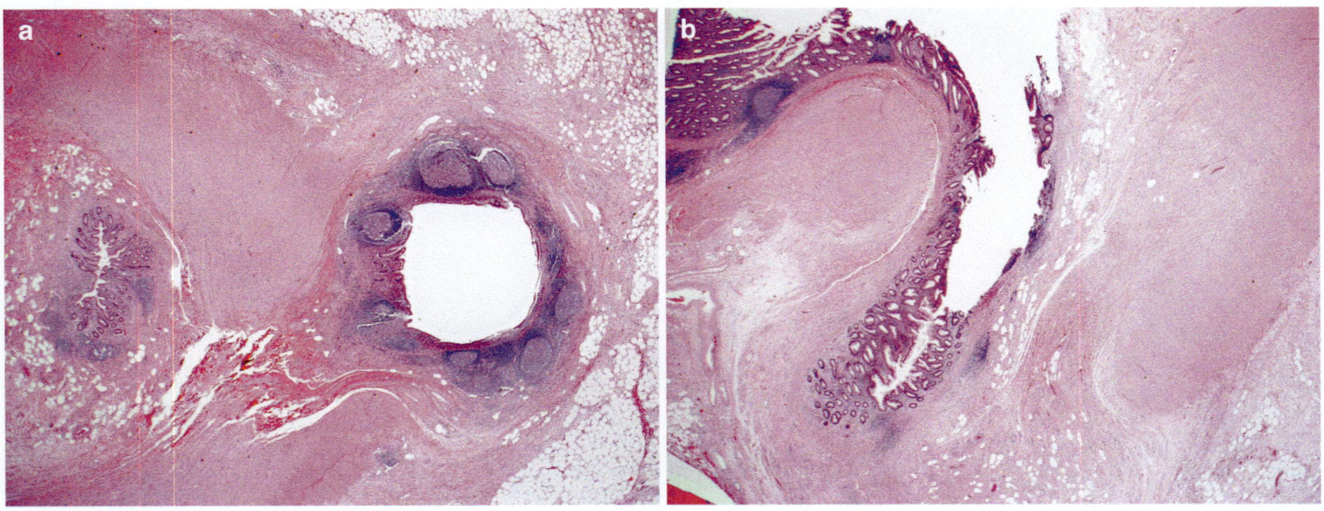

Fig. 19.16 Appendiceal diverticulum. (**a** and **b**) Acquired diverticula with herniation of the appendiceal epithelium through the muscularis propria, typically at the site of penetration arteries

cells, and axons within a collagenous or myxoid stroma (Fig. 19.17). Admixed mast cells, eosinophils, and endocrine cells may be present. The findings can be confined to the mucosa or replace the entire lumen and underlying crypts. S100 and NSE immunostains highlight the neural component (Schwann cells and axon, respectively) [71, 72].

Intussusception

Predisposing conditions to intussusception include mobile mesoappendix, wide proximal appendiceal lumen, endometriosis, parasites, lymphoid hyperplasia, tumors, and polyps. Appendiceal intussusception may act as a lead point for ileocolic intussusception. Histologic findings may show mucosal prolapse-like changes with crypt architectural distortion, ingrowth of the smooth muscle into the lamina propria, and fibrosis [73, 74].

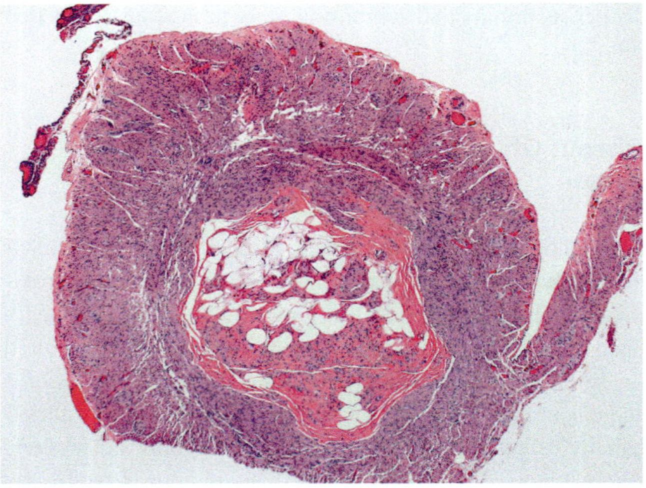

Fig. 19.17 Fibrous obliteration of the appendiceal lumen. Cross-section from the appendix showing absence of the lumen which is replaced by spindle cells with adipose tissue

Torsion

Risk factors for appendiceal torsion include long appendix (more than 7–10 cm), obstruction, inflammation, and malformation. Grossly, the appendix is twisted and may show luminal dilatation distal to the torsion site, congestion, hemorrhage, and/or necrosis. Histologic examination shows edema, inflammation, hemorrhage, ulceration, and/or infarction [75].

Inverted Appendix

This term describes inversion of the appendix into the cecum where it appears as a polyp. It could be congenital or due to intussusception. Histologic examination may be unremarkable or may show inflammation and lymphoid follicles (Fig. 19.18a, b) [76, 77].

Mucocele

The term "mucocele" is used when there is a gross dilatation of appendiceal lumen due to accumulation of mucin. The lesion can be associated with obstructive, inflammatory, or neoplastic processes. Grossly, the appendix is dilated and shows mucin accumulation. Histologically, the lesion is composed of mucin accumulation that can extravasate into the tissue with associated inflammatory infiltrate composed

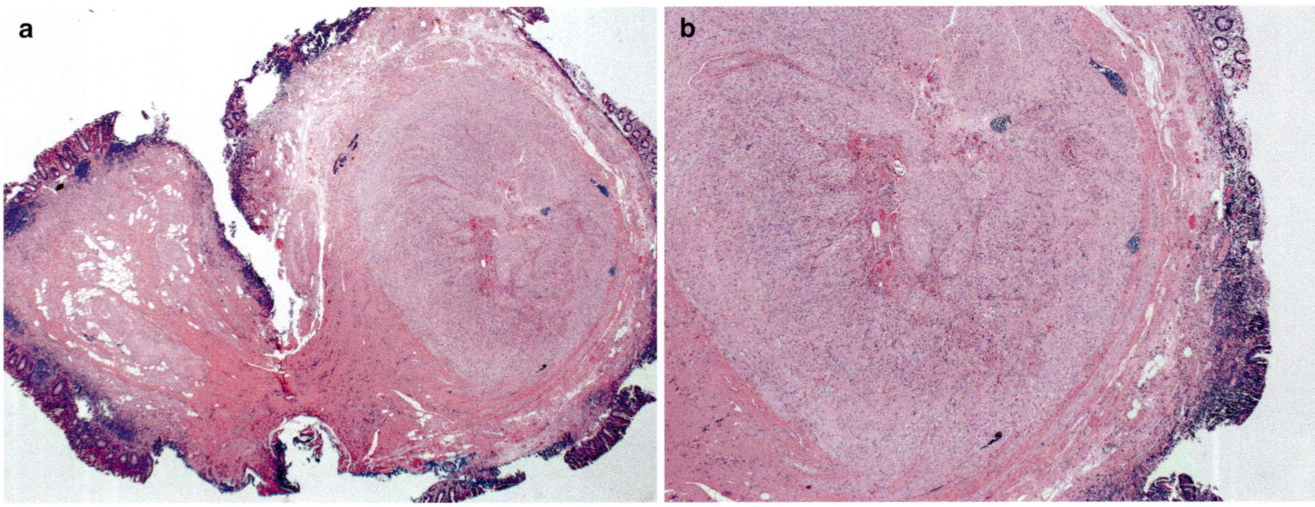

Fig. 19.18 Inverted appendix (specimen submitted as cecal polyp resected during colonoscopy). (**a**) Section from the polyp shows muscular wall and benign lining epithelium with lymphoid aggregates. (**b**) Higher-power picture highlighting the muscularis propria and absence of epithelial dysplasia

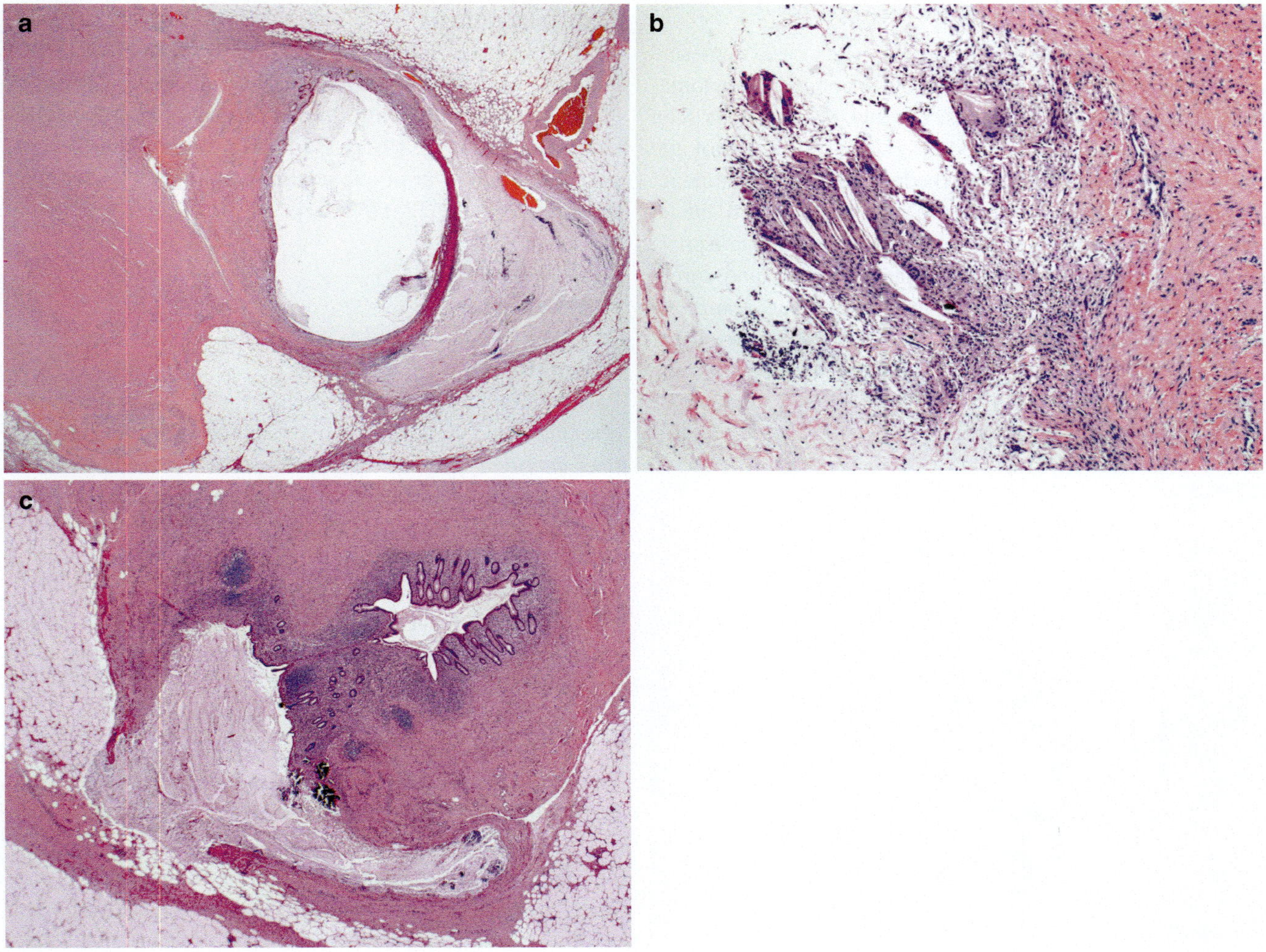

Fig. 19.19 Appendiceal mucocele. (**a**) Cystically dilated appendix lumen lined by partially attenuated benign mucosa with a collection of mucin within the lumen and wall. (**b**) The mucin is associated with histiocytes, calcifications, cholesterol clefts, and giant cells. (**c**) A ruptured mucocele with mucin extravasation mimicking appendiceal mucinous neoplasm. Note the absence of epithelial dysplasia and preserved lamina propria, muscularis mucosae, and submucosa

of mainly histiocytes, (Fig. 19.18a). The epithelium can be partially or completely denuded. Calcifications and cholesterol clefts with giant cells can be seen (Fig. 19.19b) [78, 79]. Lack of epithelial dysplasia and preserved mucosal layers help to distinguish mucocele (Fig. 19.18c) from appendiceal mucinous neoplasm.

Miscellaneous Disorders

Unremarkable Appendices Removed for a Clinical Suspicion of Acute Appendicitis

Possible etiologies for the patients' symptoms in these cases include *Yersinia ileitis*, mesenteric adenitis, cystic fibrosis, endometriosis, and other intra-abdominal pathologies.

Mullerian Rests

Endometriosis

Appendiceal endometriosis usually affects the serosa and/or muscularis propria of the appendix; however, submucosal cases have been reported. Gross examination may show cysts filled with hemorrhagic debris. Histologic examination shows endometrial-type glands and stroma that undergo changes in response to the menstrual cycle with accompanied hemosiderin deposition and a fibroblastic reaction (Fig. 19.20). Intestinal metaplasia may occur. There are also fibrosis and adhesions that can lead to complications such as infertility, intestinal obstruction, chronic pain, and appendiceal intussusception. Rarely, clear cell carcinoma or other mullerian carcinomas may arise in endometriotic foci [71, 80, 81].

Deciduosis

Deciduosis results from progesterone effect on extrauterine mesenchymal cells during pregnancy. In contrast to endometriosis, deciduosis lacks glands. Grossly, deciduosis is seen as a white plaques or small nodules on the serosa. Histologic examination shows large polyhedral cells with abundant granular eosinophilic cytoplasm and small, round nuclei with distinct nucleoli arranged in sheets in the serosa (Fig. 19.21a, b) or outer muscularis propria, and rarely mucosa. The cells of the deciduosis may show desmin or muscle actin positivity, and it is usually negative for cytokeratins, epithelial membrane antigen, carcinoembryonic antigen, and S100 [82, 83].

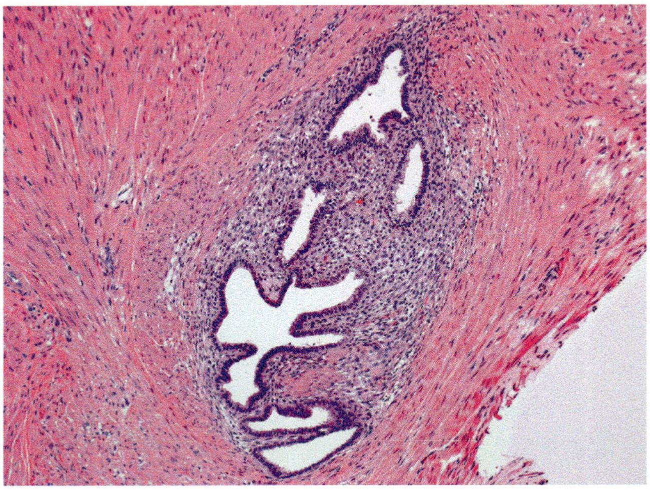

Fig. 19.20 Endometriosis of the appendix. Endometrial-type glands and stroma are present in the appendiceal muscularis propria

Endosalpingiosis

Endosalpingiosis might be seen grossly as solid or cystic nodules. Histologic examination demonstrates cysts or glands in association with fibrous stroma, but not the endometrial stroma (Fig. 19.22a). The lining epithelium is composed of a one layer of cuboidal or columnar cells that may have cilia (Fig. 19.22b) [84, 85].

Heterotopias

Gliomatosis

Pelvic gliomatosis can affect the serosal aspect of the appendix. It is found in patients with ovarian teratoma and also has been reported as a rare complication of ventricular shunts. Mature glial tissue is seen histologically. Malignant transformation has been reported [86–88].

Ectopic Tissue

Gastric and esophageal tissues have been reported in the appendix. Ectopic spleen after splenic rupture has also been reported [89].

Rosai-Dorfman Disease (Sinus Histiocytosis with Massive Lymphadenopathy)

Appendiceal involvement by Rosai-Dorfman disease is rare. There is usually nodal involvement as well. On histologic examination, histiocytes with abundant cytoplasm that show emperipolesis (engulfed inflammatory cells) are seen (Fig. 19.23a, b). Mixed inflammatory infiltrate with fibrosis

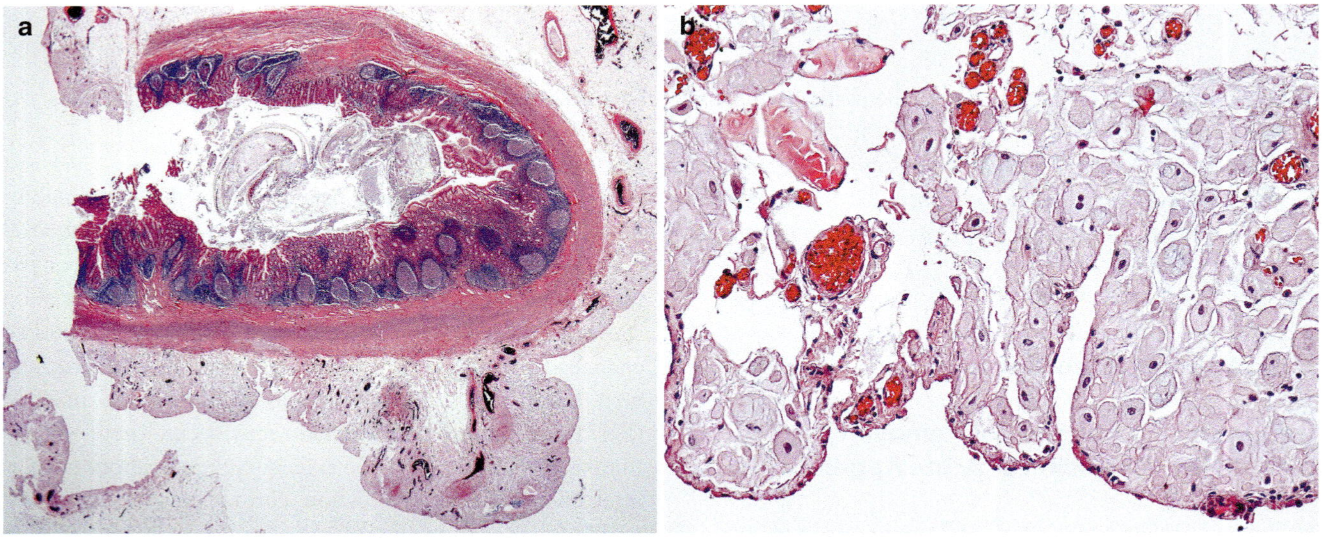

Fig. 19.21 Deciduosis of the appendix. (**a**) Involvement of the outer aspect of the appendix by deciduosis. (**b**) Sheets of large polyhedral cells with abundant eosinophilic cytoplasm and small nuclei

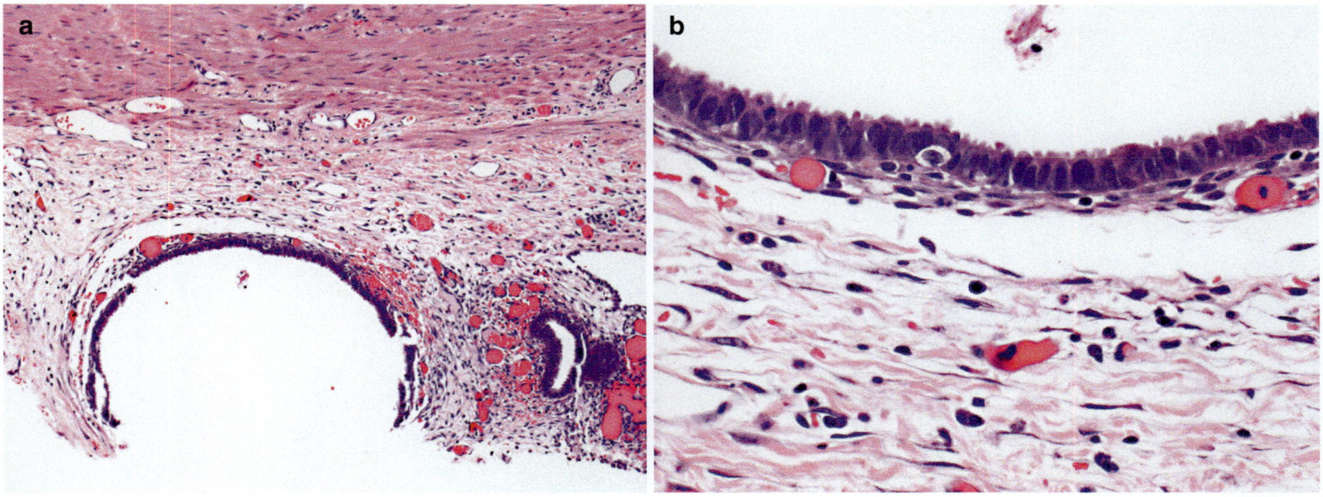

Fig. 19.22 Endosalpingiosis of the appendix. (**a**) Involvement of the outer aspect of the appendix by salpingiosis. (**b**) The gland is lined by one layer of cuboidal to low columnar ciliated epithelial cells. Note the absence of endometrial stroma

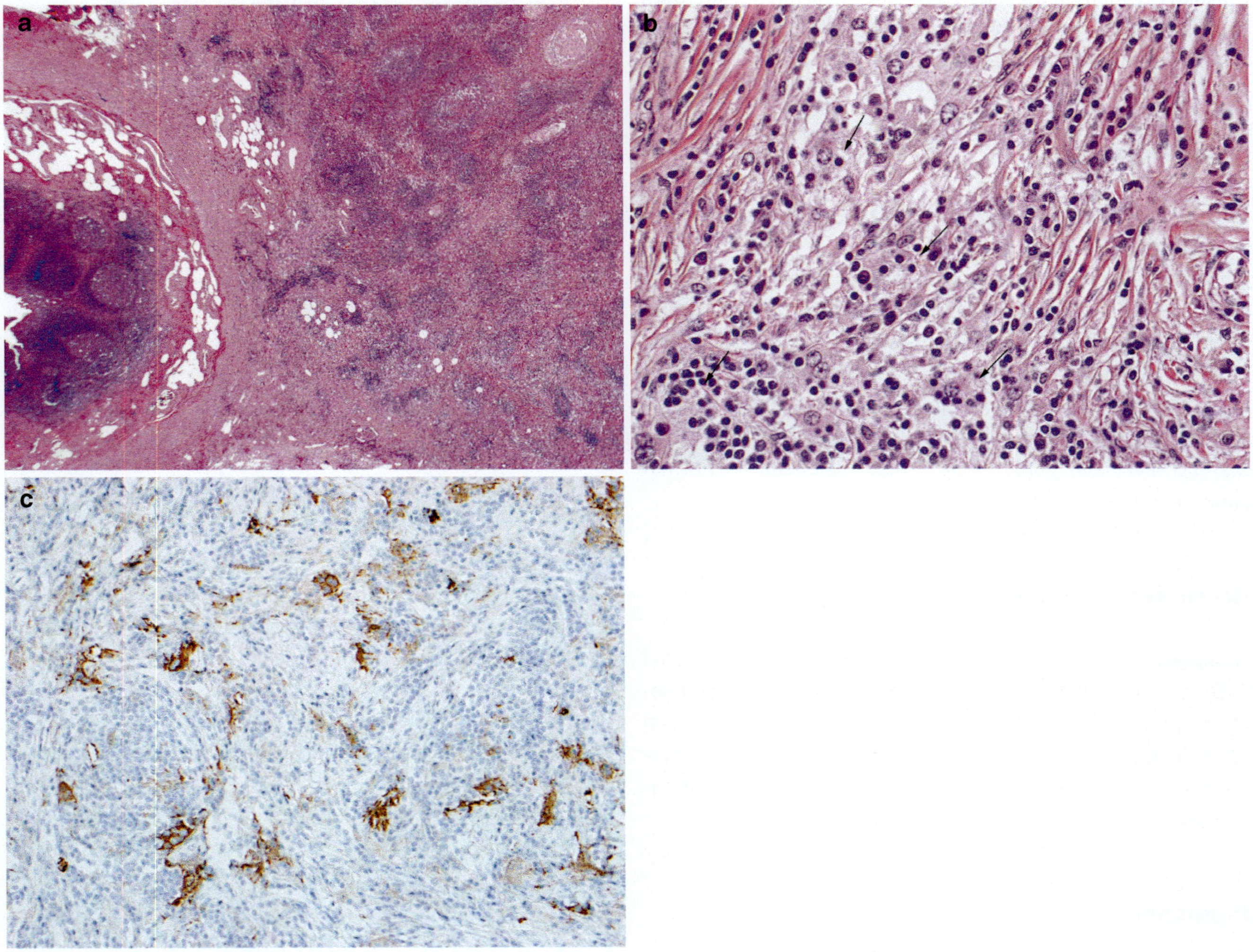

Fig. 19.23 Rosai-Dorfman disease of the appendix. (**a**) Inflammation of the appendiceal wall. (**b**) Emperipolesis with engulfed inflammatory cells by large histiocytes (arrows) in background of lymphocytes and plasma cells. (**c**) S100 immunostain highlights the large histiocytes with emperipolesis

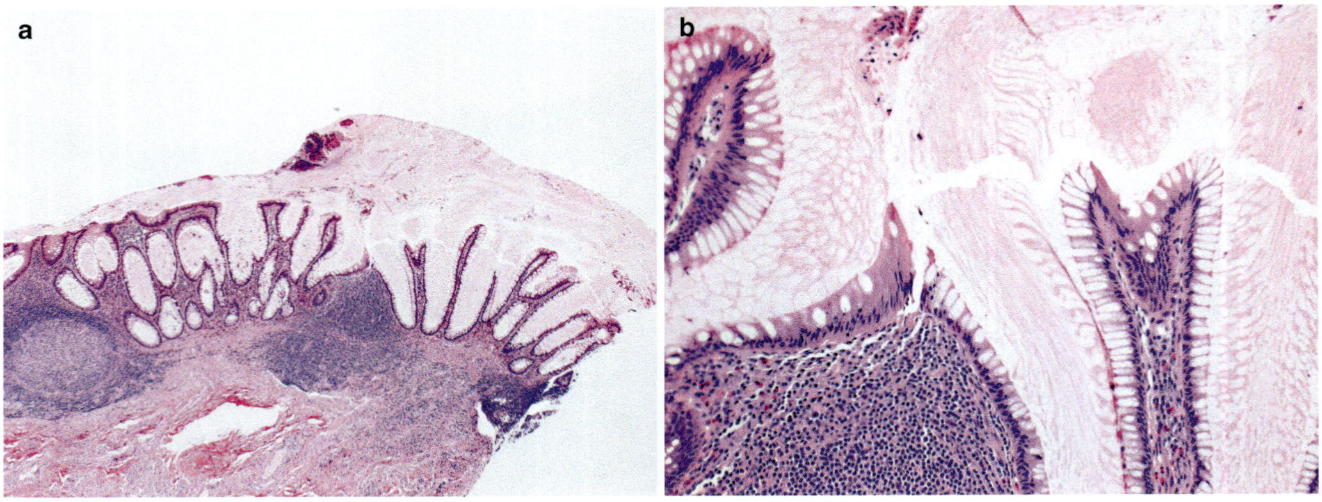

Fig. 19.24 Cystic fibrosis of the appendix. (**a**) Thick eosinophilic mucin in the appendix lumen and dilated crypts. (**b**) Prominent goblet cells and luminal eosinophilic mucin

is usually present in the background. S100 immunostain may help in identifying the emperipolesis (Fig. 19.23c) in questionable cases [90, 91].

Cystic Fibrosis

Cystic fibrosis is an inherited autosomal-recessive disease. Thick mucous secretions are the hallmark of the disease, and multiple organs can be affected. The incidence of appendiceal acquired diverticula is increased in these patients, while the incidence of acute appendicitis is decreased. Grossly, the affected appendix appears enlarged and filled with thick inspissated mucin. On histologic examination, dilated glands with luminal eosinophilic inspissated mucin (Fig. 19.24a) may be seen, and goblet cells appear distended by normal appearing mucin (Fig. 19.24b) [92, 93].

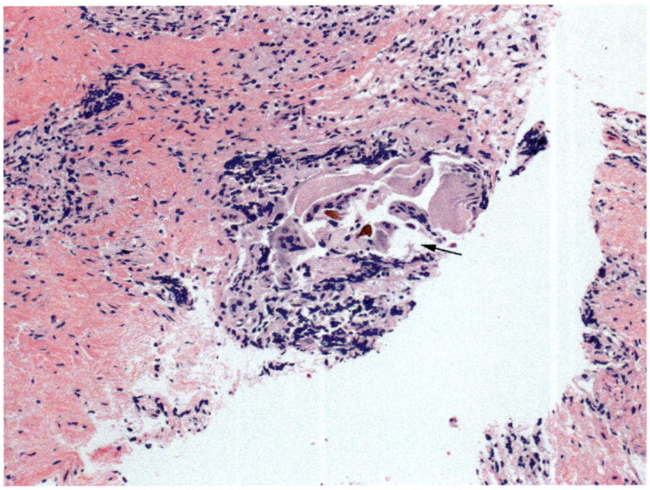

Fig. 19.25 Appendix with a foreign body. Foreign body with associated giant cell reaction (arrow)

Acute Necrotizing Arteritis

Acute necrotizing arteritis of the appendix is rare and limited to the appendix in most cases; however, widespread involvement in a pattern similar to polyarteritis nodosa can occur in up to a third of cases. On histologic examination, arteries show fibrinoid necrosis of their wall with or without inflammation [94, 95].

Pigments

Melanosis

Appendiceal melanosis in adults is usually due to laxative use, while in children, it is thought to be secondary to infection. Histologic findings include the presence of brown or yellow pigmented macrophages in the lamina propria [96, 97].

Barium

Barium is a light green nonpolarizable crystalline material that can be present in the lumen of the appendix. Occasionally, the barium extravagates into the mucosa and causes granulomatous reaction [98].

Fecalith and Foreign Body Appendicitis

Variable swallowed objects can be trapped in the appendix, and they represent a rare potential cause of appendicitis, which can

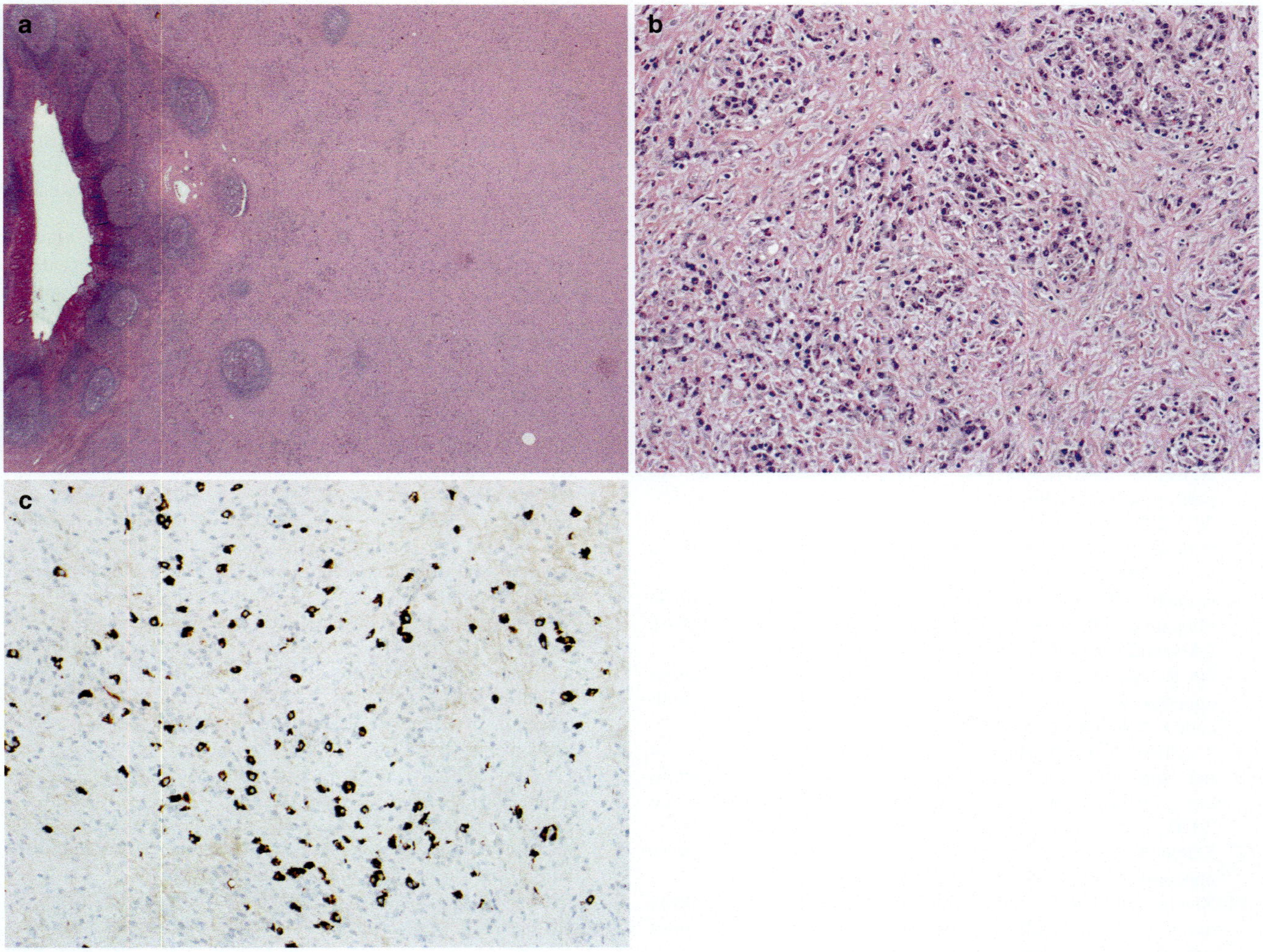

Fig. 19.26 IgG4-related disease involving appendix. (**a**) The appendiceal wall is thickened by fibroinflammation. Note the mucosa is not involved. (**b**) High-power view reveals lymphoplasmacytic infiltrate admixed with some eosinophils, fibroblast proliferation, and fine collagen deposit, giving a storiform appearance. (**c**) The immunostain highlights numerous IgG4-positive plasma cells

occur years after ingestion. The risk of appendicitis increases with the stiff and pointed agents. Acute appendicitis results from occlusion of the appendix lumen by the foreign material or fecalith. Granulomatous inflammation with giant cells may also be seen around the foreign material (Fig. 19.25) [99–101].

IgG4-Related Disease

The diagnosis requires the presence of appropriate histologic findings and increased IgG4-positive plasma cells (or IgG4/IgG ratio of more than 40%). The histologic findings are similar to those seen in other organs and include plasma-cell-rich inflammation, fibrosis (usually storiform at least focally), and obliterative phlebitis (Fig. 19.26a–c). Increased number of eosinophils can also be seen [102–104].

References

1. Yaeger AA, Cheng PM, Tatishchev S, Whang G. Acute eosinophilic appendicitis: a radiologic-pathologic correlation. Clin Imaging. 2018;51:337–40.
2. Rautio M, Saxén H, Siitonen A, Nikku R, Jousimies-Somer H. Bacteriology of histopathologically defined appendicitis in children. Pediatr Infect Dis J. 2000;19(11):1078–83.
3. Song DW, Park BK, Suh SW, Lee SE, Kim JW, Park JM, Kim HR, Lee MK, Choi YS, Kim BG, Park YG. Bacterial culture and antibiotic susceptibility in patients with acute appendicitis. Int J Color Dis. 2018;33(4):441–7.
4. Carr NJ. The pathology of acute appendicitis. Ann Diagn Pathol. 2000;4(1):46–58.
5. Gigabhoy R, Cheddie S, Singh B. Appendicitis in the HIV Era: a South African perspective. Indian J Surg. 2018;80(3):207–10.
6. Dikicier E, Altintoprak F, Ozdemir K, Gundogdu K, Uzunoglu MY, Cakmak G, Onuray F, Capoglu R. Stump appendicitis: a

retrospective review of 3130 consecutive appendectomy cases. World J Emerg Surg. 2018;13:22.
7. Subramanian A, Liang MK. A 60-year literature review of stump appendicitis: the need for a critical view. Am J Surg. 2012;203(4):503–7.
8. Al-Mansour M, Watch L. Granulomatous stump appendicitis mimicking Crohn's disease. Am Surg. 2011;77(8):172–4.
9. Guo G, Greenson JK. Histopathology of interval (delayed) appendectomy specimens: strong association with granulomatous and xanthogranulomatous appendicitis. Am J Surg Pathol. 2003;27(8):1147–51.
10. Singh V, John KM, Malik A, Pareek T, Dutta V. Xanthogranulomatous appendicitis: uncommon histological variant of a common entity. Med J Armed Forces India. 2015;71(Suppl 1):S19–21.
11. AbdullGaffar B. Granulomatous diseases and granulomas of the appendix. Int J Surg Pathol. 2010;18(1):14–20.
12. Al-Kurd A, Mizrahi I, Siam B, Kupietzky A, Hiller N, Beglaibter N, Eid A, Mazeh H. Outcomes of interval appendectomy in comparison with appendectomy for acute appendicitis. J Surg Res. 2018;225:90–4.
13. Park SH, Loftus EV Jr, Yang SK. Appendiceal skip inflammation and ulcerative colitis. Dig Dis Sci. 2014;59(9):2050–7.
14. Bronner MP. Granulomatous appendicitis and the appendix in idiopathic inflammatory bowel disease. Semin Diagn Pathol. 2004;21(2):98–107.
15. Ho P, Law WL, Choy C, Chan GS, Chu KW. Granulomatous appendicitis progressing to Crohn's disease with bleeding complication. ANZ J Surg. 2003;73(7):554–6.
16. Machado NO, Chopra PJ, Hamdani AA. Crohn's disease of the appendix with enterocutaneous fistula post-appendicectomy: an approach to management. N Am J Med Sci. 2010;2(3):158–61.
17. Stangl PC, Herbst F, Birner P, Oberhuber G. Crohn's disease of the appendix. Virchows Arch. 2002;440(4):397–403.
18. Rha B, Kelly DR, Shimamura M. Eosinophilic appendicitis attributable to Strongyloides infection in a pediatric renal transplant patient. J Pediatric Infect Dis Soc. 2013;2(3):274–7.
19. Cruz DB, Friedrisch BK, Fontanive Junior V, da Rocha VW. Eosinophilic acute appendicitis caused by Strongyloides stercoralis and Enterobius vermicularis in an HIV-positive patient. BMJ Case Rep. 2012;2012:bcr0120125670.
20. Kanoksil W, Larbcharoensub N, Soontrapa P, Phongkitkarun S, Sriphojanart S, Nitiyanant P. Eosinophilic appendicitis caused by Schistosoma japonicum: a case report and review of the literature. Southeast Asian J Trop Med Public Health. 2010;41(5):1065–70.
21. Akbulut S, Tas M, Sogutcu N, Arikanoglu Z, Basbug M, Ulku A, Semur H, Yagmur Y. Unusual histopathological findings in appendectomy specimens: a retrospective analysis and literature review. World J Gastroenterol. 2011;17(15):1961–70.
22. Tucker ON, Healy V, Jeffers M, Keane FB. Granulomatous appendicitis. Surgeon. 2003;1(5):286–9.
23. Pal K. Granulomatous appendicitis in children: a single institutional experience. Afr J Paediatr Surg. 2014;11(1):26–31.
24. Richards ML, Aberger FJ, Landercasper J. Granulomatous appendicitis: Crohn's disease, atypical Crohn's or not Crohn's at all? J Am Coll Surg. 1997;185(1):13–7.
25. Iida T, Yamashita K, Arimura Y, Shinomura Y. Colonic sarcoidosis presenting as granulomatous appendicitis. J Gastrointestin Liver Dis. 2016;25(1):8.
26. Tapia EO. Granulomatous appendicitis caused by sarcoidosis: report of one case. Rev Med Chil. 2014;142(4):526–8.
27. Hunjan T, Chaudery M, Zaidi A, Beggs AD. Appendicular sarcoidosis mimicking acute appendicitis. BMJ Case Rep. 2012;2012:pii: bcr2012006825. https://doi.org/10.1136/bcr-2012–006825.
28. Lamps LW. Infectious causes of appendicitis. Infect Dis Clin N Am. 2010;24(4):995–1018, ix–x
29. Barayan SS, Al-Anazi AR. Malakoplakia in the appendix: unusual association with mucinous cystadenoma: case report and review of literature. Saudi J Gastroenterol. 2002;8(1):28–30.
30. Kojima M, Morita Y, Shimizu K, Yoshida T, Yamada I, Togo T, Johshita T. Immunohistological findings of suppurative granulomas of Yersinia enterocolitica appendicitis: a report of two cases. Pathol Res Pract. 2007;203(2):115–9.
31. Lamps LW, Madhusudhan KT, Greenson JK, Pierce RH, Massoll NA, Chiles MC, Dean PJ, Scott MA. The role of Yersinia enterocolitica and Yersinia pseudotuberculosis in granulomatous appendicitis: a histologic and molecular study. Am J Surg Pathol. 2001;25(4):508–15.
32. Gómez-Torres GA, Ortega-Gárcia OS, Gutierrez-López EG, Carballido-Murguía CA, Flores-Rios JA, López-Lizarraga CR, Bautista López CA, Ploneda-Valencia CF. A rare case of subacute appendicitis, actinomycosis as the final pathology reports: a case report and literature review. Int J Surg Case Rep. 2017;36:46–9.
33. Karateke F, Ozyazıcı S, Menekşe E, Daş K, Ozdoğan M. Unusual presentations of actinomycosis; anterior abdominal wall and appendix: report of three cases. Balkan Med J. 2013;30(3):315–7.
34. van Spreeuwel JP, Lindeman J, Bax R, Elbers HJ, Sybrandy R, Meijer CJ. Campylobacter-associated appendicitis: prevalence and clinicopathologic features. Pathol Annu. 1987;22(Pt 1):55–65.
35. Campbell LK, Havens JM, Scott MA, Lamps LW. Molecular detection of Campylobacter jejuni in archival cases of acute appendicitis. Mod Pathol. 2006;19(8):1042–6.
36. Chiş B, Dudric V, Fodor D. Tuberculous appendicitis. A case report. Med Ultrason. 2017;19(3):333–5.
37. Ridha A, Safiullah SM, Al-Abayechi S, Nadeem AUR. Acute appendicitis: an extracolonic manifestation of Clostridium difficile colitis. Case Rep Med. 2017;2017:5083535.
38. Brown TA, Rajappannair L, Dalton AB, Bandi R, Myers JP, Kefalas CH. Acute appendicitis in the setting of Clostridium difficile colitis: case report and review of the literature. Clin Gastroenterol Hepatol. 2007;5(8):969–71.
39. Gan J, Bryant C, Arul D, Parmar C. Intestinal spirochaetosis mimicking acute appendicitis with review of the literature. BMJ Case Rep. 2017;2017:pii: bcr-2017–221574.
40. Grynspan D, Rabah R. Adenoviral appendicitis presenting clinically as acute appendicitis. Pediatr Dev Pathol. 2008;11(2):138–41.
41. Berrebi D, Ferkdadji L, Delagausie P, Aigrain Y, Peuchmaur M. Adenovirus and intranuclear inclusions in the appendix in children with acute intussusception. Ann Pathol. 1997;17(2):89–93.
42. Kothari A, Caradine KD, Rico Crescencio JC, Sasapu A, Veeraputhiran MK, Jethava Y, Burgess MJ. Cytomegalovirus appendicitis after hematopoietic stem cell transplantation. Transpl Infect Dis. 2017;19(5):e12747.
43. Katzoli P, Sakellaris G, Ergazaki M, Charissis G, Spandidos DA, Sourvinos G. Detection of herpes viruses in children with acute appendicitis. J Clin Virol. 2009;44(4):282–6.
44. Lopez-Navidad A, Domingo P, Cadafalch J, Farrerons J, Allende L, Bordes R. Acute appendicitis complicating infectious mononucleosis: case report and review. Rev Infect Dis. 1990;12(2):297–302.
45. Stadlmann S, Lenggenhager DM, Alves VA, Nonogaki S, Kocher TM, Schmid HR, Singer G. Histopathologic characteristics of the transitional stage of measles-associated appendicitis: case report and review of the literature. Hum Pathol. 2011;42(2):285–90.
46. Smedegaard LM, Christiansen CB, Melchior LC, Poulsen A. Appendicitis caused by primary varicella zoster virus infection in a child with DiGeorge syndrome. Case Rep Pediatr. 2017;2017:6708046.

47. Lukšić B, Mladinov S, Goić-Barišić I, Srzić A, Brizić I, Perić L. Acute appendicitis, a rare complication of varicella: a report of three cases. J Infect. 2012;64(4):430–3.
48. Kim HS, Yeo HJ, Shin DH, Cho WH, Kim D. Isolated acute appendicitis caused by Aspergillus in a patient who underwent lung transplantation: a case report. Transplant Proc. 2018;50(4):1199–201.
49. ter Borg F, Kuijper EJ, van der Lelie H. Fatal mucormycosis presenting as an appendiceal mass with metastatic spread to the liver during chemotherapy-induced granulocytopenia. Scand J Infect Dis. 1990;22(4):499–501.
50. Moyana TN, Kulaga A, Xiang J. Granulomatous appendicitis in acute myeloblastic leukemia: expanding the clinicopathologic spectrum of invasive candidiasis. Arch Pathol Lab Med. 1996;120(2):203–5.
51. Zouari M, Louati H, Abid I, Trabelsi F, Ben Dhaou M, Jallouli M, Mhiri R. Enterobius vermicularis: a cause of abdominal pain mimicking acute appendicitis in children. A retrospective cohort study. Arch Iran Med. 2018;21(2):67–72.
52. Hamdona SM, Lubbad AM, Al-Hindi AI. Histopathological study of Enterobius vermicularis among appendicitis patients in Gaza strip, Palestine. J Parasit Dis. 2016;40(1):176–83.
53. Ahmed SA, Mohammed U, Sanda RB, Makama J, Shehu MS, Ameh EA, Mayun AA. Schistosomiasis of the appendix in a tertiary hospital in northern Nigeria: a 22-year review. J Lab Physicians. 2014;6(1):18–21.
54. Meshikhes AW, Chandrashekar CJ, Al-Daolah Q, Al-Saif O, Al-Joaib AS, Al-Habib SS, Gomaa RA. Schistosomal appendicitis in the Eastern Province of Saudi Arabia: a clinicopathological study. Ann Saudi Med. 1999;19(1):12–4.
55. Ramsden K, Freeth M. Cryptosporidial infection presenting as an acute appendicitis. Histopathology. 1989;14(2):209–11.
56. Dorfman S, Cardozo J, Dorfman D, Del Villar A. The role of parasites in acute appendicitis of pediatric patients. Investig Clin. 2003;44(4):337–40.
57. Kobayashi T, Watanabe K, Yano H, Murata Y, Igari T, Nakada-Tsukui K, Yagita K, Nozaki T, Kaku M, Tsukada K, Gatanaga H, Kikuchi Y, Oka S. Underestimated amoebic appendicitis among HIV-1-infected individuals in Japan. J Clin Microbiol. 2016;55(1):313–20.
58. Karagin PH, Stenram U, Wadström T, Ljungh A. Helicobacter species and gut bacterial DNA in Meckel's diverticulum and the appendix. World J Gastroenterol. 2011;17(36):4104–8.
59. Naganathan G, Amin NK. Raoultella Planticola associated necrotizing appendicitis: a novel case report. Int J Surg Case Rep. 2018;44:38–41.
60. Sandermann J, Glenthøj A, Nielsen KK. Peroperative mechanical manipulation of the appendix. A cause of periappendicitis? Ann Chir Gynaecol. 1989;78(2):127–9.
61. Chaudhary P, Nabi I, Arora MP. Periappendicitis: our 13 year experience. Int J Surg. 2014;12(9):1010–3.
62. Fink AS, Kosakowski CA, Hiatt JR, Cochran AJ. Periappendicitis is a significant clinical finding. Am J Surg. 1990;159(6):564–8.
63. Kim S, Lim HK, Lee JY, Lee J, Kim MJ, Lee AS. Ascending retrocecal appendicitis: clinical and computed tomographic findings. J Comput Assist Tomogr. 2006;30(5):772–6.
64. Nageswaran H, Khan U, Hill F, Maw A. Appendiceal duplication: a comprehensive review of published cases and clinical recommendations. World J Surg. 2018;42(2):574–81.
65. Host WH, Rush B, Lazaro EJ. Congenital absence of the vermiform appendix. Am Surg. 1972;38(6):355–6.
66. Lima M, Antonellini C, Aquino A, Dòmini M, Libri M, Centonze N, Ruggeri G, Pigna A. Agenesis of the appendix vermiformis. Pediatr Med Chir. 2003;25(5):370–2.
67. de la Fuente AA. Septa in the appendix: a previously undescribed condition. Histopathology. 1985;9(12):1329–37.
68. Abdullgaffar B. Diverticulosis and diverticulitis of the appendix. Int J Surg Pathol. 2009;17(3):231–7.
69. Deschênes L, Couture J, Garneau R. Diverticulitis of the appendix. Report of sixty-one cases. Am J Surg. 1971;121(6):706–9.
70. Hsu M, Young RH, Misdraji J. Ruptured appendiceal diverticula mimicking low-grade appendiceal mucinous neoplasms. Am J Surg Pathol. 2009;33(10):1515–21.
71. Dincel O, Göksu M, Türk BA, Pehlivanoğlu B, İşler S. Incidental findings in routine histopathological examination of appendectomy specimens; retrospective analysis of 1970 patients. Indian J Surg. 2018;80(1):48–53.
72. Olsen BS, Holck S. Neurogenous hyperplasia leading to appendiceal obliteration: an immunohistochemical study of 237 cases. Histopathology. 1987;11(8):843–9.
73. Samuk I, Nica A, Lakovski Y, Freud E. Appendiceal intussusception: a diagnostic challenge. Eur J Pediatr Surg. 2018;28(1):30–3.
74. Ozuner G, Davidson P, Church J. Intussusception of the vermiform appendix: preoperative colonoscopic diagnosis of two cases and review of the literature. Int J Color Dis. 2000;15(3):185–7.
75. Wan Hassan WA, Tay YK, Ghadiri M. Torsion of the vermiform appendix: a case report and review of literature. Am J Case Rep. 2018;19:365–8.
76. Yan SL, Yeh YH, Lai MT, Lee YT. Inverted appendix in an asymptomatic patient without intussusception or previous appendectomy. Color Dis. 2010;12(10 Online):e339–40.
77. Matsushita M, Nishio A, Seki T, Okazaki K. Inverted appendix: final diagnosis or endometriosis? Am J Gastroenterol. 2016;111(5):746.
78. Orcutt ST, Anaya DA, Malafa M. Minimally invasive appendectomy for resection of appendiceal mucocele: case series and review of the literature. Int J Surg Case Rep. 2017;37:13–6.
79. Pai RK, Longacre TA. Appendiceal mucinous tumors and pseudomyxoma peritonei: histologic features, diagnostic problems, and proposed classification. Adv Anat Pathol. 2005;12(6):291–311.
80. Gustofson RL, Kim N, Liu S, Stratton P. Endometriosis and the appendix: a case series and comprehensive review of the literature. Fertil Steril. 2006;86(2):298–303.
81. Vyas M, Wong S, Zhang X. Intestinal metaplasia of appendiceal endometriosis is not uncommon and may mimic appendiceal mucinous neoplasm. Pathol Res Pract. 2017;213(1):39–44.
82. Suster S, Moran CA. Deciduosis of the appendix. Am J Gastroenterol. 1990;85(7):841–5.
83. Chai D, Wijesuriya R. Deciduosis of the appendix: diagnostic dilemma continues despite MRI evidence. Ann R Coll Surg Engl. 2016;98(8):e200–2.
84. Pollheimer MJ, Leibl S, Pollheimer VS, Ratschek M, Langner C. Cystic endosalpingiosis of the appendix. Virchows Arch. 2007;450(2):239–41.
85. Chakhtoura G, Nassereddine H, Gharios J, Khaddage A. Isolated endosalpingiosis of the appendix in an adolescent girl. Gynecol Obstet Fertil. 2016;44(11):669–71.
86. Harms D, Jänig U, Göbel U. Gliomatosis peritonei in childhood and adolescence. Clinicopathological study of 13 cases including immunohistochemical findings. Pathol Res Pract. 1989;184(4):422–30
87. Hill DA, Dehner LP, White FV, Langer JC. Gliomatosis peritonei as a complication of a ventriculoperitoneal shunt: case report and review of the literature. J Pediatr Surg. 2000;35(3):497–9.
88. Dadmanesh F, Miller DM, Swenerton KD, Clement PB. Gliomatosis peritonei with malignant transformation. Mod Pathol. 1997;10(6):597–601.
89. Droga BW, Levine S, Baber JJ. Heterotopic gastric and esophageal tissue in the vermiform appendix. Am J Clin Pathol. 1963;40:190–3.
90. Zhao M, Li C, Zheng J, Yu J, Sha H, Yan M, Jin J, Sun K, Wang Z. Extranodal Rosai-Dorfman disease involving

appendix and mesenteric nodes with a protracted course: report of a rare case lacking relationship to IgG4-related disease and review of the literature. Int J Clin Exp Pathol. 2013;6(11):2569–77.

91. Lauwers GY, Perez-Atayde A, Dorfman RF, Rosai J. The digestive system manifestations of Rosai-Dorfman disease (sinus histiocytosis with massive lymphadenopathy): review of 11 cases. Hum Pathol. 2000;31(3):380–5.
92. George DH. Diverticulosis of the vermiform appendix in patients with cystic fibrosis. Hum Pathol. 1987;18(1):75–9.
93. Coughlin JP, Gauderer MW, Stern RC, Doershuk CF, Izant RJ Jr, Zollinger RM Jr. The spectrum of appendiceal disease in cystic fibrosis. J Pediatr Surg. 1990;25(8):835–9.
94. Daniels J, Deshpande V, Serra S, Chetty R. Incidental single-organ vasculitis of the gastrointestinal tract: an unusual form of single-organ vasculitis with coexistent pathology. Pathology. 2017;49:661–5.
95. Moyana TN. Necrotizing arteritis of the vermiform appendix: a clinicopathologic study of 12 cases. Arch Pathol Lab Med. 1988;112:738–41.
96. Graf NS, Arbuckle S. Melanosis of the appendix: common in the paediatric age group. Histopathology. 2001;39(3):243–9.
97. Rutty GN, Shaw PA. Melanosis of the appendix: prevalence, distribution and review of the pathogenesis of 47 cases. Histopathology. 1997;30(4):319–23.
98. Katagiri H, Lefor AK, Kubota T, Mizokami K. Barium appendicitis: a single institution review in Japan. World J Gastrointest Surg. 2016;8(9):651–5.
99. Klingler PJ, Seelig MH, DeVault KR, Wetscher GJ, Floch NR, Branton SA, Hinder RA. Ingested foreign bodies within the appendix: a 100-year review of the literature. Dig Dis. 1998;16(5):308–14.
100. Green SM, Schmidt SP, Rothrock SG. Delayed appendicitis from an ingested foreign body. Am J Emerg Med. 1994;12(1):53–6.
101. Ramdass MJ, Young Sing Q, Milne D, Mooteeram J, Barrow S. Association between the appendix and the fecalith in adults. Can J Surg. 2015;58(1):10–4. https://doi.org/10.1503/cjs.002014.
102. Kim HS, Kang WK, Chung DJ. Appendiceal immunoglobulin G4-related disease mimicking appendiceal tumor or appendicitis: a case report. Korean J Radiol. 2016;17(1):56–8.
103. Veerankutty FH, Saleem S, Chacko S, Sreekumar VI, Krishnan P, Varma D, Kurumboor P. IgG4-related disease of the appendix. J Gastrointest Surg. 2018;22(6):1124–6.
104. Kwon DH, Kallakury BV. RE: Appendiceal immunoglobulin G4-related disease mimicking appendiceal tumor or appendicitis: a case report. Korean J Radiol. 2017;18(6):1012–3.

Non-neoplastic Diseases of Anus

20

Sejal Subhash Shah

Infections

Anorectal infections are most often caused by sexually transmitted pathogens in patients who participate in anal-receptive intercourse and men who have sex with men (MSM). In this population, the common etiological agents include *Neisseria gonorrhoeae*, *Chlamydia trachomatis*, herpes simplex virus (HSV) type 2, and *Treponema pallidum* [1]. Patients with sexually transmitted infections (STI) most commonly present with proctitis and anal or perianal ulcers. The other manifestations include anal discharge (mucous, bloody, or purulent), pain, and tenesmus [2].

Herpes Simplex Virus

Anogenital herpetic infections are caused by HSV types 1 and 2. Though HSV type 2 accounts for most cases of infection, an increased proportion of HSV type 1 infection is observed especially in young women and MSM [3]. HSV infects the squamous epithelial cells of the anal canal and perianal skin. Clinically, the patients present with vesicles which later break down to form ulcers. The initial outbreak may be associated with systemic manifestations such as fever, lymphadenopathy, and body aches [2, 4].

Histologic examination reveals ulcerated squamous mucosa with acute and chronic inflammation and granulation tissue. Epithelial cells infected by HSV show characteristic intranuclear inclusions with multinucleation, nuclear molding, and chromatin margination (3 Ms of herpes). These are best seen in the squamous epithelium at the edge of ulcer. Herpes immunohistochemical (IHC) stain can be useful to highlight and confirm the presence of viral particles (see Fig. 5.11).

S. S. Shah (✉)
Department of Pathology, Kaiser Permanente Southern California, Irvine, CA, USA

Treponema Pallidum

Syphilis is a systemic disease caused by spirochete bacterium *Treponema pallidum* (*T. pallidum*). The disease has multiple stages including primary, secondary, latent, and tertiary. In the primary stage, single or multiple sores (chancre) develop at the site of inoculation. These are generally firm, round, and painless, last for 3–6 weeks, and later resolve irrespective of whether treatment is received or not [2]. In a subset of patients, the lesions are painful and multiple and may be clinically misdiagnosed as HSV infection [5]. A quarter of untreated patients develop secondary syphilis which occurs following hematogenous dissemination of *T. pallidum* [2]. These patients show systemic symptoms such as fever, maculopapular rash, malaise, and lymphadenopathy. The anorectal region shows presence of mucous membrane lesions and snail track ulcers and may show presence of condyloma lata which are wartlike, gray, raised, flat, and broad-based papular lesions which occur in moist areas. Transmission of infection occurs in one-third of patients exposed to the early lesions of syphilis [6]. In the latent stage of syphilis, patients show no visible signs or symptoms. Fifteen percent of untreated patients develop tertiary syphilis, approximately 10–30 years after initial infection, resulting in damage to the internal organs, brain, and nervous system and may result in death [7].

On endoscopic examination, patients with anorectal syphilis may show ulcerative proctitis with mucosal friability, anal canal ulcers, or ulcerated mass mimicking malignancy [8–10]. On histologic examination, different patterns of inflammatory response to syphilis may be seen [9, 11, 12]. The squamous mucosa may show hyperplasia, erosion, or ulceration with granulation tissue (Fig. 20.1a, b). In the plasma-cell-rich type, a thick band of dense plasma-cell-rich chronic inflammatory infiltrate is present predominantly at the junction of squamous epithelium and lamina propria (Fig. 20.2) [9, 11]. Additionally, perineural plasma cells may also be identified. A smaller sub-

L. Zhang et al. (eds.), *Surgical Pathology of Non-neoplastic Gastrointestinal Diseases*,
https://doi.org/10.1007/978-3-030-15573-5_20

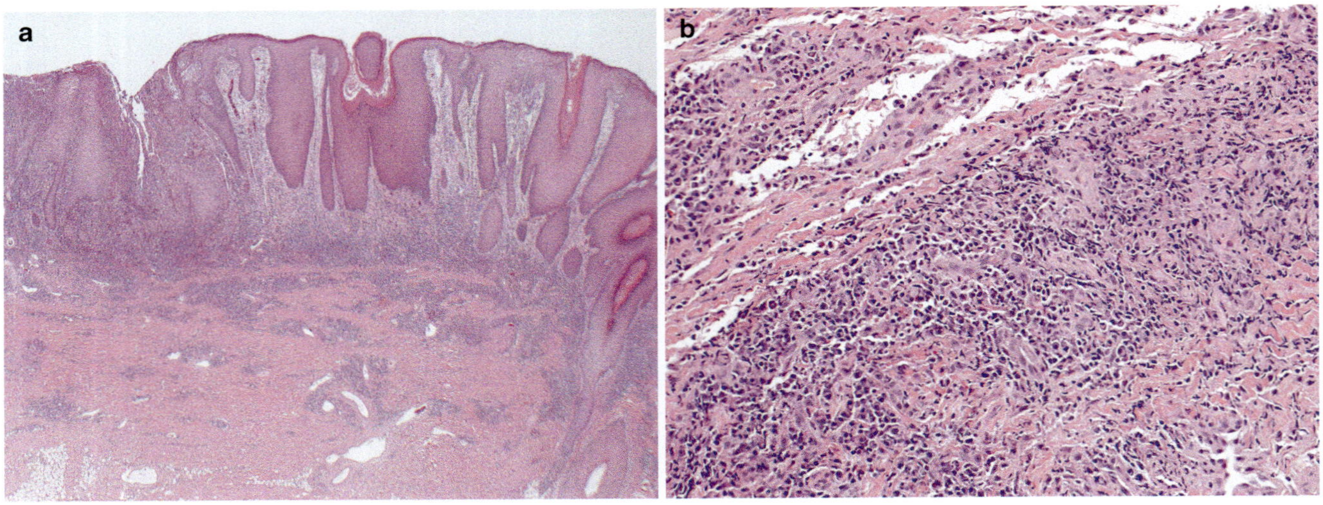

Fig. 20.1 Anal syphilis presented as a mass lesion. Hyperplastic squamous mucosa with focal ulceration and dense band-like chronic inflammatory infiltrate at the junction of squamous epithelium, lamina propria, and submucosa (**a**). An area of ulceration with chronic inflammatory infiltrate composed predominantly of plasma cells (**b**)

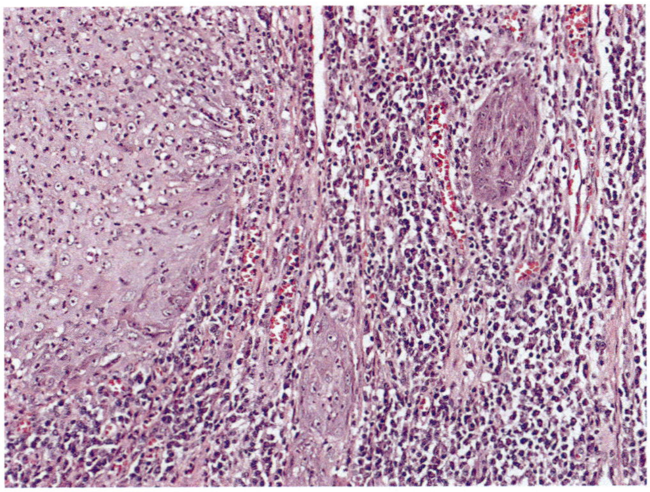

Fig. 20.2 Anal syphilis. Prominent plasma cells infiltrates at the junction of the epithelium and lamina propria

set of cases show lymphohistiocytic pattern characterized by presence of numerous histiocytes in addition to lymphocytes and plasma cells [11]. Associated poorly formed granulomas may or may not be seen. The third pattern is lymphoma-like pattern showing activated lymphocytes in a background of polymorphous inflammatory infiltrate composed of lymphocytes, histiocytes, plasma cells, neutrophils, and eosinophils [11]. An eosinophil-rich pattern of inflammation with eosinophils ranging from 8 to >200 eosinophils per 10 high-power fields has also been described [12]. The silver stains may or may not identify the spirochetes. IHC stain for *T. pallidum* can be useful to highlight the corkscrew-shaped organisms and confirm the diagnosis (Fig. 20.3a–c). A diagnostic pitfall is cross-reaction of *T. pallidum* immunostain with *Brachyspira* species which are causative agents of human intestinal spirochetosis [13]. For definitive diagnosis of syphilis, the patient can undergo screening with venereal disease research laboratory (VDRL) test and rapid plasma regain (RPR) test which are non-treponemal serological tests, followed by more specific treponemal tests including fluorescent treponemal antibody absorption tests and immunoassays.

It is crucial to detect and treat syphilis in the early stages to prevent the disease progression to tertiary syphilis. Hence, in the pathologic assessment of inflammatory and ulcerative lesions of the anal canal, the differential of syphilis should be considered when characteristic morphological features are present.

Chlamydia

Lymphogranuloma venereum (LGV) is a systemic disease caused by *Chlamydia trachomatis* serotypes L1, L2, and L3. Infection with *Chlamydia trachomatis*, *serovars* D–K (non-LGV strains), may be either asymptomatic or may cause mild proctitis. Recently, resurgence of LGV has been reported in patients who are MSM and human immunodeficiency virus (HIV)-positive, and hence early diagnosis to prevent complications and further transmission of infection is important [14–18].

The initial stage is characterized by development of a pustule or ulcer at the site of inoculation. In the secondary stage, patient presents with systemic symptoms such as fever, arthralgia, and malaise. They may develop inguinal syn-

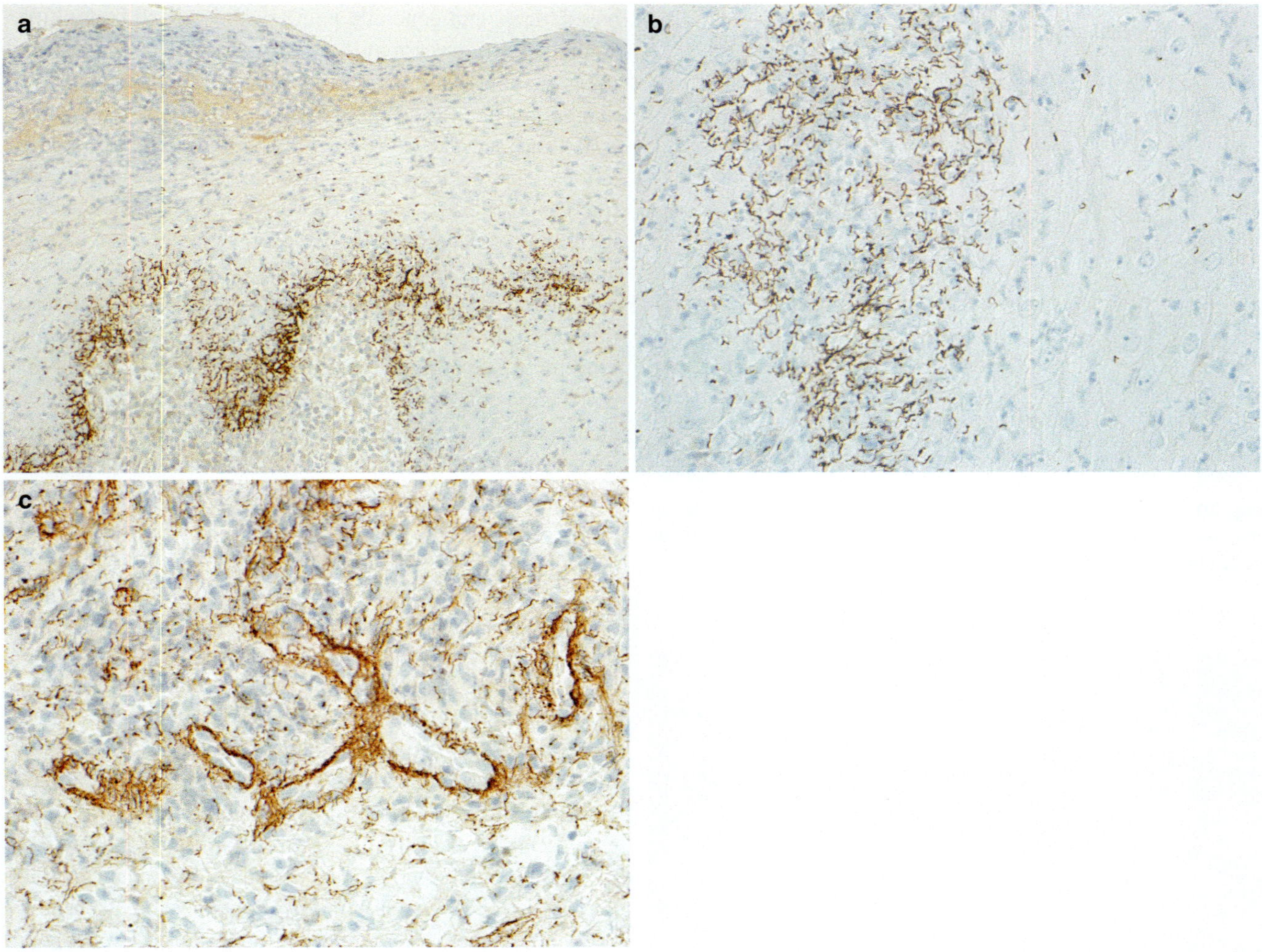

Fig. 20.3 *Treponema pallidum* immunohistochemical stain highlights organisms prominent at the junction of the epithelium and lamina propria (**a**). On higher power, characteristic corkscrew-shaped organisms are identified (**b**) and especially concentrated around blood vessels (**c**)

drome characterized by inguinal lymphadenopathy with suppuration and ulceration or anogenitorectal syndrome characterized by proctitis or proctocolitis with anorectal pain, discharge, and bleeding [4]. Untreated patients progress to form anal fistulas, strictures, and perianal abscesses, features mimicking Crohn's disease.

The histological features include lymphohistiocytic infiltrate, presence of plasma cells, lymphoid aggregates, mild to moderate acute inflammation with cryptitis and crypt abscess formation, and fibrosis [19]. The differential diagnoses for these findings include syphilitic proctitis and inflammatory bowel disease. In the appropriate clinical setting, the possibility of LGV should be raised. Additionally, it should be noted that syphilis and LGV infection can coexist, particularly in HIV-positive MSM patients. Diagnosis of *C. trachomatis* infection can be confirmed by culture, nucleic acid amplification testing (NAAT), and PCR-based genotyping.

Inflammatory Bowel Disease

Crohn's disease is a chronic and relapsing inflammatory bowel disease. Anal and perianal involvement is a significant cause of morbidity and can be seen in 22–56% of patients with Crohn's disease with the incidence being greater than 90% for patients showing large bowel and rectal involvement [20–25]. In a small subset of patients (5%), anal involvement is the sole clinical manifestation of the disease [21, 26]. In contrast to Crohn's disease, anal involvement in ulcerative colitis is generally non-specific and not related to the inflammatory bowel disease.

In ulcerative colitis, histological changes of active chronic inflammation are predominantly seen in the proximal anal canal, with the distal anal canal showing mostly non-specific submucosal chronic inflammation. In Crohn's disease, variable histological features may be seen which include patchy active chronic inflammation. The fistulas and fissures are

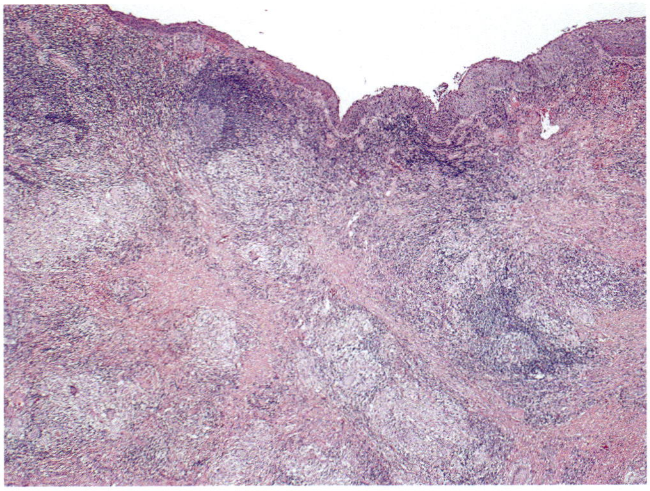

Fig. 20.4 Anal involvement by Crohn's disease showing squamous mucosa with marked subepithelial chronic inflammation and multiple noncaseating granulomas

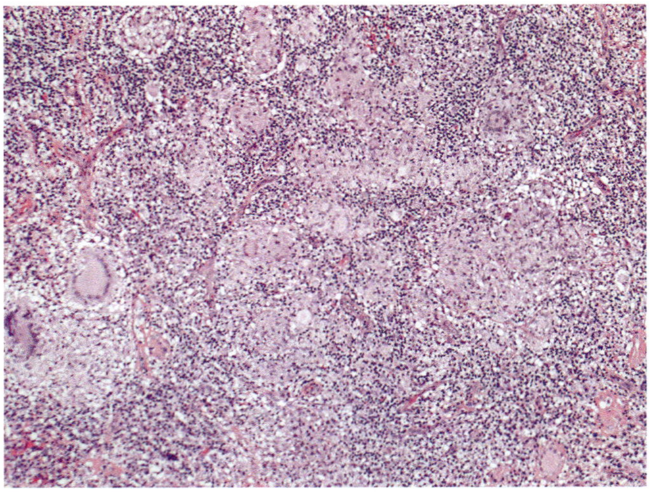

Fig. 20.5 Multiple ill-defined non-necrotizing granulomas composed of epithelioid histiocytes and giant cells in Crohn's disease

generally associated with marked chronic inflammation. The presence of ill-defined non-necrotizing granulomas supports the diagnosis of Crohn's disease (Figs. 20.4 and 20.5). The possibility of foreign body granulomas associated with fistulas, sarcoidosis, and infectious processes such as tuberculosis which show necrotizing granulomas, *Chlamydia trachomatis* infection, and granuloma inguinale should be excluded. Stains to identify mycobacterial and fungal organisms are useful.

Perianal manifestations of Crohn's disease include a wide range of entities including skin tags, hemorrhoids, perianal fistulas, rectovaginal fistulas, perianal abscesses, anal ulcers, anogenital strictures and stenosis, anal fissures, and anorectal carcinoma. In Crohn's disease, anal fissures are broad-based, deep, and generally painless and tend to be multiple. Anorectal strictures may be long and tubular arising from inflammation of the rectum or may be short, annular, and diaphragm-like [27]. Surgical management for patients with anal fissures and strictures includes sphincterotomy and dilatation of anorectal strictures. Two types of skin tags are identified in Crohn's disease. The first type is large, cyanotic, hard, and edematous, and the second type is narrow or flat and broad, soft, and painless.

Perianal fistulas are common and debilitating manifestation of Crohn's disease that are associated with significant morbidity. The etiology of Crohn's fistula is unclear but may represent fistula in the anus arising from inflamed or infected anal glands and/or penetration of fissure or ulcers in the rectum or anal canal [27]. These are classified as simple or complex based on physical examination of perianal area and endoscopic evaluation. A simple fistula is low (superficial or low intersphincteric or low transsphincteric origin of the fistula tract), has a single external opening, and has no evidence of pain, fluctuation, rectovaginal fistula, or anorectal stricture. In contrast, a complex fistula is high (high intersphincteric or high transsphincteric or extrasphincteric or suprasphincteric origin of the fistula tract), may have multiple external openings, and may be associated with pain, fluctuation, presence of rectovaginal fistula, presence of anorectal stricture, and/or presence of active rectal disease on endoscopy [27]. Perianal fistulizing Crohn's disease is less likely to heal without intervention. Medical treatment includes antibiotics, steroids, immunomodulators such as azathioprine and 6-mercaptopurine, and antitumor necrosis factor agents. Surgical treatment includes incision and drainage of perianal abscess, simple fistulotomy, non-cutting seton placement, endorectal advancement flap, diverting procedures with ostomy, and proctectomy.

Hemorrhoids

Hemorrhoids are cushions within the submucosal tissue of the anal canal. These cushions surround direct arteriovenous communication between terminal branches of superior rectal arteries and the superior, middle, and inferior rectal veins [28, 29]. These cushions are typically present in the right anterior, right posterior, and left lateral regions of the anal canal, and their presence is essential for complete closure of the anal canal. A large epidemiologic study showed that prevalence rate of hemorrhoids was 4.4% in the United States [30]. The peak in prevalence was noted from ages 45 to 65 years. Additionally, whites were affected more and the prevalence was associated with higher socioeconomic status.

The exact pathogenesis of hemorrhoids is not known. The possible theories suggest that they represent abnormal

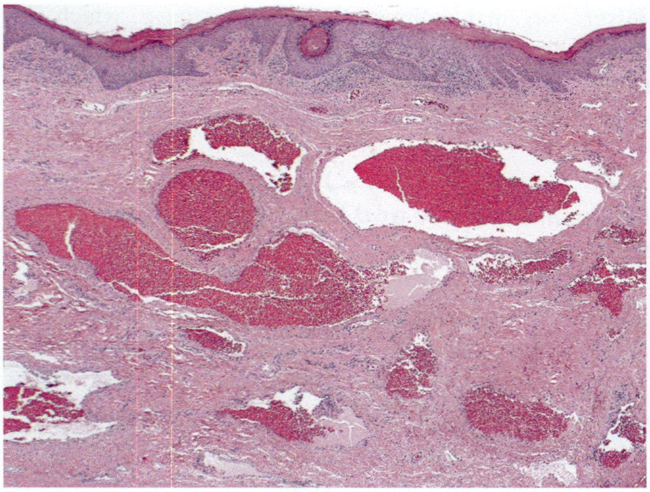

Fig. 20.6 Hemorrhoid showing thick-walled and dilated submucosal blood vessels

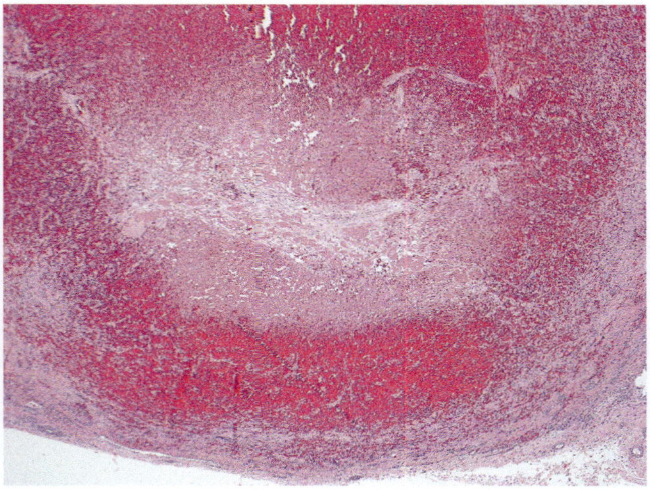

Fig. 20.7 Organizing thrombus within a blood vessel in a hemorrhoid

dilatation of veins of internal hemorrhoidal venous plexus, abnormal distention of the arteriovenous anastomosis, prolapse of the cushions and the surrounding connective tissue, and elevated anal sphincter pressure [31, 32]. An increase in intra-abdominal pressure due to constipation, diarrhea, straining at defecation, inadequate fiber intake, ascites, and pregnancy may contribute to the development of the disease. Hemorrhoids are classified as external or internal. The external hemorrhoids originate from the inferior hemorrhoidal plexus, arise distal to the dentate line, and are lined by squamous epithelium. The internal hemorrhoids originate from the superior hemorrhoidal plexus, arise proximal to the dentate line, and are lined by rectal or transitional mucosa. The clinical symptoms include painless bleeding, mucus discharge, discomfort, pain, prolapse, pruritus, and soiling. Thrombosis, strangulation, and ulceration of hemorrhoids can result in acute pain with mass formation and bleeding.

Excision specimens of hemorrhoids show presence of prominent, dilated, and thick-walled submucosal vessels (Fig. 20.6) which may show presence of organizing thrombi (Fig. 20.7). Recent or remote hemorrhage may be seen in the surrounding soft tissue, and the mucosa may show prolapse-type changes. The overlying squamous mucosa should also be carefully inspected for squamous neoplasia and melanocytic lesions. In one study, pagetoid dyskeratosis, which is presence of pale cells in the epidermis, was identified in 68% of hemorrhoidectomy specimens [33]. This is considered to be a reactive process which is possibly stimulated by friction. This finding must be distinguished from human papilloma virus (HPV)-associated cytopathic effect, extramammary Paget disease, pagetoid spread of carcinoma cells, pagetoid Bowen disease, and pagetoid melanoma.

Treatment of symptomatic hemorrhoids can be varied [34]. A conservative approach includes dietary and lifestyle changes which include high-fiber diet and increased fluid intake, topical anesthetics, steroids, suppositories, and sitz baths. Office-based procedures include rubber band ligation, sclerotherapy, bipolar diathermy, and infrared photocoagulation. Surgical management including open or closed excision is also available.

Fibroepithelial Polyps

Fibroepithelial polyps are synonymous with hypertrophied anal papillae and anal tags. These are benign polypoid projections of anal mucosa and submucosa. They are generally small, ranging in greatest dimension from 0.5 to 4 cm, with a mean size of 0.9 cm [35]. Rarely, they can present as large masses [36, 37]. These may be found incidentally during digital examination or may be associated with chronic fissure, fistula, anal ulcer, irritation, or infection. The patients may be asymptomatic or may present with discharge, discomfort, pruritus, or sensation of incomplete evacuation [38].

Fibroepithelial polyps consist of fibrous, myxoid, or collagenous stroma covered by squamous epithelium (Figs. 20.8 and 20.9). The stroma shows spindled or stellate stromal cells (Fig. 20.10) which are CD34 positive. The stromal cells may show multinucleation and appear enlarged, atypical, or bizarre. The stroma also shows a variable number of inflammatory cells, mast cells, and smooth muscle cells. The stromal vessels may show hyalinization, particularly at the base of the polyp. Fibroepithelial polyps can have clinical appearance of hemorrhoids and may be submitted as such to the pathologists. These lesions lack the presence of dilated blood

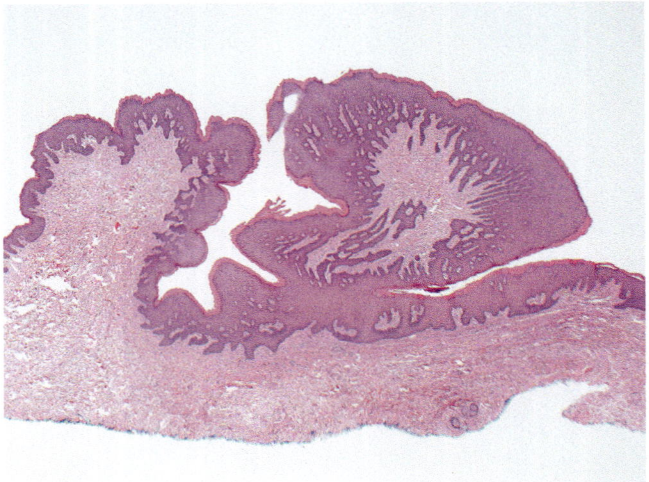

Fig. 20.8 Fibroepithelial polyp showing fibrous stroma covered by squamous epithelium

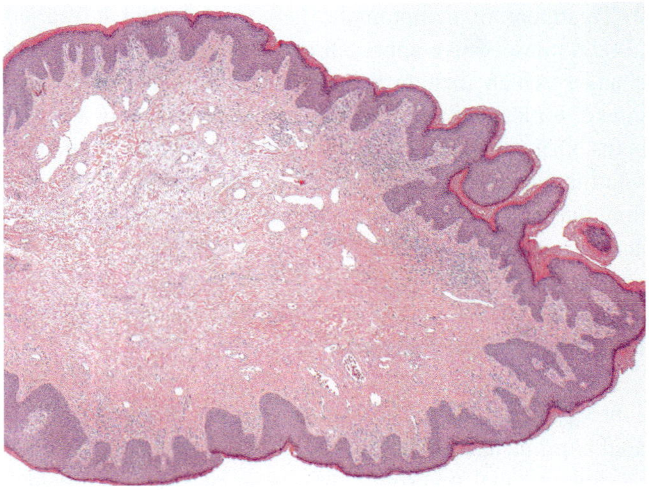

Fig. 20.9 Fibroepithelial polyp with mild chronic inflammation

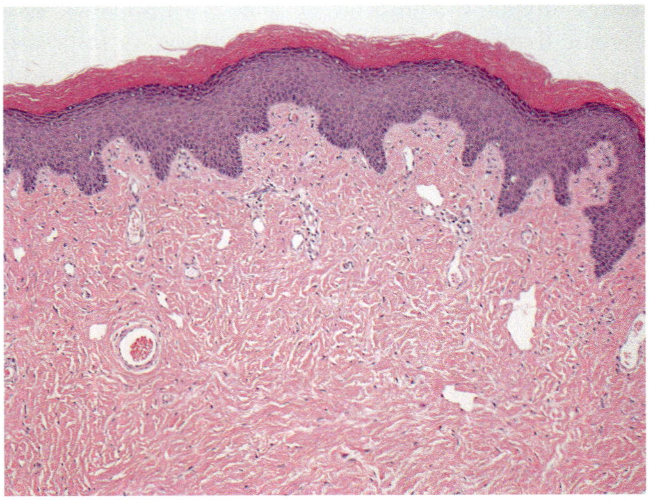

Fig. 20.10 Fibroepithelial polyp with stroma containing blood vessels and spindled stromal cells

vessels, organizing thrombi, and hemorrhage, which are typically seen in hemorrhoids. The overlying squamous epithelium should be carefully evaluated for unsuspected HPV viral cytopathic effect and neoplasia.

Mucosal Prolapse and Inflammatory Cloacogenic Polyp

Inflammatory cloacogenic polyps (ICPs) are inflammatory polyps that arise at the anorectal junction. They may be single or multiple and are generally located in the anterior anal canal [39, 40]. They tend to occur in the middle age but have also been reported in children [41]. The patients most commonly present with hematochezia.

ICPs occur due to mucosal prolapse, and hence these lesions show histological findings similar to other mucosal prolapse disorders such as solitary rectal ulcer syndrome (SRUS). Since these polyps arise from the anorectal junction, they are lined by squamous, transitional, and columnar epithelia. These polyps show tubulovillous architecture with surface erosion and ulceration (Figs. 20.11 and 20.12). The epithelium may show hyperplastic, serrated, and reactive changes. The mucosal glands are hyperplastic with distortion and displacement/herniation into the submucosa. These glands have bland cytological features, maintain a lobular architecture, and are accompanied by a variable amount of lamina propria. The muscularis mucosae is hyperplastic and irregular and shows radial extension of fibromuscular strands into the lamina propria, which causes distortion of crypts, resulting in "diamond-shaped" crypts. Deposition of elastin may also be seen in the mucosa.

It should be noted that adenomatous polyps may show associated mucosal prolapse-like changes. These changes may also be seen overlying a neoplastic process, and hence if

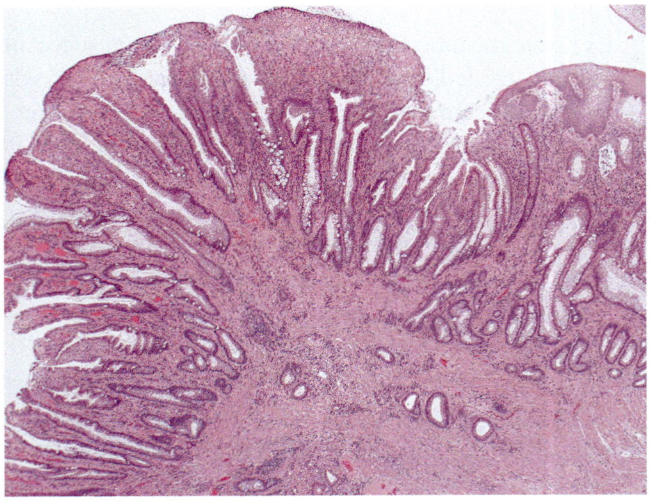

Fig. 20.11 Inflammatory cloacogenic polyp lined by squamous and columnar epithelia showing thickened muscularis mucosa with radial extension into the lamina propria

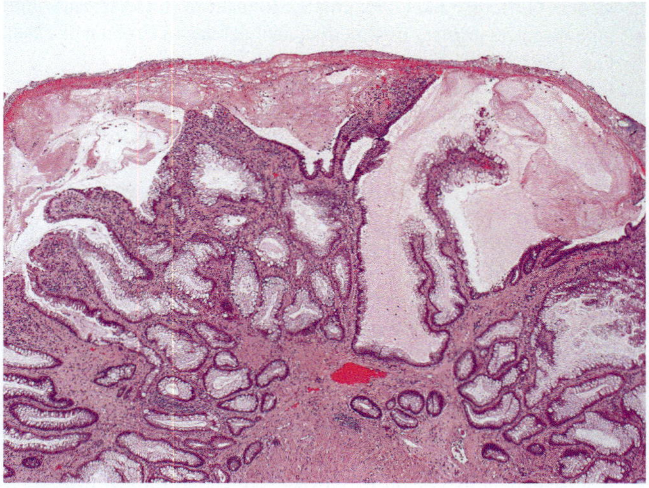

Fig. 20.12 Inflammatory cloacogenic polyp. Columnar epithelium showing erosion with hyperplasia and distortion of mucosal glands

there is clinical suspicion of neoplasm, a repeat biopsy to evaluate for underlying neoplasm may be indicated. ICPs show herniation and displacement of mucosal glands into the submucosa, so-called cystica colitis profunda, and this may be concerning for malignancy. The presence of nonneoplastic epithelium, lobular configuration, and associated lamina propria is useful to support the diagnosis of ICP.

Anal Fissures and Ulcers

An anal fissure is a linear or elliptical tear or defect in the skin of the anal canal. They occur distal to the dentate line and are most commonly located in the posterior midline. The most common presentation is sharp or tearing pain during and after defecation. Other symptoms include bleeding and discomfort. Anal fissures may be acute or chronic [42, 43]. Acute fissures are sharply demarcated, have granulation tissue at the base, and often heal spontaneously. Anal fissures that persist for a period longer than 4–6 weeks or are recurrent are classified as chronic fissures. Chronic fissures have indurated raised edges, show presence of internal sphincter muscle fibers at the base, and may be associated with hypertrophied anal papilla at the proximal end and external skin tag (sentinel pile) at the distal end. Chronic fissures are associated with history of cyclical pain and intermittent healing followed by recurrence. Fissures that are multiple, large, irregular, and not located in the midline are considered atypical. These atypical fissures tend to be associated with STIs (syphilis, herpes, and HIV), granulomatous diseases (tuberculosis and sarcoidosis), inflammatory bowel disease (Crohn's disease), and an underlying malignancy [44].

The exact etiology of anal fissure is not known. The possible etiologies include low-fiber diet and constipation leading to trauma by passage of hard stool, trauma during pregnancy, spasm or hypertonicity of internal anal sphincter, and anoreceptive intercourse [43, 45]. Histological features include ulceration, acute and chronic inflammation, presence of granulation tissue, and reactive epithelial changes.

Conservative management includes increased fiber intake, sitz baths, topical nitrates (glyceryl trinitrate), topical and oral calcium channel blocker, and botulinum toxin injection. Patients not responding to conservative treatment may need surgical intervention. The gold standard surgical procedure is lateral internal sphincterotomy. Other approaches include anal dilation, endorectal advancement flaps, and fissurectomy.

Anal Fistula and Abscess

Anorectal abscesses arise following infection of the anal glands [46]. The abscess tracks along the path of least resistance and accumulates where the gland terminates resulting in perianal, ischiorectal, intersphincteric, supralevator, or horseshoe abscess [47]. In approximately 30–40% of cases, the infection then spreads into adjacent spaces resulting in formation of fistulas [48, 49]. An anal abscess is the acute phase of an anorectal infection, and a fistula is considered to be the chronic phase of the same infection. Clinical symptoms include pain, swelling, redness, and systemic symptoms such as fever and malaise. Abscesses and fistulas are idiopathic in most cases and occur in healthy subjects. In a small subset of patients, these may be associated with Crohn's disease and malignancy and may be seen in patients with hidradenitis suppurativa.

On histologic examination, non-specific acute and chronic inflammation, granulation tissue, and fibrosis are identified. Foreign body giant cell reaction may also be seen. Careful evaluation for granulomatous inflammation should be performed, the presence of which may suggest the possibility of Crohn's disease or infectious etiology. In these cases, special stains for acid-fast bacilli and fungal organisms will be helpful. Careful examination for any coexistent malignancy should also be performed.

The surgical management includes incision and drainage of the abscess, fistulotomy, fistulectomy, cutting seton placement, fibrin glue, fistula plug, endorectal advancement flap, and ligation of the intersphincteric fistula tract.

References

1. Klausner JD, Kohn R, Kent C. Etiology of clinical proctitis among men who have sex with men. Clin Infect Dis. 2004;38(2):300–2.
2. Cone MM, Whitlow CB. Sexually transmitted and anorectal infectious diseases. Gastroenterol Clin N Am. 2013;42(4):877–92.
3. Ryder N, Jin F, McNulty AM, Grulich AE, Donovan B. Increasing role of herpes simplex virus type 1 in first-episode anogenital herpes in heterosexual women and younger men who have sex with men, 1992–2006. Sex Transm Infect. 2009;85(6):416–9.
4. Hamlyn E, Taylor C. Sexually transmitted proctitis. Postgrad Med J. 2006;82(973):733–6.

5. Towns JM, Leslie DE, Denham I, Azzato F, Fairley CK, Chen M. Painful and multiple anogenital lesions are common in men with Treponema pallidum PCR-positive primary syphilis without herpes simplex virus coinfection: a cross-sectional clinic-based study. Sex Transm Infect. 2016;92(2):110–5.
6. Hook EW 3rd, Marra CM. Acquired syphilis in adults. N Engl J Med. 1992;326(16):1060–9.
7. Center for Disease Control and Prevention (CDC). Syphilis: CDC fact sheet. http://www.cdc.gov/std/syphilis/STDFact-Syphilis.htm. Accessed 1 Aug 2018.
8. Furman DL, Patel SK, Arluk GM. Endoscopic and histologic appearance of rectal syphilis. Gastrointest Endosc. 2008;67(1):161.
9. Gopal P, Shah RB. Primary anal canal syphilis in men: the clinicopathologic spectrum of an easily overlooked diagnosis. Arch Pathol Lab Med. 2015;139(9):1156–60.
10. Zhao WT, Liu J, Li YY. Syphilitic proctitis mimicking rectal cancer: a case report. World J Gastrointest Pathophysiol. 2010;1(3):112–4.
11. Tse JY, Chan MP, Ferry JA, Deshpande V, Sohani AR, Nardi V, Schaffer A, Nazarian RM, Zukerberg LR. Syphilis of the aerodigestive tract. Am J Surg Pathol. 2018;42(4):472–8.
12. Rosa G, Bennett D, Piliang MP. Eosinophil-rich syphilis: a report of four cases. J Cutan Pathol. 2015;42(8):554–8.
13. Graham RP, Naini BV, Shah SS, Arnold CA, Kannangai R, Torbenson MS, Lam-Himlin DM. Treponema pallidum immunohistochemistry is positive in human intestinal spirochetosis. Diagn Pathol. 2018;13(1):7.
14. Nieuwenhuis RF, Ossewaarde JM, Götz HM, Dees J, Thio HB, Thomeer MG, den Hollander JC, Neumann MH, van der Meijden WI. Resurgence of lymphogranuloma venereum in Western Europe: an outbreak of Chlamydia trachomatis serovar l2 proctitis in the Netherlands among men who have sex with men. Clin Infect Dis. 2004;39(7):996–1003.
15. Van der Bij AK, Spaargaren J, Morré SA, Fennema HS, Mindel A, Coutinho RA, de Vries HJ. Diagnostic and clinical implications of anorectal lymphogranuloma venereum in men who have sex with men: a retrospective case-control study. Clin Infect Dis. 2006;42(2):186–94.
16. de Vrieze NH, de Vries HJ. Lymphogranuloma venereum among men who have sex with men. An epidemiological and clinical review. Expert Rev Anti-Infect Ther. 2014;12(6):697–704.
17. Reyes-Urueña JM, Garcia De Olalla P, Vall-Mayans M, Arando M, Caballero E, Cayla JA, Barcelona STI Group. Lymphogranuloma venereum in Barcelona, 2007–2012: the role of seroadaptation in men who have sex with men. Epidemiol Infect. 2015;143(1):184–8.
18. Kropp RY, Wong T, Canadian LGV Working Group. Emergence of lymphogranuloma venereum in Canada. CMAJ. 2005;172(13):1674–6.
19. Arnold CA, Limketkai BN, Illei PB, Montgomery E, Voltaggio L. Syphilitic and lymphogranuloma venereum (LGV) proctocolitis: clues to a frequently missed diagnosis. Am J Surg Pathol. 2013;37(1):38–46.
20. Williams DR, Coller JA, Corman ML, Nugent FW, Veidenheimer MC. Anal complications in Crohn's disease. Dis Colon Rectum. 1981;24(1):22–4.
21. Platell C, Mackay J, Collopy B, Fink R, Ryan P, Woods R. Anal pathology in patients with Crohn's disease. Aust N Z J Surg. 1996;66(1):5–9.
22. Rankin GB, Watts HD, Melnyk CS, Kelley ML Jr. National Cooperative Crohn's Disease Study: extraintestinal manifestations and perianal complications. Gastroenterology. 1979;77(4 Pt 2):914–20.
23. Harper PH, Fazio VW, Lavery IC, Jagelman DG, Weakley FL, Farmer RG, Easley KA. The long-term outcome in Crohn's disease. Dis Colon Rectum. 1987;30(3):174–9.
24. Schwartz DA, Loftus EV Jr, Tremaine WJ, Panaccione R, Harmsen WS, Zinsmeister AR, Sandborn WJ. The natural history of fistulizing Crohn's disease in Olmsted County, Minnesota. Gastroenterology. 2002;122(4):875–80.
25. Hellers G, Bergstrand O, Ewerth S, Holmström B. Occurrence and outcome after primary treatment of anal fistulae in Crohn's disease. Gut. 1980;21(6):525–7.
26. Ingle SB, Loftus EV Jr. The natural history of perianal Crohn's disease. Dig Liver Dis. 2007;39(10):963–9.
27. Sandborn WJ, Fazio VW, Feagan BG, Hanauer SB, American Gastroenterological Association Clinical Practice Committee. AGA technical review on perianal Crohn's disease. Gastroenterology. 2003;125(5):1508–30.
28. Thomson WH. The nature of haemorrhoids. Br J Surg. 1975;62(7):542–52.
29. Madoff RD, Fleshman JW, Clinical Practice Committee, American Gastroenterological Association. American Gastroenterological Association technical review on the diagnosis and treatment of hemorrhoids. Gastroenterology. 2004;126(5):1463–73.
30. Johanson JF, Sonnenberg A. The prevalence of hemorrhoids and chronic constipation. An epidemiologic study. Gastroenterology. 1990;98(2):380–6.
31. Kaidar-Person O, Person B, Wexner SD. Hemorrhoidal disease: a comprehensive review. J Am Coll Surg. 2007;204(1):102–17.
32. Deutsch AA, Moshkovitz M, Nudelman I, Dinari G, Reiss R. Anal pressure measurements in the study of hemorrhoid etiology and their relation to treatment. Dis Colon Rectum. 1987;30(11):855–7.
33. Val-Bernal JF, Pinto J. Pagetoid dyskeratosis is a frequent incidental finding in hemorrhoidal disease. Arch Pathol Lab Med. 2001;125(8):1058–62.
34. Sneider EB, Maykel JA. Diagnosis and management of symptomatic hemorrhoids. Surg Clin North Am. 2010;90(1):17–32.
35. Groisman GM, Polak-Charcon S. Fibroepithelial polyps of the anus: a histologic, immunohistochemical, and ultrastructural study, including comparison with the normal anal subepithelial layer. Am J Surg Pathol. 1998;22(1):70–6.
36. Yilmaz B, Coban S, Usküdar O, Unverdı H, Aktaş B, Yüksel O. Giant fibroepithelial polyp of the anus. Turk J Gastroenterol. 2011;22(6):651–2.
37. Galanis I, Dragoumis D, Tsolakis M, Zarampoukas K, Zarampoukas T, Atmatzidis K. Obstructive ileus due to a giant fibroepithelial polyp of the anus. World J Gastroenterol. 2009;15(29):3687–90.
38. Gupta PJ. Hypertrophied anal papillae and fibrous anal polyps, should they be removed during anal fissure surgery. World J Gastroenterol. 2004;10(16):2412–4.
39. Lobert PF, Appelman HD. Inflammatory cloacogenic polyp. A unique inflammatory lesion of the anal transitional zone. Am J Surg Pathol. 1981;5(8):761–6.
40. Saul SH. Inflammatory cloacogenic polyp: relationship to solitary rectal ulcer syndrome/mucosal prolapse and other bowel disorders. Hum Pathol. 1987;18(11):1120–5.
41. Poon KK, Mills S, Booth IW, Murphy MS. Inflammatory cloacogenic polyp: an unrecognized cause of hematochezia and tenesmus in childhood. J Pediatr. 1997;130(2):327–9.
42. Nelson RL. Anal fissure (chronic). BMJ Clin Evid. 2014;2014: pii 0407.
43. Shawki S, Costedio M. Anal fissure and stenosis. Gastroenterol Clin N Am. 2013;42(4):729–58.
44. Schlichtemeier S, Engel A. Anal fissure. Aust Prescr. 2016;39(1):14–7.
45. Beaty JS, Shashidharan M. Anal fissure. Clin Colon Rectal Surg. 2016;29(1):30–7.
46. Abcarian H. Anorectal infection: abscess-fistula. Clin Colon Rectal Surg. 2011;24(1):14–21.
47. Sneider EB, Maykel JA. Anal abscess and fistula. Gastroenterol Clin N Am. 2013;42(4):773–84.
48. Ramanujam PS, Prasad ML, Abcarian H, Tan AB. Perianal abscesses and fistulas. A study of 1023 patients. Dis Colon Rectum. 1984;27(9):593–7.
49. Vasilevsky CA, Gordon PH. The incidence of recurrent abscesses or fistula-in-ano following anorectal suppuration. Dis Colon Rectum. 1984;27(2):126–30.

Index

L. Zhang et al. (eds.), *Surgical Pathology of Non-neoplastic Gastrointestinal Diseases*,
https://doi.org/10.1007/978-3-030-15573-5

Printed by Printforce, the Netherlands